AF573949

Pediatric Hematopathology

Pediatric Hematopathology

Robert D. Collins, MD
Professor of Pathology
Department of Pathology
Vanderbilt University School of Medicine
Nashville, Tennessee

Steven H. Swerdlow, MD
Professor of Pathology
Department of Pathology
University of Pittsburgh School of Medicine
Pittsburgh, Pennsylvania

CHURCHILL LIVINGSTONE
A Harcourt Health Sciences Company
New York Edinburgh London Philadelphia

CHURCHILL LIVINGSTONE
A Harcourt Health Sciences Company
The Curtis Center
Independence Square West
Philadelphia, Pennsylvania 19106

Library of Congress Cataloging-in-Publication Data

Pediatric hematopathology/
[edited by] Robert D. Collins, Steven H. Swerdlow.–1st ed.

p. cm.

ISBN 0–443–07566–2

1. Pediatric hematology. 2. Hematopoietic system–Cancer. 3. Blood–Diseases. 4. Children–Diseases. I. Collins, Robert D., M.D. II. Swerdlow, Steven H., M.D.

RJ411.P42 2001 618.92′15–dc21 00–059639

Editor-in-Chief: Richard Zorab
Acquisitions Editor: Marc Strauss
Production Manager: Natalie Ware
Illustration Specialist: Peg Shaw
Book Designer: Ellen Zanolle

Dedication art courtesy of Wendy Leonard.

Pediatric Hematopathology ISBN 0–443–07566–2

Printed in the United States of America.

Last digit is the print number: 9 8 7 6 5 4 3 2 1

To the welfare of children

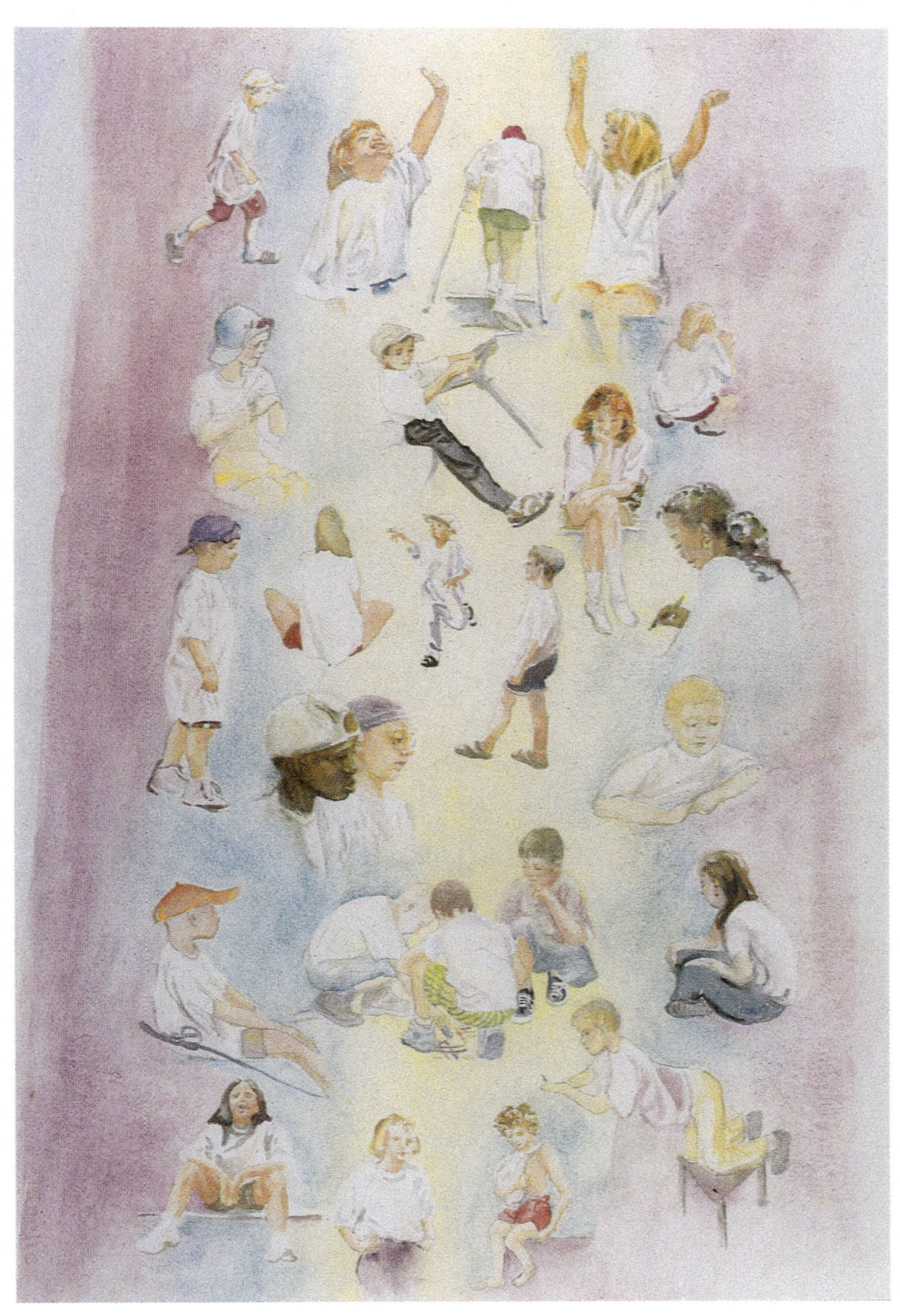

Contributors

Robert D. Collins, MD
Professor of Pathology
Department of Pathology
Vanderbilt University School of Medicine
Nashville, Tennessee

John B. Cousar, MD
Clinical Professor of Pathology
Medical College of Virginia at
Virginia Commonwealth University
Richmond, Virginia

Kathy Foucar, MD
Professor of Pathology and Vice Chair for Clinical Affairs
Department of Pathology
University of New Mexico School of Medicine
Albuquerque, New Mexico

Kathy Hamilton, MD
Fellow, Anatomical Pathology
Vanderbilt University School of Medicine
Nashville, Tennessee

Andras Khoor, MD
Senior Associate Consultant
Mayo Clinic
Jacksonville, Florida

Marsha C. Kinney, MD
Associate Professor of Pathology
Vanderbilt University School of Medicine
Director, Hematology Laboratory
Vanderbilt University Medical Center
Nashville, Tennessee

Carl R. Kjeldsberg, MD
Professor and Chair
Department of Pathology
University of Utah School of Medicine
Salt Lake City, Utah

Paul J. Kurtin, MD
Associate Professor of Pathology
Mayo Medical School
Rochester, Minnesota

Laura W. Lamps, MD
Assistant Professor of Pathology
University of Arkansas College of Medicine
Little Rock, Arkansas

Richard S. Larson, MD, PhD
Assistant Professor of Pathology
University of New Mexico School of Medicine
Albuquerque, New Mexico

Catherine Leith, MB, BChir
Associate Professor
Department of Pathology and Laboratory Medicine
University of Wisconsin Medical School
Madison, Wisconsin

Todd C. Murry, MD, PhD
Fellow of Dermatopathology
Joan and Sanford I. Weill Medical College of Cornell University
New York, New York

Sherrie Perkins, MD, PhD
Associate Professor of Pathology
University of Utah School of Medicine
Director of Hematopathology
University of Utah Health Sciences
ARUP Laboratories
Salt Lake City, Utah

Kevin Salhany, MD
Associate Professor of Pathology
University of Pennsylvania Medical Center
Philadelphia, Pennsylvania
Deceased

Margie A. Scott, MD
Associate Professor of Pathology
University of Arkansas College of Medicine
Assistant Chief of Pathology and Laboratory Medicine
Medical Director of Clinical Laboratories
Central Arkansas Veterans HealthCare System
Little Rock, Arkansas

Sanya Sukpanichnant, MD
Associate Professor of Pathology
Faculty of Medicine
Mahidol University
Siriraj Hospital
Bangkok, Thailand

Steven H. Swerdlow, MD
Professor of Pathology
University of Pittsburgh School of Medicine
Director
Division of Hematopathology
UPMC–Presbyterian Hospital
Pittsburgh, Pennsylvania

Paul E. Wakely, Jr, MD
Professor of Pathology
The Ohio State University College of Medicine
Columbus, Ohio

Kay Washington, MD, PhD
Associate Professor of Pathology
Vanderbilt University School of Medicine
Nashville, Tennessee

Preface

The goal of *Pediatric Hematopathology* is to provide in a single text the essential diagnostic and biologic information about the diseases that affect the lymphatic tissues and marrow in children. Our presentation is oriented toward the diagnostic laboratory in a general hospital or in one dedicated to the care of children. We hope that pathologists find our approach to diagnostic hematopathology useful. Clinicians and students may use this text to facilitate their understanding of certain childhood diseases.

This is the first pediatric hematopathology text. Its publication is justified although only a few marrow and lymphatic diseases are unique to children, and several other texts describe the hematopathologic diseases of adults. However, mistakes are easily made in the diagnosis of reactive states in children, particularly if pathologists have had limited experience with these reactions and are not aware of the relevant differential diagnoses. Furthermore, it is possible in this text to highlight the most important clinical and pathologic syndromes of children, thereby providing illustrations and information not available in other texts.

Pediatric Hematopathology is being published at a time when the burgeoning complexity of hematopathology, particularly lymphoma classification, is legendary and when specialties are evolving for single-organ systems, specific diseases, and individual diagnostic methods. Although the basic approach in pediatric hematopathology must be similar to that in adult hematopathology, the emphasis is quite different, simply because many diseases common in adults are rare in children. Alternatively, certain inherited diseases and infections are far more common in children than in adults.

As an example of focused emphasis, the lymphoma section herein is relatively brief compared with most adult hematopathology texts. Sections on inherited diseases and infections, however, are considerably more detailed. Whatever the disease or clinical presentation, our goal is to be sufficiently encyclopedic so that pathologists involved with hematic or lymphatic problems in children can find solutions herein.

The conceptual approach of *Pediatric Hematopathology* also differs from other similar texts. We emphasize the organs affected at clinical presentation, as, in every case, the source of sampled tissue should be known by the pathologist. When the presenting lesion is in fact a secondary phenomenon as in leukemia cutis, the major discussion is in the marrow/leukemia section, and there is a secondary discussion with appropriate cross referencing under skin. We also emphasize that the most important diagnostic information for many diseases is clinical and/or histopathologic, although we recognize that some lymphatic and marrow diseases in children are precisely diagnosed only by utilizing multiparameter analyses.

Major mistakes may be made when pathologists are not aware of clinical data or previous diagnoses. The most complex histopathologic problem, in comparison, is often easily resolved by having basic clinical information. Our emphasis on important clinical and pathologic syndromes and their frequency should help minimize errors.

Several diseases of the neonate do not occur in the adult. These include severe leukoerythroblastic reactions observed with congenital infections, hemolytic disease, and cyanotic heart disease, and transient myeloproliferative disorders of Down syndrome and congenital leukemia, to name a few. For these and similar pediatric problems, it is useful for generalists and specialists to have available the detailed differential diagnosis and diagnostic criteria as provided in this text.

Robert D. Collins, MD
Steven H. Swerdlow, MD

Acknowledgments

The contributors to *Pediatric Hematopathology* wish to express their appreciation to the physicians responsible for submitting patient samples in consultation, to the professional and staff personnel involved in patient care in their medical centers, and to their colleagues specializing in the field of hematopathology. We especially thank our students and mentors. Our students have provided an essential element of continuity to the educational activities in which we are involved, and our mentors have shared freely their wisdom and experience. We hereby express our appreciation to the many other people involved in specimen handling, photography, and manuscript preparation. Major projects of this type are completed only through the support of family, friends, and colleagues, who provide essential "behind-the-scenes" sustenance and assistance.

The contributors and editors are also very appreciative of the professional editorial assistance of the W.B. Saunders Company staff, particularly Marc Strauss, Natalie Ware, Ellen Zanolle, Peg Shaw, and Ethel Cathers. Expert copy editing was provided by Pamela Ann Lloyd.

We are indebted to Greg Kinney for the photographs of patients, to Brent Weedman for the photographs of textbooks, to Wendy Leonard for the montage used as background for the dedication, and to Dr. Karen Wasilewski for facilitating visits to Camp Horizon.

The editors wish specifically to recognize Dr. Robert J. Lukes, Dr. Alfred G. Stansfeld, and Professor Karl Lennert for their guidance and support. *Pediatric Hematopathology* reflects in many ways the revolutionary insights of Dr. Lukes and Professor Lennert into the relationships between the immune system, its deficiencies, and its neoplasms. We also wish to acknowledge with gratitude the friendship of Professor Alistair Robb-Smith, who was far ahead of his time in anticipating the complexities of lymphomas.

Contents

1 **Status of Pediatric Hematopathology** 1
Robert D. Collins

2 **General Approach to Diagnostic Hematopathology** 5
Robert D. Collins

Body Fluid Examination 5
Carl R. Kjeldsberg

Lymph Node Aspiration Cytopathology 12
Paul E. Wakely, Jr.

Appendix
Technique of Fine-Needle Aspiration Biopsy 19

3 **Immunodeficiency Disorders** 21
Richard S. Larson

X-Linked Lymphoproliferative Disorder 42
Richard S. Larson, Robert D. Collins, and Steven H. Swerdlow

Posttransplant Lymphoproliferative Disorders 48
Steven H. Swerdlow

4 **Acute Leukemias** 61
Kathy Foucar and Catherine Leith

5 **Chronic Leukemias** 95
Kathy Foucar

6 **Disorders of Hematopoiesis** 105
Sherrie Perkins

Thalassemia 140
Sanya Sukpanichnant

7 **Myeloproliferative and Myelodysplastic Disorders** 147
Sherrie Perkins

8 **Blood and Marrow Pathology in Infections, Systemic Diseases, and Metastatic Neoplasms and Following Therapy** 157
Sherrie Perkins

Dengue and Malaria 169
Sanya Sukpanichnant

9 **Neonatal Hematopathology: Special Considerations** 173
Kathy Foucar

10 **Histiocytoses** 185
Steven H. Swerdlow, Kevin Salhany, and Robert D. Collins

11 **Diagnosis and Classification of Lymphomas** 195
Robert D. Collins

12 **Lymphomas: Epidemiologic, Biologic, and Pathogenetic Features** 199
Steven H. Swerdlow

13 **Hodgkin Diseases** 211
Paul J. Kurtin

14 **B Cell Lymphomas** 235
John B. Cousar

15 T Cell Lymphomas and Natural Killer Cell Neoplasms 245
Marsha C. Kinney

16 Lymph Nodes: Other Pathologic Conditions 277
Steven H. Swerdlow

Infections Involving Lymph Nodes 289
Margie A. Scott

Leishmaniasis, Melioidosis, Penicilliosis, and Typhoid Fever 312
Sanya Sukpanichnant

Neoplasms Other Than Lymphomas in Lymph Nodes 317
John B. Cousar

17 Thymus Gland 323
Paul J. Kurtin

18 Spleen 343
Robert D. Collins

19 Gastrointestinal Tract and Liver 361
Laura W. Lamps and Kay Washington

20 Lung 381
Andras Khoor

21 Skin and Subcutaneous Tissue 389
Todd C. Murry, Kathy Hamilton, and Robert D. Collins

22 Other Extranodal Sites 403
Sanya Sukpanichnant

Index 411

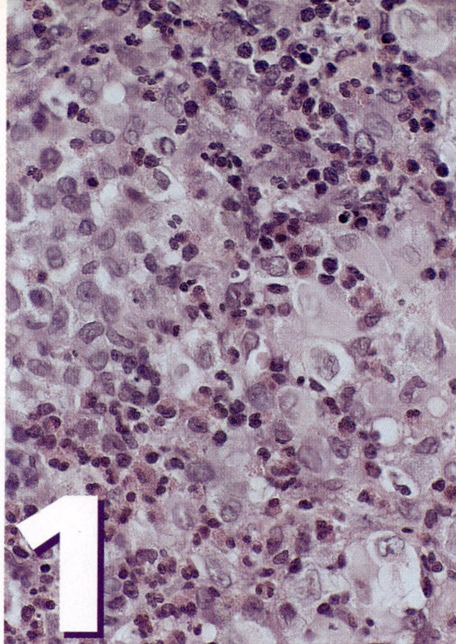

Robert D. Collins

Status of Pediatric Hematopathology

We choose to introduce this book by emphasizing the reason for our existence as professionals. Most pathologists do not see patients and can only imagine the perturbations in daily life and outlook engendered by some diagnoses. The diagnosis most dreaded is that of cancer. It is therefore appropriate for us to begin with a few pictures taken at Camp Horizon, a summer camp for children with cancer, located near Nashville, Tennessee (Figs. 1–1 and 1–2). This camp is funded by the American Cancer Society and attended by children 7 to 17 years of age. Most are under treatment at Vanderbilt University Medical Center in Nashville or at St. Jude Children's Research Hospital in Memphis. There are 2 weeks of camp each summer, with 50 to 60 children attending each week. Approximately 75% return for more than 1 year, but there are usually 1 or 2 deaths each year among the campers. Camps of this type are held across this country and around the world. They have become very effective support groups for patients, siblings, and families. Back at the hospital, there are needles, catheters, injections, procedures, and treatments (Figs. 1–3 and 1–4). The pictures in this chapter and scattered throughout the text are powerful images of the courage and vulnerability of children; these photographs also serve to remind us of our most fundamental responsibility as physicians.

The status of pediatric hematopathology in the twentieth century is reflected in the contents of this book. The timing of its publication affords a unique opportunity to speculate on the prospects for pediatric hematopathology and pathology in the twenty-first century.

SUPERSPECIALIZATION IS INEVITABLE

The watershed event in the twentieth century in hematopathology as well as oncology was, by many measures, the discovery of Burkitt lymphoma. Its recognition by Denis Burkitt on the basis of clinical features and, subsequently, its histopathologic definition spawned an enormous literature representing work from around the world. This work culminated in the discovery of the Epstein-Barr virus, the characteristic karyotypic abnormalities associated with Burkitt lymphoma, the mechanism of oncogene activation leading to this lymphoma, and the fact that chemotherapy was useful or curative as treatment; furthermore, the relationship of this human lymphoma to climate and viral infection was of enormous significance. To understand why some years passed before this lymphoma was proved to have B cell features, one should read the section on immunity in a standard pathology text of that time (e.g., Anderson, 1948). In that text immunity was covered in less than one page, lymphocytes were assigned no specific functions other than possibly being the source of gamma globulins, and it was assumed that lymphocytes might transform into macrophages. Plasma cells were recognized in areas of chronic inflammation, but their histogenesis was unknown. In short, 50 years ago we had only the most rudimentary information about this important host defense system and its diseases. In view of the state of our knowledge and the extent of our ignorance, it is all the more remarkable that so much has been learned by studying this particular disease of the immune system.

Now, a standard text on immunology (Paul, 1999) is 1616 pages in length (Fig. 1–5); even the first edition (1984) contained 809 pages. Detailed information about specific diseases of the immune system is also available; Figure 1-5 shows a tome on infectious diseases in children with immunodeficiency (Patrick, 1992), emphasizing the emerging clinical importance of infections in this population of patients. The volume and detail of the information available about the immune system is further exemplified by the publication in 1999 of *Dendritic Cells: Biology and Clinical Applications* and, in 1998, the third edition of *The Cytokine Handbook* (Fig. 1–6). Most pathologists and clinicians are barely familiar with dendritic cells, yet the former book documents their important role in immunity. The latter text describes a bewildering array of peptides responsible for signaling among cells of the immune system: the cytokines. It is evident that the study of just one of these topics of great current interest—dendritic cells or cytokines—may require a lifetime. It is paradoxical that, within the last 50 years, we have progressed from having scant information about immunity to having such a surfeit that single individuals cannot master the field and are just as ignorant in some respects as we were in 1950. Consequently, there will be superspecialists in the field of pediatric hematopathology, with some pathologists fully qualified to diagnose leukemia, perhaps only certain types of leukemia, and others to diagnose lymphomas.

DISEASES WILL BE RECOGNIZED EARLIER

Senior pathologists now practicing have witnessed dramatic changes in their concepts of breast, colon, and prostate cancer. Development of mammography, colonoscopy, and prostate-specific antigen tests has led to the routine recognition of microscopic cancers, rather than the bulky tumors seen previously, in these sites and have caused major changes in concepts of treatment as well as of pathogenesis. We should anticipate the probability of similar early diagnoses in patients with leukemias and lymphomas. The diagnosis of acute leukemia is now made

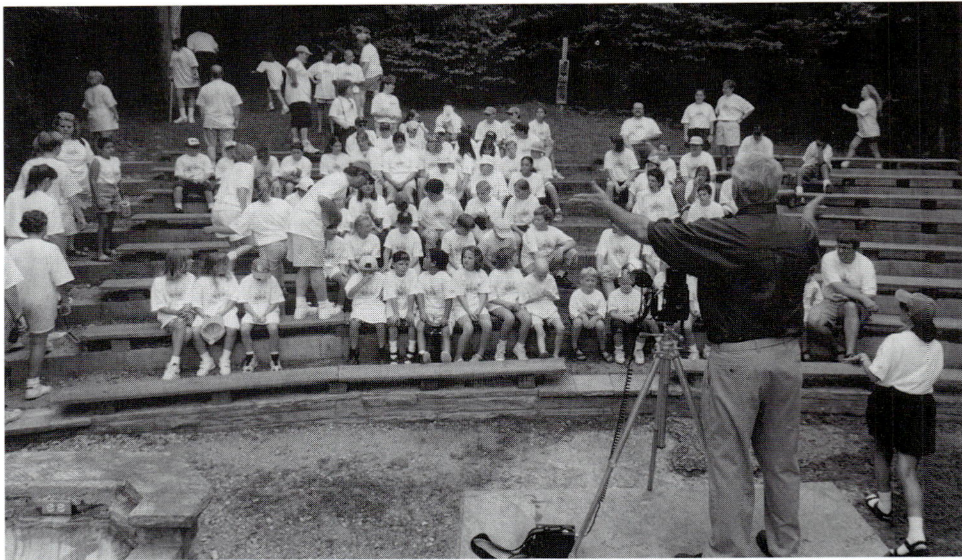

Figure 1–1

Camp Horizon, near Nashville. Campers assembling for the group photograph in the 1998 session. Courtesy of Greg Kinney.

only when the marrow is essentially replaced by tumor, with patients progressing rapidly through manifestations of marrow insufficiency to marrow failure. To understand acute leukemia, we must define biologic subsets of leukemia by multiparameter studies rather than by the current emphasis on descriptive features that reflect the appearance of the predominant cell. Identification of biologic subsets, that is, specific clinical or pathologic entities, will enable us to acquire the same type of information as derived from the study of Burkitt lymphoma, information that is useful in identifying populations of patients at risk and mechanisms of pathogenesis. Then it should be possible to perform appropriate screening tests—perhaps looking for circulating tumor products—on members of the risk groups.

DIAGNOSTIC METHODS WILL CHANGE

If experience is a guide, the size and nature of diagnostic biopsies and samples will change dramatically in the twenty-first

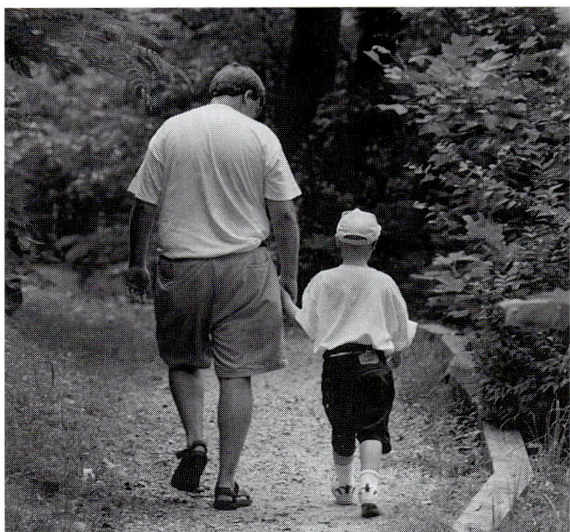

Figure 1–2

Camp Horizon, near Nashville. A physician and a camper taking a short hike. The camper had acute lymphocytic leukemia with multiple relapses. This picture was taken 1 year after a marrow transplantation from an unrelated donor, and this child was apparently free of disease 2 years later. Courtesy of Greg Kinney.

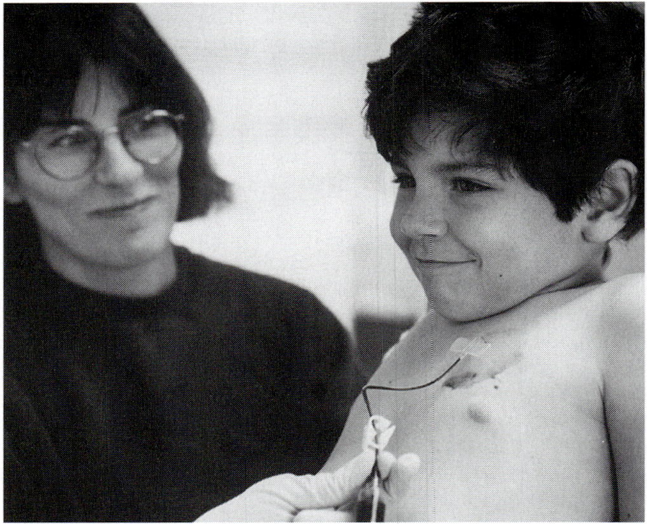

Figure 1–3

Hematology-Oncology Treatment Center, Vanderbilt University. This 8-year-old girl with a port-a-cath was just beginning therapy after relapse of acute lymphocytic leukemia. Courtesy of Greg Kinney.

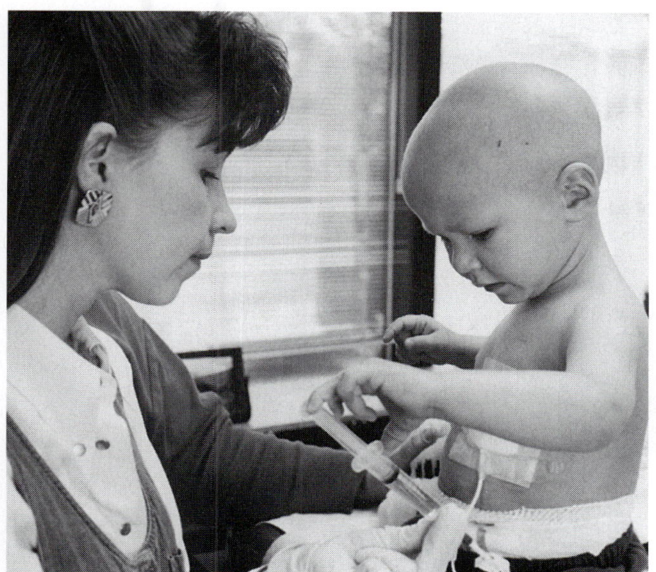

Figure 1–4

Hematology-Oncology Treatment Center, Vanderbilt University. This 3-year-old boy was self-injecting medications via a Hickman catheter for a hepatoblastoma that had relapsed with a pulmonary metastasis. He was apparently disease free 2 years later. Courtesy of Greg Kinney.

century. Directed needle biopsies of tumorous masses are likely to become routine, with cytologic examinations as well as multiparameter studies using flow cytometry, detection of genetic abnormalities, detection of oncogenes, and chemotherapy susceptibility profiles being part of the standard studies. Specialized tests available in only a few reference laboratories may be requested for certain tumors. Clinical features and microscopic examination will be more useful for triage of samples than for establishment of a final diagnosis. Sampling of recurrent disease or evaluating of relapse will be much more complicated than at present. Treatment of relapses is likely to be very specific, with its type determined by the clonal evolution of a neoplastic process in terms of resistance to drugs or biologic agents.

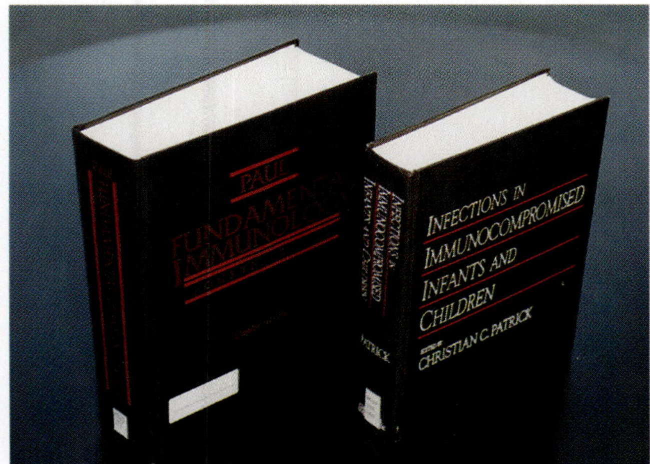

Figure 1–5

A 1999 text on immunology and a 1992 text on infections in immunocompromised children.

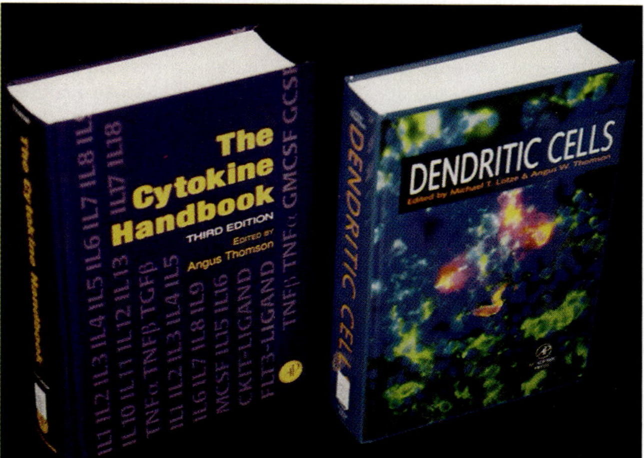

Figure 1–6

These 1998 and 1999 texts deal with cytokines and dendritic cells, respectively.

ENDANGERED COMMUNICATIONS

Pathologists are often perceived by their fellow physicians to be insulated from the grit, demands, and rewards of patients' care. Some of this insulation reflects a choice by pathologists to focus on laboratory work and/or a choice to be shielded from the immediate concerns of patients. Some of the insulation is due to the physical separation of pathologists from patients as well as the separation of pathologists from their fellow physicians. Pathology laboratories are usually a distance away from the major clinical traffic in a hospital. Specimen samples, including surgical specimens, are often delivered with inadequate, garbled, or irrelevant information about the patient's clinical problem, although billing data and ICD-9 codes are always present. Since reports are available by computer, fax, or phone, the most essential information in many cases—the diagnosis—is often established in a vacuum, without discussion of the primary diagnostic data with the responsible clinician.

This practice is perhaps the most damaging legacy of the twentieth century in terms of its implications for patients' care and represents a serious impediment to the proper practice of pathology in the twenty-first. This legacy may be attributed to withering of communication skills in complex medical centers. It seems paradoxical that it is so difficult to speak to our colleagues down the hall and yet so easy to direct-dial a colleague in Bangkok. It is also paradoxical that essential clinical information is often not readily available on our patients when we are immersed in a tidal wave of biologic data from around the world, pouring in electronically as well as on the printed page.

In the twenty-first century, many diagnoses will be made and treatments rendered on the basis of automated or semiautomated analyses rather than microscopic examination. Microscopy has an advantage beyond its extraordinary usefulness and accuracy when properly applied: microscopy makes it possible for two physicians to look at the same sample together and then to discuss the case and the diagnostic possibilities in a collegial atmosphere. This kind of interaction is far more difficult when automated data flow in from various specialty laboratories, perhaps with conflicting interpretations. In this worst-case scenario of conflicting interpretations, which pathologist or laboratorian will be responsible for resolving the discrepancies and generating a cumulative report in which a final diagnosis is rendered?

PROSPECTS

If pathologists assume responsibility for the proper triage of diagnostic materials and for the collation of data to provide an integrated diagnosis, the profession has a bright future with a continued central responsibility in patients' care. This optimism is particularly warranted if some specialty laboratory work is performed locally. If triage becomes an automatic process and if pathologists assume minimal responsibility for integrating the data from sophisticated laboratories, we may be relegated to a technical role in the care of patients.

REFERENCES

Anderson WAD (ed): Pathology. CV Mosby, St. Louis, 1948.

Lotze MT, Thomson AW (eds): Dendritic Cells: Biology and Clinical Applications. Academic Press, San Diego, 1999.

Patrick CC (ed): Infections in Immunocompromised Infants and Children. Churchill Livingstone, New York, 1992.

Paul WE (ed): Fundamental Immunology, 4th ed. Lippincott-Raven, Philadelphia, 1999.

Thomson AW (ed): The Cytokine Handbook, 3rd ed. Academic Press, San Diego, 1998.

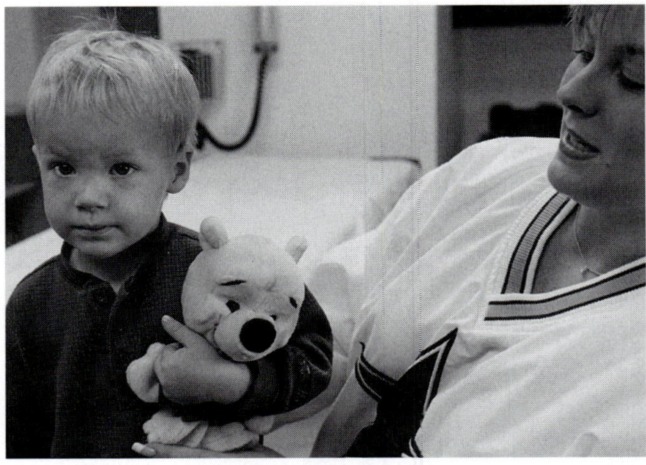

Hematology-Oncology Treatment Center, Vanderbilt University. This 3-year-old was ready to come off treatment. He had acute lymphocytic leukemia with high-risk features (white cell count >50,000/dl). Courtesy of Greg Kinney.

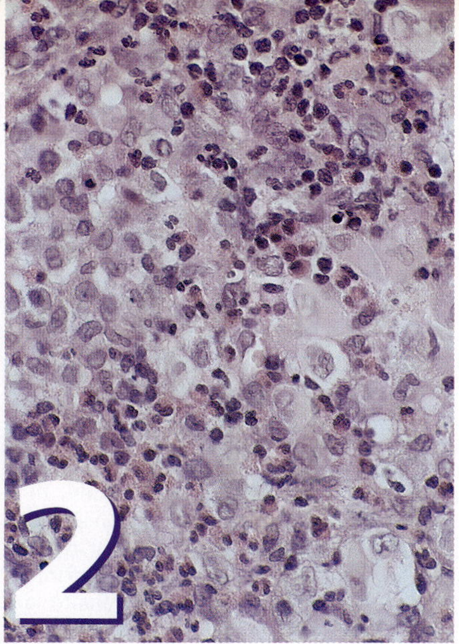

Robert D. Collins

General Approach to Diagnostic Hematopathology

Hematopathology is generally regarded as a complex discipline, a reputation that is well deserved. The principal organs directly affected by hematic or lymphatic diseases include marrow, nodes, spleen, tonsils, thymus, gut, respiratory tract, and skin. In these organs, complex systems of cell production, interaction, destruction, and traffic occur. Furthermore, the functional subpopulations of these various cell types are incompletely defined or imprecisely identified by current techniques. These intrinsic biologic complexities are compounded by terminologic confusion and imprecision that persist in certain disease categories because of conceptual inconsistencies. In addition, diseases often reflect the multitudinous environmental stimulations or injuries possible in this germ- and toxin-rich world.

Some diseases may be recognized only by experts and only by integrating histopathologic, immunophenotypic, and karyotypic information. However, general pathologists will be comforted to know that there is the same order and predictability in hematopathology as in other fields. Common diseases do occur commonly, and the general principles applicable in other fields of pathology are relevant in hematopathology. For many diseases, precise diagnostic criteria have been established and are easily employed by general pathologists as well as specialists. A conceptual framework for lymphoma and leukemia classification, although not widely publicized, nevertheless exists and is herein used.

The *modus operandi* we recommend in pediatric hematopathology is based on the following precepts:

1. Clinical information about symptoms, distribution of disease, and pace of illness is invaluable in diagnosis and should always be in harmony with diagnostic considerations.
2. Microscopic examination of tissue or body fluids is the cornerstone of pathology. Preparation of high-quality sections and blood or marrow films is crucial.
3. Approximately 25 important diseases should be diagnosed with assurance by general pathologists because diagnostic criteria are well established. These are the most frequent neoplasms and reactive processes in various organ systems or are diseases in which immediate recognition is crucial to clinical outcome. These diseases are emphasized throughout this book.
4. Finally, we believe pathologists are responsible for integrating information obtained from biopsies in a single final report, in which multiparameter data are analyzed, discrepancies (between clinical information and histopathologic diagnosis, or between flow cytometric results and histopathologic studies) discussed, and possibilities for further studies outlined. This responsibility is cumulative and should extend to review of previous biopsies. By this approach, we may be of greatest help in guiding diagnosis and treatment of the patients from whom samples have been obtained for our examination.

Carl R. Kjeldsberg

Body Fluid Examination

Hematopathologic diagnoses in pediatrics are usually made by histologic examinations of tissue or microscopic examinations of blood or marrow samples. Occasionally, the primary diagnoses come from examination of cerebrospinal, pleural, peritoneal, or, rarely, pericardial fluid. More frequently, fluid specimens, especially cerebrospinal fluid (CSF), are examined as a staging procedure, in follow-up, or to rule out relapse of disease.

SPECIMEN HANDLING

Body fluid specimens as well as tissue biopsies must be handled appropriately to obtain maximum information from the laboratory studies. Ideal specimen handling begins with detailed clinical information about previous diagnoses, and the patient's current status, diagnostic considerations, and current therapy. Prompt transport to the laboratory is essential. Advance notification from the clinical services is particularly useful in emergent circumstances, when the clinical problems are particularly complex, and when the samples are difficult to collect.

Cerebrospinal Fluid

CSF specimens should be collected sequentially in three sterile tubes: tube 1 is used for chemical and immunologic studies, tube 2 for microbiologic studies, and tube 3 for cell count and morphologic or cytologic examination. Sequential collection minimizes blood contamination in the third tube. CSF containing any blood may not be suitable for evaluating central nervous system (CNS) involvement if there are circulating blasts. CSF specimens should be sent to the laboratory promptly and examined there immediately. The urgency is due to the fact that lysis of cells in CSF takes place soon after removal of the fluid. In order to minimize cell loss, CSF intended for flow cytometric analysis should be transferred on ice, and the cells should be separated by centrifugation at 4°C and suspended in phosphate-buffered saline solution with 1% bovine serum albumin and 5% fetal calf serum. Aliquots are then incubated on ice with labeled monoclonal antibodies (Dux et al, 1994).

CSF cells may be concentrated and deposited on slides by sedimentation methods, filter techniques, and cytocentrifugation. Filter techniques and cytocentrifugation are the most popular. The initial low cell count mandates maximal cell recovery in the laboratory, which is dependent on careful attention to the technical aspects of fluid handling (Kjeldsberg & Knight, 1993). Cells collected on filters are Papanicolaou-stained. Cytocentrifuged preparations are stained with Wright-Giemsa stain and/or Papanicolaou stain. Papanicolaou staining requires wet fixation of the cells in ethanol, whereas Wright-Giemsa–stained slides are air-dried and subsequently fixed in methanol. In cases of suspected malignancy, extra cytocentrifuged slides should be prepared and left unstained for later use in cytochemical or immunocytochemical procedures, which cannot be done on filter preparations. Papanicolaou and Wright-Giemsa stains are both popular in cytologic examination of body fluids. Wright-Giemsa stains have the advantage in hematopoietic disorders, since the appearance of cells in body fluids may be directly compared with that in marrow and/or peripheral blood.

Serous (Pleural, Peritoneal, and Pericardial) Effusions

Serous fluid specimens should be divided at the time of collection into several tubes, the number depending upon the type of laboratory tests to be performed. Fluid from the last tube should be used for cell counts and morphologic examination. Specimens should be examined promptly. If processing is delayed, storage at 4°C is advised to minimize deterioration of cells. In contrast to CSF specimens, serous fluid specimens maintain satisfactory morphologic qualities up to 24 h after fluid collection. One-percent heparin in saline solution is often added in the laboratory to reduce clotting. Some pleural and peritoneal effusions clot unless fluid is drawn into syringes containing 1 ml of 1% heparin in saline solution. In addition to their usefulness in morphologic examination, serous fluid specimens are well suited for immunocytochemical, flow cytometric, molecular pathologic, and cytogenetic studies.

Cell concentration methods include cytocentrifugation and filter techniques (Kjeldsberg & Knight, 1993). Additional cytocentrifuged slides should always be made for possible cytochemical and/or immunocytochemical studies. Papanicolaou stain and Wright-Giemsa stain have been used successfully. Both stains are frequently used because each has advantages and disadvantages (Venrick & Sidawy, 1993).

If malignant lymphomas are suspected, cell blocks should be prepared in addition to cytocentrifuged or filtered specimens, particularly since immunocytochemical studies of paraffin-embedded specimens are so valuable in hematopathology.

HEMATOLOGIC DISORDERS IN BODY FLUIDS

Cerebrospinal Fluid

Leukemia

Leukemic cells may reach the CNS by hematogenous spread or by direct extension from involved cranial marrow (Bleyer, 1989). A few patients with leukemia present with CNS disease without demonstrated marrow or blood involvement (Ganick et al, 1983). CNS prophylaxis with cranial irradiation and intrathecal chemotherapy has reduced the incidence of CNS leukemia in acute lymphoblastic leukemia (ALL) to less than 10%. Patients rarely present with neurologic symptoms. More often, the diagnosis of CSF leukemia is made during routine examinations of CSF. A lumbar puncture is usually performed at the time of diagnostic marrow aspiration to evaluate the CSF. During remission, CSF is examined for blasts whenever intrathecal therapy is given. CSF is also examined at cessation of therapy.

Leukemic cells are most precisely identified in CSF in Wright-Giemsa–stained slide preparations, since their morphologic features may be compared with those of the blasts in the blood and marrow. Leukemic blasts in Papanicolaou-stained specimens are smaller than those in Wright-Giemsa–stained preparations. Lymphoblasts in ALL characteristically have nuclear chromatin that is delicate and evenly distributed and one or several nucleoli. The cytoplasm is scant, gray, or basophilic (Fig. 2–1). The blasts may appear larger, with more cytoplasm, more irregularity in nuclear contours, and more prominent nucleoli than the concurrent blasts in the blood or marrow (Fig. 2–2). Leukemic cells may be considerably distorted in cytocentrifuged preparations, and advanced degenerative changes occur if the CSF is not processed immediately. Morphologic changes also occur in leukemic cells as a result of chemotherapy and/or infections (Fig. 2–3). CSF involvement is less common in acute myelogenous leukemia (AML). Blasts in AML in CSF and marrow may have more cytoplasm and more prominent nucleoli than those in ALL (Fig. 2–4). Accurate diagnoses of CNS involvement have major clinical implications. The accuracy of diagnosis is clearly dependent on the experience and judgment of the morphologist, the adequacy of the specimen, and the appropriate technical preparation of the specimen.

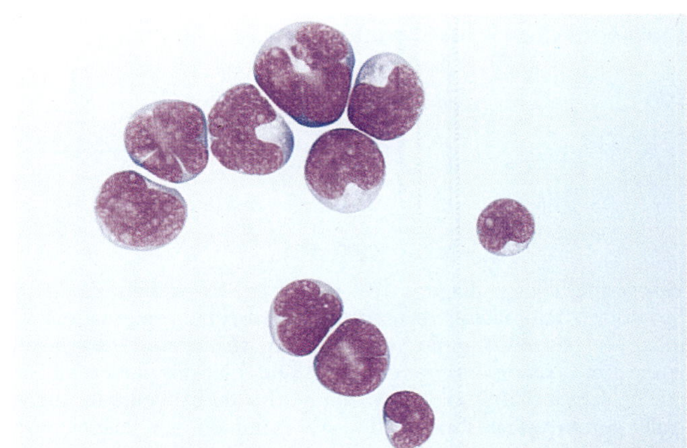

Figure 2–1

Acute lymphoblastic leukemia, CSF. The blasts vary considerably in size, but all have a characteristic fine nuclear chromatin pattern. The nuclear indentations in several blasts are probably due to cytocentrifugation artifact.

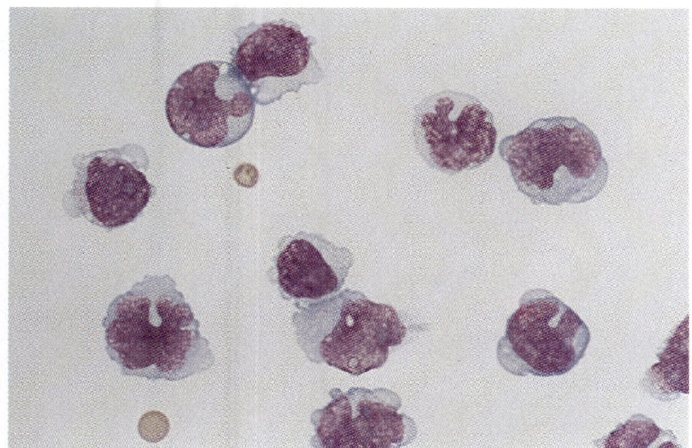

Figure 2–2

Acute lymphoblastic leukemia, CSF. Considerable distortion of the cytomorphologic features is seen. However, a monotonous cell population characteristic of acute leukemia is present.

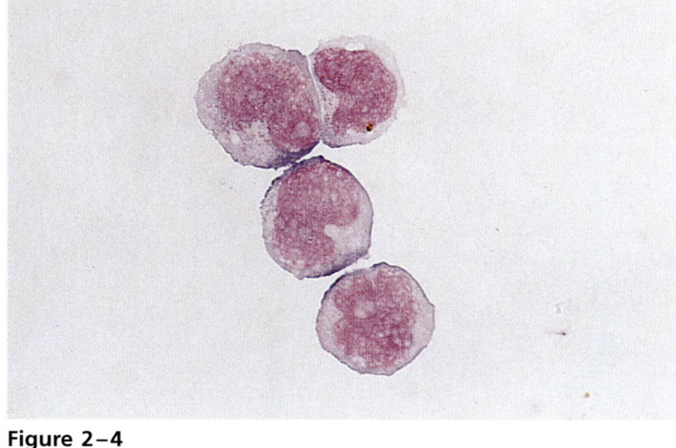

Figure 2–4

Acute myeloblastic leukemia, CSF. The blasts usually have more abundant cytoplasm and more prominent nucleoli than in acute lymphoblastic leukemia.

Cases are particularly challenging when only a few cells are present. It is surprising that there are no uniform criteria for diagnosing CNS leukemia, and the criteria for diagnosis have been modified over the years (Lauer et al, 1989). The changes in the criteria are probably due to improvement in the cytologic preparations and changes in the CNS prophylaxis. The current criteria for CNS involvement in ALL are >5 leukocytes/μl and one or more unequivocal blasts on cytocentrifuged preparations (Mastrangelo et al, 1986).

The diagnosis of CNS leukemia is relatively simple when a monotonous population of numerous blasts is present, but a diagnosis may be extremely difficult if blasts are rare. Based on the current criteria, the identification of unequivocal blasts in the CSF in a patient with acute leukemia with <5 leukocytes/μl poses a diagnostic dilemma as to whether the patient has had a relapse and needs therapy. In one study, CNS relapse in a child with ALL was predicted by five blasts with <6 leukocytes/μl (Odom et al, 1990), whereas other studies have taken the position that blasts on a cytocentrifuged preparation do not predict a CNS relapse if the leukeocyte count is <6/μl (Gilchrist et al, 1990). There is agreement, however, that patients with unequivocal blasts in the CSF, irrespective of the leukocyte count, should have repeat CSF examination within 2 to 3 weeks.

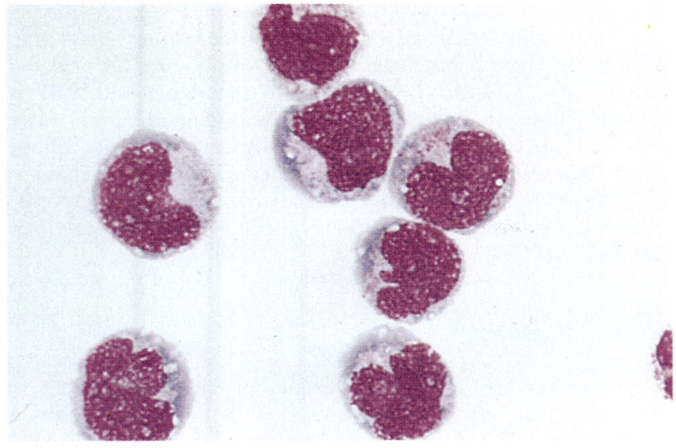

Figure 2–3

Acute lymphoblastic leukemia, CSF. Nuclear degenerative changes are seen.

In addition to cytomorphologic studies, other methods may help identify leukemic cells in the CSF. Cytochemical studies using myeloperoxidase and esterase stains may be helpful in the diagnosis of AML. Immunocytochemical studies of CSF allow typing of the cells and comparison with the leukemic phenotype. Immunophenotyping using cytocentrifuge preparation is limited by the usual paucity of test cells in CSF. Since terminal deoxynucleotidyl transferase (TdT) is present in lymphoblasts in more than 90% of ALL cases, immunofluorescent and immunoperoxidase methods for detecting TdT have been used to study CSF. The presence of TdT-positive cells in CSF free of contaminated blood may predict the development of CNS leukemia even with negative cytomorphologic study results (Hooijkas et al, 1989). This TdT testing may be of value even on paucicellular samples. TdT- and CD10-positive cells have been demonstrated in morphologically negative CSF samples (Homans et al, 1990). More children with ALL may have occult CNS leukemia at initial diagnosis than are currently recognized. However, immunophenotypically abnormal cells in the CSF at diagnosis are not clearly associated with an increased incidence of CNS relapse. Expression of CD22, CD23, and/or IgM markers by leukemic cells in the marrow is apparently associated with CSF involvement (Donskoy et al, 1997), indicating that maturing B-lineage leukemic blasts may have enhanced capabilities to localize in CSF.

Contamination of the CSF by peripheral blood containing blasts may lead to a false-positive diagnosis of CNS leukemia. Contamination with peripheral blood may have occurred even when the CSF appears clear. Since this possibility is of particular concern when the blast count in the peripheral blood is high, counts should be known when CSF is examined.

"Nonspecific" pleocytosis may be seen in 30% of patients with ALL (McIntosh & Ritchey, 1986; Lauer et al, 1989). Cell counts range from 5 to 60 leukocytes/μl and consist predominantly of lymphocytes with variable numbers of monocytes. These reactive cells may resemble leukemic blasts (Fig. 2–5). "Nonspecific" pleocytosis follows intrathecal chemotherapy and

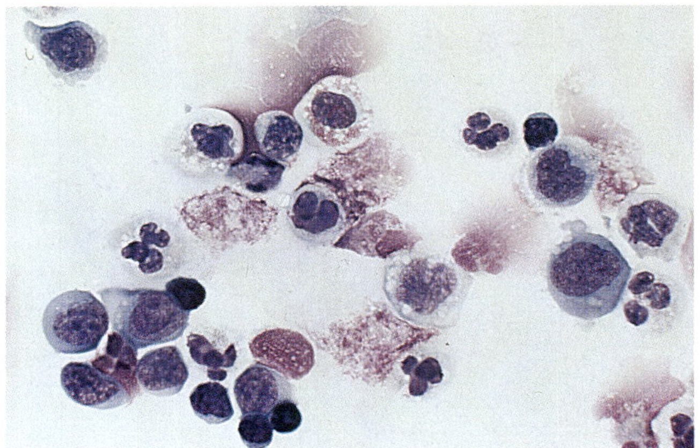

Figure 2–5

Nonspecific pleocytosis, CSF. Polymorphonuclear leukocytes, lymphocytes, and monocytes are seen. Some of the mononuclear cells could be mistaken for leukemic blasts.

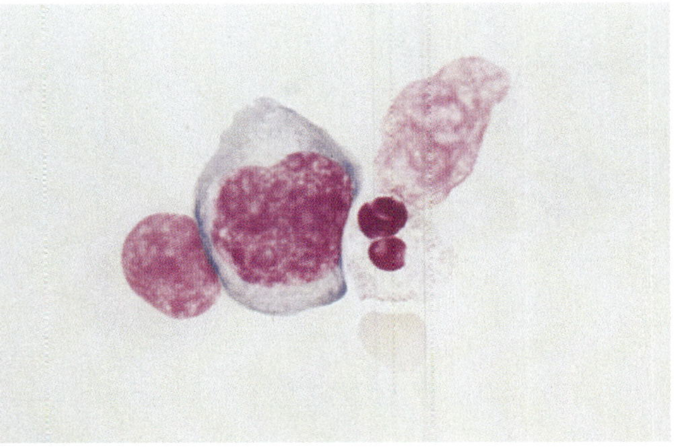

Figure 2–7

Viral meningitis, CSF. A large transformed lymphocyte (immunoblast) is seen between a lymphocyte and a polymorphonuclear leukocyte.

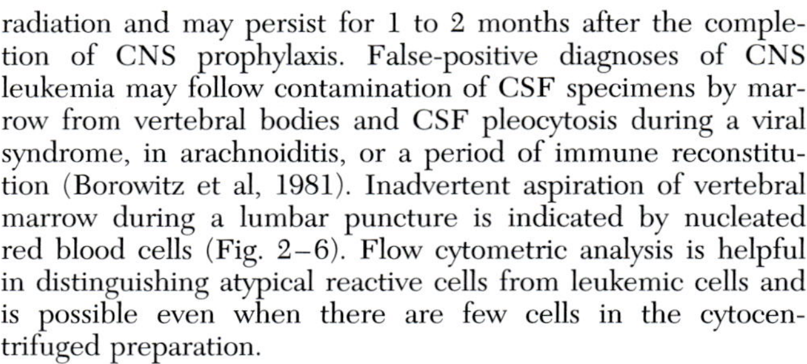

radiation and may persist for 1 to 2 months after the completion of CNS prophylaxis. False-positive diagnoses of CNS leukemia may follow contamination of CSF specimens by marrow from vertebral bodies and CSF pleocytosis during a viral syndrome, in arachnoiditis, or a period of immune reconstitution (Borowitz et al, 1981). Inadvertent aspiration of vertebral marrow during a lumbar puncture is indicated by nucleated red blood cells (Fig. 2–6). Flow cytometric analysis is helpful in distinguishing atypical reactive cells from leukemic cells and is possible even when there are few cells in the cytocentrifuged preparation.

Lymphomas

Primary CNS lymphomas are rare in children. It is also rare for lymphomas in other sites to involve the CNS at the time of diagnosis. Examination of CSF is part of the initial diagnostic work-up of children with B and T lymphomas and is of special importance in Burkitt lymphoma and lymphoblastic lymphoma. Detection of lymphoma in CSF is more likely when the marrow is involved. The CNS is a common site of relapse in lymphoblastic lymphomas. Lymphoblastic lymphoma involving the CSF has an appearance similar to that of ALL (L1 or L2). Burkitt lymphoma in the CSF is characterized by intermediate-sized cells having moderately abundant, deep-blue cytoplasm (with a Wright-Giemsa stain), multiple cytoplasmic vacuoles, and nuclei with slightly coarse chromatin and one or several prominent nucleoli.

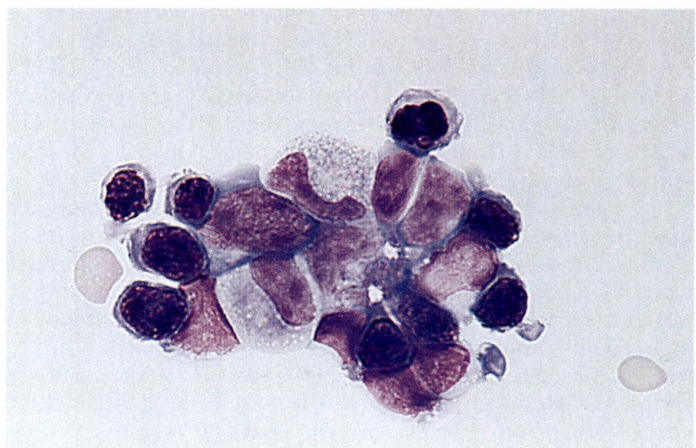

Figure 2–6

Marrow contamination, CSF. Nucleated red blood cells surrounding immature myeloid cells are seen.

In patients undergoing CNS staging for B and T cell lymphoma (or leukemias), a false-positive diagnosis may be made when only a few cells are present. Reactive or transformed lymphocytes in viral meningitis may be mistaken for malignant cells (Fig. 2–7). Viral meningitides typically evoke a spectrum of lymphocytes, including those with low nuclear-cytoplasmic ratios, eccentric and oval nuclei, and prominent nucleoli; plasmacytoid or immunoblastic lymphocytes are often present. The distinction between "atypical" reactive lymphocytes and lymphoma may be extremely difficult to make in immunosuppressed patients with predisposition to infection and Epstein-Barr–associated lymphoproliferative disorders (Kappel et al, 1994). Cytochemical, immunocytochemical, and flow cytometric studies may be useful in difficult cases. Flow cytometric analysis may be particularly helpful, since Burkitt lymphoma cells are monoclonal B cells, whereas lymphoblastic lymphomas are usually TdT positive and have a T cell phenotype.

Polymerase chain reaction (PCR) techniques may help differentiate lymphoma from atypical lymphocytes in selected patients (Rhodes et al, 1996), although experience with CSF is limited. Tumor-derived DNA may be obtained from intact cells, nuclear debris, and soluble DNA released from tumor cells. Demonstration of clonality is not proof of malignancy, since clonal processes are seen in posttransplant lymphoproliferative disorders and conditions such as multiple sclerosis (Young et al, 1996).

Serous Effusions

The great majority of serous effusions in children are benign. Most malignant effusions are caused by lymphomas (Hallman & Geisinger, 1994). Malignant serous effusions are usually clear or slightly bloodstained; rarely, the effusions are chylous due to damage to thoracic duct or cisterna chyli by lymphoma. Most lymphomatous effusions are secondary, but occasionally primary diagnoses of lymphoma are made by cytologic exami-

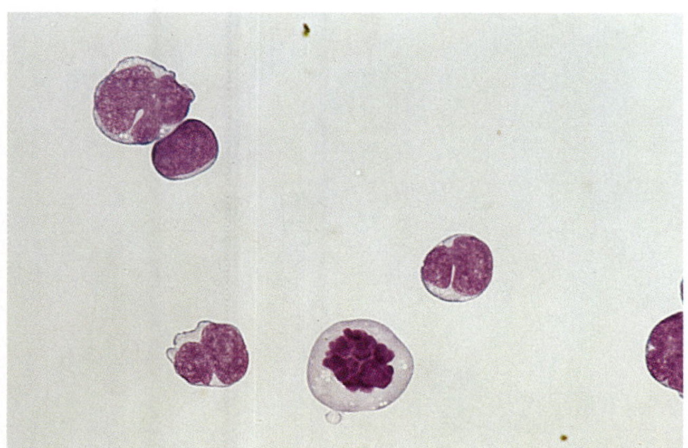

Figure 2–8

Lymphoblastic lymphoma, pleural fluid. Lymphoblasts have prominent nuclear cleavage, and a mitotic figure is seen.

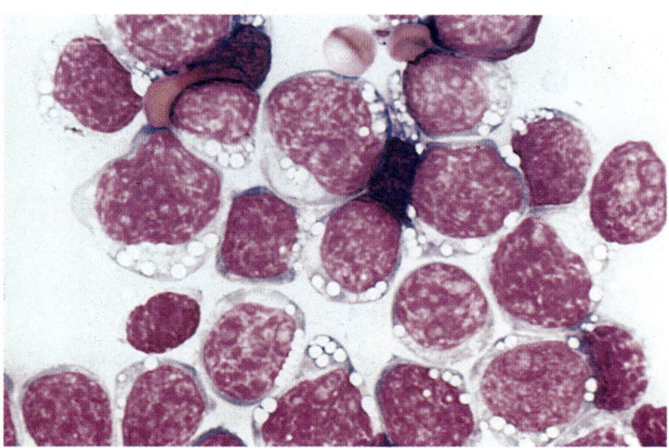

Figure 2–10

Neuroblastoma, pleural fluid. The malignant cells resemble large-cell lymphoma.

nation of serous fluid. Some children with mediastinal lymphoblastic lymphoma may present with a massive pleural effusion, causing respiratory difficulties; the diagnosis of lymphoma in these patients may be made by examination of thoracentesis fluid, thereby avoiding dangerous surgical biopsies in airway-compromised patients. Burkitt lymphoma may present with a peritoneal effusion associated with intestinal obstruction. A primary diagnosis may be made by examination of the peritoneal fluid. Burkitt lymphoma rarely produces pleural effusions (Haddad et al, 1995).

Lymphomatous pleural effusions are usually from lymphoblastic lymphoma (Fig. 2–8) and large-cell lymphoma (Fig. 2–9). Hodgkin disease frequently involves the mediastinum, but pleural effusions are uncommon. Differential diagnosis of malignant pleural effusion includes acute leukemia; pleural effusions are rarely the presenting features. Pleural involvement may be encountered, however, during its course. Pleural effusion is a rare presenting feature of acute leukemia. It may be encountered during the course of the disease, however.

Other tumors in the differential diagnosis are neuroblastoma (Fig. 2–10), nephroblastoma (Wilms tumor), and rhabdomyosarcoma (Geisinger et al, 1994).

Leukemia and lymphoma in children may rarely occur with unexplained pericardial effusions, and a diagnosis may be made by cytologic examination of the pericardial fluid (Spottswood, et al, 1994). Pericardial effusions in leukemia and lymphoma are usually due to infection or radiation-induced pericarditis or myocarditis (Shafer et al, 1993).

Malignant lymphomas associated with peritoneal effusions are usually Burkitt lymphoma (Fig. 2–11) and large-cell lymphoma. Other malignancies to consider in children are neuroblastomas and malignant germ cell tumors (Helson et al, 1975).

Lymphoma and leukemia cells in serous effusions are characteristically monomorphic and usually noncohesive, but these cells may clump in cytocentrifuged preparations. Individual cell necrosis and karyorrhexis are frequent. The lymphoblastic lymphomas are characterized by a monotonous population of medium-sized cells with delicate nuclear chromatin, small

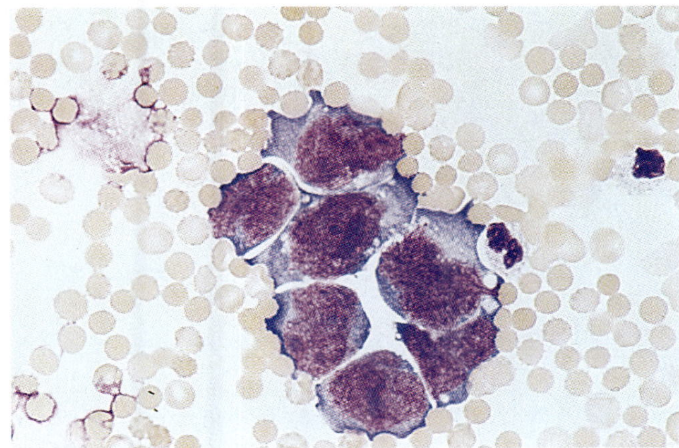

Figure 2–9

Large-cell lymphoma, pleural fluid. The malignant cells have abundant cytoplasm and are many times larger than the benign small lymphocytes present.

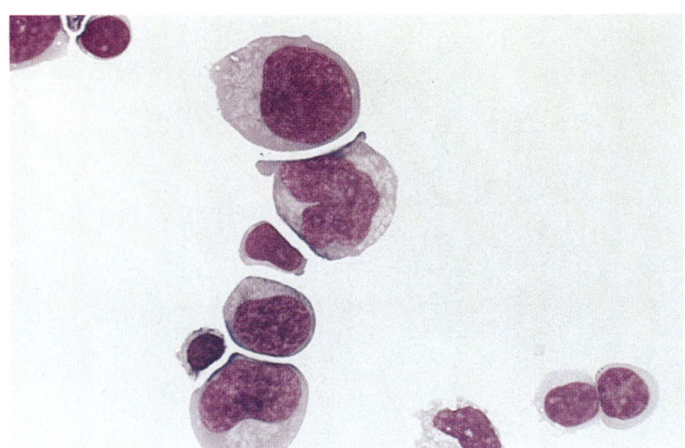

Figure 2–11

Burkitt lymphoma, peritoneal fluid. Cytoplasm of the malignant cells typically contains multiple vacuoles.

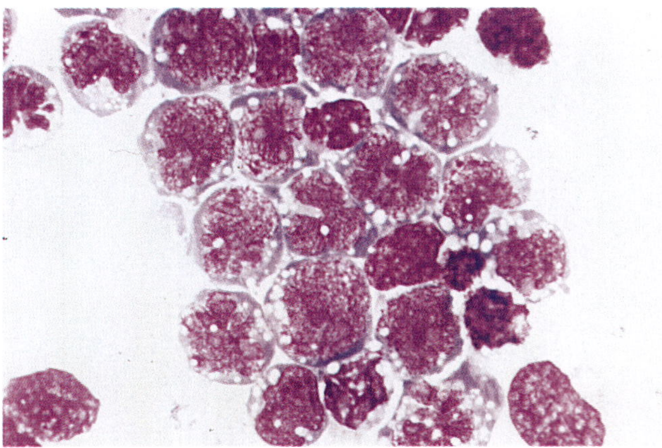

Figure 2–12

Large-cell lymphoma, peritoneal fluid. Cytoplasmic vacuoles are demonstrated.

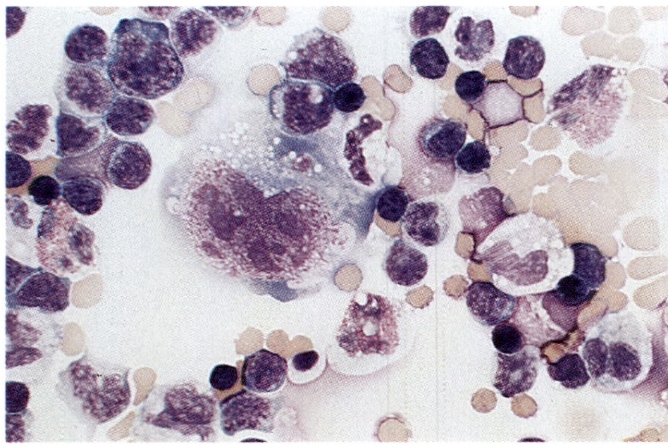

Figure 2–14

Hodgkin disease, pleural fluid. A mononuclear variant of a Reed-Sternberg cell is surrounded by lymphocytes, granulocytes, and eosinophils.

indistinct nucleoli, and scant cytoplasm. Nuclei may be convoluted or nonconvoluted (Fig. 2–8).

Burkitt lymphoma cells are of medium size but have more abundant cytoplasm (deep blue with Wright-Giemsa stain) with characteristic vacuoles (Fig. 2–11). The nuclei in Burkitt lymphoma have coarser chromatin than the cells in lymphoblastic lymphomas. Several prominent nucleoli are usually seen in the former. Cytoplasmic vacuoles are a characteristic feature of Burkitt lymphoma, but similar vacuoles may be seen in other types of lymphoma in serous effusions (Fig. 2–12). Cells in large-cell lymphomas are larger than those in Burkitt and lymphoblastic lymphomas, cytoplasm is more abundant, nuclei have moderately clumped chromatin, and several prominent nucleoli are usual. The cells in anaplastic large-cell lymphoma are usually pleomorphic and may resemble those of carcinoma (Fig. 2–13).

Hodgkin disease occasionally involves the pleural cavity, but it may be difficult to find binucleated Reed-Sternberg cells in serous effusions. Usually there is a mixed cell population of lymphocytes, neutrophils, eosinophils, and mononuclear cells with large nucleoli (mononuclear variants of Reed-Sternberg cells) (Fig. 2–14).

In addition to the distortion from slide preparation, artifactual morphologic variation may be seen in the malignant cells in serous effusions. Nuclei may have markedly irregular nuclear contours (Figs. 2–12 and 2–15), or cells may be larger than expected, for example, if tissue sections are available for comparison.

Primary lymphomas involving the pleural, pericardial, or peritoneal cavities (body cavity–based or serous lymphoma) are extremely uncommon. These lymphomas arise in patients infected with HIV or with chronic tuberculous pleuritis (Jones et al, 1996; Cesarman et al, 1995; Jaffe, 1996). This type of lymphoma has been described only in adults but may occur in children if they have the appropriate risk factors.

Benign lymphocytes in serous fluids may transform in response to various stimuli (Fig. 2–16) and closely simulate malignant lymphoma. Varying proportions of transformed and reactive lymphocytes (immunoblasts and immunocytes, respectively) are seen in infections and a variety of other conditions. In

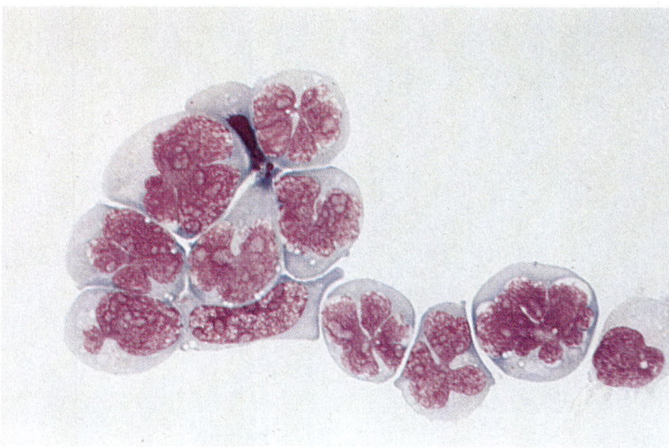

Figure 2–13

Anaplastic large-cell lymphoma, pleural fluid. The malignant cells are pleomorphic.

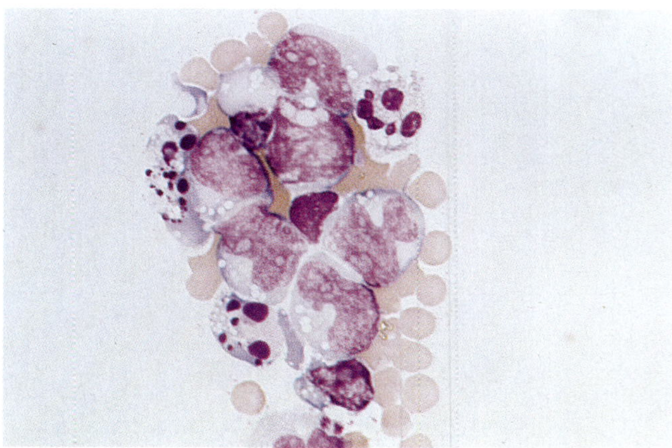

Figure 2–15

Large-cell lymphoma, pleural fluid. The malignant cells are surrounded by degenerative polymorphonuclear leukocytes and have markedly irregular nuclear contours and cytoplasmic vacuoles.

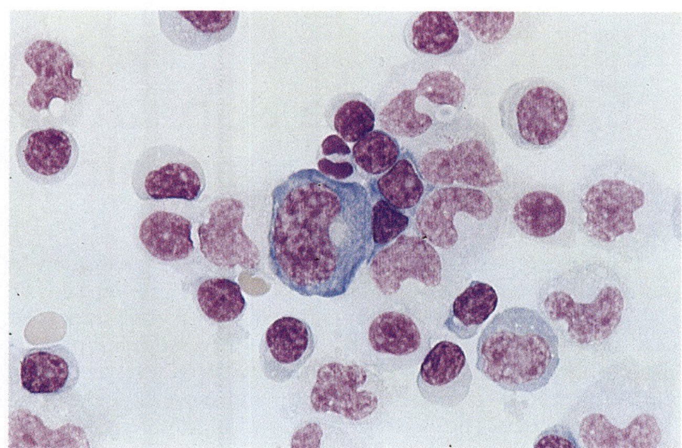

Figure 2–16

Reactive pleural fluid. Lymphocytes and monocytes are noted.

transformed lymphocytes, nucleoli may be prominent, nuclei may have irregular nuclear contours (partly from centrifugation), and mitoses are common.

Serous fluid is an excellent medium for preserving benign and malignant cells and is well suited for immunophenotyping and molecular pathologic studies (Katz et al, 1987). Flow cytometric analysis is the method of choice for differentiating atypical lymphocytosis from malignant lymphoma. Immunophenotypic studies utilizing immunocytochemical studies performed on cytocentrifuged specimens may distinguish among lymphomas, undifferentiated carcinomas, and small, round-cell tumors (Shield et al., 1996). Immunocytochemical studies of cytocentrifuged preparations are associated with the usual problems of background staining and false-positive and false-negative results. Considerable experience and expertise both in the technical preparation and in the interpretation are required (Kjeldsberg & Knight, 1993; Leong, 1996). Cell blocks are prepared when enough fluid is available for paraffin immunoperoxidase study if necessary. Immunostaining may be done on previous Papanicolaou-stained slides (Abendroth & Dabbs, 1995).

B-cell and T-cell gene rearrangement studies with either the classic Southern analysis method or PCR may be used to establish a diagnosis of malignant lymphoma. Cells for these studies may come from frozen pellets or paraffin blocks.

REFERENCES

Abendroth CS, Dabbs DJ: Immunocytochemical staining of unstained versus previously stained cytologic preparations. Acta Cytol 39:379–386, 1995.

Bleyer WA: Biology and pathogenesis of CNS leukemia. Am J Pediatr Hematol Oncol 11:57–63, 1989.

Borowitz M, Bigner SH, Johnston WW: Diagnostic problems in the cytologic evaluation of cerebrospinal fluid for lymphoma and leukemia. Acta Cytol 25:665–674, 1981.

Cesarman E, Chang Y, Moore PS, et al: Kaposi's sarcoma associated herpes virus like DNA sequences in AIDS-related body cavity based lymphomas. N Engl J Med 332:1186–1191, 1995.

Donskoy E, Tausche F, Altman A, et al: Association of immunophenotype with cerebrospinal fluid involvement in childhood B-lineage acute lymphoblastic leukemia. Am J Clin Pathol 107:608–616, 1997.

Dux R, Kindler-Röhrborn A, Annas M, et al: A standardized protocol for flow cytometric analysis of cells isolated from cerebrospinal fluid. J Neurol Sci 121:74–78, 1994.

Ganick DJ, Sondel PM, Gilbert EF, et al: Leukemia presenting as central nervous disease without bone marrow involvement. Med Pediatr Oncol 11:229–232, 1983.

Geisinger KR, Silverman JF, Wakely PE: Pediatric Cytopathology. ASCP Press, Chicago, pp 161–202, 231–254, 1994.

Gilchrist G, Tubergen P, Coccia P, et al: Cerebrospinal fluid blasts (CSFB) on cytocentrifuge do not predict for central nervous system leukemia (CNSL) in children with intermediate risk acute lymphoblastic leukemia (ALL). Children's Cancer Group-105 Proc Am Soc Clin Oncol 9:217, 1990.

Haddad MG, Silverman JF, Joshi VV, et al: Effusion cytology in Burkitt's lymphoma. Diagn Cytopathol 12:3–7, 1995.

Hallman JR, Geisinger KR: Cytology of fluids from pleural, peritoneal and pericardial cavities in children: a comprehensive survey. Acta Cytol 38:209–217, 1994.

Helson L, Krochnal P, Hajdu SI: Diagnostic value of cytologic specimens obtained from children with cancer. Ann Clin Lab Sci 5:294–297, 1975.

Homans AC, Barker BE, Forman EW, et al: Immunophenotypic characterizations of cerebrospinal fluid cells in children with acute lymphoblastic leukemia at diagnosis. Blood 76:1807–1811, 1990.

Hooijkaas H, Hählen KK, Adriaansen HJ, et al: Terminal deoxynucleotidyl transferase (TdT) positive cells in cerebrospinal fluid and development of overt CNS leukemia: a 5-year follow-up study of 113 children with a TdT-positive leukemia or non-Hodgkin's lymphoma. Blood 74:416–422, 1989.

Jaffe ES: Primary body cavity-based AIDS-related lymphomas. Am J Clin Pathol 105:141–143, 1996.

Jones D, Weinberg DS, Pinkus GS, et al: Cytologic diagnosis of primary serous lymphoma. Am J Clin Pathol 106:359–364, 1996.

Kappel TJ, Manivel JC, Goswitz JJ: Atypical lymphocytes in spinal fluid resembling posttransplant lymphoma in a cardiac transplant recipient: a case report. Acta Cytol 38:470–474, 1994.

Katz RL, Raval P, Manning JT, et al: A morphologic, immunologic, and cytometric approach to the classification of non-Hodgkin's lymphoma in effusions. Diagn Cytopathol 3:91–101, 1987.

Kjeldsberg C, Knight J: Body Fluids. ASCP Press, Chicago, pp 303–348, 1993.

Lauer SJ, Kirchner PA, Camitta BM: Identification of leukemic cells in the cerebrospinal fluid from children with acute lymphoblastic leukemia: advances and dilemmas. Am J Pediatr Hematol Oncol 11:64–73, 1989.

Leong AS-Y: Immunostaining of cytologic specimens. Am J Clin Pathol 105:139–140, 1996.

Mastrangelo R, Poplack D, Bleyer A, et al: Report and recommendations of the Rome Workshop concerning poor prognosis acute lymphoblastic leukemia in children: biologic bases for staging, stratification, and treatment. Med Pediatr Oncol 14:191–194, 1986.

McIntosh S, Ritchey AK: Diagnostic problems in cerebrospinal fluid of children with lymphoid malignancies. Am J Pediatr Hematol Oncol 8:28–31, 1986.

Odom LF, Wilson H, Cullen J, et al: Significance of blasts in low-cell-count cerebrospinal fluid specimens from children with acute lymphoblastic leukemia. Cancer 66:1748–1754, 1990.

Rhodes CH, Glantz MJ, Glantz L, et al: A comparison of polymerase chain reaction examination of cerebrospinal fluid and conventional cytology in the diagnosis of lymphomatous meningitis. Cancer 77:543–548, 1996.

Shafer FE, Martin GR, Duval-Arnold B, et al: Cardiac lymphoma presenting with pericardial effusion in a pediatric patient: case report, management, and literature review. Pediatr Hematol Oncol 10:211–213, 1993.

Shield PW, Perkins G, Wright RG: Immunocytochemical staining of cytologic specimens: How helpful is it? Am J Clin Pathol 105:157–162, 1996.

Spottswood SE, Goble MM, Massey GV, et al: Acute monoblastic leukemia presenting with pericardial effusion and cardiac tamponade. Pediatr Radiol 24:494–495, 1994.

Venrick MG, Sidawy MK: Cytologic evaluation of serous effusions: processing techniques and optimal number of smears for routine preparation. Am J Clin Pathol 99:182–186, 1993.

Young C, Gordon N, Safran HP, et al: Monoclonal B-cell population mimicking lymphoma in a patient with multiple sclerosis. Arch Pathol Lab Med 120:275–278, 1996.

Paul E. Wakely, Jr.

Lymph Node Aspiration Cytopathology

Fine-needle aspiration (FNA) biopsy is an excellent technique to determine the nature of lymph node enlargement in children—a fact not generally recognized by physicians' caring for these patients. As a consequence, FNA remains underutilized, even in major centers, for the evaluation of lymphadenopathy in childhood as well as for the assessment of mass lesions.

Persistently enlarged lymph nodes of children are worrisome to parents and pediatricians alike. Lymph node enlargement in children is often watched for a few weeks and even treated empirically with antibiotics. If adenopathy persists, physicians experience the clinical dilemma of continuing observation with the risk of delaying treatment for a serious illness, performing an open biopsy with its attendant risks and costs, or having an FNA procedure.

Sampling an enlarged lymph node with a thin-gauge needle has similarities to incisional or excisional biopsies to determine the cause of adenopathy. In contrast to the surgical procedure, FNA does not involve a skin incision, nor does it require the trappings necessary for a surgical procedure. Obviously, the intent is not to remove an entire lymph node or even to obtain tissue fragments but to obtain cells that are then spread onto glass slides for microscopic evaluation as well as to collect cells for possible ancillary immunophenotyping or molecular studies. FNA as a method of tissue sampling has its own limitations, which are discussed later. Table 2–1 outlines some of the similarities and differences between FNA and surgical biopsy.

Pathologists interpreting aspiration smears must amalgamate the clinical picture, the microscopic details seen on the glass slide, and the ancillary studies, if necessary, to generate a diagnosis (Frable, 1989). Aspiration cytopathologic analysis is nearly always diagnostic, unlike exfoliative cytopathologic study, which often functions as a screening procedure.

Table 2–1
Comparison of Surgical and Fine-Needle Aspiration Biopsies of Lymph Nodes

	Surgery	FNA
Material obtained	Tissue	Cells
Cost	Relatively expensive	Much less expensive
General anesthesia	Sometimes necessary	Unnecessary
Equipment needed	Variable, can be extensive	Minimal
Sampling error	Rarely a problem	Always a possibility
Complications	Uncommon	Rare
Scar or sutures	Normal consequence	Never occurs
Pathologist's confidence	Expertise widespread	Expertise more limited
Insufficient material for diagnosis	Almost never	Sometimes
Immunophenotyping or molecular studies of pathologic material	Possible	Possible

If the lymphadenopathy is deep, FNAs are performed by interventional radiologists. The physicians performing superficial node FNAs vary with local conditions, traditions, expertise, and interests. Pathologists actually performing aspirations are necessarily more informed about clinical circumstances, more directly involved in processing tissue, and more timely in providing diagnoses. The downside of time commitment is generally outweighed by the aforementioned advantages, provided pathologists have the training to maximize the utility of FNA procedures.

ADVANTAGES AND LIMITATIONS

Some masses in children, particularly those in the head and neck, are clinically thought to represent lymph nodes but are lymphangiomas, abscesses, branchial cleft cysts, or soft tissue tumors. This fact partially accounts for decreased sensitivity of FNA in comparison with tissue pathologic studies; such comparisons are faulted by inaccurate clinical diagnoses and are beside the point. In many instances the tissue diagnosis remains the "gold standard," but in some diseases (e.g., lymphoblastic lymphoma) aspiration cytopathologic analysis is superior to tissue examination, in part because it is safer. In other circumstances (outlined later) FNA offers a rapid, convenient, and economical approach to diagnosis in children. FNAs are particularly useful in directing the management of children with lymphadenopathy, providing material for culture and sampling enlarged lymph nodes for staging purposes in those known to have cancer. Smears may be evaluated in minutes for a diagnosis while the patient is in the room. Clinicians may be informed shortly after an FNA, reducing the anxiety of parents if the condition is benign or facilitating immediate therapy or further procedures if it is not. In our institution, a preliminary interpretation is usually available within 20 min after completing the FNA. Advantages provided by FNA are listed in Table 2–2.

The major contraindication to FNA of a superficial lymph node is a severe coagulation disorder. This condition is a relative contraindication, since FNA may be performed if blood products temporarily correct the coagulopathy. Hematoma formation is the only significant complication of superficial FNA. Hemorrhage, fibrosis, and partial or total infarction of lymph nodes occur but are rare. FNA of a deep axillary or supraclavicular lymph node may cause pneumothorax, which is also a possibility when FNA of an enlarged mediastinal lymph node or a mediastinal mass is attempted.

The major shortcomings of FNA may be attributed to sampling errors from improper technique or partial lymph node involvement by a malignancy. Sampling errors should be expected when FNA is performed on nodes partially or extensively fibrosed from lymphoma. Such fibrosis often prevents the extraction of diagnostic cells from their collagen bed.

Aspiration cytologic preparations do not preserve growth patterns, but evaluation of lymph node architecture is not as crucial in pediatric lymphomas as it is in adult lymphomas. The vast majority of pediatric B- and T-cell lymphomas have a diffuse pattern.

Various causes for inconclusive or incorrect results from FNA are listed in Table 2–3. Clinical judgment must override

Table 2–2

Advantages of Fine-Needle Aspiration Biopsy of Lymph Node

Triaging Children with Lymphadenopathy

Confirms that a mass is lymphatic tissue
Helps identify patients who require surgery (e.g., Hodgkin disease) and those for whom surgical biopsy is not indicated (e.g., reactive hyperplasia)
Helps focus laboratory testing, resulting in a more informed and economical work-up (e.g., granulomatous disease)
May suggest the primary site if metastatic tumor is found
Provides material for culture if infectious process is suspected

FNA as a Diagnostic Tool

Rapid turnaround time (minutes for a preliminary interpretation)
High diagnostic sensitivity and specificity for experienced observers
Ability to sample multiple nodes if necessary
Minimal trauma, complications rare
Low cost
Capable of obtaining cells for immunotyping and other ancillary tests

FNA Value for Patients with Cancer

Preserves lymph node architecture if surgical biopsy is required
Documents metastases
Helps in staging

FNA Preferred to Surgical Biopsy

With unacceptable surgical candidate (e.g., paratracheal or mediastinal adenopathy or respiratory compromise)
When conservative management is more appropriate
When cytomorphologic study plus immunophenotyping is diagnostic (e.g., lymphoblastic lymphoma)

negative FNA results. Any clinically suspect lymph node that is interpreted cytopathologically as benign requires further evaluation and possible surgical excision. FNA is rarely informative when performed on patients with only a vague "swelling" or induration of an area. FNA yield is high, however, when discrete masses are present.

ACCURACY DATA

Sensitivity and specificity data for pediatric FNA are flawed by lack of uniformity in definition of childhood (the age of the oldest patients in studies varies from 16 to 19 years), by including young adults who had a higher percentage of malignancies (Kardos et al, 1989) and by including immunophenotyping as an adjunct to cytomorphologic analysis in some studies.

Table 2–3

Sources of Error in Fine-Needle Aspiration

Sampling error due to:
  Improper technique, or operator-dependent error
  Lymph node fibrosis
  Lymph node necrosis
  Partial involvement of lymph node by malignancy
  Small or deep-seated lymph node
Inability to evaluate architecture or vascular pattern
  Subtyping of some lymphocytic disorders not possible
Interpretation error
  Limited experience or expertise

Table 2–4 contains data about the accuracy of pediatric lymph node aspirates. In some studies all anatomic sites, including the lymph nodes, were sampled (Eisenhut et al, 1996; Silverman et al, 1991; Wakely et al, 1988), while others were restricted to FNA of nodes only (Buchino & Jones, 1994; Kardos et al, 1989). In contrast to similar studies in adults, there are very few cases in children, emphasizing the limited use of FNA in children and infrequent clinically disturbing adenopathy in children. Collective experience shows that the sensitivity and specificity of pediatric lymph node FNA are very high in centers where the goal is to distinguish a benign from a malignant condition. Accuracy data for distinct entities such as a particular lymphoma are discussed later under individual diseases.

TECHNIQUE

Children old enough to understand the procedure generally are cooperative, but restraints are needed for infants or toddlers by swaddling in a sheet to immobilize the arms. Anesthesia is not required, but some centers obtain local anesthesia with a topical cream or superficial lidocaine injection. Anesthetics should be injected at the periphery of the mass to avoid subsequent aspiration with sample dilution. Children are routinely sedated when undergoing radiographically guided (usually computerized tomography [CT]) FNA of deep lymph nodes or masses. FNA is not a surgical procedure and may be described to parents as being similar to a needle puncture for blood tests. Young children should not be shown the equipment and needle before the procedure, since their seeing the needle inevitably produces fear and anxiety.

For superficial aspirates, diligent cleansing of the skin surface is not necessary, nor are sterile towels and expensive prepackaged equipment trays. It is more economical and just as efficacious to use alcohol swabs for cleansing and generally

Table 2–4

Sensitivity and Specificity of Fine-Needle Aspiration of Lymph Nodes, Selected Studies

Total	Benign	Malignant	Unsatisfactory	Sensitivity (%)	Specificity (%)	Reference
168	159	8	1	100	100	Eisenhut et al, 1996
123	105	5	13	100	97	Buchino & Jones,1994
41	35	6	0	100	100	Silverman et al, 1991
127	87	40	0	93	95	Kardos et al, 1989
44	31	12	0	100	97	Wakely et al, 1988

only a Band-Aid for closure. Surgical skin disinfectant and sterile procedures are necessary for deep aspirates. FNA may be performed using a syringe for vacuum or with a needle alone. For lymph node aspirates both methods are probably equally effective. The needle-only technique is particularly useful for small (< 1 cm) or excessively mobile lymph nodes. More cells are generally obtained with a syringe.

Three separate aspirating passes into a mass are routine. One aspiration involves inserting the needle, moving it back and forth in the mass, removing it, making smears, and rinsing the needle in balanced saline solution. The procedure is repeated in a slightly different area. Cysts are aspirated entirely, followed by palpation. Residual masses should be reaspirated. The first aspiration generally has the highest yield, and subsequent ones are often contaminated with blood.

A modified Romanovsky stain commonly known as Diff-Quik is often used for most lymph node FNA in preference to a modified Papanicolaou stain. The Diff-Quik stain better highlights cytoplasmic details of lymphocytes, accentuates the presence of lymphoglandular bodies (cell fragments), and is directly comparable to marrow aspirates and peripheral blood films. Details of the FNA procedure are given in Appendix 1. For further details and illustrations, please consult the excellent monograph by Stanley and Löwhagen (1993).

SPECIFIC LESIONS

The remainder of this section deals with specific entities that may be diagnosed when performing FNA in a pediatric population. Certain diagnoses may be made with confidence using FNA. Pathologists should also know the pitfalls in this population of patients. Cytomorphologic analysis and adjunctive immunophenotyping are stressed herein. Clinical features, pathogeneses, and tissue pathologic characteristics of specific lesions are described elsewhere.

Methodical assessment is just as critical in FNA as it is in tissue pathologic studies. The cellularity of smears, cell distribution and arrangement (single cells and cell clusters), cell mixture, and presence of acellular background material are all evaluated in addition to individual cell morphologic features.

Benign Lymphadenopathy

Reactive Lymph Node Hyperplasia

Lymphadenopathy is common in children because lymph nodes are subject to repeated antigenic stimulation. Reactive hyperplasia predominates in pediatric lymph node aspirates in most general hospitals.

Once the cells in an aspirate are recognized as lymphocytes, the major issue is differentiating a reactive process from a lymphoma, a problem exacerbated by the inability to evaluate tissue architecture. The basic tenets used in recognizing lymphocytes, benign or malignant, are their distribution predominantly as discohesive, individual cells (single-cell pattern) and the presence of isolated globular or flakelike cytoplasmic fragments in the background. These fragments (lymphoglandular bodies) are attributed to disruption of fragile lymphocytes in smear preparations. Lymphocytes usually are not cohesive, but the smear thickness, the spreading technique, and the nature of the lesion may produce clusters in some foci of the aspirate. These important features of single-cell pattern and lymphoglandular bodies are seen in the smears of every entity discussed in this section except metastatic tumors (if reacting lymphocytes are not present).

Because there is little stroma in reactive hyperplasia, large numbers of cells are usually obtained, and smears are moderately to highly cellular. The degree of cellularity in FNA does not correlate with the benign or malignant nature of lymphocytic processes.

Small, round lymphocytes predominate in most reactive lymphocytic hyperplasias, but these smears are characteristically polymorphic in distinction to most B- and T-cell lymphomas. Small lymphocytes exhibit coarse, condensed chromatin and meager cytoplasm; cells with plasmacytoid features (eccentric nuclei and moderate amounts of cytoplasm with slight perinuclear clearing); and variable numbers of immunoblasts (large cells with nucleoli and moderate amounts of peripheral basophilic cytoplasm) (Fig. 2–17). Mast cells, neutrophils, and eosinophils appear infrequently, but macrophages usually appear. Cellular polymorphism in FNA narrows the differential diagnosis in childhood to reactive hyperplasia, Hodgkin lymphoma, and partial node involvement by a malignancy regardless of cell type. Minimally reactive lymph nodes in children, ones usually < 1 cm in greatest dimension, may contain a monomorphic population of small, round lymphocytes. The possibility of small-cell lymphoma is not an issue, since these lymphomas are restricted to adults.

A central component of most cases of reactive hyperplasia is proliferation and enlargement of secondary follicles. Certain components of these structures—tingible-body macrophages and follicular center fragments—are generally scattered throughout the smear. Their presence on the smear is not proof of a benign condition, since most high-grade lymphomas contain tingible-body macrophages, and follicular fragments may be found in smears from nodes partially involved by a malignancy. Fragmentation of follicles characteristically produces clusters of cells that contain delicate branching capillaries as well as lymphocytes of various sizes mixed with histiocytes and dendritic follicular cells. The latter may reliably be identified on smears only by immunophenotyping. Loose clusters of lymphocytes and histiocytes (lymphohistiocytic aggregates) may be found in smears from reactive nodes. Features not seen in reactive lymph nodes are markedly pleomorphic cells, atypical mitoses, individual cell necrosis, and a background of cellular debris.

Reactive-appearing processes must be carefully examined for large uninucleated or binucleated cells of the Reed-

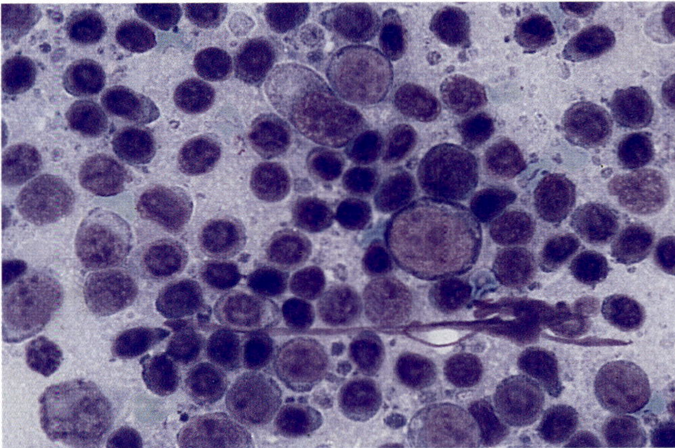

Figure 2–17

Reactive hyperplasia, lymph node. A polymorphous population of nonclustering lymphocytes is highlighted by the immunoblast just to the right of center. Note that the field is dominated by small lymphocytes, but plasmacytoid lymphocytes are also seen. Lymphoglandular bodies are the tiny gray-blue cytoplasmic globules haphazardly scattered in the background. Romanovsky stain.

Sternberg (RS) type. Hodgkin lymphoma is a major consideration in the differential diagnosis of pleomorphic processes in children, a consideration that may be heightened by clinical suspicion before the FNA is performed. Immunophenotyping, by flow cytometric or immunohistochemical techniques, is rarely required to diagnose reactive lymphoid hyperplasia. Material is available, if necessary, since every needle pass is rinsed in a balanced saline solution.

Lymphadenitis

In acute lymphadenitis, smears are hypercellular, and many neutrophils are admixed with lymphocytes. If an abscess exists, pus is noted either in the hub or in the barrel of the syringe during the FNA. The smear consists of a pure population of neutrophils. Part of obviously purulent material should be submitted for culture by expelling it into a sterile container or a culturette device. Cultures should be attempted even if a child is being treated, since antibiotic resistance is an increasing problem.

Fungi and occasionally bacteria may be identified on Romanovsky-stained smears, or these organisms may be identified by special stains on aspirate smears or cytocentrifuged preparations from balanced saline solution. Immunosuppressed children are often unable to mount a granulomatous response. Stains for mycobacteria are particularly appropriate in patients with AIDS, since the smear examination often suggests acute lymphadenitis (Fig. 2–18).

Presumably because of their lipid coating, mycobacteria in Romanovsky-stained smears appear as unstained linear "negative images" and may be found extracellularly or within macrophages, where they resemble Gaucher cells because of their linear striations.

Granulomatous Lymphadenitis

Granulomas are recognized in aspirate smears as either loose or tight clusters of epithelioid histiocytes. Granulomas may be distinguished from lymphohistiocytic aggregates by concentrating on the nuclear features of cells in the group, since epithelioid histiocyte nuclei in smears display an elongated, almost elliptical outline and often project away from the granuloma center in a star-burst pattern. A slight nuclear indentation on one side may produce a shape that has been compared with a boomerang or footprint in the sand.

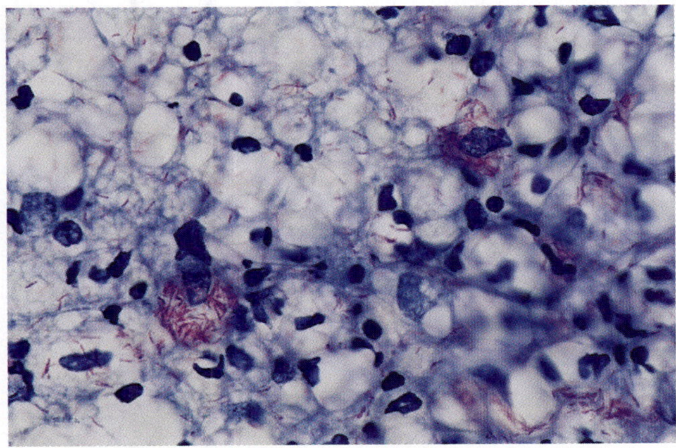

Figure 2–18

Tuberculous lymphadenitis, lymph node. Stained acid-fast bacilli are found in the background as well as engulfed by the two histiocytes in this field. Ziehl-Neelsen stain.

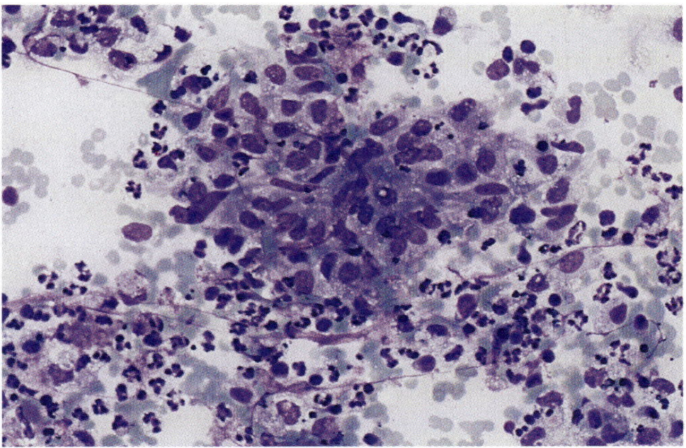

Figure 2–19

Acute granulomatous lymphadenitis, consistent with cat-scratch disease, lymph node. A tight cluster of epithelioid histiocytes is surrounded by many neutrophils and karyopyknotic nuclear debris. Some of the histiocytes display a characteristic elongation of cell nuclei. Romanovsky stain.

Cat-scratch disease is the cause of most cases of suppurative granulomatous lymphadenitis in childhood. Smears are moderately to highly cellular and contain neutrophils, a variable degree of background necrosis, and occasional multinucleated giant cells. Granulomas vary in number, and their presence is often obscured by the acute inflammation and karyorrhectic debris (Fig. 2–19). Samples in early stages of cat-scratch disease contain few granulomas and are easily mistaken for reactive hyperplasia. Confirmation of cytomorphologic impressions are obtained by polymerase chain reaction (PCR) for the genomic fragments of the responsible organism, *Bartonella henselae*, and silver stains are rarely worthwhile.

Most examples of mycobacterial lymphadenitis contain neutrophils, lymphocytes, or plasma cells in addition to granulomas. Caseation necrosis may not be present, particularly in immunosuppressed patients.

Lymphadenitis caused by toxoplasmosis is difficult to diagnose by FNA. The small collections of intra- and parafollicular epithelioid histiocytes seen in tissue sections cannot be seen in aspirate smears, and the cysts of *Toxoplasma gondii* are rarely found in aspirates. Serologic testing is therefore necessary for diagnosis.

Sinus Histiocytosis with Massive Lymphadenopathy (Rosai-Dorfman Disease)

There are few reports about recognizing this entity by FNA (Trautman et al, 1991), but the key cytopathologic feature is histiocytes that have engulfed viable lymphocytes (Fig. 2–20). Histiocyte immunostaining for S-100 may be performed directly on smears. The S-100–positive cells of sinus histiocytosis differ morphologically from those in Langerhans cell histiocytosis, which have an irregular and sometimes reniform border and often contain linear nuclear grooves. This entity, which is readily recognized in tissue sections because of the distended sinuses, may be overlooked in FNA because the spectrum of lymphocyte morphologic features described earlier for reactive hyperplasia may be seen. Smears may be misleading, in that collections of engulfed lymphocytes may obscure the underlying histiocyte nucleus. Small lymphocytes may be shown to be intracytoplasmic by their thin halo. This manifestation of lymphocytic phagocytosis distinguishes this process from lymphohistiocytic aggregates of a nonspecific reactive lymph node hyperplasia.

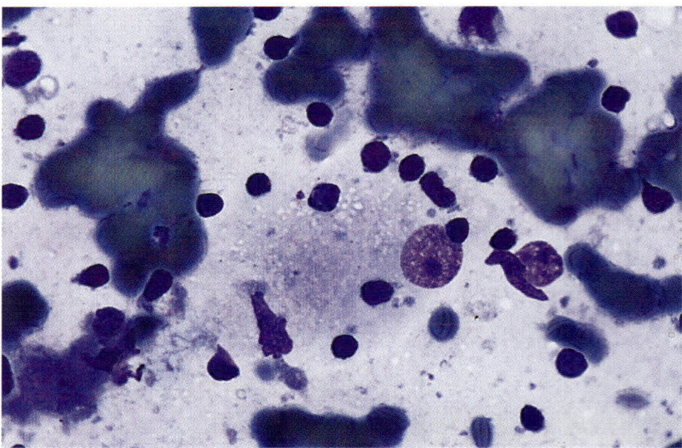

Figure 2–20

Rosai-Dorfman disease, lymph node. A single histiocyte with an eccentric nucleus and prominent nucleolus has phagocytosed eight small lymphocytes. The cell border is difficult to appreciate in Romanovsky-stained smears. Histiocytes were revealed on S-100 immunostaining (not shown). Romanovsky stain.

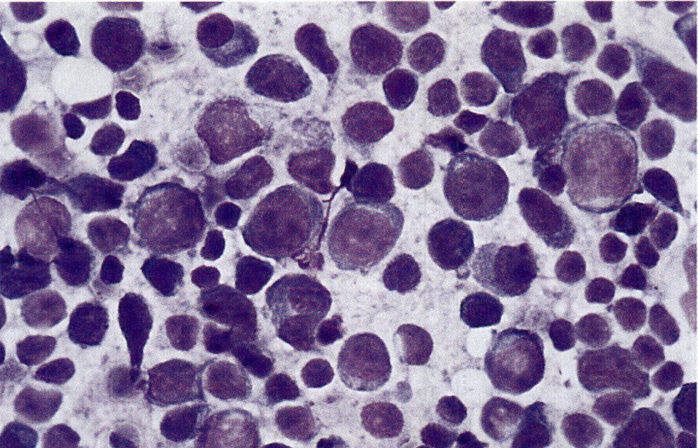

Figure 2–21

Infectious mononucleosis, lymph node. Numerous immunoblasts make this smear highly suspicious for mononucleosis. Lymphocyte heterogeneity is considerably more marked than in large-cell lymphoma. Note the plasmacytoid lymphocyte at the top of the field. Romanovsky stain.

Angiofollicular Hyperplasia (Castleman Disease)

There are few if any reports showing that angiofollicular hyperplasia may be diagnosed with confidence by FNA. Aspirates in this disease appear reactive, but the vascular pattern seen in tissue sections becomes unrecognizable after aspiration. Hyalinized germinal centers are not confidently appreciated in smears.

Infectious Mononucleosis

The diagnosis of infectious mononucleosis is usually based on combined clinical and serologic features. FNA may suggest or exclude this diagnosis in a child who has not undergone serologic testing or who has negative serologic test results. FNA is also occasionally used to exclude or diagnose a malignant lymphoma in children with mononucleosis-like clinical symptoms.

Aspiration smears are hypercellular, containing a polymorphous lymphocytic population with numerous plasmacytoid lymphocytes and numerous immunoblasts. These are large cells with fine nuclear chromatin, prominent nucleoli, and ample basophilic cytoplasm (Fig. 2–21) (Kardos et al, 1988). Pleomorphic binucleate immunoblasts resembling RS cells may rarely be found.

Aspirates in patients with mononucleosis contain numerous immunoblasts and plasmacytoid lymphocytes and few tingible-body macrophages or follicular fragments. These features favor a diagnosis of mononucleosis over other causes of reactive hyperplasia. The prevalence of immunoblasts and large cells may be misinterpreted as large-cell lymphoma unless the range of lymphocytes in mononucleosis is recognized. Flow cytometric analysis is generally not needed for diagnosis but may help by showing polyclonal B cells and a predominance of T cells with a suppressor or cytotoxic phenotype.

Neoplastic Lymphadenopathy

Lymphoblastic Lymphoma

Experience over the last decades in several centers has shown that aspiration cytopathologic study has supplanted tissue biopsy as the best method of diagnosis of lymphoblastic lymphoma, since FNA diagnosis in this disease appears infallible (Jacobs et al, 1992; Kardos et al, 1987; Tani et al, 1993; Wakely & Kornstein, 1996). Patients often have a palpable neck mass and are critically ill from some degree of respiratory compromise. FNA should be the first procedure for diagnosis because it is expedient, minimally invasive, reliable, and, as mentioned, does not require sedation or general anesthesia. Furthermore, cells are readily obtained for ancillary studies. Cytomorphologic evaluation and immunotyping may be performed in 1 to 2 h.

Aspirates in lymphoblastic lymphoma are hypercellular, and smears are thick. Monomorphic lymphoblasts cover the smear in a single-cell pattern with clumping, particularly at the edges of the smear (Fig. 2–22). There is little variation in cellular appearance, although a dimorphic pattern may be seen if the predominant lymphoblast is admixed with smaller hyperchromatic degenerating blasts. Lymphoblasts are about twice the size of small lymphocytes. Their nuclei conform to the L1 or L2 morphologic characteristics of the French-American-British (FAB) classification for acute lymphoblastic leukemia (Geisinger et al, 1994). Cytoplasm, with or without tiny indistinct vacuoles, is sparse. Mitotic figures are usually numerous. Lymphoglandular

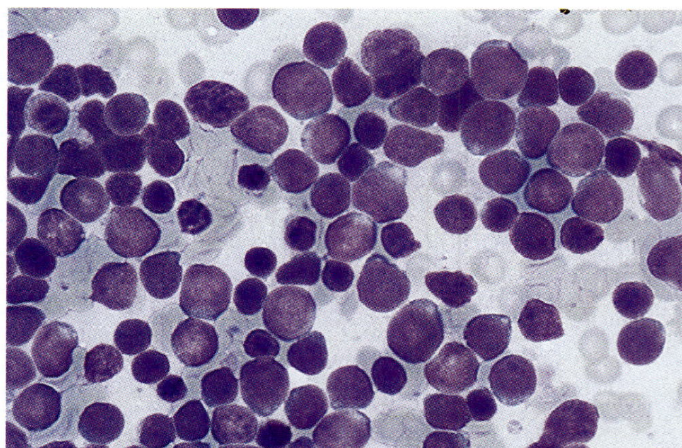

Figure 2–22

Lymphoblastic lymphoma, lymph node. Singly dispersed blasts have very finely granular chromatin and meager cytoplasm. There is a monomorphous population of cells, but the degenerating blasts exhibiting more darkly staining and smaller nuclei give a false impression of a dimorphic population of cells. Romanovsky stain.

bodies vary in amount but may be found in every case, and tingible-body macrophages are also easily identified.

Immunocytochemical study is mandatory if the cytopathologic diagnosis is lymphoma or "suspicious for lymphoma" in children. The proper morphologic features, combined with corroborating immunologic typing are diagnostic. Nearly all cases of lymphoblastic lymphoma are positive for terminal deoxynucleotidyl transferase (TdT), a nuclear marker that can be recognized in cytocentrifuged preparations. More than 90% of cases are of the T cell phenotype.

The differential diagnosis involves other lymphomas. The monomorphic appearance excludes reactive hyperplasia from consideration. FNA performed on mediastinal masses of any type may obtain normal thymocytes that are also TdT positive. The differences between lymphoblastic lymphoma and Burkitt lymphoma are described in the next section. Large-cell lymphomas are not a consideration because of the size of the cell.

Burkitt Lymphoma

Burkitt lymphoma is high-grade, and diagnoses may be made by coupling cytomorphologic with immunocytochemical analysis without the need for tissue biopsy. Both of the most common and serious lymphomas in children may therefore be diagnosed using FNA procedures with immunophenotyping. Children with large intra-abdominal tumors may have planned surgical debulking after diagnosis of Burkitt lymphoma by FNA, a sequence of some advantage to these patients. Reports on the diagnostic accuracy of FNA in Burkitt lymphoma are few in number, but sensitivity and specificity approach 100% (Das et al, 1987; Stastny et al, 1995). Since Burkitt lymphoma is usually infradiaphragmatic, FNAs are often radiographically guided.

Aspirate smears are highly cellular and consist of discohesive, monomorphic lymphocytes two to three times the size of small lymphocytes. Nuclei conform to the L3 morphologic features of the FAB system; they are round, with coarsely clumped chromatin and one to several discrete nucleoli that are more conspicuous and discrete in Papanicolaou-stained smears (Geisinger et al, 1994) (Fig. 2–23). Cytoplasm is deeply basophilic in Romanovsky-stained preparations, is moderate in amount, and typically contains coarse lipid vacuoles. Background lymphoglandular bodies may also show vacuolization. Tingible-body macrophages are randomly dispersed throughout the smear, mimicking the "starry sky" pattern in histologic sections. Individual cell necrosis is common, and there are many mitoses. Burkitt lymphoma is a B cell malignancy that readily demonstrates light-chain restriction, reactivity with pan–B cell markers, and CD10 positivity. Results of staining for TdT are negative in virtually all cases.

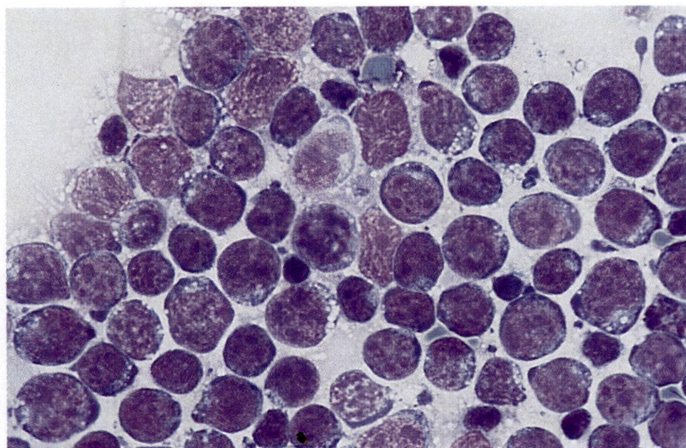

Figure 2–23

Burkitt lymphoma, lymph node. Even in air-dried smears, the coarse nuclear chromatin and multiple nucleoli of Burkitt lymphoma cells are usually appreciated. Small, delicate cytoplasmic vacuoles exist in most cells. A few pyknotic nuclei are also present. Romanovsky stain.

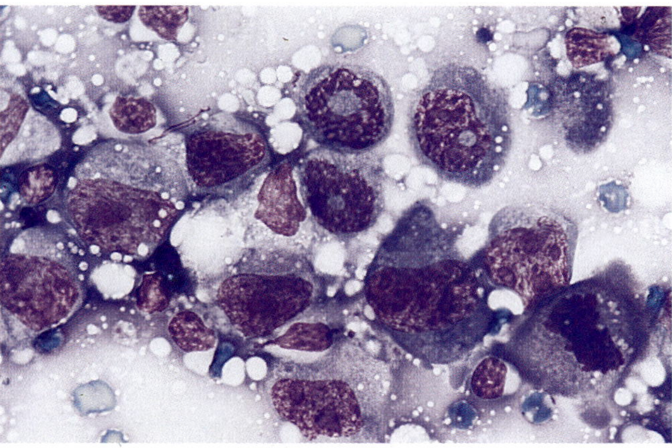

Figure 2–24

Anaplastic large-cell lymphoma (CD30+), lymph node. Very large and unquestionably pleomorphic nuclei contain a moderate amount of cytoplasm that is vacuolated. Ringlike nuclei in a cell at the top of the field are characteristic of this lymphoma in aspirate smears. A mitotic figure is seen at the lower right. Romanovsky stain.

Burkitt lymphoma is simply differentiated from other childhood lymphomas, since the features of cell size, chromatin pattern, vacuolization, and immunophenotype are characteristic. The most difficult cases cytologically are those in which cellularity is less than optimal, vacuoles are not abundant, and cells are insufficient for immunophenotyping. CT-guided procedures are more effective when pathologists are on hand to inform the radiologists as to the amount and quality of material aspirated.

Large-Cell Lymphoma

Large-cell lymphoma in children may occur in the mediastinum as in the retroperitoneum, and as superficial lymphadenopathy. Cellularity of smears is variable, particularly in deep aspirates using CT guidance. Tumor cells are generally three or more times the size of small lymphocytes. Nuclei are large and vary in shape. Nucleoli are generally conspicuous and may be multiple. Cytoplasm is moderate to abundant and may include small vacuoles. Immunoblasts may be present on smears, along with tingible-body macrophages and necrosis.

Anaplastic large-cell (CD30+) lymphoma is a special type of large-cell lymphoma with a predilection for teenagers and young adults. Aspirate smears show moderate to high cellularity, with large malignant cells that display obvious pleomorphism (Akhtar et al, 1992). Multinucleated forms are common. Nuclei are often arranged in a concentric "wreathlike" fashion in the cell (Fig. 2–24). The cytopathologic diagnosis of anaplastic large-cell lymphoma is difficult without immunophenotyping because it may be confused with a nonlymphocytic malignancy, such as anaplastic carcinoma, melanoma, or sarcoma.

Hodgkin disease (HD) may be difficult to differentiate from anaplastic large-cell lymphoma. The latter may have mirror-image nuclei with large nucleoli but lacks a population of reactive lymphocytes and eosinophils. The accuracy of FNA in the diagnosis of a large series of anaplastic large-cell lymphoma has not been established, but the cytomorphologic features coupled with immunophenotyping allows for a diagnosis in many childhood cases. Immunocytochemical analysis is useful in making this distinction, since most anaplastic large-cell lymphomas are CD45+, are epithelial membrane antigen positive, and have a T-cell phenotype unlike classic HD. More specifically, the 2;5 translocation clearly identifies this neoplasm, or the gene product of the translocation may be visualized with antibody to p80.

Hodgkin Disease

The diagnosis of HD by FNA may be quite difficult. Binucleated RS cells are rarely seen, but mononuclear RS cells are distinctive (Fig. 2–25). These cells are large, are often apparent at medium magnification, and have lobated nuclear contours. RS cells may be hidden in a sea of lymphocytes when the smear is cellular. The spectrum of large lymphocytes and immunoblasts in HD may mimic reactive hyperplasia, particularly in partially involved nodes. Nuclear chromatin may be fine or coarse in RS variants, and nucleoli are generally large and distinct. Nucleoli may be seen in Romanovsky-stained smears if they are not overstained but are best identified in Papanicolaou-stained preparations. Bare nuclei of these RS variants may also be present.

Since nodular sclerosis is the most common subtype of HD, FNA often results in hypocellular smears. Fibrosis interferes with aspiration of RS cells, and a concentrated search may be needed to find these cells in hypocellular aspirates. Such searches are particularly indicated when nodes are firm and thus clinically suspect. Aspirates in HD may contain fibrous stroma, eosinophils, necrosis, plasma cells, neutrophils, and granulomas, with some variation from case to case. Subtyping HD by FNA is not reliable. Excisional biopsy should be obtained to confirm the FNA impression prior to therapy whenever possible. Immunostaining of smears or cytocentrifuged preparations may occasionally be helpful in differentiating HD from other lymphomas.

Metastatic Tumor

The value of FNA in confirming the presence of metastatic tumor in children is well established. Diagnoses are usually uncomplicated and highly accurate because smears contain cells that are recognizable as neoplastic, in addition to having features, described subsequently, that are not usually found in lymphoma cells. Furthermore, the tissue slides from the primary tumor should be available for comparison with the aspirate.

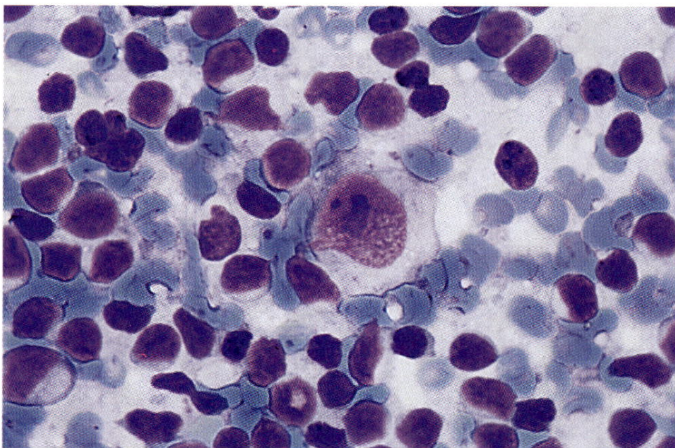

Figure 2–25

Hodgkin disease, lymph node. Mononuclear Reed-Sternberg variants with large nuclei and large, misshapen nucleoli are consistently found in Hodgkin disease, while "classic" binucleated Reed-Sternberg cells are rare. Mononuclear cells may "hide" among small lymphocytes and are easily overlooked. Romanovsky stain.

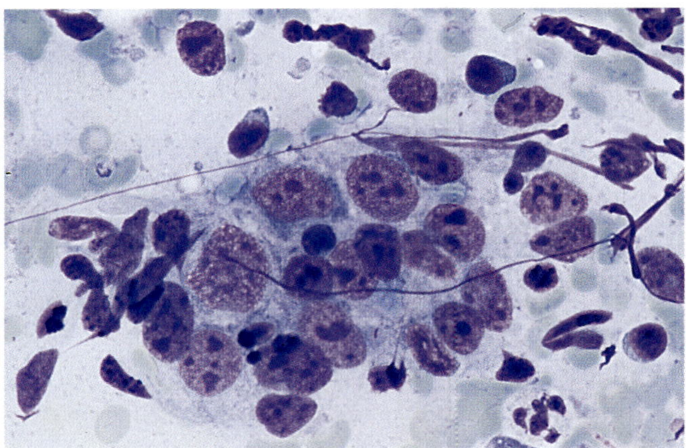

Figure 2–26

Nasopharyngeal carcinoma, metastatic, lymph node. Small lymphocytes with slight cytoplasmic elongation are dispersed in and around this oval aggregate of malignant epithelial cells. Multiple irregular nuclei are conspicuous in these cells. Romanovsky stain.

Metastases to lymph nodes are uncommon in children but are sufficiently frequent in rhabdomyosarcoma, neuroblastoma, and nasopharyngeal carcinoma that pathologists should be familiar with the cytomorphologic features of these neoplasms. Smears of both rhabdomyosarcoma and neuroblastoma are hypercellular and have cells scattered in both single cells and clusters. The absence of numerous lymphoglandular bodies in the smear background is very good evidence that one has not aspirated lymphocytes. Tumor cells are two to three times the size of small lymphocytes. Differentiating rhabdomyoblasts have a distinctive morphologic feature: they are cells with two or more nuclei and abundant cytoplasm (Almeida et al, 1994). Nucleoli and tapering of cell cytoplasm may be seen in rhabdomyosarcomas.

Neuroblastoma has the same high nuclear-cytoplasmic ratio as rhabdomyosarcoma and many lymphomas. Nuclear molding and clustering is common in neuroblastoma—a difference from lymphomas. Nuclei are oval to minimally irregular with inconspicuous nucleoli. Background neuropil, a delicate fibrillary tangle of cell processes, is the most helpful feature in recognizing neuroblastoma. Occasionally, neuropil is nodular and encircled by cells forming classic Homer-Wright rosettes. Just as often, however, neuropil is a variably shaped fibrillary web that may have only a few nuclei around it.

Nasopharyngeal carcinoma (lymphoepithelioma) affects adolescents and young adults, and usually arises in the roof and lateral walls of the nasopharynx. Presentation is often as an enlarged unilateral or bilateral cervical lymph node. Smears are moderately cellular but may be hypocellular. Malignant epithelial cells form tight clusters and display large nuclei; single, prominent nucleoli; and moderate amounts of cytoplasm with indistinct cell borders (Fig. 2–26). Cytologic evidence of reactive lymphocytic hyperplasia is almost always present. Eosinophils and macrophages may suggest HD. Lymphocytes may greatly outnumber the syncytia of malignant cells, which may be mistaken for follicular center fragments.

In clinically suspect cases, all smears must be reviewed carefully, since epithelial cells may be very difficult to find. Immunostaining may be very helpful in highlighting cytokeratin-positive cells in smear or cytocentrifuged preparations. Papanicolaou stains to show keratin differentiation are not useful, since most of these tumors have scant amounts of keratin.

REFERENCES

Akhtar M, Ali MA, Haider A, et al: Fine-needle aspiration biopsy of Ki-1-positive anaplastic large-cell lymphoma. Diagn Cytopathol 8:242–247, 1992.

Almeida M, Stastny JF, Wakely PE Jr, et al: Fine-needle aspiration biopsy of childhood rhabdomyosarcoma: reevaluation of the cytologic criteria for diagnosis. Diagn Cytopathol 11:231–236, 1994.

Buchino JJ, Jones VF: Fine needle aspiration in the evaluation of children with lymphadenopathy. Arch Pediatr Adolesc Med 148:1327–1330, 1994.

Das DK, Gupta SK, Pathak IC, et al: Burkitt-type lymphoma: diagnosis by fine needle aspiration cytology. Acta Cytol 31:1–7, 1987.

Eisenhut CC, King DE, Nelson WA, et al: Fine-needle biopsy of pediatric lesions: a three-year study in an outpatient biopsy clinic. Diagn Cytopathol 14:43–50, 1996.

Frable WJ: Needle aspiration biopsy: past, present, future. Hum Pathol 20:504–517, 1989.

Geisinger KR, Silverman JF, Wakely PE Jr: Pediatric Cytopathology. ASCP Press, Chicago, pp 201–228, 1994.

Jacobs JC, Katz RL, Shabb N, et al: Fine needle aspiration of lymphoblastic lymphoma: multiparameter diagnostic approach. Acta Cytol 36:887–894, 1992.

Kardos TF, Kornstein MJ, Frable WJ: Cytopathology and immunopathology of infectious mononucleosis. Acta Cytol 32:722–726, 1988.

Kardos TF, Maygarden SJ, Blumberg AK, et al: Fine needle aspiration biopsy in the management of children and young adults with peripheral lymphadenopathy. Cancer 63:703–707, 1989.

Kardos TF, Sprague RI, Wakely PE Jr, et al: Fine needle aspiration biopsy of lymphoblastic lymphoma and leukemia: a clinical, cytologic, and immunologic study. Cancer 60:2448–2453, 1987.

Silverman JF, Gurley AM, Holbrook CT, et al: Pediatric fine-needle aspiration biopsy. Am J Clin Pathol 95:653–659, 1991.

Stanley MW, Löwhagen T: Fine Needle Aspiration of Palpable Masses. Butterworth-Heinemann, Boston, pp 1–57, 1993.

Stastny JF, Almeida MM, Wakely PE Jr, et al: Fine needle aspiration biopsy and imprint cytology of small non-cleaved cell (Burkitt's) lymphoma. Diagn Cytopathol 12:201–207, 1995.

Tani E, Maeda S, Fröstad B, et al: Aspiration cytology with phenotyping and clinical presentation of childhood lymphomas. Diagn Oncol 3:294–301, 1993.

Trautman BC, Stanley MW, Goding GS et al: Sinus histiocytosis with massive lymphadenopathy (Rosai-Dorfman disease): diagnosis by fine needle aspiration. Diagn Cytopathol 7:513–516, 1991.

Wakely PE Jr, Kardos TF, Frable WJ: Application of fine needle aspiration biopsy to pediatrics. Hum Pathol 19:1383–1386, 1988.

Wakely PE Jr, Kornstein MJ: Aspiration cytopathology of lymphoblastic lymphoma and leukemia: the MCV experience. Pediatr Pathol Lab Med 16:243–252, 1996.

Appendix

Technique of Fine-Needle Aspiration Biopsy

EQUIPMENT

- ☐ Disposable 10- or 20-ml syringes.
- ☐ Disposable fine needles: 22-, 23-, 25-, or 27-gauge needles, 1–1.5 inches in length for each gauge. We use mainly a 25-gauge, 1-inch needle in small children.
- ☐ Syringe holder (multiple commercial manufacturers).
- ☐ Nonfrosted, nonalbuminized glass slides. Alcohol swabs. Gauze pads.

THE ASPIRATION PROCEDURE

Verbal consent or written consent from the parent may be required. The procedure is explained to the parents; children are told there will be a slight sting. Older children and adolescents are fully informed in the presence of the parent or parents, and their cooperation is requested. Positioning of the patient depends on the location of the mass. Most young children are swaddled with bed linen in a "papoose" fashion if the procedure is in the head and neck region.

The skin is cleansed with alcohol; the mass is firmly fixed with the thumb and index finger or between the index finger and third finger of one hand, while the syringe–syringe holder–needle apparatus is held in the other. The needle is quickly inserted into the mass, and the syringe plunger is retracted to create a vacuum, drawing cells and fluid into the barrel of the needle. Multiple back-and-forth excursions are made into the mass with quick jackhammer-like strokes. Once material appears in the hub of the syringe, the plunger is released and allowed to return to its normal position. The negative pressure in the syringe must be released before the needle is removed, otherwise cellular material is aspirated into the barrel of the syringe and becomes irretrievable. Once the needle is removed, an assistant or a nurse takes a gauze pad and presses the puncture site to minimize oozing and hematoma development.

With the needle-only technique, the needle is passed back and forth in the mass as described. After its removal, the needle is attached to a syringe to expel the material in its barrel, as detailed next.

HANDLING THE ASPIRATE

After removing the needle from the syringe, air is drawn into the barrel of the syringe and the needle reattached. Needle contents are then quickly expelled onto a glass slide, sometimes forcefully. Repeat this process with different slides until all fluid is expressed. Delays in expelling fluid may cause the cellular material to dry or clot in the barrel of the needle. The bevel of the needle should be placed directly against the glass slide to minimize splattering.

The simplest slide preparation involves placing a second glass slide on top of the first one, on which there is a droplet of cellular material. The weight of the second slide causes the material to spread on both slides, which are then gently pulled apart. Other methods of slide preparation are detailed in the monograph by Stanley and Löwhagen (1993).

Once slides are made, the needle is inserted into a small test tube filled with sterile balanced saline solution. This solution is aspirated into the needle and syringe barrel and then expelled. The lymphocytes collected in this solution may be used for flow cytometric studies, cytocentrifuged preparations, or molecular studies.

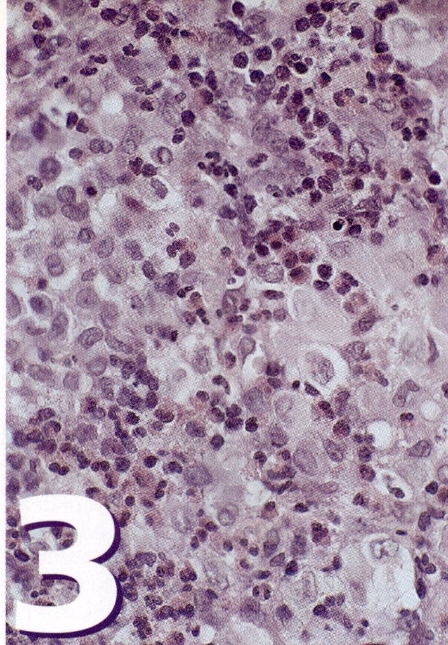

Richard S. Larson

Immunodeficiency Disorders

GENERAL CONSIDERATIONS

Classification of Primary Immunodeficiency Disorders

Immunodeficiency disorders are a diverse group of illnesses in which there are increased susceptibility to infections, autoimmune diseases, and neoplasms. Disorders of the immune system may occur as either primary or secondary processes. Primary immunodeficiencies are inherited diseases. Recurrent infections during childhood are the hallmark of primary immunodeficiencies, with the types of infections related to the nature of the immune defect. Secondary immunodeficiencies are acquired by nutritional defects, immunosuppressive therapy, metabolic disorders, or infections. Autoimmune disorders and neoplasms, including those of hematopoietic origin, occur more frequently in immunodeficiencies. The nature and frequency of autoimmunity or neoplasm vary among specific immunodeficiencies. Many of the infections, autoimmune disorders, and hematopoietic tumors that occur in immunodeficient patients are discussed elsewhere in this book in more detail. This chapter focuses on the clinical presentations, abnormal laboratory test results, and histologic findings seen in primary immunodeficiencies.

Phenotypic syndromes were the first described immunodeficiencies (Table 3–1) and include ataxia-telangiectasia (Syllaba & Henner, 1926), mucocutaneous candidiasis (Thorpe & Handley, 1929), and Wiskott-Aldrich syndrome (Wiskott, 1937). After the introduction of antibiotics reduced the morbidity and mortality rates of infection, several primary immunodeficiency states became apparent in the 1950s and 1960s: Swiss-type agammaglobulinemia (severe combined immunodeficiency [SCID]) (Hitzig et al, 1958), Bruton congenital agammaglobulinemia (X-linked agammaglobulinemia [XLA]) (Bruton, 1952), combined variable immunodeficiency (CVID) (Sanford et al, 1954), and chronic granulomatous disease (CGD) (Berendes et al, 1957). The number of recognized immunodeficiency disorders has expanded rapidly since these initial descriptions. In 1995 the World Health Organization (WHO) listed 82 distinct entities (Rosen et al, 1995) (Table 3–2).

To hematopathologists and hematologists accustomed to the evolution of lymphoma classification systems, it is not surprising that there are various classification systems for immunodeficiency disorders. The problem is made more difficult by the multiple names applied to similar entities. Classifications have generally been based on the observation that the immune system is divisible into distinct functional components of B lymphocytes, T lymphocytes, phagocytes (neutrophils and monocytes), and complement system. According to this framework, disorders of antibody production were equated with B lymphocyte defects, and many defects of cellular immunity were presumed to be T lymphocyte defects. Some later insights into the biologic basis of immunodeficiency disorders have altered these assumptions. For instance, the clinical manifestations and diagnosis of X-linked hyper-IgM syndrome are related to the inability of B lymphocytes to switch from IgM to IgG production. The B lymphocytes in these patients are normal, however, and it is a T lymphocyte defect (the lack of surface expression of CD40L) that prevents appropriate T and B lymphocyte cooperation. B lymphocytes are thereby unable to produce IgG. The biologic defect is related to T lymphocytes in these patients, whereas the clinical manifestation appears as a B lymphocyte disorder (Allen et al, 1993).

In order to address these difficulties, the WHO in 1995 recommended a classification scheme that standardizes terminology (Rosen et al, 1995) (see Table 3–2). The WHO classification appears complicated at first but has the potential of accommodating later observations on the pathogenesis of these diseases. This classification system defines distinct clinicopathologic entities, grouped by their predominant clinical and pathologic manifestations. It also minimizes eponyms and hypothetical pathogenetic mechanisms. The WHO classification is thus used in this chapter. This classification will inevitably be revised as "new" immunodeficiency disorders are defined and as our understanding of the pathogenesis of these diseases is enhanced. This chapter focuses on the more common disorders. Rare immunodeficiencies, complement disorders, IgE-related defects, and immunodeficiencies associated with or secondary to other diseases have been omitted.

Epidemiology

In 1969 the incidence of primary immunodeficiencies was estimated at 1 in 100,000 (Medical Research Council Working Party, 1969). The incidence is now estimated at approximately 1 in 10,000 due to the increased identification of patients with primary immunodeficiencies and the increased number of recognized disorders (Hayakawa et al, 1981; Hosking & Roberton, 1983; Pappas, 1999). Among hospitalized patients, the incidence of immunodeficiency is estimated at 0.3–2.3%, whereas among outpatients the incidence is 7 in 1000 (0.7%) (Hobbs, 1966). Approximately 400 new cases of primary immunodeficiency are predicted for the United States per year, using an estimate of one immunodeficiency per 10,000 births.

Selective IgA deficiency is the most common primary immunodeficiency disorder. One in 333 blood donors in

Table 3–1

Recognition of Primary Immunodeficiency Disorders by Year, Showing Influence of Antibiotics and Current Sophisticated Testing

Disorder	Year
Immunodeficiencies associated with phenotypic abnormalities	
Ataxia-telangiectasia	1926
Chronic mucocutaneous candidiasis	1929
Wiskott-Aldrich syndrome	1937
DiGeorge anomaly	1965
Immunodeficiencies described with the advent of antibiotics	
Severe combined immunodeficiency	1950, 1953, 1958
X-linked agammaglobulinemia	1952
Common variable immunodeficiency	1954
Chronic granulomatous disease	1957
WHO classification, 82 entities	1995

Tennessee demonstrated IgA deficiency (Cassidy & Nordby, 1975). Selective IgA deficiency is common, but it is usually asymptomatic, for reasons unknown. Even if selective IgA deficiency is excluded, disorders predominantly affecting antibody production form the second largest group of immunodeficiencies, occurring twice as frequently as all other primary immunodeficiencies combined. Combined immunodeficiencies are a common group; approximately one third are T cell defects, and two thirds have combined B and T cell defects. Neutrophil and monocyte disorders and complement deficiencies occur at very low frequencies, but their molecular basis is probably the most clearly defined (Hayakawa et al, 1981; Ryser et al, 1988) (Fig. 3–1).

Primary immunodeficiency disorders usually become apparent during childhood. It has been estimated that 40% of cases are diagnosed in the first year of life, another 40% by 5 years of age, and only 5% in adulthood (Hayakawa et al, 1981; Medical Research Council Working Party, 1969; Ryser et al, 1988). Most of the late-onset cases are in patients with CVID. There is a strong male predominance (estimates range from 62 to 83%) among children diagnosed with immunodeficiency. The differences in age of onset and gender are mainly accounted for by the large number of boys with X-linked immunodeficiencies and early-onset disease.

Primary immunodeficiency disorders are heterogeneous in their pattern of inheritance and type of genetic aberration, in that they may result from single gene defects, multigene defects, or multifactorial disorders with genetic susceptibility. Given the genetic pattern of inheritance, it is somewhat surprising that a family history of a similar primary immunodeficiency occurs in only 25% of patients (Hayakawa et al, 1981; Medical Research Council Working Party, 1969; Ryser et al, 1988).

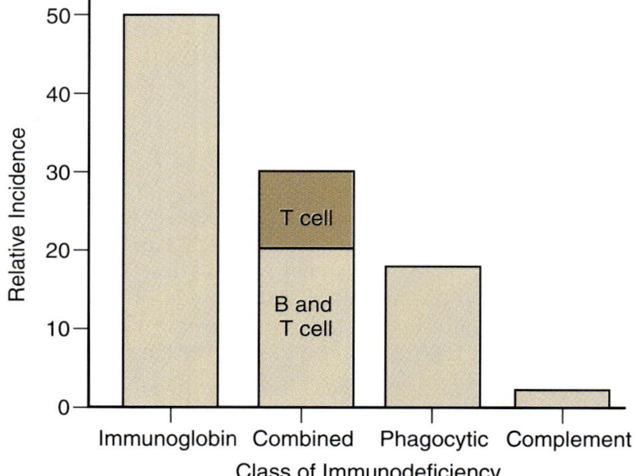

Figure 3–1

Relative incidence of immunodeficiencies in relationship to the class of immunodeficiency.

Approach to Diagnosis

Clinical findings are rarely diagnostic of immunodeficiency disorders but provide guidance as to the necessity for an immunodeficiency evaluation and its type. Patients with immunodeficiencies frequently have recurrent or chronic infection, although, in some, infections are acute and life-threatening. The location of infections and the specific etiologic agents provide insight as to the underlying immunodeficiency. A family history of immunodeficiency (types of infection, early deaths, and relationship of affected members) is also helpful in diagnosis. The presence of skeletal or other phenotypic abnormalities that are associated with immunodeficiencies may be useful for diagnosis.

The initial screening for a suspected immunodeficiency includes complete blood count; quantitation of serum IgG, IgM, and IgA levels; assessment of antibody function; and infection evaluation. Measurement of total hemolytic complement, phagocytic capability, and T-cell enumeration and function should generally be reserved for secondary testing because of the rarity of complement, phagocytic, and combined immunodeficiency disorders. Biopsy is rarely performed for diagnosis, but tissue examinations may provide important clues by the type of inflammatory reaction provoked, the nature of infectious agents, and the predominance or absence of certain inflammatory cells. Autopsies of those with acute illnesses may indicate the possibility of familial immunodeficiencies.

Determination of the white blood cell count and examination of the peripheral blood film may suggest a primary immunodeficiency. Persistent lymphopenia (defined as an absolute lymphocyte count $<1500/\mu l$) occurs in many types of primary immunodeficiency. An absolute count between 1500 and $2000/\mu l$ is suggestive of lymphopenia, and evaluation should be repeated over several weeks. "Atypical" or activated lymphocytes with abundant cytoplasm associated with viral infection are unusual in immunodeficiencies. Granulocyte and monocyte morphologic features may be diagnostic or suggestive of an immunodeficiency such as Chédiak-Higashi syndrome.

Serum immunoglobulin levels (IgG, IgM, IgA, and IgE) should be measured. Results are interpreted in part on the basis of age. Premature infants have particularly low levels of immunoglobulin during their first year of life. In older children or adults, a total immunoglobulin (IgG + IgM + IgA) level >600 mg/dl makes an immunoglobulin deficiency very unlikely.

Humoral response may in part be tested by obtaining various antibody titers. An immunodeficiency of antibody production probably exists if isoagglutinin and other antibody titers are abnormal. Saline isoagglutination titers measure IgM function and production. In individuals over 6 months of age, the ratio of A1 to B should be at least 1:8. IgG production may be evaluated (if the patient has been previously immunized) by tetanus, rubella, measles, diphtheria, or *Haemophilus influenzae* B titers. In vitro assays of B cell proliferation and antibody production are most useful in defining the precise immunodeficiency but are not usually necessary as part of an initial evaluation.

Abnormal T cell function (expected in cellular or combined immunodeficiency disorders) may be evaluated by skin tests for delayed-type hypersensitivity reactions. Intradermal injections of fluid tetanus, *Candida albicans*, mumps antigen, measles antigen, or purified protein derivative are commonly employed.

Table 3–2

1995 WHO Classification of Primary and Secondary Immunodeficiencies

Groups Discussed in Chapter

Predominantly Antibody Deficiencies

1. X-linked agammaglobulinemia
2. Hyper-IgM syndrome
   a. X-linked
   b. Other
3. Ig heavy-chain gene deletions
4. κ-chain deficiency
5. Selective deficiency of IgG subclasses (with or without IgA deficiency)
6. Antibody deficiency with normal immunoglobulins
7. Common variable immunodeficiency
8. IgA deficiency
9. Transient hypogammaglobulinemia of infancy

Combined Immunodeficiencies

10. Severe combined immunodeficiency (SCID)
   a. X-linked
   b. Autosomal recessive
11. Adenosine deaminase (ADA) deficiency
12. Purine nucleoside phosphoryfase (PNP) deficiency
13. MHC class II deficiency
14. Reticular dysgenesis
15. CD3γ or DC3$_6$ deficiency
16. CD8 deficiency
17. Primary CD4 deficiency
18. Primary CD7 deficiency
19. IL-2 deficiency
20. Multiple cytokine deficiency
21. Signal transduction deficiency

Immunodeficiency Syndrome–Associated Phenotypic Anomalies

22. Wiskott-Aldrich syndrome
23. Ataxia-telangiectasla
24. DiGeorge anomaly

Defects of Phagocytic Function

25. Chronic granulomatous disease (CGD)
   a. X-linked CGD (deficiency of 91-kD binding chain of cytochrome b)
   b. Autosomal recessive CGD
      (1) p22 phox
      (2) p47 phox
      (3) p67 phox
26. Leukocyte adhesion defect, type 1 (deficiency of β chain (CD18) of LFA-1, Mac-1, p150,95)
27. Leukocyte adhesion defect, type 2 (failure to convert GDP mannose to fucose)
28. Neutrophil G6PD deficiency
29. Myeloperoxidase deficiency
30. Secondary granule deficiency
31. Shwachman syndrome
32. Chédiak-Higashi syndrome

Additional Groups

Complement Deficiencies

33. C1q deficiency
34. C1r deficiency
35. C4 deficiency
36. C2 deficiency
37. C3 deficiency
38. C5 deficiency
39. C6 deficiency
40. C7 deficiency
41. C8α + C8γ deficiency
42. C8β deficiency
43. C9 deficiency
44. C1 inhibitor deficiency
45. Factor I deficiency
46. Factor H deficiency
47. Factor D deficiency
48. Properdin deficiency

Immunodeficiency Associated with or Secondary to Other Diseases

Chromosomal Instability or Defective Repair

49. Bloom syndrome
50. Fanconi anemia
51. ICF (Immunodeficiency, Centromeric instability, and Facial anomalies) syndrome
52. Nijmegen breakage syndrome
53. Seckel syndrome
54. Xeroderma syndrome

Chromosomal Defects

55. Down syndrome
56. Tumer syndrome
57. Chromosome 18 rings and deletions

Skeletal Abnormalities

58. Short-limbed skeletal dysplasia
59. Cartilage-hair hypoplasia

Immunodeficiency with Generalized Growth Retardation

60. Schimke immuno-osseous dysplasia
61. Immunodeficiency with absent thumbs
62. Dubowitz syndrome
63. Growth retardation, facial anomalies, and immunodeficiency
64. Progeria (Hutchinson-Gilford syndrome)

Immunodeficiency with Dermatologic Defects

65. Partial albinism
66. Dyskeratosis congenita
67. Netherton syndrome
68. Acrodermatitis enteropethica
69. Anhidrotic ectodermal dysplasia
70. Papillon-Lefèvre syndrome

Hereditary Metabolic Defects

71. Transcobalamin 2 deficiency
72. Methylmalonic acidemia
73. Type 1 hereditary orotic aciduria
74. Blotin-dependent carboxylase deficiency
75. Mannosidosis
76. Glycogen storage disease, type 1b

Hypercatabolism of Immunoglobulin

77. Familial hypercatabolism
78. Intestinal lymphangiectasia

Other

79. Hper-IgE syndrome
80. Chronic mucocutaneous candidiasis
81. Hereditary or congenital hyposplenia or asplenia
82. Ivermark syndrome

Source: Rosen FS, Wedgwood RJP, Eibl M, et al: Clin Exp Immunol 1 (suppl. 99):1, 1995.

Results of skin tests in normal adults and children older than 2 years of age are positive. Under 2 years of age, normal and immunodeficient children may be anergic, which limits the value of this test in infants. T cell subset enumeration by flow cytometric analysis may be helpful. Specialized in vitro functional assays of T cell proliferation and function are also available. Patients with primary complement deficiency have low total hemolytic complement activity, as measured by low CH_{50}.

If results of the aforementioned screening tests are normal, immunodeficiency is essentially excluded. Further evaluation and testing are warranted, however, if a screening test result is positive or if a chronic infection is unexplained. These tests and their expected results are detailed in the discussion of each entity.

PREDOMINANTLY IMMUNOGLOBULIN DISORDERS

Selective IgA Deficiency

Definition

Selective IgA deficiency is a primary immunodeficiency characterized by decreased (<5 mg/dl) or absent serum levels of IgA with nomal serum levels of other immunoglobulin subtypes.

Clinical Features

Selective IgA deficiency is the most common as well as the mildest form of primary immunodeficiency. First described in children with ataxia-telangiectasia, IgA deficiency was later found in patients with other illnesses as well as asymptomatic "normal" subjects (Rockey et al, 1964; Thieffry et al, 1961; West et al, 1962). The biologic and clinical manifestations of selective IgA deficiency are extraordinarily heterogeneous. Selective IgA deficiency involves 1 in 333 to 1 in 3000 people, depending on the population studied (Bachman, 1965; Cassidy & Nordby, 1975; Grundbacher, 1972), with the various incidence rates a result in part of case definition. Some authors have used 10 mg/dl, but 5 mg/dl is the usual value (Buckley & Dees, 1969; Hong & Amman, 1989). Patients with IgA levels between 5 and 10 mg/dl may be diagnosed as having "partial" IgA deficiency, but such levels likely reflect immaturity of the immune system. "Spontaneous" remission of selective IgA deficiency is most likely in children under 5 years of age and usually occurs in those individuals with "partial" deficiency (Ammann & Hong, 1970).

IgA deficiency has been associated with a legion of illnesses, but most IgA-deficient individuals remain healthy (Table 3–3) (Ammann & Hong, 1970; Burks & Steele, 1986; Cunningham-Rundles, 1990; Hanson, 1983; Rockey et al, 1964; Strober & Sneller, 1991). Recurrent sinopulmonary bacterial infection is the most frequent illness associated with IgA deficiency. Patients with coincident deficiency of IgG2 are more likely to have serious or life-threatening infections. Allergies are also more common in IgA-deficient individuals (Kaufman & Hobbs, 1970). Food allergy is frequent, but the most common disorders are allergic conjunctivitis, rhinitis, urticaria, atopic eczema, and bronchial asthma (Hanson, 1983; Plebani et al, 1987; Strober & Sneller, 1991). Neurologic disorders, including mental retardation, have been reported. Anticonvulsant therapy may reduce IgA levels (Haddow et al, 1970; Ruff et al, 1987; Sorrell et al, 1971).

Table 3–3
Some Diseases Associated with Selective IgA Deficiency

Recurrent infections
Allergies
Numerous autoimmune disorders
Numerous gastrointestinal disorders
Chromosomal abnormalities
Neurologic disorders
Familial history of pulmonary fibrosis
Other immunodeficiencies
Endocrinopathies

Several gastrointestinal illnesses are associated with IgA deficiency. Patients with celiac disease have a high incidence (approximately 1 in 200 patients) of IgA deficiency (Ammann & Hong, 1970; Crabbe & Heremans, 1966; Hanson, 1983; Gillett et al, 1997); celiac disease is not associated with other immunodeficiencies. One of the best-documented gastrointestinal associations with IgA deficiency is malabsorption from infection with *Giardia lamblia* (Zinneman & Kaplan, 1975). Autoimmune disorders, including gastrointestinal autoimmunity, have also been associated with IgA deficiency (Ammann & Hong, 1971a; Ammann & Hong, 1970; Hong & Amman, 1989). Gastric carcinomas and lymphomas are seen at increased frequency in individuals with IgA deficiency (Cunningham-Rundles et al, 1980; Kersey et al, 1988). The degree of immunodeficiency does not correlate with the risk of malignancy.

Histopathologic Features

Histopathologic changes associated with IgA deficiency are related in most cases to the infection or disease. Lymph node architecture and histologic features are normal, and IgA-bearing B lymphocytes may be found in the peripheral blood and gastrointestinal tract (Hobbs, 1968). Only a few related autopsy reports are available, and detailed information regarding other hematopoietic tissues is sparse (Krieger & Brough, 1967).

Malabsorption is common, resulting in gastrointestinal biopsies. Various histologic changes may be seen (Ammann & Hong, 1971b; Andre et al, 1978; Crabbe et al, 1965) that are consistent with the diagnosis of IgA deficiency and provide an explanation for malabsorption. There are no findings, however, diagnostic of selective IgA deficiency. As expected, villous blunting and other changes similar to those in celiac disease may be present. Follicular hyperplasia is common and has been invoked as a cause of malabsorption. Asymptomatic celiac disease or follicular hyperplasia may be found "incidentally" in patients with IgA deficiency who do not have malabsorbtion. Infection with *G. lamblia* may be responsible for malabsorption. Despite the association of villous blunting, infection, or follicular hyperplasia with malabsorption, a number of cases show minimal histologic changes. In some of the latter cases, IgM-bearing plasma cells—not IgA-bearing plasma cells—are detected in the mucosa. In some cases, normal histologic features, including plasma cells producing IgA, are found.

Follicular hyperplasia similar to that in the gastrointestinal tract may occur at other sites. The frequency of gastric epithelial tumors is increased in patients with IgA deficiency. These patients also have a higher frequency of lymphomas (Cunningham-Rundles et al, 1980; Kersey et al, 1988). The classification of these lymphomas is problematic, but most are B and T cell lymphomas and extranodal, and they involve the jejunum. Lymphomas also occur in the central nervous system at higher incidence in IgA-deficient patients. Whether follicular hyperplasia in the bowel is a precursor state to lymphoma is unknown, but follicular hyperplasia is frequently seen in association with follicular center cell lymphomas at other sites. Hodgkin disease has been rarely reported in these patients and is likely to be a coincidence.

Laboratory Findings and Diagnosis

The diagnosis rests on the demonstration of a persistently low serum IgA level. The WHO recognizes a level of <5 mg/dl as the indicator. In an otherwise healthy patient, further evaluation is not necessary. In patients with infections, IgG subclass levels should be determined, since patients with a combined IgA-IgG2 deficiency have normal total IgG levels but a history of serious or life-threatening infections. These patients also do not respond to polysaccharide vaccines (e.g., pneumococcal or meningococcal). Intravenous immunoglobulin and blood transfusions should be given cautiously, since anti-IgA antibodies are frequently present in the sera of these patients.

Pathogenesis

IgA deficiency results from heterogeneous biologic defects. Most cases are sporadic, although many familial cases have been reported (Oen et al, 1982). Modes of inheritance are autosomal recessive, autosomal dominant and multifactorial (Buckley & Dees, 1969; Koistinen, 1976). IgA deficiency is common in families with CVID ("Combined Variable Immunodeficiency"), for reasons unknown. Most IgA-deficient individuals without physical or mental disorders do not have chromosomal abnormalities (Herrmann et al, 1982). Patients with such disorders often have chromosomal abnormalities, particularly involving chromosome 18 (Lewkonia et al, 1980).

The lack of disease in IgA-deficient individuals is usually attributed to an increase in secretory IgM in the saliva and gastrointestinal fluid as well as the mucosa. IgA deficiency results from a failure in terminal differentiation of IgA-producing B cells. The favored current hypothesis supported by several lines of evidence is that, in most patients, a T cell regulatory defect results in inadequate production of IgA by plasma cells. The IgA gene and the immunoglobulin switch region in these patients are normal (Hammarstrom et al, 1985). The peripheral blood B lymphocytes expressing IgA, however, have the immature phenotype seen in newborns, in that they have IgM, IgD, and IgA surface expression (Conley & Cooper, 1981; Lawton et al, 1972). Thymectomized neonates, who lack proper T cell development, may have IgA deficiencies (Perey et al, 1970).

Despite these reasons for suspecting a T cell defect in IgA deficiency, few individuals with IgA deficiency have had identifiable T cell defects. As a result, failure of terminal B cell differentiation leading to adequate IgA production has also been attributed to an intrinsic B cell defect and/or maternal anti-IgA antibodies that suppress fetal IgA development (Cassidy et al, 1979; Inoue et al, 1984; Petty et al, 1985). IgA deficiency has also been associated with major histocompatibility complex class I, II, and III types (Hammarstrom & Smith, 1983; Lakhanpal et al, 1988; Wilton et al, 1985). This suggests that either a genetic abnormality in the area of chromosome 6 near the major histocompatibility locus confers susceptibility to IgA deficiency, or that MHC I, II, and III types are simply a marker of the genetic background in which IgA deficiency may occur.

Hyper-IgM Syndrome

Equivalent Terms

Immunoglobulin deficiency with increased IgM is its equivalent.

Definition

Hyper-IgM syndrome is a primary immunodeficiency characterized by normal or increased serum levels of IgM in association with decreased levels of other serum immunoglobulins, including IgG, IgA, and IgE.

Clinical Features

Hyper-IgM syndrome, like IgA deficiency and many primary immunodeficiencies, represents a group of distinct entities with similar clinical expressions. Seventy percent of the cases are X-linked and therefore occur in males. The remaining cases are inherited in an autosomal recessive fashion, with autosomal dominant inheritance rarely shown (Beall et al, 1980; Brahmi et al, 1983; Rosen & Janeway, 1966).

Hyper-IgM syndrome is associated with recurrent infections, with normal to elevated IgM levels and depressed IgG, IgA, and IgE levels. Infections usually first occur between 6 months and 2 years of age, coinciding with the decline in maternally derived antibodies. Sinopulmonary infection is the most common clinical presentation, and most infections have a bacterial cause. Peritonsillar and peritracheal soft tissue infections may become life-threatening. Gastrointestinal complaints and malabsorption are frequently reported. In contrast to selective IgA deficiency, *G. lamblia* is reported in only a few cases of hyper-IgM syndrome, but cryptosporidium infection may cause protracted watery diarrhea (Stiehm et al, 1986). *Pneumocystis carinii* and cryptosporidium infections are rarely seen in antibody deficiency syndromes other than hyper-IgM syndrome. Arthritis and autoimmunity leading to thrombocytopenia, hemolytic anemia, or hypothryroidism also occur in hyper-IgM syndrome. Fifty percent of patients have persistent stomatitis and recurrent oral ulcers. Extensive verruca vulgaris may also be present (Rosen & Janeway, 1966). Patients with hyper-IgM syndrome are not susceptible to enteroviral infections, as are patients with XLA (see "X-Linked Agammaglobulinemia"); but the overall prognosis is similarly poor. Hyper-IgM syndrome has an increased risk of malignancy. The incidence of B and T cell lymphomas and Hodgkin disease is much higher than in other immunodeficiencies (Table 3–4) (Filipovich et al, 1987).

Table 3–4
Distribution of Tumors and Immunodeficiencies

Immunodeficiency	Adenocarcinoma	Lymphoma	Leukemia	Hodgkin Disease	Other Tumors	Total Tumors
Severe combined immunodeficiency	1	31	5	4	1	42 (8.6%)
Hypogammaglobulinemia	3	7	7	3	1	21 (4.3%)
Common variable immunodeficiency	20	55	8	8	29	120 (24.5%)
IgA deficiency	8	6	0	3	21	38 (7.8%)
Hyper-IgM syndrome	0	9	0	4	3	16 (3.3%)
Wiskott-Aldrich syndrome	0	59	7	3	9	78 (15.9%)
Ataxia-telangiectasia	13	69	32	16	20	150 (30.6%)
Other immunodeficiencies	1	12	4	1	7	25 (5.1%)
Immunodeficiency categories	46 (9.4%)	248 (50.6%)	63 (12.9%)	42 (8.6%)	91 (18.6%)	490 (100%)

Source: Adapted from WHO Scientific Group on Immunodeficiency, 1989.

Histopathologic Features

Lymphocytic tissue is histologically abnormal in the X-linked form of hyper-IgM syndrome, and these abnormalities may help in establishing the diagnosis (Geha et al, 1979; Stiehm & Fundenberg, 1966). Germinal centers are often inapparent in lymph nodes or spleen but in some cases are hyperplastic (Fig. 3–2). B lymphocytes are present, and plasma cells are usually abundant. Although IgM-producing plasma cells are present, there is an absence of IgG- or IgA-bearing plasma cells. T lymphocytes are normal in number, distribution, and the ratio of their subsets. The histologic features of non–X-linked hyper-IgM syndrome are not well characterized. The thymus has few if any Hassall corpuscles, and atrophic thymus has been reported in two patients.

Neutropenia may be intermittent or persistent. Marrow examination in patients with neutropenia usually shows a block at the myelocyte-promyelocyte stage of differentiation or, rarely, a reduced number of the entire granulocytic series, including progenitors (Benkerrou et al, 1990; Notarangelo et al, 1992). Normal granulocyte maturation occurs in patients without neutropenia. With few exceptions, the marrow has a normal number of plasma cells.

Enlargement of tonsils, lymph nodes, spleen (see Fig. 3–2), and liver is a common feature that requires particularly careful clinical evaluation, since B and T lymphomas and Hodgkin disease occur (Filipovich et al, 1987). Fortunately, lymphadenopathy and hepatosplenomegaly are usually due to benign lymphocytic proliferation. Some lymphoproliferations, however, may be quite abnormal and very suggestive of lymphoma (see Fig. 3–2), requiring a comprehensive diagnostic evaluation.

Laboratory Findings and Diagnosis

Patients have normal or elevated serum IgM levels with low levels of or absent IgG, IgA, and IgE. The IgM level may be normal or as high as 1000 mg/dl. IgM is polyclonal and associated with both κ and λ light chains. IgG antibody titers are low. The X-linked form of the disease may be unequivocally diagnosed by demonstrating the lack of CD40L on the surface of activated CD4+ T cells using flow cytometric analysis. The diagnosis may then be further refined by demonstration of a mutation within the CD40L gene by DNA sequencing. The latter two techniques may also be used to identify female carriers (Hollenbaugh et al, 1994).

Several other immunologic abnormalities differentiate X-linked hyper-IgM syndrome from other clinically related immunodeficiencies, such as XLA (see "X-Linked Agammaglobulinemia"). Peripheral blood B cells from patients with hyper-IgM syndrome have surface expression of IgM, IgD, or both but rarely other immunoglobulin isotypes. Autoantibodies may be present, leading to thrombocytopenia, hemolytic anemia, or hypothyroidism (Notarangelo et al, 1992; Pascual-Salcedo et al, 1983).

Pathogenesis

The clinical picture of hyper-IgM syndrome is dominated by increased IgM levels, with decreased secondary immunoglobulins levels. The cellular defect in these patients involves T lymphocytes rather than B lymphocytes. The precise defect on T lymphocytes in the X-linked form of hyper-IgM syndrome is the lack of proper expression of CD40L (gp39) on the surface of T lymphocytes. Numerous genetic abnormalities have now

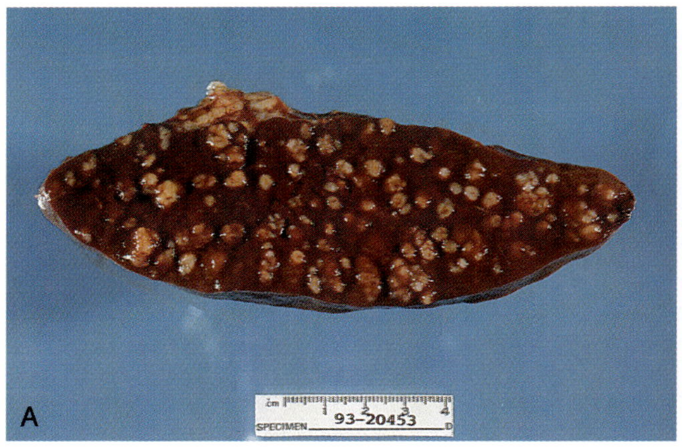

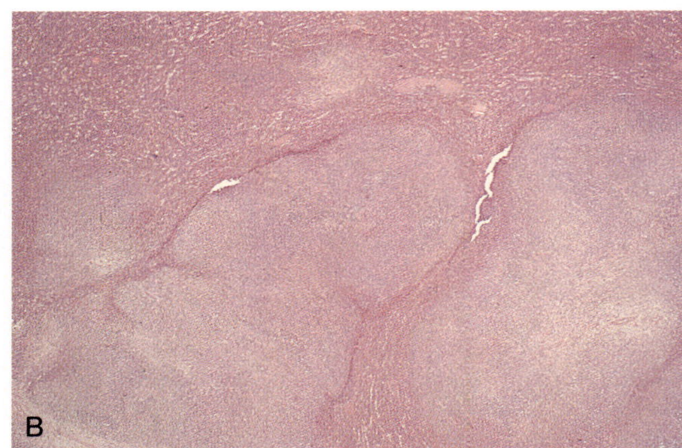

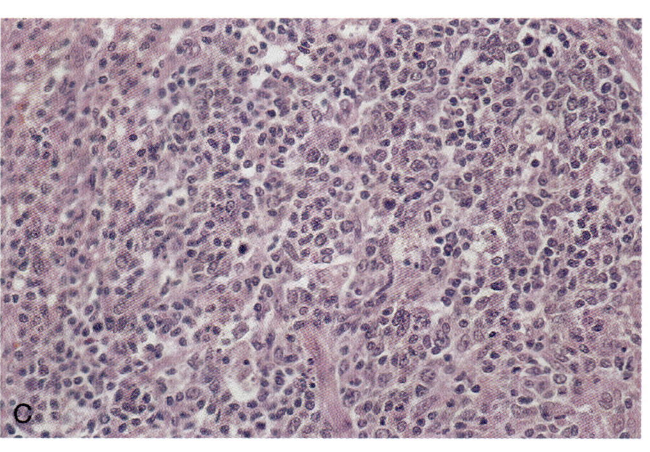

Figure 3–2

Hyper-IgM, spleen. This 12-year-old boy had a splenectomy for gradual spleen enlargement. *A*. This spleen weighed 1310 g and on cut section showed numerous pale nodules, suggestive of lymphoma. Flow cytometric studies showed 90% CD3+, 61% CD4+, 28% CD8+, and 10% CD20+ cells with polyclonality. *B*. Low magnification shows marked follicular hyperplasia, with loss of normal mantle and marginal zone compartments. CD40 ligand was present on the T cells in this patient, suggesting that the pathologic characteristics of this type of hyper-IgM (Notarangelo, 1992) may differ from those of the X-linked form of the disease. *C*. High magnification shows a mixture of small and transformed lymphocytes. Numerous plasma cells are present and were found to be polyclonal on immunoperoxidase studies (not shown).

been demonstrated within the CD40L gene of various patients with hyper-IgM syndrome, leading to inadequate expression of CD40L or expression of a nonfunctional CD40L molecule (Villa et al, 1994).

CD40L is integral to T and B lymphocyte cooperation (Lane et al, 1992; Noelle et al, 1992). CD40L is expressed on the surface of T lymphocytes, binds to CD40 on the surface of B cells, and provides one of the signals necessary for B lymphocytes to switch from IgM to IgG production. Without proper surface expression of CD40L, T lymphocytes cannot fully signal B lymphocytes to switch from IgM to IgG production during an immune response. Thus, a patient has elevated IgM levels and low IgG and IgA levels. In addition, CD40L is expressed on monocytes and follicular dendritic cells. Interactions between B cells and dendritic cells in the follicular center apparently are important to normal formation of germinal centers. Based on the hyper-IgM syndrome and several in vitro observations, it has been suggested that the CD40-CD40L pathway rescues B lymphocytes from apoptosis in the germinal center. Perturbations of the CD40-CD40L complex might also cause other clinical manisfestations of the hyper-IgM syndrome, such as neutropenia, infection with *P. carinii*, and increased risk of malignancy, by impairing other cell-cell interactions. The molecular defect in non–X-linked forms of hyper-IgM syndrome is not known.

X-Linked Agammaglobulinemia

Equivalent Terms

Bruton hypogammaglobulinemia is an equivalent.

Definition

XLA is a congenital immunodeficiency associated with a paucity of B lymphocytes.

Clinical Features

XLA was one of the first immunodeficiencies described in which there were no phenotypic abnormalities (Bruton, 1952; Lederman & Winkelstein, 1985). Patients have markedly hypoplastic or absent tonsils, adenoids, and lymph nodes. Infection is the most common clinical manifestation. As in hyper-IgM syndrome, patients are asymptomatic at birth but develop hypogammaglobulinemia as maternally derived antibodies are catabolized. Recurrent infections usually begin between 4 and 12 months of age, although 10–20% of patients present after 18 months of age. Sinopulmonary and gastrointestinal tract infections are most common, with skin, central nervous system, and joints also frequently infected. Pyogenic encapsulated bacteria, organisms for which antibody is important for biologic clearance, predominate. *Streptococcus pneumoniae, H. influenzae, Staphylococcus aureus*, and *Pseudomonas* species cause almost all the cases of sepsis, pyogenic meningitis, or septic arthritis, while *G. lamblia* or *Campylobacter* are usually responsible for gastrointestinal infections.

Viral resistance is generally intact, but there is one important exception: patients with XLA are susceptible to enteroviral infections with echovirus, coxsackievirus, and poliovirus (McKinney et al, 1987). Antibody is important in neutralizing these viruses. As a result, immunization of these patients with live attenuated poliovirus vaccine often leads to poliomyelitis, and disseminated infections with echovirus and coxsackievirus occur. Other, less common clinical manifestations include neutropenia, alopecia totalis, protein-losing enteropathy, malabsorption with disaccharridase deficiency, and amyloidosis (Dubois et al, 1970; Hermaszewski & Webster, 1993; Ipp & Gelfand, 1976).

The entity XLA with growth hormone deficiency has been described in at least four unrelated families (Fleisher et al, 1980). Subsequent studies, however, suggest that the low growth hormone level in these individuals is nonspecific and related to recurrent infections (Haraldsson et al, 1993; Ohzeki et al, 1993).

Histopathologic Features

The histopathologic features of XLA are distinctive. Patients have hypoplastic lymphatic organs, such as lymph nodes, adenoids, and tonsils. The lymph nodes have absent or markedly atretic germinal centers, and there are decreased numbers of B lymphocytes. Plasma cells are absent in lymph nodes, marrow, and extranodal sites, including gastrointestinal sites.

Laboratory Findings and Diagnosis

Diagnosis rests on the demonstration of markedly reduced serum levels of IgM, IgG, and IgA (<100 mg/dl) (Lederman & Winkelstein, 1985; Rosen et al, 1984). Following immunization, patients with XLA still fail to make IgG. Thus, antibody titers are reduced or undetectable after vaccination. Antibody to ubiquitous IgM antigens (anti–A and anti–B isohemagglutinins) is also absent. In the first few months of life it may be difficult to accurately detect immunoglobulin levels, since maternally derived antibodies may obscure the panhypogammaglobulinemia.

With the use of immunophenotyping techniques, B lymphocytes may be demonstrated in marrow, but few, if any, B lymphocytes are demonstrated in the peripheral blood (Schiff et al, 1974). Plasma cells are not present in either the marrow or the peripheral blood (Ament et al, 1973b). T lymphocyte numbers and function are normal. Molecular tests may detect a carrier state or may enable prenatal diagnosis (Zhu et al, 1994a; Zhu et al, 1994b).

Pathogenesis

The underlying defect in XLA is limited to B lymphocytes. A profound deficiency in B lymphocytes causes hypogammaglobulinemia. Mutations in a B lymphocyte–specific tyrosine kinase gene, *BTK*, are responsible for the disease (Tsukada et al, 1993; Vetrie et al, 1993; Zhu et al, 1994a; Zhu et al, 1994b). The name *BTK* recognizes, Dr. Bruton, who first described this disease (*B*ruton agammaglobulinemia *t*yrosine *k*inase). The *BTK* gene is located on the X chromosome, and its expression is restricted to B cells. *BTK* mutations appear to inhibit or block differentiation of pre–B lymphocytes to B lymphocytes. As a result, patients have B cell precursors in marrow but have few in lymphatic tissue, extranodal sites, and blood. Predictably, plasma cells are rare or absent in all tissues. Mutational analysis has shown heterogeneous gene alterations in patients with XLA. Studies have indicated that the location and type of mutation do not correlate with a clinical phenotype or prognosis of XLA (Zhu et al, 1994a; Zhu et al, 1994b).

The block in B-lymphocyte differentiation is incomplete, since most patients have some immunoglobulin of one or another isotype in their serum (Lederman & Winkelstein, 1985). Immunoglobulin rearrangements in B lymphocytes from patients with XLA are normal (Milili et al, 1993). Furthermore, the block in B lymphocyte differentiation is principally at the pre–B lymphocyte stage, although there are effects at other stages of development. For instance, marrow samples from patients with XLA have early and pre–B lymphocytes; however, the ratio of pre–B to early B lymphocytes is lower than in normal marrow (Campana et al, 1990).

Combined Variable Immunodeficiency Disorder

Equivalent Terms

Swiss-type immunodeficiency is its equivalent.

Definition

CVID is a heterogeneous group of congenital immunodeficiencies characterized predominantly by antibody deficiency.

Clinical Features

Patients may present with CVID at all ages, in contrast to those with other antibody deficiencies, who usually develop illnesses during early childhood. CVID is usually diagnosed in the second or third decades (Cunningham-Rundles et al, 1987; Hermaszewski & Webster, 1993; Rosen & Janeway, 1966; Sneller et al, 1993). These patients suffer recurrent sinopulmonary symptoms similar to those of other antibody deficiencies and are occasionally identified in pulmonary clinics, since they develop bronchiectasis after chronic or recurrent lung infections. Pyogenic bacteria cleared by opsonins are usually involved in these infections, particularly *H. influenzae, S. pneumoniae*, and staphylococci. Mycoplasma pneumonia is also frequent, while in contrast to hyper-IgM syndrome *P. carinii* infection rarely occurs. Mycobacterial and fungal infections are rare. Noncaseating granulomas of the lung, liver, and spleen may develop, and a condition resembling sarcoidosis has been described in patients with CVID in the southeastern United States (Sharma & James, 1971).

Gastrointestinal complaints, including malabsorption, are common. *G. lamblia* is responsible for malabsorption in a small cohort of CVID patients. Herpes zoster infection eventually develops in 20% of patients. Autoimmune disorders are also frequent in CVID patients. There is an unusually high incidence of gastric carcinoma and lymphoma in older patients with CVID. Chronic lung disease, malignancy, chronic gastroenteritis, and virally induced liver failure may cause early death. The life expectancy of males is 29 years, and that of females 55 years. This dramatic gender difference in survival is not explained. Prophylactic use of immunoglobulin as well as antibiotic therapy for acute infections has greatly improved the prognosis in CVID.

Histopathologic Features

Lymph node architecture and cellular distribution are normal, but germinal centers may be hyperplastic in the nodes and spleen (Fig. 3–3). Hyperplasia of follicular centers is frequently observed in gastrointestinal biopsies. This hyperplasia may be so pronounced that protrusions of the mucosa are seen on radiographs (Hermans et al, 1966). Plasma cells in the lamina propria are absent or markedly reduced. Patients with follicular hyperplasia are often asymptomatic unless infected by *G. lamblia*. Eradication of the parasites with appropriate therapy may cure the malabsorption and normalize villous architecture (Ament et al, 1973b); however, follicular hyperplasia often persists. Carcinomas as well as B cell and T cell lymphomas develop at higher frequency in older individuals with CVID, indicating that lymphadenopathy be fully evaluated.

Laboratory Findings and Diagnosis

Serum immunoglobulin levels are decreased. IgG levels rarely exceed 300 mg/dl, whereas IgM and IgA levels are low or undetectable. Isohemagglutinin titers and specific antibody titers after vaccination are depressed or indicate an absence of isohemagglutinin or antibody. Although antibody levels are decreased, most patients have normal or moderately decreased numbers of circulating B lymphocytes. Plasma cells are absent. T lymphocyte subsets are normal in number, although one third of patients have a low CD4:CD8 ratio, usually from increased CD8+ T cells. Lymphocyte surface markers are usually normal. Approximately 50% of cases have subnormal T cell proliferation. A significant proportion of patients have a depressed switch from IgM to IgG production.

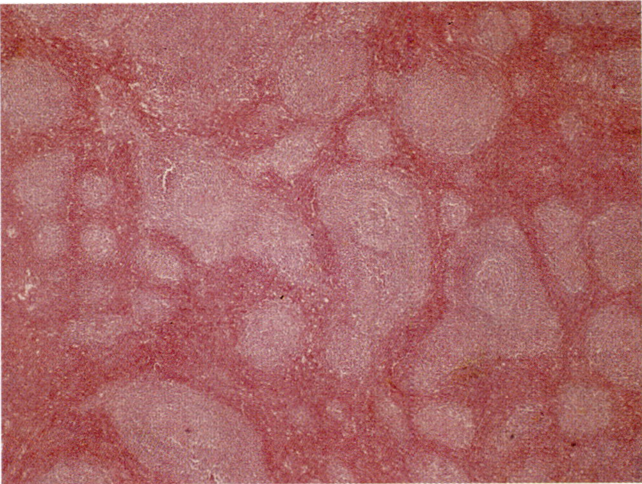

Figure 3–3

Common variable immunodeficiency, spleen. Moderate splenomegaly may occur, with marked hyperplasia of germinal centers, as in this photomicrograph.

Features of CVID may overlap considerably with those of other immunodeficiencies, including XLA and hyper-IgM syndrome. The molecular defect of CVID is not known, and its diagnosis rests on the exclusion of other well-defined immunodeficiency syndromes. Patients with hyper-IgM syndrome or XLA may be identified by specific molecular defects (see "Hyper-IgM Syndrome" and "X-Linked Agammaglobulinemia") IgA deficiencies are also in the differential diagnosis, since patients have clinical features overlapping with those of CVID. The rare CVID patients with low or undetectable numbers of B lymphocytes in the peripheral blood may have a form of XLA. Studies for *BTK* mutations have not been performed in these cases (Vorechovsky et al, 1993; Zhu et al, 1994a).

Pathogenesis

CVID is a heterogeneous group of disorders in which a wide variety of B and T lymphocyte defects have been demonstrated. B lymphocyte dysfunction in most cases is probably caused by a primary T lymphocyte defect resulting in abnormal B and T lymphocyte interaction. The precise molecular mechanisms are unknown. There are normal numbers of B lymphocytes in the peripheral blood and lymphatic tissue in most patients, without differentiation into functional plasma cells. Appropriate B lymphocyte differentiation is affected by T lymphocyte contact and cytokine secretion. Defects intrinsic to B lymphocytes as well as T lymphocyte abnormalities have been described and proposed as causes of CVID.

Early studies suggested that most patients with CVID had an intrinsic B lymphocyte defect. This conclusion was based on the observations that CVID B lymphocytes cocultured with normal T lymphocytes did not produce immunoglobulin; immunoglobulin was produced if CVID T lymphocytes were cocultured with normal B lymphocytes (De la Concha et al, 1982). Furthermore, B lymphocytes from most patients with

CVID produced immunoglobulin (usually IgM) when mitogens and soluble factors were employed (Bryant et al, 1990). It appears that B lymphocytes in most patients may produce immunoglobulin if the appropriate signals are present.

Careful analysis of T lymphocyte function has revealed various abnormalities in a large number of patients with CVID. Patients with CVID usually have normal T-lymphocyte subsets; a small cohort has increased numbers of CD8+ T lymphocytes, with normal or decreased CD4+ T lymphocytes, resulting in a reduced CD4/CD8 ratio (Jaffe et al, 1993). Defects in T lymphocyte proliferation have been described in some patients (Cunningham-Rundles et al, 1981). Other cohorts have defective cytokine production (Paganelli et al, 1988; Pastorelli et al, 1989). Of special interest is a group of CVID patients with splenomegaly and lymphadenopathy who have elevated levels of serum T lymphocyte–produced cytokines, suggestive of chronic immune stimulation (Aukrust et al, 1994). In this group the increase in the T lymphocyte–produced cytokine IL-4 may be physiologically significant, since IL-4 suppresses immunoglobulin production in vitro.

CVID is not usually inherited as a single gene defect, but there is evidence for a genetic component in some patients. A small group of CVID patients have a positive family history. Interestingly, in these families some members may have IgA deficiency and others CVID. There is also an association of CVID with certain HLA haplotypes (Ashman et al, 1992; Volanakis et al, 1992).

Other Immunoglobulin Deficiencies

A number of unusual immunoglobulin deficiencies have also been reported, including selective immunoglobulin deficiencies of IgM and IgE and each subclass of IgG (IgG1, IgG2, IgG3, and IgG4) (Hobbs et al, 1967; Hong, 1971; Schur et al, 1970). Recurrent infections have been reported in IgM and IgG subclass deficiencies. The clinical significance of IgE deficiency has been difficult to determine. Antibody deficiencies have also been described in association with Down syndrome and transcobalamin II deficiency (Hitzig & Kenny, 1975; Miller et al, 1969). Patients with increased levels of IgD (hyper-IgD syndrome), the least understood of immunoglobulins, have also been described. These patients have a history of adverse reactions to vaccinations (Haraldsson et al, 1992). Because of the rarity of the diseases, their histologic and pathologic characteristics are not well defined and are not be discussed here.

COMBINED IMMUNODEFICIENCIES

Severe Combined Immunodeficiency

Equivalent Terms

Swiss-type agammaglobulinemia, lymphopenic agammaglobulinemia, thymic alymphoplasia, hereditary thymic dysplasia, cellular immunodeficiency with abnormal immunoglobulin synthesis, and Nezelof syndrome are equivalents.

Definition

SCIDs comprise a heterogeneous group of disorders associated with defective T and B lymphocyte function.

Clinical Features

The term *SCID* refers to a diverse group of diseases in which patients have significant defects in both T and B lymphocytes. Several subtypes of SCID with different genetic defects have been recognized. These subtypes have different clinical presentations and laboratory findings (Table 3–5) but generally patients receive similar therapy. Several "new" combined immunodeficiencies have been recognized. Further variations in subclassification is expected, since the pathogenesis of subtypes is so diverse. SCID is more common in males than in females as the most common form is X linked. The remainder of the cases result from autosomal recessive inheritance.

Patients commonly present with "thrush" (moniliasis) or extensive "diaper rash" (from candidal infection) that does not respond to antibiotic therapy owing to its T lymphocyte defect. The infection may recur at the cessation of therapy or may never clear. Some infants have a rash shortly after birth due to transplacental passage of lymphocytes that mount a graft-versus-host reaction. Freedom from infection during the first year of life does not necessarily indicate a milder defect, since exposure often determines the frequency of infection. Ultimately, all these patients experience serious infections. The B lymphocyte deficiency causes bacterial infections, whereas the T lymphocyte deficiency results in viral infections (varicella and cytomegalovirus [CMV] pneumonia) as well as opportunistic infections (e.g., *P. carinii*). Life-threatening infections may occur when attenuated viruses are used for vaccination.

Skin disorders are common, and patients may have total alopecia, seborrheic dermatitis, or hanging, loose folds. Gastrointestinal manifestations, such as diarrhea, may be severe. Chronic hepatitis secondary to CMV or other viral agents is common. Patients without antibody are more likely to have enlarged lymph nodes. The prognosis is poor and rapidly fatal if untreated. Marrow transplantation may be curative.

Histopathologic Features

The histopathologic findings in SCID are not clearly defined. Nevertheless, thymic biospies have been advocated for diagnoses, since findings in some patients may be distinctive. In the most dramatic cases, thymic lobules are small and consist of small, spindle-shaped epithelial cells. No lymphocytes or Hassall corpuscles are present. Corticomedullary differentiation is lacking. In less severe cases, minor amounts of corticomedullary differentiation may be present, but lymphocytes are decreased and Hassall corpuscles are absent.

Laboratory Findings and Diagnosis

The laboratory findings in SCID vary with the underlying genetic defect. Certain common findings, however, are summarized here. Patients have a profound lymphopenia and do not show antibody response to vaccines. Immunoglobulin levels are usually extremely low in SCID. IgA and IgM may be undetectable by routine assays. Rarely, patients may have elevated IgM levels and monoclonal paraprotein.

Assessment of the T lymphocyte system by flow cytometric analysis is particularly helpful in X-linked SCID, since there is a marked lymphopenia. Cells with a mature T lymphocyte phenotype (CD3+/CD4+ or CD3+/CD8+) are not present. Measurements of T lymphocyte function correlate more closely with analyses of the potential protective capability of T lymphocytes. The most informative test is the in vitro proliferative response to specific antigen. T lymphocytes are exposed to a mitogen that in normal subjects stimulates T lymphocytes in a global manner and induces proliferation. Absent mitogen responses indicate a severe T lymphocyte defect. Since this test requires previous sensitization, in vitro proliferation assays are not useful early in life. Further, its specialized nature limits availability to a few reference laboratories. Skin testing for delayed hypersensitivity is the in vivo analogue of these antigen proliferation assays. Skin tests are less sensitive than the in vitro assays, and they may be nonreactive in 2- to 3-year-old normal children. T

Table 3–5
Clinical Features and Laboratory Findings in Combined Immunodeficiency Disorders

Disease	Clinical Features	T Cells	B Cells
"Typical" SCID	X-linked Thrush Bacterial and viral infection	CD3+ CD4 + low CD3+ CD8 + low Mitogen response low IL-2 production low	CD19/20 normal Total Ig levels normal IgG antibody responses low IgM, IgA antibody responses normal
New X-linked immunodeficiency	X-linked Intractable diarrhea Overwhelming sepsis	CD3+ CD4 + normal CD3+ CD8 + normal CD45+ normal Mitogen response slightly low	SIg + cells normal Total Ig levels high Specific antibody formation poor
CID associated with cyclic hematopoietic defect	Cyclic hematopoiesis *Pneumocystis* pneumonia	T cell count low to normal Mitogen response low to normal	Total number of B cells normal Total Ig levels very low
CD4 decrease without AIDS, idiopathic CD4 lymphocytopenia	HIV negative; risk factors positive in <50% Immunologic studies tend to remain stable Age 16 years or over Wasting syndrome Extrapulmonary cryptococcosis Atypical *Mycobacterium* infection Kaposi sarcoma Some asymptomatic	CD4+ <300/ml or <20% of total	Total Ig levels normal to low
IL-1 defect	Failure to thrive Severe herpes zoster	Lymphocytosis (8470/ml) CD3+ CD4 + high CD3+ CD8 + high	Total Ig levels normal
Multiple cytokine defects, IL-2 defect	Oral thrush	Lymphocytes normal to high CD2+ normal CD3+ CD4 + low to normal CD3+ CD8 + low to normal Mitogen and antigen response low, correctable by exogenous IL-2	CD20+ normal All Ig levels very low
Calcium flux defect	Protracted diarrhea CMV pneumonia	Lymphocytes normal	IgA elevated IgM elevated IgG restricted heterogeneity

Source: Adapted from Hong R: Disorders of T-cell System in Immunologic Disorders in Infants and Children. WB Saunders, Philadelphia, p 347, 1996.

lymphocyte function may also be assessed by cytokine levels, which are usually low in patients with SCID. C1q levels are typically one third of normal in patients with SCID. This serum defect is consistent but unexplained.

Pathogenesis

There are many recognized causes of combined immunodeficiencies, and the list is growing rapidly. The clinical presentations of SCID patients do not correlate with precise defects delineated by in vitro T cell assessment or other tests. For instance, oral candidiasis that is highly resistant to therapy is observed in only some of the patients with functional T cell defects. Clinical manifestations in SCID are not predictive of laboratory findings, probably indicating imprecision in current laboratory evaluation and/or complex clinical expression.

Defects in SCID have been identified at all steps of T cell development, including stem cell generation, thymic differentiation, surface receptor expression, cytokine response or production, lymphocyte homing, and maintenance of cell numbers.

A failure in stem cell generation is probably the cause of reticular dysgenesis (see "Reticular Dysgenesis"). In stem cell defects, the thymus contains no lymphocytes. In DiGeorge syndrome, there may be a lack of thymic development (see "DiGeorge Syndrome") or aberrant thymic differentiation resulting from a problem in negative and positive selection of T lymphocytes in the thymus. Two examples have been described in humans: a deficiency of CD8+ cells and a deficiency in molecular components of the T cell receptor (TCR). A selective deficiency in CD8+ cells appears to be caused by a mutation in a kinase gene *ZAP70*, involved in cytoplasmic signaling after engagement of the TCR. This receptor has two polypeptide subunits that associate with at least four subunits that compose CD3. Deficiencies in several of these subunits lead to abnormal or absent expression of the TCR. In these cases, TCR-positive cells are detectable, but only at 10–20% of normal levels.

Cytokines enhance the proliferation of lymphocytes necessary for immunologic responses. Defective IL-1 synthesis has been described in SCID. Lymphocytes may also lack receptors for cytokines (e.g., IL-2 receptor). The patients have marked lymphopenia with an X-linked inheritance. The disease is called X-linked SCID and is the result of mutations in the γ chain of the IL-2 receptor. IL-2 receptors are also expressed on myelocytes, which explains the high incidence of other types of hematopoietic defects in these patients. Defects in the surface expression of CD4 and CD7 may also lead to SCID. Defects in CD4 expression on lymphocytes must be distinguished from idiopathic CD4 lymphopenia (see "Idiopathic CD4 Lymphopenia").

Immunodeficiency with Enzyme Deficiency

Equivalent Terms

Adenosine deaminase and nucleoside phosphorylase deficiencies are equivalents.

Definition

Congenital immunodeficiencies may be associated with one of two enzyme deficiencies of the purine nucleotide pathway: adenosine deaminase activity (ADA) deficiency and purine nucleoside phosphorylase (PNP) deficiency.

Clinical Features

ADA Deficiency. Four types of ADA deficiency have been described: ADA-SCID, delayed-onset ADA deficiency, late-onset ADA deficiency, and partial ADA deficiency (Hirschhorn, 1993; Santisteban et al, 1993). Eighty to 90% of patients are in the first group, presenting with early onset of life-threatening infection and marked lymphopenia. Serious infections begin in the latter part of the first year in the second group. The third group presents even later, with the diagnosis often made after 4 years of age. This group is likely underdiagnosed, since ADA-SCID deficiency may not be considered clinically. Autoimmunity is more common in the second and third groups. Approximately a dozen patients found to have ADA deficiency incidentally as a result of population screening appear to have normal immunity.

PNP Deficiency. All patients with PNP deficiency are symptomatic (Markert, 1991), presenting with recurrent viral, bacterial, and fungal infections. The development of symptoms attributable to immunodeficiency may be delayed for years. Two thirds of patients have neurologic disorders, including mental retardation and muscle spasticity. Autoimmune processes have also been reported.

Histopathologic Features

Marked lymphocyte depletion is seen in the thymus, spleen, and lymph nodes (Ratech et al, 1989; Ratech et al, 1985), although a pattern unique to enzyme deficiency has not been observed. In addition to lymphocyte depletion, atrophy and sclerosis of the adrenal and pituitary glands has been reported in a group of ADA-deficient cases at autopsy.

Laboratory Findings and Diagnosis

ADA deficiency is associated with B and T lymphocyte defects, while PNP deficiency is associated with normal B lymphocyte immunity and absent or severely impaired T lymphocyte immunity. ADA and PNP deficiency are established by documenting low and absent levels of ADA and PNP, respectively, in erythrocytes, lymphocytes, or fibroblasts (Makrynikola & Bradstock, 1993). Carrier states may be identified by finding approximately half-normal levels. In addition, patients with PNP deficiency have decreased uric acid levels. Characteristic x-ray findings seen in about half the cases of ADA deficiency include cupping and flattening of the ribs as well as abnormalities of the transverse processes of the vertebrae and scapula (Cederbaum et al, 1976).

Pathogenesis

ADA and PNP deficiencies are usually inherited in an autosomal recessive manner (Sandman et al, 1977). These enzymes are involved in the purine salvage pathway and are necessary for proper DNA production. Although present in all cells, the primary effect of their deficiencies is on lymphocytes. B lymphocytes are relatively spared in PNP deficiency, a seeming paradox perhaps due to selective toxicity from variation in intracellular accumulation of toxic metabolites (Hirschhorn, 1993; Hirschhorn, 1990; Kredich & Martin, 1977). T lymphocytes may have enhanced susceptibility to accumulate metabolites because of their high turnover. In addition to its involvement in DNA metabolism, ADA is expressed on the surface of lymphocytes, where it binds to CD26 (Kameoka et al, 1993). The biologic significance of ADA-CD26 interaction is unknown, and subsequent insight in this area may explain the extensive impact that ADA deficiency has on immune functions. Elevated adenosine in ADA deficiency may cause the neurologic symptoms seen in ADA (but not PNP) deficiency.

Only small amounts (1–5%) of normal ADA production are necessary for competent immunity. Carriers are asymptomatic, since they usually express 50% of normal levels. A number of mutations in the ADA gene locus, including point mutation, novel splicing defects, and deletions, lead to complete ADA deficiency (Hirschhorn, 1993; Hirschhorn, 1990; Santisteban et al, 1993). It is unclear how the various mutations cause observed heterogeneity in clinical presentation but is possible that these are related to small (<2% of normal) yet functional amounts of ADA produced in some cases. PNP deficiency may be related to point mutations in the PNP gene on chromosome 14 (Andrews & Markert, 1992).

Bare Lymphocyte Syndrome

Equivalent Terms

Major histocompatiblity complex class I or class II antigen deficiency is the equivalent.

Definition

Bare lymphocyte syndrome refers to several immunodeficiencies associated with inadequate expression of major histocompatibility complex (MHC) class I or class II antigens.

Clinical Features

This syndrome was originally reported in North American and Turkish families but has now been identified in other groups (Hadam et al, 1984; Touraine et al, 1985). Patients were first recognized when screening for marrow transplantation revealed an absence of MHC molecules on their lymphocytes, engendering the term *bare lymphocyte syndrome*. Most of the initial cases had an autosomal recessive pattern of inheritance resulting from consanguinity, but many sporadic cases (i.e., negative family history) have now been described.

In the fulminant form, patients with bare lymphocyte syndrome typically have severe or recurrent systemic infections within the first 8 months of life. Infectious agents are bacterial, viral, protozoan, and fungal organisms, particularly *Candida*, *P. carinii*, and herpes. The infections in these patients are similar in course to those in most other combined immunodeficiencies.

Chronic, severe diarrhea and malabsorption often result from *Giardia lamblia* infection. A thymus shadow is usually seen on chest x-ray. Peripheral lymphadenopathy is a variable finding. A few patients appear less susceptible to life-threatening infections, and they have partial deficiency of MHC expression (Rijkers et al, 1987).

Histopathologic Features

Follicle development in lymph nodes is poor, and germinal centers are small, decreased in number, or absent. Virtually no plasma cells are found in tissues or marrow. Changes in thymus morphologic features are subtle, but there are decreased levels of lymphocytes in the cortical areas and fewer Hassall corpuscles (Schuurman et al, 1985).

Laboratory Findings and Diagnosis

Markedly diminished or absent MHC class I or II antigens on the surface of lymphocytes, most readily demonstrated by flow cytometric analysis, establishes the diagnosis of bare lymphocyte syndrome.

The total number of B and T lymphocytes is normal or only slightly reduced. Plasma cells are not present in marrow or lymphatic tissue (Hadam et al, 1984; Rijkers et al, 1987), leading to panhypogammaglobulinemia in virtually all individuals. In MHC class II deficiency the number of helper (CD4+) T cells is also significantly reduced due to an absence of CD45RA+ helper T cells (Kruisbeek et al, 1985). The lack of CD4+ cells is usually accompanied by an increase in CD8+ cells, resulting in a normal total T lymphocyte count but an inverted CD4:CD8 cell ratio.

Discordance between in vivo and in vitro functional testing is often present in these so-affected patients (Hadam et al, 1984; Rijkers et al, 1987; Touraine et al, 1985). Specific antibody production following immunization is severely decreased—a mitigation of antibody response that may not correlate with in vitro assays of antibody production. Such discordances are presumably due to variability in the magnitude of the class II deficiency and the B cell functional impairment. Delayed-type hypersensitivity skin test reactions are weak to absent, and yet in vitro T cell proliferation responses are normal or only modestly reduced.

Pathogenesis

The inability of cells to recognize foreign antigens in the context of MHC molecules is the primary basis for the immunodeficiency in this syndrome. Defects in lymphocyte differentiation and function caused by lack of MHC antigens compound the defects in cellular and humoral immunity.

Class I MHC antigens are expressed on all cells. In contrast, class II MHC antigens are constitutively expressed only on B lymphocytes and myelocyte or monocyte lineage cells. Class II MHC antigens may be induced on a variety of cell types. Class I and class II MHC antigens serve as recognition structures for the interactions among immunocompetent cells and are vital for initiating immune responses. In addition to their essential role in immune responses, MHC molecules are also critical in lymphocyte maturation and differentiation (Kruisbeek et al, 1985; Blue et al, 1985). For example, deficiency in intrathymic class I antigens results in diminished numbers of CD4+ cells emerging from the thymus. Class II MHC antigen–expressing cells are involved in intrathymic differentiation and "education" of T cells. As a result of defects in class II antigen expression, the CD4+ cells that do emerge from the thymus do not mature into CD4+CD45RA+ cells (i.e., helper cells with antigenic memory).

There are many molecular anomalies responsible for defective MHC expression, all inherited in an autosomal recessive manner. The lack of MHC antigen expression is the result of a failure in the transcription of MHC genes, since the genes encoding MHC antigens are intact (de Preval et al, 1988; Lisowska-Grospierre et al, 1985). At least four different defects are responsible for the failure of transcription, but the precise nature of these defects is not yet defined (Benichou & Strominger, 1991).

Other Combined Immunodeficiencies

Reticular Dysgenesis

Reticular dysgenesis, a congenital cellular and antibody deficiency associated with agenesis of granulocyte precursors in the marrow (Haas et al, 1986; Haas et al, 1977; Ownby et al, 1976), leads to death shortly after birth. Within the first few days of life, patients develop failure to thrive, vomiting, diarrhea, localized infections, and a rapidly deteriorating course. Patients have not lived beyond 90 days. The most recognizable laboratory finding is marked leukopenia. Hemoglobin and platelet levels are normal or slightly depressed. At autopsy, the thymus is small and without Hassall corpuscles. Lymphocytes are depleted in lymph nodes, spleen, and gastrointestinal tract. There is an absence of granulocyte precursors in the marrow. The marrow does contain megakaryocytes and erythrocytes. Reticular dysgenesis is apparently caused by a stem cell defect, with the manifestation beginning at about 10 weeks of gestation. This disorder may be treated by marrow transplantation.

Idiopathic CD4 Lymphopenia

Idiopathic CD4 lymphopenia refers to a small cohort of individuals in whom CD4+ T lymphocytes are profoundly decreased but HIV infection cannot be proved (Duncan et al, 1993; Fauci, 1993; Ho et al, 1993; Smith et al, 1993; Spira et al, 1993). Most cases occur in adults, but rare cases occur in children. The geographic and age distribution are much broader than for AIDS, but approximately 40% of these patients have some risk factor for AIDS. Levels of CD4+ lymphocytes below the 95th percentile for age or less than 20% of the total T lymphocyte count define the disease. Infection with opportunistic agents is common, and no definitive cause has been determined.

Griscelli Syndrome

This syndrome manifests itself as a combined immunodeficiency resembling Chédiak-Higashi syndrome (see "Chédiak-Higashi Syndrome") (Griscelli et al, 1978; Siccardi et al, 1978). Individuals with Griscelli syndrome have characteristic silvery hair, and leukocytes lack the Chédiak-Higashi–type cytoplasmic granules. Patients have widespread histiocytic infiltrations, resulting in hepatosplenomegaly, lymphadenopathy, and pulmonary infiltration. Lymph node architecture may be obliterated. Immune dysfunctions include decreased CD3+ cell counts, although lymphocyte counts are normal. Mitogen responses of T lymphocytes are normal to minimally depressed. Serum immunoglobulin levels may be normal or low. Marrow transplantation is curative.

Nezelof Syndrome

Nezelof syndrome, also known as cellular immunodeficiency with abnormal immunoglobulin synthesis (Lawlor et al, 1974; Nezelof, 1968), is associated with profound T lymphocyte deficiency and decreased or absent antibody function. Immunoglobulin levels are normal or mildly depressed, but immunoglobulins are functionally incompetent. Despite these abnormalities, patients may have a mild course relative to that of other combined immunodeficiencies.

COMBINED IMMUNODEFICIENCIES WITH PHENOTYPIC FINDINGS

DiGeorge Anomaly

Equivalent Terms

Thymic hypoplasia, third and fourth pouch/arch syndrome, cellular immunodeficiency with hypoparathyroidism are the equivalents.

Definition

DiGeorge anomaly is a congenital immunodeficiency characterized clinically by hypocalcemia, cardiac defects, and increased susceptibility to infections.

Clinical Features

DiGeorge anomaly may be considered a field defect, that is, a malformation consistently involving a group of tissues (the field) that develop as a unit during normal embryogenesis. All tissues in the field are not equally affected in all patients, causing variation in clinical manifestations. The clinical presentation is varied, although most if not all cases have a similar pathogenesis.

DiGeorge anomaly results in part from a defect in structures that develop from the third and fourth pharyngeal pouches, explaining the frequent absence of parathryoid glands and thymus as well as cardiac defects (Conley et al, 1990; Conley et al, 1979). Most patients may be recognized by their external features, including their distinctive facies. An absent thymus causes an immune system defect in only 25% of patients (Bastian et al, 1989). These patients experience chronic rhinitis, recurrent pneumonia (often from *P. carinii*), and oral candidiasis. The absence of parathyroid glands leads to hypocalcemic tetany within the first 24–48 h of life. Fortunately, tetany is rare and frequently transient. Cardiac defects are quite heterogeneous, but an interrupted aortic arch and truncus arteriosus are most common (Conley et al, 1990). The T lymphocyte deficiency causing infection may also lead to autoimmune disorders, such as Graves disease and intractable eczema.

The term *partial DiGeorge anomaly* refers to patients with a small but histologically normal thymus. T cell function gradually improves in these children. The combination of parathyroid and thymic deficiencies has also been referred to as Zellweger syndrome. Most cases of DiGeorge anomaly and Zellweger syndrome are part of a much larger group of entities that have a microdeletion of chromosome 22 (see "Pathogenesis").

Laboratory Findings and Diagnosis

A constellation of clinical, pathologic, and laboratory findings defines DiGeorge anomaly. Histologic evaluation is usually not needed. Changes are not well documented. The combination of facial and cardiac defects is distinctive. A low serum calcium level, an elevated phosphorus level, and an absent to low parathyroid hormone level confirm a parathyroid deficiency. Chest x-ray findings may show an absent thymic shadow. A hypoplastic or an undescended thymus gland may provide for adequate T lymphocyte function in most patients. An undescended thymus may be difficult to find, since it may reside under the tongue, in the thyroid, or in the middle ear (Borzy et al, 1979) (Fig. 3–4).

There is confusion regarding the degree and permanence of the immune defect in DiGeorge anomaly, due in part to older methods for assessing T lymphocyte function. Currently, a CD4 count <400/dl and a mitogen proliferative response of less than 10 times background are reliable indications of immunodeficiency (Conley et al, 1990).

Karyotyping is warranted in all suspected cases (Lammer & Opitz, 1986), since approximately 90% of DiGeorge anomaly patients show chromosomal abnormalities. The most common chromosomal abnormality, microdeletion of chromosome 22q11.2, is not detectable by normal karyotypic analysis (Larson & Butler, 1995). Fluorescent in situ hybridization techniques do provide a rapid and reliable means of detecting these deletions. Defects in chromosomes 1, 5, 10, 12, 17, and 18 have also been described.

Pathogenesis

The field defect involving the third and fourth pharyngeal pouches in DiGeorge anomaly explains the abnormal facies, absent parathyroid glands, absent or hypoplastic thymus, and cardiac defects. The disease is usually sporadic but may be inherited.

The T lymphocyte defect was initially considered the result of a small or absent thymic mass, but this explanation appears

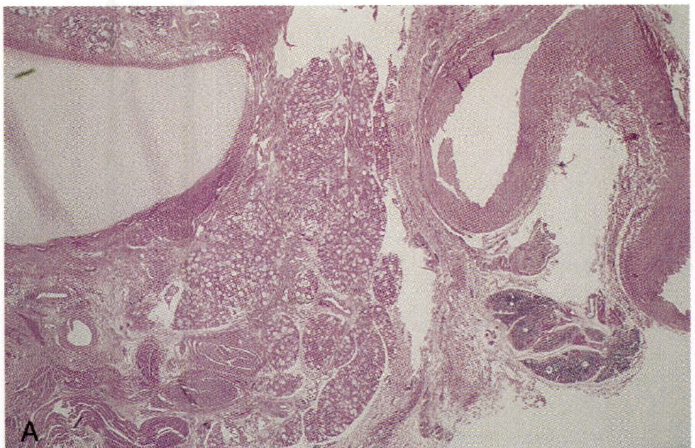

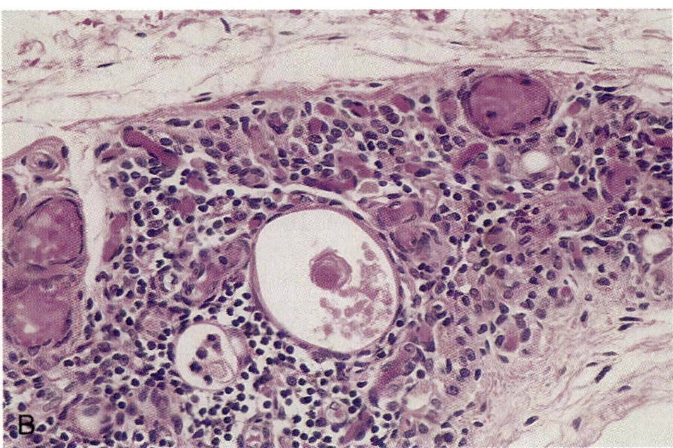

Figure 3–4

DiGeorge anomaly, undescended thymus. This $2\frac{1}{2}$-month-old child died from complications of cardiac surgery for a complex cardiac defect. Thymic tissue was not found in the anterior mediastinum or mediastinum at surgery or autopsy. *A*. Multiple sections of the neck showed undeveloped thymic tissue lateral to the trachea and just below the thyroid gland. *B*. High magnification shows no corticomedullary differentiation. An ill-formed Hassall corpuscle is present.

to be incorrect. Small amounts of thymic tissue are present in many patients, explaining why an immune defect is present in only 25% of patients even though thymic shadow is absent in most cases. In addition, the T lymphocyte defect may be partial or transient. In most cases, the thymus is small, undeveloped, and undescended (Borzy et al, 1979) (see Fig. 3–4). These observations all indicate that a small gland is present (albeit misplaced) in most patients and that it is stunted in development but with time provides normal T lymphocyte function.

A microdeletion of the proximal portion of chromosome 22q seems to be involved in the pathogenesis of many DiGeorge anomaly cases (Larson & Butler, 1995). Most familial and many sporadic cases are associated with chromosome 22q11.2 microdeletion. The same microdeletion has been implicated in the pathogenesis of various developmental disorders, including Shprintzen syndrome (cardiac and facial anomalies), isolated conotruncal heart defects, and CHARGE syndrome (coloboma, heart defects, atresia of cloanus, retardation, genial defects, and ear abnormalities) (Burn et al, 1993; Emanual et al, 1992; Goldmuntz et al, 1993). Since there is overlap in the clinical presentation of these syndromes and since microdeletions of chromosome 22 have been demonstrated in each disorder, the acronym CATCH 22 (cardiac defects, abnormal facies, thymic hypoplasia, cleft palate, and hypocalcemia) has been proposed as an encompassing term for this group of disorders (Scambler et al, 1991; Wilson et al, 1993). Alternatively, some investigators have proposed that microdeletions of chromosome 22 explain only the cardiac defects and that additional molecular defects may cause other abnormalities.

Ataxia-Telangiectasia

Definition

Ataxia-telangiectasia is an immunodeficiency associated with sinopulmonary infections, telangiectasia, progressive ataxia, and hypersensitivity to ionizing radiation.

Clinical Features

The distinguishing clinical characteristics are ataxia and telangiectasia. The onset of these symptoms is variable but generally occurs before 5 years of age (Fiorilli et al, 1983; Swift, 1984; Boder, 1985). In most patients cerebellar ataxia develops during infancy; it is progressive and unrelenting. Eye movements provide a reliable diagnostic finding. Poor coordination with movement is almost always observed. Telangiectasia, initially of the bulbar conjunctivae, may be seen as early as 1 year or as late as 6 years of age. Telangiectasia is also progressive, ultimately involving lateral aspects of the nose, the ears, the antecubital and the popliteal areas, and the dorsa of the hands and feet.

Patients are susceptible to viral and bacterial infections before or after ataxia, and telangiectasia appear (Boder, 1985). In contrast to many other immunodeficiencies, individuals with ataxia-telangiectasia are not at increased susceptibility to opportunistic infections. There is considerable variation in the cause and severity of infections among patients in different countries, suggesting that exposure, hygiene, and medical care may influence the outcome for these patients (Roifman & Gelfand, 1985). B and T cell lymphomas, Hodgkin disease, and other malignancies occur at higher rates. Family members may also be at risk of malignancy (Swift et al, 1991; Swift, 1984; Boder, 1985).

Histopathologic Features

Pathologic studies on the central nervous system have shown a progressive loss of Purkinje cells and granular cell layer in the cerebellum (Aguilar et al, 1968), correlating with the increasing severity of cerebellar ataxia and dysarthria. Spinal cord abnormalities are also common. Bronchiectasis is frequent and is usually associated with pneumonia. Histologic changes in the liver, such as chronic hepatitis or fibrosis, that might explain elevated α-fetoprotein levels are not found (see "Laboratory Findings and Diagnosis"). Atrophy of the ovaries or testes has been observed in postmortem examinations.

Lymph nodes may be hypoplastic, with depletion of B lymphocytes in follicles. In some patients follicular hyperplasia does not occur after antigenic stimulation (Peterson et al, 1966). Abnormalities in the thymus vary from atrophy in some cases to hypoplasia with an absence of Hassall corpuscles.

Laboratory Findings and Diagnosis

The diagnosis is usually made in infants by demonstrating the combination of ataxia, telangiectasia, and immune deficits (Feigin et al, 1970; Fiorilli et al, 1983; Gropp & Flatz, 1967; Oppenheim et al, 1973; Peterson et al, 1966). In addition to the manifestations discussed earlier, the peripheral blood usually shows lymphopenia and eosinophilia. Granulocytopenia has also been described. A decreased proportion of CD4+ lymphocytes may be observed. Immunoglobulin abnormalities of various types are observed in these patients. IgA deficiency, the most common abnormality, is found in approximately 70% of patients. IgA deficiency may occur coincidentally with a decreased IgG level or decreased specific IgG subclass levels (usually IgG2) as well. Titers of antibody to viral and bacterial antigens may also be deficient. Abnormal T cell immunity (negative skin hypersensitivity test results or decreased response of lymphocytes to phytohemagglutinin in vitro) is demonstrated in about 60% of patients.

Excessive chromosome breakage has been reported. Since lymphocytes from patients with ataxia-telangiectasia proliferate poorly in vitro, karyotypic studies are of limited value. Radiosensitivity of chromosomes to breakage may also be tested. Many patients have extremely radiosensitive chromosomes. Some investigators group patients according to their clinical manifestations and chromosomal radiosensitivity (Lange et al, 1993). However, the clinical significance of this grouping is unclear, and the test is not widely available.

Abnormal liver function test results and abnormal 17-ketosteroid, follicle-stimulating hormone, and serum α-fetoprotein levels may be present in these patients (Ammann et al, 1969b; Ishiguro et al, 1986). The latter abnormality is a common finding in ataxia-telangiectasia not found in other immunodeficiencies. The elevation of α-fetoprotein levels occurs in the absence of chronic liver disease or malignancy.

Pathogenesis

Although there is no consistent immunologic defect in patients with ataxia-telangiectasia, a single genetic defect has been localized to chromosome 11q22-23 (Sobel et al, 1992; Savitsky et al, 1995). The function or identity of this gene is not known; therefore, it is not understood how this defect leads to multisystem dysfunction and chromosomal sensitivity to radiation. Although the chromosomal break points appear random in ataxia-telangiectasia, the genetic defect is not due to chromosomal breakage, since translocations or deletions of genetic material at the gene site have not been observed.

It has been hypothesized that the basic defect in ataxia-telangiectasia is one of organ differentiation and maturation, and that alterations in the ataxia-telangiectasia gene might prevent proper maturation of a number of tissues. In this context the immunologic, neurologic, and other organ disorders might result from progressive cellular failure. In support of this hypothesis is the observation that the immune system in patients with ataxia-telangiectasia progressively deteriorates over time (Ammann et al, 1969a). The contention that the ataxia-telangiectasia gene supports basic cellular maturation (Waldmann & McIntire, 1972) is further confirmed by the presence of α-fetoprotein in the serum, since this substance is usually produced by embryonic liver.

How the defective ataxia-telangiectasia gene leads to chromosomal breakage after exposure to ionizing radiation is unclear. However, accumulating chromosomal breaks may also contribute to cellular attrition.

Wiskott-Aldrich Syndrome

Definition

Wiskott-Aldrich syndrome is characterized by thrombocytopenia, immunodeficiency, eczema, and recurrent infections.

Clinical Features

Wiskott-Aldrich syndrome has an X-linked form of inheritance. The initial patient presentation is typically an episode of petechiae or bleeding in the first 6 months of life. An eczematoid rash accompanied by bacterial and viral infections of the sinorespiratory tract also occurs during this period. CMV, *P. carinii*, herpes simplex, and varicella may be the etiologic agents. Splenomegaly, hepatomegaly, and cervical lymphadenopathy may be present. Patients usually have severe reactions to vaccines, particularly polysaccharide antigens. These reactions may include worsening of petechiae, eczema, and purpura. Malignancies, particularly lymphomas, occur more frequently in children with Wiskott-Aldrich syndrome who are over the age of 8 years (Bensel et al, 1966; Brand & Marinkovich, 1969; Chaptal et al, 1966). Many of the lymphomas have a predilection for the central nervous system.

The clinical presentation is variable. The classic manifestations (thrombocytopenia, eczema, and infection) may occur in only 25% of patients. In addition, variant forms of Wiskott-Aldrich syndrome apparently have unusual immunologic findings in addition to the usual clinical features. The relationship of these variant forms to the "classic" disease is unclear.

Histopathologic Features

There are characteristic histologic findings in the lymphatic tissue of patients with Wiskott-Aldrich syndrome (Cooper et al, 1968; Wolff, 1967; Wolff & Bertucio, 1957), including varying degrees of lymphocyte depletion in lymph nodes, thymus, and gastrointestinal tract. Lymph nodes show progressive depletion of T lymphocytes in the interfollicular areas with age. In young patients depletion may be only slight, but older children have moderate to severe depletion of T lymphocytes. Germinal center formation is poor or absent. Paradoxically, the lymphocytic tissue of the gastrointestinal tract is often less affected than other sites. The thymus may be small, with normal histologic components (normal thymic architecture, normal corticomedullary differentiation, and Hassall corpuscles), whereas other patients have scant thymic tissue. In summary, there is considerable variation among patients of similar age in the degree of lymphatic tissue depletion, reflecting the variability in disease evolution and heterogeneity of the syndrome.

Laboratory Findings and Diagnosis

The diagnosis is made in male infants by demonstrating recurrent infections, eczema, and thrombocytopenia. In addition, there is a characteristic pattern of immunoglobulin levels: markedly elevated IgA and IgE levels and low IgM levels (Chaptal et al, 1966). This pattern may not develop until the patient is several years of age. Patients with Wiskott-Aldrich syndrome have both B and T lymphocyte defects, but the number of B and T lymphocytes is normal. There is a consistent inability to form antibody after vaccination with polysaccharide antigens. There are normal antibody responses to other bacterial, parasitic, and simple protein antigens (Cooper et al, 1968). This finding may not be helpful in the very young, since normal infants may not respond to polysaccharide vaccines until 18 months of age. Flow cytometric analysis of T lymphocytes shows absent or decreased expression of CD43 in patients of all ages (Higgins et al, 1991). T lymphocyte functional defects are manifested in some patients by failure of lymphocytes to proliferate in response to periodate. Hematologic abnormalities include anemia, lymphopenia, eosinophilia, and thrombocytopenia. Platelet sizing may be helpful; small platelets, present in a minority of patients with Wiskott-Aldrich syndrome, are rarely present in other disorders (Murphy et al, 1972). Paraproteins, usually IgG, are reported with and without an associated malignancy (Bruce & Blaese, 1974).

Pathogenesis

Wiskott-Aldrich syndrome, like the DiGeorge anomaly, appears to be a spectrum of diseases caused by a chromosomal deletion or deletions in contiguous regions. The responsible gene has been identified and named *WASP* (Wiskott-Aldrich syndrome protein) (Derry et al, 1994). It is located on Xp11.22-23 and is expressed in lymphocytes, megakaryocytes, spleen, and thymus. Additional contiguous deletions along the X chromosome may affect additional genes in some patients.

The immune defect in Wiskott-Aldrich syndrome involves both B and T lymphocytes, but the T lymphocyte defect has been more extensively studied. The patients have defective T lymphocyte function related in part to decreased or absent expression of CD43. The role of CD43 in immune system development and function is not completely understood, although it is known that CD43 is involved in lymphocyte maturation, differentiation, responsiveness of T lymphocytes to antigen, T lymphocyte activation, and T lymphocyte proliferation (Mentzer et al, 1987; Park et al, 1991; Yonemura et al, 1993). CD43 is located on chromosome 16. The gene appears intact in Wiskott-Aldrich syndrome patients. The defect on the X chromosome may cause the down-regulation of CD43 on cells of the immune system. Since the response of lymphocytes to polysaccharides and immobilized antigens is dependent on microvilli formation and proper cytoskeletal formation, the central defect in Wiskott-Aldrich syndrome may be the inability of cells to form microvilli. Although the postulated lack of microvilli formation may explain many of the selective immune defects in Wiskott-Aldrich syndrome (Molina et al, 1993; Molina et al, 1992), there is no current molecular explanation for the ezcema, malignancy, thrombocytopenia, and small platelets observed in these patients.

DISORDERS OF THE PHAGOCYTIC SYSTEM

Cells of the phagocytic system (neutrophils, monocytes, and macrophages) engulf and kill microbes. Normal host defense is dependent upon adequate numbers of these cells and their functional competence. This point is well appreciated clinically, since neutropenic patients suffer recurrent, often life-threatening infections. In addition, patients with normal numbers of phagocytic cells but defective functional capabilities have been described. Patients with some of these disorders are described in this section.

Leukocyte Adhesion Deficiency

Definition

Leukocyte adhesion deficiency is characterized by the inability of leukocytes to extravasate from the blood.

Clinical Features

Patients with leukocyte adhesion deficiency type 1 have recurrent, often life-threatening bacterial infections of the skin, mucous membranes, and intestinal tract (Anderson & Springer, 1987; Anderson et al, 1984; Arnout, 1993; Fischer et al, 1988). These patients also have neutrophilic leukocytosis, impaired pus formation, delayed wound healing, and prolonged attachment of the umbilical cord after birth. During the neonatal period, septicemia or abdominal infection usually occurs. Severe or persistent gingivitis and periodontitis are common in their childhood and may result in early loss of deciduous as well as permanent teeth. Culture of the infectious lesions of leukocyte adhesion deficiency patients reveals a wide spectrum of fungi and gram-positive and gram-negative bacteria. There is normal susceptibility to viral infections, and viral vaccines do not have adverse effects. There are two clinical phenotypes of leukocyte adhesion defect type 1: one group has shorter life expectancy and has severe infections, and the second group has a longer life expectancy and less severe and less frequent infections. The genetic alterations producing these two clinical phenotypes of leukocyte adhesion deficiency type 1 are understood (see "Pathogenesis").

Only two patients with type 2 deficiency have been described (Etzioni et al, 1992). In addition to recurrent bacterial infections, periodontitis, and neutrophilia, they also had distinctive facies and mental retardation. The genetic and biologic alterations leading to type 2 disease are described later (see "Pathogenesis").

Histopathologic Features

The architecture and cell distribution of lymphatic tissue are normal in leukocyte adhesion deficiency type 1 (Anderson et al, 1984; Anderson & Springer, 1987; Fischer et al, 1988; Todd & Fryer, 1988). Patients have peripheral neutrophilia and corresponding myelocytic predominance in the marrow. Neutrophils are absent in sites of infection (Fig. 3–5), and bacterial overgrowth may be seen. Eosinophils may be seen within these infectious sites. The histologic findings in type 2 deficiency have not been described.

Laboratory Findings and Diagnosis

A characteristic laboratory finding in patients with leukocyte adhesion defect is marked neutrophilia. Normal blood counts essentially exclude the diagnosis in otherwise well neonates with delayed umbilical cord detachment. Flow cytometric analysis demonstrating a lack of CD11 or CD18 expression on peripheral blood neutrophils or monocytes is diagnostic (Arnout, 1993).

Other sophisticated tests of neutrophil and monocytic function (including adherence to plastic, spreading, chemotaxis, aggregation, adherence to endothelium, and phagocytosis of C3b-coated particles) show marked abnormalities (Anderson et al, 1984; Anderson & Springer, 1987; Fischer et al, 1988). There is also a deficient respiratory burst triggered by particulate phagocytosis. Serum immunoglobuin levels, antibody titers, and delayed hypersensitivity reactions are normal, although in vitro studies on T cell functions and proliferation show abnormalities.

Pathogenesis

Leukocyte adhesion disorders are associated with abnormalities of both leukocyte adhesion and motility (Anderson et al, 1984; Anderson & Springer, 1987; Fischer et al, 1988; Arnout, 1993). There are two types of adhesive interactions between leukocytes and endothelium prior to extravasation. Leukocytes first roll on endothelium (rolling adherence), using selectin molecules, and then firmly adhere, using integrin molecules. Integrin-dependent firm adherence is defective in type 1 deficiencies, and selectin-dependent rolling adherence is deficient in type 2.

Integrin-dependent firm adhesion of leukocytes to endothelium is reduced by mutations in the CD18 gene. CD18 is a shared β subunit that associates with four different α subunits and escorts the $\alpha\beta$ complex to the cell surface. Decreased or ineffective CD18 production prevents surface expression of the four $\alpha\beta$ complexes: lymphocyte function–associated antigen 1 (LFA-1, CD11a); Mac-1 (CD11b); p150,95 (CD11c); and αd (anticipated CD11d). These four molecules are integral to adhesive functions of leukocytes. As a result, decreased or absent CD18 expression results in the inability of neutrophils to adhere firmly to the endothelium and extravasate into inflamed sites.

Leukocyte adhesion defect type 1 is inherited in an autosomal recessive manner. Several mutations in the CD18 gene (Dimanche-Bortrel et al, 1988; Kishimoto et al, 1987;

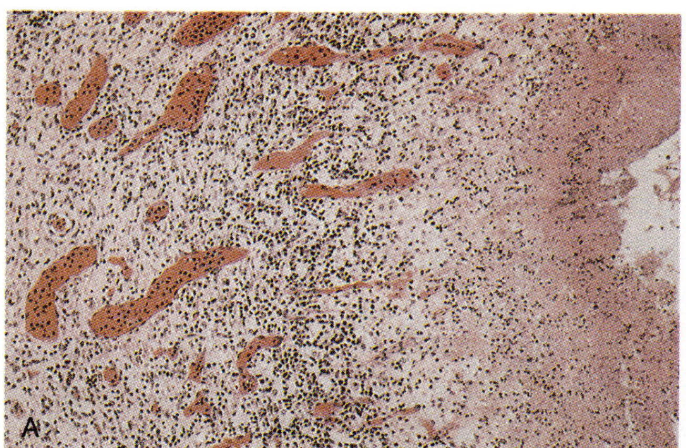

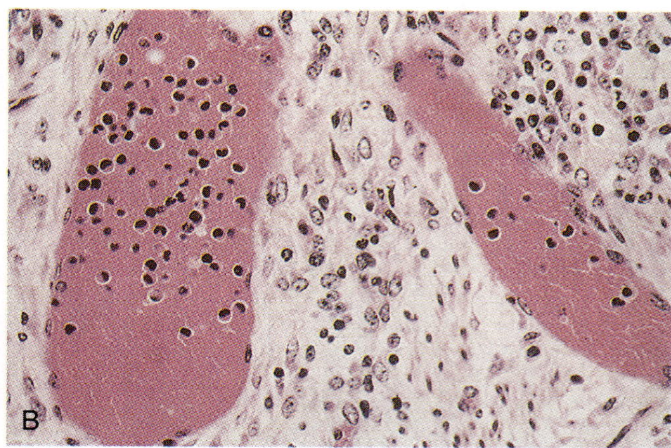

Figure 3–5

Leukocyte adhesion deficiency, gastrointestinal tract. This patient died as a neonate with enterocolitis. *A.* Low magnification of severe enterocolitis. *B.* High magnification shows a virtual absence of neutrophils from the submucosa as well as marked engorgement.

Rodriguez et al, 1993) either reduce cell surface expression of normal CD18 protein or cause expression of a structurally altered CD18 protein that is not fully functional. Heterozygotes are carriers and do not have an increased frequency of infections, although the levels of CD18 are 50% of normal. Homozygotic patients with diminished surface expression (3–10%) have a mild clinical phenotype. Patients with lower expression of CD18 have a severe phenotype.

Leukocyte adhesion defect type 2 results from lack of expression of the adhesion receptor CD15s (sialyl-Lewis X); this receptor is the counterstructure of E-selectin (CD62E) on endothelium. The receptor ligand pair of CD15s and CD62e mediates rolling adherence on endothelium at sites of inflammation, a necessary first step for neutrophil or monocyte extravasation. Only two patients with type 2 deficiency have been described; these boys were unrelated progeny of consanguineous parents.

Chronic Granulomatous Disease

Definition

Chronic granulomatous disease (CGD) is a primary immunodeficiency associated with defective microbial killing by phagocytic cells. B and T lymphocyte functions are normal.

Clinical Features

CGD may be inherited in either an X-linked or autosomal recessive manner. There are no significant differences in the site or cause of infections in CGD regardless of inheritance, but patients with X-linked inheritance have an earlier onset of infections and are hospitalized twice as frequently as patients with autosomal recessive CGD (Weening et al, 1985).

Patients with CGD have the typical responses to infection of fever, leukocytosis, and localized inflammation. Abscesses form frequently. Lymphadenopathy, hepatomegaly, and splenomegaly are common. There is incomplete clearance of the infection, ultimately resulting in a granulomatous lesion. Severe infections usually occur during the first year of life, and 80% of patients are identified by 2 years of age (Johnston & Newman, 1977). The sites principally infected are skin, mucous membranes, lung, intestines, and perianal tissue (Gallin et al, 1983). Pneumonia may be life-threatening. Gastrointestinal infection may lead to malabsorption or obstruction from gastric antral narrowing. An agent is not identified in many infections. The most common microbes are *S. aureus*, *Serratia marcescens*, *Escherichia coli*, *Pseudomonas*, *Aspergillus*, or rare fungi. Infections are often incompletely resolved by antibiotics (Gallin et al, 1983; Lazarus & Neu, 1975). It is surprising to note that septicemia and meningitis are uncommon.

Lupus erythematosus (systemic and discoid) has been reported at a high frequency (Manzi et al, 1991). This finding that may be related to CGD inheritance. Mothers of boys with X-linked CGD may have discoid lupus with and without serologic evidence of lupus (Kragballe et al, 1981; Lee & Yap, 1994).

CGD patients are short in stature (Payne et al, 1983), with some of the growth retardation likely related to serious, recurrent, and prolonged infections. Most children with CGD are shorter than normal by 2 years of age, however, and do not catch up during extended asymptomatic periods, suggesting an associated genetic abnormality.

Histopathologic Features

Uninfected organs in most patients with CGD are normal histologically, but abscesses and granulomas may involve virtually any site. The lung and gastrointestinal tract lesions are best documented (Ament & Ochs, 1973a; Fisher et al, 1987; Subramaniam et al, 1974). Abscesses, granulomas, and acute as well as chronic signs of pneumonia may all be seen in the lung. Lesions in the gastrointestinal tract may closely resemble those of Crohn disease. Granulomatous lesions have been observed in the esophagus, intestine, and ureters in both diseases, further complicating the distinction of CGD from Crohn disease. Please see Chap. 16 for additional descriptions of histopathologic changes in CGD.

Laboratory Findings and Diagnosis

The diagnosis rests on demonstrating failure of neutrophils to undergo an oxidative burst after phagocytosis. Oxidase activity is usually measured by superoxide generation in a nitroblue tetrazolium (NBT) dye test or by oxygen consumption, as measured by chemoluminescence assay.

NBT testing is sensitive and specific for the diagnosis of CGD and for identifying female carriers (Baehner & Nathan, 1968). Patients with CGD have negative test result, and female carriers are chimeric. Thus, both NBT-positive and NBT-negative cells are observed in females. This chimerism reflects the location of the genetic defect on the X chromosome as well as female lyonization. The chemoluminescence assay is a less sensitive indicator of superoxide production (Mills et al, 1980). Although useful in diagnosing CGD, it does not detect the female carrier state. Flow cytometric techniques have been found useful in diagnosis of CGD.

Western blot testing may be performed in order to differentiate the type of CGD (discussed later). X-linked and autosomal recessive subtypes cannot be accurately identified by NBT test results alone, since approximately one third of X-linked cases arise spontaneously, and carriers with extreme lyonization exist.

Pathogenesis

The hallmark of CGD is the lack of a respiratory burst in phagocytic cells. A molecular defect in the nicotinamide adenine dinucleotide phosphate (NADPH) oxidase system prevents generation of superoxide and other reactive species that participate in killing ingested microbes. At least eight genetic subtypes have been reported. X-linked CGD constitutes approximately 60% of cases (Curnutte, 1993a).

There are four major structural components of the NADPH oxidase system: gp91-phox, p22-phox, p47-phox, and p67-phox. Microbial attachment to receptors on a phagocytic cell causes assembly of these four components. Resultant NADPH oxidase activation leads to production of superoxide. Defects in any of these four components result in loss of enzymatic activity and CGD. The gene for gp91-phox is located on the short arm of the X chromosome. Mutations in this gene account for all cases of X-linked CGD. Patients with the autosomal recessive form may have defects in the p47-phox gene on chromosome 7 (33% of all CGD cases), the p67-phox gene on chromosome 21 (5% of cases), and the p22-phox gene on chromosome 16 (5% of cases) (Roos, 1994).

The specific gene defects are extemely heterogeneous and difficult to detect reliably by Southern analysis, since more than 40 different mutations have been described for the X-linked form. Thus, Western blot analysis is the test of choice for identifying the deficient gene. The causative protein will be absent on Western blots. Because gp91-phox and p22-phox form a complex, a deficiency in either of these proteins results in an absence of both proteins. Since gp91 deficiency has X-linked inheritance and p22-phox deficiency is autosomal recessive, NBT testing of family members discriminates between these two possibilities. Detection of female carriers identifies the disease as X linked and indicates that the defect is in the gp91-phox gene. An absence of p47-phox or p67-phox does not affect the production or detection of the other -phox components. There are variant forms of CGD in which one of these proteins may be diminished rather than absent. Such cases will have defective NBT testing (Roos, 1994).

Other Phagocytic Deficiencies

Myeloperoxidase and Eosinophil Peroxidase Deficiency

The absence or deficiency of myeloperoxidase causes a phagocytic defect. Some patients may have severe recurrent infections; *C. albicans* infections are particularly frequent, since the phagocytes of such patients are unable to kill *C. albicans* (Lehrer & Cline, 1969). Myeloperoxidase deficiency may be quite common. The peroxidase gene is on chromosome 17, and the incidence of defects has been estimated at 1 in 4000 (Parry et al, 1981). The diagnosis may be confirmed by demonstrating that myeloperoxidase stains of peripheral blood show that granulocytes lack myeloperoxidase.

Myeloperoxidase deficiency affects both neutrophils and eosinophils, but an isolated eosinophil peroxidase deficiency has been identified (Zabacchi et al, 1992). Most people with eosinophil peroxidase deficiency and myeloperoxidase deficiency are not ill. The diagnosis may be confirmed by lack of Sudan black or myeloperoxidase staining in eosinophils.

Glucose-6-Phosphate Dehydrogenase Deficiency

Leukocytes from patients with glucose-6-phosphate dehydrogenase deficiency have defective bactericidal ability and fail to kill *S. aureus*, *E. coli*, or *Serratia*. Patients with low ($<25\%$ of normal) or absent levels of glucose-6-phosphate dehydrogenase have severe infections. The lack of glucose-6-phosphate dehydrogenase leads to deficient NADPH and reduces hexose monophosphate shunt activity. Thus, leukocytes from these patients have defective respiratory bursts and abnormal NBT test results (Gray et al, 1973).

Glutathione Synthetase Deficiency

Several patients with glutathione synthetase deficiency have been identified (Mohler et al, 1970). These patients have reduced levels of glutathione in erythrocytes and granulocytes. As a result, intracellular killing of *S. aureus* is impaired. Therapy with the antioxidants vitamin E, ascorbate, and *N*-acetylcysteine has increased the glutathione levels in these patients, promoting the normal bactericidal activity of leukocytes.

Chédiak-Higashi Syndrome

Chédiak-Higashi syndrome is an autosomal recessive disorder characterized by recurrent pyogenic infections, partial oculocutaneous albinism, progressive neuropathy, and giant cytoplasmic granules in cells (Barak & Nir, 1987). The diagnosis is strongly suggested by the clinical presentation and confirmed by the abnormal granules in leukocytes in peripheral blood films. Large lysosomal granules may also be seen in Schwann cells and melanocytes, as well as epithelium of renal tubules, gastric mucosa, pancreas, and thyroid. Leukocytes from patients with Chédiak-Higashi syndrome have many functional defects, especially defective intracellular killing. The respiratory oxidative response, which is abnormal in a number of phagocytic disorders described earlier, is normal in Chédiak-Higashi syndrome.

Specific Granule Deficiency

Specific granule deficiency is a rare autosomal recessive disorder characterized by recurrent, severe infections of the skin, mucous membranes, and lungs (Curnutte & Boxer, 1993b). Most patients survive if infections are treated promptly and aggressively. Neutrophils are bilobed, resembling Pelger-Huët cells, and secondary granules are absent. Since these granules contain proteins (lactroferrin and vitamin B_{12}-binding protein) necessary for a normal respiratory burst, intracellular killing of bacteria is defective. The phagocytic cells have normal amounts of myeloperoxidase and lysozyme.

REFERENCES

Aguilar MJ, Kamoshita S, Landing BH, et al: Pathological observations in ataxia-telangiectasia. J Neuropathol Exp Neurol 27:659, 1968.

Allen RC, Armitage RJ, Conley ME, et al: CD40 Ligand gene defects responsible for X-linked hyper-IgM syndrome. Science 259:990, 1993.

Ament ME, Ochs HD: Gastrointestinal manifestations of chronic granulomatous disease. N Engl J Med 288:382, 1973a.

Ament ME, Ochs HD, Davis SD: Structure and function of the gastrointestinal tract in primary immunodeficiency syndromes: a study of 39 patients. Medicine 52:227, 1973b.

Ammann AJ, Cain WA, Ishizaka K, et al: Immunoglobulin E deficiency in ataxia-telangiectasia. N Engl J Med 281:469, 1969a.

Ammann AJ, DuQuesnoy RJ, Good RA: Endocrinological studies in ataxia-telangiectasia and other immunological deficiency diseases. Clin Exp Immunol 6:587, 1969b.

Ammann AJ, Hong R: Selective IgA deficiency and autoimmunity. Clin Exp Immunol 7:833, 1970.

Ammann AJ, Hong R: Selective IgA deficiency: presentation of 30 cases and a review of the literature. Medicine 60:223, 1971a.

Ammann AJ, Hong R: Unique antibody to basement membrane in patients with selective IgA deficiency and celiac disease. Lancet 1:1264, 1971b.

Anderson DC, Schmalstieg FC, Arnaout AM, et al: Abnormalities of polymorpho-nuclear leukocyte function associated with a heritable deficiency of high molecular weight surface glycoproteins (GP138): common relationship to diminished cell adherence. J Clin Invest 74:536, 1984.

Anderson DC, Springer TA: Leukocyte adhesion deficiency: an inherited defect in the Mac-1, and p150, 95 glycoproteins. Ann Rev Med 38:175, 1987.

Andre C, Andre F, Fargier MC: Distribution of IgA1 and IgA2 plasma cells in various normal human tissues and in the jejunum of plasma IgA deficient patients. Clin Exp Immunol 33:327, 1978.

Andrews LG, Markert ML: Exon skipping in purine nucleoside phosphorylase mRNA processing leading to severe immunodeficiency. J Biol Chem 267:7834, 1992.

Arnout MA: Molecular basis for leukocyte adhesion deficiency. Biochem Macrophages Relat Types 335, 1993.

Ashman RF, Schaffer FM, Kemp JD, et al: Genetic and immunologic analysis of a family containing five patients with common-variable immune deficiency or selective IgA deficiency. J Clin Immunol 12:406, 1992.

Aukrust P, Muller F, Froland SS: Elevated serum levels of interleukin-4 and interleukin-6 in patients with common variable immunodeficiency (CVI) are associated with chronic immune activation and low numbers of CD4 + lymphocytes. Clin Immunol Immunopathol 70:217, 1994.

Bachman R: Studies on the serum gamma A-globulin level: III the frequency of A-gamma-A-globulinemia. Scand J Clin Lab Invest 17:316, 1965.

Baehner RL, Nathan DG: Quantitative nitroblue tetrazolium test in chronic granulomatous disease. N Engl J Med 287:971, 1968.

Barak Y, Nir E: Chédiak-Higashi syndrome. Am J Pediatr Hematol Oncol 9:42, 1987.

Bastian J, Law S, Vogler L, et al: Prediction of persistent immunodeficiency in the DiGeorge anomaly. J Pediatr 115:391, 1989.

Beall GN, Ashman RF, Miller ME, et al: Hypogammaglobulinemia in mother and son. J Allergy Clin Immunol 65: 471, 1980.

Benichou B, Strominger JL: Class II antigen-negative patients and mutant B cell lines represent at least three, and probably four, distinct genetic defects defined by complementation analysis. Proc Natl Acad Sci USA 88:4285, 1991.

Benkerrou M, Gougeon ML, Griscelli C, et al: Hypogammaglobulinemie G et A avec hypergammaglobulinemie M: a propos de 12 observations. Arch Fr Pediatr 47:345, 1990.

Bensel TRW, Stadlan EM, Krivit W: The development of malignancy in the course of the Aldrich syndrome. J Pediatr 68:761, 1966.

Berendes H, Bridges RA, Good RA: A fatal granulomatous disease of childhood: the clinical study of a new syndrome. Minn Med 40:309, 1957.

Blue ML, Daley JF, Levine H, et al: Class II major histocompatibility complex molecules regulate the development of T4+T8 − inducer phenotype of cultured human thymocytes. Proc Natl Acad Sci USA 82:8178, 1985.

Boder E: Ataxia-telangiectasia: an overview. Kroc Found Ser 19:1, 1985.

Borzy MS, Schulte-Wissermann H, Gilbert E, et al: Thymic morphology in immunodeficiency diseases: results of thymic biopsies. Clin Immunol Immunopathol 12:31, 1979.

Brahmi Z, Lazarus KH, Hodes ME, et al: Immunologic studies of three family members with the immunodeficiency with hyper-IgM syndrome. J Clin Immunol 3:127, 1983.

Brand MM, Marinkovich VA: Primary malignant reticulosis of the brain in Wiskott-Aldrich syndrome. Arch Dis Child 44:536, 1969.

Bruce RM, Blaese RM: Monoclonal gammopathy in the Wiskott-Aldrich syndrome. J Pediatr 85:204, 1974.

Bruton OC: Agammaglobulinemia. Pediatrics 9:722, 1952.

Bryant A, Calver NC, Toubi E, et al: Classification of patients with common variable immunodeficiency by B cell secretion of IgM and IgG in response to anti-IgM and interleukin-2. Clin Immunol Immunopathol 56:239, 1990.

Buckley RH, Dees SC: Correlation of milk precipitins with IgA deficiency. N Engl J Med 281:465, 1969.

Burks AW Jr, Steele RW: Selective IgA deficiency. Ann Allergy 57:3, 1986.

Burn J, Takao A, Wilson D, et al: Conotruncal anomaly face syndrome is associated with a deletion with chromosome 22q11. J Med Genet 30:822, 1993.

Campana D, Farrant J, Inamdar N, et al: Phenotypic features and proliferative activity of B cell progenitors in X-linked agammaglobulinemia. J Immunol 145:1675, 1990.

Cassidy JT, Nordby GL: Human serum immunoglobulin concentrations: prevalence of immunoglobulin deficiencies. J Allergy Clin Immunol 55:35, 1975.

Cassidy JT, Oldham G, Platts-Mills TAE: Functional assessment of a B cell defect in patients with selective IgA deficiency. Clin Exp Immunol 35:296, 1979.

Cederbaum SD, Kaitila I, Rimoin DL, et al: The chondroosseous dysplasia of adenosine deaminase deficiency with severe combined immunodeficiency. J Pediatr 89:737, 1976.

Chaptal J, Royer P, Jean R, et al: Syndrome de Wiskott-Aldrich avec survie prolonge (9 ans): evolution mortelle par thymosarcoma. Arch Fr Pediatr 23:907, 1966.

Conley ME, Beckwith JB, Mancer JFK, et al: The spectrum of the DiGeorge syndrome. J Pediatr 94:883, 1979.

Conley ME, Buckley RH, Hong R, et al: X-linked severe combined immunodeficiency: diagnosis in males with sporadic severe combined immunodeficiency and clarification of clinical findings. J Clin Invest 85:1548, 1990.

Conley ME, Cooper MD: Immature IgA B cells in IgA-deficient patients. N Engl J Med 305:495, 1981.

Cooper MD, Chase HP, Lowman JT, et al: Wiskott-Aldrich syndrome: immunologic deficiency disease involving the afferent limb of immunity. Am J Med 44:499, 1968.

Crabbe PA, Carbonara AO, Heremans JF: The normal human intestinal mucosa as a major source of plasma cells containing gamma-A immunoglobulin. Lab Invest 14:235, 1965.

Crabbe PA, Heremans JF: Lack of gamma A-immunoglobulin in serum of patients with steatorrhea. Gut 7:119, 1966.

Cunningham-Rundles C: Genetic aspects of immunoglobulin A deficiency. Adv Hum Genet 19:234, 1990.

Cunningham-Rundles C, Pudifin DJ, Armstrong D, et al: Selective IgA deficiency and neoplasia. Vox Sang 38:61, 1980.

Cunningham-Rundles C, Siegal FP, Cunningham-Rundles S, et al: Incidence of cancer in 98 patients with common varied immunodeficiency. J Clin Immunol 7:294, 1987.

Cunningham-Rundles S, Cunningham-Rundles C, Ma DI, et al: Impaired proliferative response to B lymphocyte activators in common variable immunodeficiency. J Clin Immunol 1:65, 1981.

Curnutte JT: Chronic granulomatous disease: the solving of a clinical riddle at the molecular level. Clin Immunol Immunopathol 67:S2, 1993a.

Curnutte JT, Boxer LA: Disorders of granulopoiesis and granulocyte function. In: Hematology of Infancy and Childhood, 3rd ed. WB Saunders, Philadelphia, p 797, 1993b.

de la Concha EG, Garcia-Rodriguez MC, Zabay JM, et al: Functional assessment of T and B lymphocytes in patients with selective IgM deficiency. Clin Exp Immunol 49:670, 1982.

de Preval C, Hadam MR, Mach B: Regulation of genes for HLA class II antigens in cell lines from patients with severe combined immunodeficiency. N Engl J Med 318:1295, 1988.

Derry JMJ, Ochs HD, Francke U: Isolation of a novel gene mutated in Wiskott-Aldrich syndrome. Cell 78:635, 1994.

Dimanche-Bortrel MT, Guyot A, de Saint-Basile G, et al: Heterogeneity in the molecular defect leading to the leukocyte adhesion deficiency. Eur J Immunol 18:1575, 1988.

Dubois RS, Roy CC, Fulginiti VA, et al: Disaccharidase deficiency in children with immunologic deficits. J Pediatr 76:377, 1970.

Duncan RA, von Reyn C, Alliegro GM, et al: Idiopathic CD4+ T-lymphocytopenia: four patients with opportunistic infections and no evidence of HIV infection. N Engl J Med 328:393, 1993.

Emanual BS, Budarf ML, Sellinger B, et al: Detection of microdeletions of 22q11.2 with fluorescence in situ hybridization (FISH): diagnosis of DiGeorge syndrome (DGS), velo-cardio-facial syndrome (VCF), CHARGE association and conotruncal cardiac malformations. Am J Hum Genet 51:1992.

Etzioni A, Frydman M, Pollack S, et al: Recurrent severe infections caused by a novel leukocyte adhesion deficiency. N Engl J Med 327:1789, 1992.

Fauci AS:CD4+ T-lymphocytopenia without HIV infection: No lights, no camera, just facts. N Engl J Med 328:429, 1993.

Feigin RD, Vietti TJ, Wyatt RG, et al: Ataxia-telangiectasia with granulocytopenia. J Pediatr 77:431, 1970.

Filipovich AH, Heinitz KJ, Robinson LL, et al: The immunodeficiency cancer registry: a research resource. Am J Pediatr Hematol Oncol 9:183, 1987.

Fiorilli M, Businco L, Pandolfi F, et al: Heterogeneity of immunological abnormalities in ataxia-telangiectasia. J Clin Immunol 3:135, 1983.

Fischer A, Lisowka-Cropierre B, Anderson DC, et al: Leukocyte adhesion deficiency: molecular basis and functional consequences. Immunodefic Rev 1:39, 1988.

Fisher JE, Khan AR, Heitlinger L, et al: Chronic granulomatous disease of childhood with acute ulcerative colitis: a unique association. Pediatr Pathol 7:91, 1987.

Fleisher TA, White RM, Broder S, et al: X-linked hypogammaglobulinemia and isolated growth hormone deficiency. N Engl J Med 302:1429, 1980.

Gallin JI, Buescher ES, Seligmann M, et al: Recent advances in chronic granulomatous disease. Ann Intern Med 99:657, 1983.

Geha RS, Hyslop N, Alami S, et al: Hyperimmunoglobulin M immunodeficiency (dysgammaglobulinemia). J Clin Invest 64:385, 1979.

Gillett HR, Gillett PM, Kingstone K, et al: IgA deficiency and coeliac disease. J Pediatr Gastroenterol Nutr 25:366, 1997.

Goldmuntz E, Driscoll DA, Budarf ML, et al: Microdeletions of chromosomal region 22q11 in patients with congenital conotruncal cardiac defects. J Med Genet 30:807, 1997.

Gray GR, Stamatoyannopoulos G, Naiman GC, et al: Neutrophil dysfunction, chronic granulomatous disease and non-spherocytic haemolytic anemia caused by complete deficiency of glucose-6-phosphate dehydrogenase. Lancet 2:530, 1973.

Griscelli C, Durandy A, Guy-Grand D, et al: A syndrome associating partial albinism and immunodeficiency. Am J Med 65:691, 1978.

Gropp A, Flatz G: Chromosome breakage and blastic transformation of lymphocytes in ataxia-telangiectasia. Humangenetik 5:77, 1967.

Grundbacher FJ: Genetic aspects of selective immunoglobulin A deficiency. J Med Genet 9:344, 1972.

Haas A, Wells J, Chin T, et al: Successful treatment of reticular dysgenesis with haploidentical bone marrow transplantation (BMT). Clin Res 34:127A, 1986.

Haas RJ, Neithammer D, Goldman SF, et al: Congenital immunodeficiency and agranulocytosis (reticular dysgenesis). Acta Paediatr Scand 66:279, 1977.

Hadam MR, Dopfer R, Niethammer D: Congenital agammaglobulinemia associated with lack of expression of HLA-D region antigens. Prog Immunodefic Res Therapy 1:43, 1984.

Haddow JE, Shapiro SR, Gall DG: Congenital sensory neuropathy in siblings. Pediatrics 45:651, 1970.

Hammarstrom L, Carlsson B, Smith CIE, et al: Detection of IgA heavy chain constant region genes in IgA deficient donors: evidence against gene deletions. Clin Exp Immunol 60:661, 1985.

Hammarstrom L, Smith CIE: HLA-A, B, C, and DR antigens in immunogloblin A deficiency. Tissue Antigens 21:75, 1983.

Hanson LA: Selective IgA-deficiency. Primary and Secondary Immunodeficiency Disorders 62. Churchill Livingstone, New York, 1983.

Haraldsson A, van der Burgt CJAM, Weemaes CMR, et al: Antibody deficiency and isolated growth hormone deficiency in a girl with Mulibrey nanism. Eur J Pediatr 152:509, 1993.

Haraldsson A, Weemaes CMR, De Boer AW, et al: Immunological studies in the hyperimmunoglobulin d syndrome. J Clin Immunol 12:424, 1992.

Hayakawa H, Iwata T, Yata J, et al: Primary immunodeficiency syndrome in Japan: I. Overview of a nationwide survey on primary immunodeficiency syndrome. J Clin Immunol 1:31, 1981.

Hermans PE, Huizenga KA, Hoffman HN, et al: Dysgammaglobulinemia associated with nodular lymphoid hyperplasia of the small intestine. Am J Med 40:78, 1966.

Hermaszewski RA, Webster ADB: Primary hypgammaglobulinaemia: a survey of clinical manifestations and complicaitons. Q J Med 86:31, 1993.

Herrmann RP, Chipper L, Bell S: Chromosome studies in healthy blood donors with IgA deficiency. Clin Genet 22:231, 1982.

Higgins EA, Siminovitch KA, Zhuang D, et al: Aberrant O-linked oligosaccharide biosynthesis in lymphocytes and platelets from patients with the Wiskott-Aldrich syndrome. J Biol Chem 266:6280, 1991.

Hirschhorn R: Adenosine deaminase deficiency. Immunodefic Rev 2:175, 1990.

Hirschhorn R: Overview of biochemical abnormalities and molecular genetics of adenosine deaminase deficiency. Pediatr Res 3(suppl): S35, 1993.

Hitzig WH, Biro A, Bosch H, et al: Agammaglobulinamie und Almphozytose mit Schwund des lymphatischen Gewebes. Helv Paediatr Acta 13:551, 1958.

Hitzig WH, Kenny AB: The role of vitamin B12 and its transport globulins in the production of antibodies. Clin Exp Immunol 20:105, 1975.

Ho DD, Cao Y, Zhu T, et al: Idiopathic CD4 + lymphocytopenia-immunodeficiency without evidence of HIV infection. N Engl J Med 328:380, 1993.

Hobbs JR: Disturbances of the immunoglobulins. Sci Basis Med 106, 1966

Hobbs JR: Immune imbalance in dysgammaglobulinemia type IV. Lancet 1:110, 1968

Hobbs JR, Milner RDG, Watt PJ: Gamma-M deficiency predisposing to meningococcal septicaemia. Br Med J 4:583, 1967.

Hollenbaugh D, Wu LH, Ochs HD, et al: The random inactivation of the X chromosome carrying the defective gene responsible for X-linked hyper IgM syndrome (X-HIM) in female carriers of HIGM1. J Clin Invest 94:616, 1994.

Hong R: The biological significance of IgE in chronic respiratory infections. The Secretory Immunologic System 433, US National Institute of Child Health and Human Development, Bethesda, MD, 1971.

Hong R, Ammann AJ: Disorders of the IgA system. Immunologic Disorders in Infants and Children 3rd ed. WB Saunders, Philadelphia, 329, 1989.

Hosking CS, Roberton DM: Epidemiology and treatment of hypogammaglobulinemia. Birth Defects, Original Articles Series 19:223, 1983.

Inoue T, Okubo H, Kudo J, et al: Selective IgA deficiency: analysis of Ig production in vitro. J Clin Immunol 4:235, 1984.

Ipp MM, Gelfand EW: Antibody deficiency and alopecia. J Pediatr 89:728, 1976.

Ishiguro T, Taketa K, Gatti RA: Tissue of origin of elevated alphafetoprotein in ataxia-telangiectasia. Dis Markers 4:293, 1986.

Jaffe JS, Eisenstein E, Sneller MC, et al: T-cell abnormalities in common variable immunodeficiency. Pediatr Res 33(suppl):S24–S28, 1993.

Johnston RB, Newman SL: Chronic granulomatous disease. Pediatr Clin North Am 24:365, 1977.

Kameoka J, Tanaka T, Nojima Y, et al: Direct association of adenosine deaminase with a T cell activation antigen, CD26. Science 261: 466, 1993.

Kaufman HS, Hobbs JR: Immunoglobulin deficiencies in an atopic population. Lancet 2:1061, 1970.

Kersey JH, Shapiro RS, Filipovich AH: Relationship of immunodeficiency to lymphoid malignancy. Pediatr Infect Dis J (suppl)7:S10, 1988.

Kishimoto TK, Hollander N, Roberts TM, et al: Heterogeneous mutations in the B subunit common to the LFA-1, Mac-1, and p150,95 glycoproteins cause leukocyte adhesion deficiency. Cell 50:193, 1987.

Koistinen J: Familial clustering of selective IgA deficiency. Vox Sang 30:181, 1976.

Kragballe K, Borregaard N, Brandrup F, et al: Relation of monocyte and neutrophil oxidative metabolism to skin and oral lesions in carriers of chronic granulomatous disease. Clin Exp Immunol 43: 390, 1981.

Kredich NM, Martin DW Jr: Role of S-adenosylhomocysteine in adenosine-mediated toxicity in cultured mouse T lymphoma cells. Cell 12:931, 1977.

Krieger I, Brough JA: Gamma-A deficiency and hypochromic anemia due to defective iron mobilization. N Engl J Med 269:886, 1967.

Kruisbeek AM, Mond JJ, Fowlkes BJ, et al: Absence of the Lyt-2, L3T4 + lineage of T cells in mice treated neonatally with anti-I-A correlates with absence of intrathymic I-A-bearing antigen-presenting cell function. J Exp Med 161:1029, 1985.

Lakhanpal S, O'Duffy JD, Homburg HA, et al: Evidence for linkage of IgA deficiency with the major histocompatibility complex. Mayo Clinic Proc 63:461, 1988.

Lammer EJ, Opitz JM: The DiGeorge anomaly as a developmental field defect. Am J Med Genet 2(suppl):113, 1986.

Lane P, Traunecker A, Hubele S, et al: Activated human T cells express a ligand for the human B cell-associated antigen CD40 which participates in T cell-dependent activation of B lymphocytes. Eur J Immunol 22:2573, 1992.

Larson RS, Butler MG: Use of fluorescence in situ hybridization (FISH) in the diagnosis of DiGeorge sequence and related diseases. Diag Mol Pathol 4:274, 1995.

Lawlor GR Jr, Amman AJ, Wright WC, et al: The syndrome of cellular immunodeficiency with immunoglobulins. J Pediatr 84:183, 1974.

Lawton AR, Royal SA, Self KS, et al: IgA determinants on B lymphocytes in patients with deficiency of circulating IgA. J Lab Clin Med 80:26, 1972.

Lazarus GM, Neu HC: Agents responsible for infection in chronic granulomatous disease of childhood. J Pediatr 86:415, 1975.

Lederman HM, Winkelstein JA: X-linked agammaglobulinemia: an analysis of 96 patients. Medicine 64:145, 1985.

Lee BW, Yap HK: Polyarthritis resembling juvenile rheumatoid arthritis in a girl with chronic granulomatous disease. Arthritis Rheum 37:773, 1994.

Lehrer RI, Cline MJ: Leukocyte myeloperoxidase deficiency and disseminated candidiasis: the role of myeloperoxidase in resistance to *Candida* infection. J Clin Invest 48:1478, 1969.

Lewkonia RM, Lin CC, Haslam RHA: Selective IgA deficiency with 18q+ and 18q− karyotypic anomalies. J Med Genet 17:453, 1980.

Lisowska-Grospierre B, Charron DJ, de Preval C, et al: A defect in the regulation of major histocompatibility complex class II gene expression in human HLA-DR negative lymphocytes from patients with combined immunodeficiency syndrome. J Clin Invest 76:381, 1985.

Makrynikola V, Bradstock KF: Adhesion of precursor-B acute lymphoblastic leukaemia cells to bone marrow stromal proteins. Leukemia 7:86, 1993.

Manzi S, Urbach AH, McCune AB, et al: Systemic lupus erythematosus in a boy with chronic granulomatous disease: case report and review of the literature. Arthritis Rheum 34:101, 1991.

Markert ML: Purine nucleoside phosphorylase deficiency. Immunodefic Rev 3:45, 1991.

McKinney RE, Katz SL, Wilfert CM: Chronic enteroviral meningoencephalitis in agammaglobulinemic patients. Rev Infect Dis 9:334, 1987.

Medical Research Council Working Party: Hypogammaglobulinemia in the United Kingdom. Lancet 1:163, 1969.

Mentzer SJ, Remold-O'Donnell E, Crimmins MAV, et al: Sialophorin, a surface sialoglycoprotein defective in the Wiskott-Aldrich syndrome, is involved in human T-lymphocyte proliferation. J Exp Med 165:1383, 1987.

Milili M, Le Deist F, de Saint-Basile G, et al: Bone marrow cells in X-linked agammaglobulinemia express pre-B-specific genes (lambda-like and V pre-B) and present immunoglobulin V-D-J gene usage strongly biased to a fetal-like repertoire. J Clin Invest 91:1616, 1993.

Miller ME, Mellman WJ, Cohen MM, et al: Depressed immunoglobulin G in newborn infants with Down's syndrome. J Pediatr 75:996, 1969.

Mills EL, Rhool KS, Quie PG: X-linked inheritance in females with chronic granulomatous disease. J Clin Invest 66:332, 1980.

Mohler DN, Majerus PW, Minnuch V, et al: Glutathione synthetase deficiency as a cause of hereditary hemolytic disease. N Engl J Med 283:1253, 1970.

Molina IJ, Kenney DM, Rosen FS, et al: T cell lines characterize events in the pathogenesis of the Wiskott-Aldrich syndrome. J Exp Med 176:867, 1992.

Molina IJ, Sancho J, Terhorst C, et al: T cells of patients with the Wiskott-Aldrich syndrome have a restricted defect in proliferative responses. J Immunol 151:4383, 1993.

Murphy S, Oski FA, Haimar JL, et al: Platelet size and kinetics in hereditary and acquired thrombocytopenia. N Engl J Med 286:499, 1972.

Nezelof C: Classification of immunodeficiency diseases. Arch Fr Pediatr 25:781, 1968.

Noelle RJ, Meenakshi R, Shepherd DM, et al: 39-kDa protein on activated helper T cells binds CD40 and transduces the signal for cognate activation of B cells. Proc Natl Acad Sci USA 89:6550, 1992.

Notarangelo LD, Duse M, Ugazio AG: Immunodeficiency with hyper-IgM (HIM). Immunodefic Rev 3:101, 1992.

Oen K, Petty RE, Schroeder ML: Immunoglobulin A deficiency in genetic studies. Tissue Antigens 19:174, 1982.

Ohzeki T, Hanaki K, Motozumi H, et al: Immunodeficiency with increased immunoglobulin M associated with growth hormone insufficiency. Acta Paediatr 82:620, 1993

Oppenheim JJ, Blaese RM, Horton JE, et al: Production of macrophage migration inhibition factor and lymphotoxin by leukocytes from normal and Wiskott-Aldrich syndrome patients. Cell Immunol 8:63, 1973.

Ownby DR, Pizzo S, Blackmon L, et al: Severe combined immunodeficiency with leukopenia (reticular dysgenesis) in siblings: immunologic and histopathologic findings. J Pediatr 89:382, 1976.

Paganelli R, Capobianchi MR, Ensoli B, et al: Evidence that defective gamma interferon production in patients with primary immunodeficiencies is due to intrinsic incompetence of lymphocytes. Clin Exp Immunol 72:124, 1988.

Pappas BE: Primary immunodeficiency disorders in infancy. Neonatal Netw 18:13, 1999.

Park JK, Rosenstein YJ, Remold-O'Donnell E, et al: Enhancement of T-cell activation by the CD43 molecule whose expression is defective in Wiskott-Aldrich syndrome. Nature 350:706, 1991.

Parry MF, Root RK, Metcalf JA, et al: Myeloperoxidase deficiency. Ann Intern Med 95:293, 1981.

Pascual-Salcedo D, De la Concha EG, Garcia-Rodriguez MC, et al: Cellular basis of hyper IgM immunodeficiency. J Clin Lab Immunol 10:29, 1983.

Pastorelli G, Roncarolo MG, Touraine JL, et al: Peripheral blood lymphocytes of patients with common variable immunodeficiency (CVI) produce reduced levels of interleukin-4, interleukin-2 and interferon-gamma, but proliferate normally upon activation by mitogens. Clin Exp Immunol 78:334, 1989.

Payne NR, Hays NT, Regelmann WE, et al: Growth in patients with chronic granulomatous disease. J Pediatr 102:397, 1983.

Perey DYE, Frommel D, Hong R, et al: The mammalian homologue of the avian bursa of Fabricius. Lab Invest 22:212, 1970.

Peterson RDA, Cooper MD, Good RA: Lymphoid tissue abnormalities associated with ataxia-telangiectasia. Am J Med 41:342, 1966.

Petty RE, Sherry DD, Johannson J: Anti-IgA antibodies in pregnancy. N Engl J Med 313:1620, 1985.

Plebani A, Monafo V, Ugazio AG, et al: Comparison of the frequency of atopic disease in children with severe and partial IgA deficiency. Int Arch Allergy Appl Immunol 82:485, 1987.

Ratech H, Alba Greco M, Gallo G, et al: Pathologic findings in adenosine deaminase-deficient severe combined immunodeficiency. I. Kidney, adrenal and chondroosseous tissue alterations. Am J Pathol 120:157, 1985.

Ratech H, Hirschhorn R, Alba Greco M: Pathologic findings in adenosine deaminase deficient-severe combined immunodeficiency. II. Thymus, spleen, lymph node, and gastrointestinal tract lymphoid tissue alterations. Am J Pathol 135:1145, 1989.

Rijkers GT, Roord JJ, Koning F, et al: Phenotypical and functional analysis of B lymphocytes of two siblings with combined immunodeficiency and defective expression of major histocompatibility complex (MHC) class II antigens on mononuclear cells. J Clin Immunol 7:98, 1987.

Rockey JH, Hanson LA, Heremans JF, et al: Beta-2A-agammaglobulinemia in two healthy men. J Lab Clin Med 63:205, 1964.

Rodriguez CR, Nueda A, Grospierre B, et al: Characterization of two new CD18 alleles causing severe leukocyte adhesion deficiency. Eur J Immunol 23:2792, 1993.

Roifman CM, Gelfand EW: Heterogeneity of the immunological deficiency in ataxia-telangiectasia: absence of a clinical-pathological correlation. Kroc Found Ser 19:273, 1985.

Roos D: The genetic basis of chronic granulomatous disease. Immunol Rev 138:121, 1994.

Rosen FS, Cooper MD, Wedgwood RJP: The primary immunodeficiencies. N Engl J Med 311:300, 1984.

Rosen FS, Janeway CA: The gamma globulins: III. The antibody deficiency syndromes. N Engl J Med 275:769, 1966.

Rosen FS, Wedgwood RJP, Eibl M, et al: Primary immunodeficiency diseases: report of a WHO Scientific Group. Clin Exp Immunol 1 (suppl 99):1, 1995.

Ruff ME, Pincus LG, Sampson HA: Phenytoin-induced IgA depression. Am J Dis Child 141:858, 1987.

Ryser O, Morell A, Hitzig WH: Primary immunodeficiencies in Switzerland: first report of the national registry in adults and children. J Clin Immunol 8:479, 1988.

Sandman R, Amman AJ, Grose C, et al: Cellular immunodeficiency associated with nucleoside phosphorylase deficiency. Clin Immunol Immunopathol 8:247, 1977.

Sanford JP, Favour CB, Tribeman MS: Absence of serum gamma globulins in an adult. N Engl J Med 250:1027, 1954.

Santisteban I, Arrendondo-Vega FX, Kelly S, et al: Novel splicing, missense, and deletion mutations in seven adenosine deaminase-deficient patients with late/delayed onset of combined immunodeficiency disease. J Clin Invest 92:2291, 1993.

Savitsky K, Bar-Shira A, Gilad S, et al: A single ataxia telangiectasia gene with a product similar to PI-3 kinase. Science 268:1749, 1995.

Scambler PJ, Carey AH, Wyse RKH, et al: Microdeletions within 22q11 associated with sporadic and familial and DiGeorge syndrome. Genomics 10:201, 1991.

Schiff RI, Buckley RH, Gilbertsen RB, et al: Membrane receptors and in vitro responsiveness of lymphocytes in human immunodeficiency. J Immunol 112:376, 1974.

Schur PH, Borel H, Gelfand EW, et al: Selective gamma-G globulin deficiencies in patients with recurrent pyogenic infections. N Engl J Med 283:631, 1970.

Schuurman HJ, van de Wijngaert FP, Huber J, et al: The thymus in "bare lymphocyte" syndrome: significance of expression of major histocompatibility complex antigens on thymic epithelial cells in intrathymic T-cell maturation. Hum Immunol 13:69, 1985.

Sharma OP, James DG: Hypogammaglobulinemia, depression of delayed type hypersensivity and granuloma formation. Am Rev Resp Dis 104:228, 1971.

Siccardi A, Bianchi E, Calligari A, et al: A new familial defect in neutrophil bactericidal activity. Helv Paediatr Acta 33:401, 1978.

Smith DK, Neal JJ, Holmber SD, et al: Unexplained opportunistic infections and CD4 + T-lymphopenia with HIV infection: an investigation of cases in the United States. N Engl J Med 328:373, 1993.

Sneller MC, Strober W, Eisenstein E, et al: New insights into common variable immunodeficiency. Ann Intern Med 118:720, 1993.

Sobel E, Lange E, Jaspers NG, et al: Ataxia-telangiectasia: linkage evidence for genetic heterogeneity. Am J Hum Genet 50:1343, 1992.

Sorrell TC, Forbes IJ, Burness FR, et al: Depression of immunological function in patients treated with phenytoin sodium (sodium diphenylhydantoin). Lancet 2:1233, 1971.

Spira TJ, Jones BM, Nicholson JKA et al: Idiopathic CD4+ T-lymphocytopenia: an analysis of five patients with unexplained opportunistic infections. N Engl J Med 328:386, 1993.

Stiehm ER, Chin TW, Haas A, et al: Infectious complications of the primary immunodeficiencies. Clin Immunol Immunopathol 40:69, 1986.

Stiehm ER, Fundenberg HH: Clinical and immunologic features of dysgammaglobulinemia type I: a report of a case diagnosed in the first year of life. Am J Med 40:805, 1966.

Strober W, Sneller MC: IgA Deficiency Ann Allergy 66:363, 1991.

Subramaniam S, Tuman D, Rausen AR, et al: "Ascites" and inguinal hernias: unusual presentation for chronic granulomatous disease of childhood. Mt Sinai J Med 41:566, 1974.

Swift A, Morrell D, Massey RB, et al: Incidence of cancer in 161 families affected by ataxia-telangiectasia. N Eng J Med 325:1831, 1991.

Swift M: Genetics and epidemiology of ataxia-telangiectasia. Ataxia-telangiectasia: genetics, neuropathology, and immunology of a degenerative disease of childhood. Kroc Found Ser 19:133, 1984.

Syllaba L, Henner, K: Contribution a l'independance de l'athetose double idiopathique et congenitale: atteinte familiale, syndrome dystrophique, signe du reseau vasculaire conjonctival, integrite psychique. Rev Neurol 1:541, 1926.

Thieffry S, Arthuis M, Aicardi J, et al: L'ataxie-telangiectasie (7 observations personnelles). Rev Neurol 105:390, 1961.

Thorpe ES, Handley HE: Chronic tetany and chronic mycelial stomatitis in a child aged four and one-half years. Am J Dis Child 38:328, 1929.

Todd RF, Fryer DR: The CD11/CD18 leukocyte glycoprotein deficiency. Hematol Oncol Clin North Am 2:13, 1988.

Touraine J-L, Marseglia GLL, Betuel H: Thirty international cases of bare lymphocyte syndrome: biological significance of HLA antigens. Exp Hematol 13(suppl):86, 1985.

Tsukada S, Saffran DC, Rawlings DJ, et al: Deficient expression of a B cell cytoplasmic tyrosine kinase in human X-linked agammaglobulinemia. Cell 72:279, 1993.

Vetrie D, Vorechovsky I, Sideras P, et al: The gene involved in X-linked agammaglobulinaemia is a member of the src family of protein-tyrosine kinases. Nature 361:226, 1993.

Villa A, Notarangelo LD, Di Santo JP, et al: Organization of the human CD40L gene: implications for molecular defects in X chromosome-linked hyper-IgM syndrome and prenatal diagnosis. Proc Natl Acad Sci USA 91:2110, 1994.

Volanakis JE, Zhu Z-B, Schaffer FM, et al: Major histocompatibility complex class III genes and susceptibility to immunoglobulin A deficiency and common variable immunodeficiency. J Clin Invest 89:1914, 1992.

Vorechovsky I, Zhou JN, Vetrie D, et al: Molecular diagnosis of X-linked agammaglobulinemia [letter]. Lancet 341:1153, 1993.

Waldmann TA, McIntire KR: Serum alpha-fetoprotein levels in patients with ataxia-telangiectasia. Lancet 2:1112, 1972.

Weening RS, Adriaansz LH, Weemaes CMR, et al: Clinical differences in chronic granulomatous disease in patients with cytochrome b-negative or cytochrome b-positive neutrophils. J Pediatr 107:102, 1985.

West CD, Hong R, Holland NH: Immunoglobulin levels from the newborn period to adulthood and in immunoglobulin deficiency states. J Clin Invest 41:2054, 1962.

Wilson DI, Burn J, Scambler P, et al: DiGeorge syndrome: part of CATCH 22. J Med Genet 30:852, 1993.

Wilton AN, Cobain TJ, Dawkins RL: Family studies of IgA deficiency. Immunogenetics 21:333, 1985.

Wiskott A: Familiarer, angeborener Morbus Werihofii? Aschr Kinderheilkd 68:212, 1937.

Wolff JA: Wiskott-Aldrich syndrome: clinical, immunologic and pathologic observations. J Pediatr 70:221, 1967.

Wolff JA, Bertucio M: A sex-linked genetic syndrome in a Negro family manifested by thrombocytopenia, eczema, blood diarrhea, recurrent infection, anemia and epistaxis. Am J Dis Child 93:74, 1957.

Yonemura S, Nagafuchi A, Sato N, et al: Concentration of an integral membrane protein, CD43 (leukosialin, sialophorin), in the cleavage furrow through the interaction of its cytoplasmic domain with actin-based cytoskeletons. J Cell Biol 120:437, 1993.

Zabacchi G, Soranzo MR, Menegazzi R, et al: Eosinophil peroxidase deficiency: morphological and immunocyto-chemical studies of the eosinophil-specific granules. Blood 80:2903, 1992.

Zhu Q, Zhang M, Rawlings DR, et al: Deletion within the Src homology domain 3 of Bruton's tyrosine kinase resulting in X-linked agammaglobulinemia (XLA). J Exp Med 180:461, 1994a.

Zhu Q, Zhang M, Winkelstein J, et al: Unique mutations of Bruton's tyrosine kinase in fourteen unrelated X-linked agammaglobulinemia families. Hum Mol Genet 3:1899, 1994b.

Zinneman HH, Kaplan AP: The association of giardiasis with reduced intestinal secretory immunoglobulin A. Dig Dis Sci 125:207, 1975.

Richard S. Larson
Robert D. Collins
Steven H. Swerdlow

X-Linked Lymphoproliferative Disorder

DEFINITION

X-linked lymphoproliferative disorder (XLPD) is a heritable disease in which males have life-threatening Epstein-Barr virus (EBV) infections.

CLINICAL FEATURES

The clinical features of XLPD are surprisingly diverse. Although the overall pattern of presentation and outcome seem somewhat defined, it is much simpler to make the diagnosis when one is treating a patient from a family known to be affected. This is a disease of males, as indicated by its name. Approximately 75% of patients present with an acute, lethal illness resembling infectious mononucleosis. The mean age of onset is 2.7 years, a curiosity in itself, since EBV mononucleosis usually produces severe illness in teenagers and young adults. Initial illnesses have been recorded in 20-year-old patients with XLPD. Fever, superficial adenopathy, pharyngeal edema, rash, and aseptic meningitis are accompanied by peripheral lymphocytosis (activated lymphocytes or virocytes are detected) and serologic evidence of acute EBV infection. Patients may experience hepatic failure despite antiviral

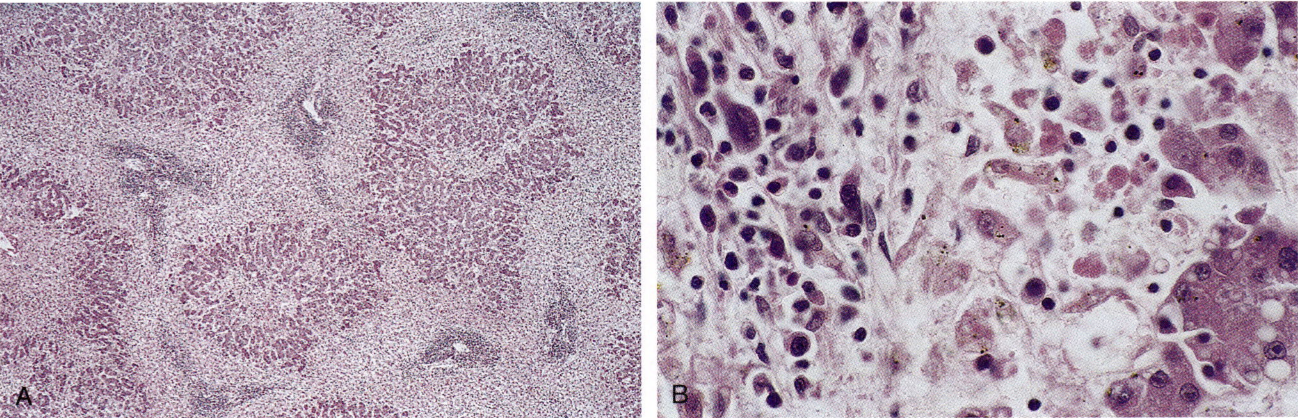

Figure 3–6

Liver, XLPD. *A*. At low magnification the extensive portal infiltrate and hepatic necrosis are evident. *B*. At high magnification necrotic hepatocytes are seen in the peripheral portion of the lobule, where the most extensive hepatic necrosis was found. The adjacent polymorphous portal infiltrate is apparent.

medication and aggressive support or may die from coagulopathy or secondary bacterial infection.

The remaining 25% of patients show considerable variation in presentation. Some develop malignant lymphomas without a clear history of an acute mononucleosis syndrome (Sullivan, 1988). These lymphomas are high grade and are often in the ileum. Others develop common variable immunodeficiency syndromes after their acute illness, with recurrent infections and hypogammaglobulinemia as prominent features. Thirty-five to 50% of the patients with the hypogammaglobulinemic presentation develop aggressive lymphomas.

The clinical course and autopsy findings of three brothers with XLPD are described next. The illnesses are of the type seen in approximately 75% of patients with XLPD. The first brother died in the late 1970; the mother remarried, and the two sons from the second marriage died in the early 1980s.

Patient AA was admitted to the hospital at age 2.5 years, 2 weeks after the onset of rash and fever attributed to a viral upper respiratory infection. The illness progressed despite ampicillin and was complicated by marked facial and scalp swelling, possibly due to staphylococcal cellulitis. The hospital course was marked by hepatic failure, bleeding diathesis, cardiopulmonary arrest during a marrow procedure, and fungal and bacterial pulmonary superinfections. Death was 3 weeks after the onset of illness. Monospot test results were repeatedly negative. The IgM level was 732 mg/dl, the IgA level 230 mg/dl, and the IgG level 440 mg/dl. Peripheral blood films showed granulocytopenia, lymphocytosis, and numerous activated lymphocytes.

Autopsy findings did not reveal the cause of the marked facial swelling. The superior vena cava was patent. Massive *Aspergillus* and *Pseudomonas* superinfection was demonstrated in the lungs. The liver, in particular, showed immunoblastic and plasmacytic proliferation in the portal areas, with extensive necrosis (Fig. 3–6). The splenic white pulp was extensively necrotic, with surrounding immunoblastic and plasmacytic proliferation (Fig. 3–7). All lymphatic tissue showed reactive changes, with immunoblasts and plasma cells (Fig. 3–8). The marrow was moderately hypocellular (Fig. 3–9). The thymus was not identified grossly or on several sections through the anterior mediastinum.

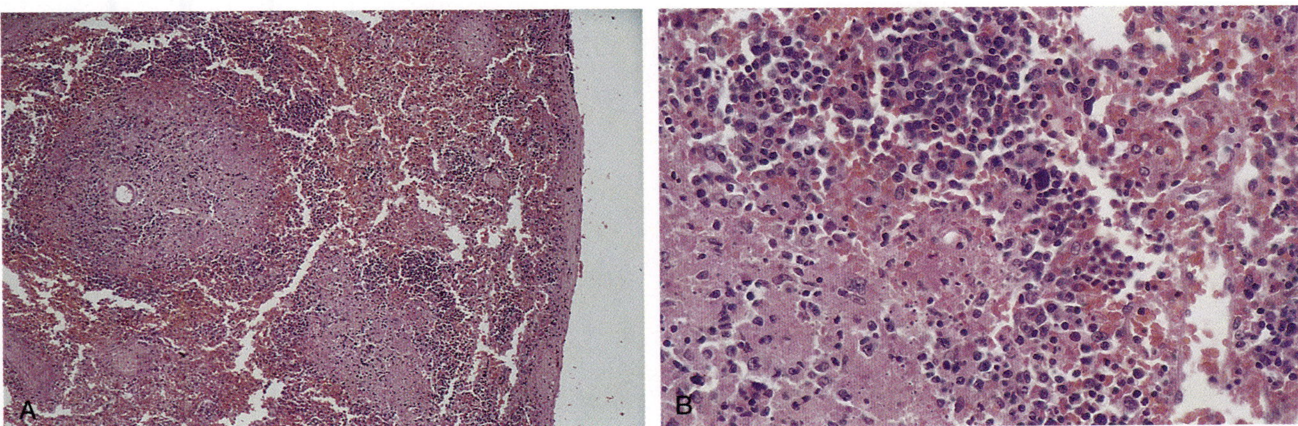

Figure 3–7

Spleen, XLPD. *A*. There is widespread necrosis of the white pulp, with a surrounding immunoblastic proliferation. *B*. At high magnification the immunoblastic proliferation, small lymphocytes, and plasma cells are detected.

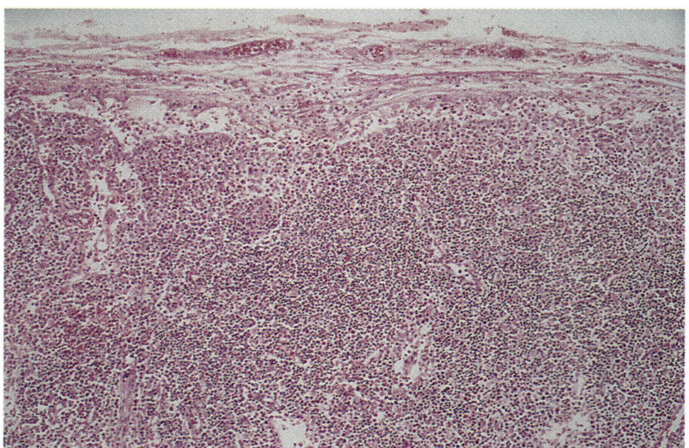

Figure 3–8

Lymph node, XLPD. There is significant architectural distortion, with loss of follicular centers as well as a diffuse proliferation of lymphocytes, plasma cells, and macrophages.

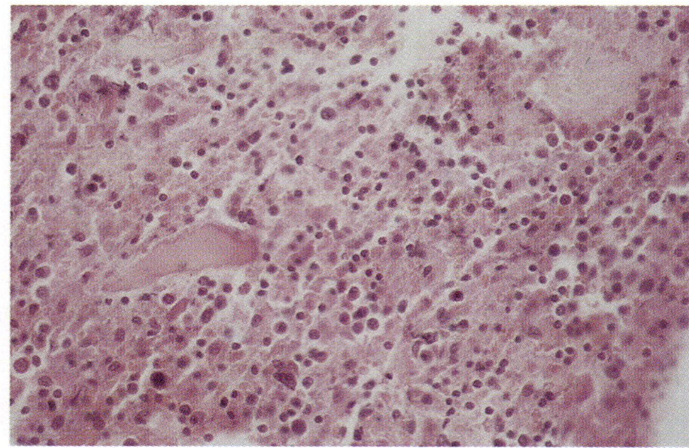

Figure 3–9

Marrow, XLPD. High magnification shows marrow depletion with scattered megakaryocytes and a few immature erythrocytic and myelocytic precursors. Figures 3–6 through 3–9 are from patient AA.

Patient BB was 1 year old at the time of death. He had the usual childhood infections, including oral thrush and pneumonia at 2 months of age. Three weeks before hospital admission, he developed an upper respiratory infection with cough and coryza. Right cervical adenopathy and fever to 102–103°F prompted treatment with amoxicillin, complicated by a maculopapular rash and blistering. On admission to the hospital, the liver was enlarged 2 cm below the right costal margin, and there was a diffuse maculopapular rash. The white blood cell count ranged from 10,000 to 25,000/mm^3, with 85% activated lymphocytes. Monospot test results were repeatedly negative. Hepatic failure, thrombocytopenia and hemorrhagic diathesis led to death on the eleventh hospital day.

Autopsy finding showed hepatomegaly, portal immunoblastic and plasmacytic infiltrates, and hepatocyte necrosis (Fig. 3–10). Spleen sections showed focal necrosis, with slight immunoblastic proliferation (Fig. 3–11). Lymph nodes were hypercellular, but follicular centers were not seen (Fig. 3–12*A*). Numerous immunoblasts and plasma cells were noted (Fig. 3–12*B*). The marrow was hypocellular (Fig. 3–13), and the thymus was atrophic (Fig. 3–14).

Patient CC was 2 years and 9 months old at the time of death. A fever of 103°F without nausea, vomiting, cough, or rhinorrhea precipitated admission to the hospital. He had an erythematous maculopapular rash over the neck and extremities as well as shotty cervical and inguinal adenopathy. There was moderate hepatosplenomegaly. The white blood cell count was 14,300/mm^3, with 37% activated lymphocytes. A Monospot test result was positive. He had a progressively adverse course, developing liver failure, thrombocytopenia, and respiratory failure, with death after 3 weeks of illness.

Autopsy findings showed that the liver was enlarged, weighing 850 g. There was moderate portal immunoblastic and plasmacytic infiltrate (Fig. 3–15). The spleen in this case showed evidence of remote necrosis of follicular centers (Fig. 3–16*A*) and overall a depleted white pulp (Fig. 3–16*B*). Lymph nodes revealed an absence of germinal centers (Fig. 3–17*A*) and erythrophagocytosis by sinus histiocytes (Fig. 3–17*B*). The marrow was hypocellular, and the thymus was depleted.

HISTOPATHOLOGIC FEATURES

Fatal infectious mononucleosis is associated with widely disseminated, destructive lymphocytic proliferations in lymph nodes and extranodal sites (Grierson & Purtilo, 1987 Purtilo &

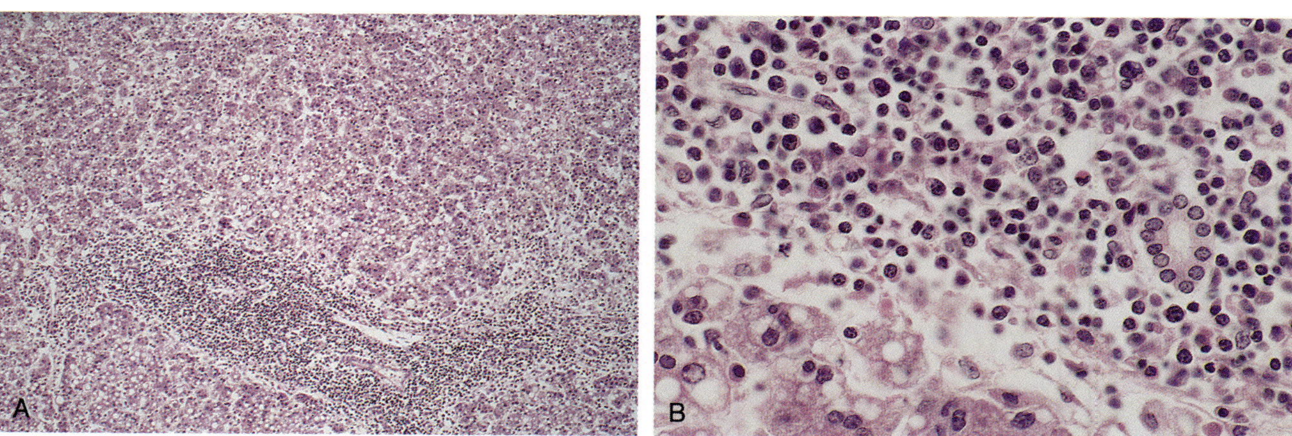

Figure 3–10

Liver, XLPD. *A*. In this case there is less hepatic necrosis, and the portal infiltrate is not as striking as in the case depicted in Figure 3–6. *B*. High magnification shows the polymorphous nature of the periportal infiltrate and the absence of significant hepatocyte necrosis. There is extensive steatosis.

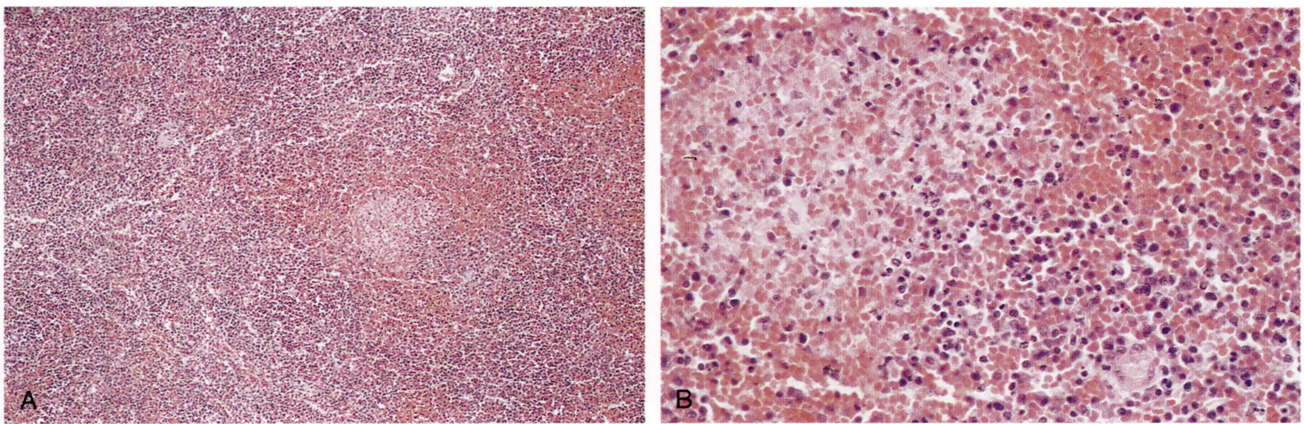

Figure 3–11

Spleen, XLPD. *A*. In this child the splenic white pulp shows alteration of architecture due to hemorrhage and focal necrosis. *B*. The immunoblastic proliferation is less apparent than in the previous case.

Grierson, 1991;). Lymph nodes demonstrate architectural preservation, with a polyclonal and polymorphous immunoblastic proliferation and necrosis (Grierson & Purtilo, 1987; Harrington et al, 1987). Later lesions have abundant plasmacytoid forms. Patients surviving more than 4 weeks show lymphocytic depletion (Grierson & Purtilo, 1987). Depleted lymph nodes contain many immunoblasts, plasma cells, and histiocytes (with prominent erythrophagocytosis) as well as single-cell and focal confluent necrosis and edema (Harrington et al, 1987). Long-term survivors may have large calcified regions in lymph nodes. Ancillary studies demonstrate EBV-infected cells mixed with T cells and natural killer cells (Grierson & Purtilo, 1987). EBV nuclear antigen is often demonstrable (Harrington et al, 1987).

At extranodal sites, the destructive polymorphous infiltrates are typically perivascular, with surrounding edematous parenchyma having foci of necrosis (Harrington et al, 1987). Fulminant hepatitis, a frequent cause of death in infectious mononucleosis, is associated with a marked periportal EBV-positive B cell infiltrate surrounded by T cells that mostly have a "suppressor/lytic" phenotype (Grierson & Purtilo, 1987). Small numbers of inflammatory cells are seen near necrotic hepatocytes. About two thirds of cases show periportal necrosis. Massive necrosis is described in a variable proportion of patients. Splenic lesions parallel those in nodes. There are immunoblastic hyperplasia and necrosis, followed by plasmacytoid proliferation and lymphocytic depletion in those surviving at least 4 weeks. The thymus, hyperplastic initially, later shows lymphocytic depletion. Necrosis may be present.

Another pathologic finding, reported in about 90% of fatal infectious mononucleosis cases, is evidence of a hemophagocytic syndrome (Purtilo & Grierson, 1991). Marrows initially show myelocytic hyperplasia for 1 to 2 weeks, followed by lymphocytic infiltrate, macrophage activation with hemophagocytosis, and destruction of hematopoietic elements (Grierson & Purtilo, 1987). Variable amounts of marrow necrosis and hemorrhage are also seen.

About 25% of patients with XLPD develop extranodal lymphoma, usually a localized mass lesion in the ileocecal region (Harrington et al, 1987). Regional lymph nodes may also be involved. About one half of the lymphomas are of small transformed (noncleaved) follicular center cell type, almost one third of either diffuse large transformed (noncleaved) or immunoblastic type, and the remainder "small cleaved," "mixed," or unclassifiable type (Harrington et al, 1987). The lymphomas are usually EBV associated (Grierson & Purtilo, 1987).

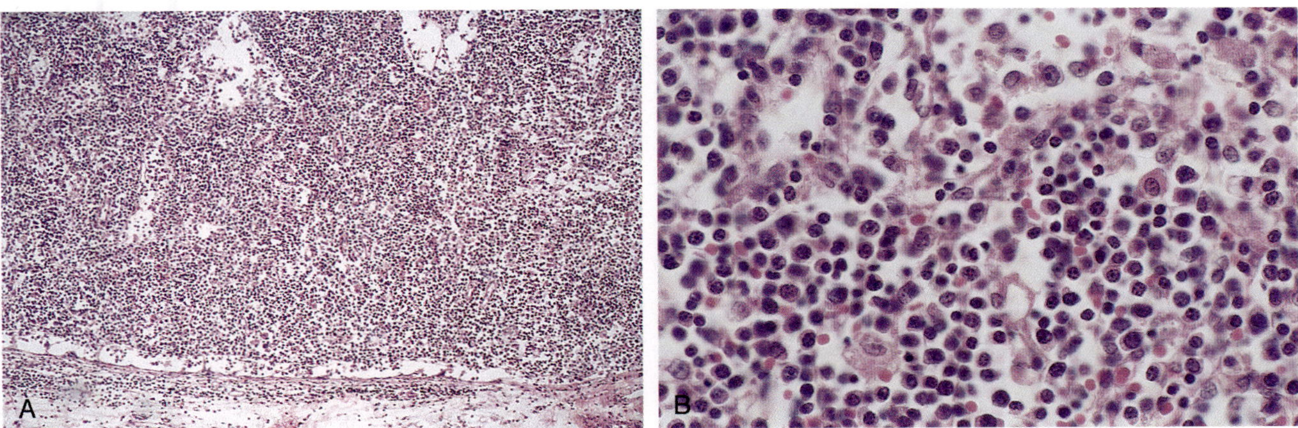

Figure 3–12

Lymph node, XLPD. *A*. Follicular centers are absent in this case, as in Figure 3–8. *B*. The polymorphous proliferation of lymphocytes, immunoblasts, plasma cells, and histiocytes is seen at high magnification.

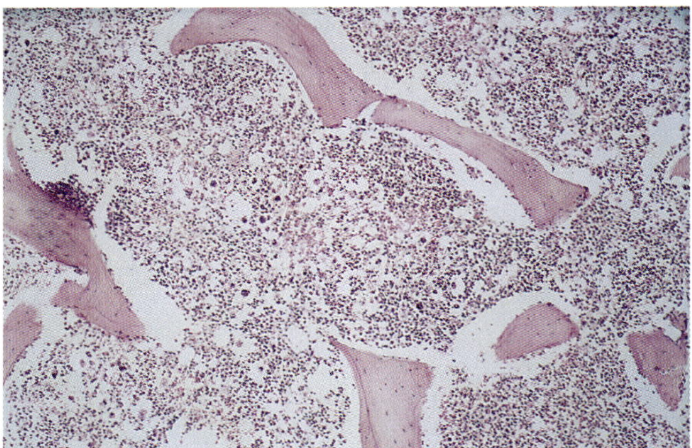

Figure 3–13

Marrow, XLPD. The marrow fills the medullary space but overall is less cellular than normal.

Infrequent histopathologic findings include marrow aplasia or hypoplasia, red blood cell aplasia, and necrotizing vasculitis in nodes.

LABORATORY FINDINGS

Patients with fatal infectious mononucleosis typically present with atypical lymphocytosis usually demonstrating predominance of plasmacytoid lymphocytes (Grierson & Purtilo, 1987; Purtilo et al, 1982; Purtilo et al, 1975). About two thirds have positive heterophile or Monospot test results. Polyclonal hypergammaglobulinemia and elevated transaminase levels are also described. Pancytopenic patients most typically have a virus-associated hemophagocytic syndrome. Patients presenting with lymphoma are often anemic but have normal white blood cell counts and usually no thrombocytopenia (Harrington et al, 1987). Mild lymphocytosis without atypical features was described in 1 of 14 patients.

Those initially surviving EBV infection typically show low titers to EBV-specific antigens (Purtilo et al, 1982). In particular, many patients with XLPD have a deficient anti–EBV nuclear antigen response (<1:10). Such a response may be delayed up to 3 years in normal males (Purtilo et al, 1982; Purtilo & Grierson, 1991). Some patients remain completely seronegative for EBV (Harrington et al, 1987). Many female carriers also have abnormal antibody responses to EBV, including markedly elevated anti-VCA titers (Grierson & Purtilo, 1987).

Patients and female carriers may be identified with 99% accuracy using restriction fragment length polymorphism to the *DXS42* region on the X chromosome (Purtilo et al, 1989; Purtilo & Grierson, 1991). Thirty-one percent of patients have hypogammaglobulinemia. About one third are hypogammaglobulinemic prior to the EBV infection (Purtilo & Grierson, 1991). A small proportion of female carriers have low IgG or IgM levels (Grierson & Purtilo, 1987). In one series, almost all affected males had decreased IgG levels and/or decreased levels of IgG1, IgG2, and/or IgG3 prior to documentable EBV infection (Grierson et al, 1991). Elevated IgM levels were also often found with elevated IgA levels in some. IgA deficiency is uncommon. Patients with IgG subclass deficiency may have a defect in the ability to switch from IgM to IgG. Failure to switch from IgM to IgG antibody production on secondary challenge with the bacteriophage X174 may identify boys with XLPD prior to EBV infection (Purtilo et al, 1989). This test, combined with linkage analysis, has the highest yield in identifying affected males. Six percent of patients have elevated IgM levels not directly associated with infectious mononucleosis (Purtilo & Grierson, 1991). About 4% of female carriers have elevated IgM levels (Grierson & Purtilo, 1987).

Survivors with XLPD demonstrate various B and T cell defects, which are described in part earlier and include low CD4:CD8 ratios and defective natural killer function. The latter may be seen only after EBV infection (Purtilo et al, 1982).

PATHOGENESIS

The gene defect that leads to XLPD has been mapped to Xq24-25 (Skare et al, 1993; Schuster et al, 1994; Lanyi et al, 1997), and it is likely that the protein structure and the function of the deleted gene will soon be known. Most males with XLPD are healthy until they become infected with EBV. Previous studies have shown that the immune system is essentially normal before EBV infection, but immunologic abnormalities develop during the course of and in response to viral infection (Sullivan et al, 1983). Thus, XLPD patients may die from infectious mononucleosis or may acquire hypogamma-

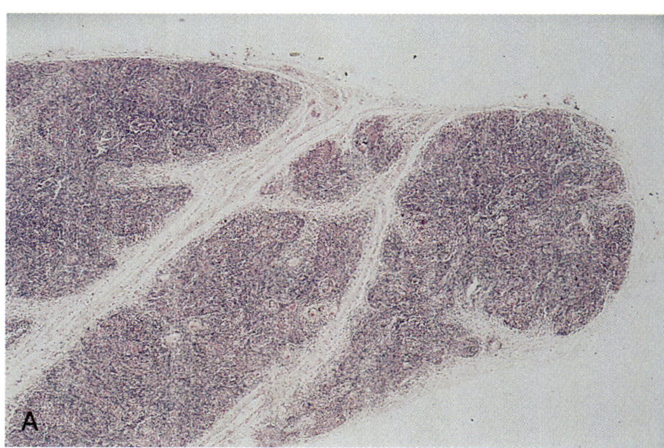

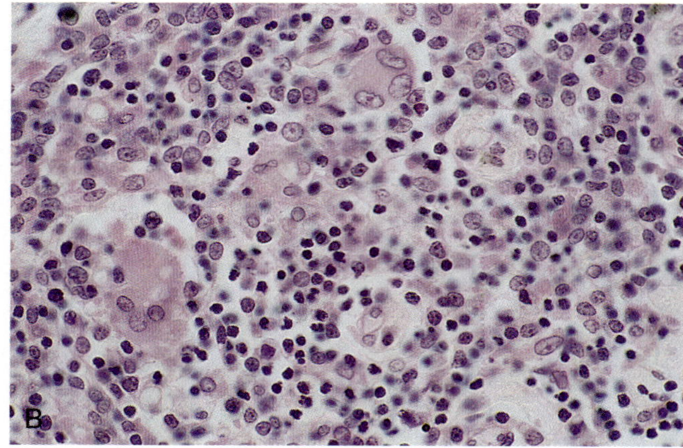

Figure 3–14

Thymus, XLPD. *A*. The thymus is depleted, and Hassall corpuscles are poorly formed. *B*. Rare giant cells are present in the depleted gland. Figures 3–10 through 3–14 are from patient BB.

globulinemia and/or virus-associated hemophagocytic syndrome following EBV infection. An extensive and particularly informative study of two males characterized their immune systems before either had acquired EBV infection (Sullivan et al, 1983). Comprehensive analysis of the immune response of these two patients showed normal B and T cell capability. Moreover, appropriate antibody and cytotoxic T cell responses to EBV occurred at the time of infection, leading to the proposal that the generation of an uncontrolled, proliferative immune response results in the adverse clinical manifestations of XLPD (Grimm et al, 1982; Seeley and Golub, 1978; Sullivan et al, 1983).

Several observations have suggested that the genetic defect in XLPD leads to deficient T cell function (Purtilo, 1991). Clinical findings (particularly aplastic anemia and hepatocytolysis) reflect abnormalities in cellular immunity that are usually mediated by T cells. Furthermore, analysis of T cell subset distribution in affected males usually shows a mild decrease in CD4 cells and a decrease in vitro synthesis of immunoglobulins. Peripheral blood lymphocytes fail to induce graft-versus-host disease in immunodeficient mice.

The ability to clear a viral infection depends on the proper balance between two types of T cell response: Th1 and Th2. Th1 responses are characterized by production of interleukin-2 (IL-2) and γ-interferon and are responsible for cell-mediated immune responses. Th2 responses are characterized by secretion of IL-4 and IL-10, which are required in humoral

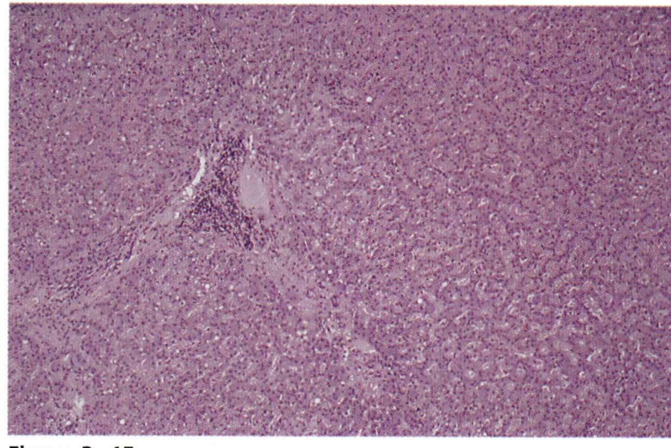

Figure 3–15

Liver, XLPD. There is less necrosis and less portal infiltrate than in the siblings.

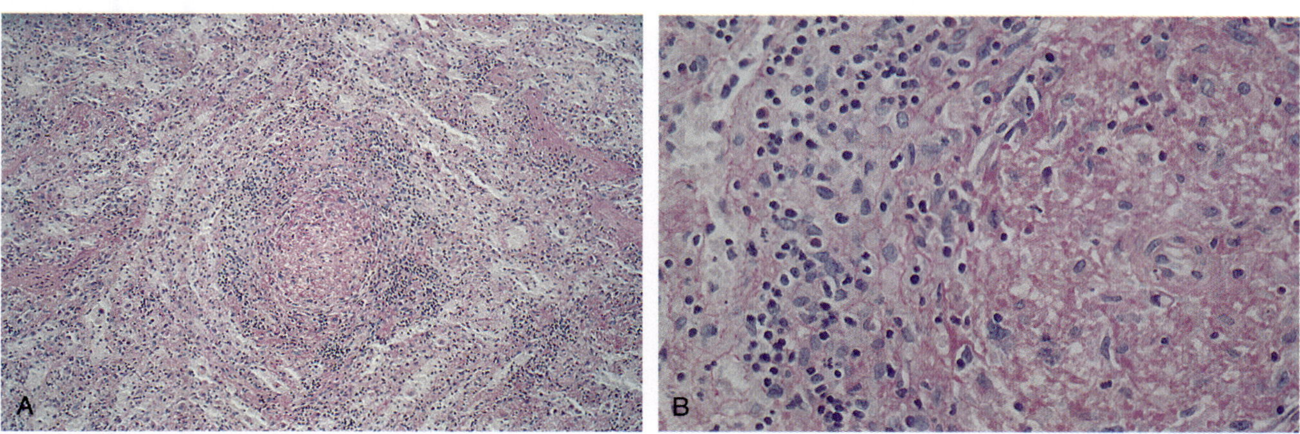

Figure 3–16

Spleen, XLPD. *A*. A PAS stain shows considerable alteration of the follicular centers, probably due to remote necrosis. *B*. At high magnification cellular debris, fibrinous exudate, and a depleted appearance of the white pulp were noted, along with the adjacent polymorphous infiltrate.

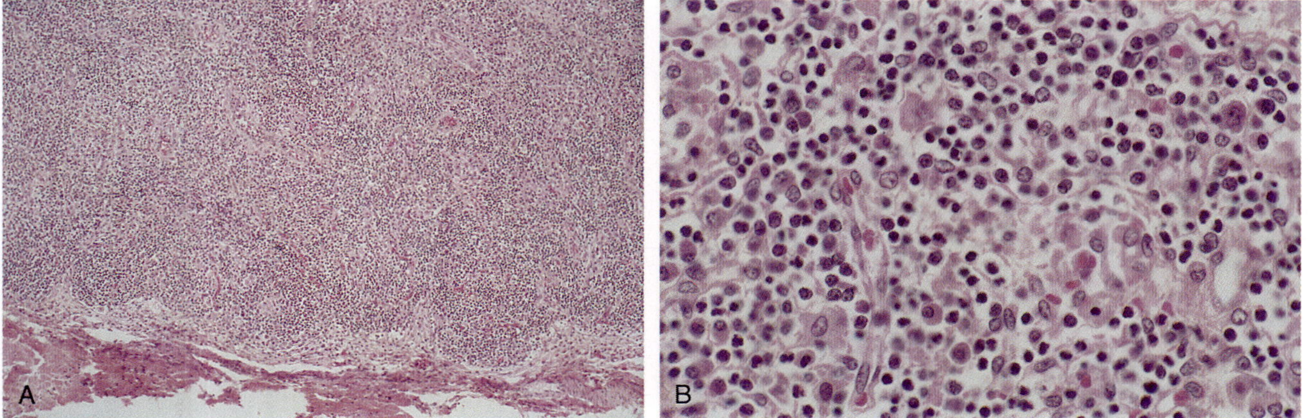

Figure 3–17

Lymph node, XLPD. *A*. General centers are absent in this case, as in Figures 3–8 and 3–12. *B*. High magnification shows a polymorphous infiltrate and evidence of erythrophagocytosis by sinus histiocytes. Figures 3–15 through 3–17 are from patient CC.

(antibody) responses. In addition, the two responses counterbalance each other, with a Th2 response down-regulating Th1 and vice versa. It is likely that an appropriate Th1 response is important in controlling EBV infections. Down-regulation by a Th2 response may result in persistent antibody production, as is frequently observed in XLPD. Characteristically, XLPD patients surviving primary infection do not mount an appropriate humoral response to EBV. They have low titers and/or absent antibodies to EBV antigens. The defect in XLPD may reside in the inability to effect an appropriate Th2 response after infection (Seemayer et al, 1995; Seemayer et al, 1993). As a result, cytotoxic T cells are produced, with their production and function unregulated. An excessively vigorous response at the time of the primary infection may lead to death from hepatocytolysis and/or aplastic anemia. Survivors, left with a weakened immune system, have variable degrees of hypogammaglobulinemia and other immune defects that predispose them to subsequent malignancy.

REFERENCES

Grierson H, Purtilo DT: Epstein-Barr virus infections in males with the X-linked lymphoproliferative syndrome. Ann Intern Med 106:538–545, 1987.

Grierson HL, Skare J, Hawk J, et al: Immunoglobulin class and subclass deficiencies prior to Epstein-Barr virus infection in males with X-linked lymphoproliferative disease. Am J Med Genet 40:294–297, 1991.

Grimm EA, Mazumder A, Zhang H, Rosenberg S: Lymphokine activated killer cell phenomenon: lysis of natural killer resistant fresh solid tumor cells by interleukin-2 activated autologous human peripheral blood lymphocytes. J Exp Med 155:1823–1841, 1982.

Harrington DS, Weisenburger DD, Purtilo DT, et al: Malignant lymphoma in the X-linked lymphoproliferative syndrome. Cancer 59: 1419–1429, 1987.

Lanyi A, Li B, Li S, et al: A yeast artificial chromosome (YAC) contig encompassing the critical region of the X-linked lymphoproliferative disease (xlp) locus. Genomics 39:55–65, 1997.

Purtilo DT: X-linked lymphoproliferative disease (XLP) as a model of Epstein-Barr virus-induced immunopathology. Springer Semin Immunopathol 13:181–197, 1991.

Purtilo DT, Cassel CK, Yang JP, et al: X-linked recessive progressive combined variable immunodeficiency (Duncan's disease). Lancet 1:935–943, 1975.

Purtilo DT, Grierson HL: Methods of detection of new families with X-linked lymphoproliferative disease. Cancer Genet Cytogenet 51:143–153, 1991.

Purtilo DT, Grierson HL, Ochs H, et al: Detection of X-linked lymphoproliferative disease using molecular and immunovirologic markers. Am J Med 87:421–424, 1989.

Purtilo DT, Sakamoto K, Barnabei V, et al: Epstein-Barr virus–induced diseases in boys with the X-linked lymphoproliferative syndrome (XLP): update on studies of the registry. Am J Med 73:49–56, 1982.

Schuster V, Seiderspinner, Grimm T, et al: Molecular genetic haplotype segregation studies in three families with X-linked lymphoproliferative disease. Eur J Pediatr 153:432–437, 1994.

Seeley JK, Golub SH: Studies on cytotoxicity generated in human mixed lymphocyte cultures: I. Time course and target spectrum of several distinct concomitant cytotoxic activities. J Immunol 120:1415–1422, 1978.

Seemayer TA, Grierson H, Pirruccello SJ, et al: X-linked lymphoproliferative disease. AJDC 147:1242–1245, 1993.

Seemayer TA, Gross TG, Egeler M, et al: X-linked lymphoproliferative disease: twenty-five years after the discovery. Pediatr Res 38:471–476, 1995.

Skare J, Wu B-L, Madan S, et al: Characterization of three overlapping deletions causing X-linked lymphoproliferative disease. Genomics 16:254–255, 1993.

Sullivan JL: Epstein-Barr virus and lymphoproliferative disorders. Semin Hematol 25:269, 1988.

Sullivan JL, Byron KS, Brewster FE, et al: X-linked lymphoproliferative syndrome: natural history of the immunodeficiency. J Clin Invest 71:1765, 1983.

Steven H. Swerdlow

Posttransplant Lymphoproliferative Disorders

DEFINITION

Posttransplant lymphoproliferative disorders (PTLDs) are a spectrum of destructive, frequently Epstein-Barr virus (EBV)–associated, lymphocyte or plasma cell proliferations following solid organ or marrow transplantation. EBV-negative PTLDs also occur and have some distinct clinicopathologic features. Although some authors attempt to distinguish PTLD from lymphoma and florid infectious mononucleosis, others view PTLDs as this spectrum, ranging from lesions with no features of a lymphocytic neoplasm to lesions that are indistinguishable from a conventional malignant lymphoma. This chapter takes the latter approach.

CLASSIFICATION

Because PTLDs represent a clinical, histologic, immunophenotypic, and genotypic spectrum, they require further classification for biologic and clinical purposes. The principal classifications are given in Tables 3–6 through 3–9 and have been reviewed (Swerdlow, 1997a; Swerdlow, 1997b). A new World Health Organization classification of PTLD has been published in a provisional form (Harris et al, 2000). The finalized classification is to be published in 2001. In brief, posttransplant lymphoproliferations include the following:

- ☐ Nondestructive polymorphic proliferations with variable numbers of transformed cells or immunoblasts. Some of

Table 3–6
Classification of Posttransplant Lymphoproliferative Disorders

"Nonspecific" reactive lymphoid hyperplasia[a]
Atypical lymphoid hyperplasia[b]
Polymorphic diffuse B cell hyperplasia
Atypical polymorphic diffuse B cell hyperplasia[b]
Polymorphic diffuse B cell lymphoma
Immunoblastic sarcoma of B cell type[b]

[a]Lacks architectural destruction and is not recognized as a PTLD.

[b]Recognized as a posttransplant lesion in the classification published by Shapiro et al (1988).

Source: Frizzera G, et al: Cancer Res 41:4262, 1981; Shapiro RS, et al: Blood 71: 1234, 1988.

these may represent infectious mononucleosis, some are considered infectious mononucleosis–like PTLD, and others are considered "plasma cell hyperplasia." These cases are not considered PTLDs by all authors and are the lesions most likely to respond to a decrease in immunosuppression.

- Plasma cell–rich lesions not associated with the clinicopathologic features of multiple myeloma (plasma cell–rich or plasmacytoma-like PTLD, minimally polymorphic PTLD).
- Destructive polymorphic proliferations that include lymphocytes at all developmental stages. Frizzera and coauthors (1981) distinguished polymorphic B cell hyperplasia from polymorphic B cell lymphoma because the latter also had necrosis and "atypical immunoblasts" that could resemble Reed-Sternberg cells.
- Destructive proliferations with predominantly transformed lymphocytes or immunoblasts (monomorphic PTLD, immunoblastic lymphoma or myeloma, immunoblastic sarcoma of B cells). These cases can be distinguished further based on the type of B and T cell lymphoma they most closely resemble, and some would diagnose them as such. These PTLDs are considered among the least likely to respond to a decrease in immunosuppression.
- Multiple myeloma.
- PTLDs indistinguishable from T cell leukemias or lymphomas. This is a rare and commonly aggressive type of PTLD, but some are indolent and may respond to decrease in immunosuppression.
- Hodgkin disease (HD) or HD-like lesions. These are rare, and the distinction from a PTLD more analogous to a T cell–rich B cell lymphoma may be very problematic. Some reported cases of posttransplant HD may now be reinterpreted as other PTLDs that more closely resemble B and T cell lymphomas.
- Composite PTLDs with more than one histologic pattern.

Table 3–7
Classification of Posttransplant Lymphoproliferative Disorders

Reactive diffuse plasmacytic hyperplasia without architectural effacement[a]
Polymorphic PTLD
Monomorphic PTLD
Minimally polymorphic PTLD

[a]These lesions were seen in patients with concurrent or subsequent PTLD, and their relationship to PTLD is considered undefined.

Source: Nalesnik MA, et al: Am J Pathol 133:173, 1988.

Table 3–8
Classification of Posttransplant Lymphoproliferative Disorders

Plasmacytic hyperplasia
Polymorphic PTLD (polymorphic B cell hyperplasia and polymorphic B cell lymphoma)
Immunoblastic lymphoma or multiple myeloma

Source: Knowles DM, et al: Blood 85:552, 1995.

- PTLDs not otherwise specified. This category should be used for PTLDs for which a definitive classification cannot be made, for example, because the cytologic preservation of the cells in a small biopsy is suboptimal.

CLINICAL FEATURES AND PROGNOSIS

Overall, childhood PTLDs are reported to occur in 4% of transplant patients (Ho et al, 1988). The incidence, however, varies greatly depending on the type of transplant, the length of follow-up, and other parameters, such as intensity and possibly type of immunosuppression. Pediatric patients have a reported PTLD incidence of 3.8–10.7% following liver transplantation (additional patients have "symptomatic" EBV infections), 1–13% after kidney transplantation, 6–9.2% after heart transplantation, and 26.8% after intestinal transplantation (Armitage et al, 1993; Asante-Korang et al, 1996; Gruber et al, 1994; Newell et al, 1996; Reyes et al, 1996; Reyes et al, 1991; Shapiro et al, 1996).

The incidence of PTLD following marrow transplant is generally low but very high among those receiving mismatched T cell–depleted marrows (24% including adult and pediatric patients) (Shapiro et al, 1988). The PTLD risk in pediatric liver transplant patients over the first 6 years is 2.8% per year, suggesting that some of the reported "incidences" of PTLD may be artificially low (Malatack et al, 1991). The influence of immunosuppression is illustrated by the observation that, among pediatric liver transplant patients, those treated with tacrolimus and OKT3 "rescue" had an incidence of 28.1%, compared with an overall incidence of 8.4% (Newell et al, 1996). In a series of pediatric renal transplants the "incidence of PTLD seemed to decrease as more experience was acquired with tacrolimus"

Table 3–9
Working Classification of Posttransplant Lymphoproliferative Disorders

Plasmacytic hyperplasia
PTLDs
- Infectious mononucleosis–like
- Plasma cell rich
- Polymorphic
- Monomorphic[a]
- Multiple myeloma–like
- T cell type
- Hodgkin disease–like[b]
- Composite
- Not otherwise specified
- Other

[a]See the text concerning the various histologic appearances of monomorphic PTLDs.

[b]See the text concerning the difficulty of distinguishing HD-like PTLDs from lesions more like T cell–rich B cell lymphomas.

Source: Swerdlow SH: Curr Diagn Pathol 4:29, 1997b.

(Shapiro et al, 1996). PTLDs occur more frequently in children than in adults. In part, this is believed to be the result of a much higher proportion of primary EBV infections and, in part, simply related to age (Nalesnik, 1996; Newell et al, 1996). "Lymphoma," a designator that would include many, although not all, PTLDs, is the most common "cancer" seen in pediatric transplant patients, with 85% arising during childhood (Penn, 1994a; Penn, 1994b). Of the posttransplant tumors actually arising in children, 74% were lymphomas, with two thirds in non–renal transplant patients (Penn, 1994a).

PTLDs occur from weeks to years following transplantation, with reported median or mean times for pediatric series of 2 months (marrow), 6 and 36 months (heart), 1.2 ± 0.3 years (liver). Other series that include adults report median times of 4 to 6.9 months (Armitage et al, 1993; Hanasono et al, 1995; Leblond et al, 1995; Nalesnik, 1996; Newell et al, 1996; Shapiro et al, 1988; Zutter et al, 1988). PTLD had an "early" appearance in pediatric renal transplant patients at 4 to 6 months, with two late "lymphomas" at 3.8 and 4.3 years (Shapiro et al, 1996). Penn reported a time to PTLD of 36 months for renal transplants and 15 months for non–renal transplants (Penn, 1994b). Prior to the use of cyclosporine A and tacrolimus, PTLDs occurred later than they do now.

Presentation

Patients with PTLD can present in several different ways: infectious mononucleosis–like presentations with or without adenopathy, more lymphomatous presentations with localized tumor masses, and presentations with widely disseminated disease and organ dysfunction. An otherwise asymptomatic lymphadenopathic presentation in children has also been described. Among children in the Cincinnati Transplant Registry, 35% of PTLD cases were localized and 65% widespread (Penn, 1994a).

Infectious mononucleosis–like presentations may include fever, sore throat, hepatosplenomegaly, adenopathy, and tonsillar enlargement that can lead to life-threatening upper airway obstruction requiring surgery (Fairley et al, 1990; Sculerati & Arriaga, 1990). The Monospot test and even IgM EBV titers may produce negative results (Fairley et al, 1990; Ho et al, 1988; Lones et al, 1995). A mononucleosis-like presentation is most common in those with primary EBV infections. The importance of tonsillar involvement in children has been stressed (Lones et al, 1995; Nalesnik, 1996). Upper airway obstruction is reported in 75% of children with PTLD presenting with head and neck symptoms (Sculerati & Arriaga, 1990). Uncomplicated and self-limited infectious mononucleosis with mild symptoms can also occur in children posttransplantation, with resolution sometimes even without a reduction in immunosuppression (Billiar et al, 1988). Whether the latter course is advisable is uncertain. Cox and coauthors (1995), for example, report that 39% of children less than 5 years of age with "symptomatic" EBV infection developed a lymphoproliferative disorder. Medical intervention, however, was not restricted to the PTLD patients. Others consider even the most infectious mononucleosis–like cases to be one end of the spectrum of PTLD.

Another important presentation of PTLD is with nodal or extranodal tumorous masses that may be associated with isolated organ dysfunction. Slightly more than half involve extranodal sites (Penn, 1994a). Although generally thought to appear later than the mononucleosis-type disease, more tumorous presentations are now being seen in the first posttransplant year (Nalesnik, 1996). Common sites for PTLD include the allograft (in liver and intestinal transplant patients, rarely in heart transplant patients), abdominal and peripheral lymph nodes, lung, central nervous system, gastrointestinal tract, and upper aerodigestive tract. Patients presenting with tumor masses will have symptoms related to their site. For example, in transplant patients with abdominal pain, bleeding, and constitutional symptoms, a gastrointestinal tract PTLD should be suspected. These lesions are often multiple and in the distal ileum or right colon. PTLD also occurs at unusual sites. Rare ocular involvement, for example, has been described in children (Robinson et al, 1995).

A further group of children present with fulminant and disseminated disease. They may have a preceding mononucleosis-like disorder. These patients appear "septic" and have widespread organ involvement and dysfunction, with or without adenopathy or other infections (Nalesnik, 1996).

Currently there is great interest in using peripheral blood studies to help identify patients with PTLD or at high risk for one, with the goal of early therapeutic intervention. It is well known that simple EBV serologic study has not proven useful in this regard. Most interest has focused on the quantitation of peripheral blood leukocyte and lymphocyte EBV DNA by polymerase chain reaction CP analysis. High levels of EBV DNA (e.g., ≥20,000 EBV genome copies/μg DNA or >500 copies/10^5 lymphocytes) are associated with PTLD and may precede it (Riddler et al, 1994; Rooney et al, 1995a; Rowe et al, 1997). Most patients with low levels do not have PTLD (e.g., <2000 EBV genome copies/μg DNA); however, the level in transplant patients without PTLD may overlap that found in those with PTLD (Kenagy et al, 1995). Marrow transplant patients have a higher median level of EBV DNA in their blood than do normal subjects, but the range is similar. The spontaneous transformation of peripheral blood B cells is also associated with PTLD, and a rapid rise in CD19+ B cells (>55%) is reported to precede PTLDs by days to a month (Morrissey et al, 1995; Rooney et al, 1995a).

Paraproteins, which are often transient, occur in a significant minority of patients following transplantation and are not necessarily associated with a PTLD (Joseph et al, 1994; Leblond et al, 1995; Radl et al, 1985). Monoclonal paraproteins are also found in many of the patients with plasma cell–rich (plasmacytoma) PTLD and myeloma. The frequency of posttransplant paraproteins in pediatric patients is unknown.

Prognosis

Overall, PTLD is associated with a 50–60% mortality rate, but the rate varies greatly, depending on the specific group of patients studied (Armitage et al, 1993; Nalesnik, 1996; Newell et al, 1996). One hundred percent survival has been described for "PTLD" treated with discontinuation of immunosuppression and ganciclovir in a renal transplant series, although two children with "lymphoma" required antineoplastic therapy (Shapiro et al, 1996). In contrast, children with PTLD following marrow transplants do very poorly (Shapiro et al, 1988; Zutter et al, 1988). From a clinical perspective, patients with infectious mononucleosis–like presentations do the best, and those with overwhelming fulminant disseminated disease do poorly (Ho et al, 1988; Nalesnik, 1996; Reyes et al, 1991). Children with localized disease, except, apparently, for central nervous system disease, also do better than those with extensive disease (Armitage et al, 1993).

Those who die of PTLD often do so within months (mean 2.9 ± 0.8 months in a series of pediatric liver transplants) (Newell et al, 1996). Death is usually due to PTLD and/or infection. Some report that histologic features are not of prognostic importance (Newell et al, 1996). Many consider the monomorphic lesions with large B cell clones and secondary molecular abnormalities the most aggressive of the PTLD and the least likely to respond to decreased immunosuppression (Chadburn et al, 1997; Knowles et al, 1995; Locker & Nalesnik, 1989). Monoclonality by itself cannot be equated with an adverse outcome or a definite need for chemotherapy or radiation. *BCL6* mutations are also associated with shortened survival time and a decreased likelihood of response to surgery and/or decreased immunosuppression (Cesarman et al, 1997). Those treated successfully for PTLD may develop allograft rejection (Newell et al, 1996). Insufficient numbers of children with plasma cell–rich PTLD, posttransplant HD, and T cell PTLD are reported to accurately state their prognoses. Most of the latter have not done well, although they may respond like other PTLDs (Leblond et al, 1995; Macon et al, 1996; Waller et al, 1993; Wu et al, 1996; Zutter et al, 1990).

Recurrent PTLDs or other EBV-associated lesions are reported to follow approximately 4.5% of PTLDs (children and adults) (Wu et al, 1996). One of 10 pediatric liver transplant PTLD survivors are reported to have had a recurrence at 1 year (Newell et al, 1996). The recurrent PTLD may or may not be histologically and genotypically similar to the original lesion (Goyal et al, 1996; Wu et al, 1996). Some may show progression to higher-grade lesions (Alfrey et al, 1992; Wu et al, 1996). Children with recurrent PTLD often still do well (Wu et al, 1996). Some pediatric transplant patients have developed HD after other PTLD or lymphocytic hyperplasias (Goyal et al, 1996; Smir et al, 1996). Two children with PTLD have experienced "recurrences" with EBV-positive smooth-muscle tumors (Kingma et al, 1996; Lee et al, 1995).

THERAPY

Therapy of PTLD varies widely, depending on the type of PTLD; the patient's characteristics, including age and type of transplant; and the physician's or institution's preference. Ho and coauthors (1988) stated, "The appropriate therapy for EBV-associated [lymphoproliferative syndrome] is at best empirical and remains a challenge." Although much has been learned since 1988, the statement is still true. In general, decreasing or eliminating immunosuppression is critical, with the specifics dictated in part by the patient's clinical circumstances. Patients must, of course, be monitored for rejection and therapy appropriately modified. Rejection is reported to be frequent by some and infrequent by others (Reyes et al, 1996; Reyes et al, 1991; Sculerati & Arriaga, 1990). Increasing steroid dosages in a fashion analogous to how infectious mononucleosis might be treated is "to be avoided" (Sculerati & Arriaga, 1990). "Supportive" surgery can also be important, for example, in gastrointestinal lesions that may perforate. Antiviral agents have been used, including acyclovir, ganciclovir, and α-interferon. α-Interferon also has antiproliferative activity and may modulate the immune system. Intravenous immunoglobulin may also be of utility.

The proportion of patients successfully treated with these measures alone is difficult to estimate; however, they do represent a significant minority of children with PTLD. For example, 4 of 11 pediatric small bowel transplant patients had resolution of PTLD without chemotherapy or radiation (one did have the graft removed) (Putnam et al, 1996). Overall, 31–50% of PTLDs have responded to decreased immunosuppression, a result termed "optimistic" (Nalesnik, 1996). Decreased immunosuppression and antiviral therapy in intestinal transplant patients had limited success (Reyes et al, 1996). Patients failing these measures, some with "unusually severe" disease (Newell et al, 1996) and some with one of the lymphoma-like PTLDs, especially of Burkitt type, are treated with standard chemotherapeutic regimens or radiation in a fashion analogous to the treatment of nonimmunosuppressed patients.

Results with antineoplastic therapies have varied, but they may be very rewarding, even for Burkitt-like lesions (Gallego-Melcon et al, 1996; Swinnen et al, 1995). Two teenaged patients with posttransplant HD were successfully treated with modified HD regimens, although there was less than 1 year follow-up (Goyal et al, 1996).

More experimental therapies include the use of anti–B cell antibodies (Benkerrou et al, 1993; Leblond et al, 1995) and, of great current interest, adoptive transfer of in vitro expanded EBV-specific cytotoxic T lymphocytes or autologous lymphokine activated killer cells (Nalesnik et al, 1997; Rooney et al, 1997; Rooney et al, 1995b). Responses are reported, but clinical data are currently limited. In marrow transplant recipients, infusions of donor leukocytes have also been used at least in adults (Papadopoulos et al, 1994). Any effort at reconstituting the immune system or augmenting cytotoxic T cell activity must be balanced with the risk of organ rejection and, depending on the specific protocol, graft-versus-host disease. There is also interest in the possibility of preemptive therapies for patients at greatest risk for PTLD.

HISTOPATHOLOGIC FEATURES

Histopathologic analysis of posttransplant lymphocytic and plasmacytic proliferations involves determining if they represent PTLD and, if so, how they should best be classified (see "Classification"). Not every posttransplant lymphocytic proliferation is a PTLD, even if some EBV-positive cells are identified. Classification may also be problematic, since PTLDs can vary so much within individual patients and even within individual lesions. The possibility of higher-grade or more aggressive lesions must be considered when a solitary biopsy sample shows only a low-grade PTLD or borderline lesion. Cytologic examination may also be diagnostic, particularly with the aid of ancillary studies (Davey et al, 1990; Dusenbery et al, 1997). Caution is advised, however, as non-PTLD lymphocyte-rich effusions may also be seen in patients with PTLD at other sites (Hudnall et al, 1996).

The first major category of PTLD is that which includes the "plasmacytic hyperplasia" or infectious mononucleosis–like "early" lesions (Harris et al, 1997) (Figs. 3–18 and 3–19). These lesions tend to occur in younger patients than do the other major types of PTLD (Chadburn et al, 1997). In both circumstances there is architectural preservation. Cases with principally small lymphocytes and plasma cells are considered plasmacytic hyperplasia. While considered a PTLD by some, at least in the absence of EBV positivity, nodal plasmacytic hyperplasia is indistinguishable from a completely nonspecific medullary plasmacytosis. Plasmacytic hyperplasia may be associated with more overt PTLD at other sites. Infectious mononucleosis–like PTLD is a more florid proliferation that includes at least moderate numbers of transformed lymphocytes or immunoblasts. Infectious mononucleosis–like PTLD resembles lesions seen in normal hosts with infectious mononucleosis. Lymph nodes demonstrate intact sinuses, and tonsillar lesions are compatible with infectious mononucleosis (see Fig. 3–19). Whether these lesions are simple EBV infection or a PTLD is controversial, although they may be clonal and even fatal (Fig. 3–20).

Plasma cell–rich PTLDs have a marked predominance of plasma cells but lack the clinicopathologic features of myeloma. These are most analogous to extramedullary plasmacytomas, although there may be a small lymphocytic component in some of these lesions. Immunoblasts should be infrequent. Plasma cell–rich PTLD (EBV-positive extramedullary plasmacytoma) has been reported in a $1\frac{1}{2}$-year-old, but other cases have been in adults (Joseph et al, 1994).

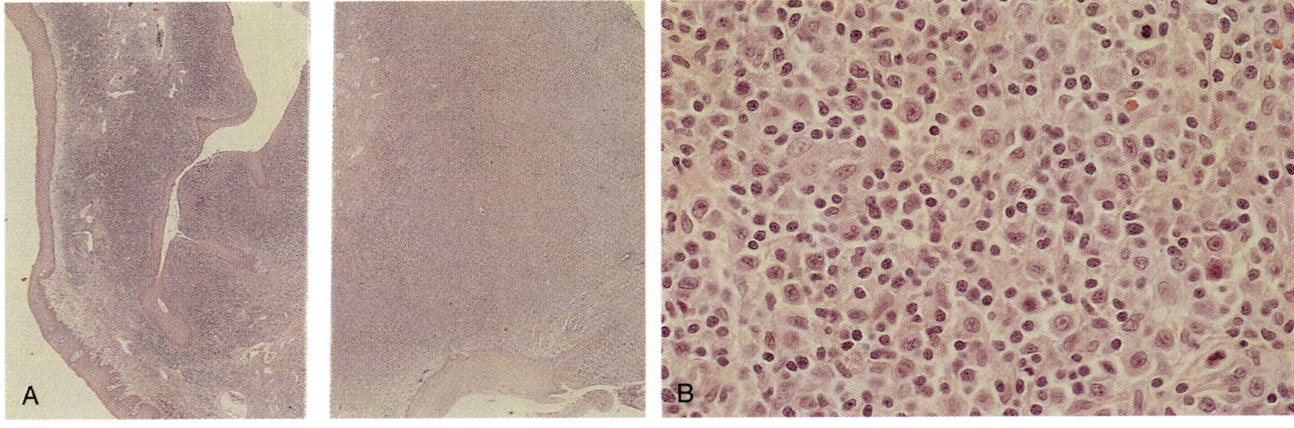

Figure 3–18

PTLD, infectious mononucleosis type. This tonsillar mass occurred in a post–kidney transplant 15-year-old boy who presented with a sore throat (patient 4 in Nalesnik et al, 1988). Genotypic studies did not demonstrate clonal B cells. The patient did well with decreased immunosuppression. This lesion was initially diagnosed as polymorphic PTLD, but others would classify it as plasmacytic hyperplasia (see the text). *A.* Although some of the tonsillar architecture is intact *(left),* follicles are absent, and other areas show a diffuse lymphocytic proliferation. The surface is partially ulcerated on the *right*. *B.* There are small and large lymphocytes. Some have clumped chromatin and angulated nuclei. Others are large and transformed (i.e., immunoblasts).

The most classic PTLDs include the polymorphic and monomorphic categories. They are invasive mass lesions that largely destroy the normal nodal architecture or underlying organ parenchyma. Polymorphic lesions are the most common type of pediatric PTLDs in some series (Lones et al, 1995; Newell et al, 1996) and are composed of a diffuse proliferation of small lymphocytes, transformed lymphocytes, immunoblasts, and plasma cells (see Fig. 3–20). Extensive bands or "swaths" of necrosis may be present, and some cases demonstrate "atypical immunoblasts" that resemble Reed-Sternberg cells (Fig. 3–21). Pleomorphic lesions with mostly transformed lymphocytes may appear polymorphic but are best

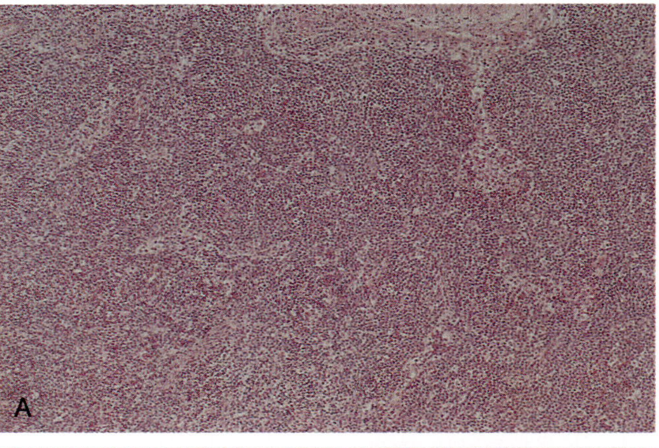

Figure 3–19

PTLD, infectious mononucleosis type. This post–liver transplant 4-year-old boy originally presented with fever, anorexia, and vague abdominal pain (patient 5 in Nalesnik et al, 1988). Genotypic studies showed a small B cell clone (1+). He did well with decreased immunosuppression. *A.* This condition was originally diagnosed as a polymorphic PTLD; however, now that infectious mononucleosis PTLD is recognized, the presence of intact sinuses in many areas of the lymph node, together with the polymorphic proliferation, supports the latter diagnosis. *B.* Note the polymorphic cell population ranging from small lymphocytes to immunoblasts. *C.* Even though a small clone was documented by genotypic studies, paraffin section immunostains showed polyclonal-appearing plasmacytoid or plasma cells (κ on the *left* and λ on the *right*).

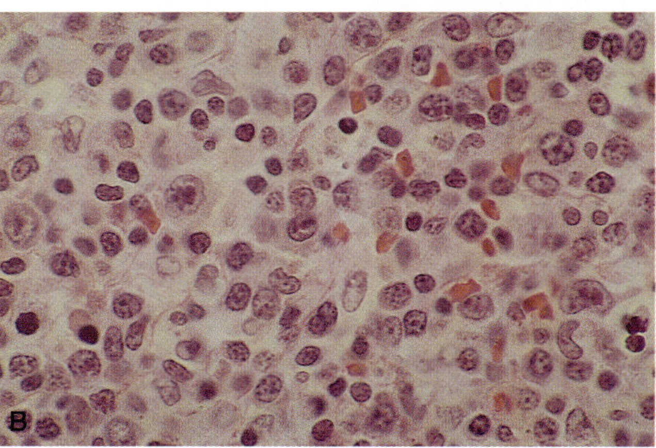

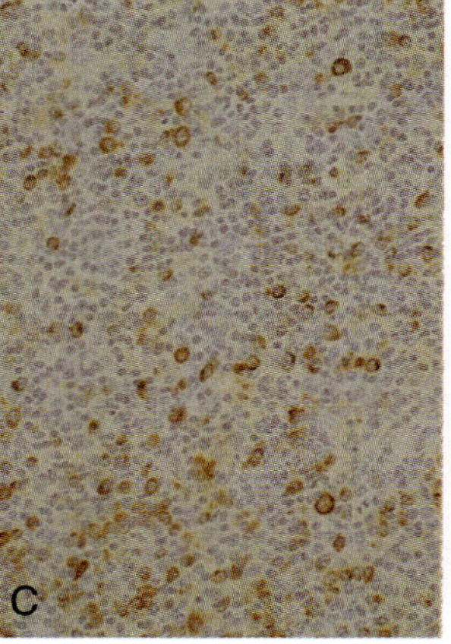

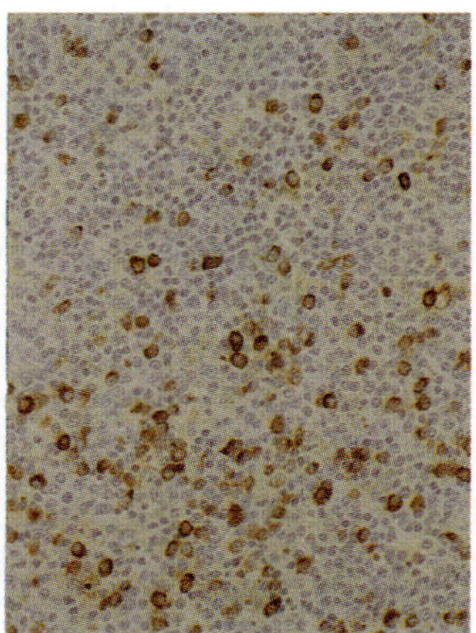

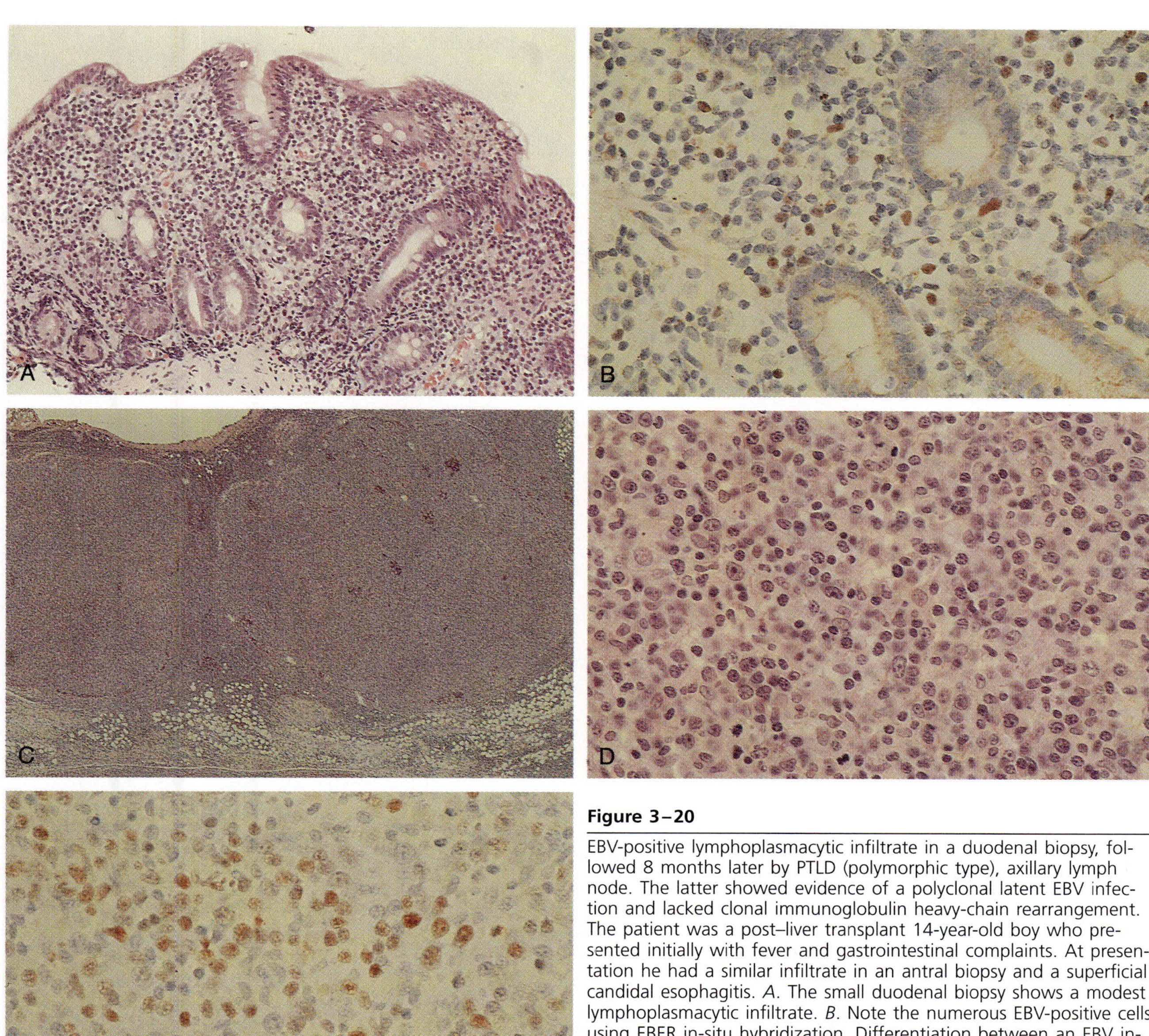

Figure 3–20

EBV-positive lymphoplasmacytic infiltrate in a duodenal biopsy, followed 8 months later by PTLD (polymorphic type), axillary lymph node. The latter showed evidence of a polyclonal latent EBV infection and lacked clonal immunoglobulin heavy-chain rearrangement. The patient was a post–liver transplant 14-year-old boy who presented initially with fever and gastrointestinal complaints. At presentation he had a similar infiltrate in an antral biopsy and a superficial candidal esophagitis. *A.* The small duodenal biopsy shows a modest lymphoplasmacytic infiltrate. *B.* Note the numerous EBV-positive cells using EBER in-situ hybridization. Differentiation between an EBV infection and early PTLD in a case such as this is controversial. *C.* Except for a peripheral sinus, the architecture of the axillary lymph node is diffusely effaced. Note the extensive perinodal infiltration. This is clearly diagnostic of a PTLD. *D.* Plasmacytoid cells are seen in moderate number in the polymorphic proliferation. *E.* The EBER in-situ hybridization again showed numerous EBV-positive cells.

considered monomorphic (Harris et al, 1997; Nelson et al, 1997) (see Fig. 3–21*C*). Monomorphic PTLDs are indistinguishable from B and T cell lymphomas. Most resemble either small, noncleaved (Burkitt) or large, noncleaved follicular center cell lymphomas, with some fulfilling the criteria for B cell immunoblastic lymphoma (Figs. 3–22 and 3–23). The latter may have admixed plasma cells and appear more polymorphic than some of the other monomorphic categories. Although many diagnose these cases as lymphomas, some cases respond to reconstitution of the immune system or to experimental therapies not traditionally used for conventional lymphomas. They should also be designated as a type of PTLD. Posttransplant myeloma is also rarely seen, at least in adults.

PTLDs fulfilling the standard criteria for a T cell neoplasm are designated separately by most authors. A T cell lineage for posttransplant "lymphomas" is reported for 9% of lymphomas arising in pediatric transplant recipients (Penn, 1994b). T cell PTLDs comprise a wide histologic spectrum with pediatric cases resembling a polymorphic mixed large and small cell lymphoma (Zutter et al, 1990), large cell lymphoma (Waller et al, 1993), peripheral T cell lymphoma, not otherwise specified (Wu et al, 1996), natural killer-like T cell lymphoma with blood and marrow involvement by large and sometimes blastic lymphocytes with azurophilic granules (Macon et al, 1996), and CD8 positive "polymorphic" PTLD involving the blood (Leblond et al, 1995) (Fig. 3–24). Other cases reported of T lymphoblastic neoplasms could have represented relapse of the original leukemia. T cell PTLD in children have occurred 1.5 months to 6 years post transplant (Zutter et al, 1990; Waller et al, 1993; Wu et al, 1996; Macon et al, 1996).

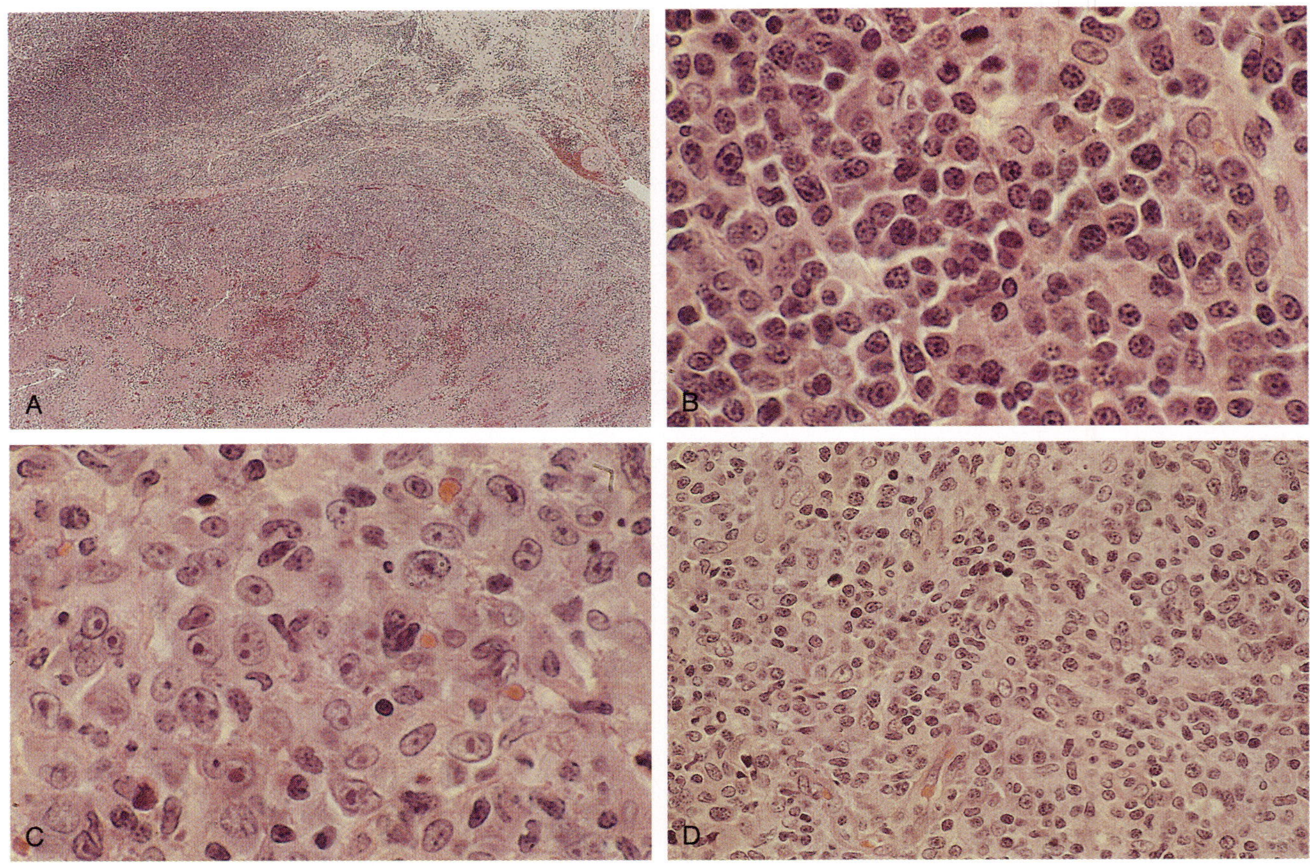

Figure 3–21

PTLD with varied histologic appearances. This tonsillar PTLD, diagnosed as being of polymorphic type, occurred in a post–liver transplant 3-year-old girl who presented with fever and upper airway obstruction (case 23 in Nalesnik et al, 1988). Genotypic studies did not demonstrate a clonal B cell population. She did well after surgery, decreased immunosuppression, and acyclovir. Classification of this case was difficult due to the various features described below. *A*. The varied histologic appearances can be appreciated even at low magnification. The darker area in the upper left is rich in small plasmacytoid cells. There are extensive swaths of necrosis, often surrounded by paler areas with numerous transformed lymphocytes/immunoblasts. *B*. Note the numerous relatively small plasmacytoid cells in this portion of the PTLD. These areas might be classified as a plasma cell–rich (or minimally polymorphic) PTLD. *C*. In this area the cells are somewhat pleomorphic but predominantly transformed. A diagnosis of a monomorphic PTLD could be rendered based on this histologic appearance. *D*. Many other areas fit the criteria for a classic polymorphic PTLD.

HD-like PTLDs are very infrequent and should fulfill the standard criteria for HD. The latter is important since Reed-Sternberg–like cells are common in many PTLDs. A nodular growth pattern and sclerosis can also help identify these cases; however, many of the reported cases are of mixed cellularity or less often lymphocyte depleted type (Garnier et al, 1996). The relationship of HD PTLDs to PTLDs that resemble conventional T cell–rich B cell lymphomas is uncertain. The pediatric patients have been in a 6-year-old and two teen-aged males who developed mixed cellularity or nodular sclerosis HD 68 months to 7 years post transplant. Two of the patients had a previous PTLD or an "atypical hyperplasia" (Goyal et al, 1996; Smir et al, 1996). A small number of other cases occurring in pediatric transplant recipients are included in the Cincinnati Transplant Tumor Registry (Penn, 1994b).

Composite PTLDs show more than one histologic pattern in clearly distinct areas. Biopsies with varying proportions of transformed cells in different regions are probably best classified based on the worst-looking areas, since many PTLDs are not completely uniform. Some pathologists do, however, require complete uniformity before making the diagnosis of monomorphic PTLD.

MARKERS

PTLDs range from polyclonal to oligoclonal to monoclonal (Knowles et al, 1995; Locker & Nalesnik, 1989; Nalesnik et al, 1988; Nelson et al, 1997; Seiden & Sklar, 1993). Paraffin section immunostains are not a sensitive tool. Clonality is best assessed in such cases using genotypic methods. Plasma cell hyperplasia is usually polyclonal, although there may be small clones as identified by EBV terminal repeat analysis. Infectious mononucleosis–like PTLDs may also be polyclonal, have only very minor clones, or sometimes exhibit more major B cell clones. Immunostains can demonstrate the expected monoclonal plasma cell population in plasma cell–rich PTLD. At least the majority of polymorphic PTLDs are monoclonal, although the size of the clonal B cell population varies. *BCL6* mutations are reported in 43%, but secondary genotypic abnormalities are not expected (Cesarman et al, 1997). Monomorphic PTLDs are uniformly monoclonal, have the most predominant B cell clones, and are the type of PTLD with secondary genotypic abnormalities, including *MYC* or *BCL6* rearrangements, *BCL6* mutations, *P53* mutations, or *NRAS* mutations (Cesarman et al, 1997; Delecluse et al, 1995;

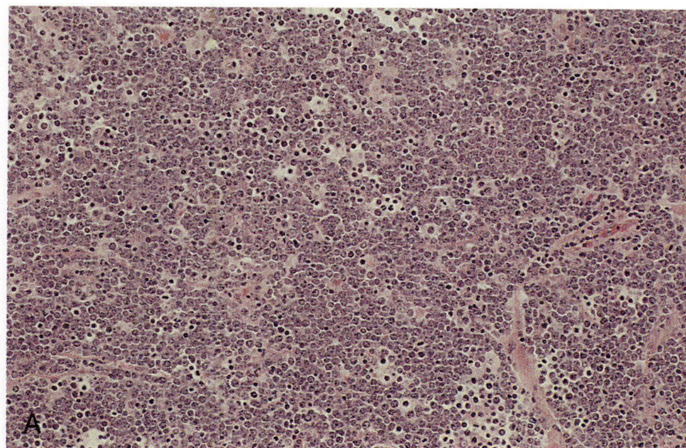

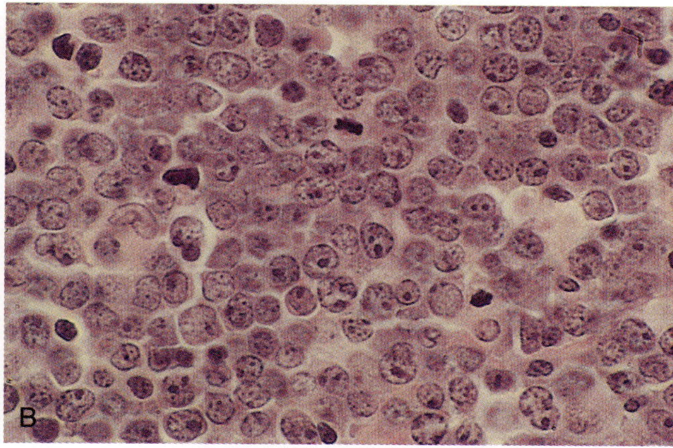

Figure 3–22

PTLD, monomorphic type (Burkitt lymphoma–like). This massive abdominal tumor occurred in a post–liver transplant 6-year-old boy (case 29 in Nalesnik et al, 1988). Immunostains demonstrated that cells in the PTLD bore monoclonal IgMλ. There was also immunoglobulin heavy-chain gene rearrangement. *A*. At low magnification the diffuse lymphocytic proliferation with a starry sky appearance suggests the diagnosis of Burkitt lymphoma. *B*. Note the relatively uniform, small transformed lymphocytes with apoptotic bodies and mitotic figures.

Knowles et al, 1995; Locker & Nalesnik, 1989; Nelson et al, 1997). All immunoblastic lymphoma and myeloma cases may have secondary genotypic abnormalities (Knowles et al, 1995). Patients can have PTLDs with multiple distinct clones at separate sites or both polyclonal and monoclonal PTLDs (Chadburn et al, 1995; Knowles et al, 1995; Locker & Nalesnik, 1989). In other patients multiple lesions may all represent the same clone, as in a conventional lymphoma. Rare cases with both immunoglobulin and T cell receptor gene rearrangements are reported (Hollingsworth et al, 1994).

Immunostains reveal variable numbers of T cells in PTLD, but B cells usually predominate. Infectious mononucleosis–like PTLD and polymorphic PTLD may have >50% admixed T cells, and HD-like cases always do. When present in conventional PTLD, Reed-Sternberg–like cells are CD45 positive, are EBV (latent membrane protein [LMP]) positive, are usually *BCL2* positive, usually mark as B cells, are often CD30 positive, but are CD15 negative (Chetty et al, 1996; Chetty et al, 1997; Murray et al, 1996).

Cases of T cell PTLD must fulfill the same criteria applied in the diagnosis of T cell lymphomas and leukemias, relying in part on immunophenotypic and/or genotypic evidence of T cell lineage. One of the pediatric cases reportedly showed a T cell phenotype but appeared polyclonal in genotypic studies (Zutter et al, 1990).

Posttransplant HD has a phenotype like that in HD in nonimmunocompromised patients, including some reported cases that have little or no CD15 positivity (Goyal et al, 1996; Swerdlow, 1997b). Pediatric cases have not been studied, but in adults Southern blot analysis may demonstrate a B cell clone, while clonal EBV-infected cells have been detected in the small number of cases studied (Swerdlow, 1997b).

Although most cases of PTLD are associated with EBV, as documented by immunostaining, EBV small nonpolyadenylated RNA (EBER) in situ hybridization, Southern blot analysis for EBV terminal repeats, or PCR analysis, some cases are clearly EBV negative. Approximately one fifth of adult PTLDs are EBV negative, based on EBER stains and/or Southern blot analysis (Nelson et al, 2000). Others report 31% EBV-negative PTLDs that, as in our experience, appear to arise later than EBV-positive cases (Leblond et al, 1995). Three pediatric T cell PTLDs have been EBV positive, and one has been EBV negative (Leblond et al, 1995; Waller et al, 1993; Wu et al, 1996; Zutter et al, 1990). In general, EBER in situ staining is considered more sensitive than EBV LMP immunostaining, although EBV-positive cells are more likely to be found in non-PTLD using the former technique (Lones et al, 1997). EBV terminal repeat Southern blot analysis offers the ability to document the clonality of the EBV infection and is a more sensitive clonal marker than is Southern blot analysis for immunoglobulin heavy-chain rearrangement (Locker & Nalesnik, 1989; Seiden & Sklar, 1993). Results of PCR analysis for EBV are frequently positive in the absence of PTLD (Lones et al, 1997).

Cytogenetic analysis is utilized much less than are immunophenotypic and genotypic analyses in PTLD. Abnormalities are found in some cases, but no consistent karyotypic

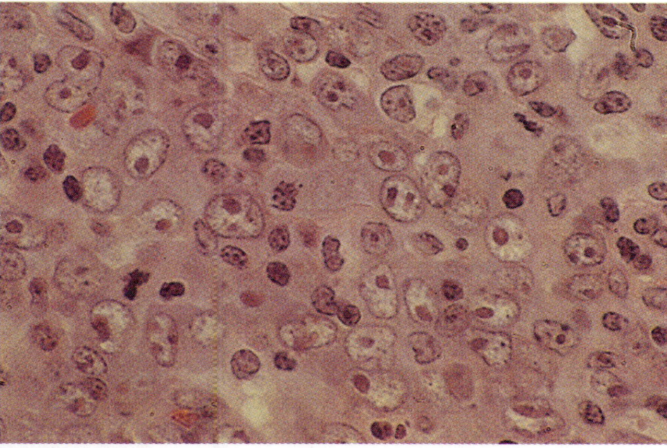

Figure 3–23

PTLD, monomorphic type (immunoblastic lymphoma-like). About 1 year earlier this post–liver transplant 11-year-old girl had a tonsillar PTLD (case 34 in Nalesnik et al, 1988). Genotypic studies were not performed. She was treated with decreased immunosuppression, acyclovir, and chemotherapy but died from her generalized PTLD. The architecture of the lymph node is diffusely effaced by numerous large transformed lymphocytes/immunoblasts. There are admixed small lymphocytes.

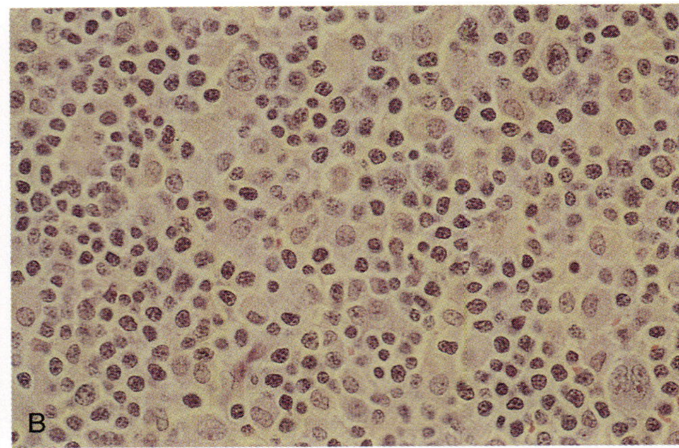

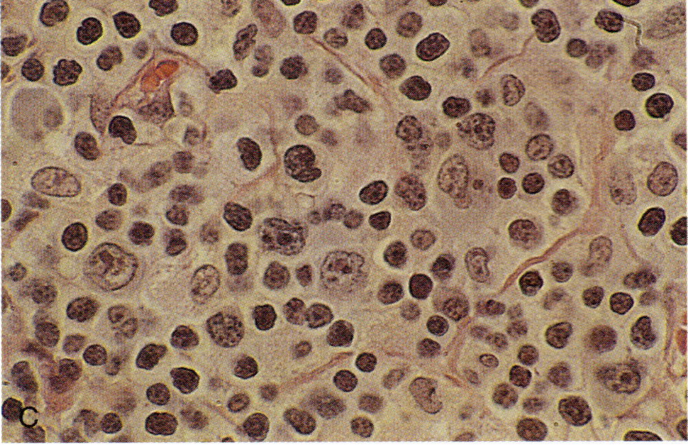

Figure 3–24

PTLD, T cell type. Five years after a heart-lung transplant and polymorphic PTLD, this 9-year-old girl presented with fever, sore throat, and cervical adenopathy. Immunophenotypic studies revealed an "aberrant" T cell phenotype (CD2+, 3+, 5−, 7−, 8+), and genotypic studies revealed a clonal T cell receptor β-chain rearrangement (case 9 in Wu et al, 1996). She did well after decreased immunosuppression. *A*. The nodal architecture is diffusely effaced except for occasional abnormal follicles. Some areas are very pale, and others demonstrate admixed small lymphocytes and prominent histiocytes. *B*. Some areas are polymorphic, with Reed-Sternberg–like cells. *C*. The paler regions resemble a typical peripheral T cell lymphoma, with packeting of small lymphocyte cells with pale cytoplasm admixed with histiocytes and some transformed lymphocytes.

abnormalities are found, except for the t(8;14) translocation observed in some Burkitt-like PTLDs.

DIAGNOSTIC CRITERIA

PTLDs are recognized in transplant patients as destructive mass-forming lymphocytic or plasmacytic proliferations (see "Classification"). Patients with lesions that lack tissue destruction or do not form a mass may be diagnosed as having PTLD based on the florid nature of the proliferation, the presence of EBV, and the lack of any other explanation for their existence. The latter lesions have also been considered to represent infectious mononucleosis.

DIFFERENTIAL DIAGNOSIS

The major differential diagnoses for PTLD include the same diffuse lymphocytic proliferations that can be present in nontransplant patients. When allografts are biopsied, rejection must be considered. In the absence of histologic features suggesting some other specific diagnosis, the presence of architectural effacement with tissue destruction and mass lesion, numerous transformed cells, nuclear atypia, and extensive necrosis favors the diagnosis of a PTLD (Randhawa et al, 1996; Rizkalla et al, 1997; Rosendale & Yousem, 1995; White et al, 1995). The presence of numerous plasma cells favors the diagnosis of PTLD, at least in the liver (Rizkalla et al, 1997).

In renal transplants the necrosis in PTLD should be serpiginous, since hemorrhagic necrosis is seen with rejection (Randhawa et al, 1996). Numerous EBV-positive cells would strongly favor the diagnosis of a PTLD, but rare EBER-positive cells do not rule out the possibility of rejection. EBV LMP positivity, however, is more significant than are scattered EBER-positive cells, since EBV LMP–positive cells reportedly are not seen with rejection (Rizkalla et al, 1997; Rosendale & Yousem, 1995). EBV LMP staining is not as sensitive as is EBER in situ hybridization in detecting EBV even in PTLD, and not all PTLDs are EBV positive. EBER-positive cells in a liver biopsy may precede an overt PTLD in the liver or elsewhere (Randhawa et al, 1992). Inflammatory infiltrates in patients with PTLD do not demonstrate EBV-positive cells (Randhawa et al, 1991).

Although not recommended as a screening tool, the finding of EBER-positive cells in a cardiac biopsy specimen, even with rejection present, should raise concern for a PTLD in the heart, or more frequently, elsewhere (Hanasono et al, 1995). The presence of numerous T cells favors the diagnosis of rejection over PTLD; however, some PTLDs can have many T cells (Lones et al, 1995; Osterhage et al, 1992; Rosendale & Yousem, 1995). Monoclonality supports the diagnosis of a PTLD, but polyclonality is nondiagnostic. Nevertheless, some cases may be very problematic. For example, "mature" PTLD may resemble rejection in intestinal biopsies, and it is difficult to assess the significance of EBV-positive cells without blatant lymphoproliferative lesions (White et al, 1995).

As discussed earlier, distinction of infectious mononucleosis from PTLD is controversial. Transplant patients do get infectious mononucleosis that can cause marked lymphocytic proliferation and hepatitis. In some, the diagnosis of infectious mononucleosis is made simply because there has not been a tissue biopsy. Criteria have been proposed for distinguishing tonsillar PTLD lesions from infectious mononucleosis, such as the latter having more intact follicles; however, many of the criteria are not absolute (Lones et al, 1995).

PATHOGENESIS

PTLDs arise in most circumstances from an EBV infection that cannot be adequately controlled. Patients with the most immunosuppression are particularly likely to develop PTLDs. In addition to decreased cellular immunity, serologic responses are blunted in transplant patients with low to absent titers of anti-EBV nuclear antigen (EBNA) antibodies and, frequently, negative Monospot test results (Ho et al, 1988; Lamy et al, 1990). If present, anti-EBNA antibodies decrease as viral load increases in patients with PTLD (Riddler et al, 1994).

EBV infections are frequently primary in children, whereas in adults they more often represent reactivation since 92% of adults are already EBV infected at the time of transplantation (Ho et al, 1988; Lamy et al, 1990; Newell et al, 1996; Reyes et al, 1991). Most PTLDs are associated with type A EBV, but a minority have type B EBV, which is endemic in Africa and more frequent in patients with AIDS (Frank et al, 1995; Smir et al, 1996).

EBV leads to transformation of the infected cells and blocks their differentiation (Seiden & Sklar, 1993). There is up-regulation of the apoptosis inhibitor *BCL2* in many PTLDs probably related to LMP-1 expression, but the EBV *BCL2* homologue *BHRF1* is not expressed (Murray et al, 1996). Although there is a body of literature discussing the presence of 30–base pair LMP-1 deletions in PTLDs and other lymphomas, Smir and coauthors (1996) report that this may be related to specific EBV substrains and that it does not have any prognostic or clear-cut biologic significance.

EBV-infected B cells in PTLD exhibit a type 3 latency pattern, with expression of six EBNAs, three LMPs, EBERs, and *BAMHIA* transcripts (Rooney et al, 1997), a pattern like that in lymphoblastic cell lines but different from that in Burkitt lymphomas, HD, and nasopharyngeal carcinomas. These cells are highly susceptible to virus–antigen-specific killing, explaining why at least some PTLDs respond to natural reconstitution of the immune system or to adoptive transfer of in vitro–expanded (EBV-specific) cytotoxic T lymphocytes (Rooney et al, 1997). Even while patients are still immunosuppressed, PTLDs show an extremely variable T cell infiltrate (Osterhage et al, 1992). The infectious mononucleosis–like, polymorphic, and HD-like categories are those most likely to show numerous T cells. In addition to latent EBV infection, a "significant proportion" of PTLDs show evidence of lytic infection (Katz et al, 1989; Montone et al, 1996; Patton et al, 1990; Rooney et al, 1997).

The EBV-driven PTLDs appear to evolve from polyclonal to oligoclonal to monoclonal proliferations, with the development of secondary genotypic or karyotypic abnormalities, as described earlier, occurring mostly in the latter cases (see the simplistic model in Swerdlow, 1997b). This clonal progression roughly correlates with the major histopathologic categories (plasmacytic hyperplasia or infectious mononucleosis–like PTLD, polymorphic PTLD, and monomorphic PTLD or multiple myeloma), although there are relatively few reported cases in which actual histologic or genotypic progression is documented. Biased use of the immunoglobulin *VH1* family in monoclonal PTLD and the pattern of *VH* gene mutations suggest that antigen selection may be important in the development and/or progression of many PTLDs (Miklos et al, 1995).

Immunoregulatory abnormalities, such as decreased levels of α-interferon, may also promote B cell proliferation and play a role in the development of PTLD (Mathur et al, 1994). Patients with PTLD have a Th2 cytokine "environment" that promotes B cell activity (Nalesnik & Starzl, 1994). Some postulate that chronic antigenic stimulation by the allograft leads to the initial proliferation of EBV-infected B cells.

As noted earlier, rare cases of EBV-positive T cell PTLD are described. Some of these cases may be analogous to the case of a 2-year-old boy with fatal infectious mononucleosis that was associated with a clonal cytotoxic T cell population and clonal EBV (Mori et al, 1992).

The nature of EBV-negative PTLDs is completely uncertain. Whereas their behavior suggests that at least a proportion are PTLDs rather than coincidental conventional lymphomas, no other inciting agent has been documented. One possibility is that, as with some cases of Burkitt lymphomas, EBV initiated the proliferation but is then "lost" (Razzouk et al, 1996).

In general, PTLDs in solid-organ recipients are usually of host origin and those in marrow recipients usually of donor origin (Weissmann et al, 1995; Zutter et al, 1988). Occasionally, PTLDs of donor origin have been reported in solid-organ recipients, including one child (Chadburn et al, 1995; Hjelle et al, 1989; Weissmann et al, 1995). These PTLDs typically arise in the allograft kidney or liver and appear to have better outcomes than do host PTLDs. A host origin for a post–marrow transplant T lymphoblastic lymphoma has been reported, but the possibility that it represented a recurrence of the previously diagnosed acute leukemia could not be ruled out (Zutter et al, 1990). In at least some cases, the EBV associated with a PTLD may be transmitted by the donor organ (Cen et al, 1991).

SUGGESTED READINGS

Ho M, Jaffe R, Miller G, et al: The frequency of Epstein-Barr virus infection and associated lymphoproliferative syndrome after transplantation and its manifestations in children. Transplantation 45:719, 1988. (Analysis of pediatric PTLD)

Knowles DM, Cesarman E, Chadburn A, et al: Correlative morphologic and molecular genetic analysis demonstrates three distinct categories of posttransplantation lymphoproliferative disorders. Blood 85:552, 1995. (One of the recent major PTLD classifications, with genotypic data)

Nalesnik MA: Posttransplantation lymphoproliferative disorders (PTLD): current perspectives. Semin Thorac Cardiovasc Surg 8:139, 1996. (A recent overview of PTLD)

Nalesnik MA, Jaffe R, Starzl TE, et al: The pathology of posttransplant lymphoproliferative disorders occurring in the setting of cyclosporine A–prednisone immunosuppression. Am J Pathol 133: 173, 1988. (A major description of the University of Pittsburgh transplant experience)

Seiden MV, Sklar J: Molecular genetic analysis of post-transplant lymphoproliferative disorders. Hematol Oncol Clin North Am 7:447, 1993. (A comprehensive review of the pathobiology of PTLD and its molecular aspects)

Swerdlow SH: Classification of the posttransplant lymphoproliferative disorders: from the past to the present. Semin Diagn Pathol 14:2, 1997. (A review of PTLD classification)

Swerdlow SH: Posttransplant lymphoproliferative disorders: a working classification. Curr Diagn Pathol 4:29, 1997. (Details of a working classification of PTLD, including a simple model of the pathophysiology)

REFERENCES

Alfrey EJ, Friedman AL, Grossman RA, et al: A recent decrease in the time to development of monomorphous and polymorphous posttransplant lymphoproliferative disorder. Transplantation 54:250, 1992.

Armitage JM, Fricker FJ, del Nido P, et al: A decade (1982–1992) of pediatric cardiac transplantation and the impact of FK506 immunosuppression. J Thorac Cardiovasc Surg 105:464, 1993.

Asante-Korang A, Boyle GJ, Webber SA, et al: Experience of FK506 immune suppression in pediatric heart transplantation: a study of long-term adverse effects. J Heart Lung Transplant 15:415, 1996.

Benkerrou M, Durandy A, Fischer A: Therapy for transplant-related lymphoproliferative diseases. Hematol Oncol Clin North Am 7:467, 1993.

Billar TR, Hanto DW, Simmons RL: Inclusion of uncomplicated infectious mononucleosis in the spectrum of Epstein-Barr virus infections in transplant recipients. Transplantation 46:159, 1988.

Cen H, Breinig MC, Atchison RW, et al: Epstein-Barr virus transmission via the donor organs in solid organ transplantation: polymerase chain reaction and restriction fragment length polymorphism analysis of IR2, IR3, and IR4. J Virol 65:976, 1991.

Cesarman E, Chadburn A, Liu YF, et al: Bcl-6 gene mutations in posttransplantation lymphoproliferative disorders (PT-LPDs) as predictors of clinical behavior [abstract]. Lab Invest 76:121A, 1997.

Chadburn A, Cesarman E, Knowles DM: Classification of post-transplantation lymphoproliferative disorders (PT-LPDs) based on morphologic and molecular genetic features has clinical relevance [abstract]. Lab Invest 76:121A, 1997.

Chadburn A, Cesarman E, YiFang L, et al: Molecular genetic analysis demonstrates that multiple posttransplant lymphoproliferative disorders occurring in one anatomic site in a single patient represent distinct primary lymphoid neoplasms. Cancer 75:2747, 1995.

Chetty R, Biddolph S, Gatter K: An immunohistochemical analysis of Reed-Sternberg–like cells in posttransplantation lymphoproliferative disorders: the possible pathogenetic relationship to Reed-Sternberg cells in Hodgkin's disease and Reed-Sternberg-like cells in non-Hodgkin's lymphomas and reactive conditions. Hum Pathol 28:493, 1997.

Chetty R, Biddolph SC, Kaklamanis L, et al: EBV latent membrane protein (LMP-1) and bcl-2 protein expression in Reed-Sternberg–like cells in post-transplant lymphoproliferative disorders. Histopathology 28:257, 1996.

Cox KL, Lawrence-Miyasaki LS, Garcia-Kennedy R, et al: An increased incidence of Epstein-Barr virus infection and lymphoproliferative disorder in young children on FK506 after liver transplantation. Transplantation 59:524, 1995.

Davey DD, Gulley ML, Walker WP, et al: Cytologic findings in post-transplant lymphoproliferative disease. Acta Cytol 34:304, 1990.

Delecluse HJ, Rouault JP, Jeammot B, et al: bcl6/Laz3 rearrangements in post-transplant lymphoproliferative disorders. Br J Haematol 91:101, 1995.

Dusenbery D, Nalesnik MA, Locker J, et al: Cytologic features of post-transplant lymphoproliferative disorder. Diagn Cytopathol 16:489, 1997.

Fairley JW, Hunt BJ, Glover GW, et al: Unusual lymphoproliferative oropharyngeal lesions in heart and heart-lung transplant recipients. J Laryngol Otol 104:720, 1990.

Frank D, Cesarman E, Liu YF, et al: Posttransplant lymphoproliferative disorders frequently contain type A and not type B Epstein-Barr virus. Blood 85:1396, 1995.

Frizzera G, Hanto DW, Gajl-Peczalska KJ, et al: Polymorphic diffuse B-cell hyperplasias and lymphomas in renal transplant recipients. Cancer Res 41:4262, 1981.

Gallego-Melcon S, de Toledo JS, Martinez V, et al: Non-Hodgkin's lymphoma after liver transplantation: response to chemotherapy. Med Pediatr Oncol 27:156, 1996.

Garnier J-L, Lebranchu Y, Dantal J, et al: Hodgkin's disease after transplantation. Transplantation 61:71, 1996.

Goyal RK, McEvoy L, Wilson DB: Hodgkin disease after renal transplantation in childhood. J Pediatr Hematol Oncol 18:392, 1996.

Gruber SA, Gillingham K, Sothern RB, et al: Cancer development in pediatric primary renal allograft recipients. Transplantation Proceedings 26:3, 1994.

Hanasono MM, Kamel OW, Chang PP, et al: Detection of Epstein-Barr virus in cardiac biopsies of heart transplant patients with lymphoproliferative disorders. Transplantation 60:471, 1995.

Harris NL, Ferry JA, Swerdlow SH: Post-transplant lymphoproliferative disorders (PTLD): Summary of Society for Hematopathology Workshop. Semin Diagn Pathol 14:8, 1997.

Harris NL, Jaffe ES, Diebold J, et al: The World Health Organization classification of neoplastic diseases of the haematopoietic and lymphoid tissues: Report of the Clinical Advisory Committee Meeting, Airlie House, Virginia, November, 1997. Histopathology 36:69, 2000.

Hjelle B, Evans-Holm M, Yen TSB, et al: A poorly differentiated lymphoma of donor origin in a renal allograft recipient. Transplantation 47:945, 1989.

Ho M, Jaffe R, Miller, et al: The frequency of Epstein-Barr virus infection and associated lymphoproliferative syndrome after transplantation and its manifestations in children. Transplantation 45:719, 1988.

Hollingsworth HC, Stetler-Stevenson M, Gagneten D, et al: Immunodeficiency-associated malignant lymphoma: three cases showing genotypic evidence of both T- and B-cell lineages. Am J Surg Pathol 18:1092, 1994.

Hudnall SD, Melez K, Galindo A, et al: Massive pseudolymphomatous pericardial effusion in the posttransplant setting mimicking posttransplant lymphoproliferative disease. Transplantation 61:1776, 1996.

Joseph G, Barker RL, Yuan B, et al: Posttransplantation plasma cell dyscrasias. Cancer 74:1959, 1994.

Katz BZ, Raab-Traub N, Miller G: Latent and replicating forms of Epstein-Barr virus DNA in lymphomas and lymphoproliferative diseases. J Infect Dis 160:589, 1989.

Kenagy DN, Schlesinger Y, Weck K, et al: Epstein-Barr virus DNA in peripheral blood leukocytes of patients with posttransplant lymphoproliferative disease. Transplantation 60:547, 1995.

Kingma DW, Shad A, Tsokos M, et al: Epstein-Barr virus (EBV)–associated smooth-muscle tumor arising in a post-transplant patient treated successfully for two PT-EBV–associated large-cell lymphomas. Am J Surg Pathol 20:1511, 1996.

Knowles DM, Cesarman E, Chadburn A, et al: Correlative morphologic and molecular genetic analysis demonstrates three distinct categories of posttransplantation lymphoproliferative disorders. Blood 85:552, 1995.

Lamy ME, Favart AM, Cornu C, et al: Epstein-Barr virus infection in 59 orthotopic liver transplant patients. Medical Microbiol Immunol 179:137, 1990.

Leblond V, Sutton L, Dorent R, et al: Lymphoproliferative disorders after organ transplantation: a report of 24 cases observed in a single center. J Clin Oncol 13:961, 1995.

Lee ES, Locker J, Nalesnik M, et al: The association of Epstein-Barr virus with smooth-muscle tumors occurring after organ transplantation. N Engl J Med 332:19, 1995.

Locker J, Nalesnik M: Molecular genetic analysis of lymphoid tumors arising after organ transplantation. Am J Pathol 135:977, 1989.

Lones MA, Mishalani S, Shintaku IP, et al: Changes in tonsils and adenoids in children with posttransplant lymphoproliferative disorder: report of three cases with early involvement of Waldeyer's ring. Hum Pathol 26:525, 1995.

Lones MA, Shintaku IP, Weiss LM, et al: Posttransplant lymphoproliferative disorder in liver allograft biopsies: a comparison of three methods for the demonstration of Epstein-Barr virus. Hum Pathol 28:533, 1997.

Macon WR, Williams ME, Greer JP, et al: Natural killer–like T-cell lymphomas: aggressive lymphomas of T–large granular lymphocytes. Blood 87:1474, 1996.

Malatack JJ, Gartner JC, Urbach AH, et al: Orthotopic liver transplantation, Epstein-Barr virus, cyclosporine, and lymphoproliferative disease: a growing concern. J Pediatr 118:667, 1991.

Mathur A, Kamat DM, Filipovich AH, et al: Immunoregulatory abnormalities in patients with Epstein-Barr virus–associated B cell lymphoproliferative disorders. Transplantation 57:1042, 1994.

Miklos JA, Locker J, Bahler DW: Evidence for antigen selection in posttransplant lymphoproliferative disorders [abstract]. Lab Invest 8:116A, 1995.

Montone KT, Hodinka RL, Salhany, et al: Identification of Epstein-Barr virus lytic activity in post-transplantation lymphoproliferative disease. Mod Pathol 9:621, 1996.

Mori M, Kurozumi H, Akagi K, et al: Monoclonal proliferation of T cells containing Epstein-Barr virus in fatal mononucleosis. N Engl J Med 327: 1992.

Morrissey PE, Lorber KM, Marcarelli M, et al: Posttransplant Epstein-Barr virus infection is associated with elevated levels of CD19+ B lymphocytes. Transplantation 59:637, 1995.

Murray PG, Swinnen IJ, Constandinou CM, et al: bcl-2 but not its Epstein-Barr virus–encoded homologue, BHRF1, is commonly expressed in posttransplantation lymphoproliferative disorders. Blood 87:706, 1996.
Nalesnik MA: Posttransplantation lymphoproliferative disorders (PTLD): current perspectives. Semin Thorac Cardiovasc Surg 8:139, 1996.
Nalesnik MA, Jaffe R, Starzl TE, et al: The pathology of posttransplant lymphoproliferative disorders occurring in the setting of cyclosporine A–prednisone immunosuppression. Am J Pathol 133: 173, 1988.
Nalesnik MA, Rao AS, Furukawa H, et al: Autologous lymphokine-activated killer cell therapy of Epstein-Barr virus–positive and –negative lymphoproliferative disorders arising in organ transplant recipients. Transplantation 63:1200, 1997.
Nalesnik MA, Starzl TE: Epstein-Barr virus, infectious mononucleosis, and posttransplant lymphoproliferative disorders. Transplantation Science 4:61, 1994.
Nelson BN, Nalesnik MA, Locker JD, et al: Posttransplant lymphoproliferative disorders (PTLD) in the adult: the Pittsburgh experience [abstract]. Lab Invest 76:131A, 1997.
Nelson BP, Locker J, Nalesnik MA, et al: Clonal and morphologic variation in a posttransplant lymphoproliferative disorder: evolution from clonal T-cell to clonal B-cell predominance. Hum Pathol 1997.
Nelson BP, Nalesnik MA, Bahler DW, et al: Epstein-Barr virus–negative post-transplant lymphoproliferative disorders: a distinct entity? Am J Surg Pathol 24:375, 2000.
Newell KA, Alonso EM, Whitington PF, et al: Posttransplant lymphoproliferative disease in pediatric liver transplantation. Transplantation 62:370, 1996.
Osterhage DA, Steele PE, Witte D, et al: T cells in posttransplant lymphoproliferative disorders (PTLD): an immunophenotypic and genotypic investigation. Lab Invest 66:85A, 1992.
Papadopoulos EB, Ladanyi M, Emanuel E: Infusions of donor leukocytes to treat Epstein-Barr virus–associated lymphoproliferative disorders after allogeneic bone marrow transplantation. N Engl J Med 330:1185, 1994.
Patton DF, Wilkowski CW, Hanson CA, et al: Epstein-Barr virus–determined clonality in posttransplant lymphoproliferative disease. Transplantation 49:1080, 1990.
Penn I: De novo malignancy in pediatric organ transplant recipients. J Pediatr Surg 29:221, 1994a.
Penn I: Posttransplant malignancies in pediatric organ transplant recipients. Transplant Proc 26:2763, 1994b.
Putnam P, Reyes J, Kocoshis S, et al: Gastrointestinal posttransplant lymphoproliferative disease in children after small intestinal transplantation. Transplant Proc 28:2777, 1996.
Radl J, Valentijn RM, Haaijman JJ, et al: Monoclonal gammopathies in patients undergoing immunosuppressive treatment after renal transplantation. Clin Immunol Immunopathol 37:98, 1985.
Randhawa P, Demetris AJ, Pietrzak B, et al: Histopathology of renal posttransplant lymphoproliferation: comparison with rejection using the Banff schema. Am J Kid Dis 28:578, 1996.
Randhawa PS, Jaffe R, Demetris AJ, et al: Expression of Epstein-Barr virus–encoded small RNA (by the EBER-1 gene) in liver specimens from transplant recipients with post-transplantation lymphoproliferative disease. N Engl J Med 327:1710, 1992.
Randhawa PS, Jaffe R, Demetris AJ, et al: The systemic distribution of Epstein-Barr virus genomes in fatal post-transplantation lymphoproliferative disorders: an in situ hybridization study. Am J Pathol 138:1027, 1991.
Razzouk BI, Srinivas S, Sample CE, et al: Epstein-Barr virus DNA recombination and loss in sporadic Burkitt's lymphoma. J Infect Dis 173:529, 1996.
Reyes J, Green M, Bueno J, et al: Epstein Barr virus associated posttransplant lymphoproliferative disease after intestinal transplantation. Transplant Proc 28:2768, 1996.
Reyes J, Tzakis A, Green M, et al: Posttransplant lymphoproliferative disorders occurring under primary FK506 immunosuppression. Transplant Proc 23:3044, 1991.
Riddler SA, Breinig MC, McKnight JLC: Increased levels of circulating Epstein-Barr virus (EBV)–infected lymphocytes and decreased EBV nuclear antigen antibody responses are associated with the development of posttransplant lymphoproliferative disease in solid-organ transplant recipients. Blood 84:972, 1994.
Rizkalla KS, Asfar SK, McLean CA, et al: Key features distinguishing post-transplantation lymphoproliferative disorders and acute liver rejection. Mod Pathol 10:708, 1997.
Robinson R, Murray PI, Willshaw HE, et al: Primary ocular posttransplant lymphoproliferative disease. J Pediatr Ophthalmol Strabismus 393, 1995.
Rooney CM, Loftin SK, Holladay MS, et al: Early identification of Epstein-Barr virus–associated post-transplantation lymphoproliferative disease. Br J Haematol 89:98, 1995a.
Rooney CM, Smith CA, Heslop HE: Control of virus-induced lymphoproliferation: Epstein-Barr virus–induced lymphoproliferation and host immunity. Mol Med 3:23, 1997.
Rooney CM, Smith CA, Ng CYC, et al: Use of gene-modified virus-specific T lymphocytes to control Epstein-Barr-virus–related lymphoproliferation. Lancet 345:9, 1995b.
Rosendale B, Yousem SA: Discrimination of Epstein-Barr virus–related posttransplant lymphoproliferations from acute rejection in lung allograft recipients. Arch Pathol Lab Med 119:418, 1995.
Rowe DT, Qu L, Reyes J, et al: Use of quantitative competitive PCR to measure Epstein-Barr virus genome load in the peripheral blood of pediatric transplant patients with lymphoproliferative disorders. J Clin Microbiol 35:1612, 1997.
Sculerati N, Arriaga M: Otolaryngologic management of posttransplant lymphoproliferative disease in children. Ann Otol Rhinol Laryngol 99:445, 1990.
Seiden MV, Sklar J: Molecular genetic analysis of post-transplant lymphoproliferative disorders. Hematol Oncol Clin North Am 7:447, 1993.
Shapiro RS, McClain K, Frizzera G, et al: Epstein-Barr virus associated B cell lymphoproliferative disorders following bone marrow transplantation. Blood 71:1234, 1988.
Shapiro R, Scantlebury VP, Jordan ML, et al: Tacrolimus in pediatric renal transplantation. Transplantation 62:1752, 1996.
Smir BN, Greiner TC, Weisenburger DD: Multicentric angiofollicular lymph node hyperplasia in children: a clinicopathologic study of eight patients. Mod Pathol 9:1135, 1996.
Swerdlow SH: Classification of the posttransplant lymphoproliferative disorders: from the past to the present. Semin Diagn Pathol 14:2, 1997a.
Swerdlow SH: Posttransplant lymphoproliferative disorders: a working classification. Curr Diagn Pathol 4:29, 1997b.
Swinnen LJ, Mullen GM, Carr TJ, et al: Aggressive treatment for post-cardiac transplant lymphoproliferation. Blood 86:3333, 1995.
Waller EK, Ziemianska M, Bangs CD, et al: Characterization of posttransplant lymphomas that express T-cell–associated markers: immunophenotypes, molecular genetics, cytogenetics, and heterotransplantation in severe combined immunodeficient mice. Blood 82:247, 1993.
Weissmann DJ, Ferry JA, Harris NL, et al: Posttransplantation lymphoproliferative disorders in solid organ recipients are predominantly aggressive tumors of host origin. Am J Clin Pathol 103:748, 1995.
White FV, Reyes J, Jaffe R, et al: Pathology of intestinal transplantation in children. Am J Surg Pathol 19:687, 1995.
Wu T-T, Swerdlow SH, Locker J, et al: Recurrent Epstein-Barr-virus associated lesions in organ transplant recipients. Hum Pathol 27:157, 1996.
Zutter MM, Durnam DM, Hackman RC, et al: Secondary T-cell lymphoproliferation after marrow transplantation. Am J Clin Pathol 94:714, 1990.
Zutter MM, Martin PJ, Sale GE, et al: Epstein-Barr virus lymphoproliferation after bone marrow transplantation. Blood 72:520, 1988.

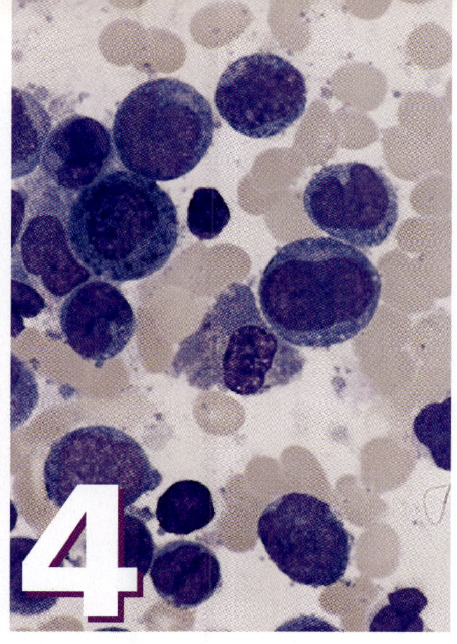

Kathy Foucar
Catherine Leith

Acute Leukemias

DEFINITIONS

Acute leukemias are hematolymphoid malignancies that arise from marrow precursor stem cells and are characterized by the loss of normal hematopoiesis as well as the predominance of immature cells in the marrow (Gale & Linch, 1998). Leukemias are classified by the state of differentiation of the predominant cell. Since acute myelogenous leukemia (AML) is derived from multipotential progenitor cells, multilineage differentiation may be present. Acute lymphoblastic leukemia (ALL) is derived from B or T lymphocyte progenitors.

EPIDEMIOLOGY AND OVERVIEW OF ACUTE LEUKEMIA

Acute leukemia may occur at any age and is even evident in neonates at a rate of 1 in 5 million births (Pui et al, 1995b). Eighty percent of childhood acute leukemias are ALL in type, whereas 80 percent of adult leukemias are AML. These acute leukemias have a prevalence of 2 to 3 cases per 100,000 population, although the incidence of AML increases substantially in the elderly (Gurney et al, 1997; Lange, 1995; Pui et al, 1995b). Various constitutional disorders are linked to an increased incidence of pediatric acute leukemia, most notably Down syndrome. Pediatric AML is increased in patients with neurofibromatosis, Bloom syndrome, and Fanconi syndrome and in monozygotic twins (Bhatia & Neglia, 1995; Cavenagh et al, 1996; Weinstein, 1996; Zack et al, 1991). Occupational exposures and paternal smoking (maternal smoking risk is less clear-cut) are also risk factors for pediatric acute leukemia (Bhatia & Neglia 1995; Pasqualetti et al, 1997; Sorahan et al, 1997).

The incidence of acute leukemia is 20 times higher in children with Down syndrome. Myelogenous leukemias, especially acute megakaryoblastic leukemia, predominate in children with Down syndrome under 4 years of age, whereas ALL predominates in those over 4 years of age (Horwitz, 1997). Compared to unaffected children, the incidence of acute megakaryoblastic leukemia is 500 times greater in infants and toddlers with Down syndrome (see "Acute Leukemia in Down Syndrome Patients") (Creutzig et al, 1996; Horwitz, 1997; Lange et al, 1998; Robison, 1992). AML is also clearly attributable to prior chemotherapy, especially alkylating agents and topoisomerase II inactivator therapy (see "Therapy-Induced AML").

GENERAL FEATURES OF ACUTE LEUKEMIA

Virtually all patients with acute leukemia present with marrow insufficiency or failure when the marrow is extensively infiltrated. Resultant cytopenias are manifest at diagnosis as profound normocytic normochromic anemia, thrombocytopenia, and neutropenia (Fig. 4–1). In some patients the thrombocytopenia is exacerbated by disseminated intravascular coagulation (DIC) which is especially prominent in patients with acute promyelocytic leukemia (APL) but also occurs infrequently in patients with acute monocytic leukemia. The white blood cell (WBC) count is highly variable in patients with acute leukemia and is a key prognostic factor in ALL. A low or normal WBC count is common in many good-risk pediatric ALL patients, whereas leukocytosis is seen in poor-risk ALL, such as neonatal and T lymphocyte ALL (T-ALL). Leukopenia is also typical of common-type APL and erythroleukemia, whereas pronounced leukocytosis characterizes many acute monocytic leukemias (Fig. 4–2) and the microgranular variant of APL.

Myeloblastic sarcomas (extramedullary tumorous masses) may develop in any location. Skin lesions are particularly common in acute monocytic leukemia, especially in neonates and infants (see "Extramedullary Disease"). Infiltrates of the gums (Fig. 4–3), nodes, and central nervous system (CNS) are common in patients with acute monocytic leukemia, likely reflecting the natural propensity of monocytic cells to migrate to solid tissues. Extramedullary manifestations are also common in ALL. In ALL patients, lymphadenopathy and hepatosplenomegaly are common at presentation, whereas relapses often involve the CNS and testes.

HISTORICAL PERSPECTIVES

Leukemia was initially recognized approximately 150 years ago by gross pathologic features at autopsy and the distinctive pus-like appearance of the blood. Medical historians now believe that the two patients initially described in 1847 as having acute leukemia actually had chronic myelogenous leukemia and chronic lymphocytic leukemia (Piller, 1993). During this premicroscopic era, acute and chronic leukemias were distinguished by survival time, whereas splenic and lymphatic forms were identified by the distribution of disease at autopsy. The first antemortem diagnosis of leukemia was made in 1876 by examination of unstained blood and marrow aspirate preparations (Henderson, 1996). In 1877, Romanovsky-type staining methods allowed a clear distinction between the nucleus and

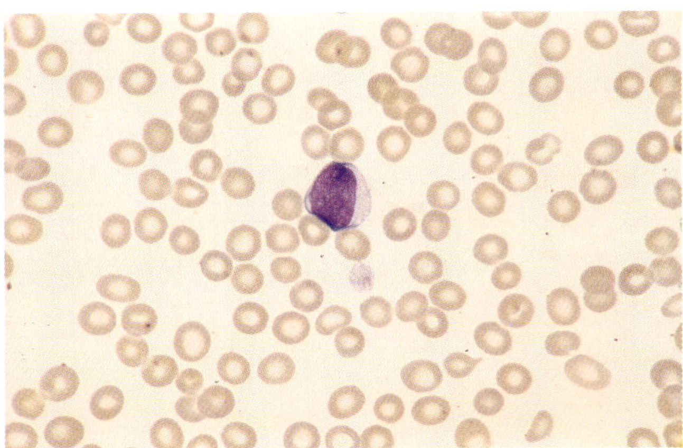

Figure 4–1

Acute leukemia, peripheral blood. This medium-power photomicrograph illustrates the striking pancytopenia that is characteristic in most cases of acute leukemia. Note the reduced number of platelets and erythrocytes and the lack of neutrophils within this field. A single blast is present. Wright stain.

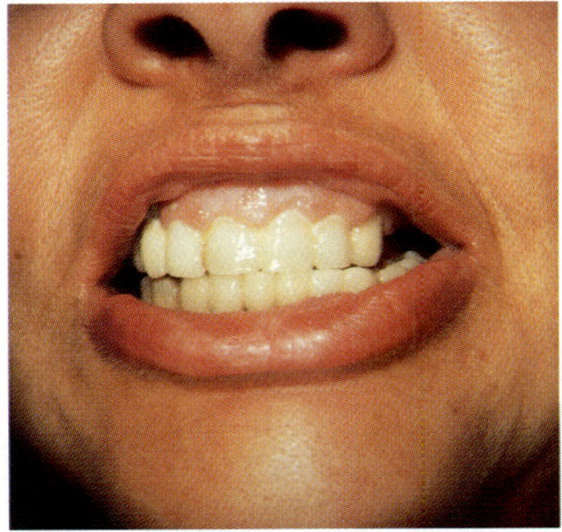

Figure 4–3

Acute monocytic leukemia. Leukemic infiltration of the gums is apparent in this young adult. (Courtesy Dr. J. Saiki.)

the cytoplasm of a cell (Fig. 4–4) (Piller, 1993). This advance prompted separation of WBCs into lymphocytic and myelocytic lineages, with subsequent proposals of stages of maturation within each lineage. In the early 1900s, morphologic descriptions of myeloblasts and lymphoblasts were published, followed shortly by descriptions of acute leukemias made up of these blastic elements. In addition to these advances in the morphologic and cytologic classification of leukemias, the early 1900s saw the development of the initial cytochemical techniques providing substantial data for lineage determination. In 1976 the first comprehensive classification system for acute leukemias was proposed by the French-American-British (FAB) Cooperative Group (Bennett et al, 1976). This system is still used worldwide, although recent progress has highlighted some limitations and deficiencies of this classification.

IDENTIFICATION OF LEUKEMIC CELLS

Leukemia diagnosis is based on determination of the phenotype and the stage of maturation of an abnormal infiltrate, usually within the blood or marrow but occasionally in extramedullary sites. Acute leukemia is diagnosed by establishing an immature (i.e., blastic) stage of maturation and identifying the predominant cell lineage (lymphocytic versus myelocytic). The modalities most useful in establishing lineage are morphologic studies, cytochemical analysis, and immunophenotyping (ideally, multicolor flow cytometric analysis), whereas the optimal methods for establishing the stage of maturation (i.e., blast versus nonblast) are morphologic studies and immunophenotyping (Table 4–1). Although variable from lineage to lineage, the morphologic features of blasts include dispersed chromatin with variably prominent nucleoli and sparse, if any, cytoplasmic granules or other features of differentiation (Fig. 4–5). By multiparameter immunophenotypic analysis, the stage of maturation is determined by assessment for expression of antigens that normally characterize immature cells within a given lineage. These antigens include CD34 and terminal deoxynucleotidyltransferase (TdT), which identify myelocytic and lymphocytic precursors, respectively, and CD1, which is a feature of immature T cells (Fig. 4–6). The broad multilineage properties of CD34, the so-called progenitor cell antigen, make it the most useful of these markers.

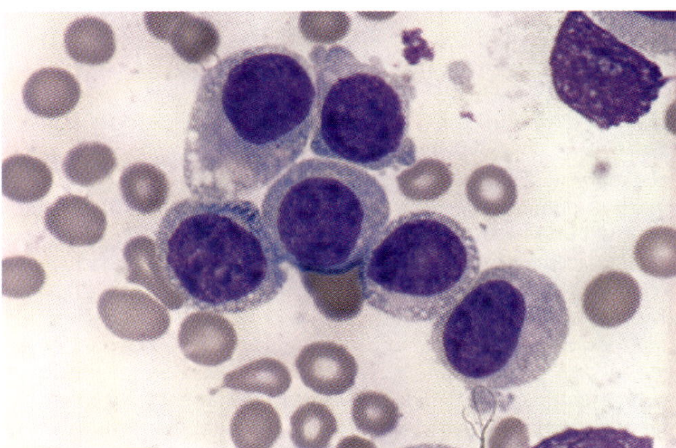

Figure 4–2

Acute monoblastic leukemia, peripheral blood. A striking leukocytosis (WBC >300,000/μl) is evident in this patient. Wright stain.

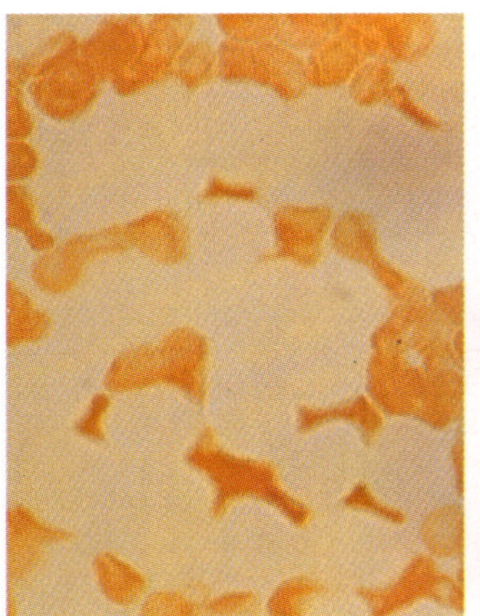

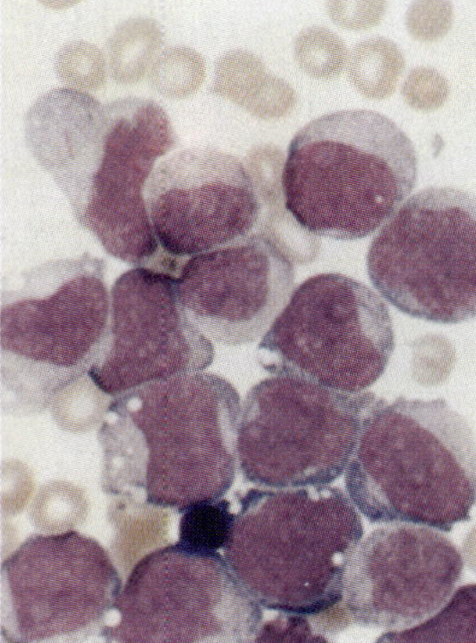

Figure 4–4

Acute leukemia, comparison of blasts in unstained and stained preparations. In unstained preparations (compare with the adjacent Wright-stained specimen), there is no clear distinction between nuclei and cytoplasm.

Table 4–1
Methods for Characterizing Leukemic Cells

Phenotypic Properties
Morphologic
Cytochemical
Immunophenotypic

Genotypic Properties
Cytogenetic
Molecular

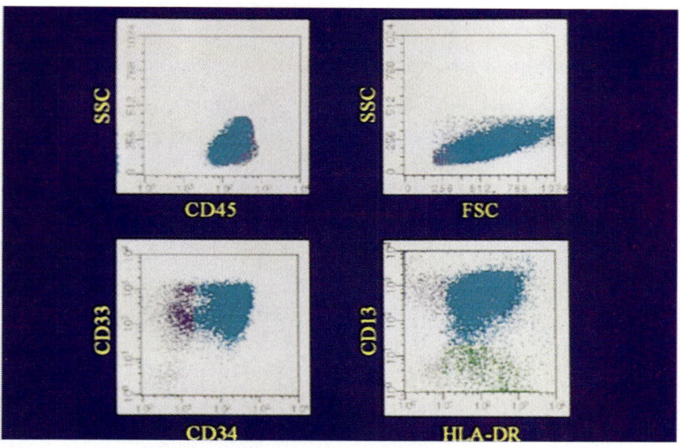

Figure 4–6

AML, flow cytometry. This composite of a flow cytometric histogram illustrates a population of blasts with weak CD45 expression and co-expression of CD33, CD13, CD34, and HLA-DR. Forward and side scatter of the blast population are also illustrated.

Cytogenetic and molecular techniques have been investigated as ways to define the genotypic features of acute leukemia (see Table 4–1). Currently, genotypic characteristics may be used to establish the diagnosis of some specific subsets of acute leukemia. In the past, these methods have most often been utilized for prognostication, assignment of biologic properties, and detection of minimal residual disease.

Morphologic Evaluation

The recognition of acute leukemia and classification of the subtypes of AML and ALL is dependent on the morphologic evaluation of blood and marrow aspirate films, imprints, clot, and biopsy sections (Table 4–2) (Foucar, 1995a; Foucar, 1995b; Taylor et al, 1996). The accurate identification of immature cells is a critical part of the process of diagnosing acute leukemia; specific blast percentages are prominent as diagnostic criteria in the FAB classification (see "Approach to the Diagnosis and Classification of Acute Leukemias") but such percentages may be viewed as problematic and arbitrary. In practice, the total picture of a case is more useful than an arbitrary blast percentage in distinguishing acute leukemia from myelodysplasia. The blasts that must be identified in blood and marrow films or imprint preparations include myeloblasts, monoblasts, erythroblasts, megakaryoblasts, and lymphoblasts (Fig. 4–7). In many AML cases, cells may have differentiated beyond the blast stage, and promyelocytes and promonocytes are often included within the "blast" population for differential cell counts (Fig. 4–8). For example, promyelocytes predominate in acute promyelocytic leukemia, and blasts are scant. In most cases of acute myelogenous leukemia, marrows contain >30% blasts, but cases of AML with t(8;21) are characterized by significant myelocytic maturation. In such cases the blast count may be <30%. In erythroleukemia the myeloblast percentage may be low at presentation because of the large number of immature erythrocyte precursors. It should be noted that maturation may be evident in AML, but the mature neutrophils are often dyspoietic and poorly functional (Fig. 4–9).

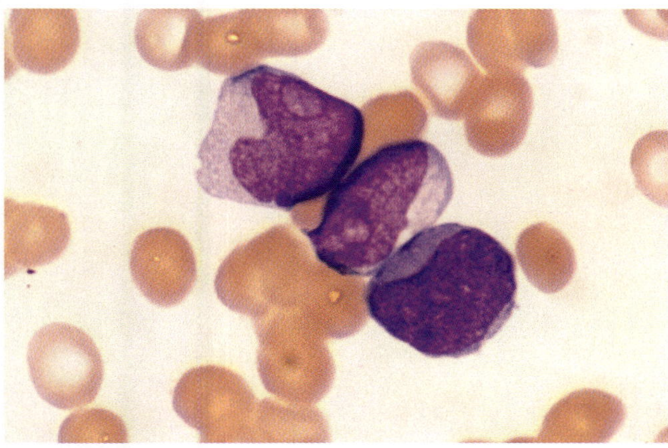

Figure 4–5

AML. Characteristic morphologic features of myeloblasts include dispersed chromatin, variably prominent nucleoli, and lack of cytoplasmic differentiation. Wright stain.

In contrast to AML, the blood and marrow in most cases of ALL contain a striking predominance of blasts (Fig. 4–10). In patients with extensive extramedullary infiltrates of lymphoblasts, an arbitrary distinction between lymphoblastic or Burkitt lymphoma and ALL may be based on the percentage of marrow blasts. Cases with >25% marrow blasts are likely to be ALL, while those cases with <25% marrow lymphoblasts are more likely to be stage IV lymphoma (Foucar, 1995a; Taylor, 1996).

Cases of AML demonstrate a highly variable appearance on marrow biopsy sections. Some cases exhibit a monomorphic infiltrate of a single cell type that completely effaces the marrow architecture, whereas others demonstrate a more heterogeneous appearance with multilineage abnormalities (Figs. 4–11 and 4–12). The proportion of blasts is also variable, reflecting the wide range of blast percentages in cases classified as AML. Fibrosis may be evident in some cases of AML, especially therapy-induced and acute megakaryoblastic leukemias (see Fig. 4–12). Necrosis may occasionally be evident on marrow biopsy sections in AML but is more common in cases of ALL. Marrow sections in AML are generally hypercellular, but hypocellular subtypes have been described, particularly in the elderly. In these cases, identification of immature myelocytic elements may be challenging and often requires special studies to confirm the diagnosis (Fig. 4–13).

In contrast, marrow biopsy sections are typically markedly hypercellular, with a striking predominance of lymphoblasts in cases of common-type ALL (Fig. 4–14). Occasionally, a normal hematopoietic lineage, most notably megakaryocytes, may be preserved. In sections, the nuclei of the lymphoblasts are generally closely spaced and round to convoluted, and exhibit finely dispersed, stippled chromatin (Fig. 4–15). Mitotic activity may be brisk, and tingible body macrophages are sometimes evident, although a "starry sky" pattern is infrequent in common-type ALL. In Burkitt lymphoma/ALL-L3, the blasts

Table 4–2
Morphologic Features of Blasts and Other Immature Cells

Type of Cell	Key Morphologic Features
Myeloblast	Large nucleus with finely dispersed chromatin and variably prominent nucleoli Moderately high nuclear-cytoplasmic ratio Variable number of cytoplasmic granules
Promyelocyte	Nuclear chromatin slightly condensed; nucleoli variably prominent; nucleus often eccentric and Golgi zone may be apparent Numerous cytoplasmic granules In APL intense cytoplasmic granularity usually present and nuclear configuration variable; in micrograular variant of APL, nuclear folding and lobulation characteristic
Monoblast	Moderate to low nuclear-cytoplasmic ratio; nuclear chromatin finely dispersed, with variably prominent nucleoli; nuclei round to folded Abundant, slightly basophilic cytoplasm containing fine granulation and occasional vacuoles
Promonocyte	Slightly condensed nuclear chromatin; variably prominent nucleoli Abundant, finely granular, blue-gray cytoplasm that may be vacuolated Very monocytic appearance, with nuclear immaturity
Erythroblast	Moderately high nuclear-cytoplasmic ratio Nucleus round with slightly condensed chromatin; nucleoli variably prominent Moderate amounts of deeply basophilic cytoplasm that may be vacuolated
Megakaryoblast	Highly variable morphologic features, often not recognizable without special studies May resemble lymphoblasts, with high nuclear-cytoplasmic ratio Nuclear chromatin fine to variably condensed Cytoplasm may be scant to moderate; usually agranular or with a few granules Possible cytoplasmic blebbing or budding may be present Possible cohesive clumps of blasts
Lymphoblast	High nuclear-cytoplasmic ratio, with scant to moderate amounts of agranular cytoplasm Variable nuclear convolutions, with dispersed chromatin and variably prominent nucleoli Blasts often small but variable in size
Burkitt leukemia/lymphoma	Moderate amount of deeply basophilic cytoplasm, with abundant distinct vacuoles Nuclear chromatin dispersed and homogeneous, with one or more generally indistinct nucleoli Blasts medium to large

Abbreviation: APL, acute promyelocytic leukemia.

on tissue sections are homogeneous and have round nuclear contours with one to three small basophilic nucleoli. Brisk mitotic activity and numerous tingible body macrophages may impart to marrow sections a starry sky appearance similar to that seen in other tissues affected by Burkitt lymphoma (Fig. 4–16).

Biopsy sections in ALL less commonly show reticulin fibrosis, necrosis, and bony abnormalities, such as osteoporosis or osteopenia (Ribeiro et al, 1988; Wallis & Reid, 1989). Mild reticulin fibrosis is present in a small proportion of cases of ALL and prevents marrow aspiration. Other than technical problems in specimen acquisition, reticulin fibrosis in ALL has no recognized special significance. Marrow necrosis is identified in approximately 1% of ALL marrow biopsy specimens. In these cases, the entire hematopoietic tissue between the bony trabeculae may be necrotic (Fig. 4–17). In rare circumstances,

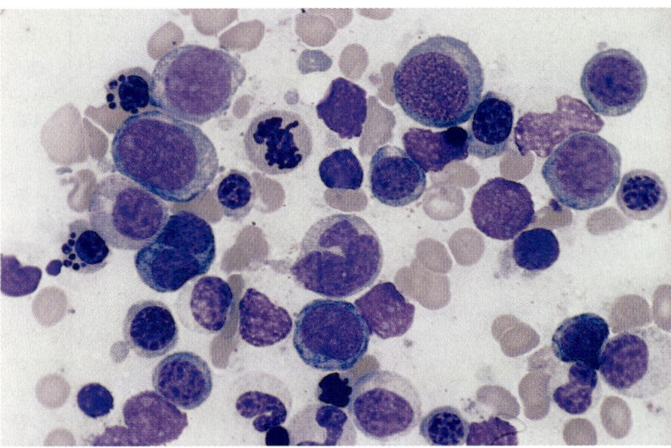

Figure 4–7

Multilineage acute leukemia, marrow aspirate. This film shows various forms, including immature myelocytic and erythrocytic elements. Wright stain.

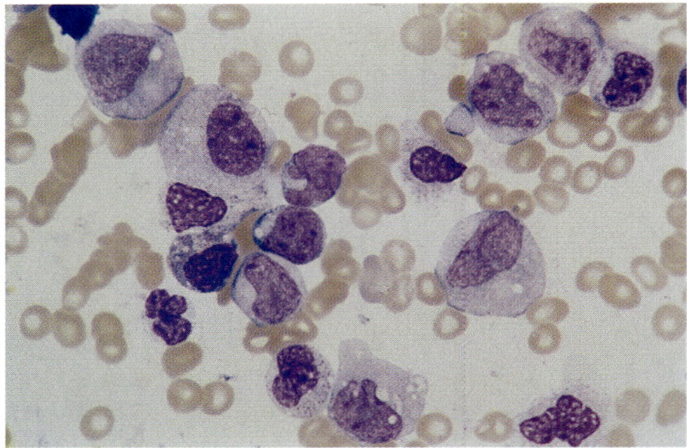

Figure 4–8

Acute monocytic leukemia, marrow aspirate. This specimen from a 4-year-old child contains blasts and immature monocytes. Wright stain.

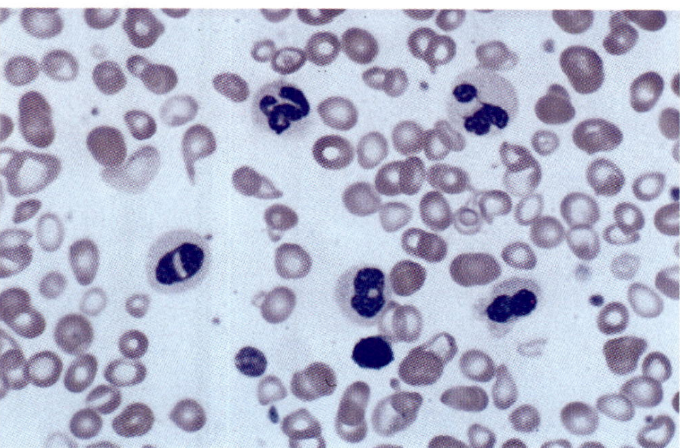

Figure 4–9

AML, peripheral blood. This film illustrates striking dyspoietic changes in mature neutrophils in a patient with AML arising from a myelodysplastic syndrome. Wright stain.

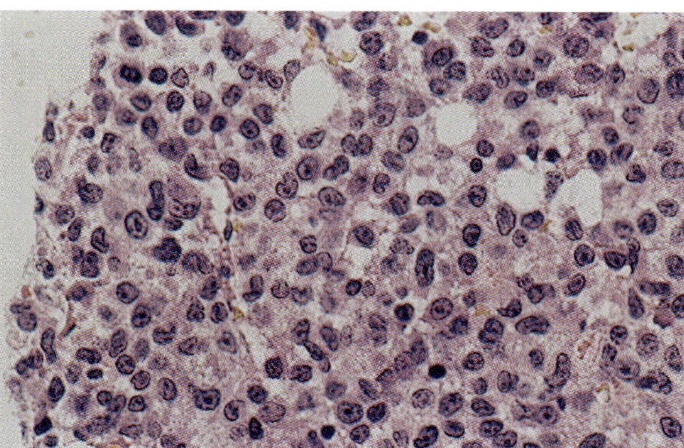

Figure 4–11

Acute monocytic leukemia, marrow biopsy. This high-magnification photomicrograph illustrates a monotonous infiltrate of uniform-appearing blasts that have abundant cytoplasm.

the bony trabeculae are also necrotic and show loss of osteocytes within lacunar spaces. The ghosts of necrotic lymphoblasts may be apparent within the eosinophilic necrotic debris that fills the marrow cavity. Extensive marrow necrosis may interfere with routine and specialized studies on the leukemia clone, but the blood may generally contain sufficient viable leukemia cells for diagnostic studies. Bony abnormalities are fairly common in childhood ALL. Osteoporosis (osteopenia) may be so pronounced that these children have severe bone pain or compression fractures. In these patients, bony trabeculae may be thin, and calcium levels are typically increased, indicating excess bone resorption. Complete resolution of bony abnormalities occurs after successful induction chemotherapy.

Cytochemical Evaluation

Immunophenotyping has generally superceded cytochemical analysis for classification of acute leukemias, but cytochemical stains are useful in subcategorizing cases of AML (Hayhoe, 1984; Li & Yam, 1987) (Table 4–3 and Fig. 4–18). In contrast, no specific cytochemical profile is diagnostic of ALL (see Table 4–3).

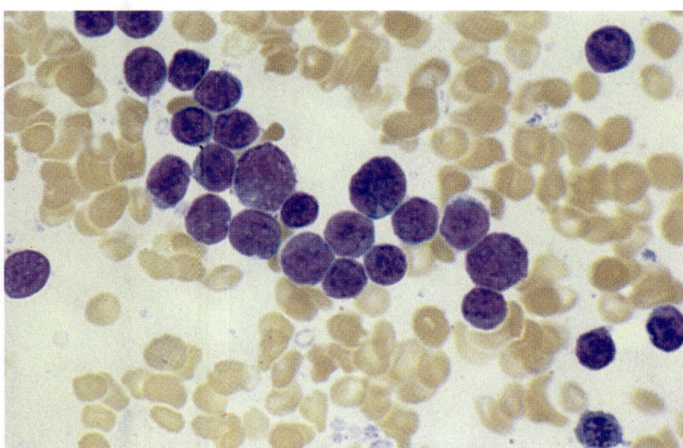

Figure 4–10

ALL, marrow aspirate. This film from a 5-year-old boy shows a monotonous population of lymphoblasts exhibiting a high nuclear-to-cytoplasm ratio, inconspicuous nucleoli, and scant cytoplasm. Wright stain.

Myeloperoxidase and chloroacetate esterase stains reveal enzymes, whereas sudan black B detects lipid in immature granulocytic elements. Despite the usefulness of the stains in identifying myeloblasts, Sudan black B and chloroacetate esterase positivity have been described in rare cases of ALL, particularly in cases of granular ALL (Cerezo et al, 1991; Keifer et al, 1985). Monocyte precursors may rarely exhibit very weak positivity for myeloperoxidase, Sudan black B, and chloroacetate esterase. Cytochemical demonstration of monocytic differentiation is largely determined by nonspecific esterase stains using either α-naphthylacetate or α-naphthylbutyrate substrates (see Fig. 4–18). Monocytic cells exhibit a variably intense diffuse cytoplasmic reaction pattern, whereas granulocytic cells may occasionally be very weakly positive. Megakaryoblasts may exhibit strong α-naphthylacetate esterase positivity that, unlike the monocytic reaction pattern, is both granular in appearance and sodium fluoride resistant. Megakaryoblasts generally lack α-naphthylbutyrate reactivity, further facilitating their distinction from monoblasts.

Periodic acid–Schiff (PAS) stains do not establish lineage, but certain patterns of PAS reactivity are characteristic of the various immature cell populations. For example, large granules and globules of cytoplasmic PAS positivity are common in both lymphoblasts of ALL and neoplastic erythroblasts. In erythroleukemia, maturing erythrocyte precursors often exhibit diffuse cytoplasmic PAS positivity, a pattern of abnormal PAS staining that may distinguish neoplastic from reactive erythrocyte precursors. A similar pattern of granular and globular PAS positivity may also occasionally be identified in megakaryoblasts, whereas weak, diffuse cytoplasmic positivity is common in granulocytic and monocytic precursors.

There is no cytochemical profile that is diagnostic of ALL, in contrast to the situation with granulocytic and monocytic leukemias (McKenna et al, 1979). All cytochemical patterns found in ALL cells overlap with those found in other leukemias, although some cytochemical staining patterns are characteristic of two subtypes of ALL (see Table 4–3). Block and globular PAS positivity is prominent in lymphoblasts (Fig. 4–19). ALL-L3/Burkitt lymphoblasts are distinct in exhibiting intense, diffuse cytoplasmic methyl green pyroninophilia, whereas the numerous cytoplasmic vacuoles (containing lipidlike material) are oil red O positive.

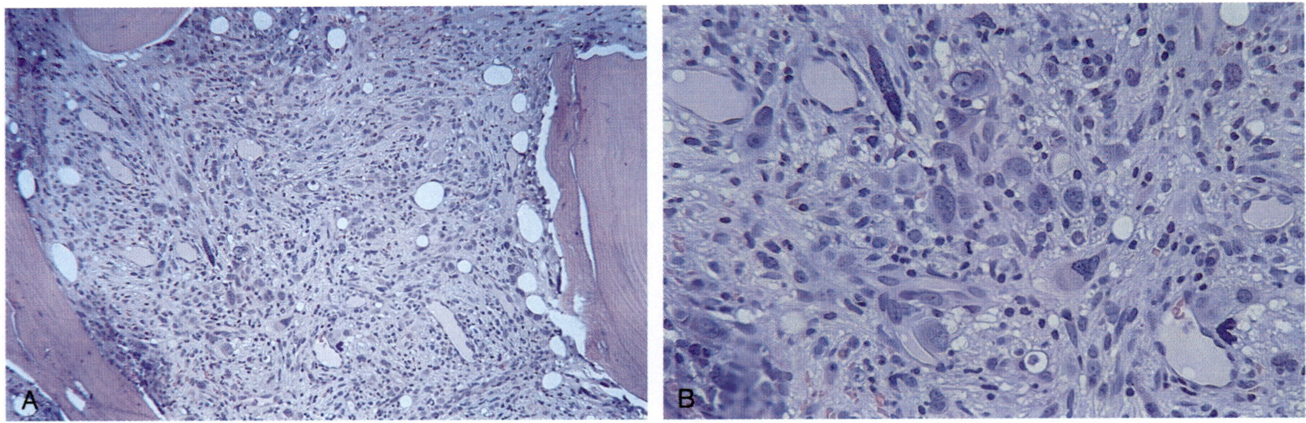

Figure 4–12

Acute megakaryoblastic leukemia, marrow biopsy. *A*. This low-magnification photomicrograph illustrates striking fibrosis and architectural distortion. *B*. At high magnification dysplastic megakaryoblasts and fibrosis are noted.

Immunophenotypic Evaluation

Various analyses may be performed on leukemic cells using flow cytometric techniques (Table 4–4). The simultaneous detection of three or more surface antigens by flow cytometric analysis facilitates assigning both lineage and stage of maturation in leukemia (Borowitz et al, 1993a; Davis et al, 1997; Traweek, 1993) (Tables 4–5 and 4–6). A panel of antibodies is required for the evaluation of cases of acute leukemia (see Table 4–6), since single antibodies do not identify adequately stage of maturation and lineage (Davis et al, 1997; Stewart et al, 1997). The immunophenotypic profile of a neoplastic population may then be compared with established antigen expression profiles of normal myelocytic and lymphocytic elements (Jennings & Foon, 1997; Rothe & Schmitz, 1996) (see Table 4–5). The DNA content of lymphoblasic leukemia cells may be measured by standard flow cytometric techniques, providing important prognostic information related to diploid, hypodiploid, or hyperdiploid subtypes of ALL. Flow cytometric techniques have been applied in drug resistance studies of acute leukemia cases to assess expression of surface antigens such as MDR1 (p-glycoprotein) and in evaluation for efflux of fluorescent dyes. This assessment of surface antigens along with efflux dyes may be used to identify cases of ALL unlikely to respond to certain chemotherapeutic modalities.

CD34, the so-called progenitor antigen, is expressed on normal cells and the most immature cells of all lineages in many acute leukemias, a feature that may distinguish these acute leukemias from marrow neoplasms in which maturation has occurred (Casasnovas et al, 1998; Creutzig et al, 1995; Khalidi et al, 1998; Lacombe et al, 1997; Sperling et al, 1995). CD13, CD33, and CD4 are expressed by immature myelocytic elements, including myeloblasts, promyelocytes, monoblasts, some promonocytes, and, occasionally, megakaryoblasts (Fig. 4–20 and Table 4–5). Cytoplasmic myeloperoxidase expression is a sensitive marker of early granulocytic maturation, whereas either glycophorin A or CD41 expression is unique to erythroblasts or megakaryoblasts. (see Table 4–5). If suspensions of viable leukemic cells are not available, antigens such as CD34, TdT, myeloperoxidase, hemoglobin A, and several B and T cell antigens may be detected in sections by immunoperoxidase techniques (Byrd et al, 1995; Quintanilla-Martinez et al, 1995; Roth et al, 1995; Soslow et al, 1997; Traweek, 1993) (Table 4–7).

There is an extensive literature on the diverse immunophenotypic features of ALL (Borowitz, 1993b; Cascavilla

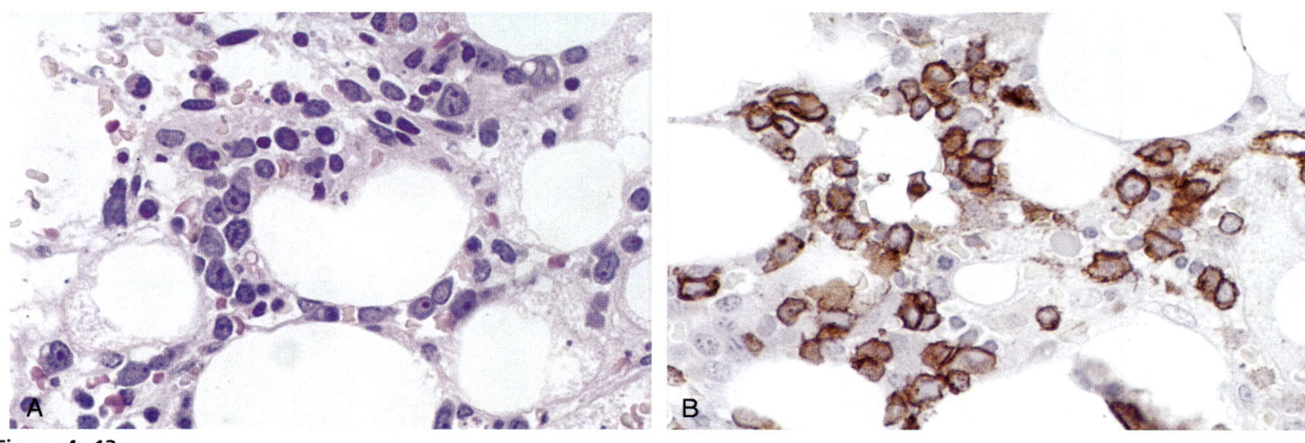

Figure 4–13

AML, hypocellular type, marrow biopsy. *A*. Increased blasts are evident. *B*. Prominent CD34 reactivity is noted on immunoperoxidase staining.

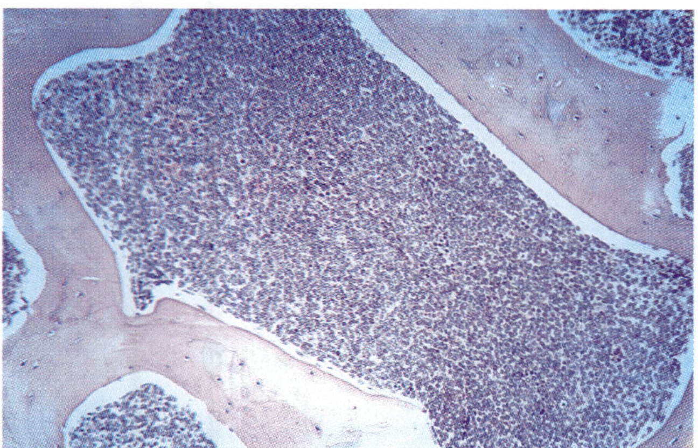

Figure 4–14

ALL, marrow biopsy. This low-magnification photomicrograph illustrates complete effacement of marrow architecture, with no residual hematopoietic elements.

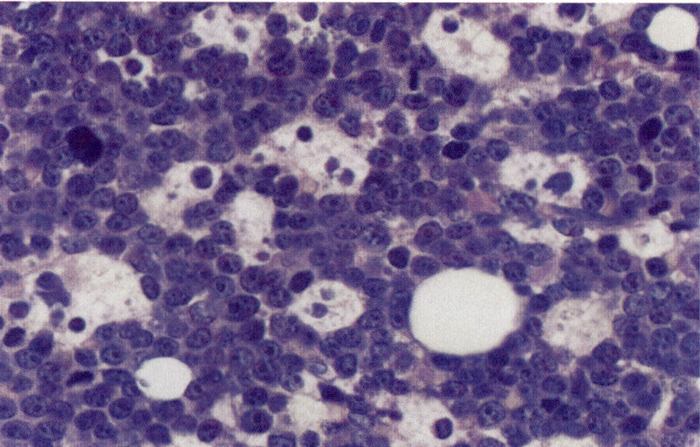

Figure 4–16

Burkitt lymphoma/ALL-L3, marrow biopsy. This marrow biopsy shows complete effacement by lymphoma. Note the "starry sky" pattern.

et al, 1997; Davis et al, 1997; Guglielmi et al, 1997; Jennings & Foon, 1997; Pui et al, 1993; Traweek, 1993; Wang et al, 1995). Immunophenotyping accurately distinguishes cases of ALL from other blastic malignancies and identifies them as B or T cell in type. The antigens characteristically expressed on B cell neoplasms include HLA-DR and CD19. Cytoplasmic CD22 expression is also very common, even in immature B cell processes (Fig. 4–21). The typical antigen profile of immature T cells includes expression of CD7 and cytoplasmic CD3. Expression of CD1, CD2, and CD5 is also fairly common. Since some of these antigens (e.g., CD2 and CD7) are also frequently expressed in AML, analysis of antibody panels is necessary for accurate lineage assignment.

Specific clinicopathologic types of ALL may be identified by integrating immunophenotypic and clinical parameters. For example, expression of CD15 and lack of CD10 are characteristic of B cell precursor ALL in infancy, a subtype associated with a high WBC count, organomegaly, and frequent cytogenetic translocations involving 11q23 (McCoy & Overton, 1995). CD34 positivity and weak or negative CD45 expression in B cell precursor ALL have been linked to hyperdiploidy, low WBC count, variable CD10 expression, and good outcome. Although flow cytometric immunophenotyping is useful in defining these clinicopathologic subtypes of ALL, immunophenotype is generally not an independent prognostic variable with current treatment regimens for high-risk ALL.

Immunophenotyping also identifies patterns of aberrant antigen expressions in acute leukemia cells. In some leukemias, this aberrant antigen profile consists of combinations of early- and late-expressed antigens that are not normally simultaneously coexpressed on developing cells. In other cases, antigens thought to be relatively specific for lymphocytes are expressed on myelocytic cells or vice versa. The aberrant phenotype found in many ALL and AML cases may be useful for identification of minimal residual disease.

Genotypic Evaluation

The genotyping of acute leukemias ranges from standard cytogenetic banding to molecular analyses for specific fusion genes, fusion gene products, or gene deletions. Clonal abnormalities

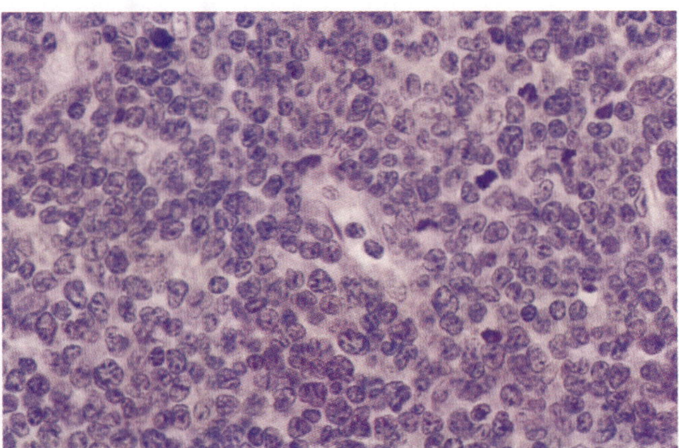

Figure 4–15

ALL, marrow biopsy. This high-magnification photomicrograph illustrates the closely packed nuclei with condensed chromatin and prominent mitotic activity, which characterize ALL on tissue sections.

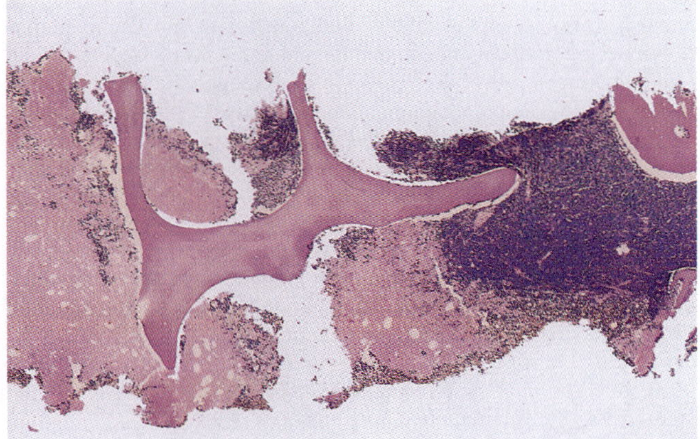

Figure 4–17

ALL, marrow biopsy. This low-magnification photomicrograph of a biopsy from a 10-year-old boy shows striking necrosis of approximately one-half of the hematopoietic space.

Table 4–3
Cytochemical Procedures Useful in Leukemia†

Cytochemical Stain	Utility and Features
Myeloperoxidase (MPO)	Most specific cytochemical stain for granulocyte precursors May be weakly positive in monocyte precursors but generally negative Mature dyspoietic granulocytes may lack MPO in some cases of AML
Sudan black B	Stains lipid membrane of primary granules and peroxisomes in granulocyte precursors May be weakly positive in monocyte precursors but generally negative Rare cases of ALL weakly positive
Naphthol ASD chloroacetate esterase (CAE)	Stains primary granules of granulocyte precursors Reports of positivity in ALL (notably granular ALL) and acute monocytic leukemias Abnormally expressed in eosinophils in patients with acute myelomonocytic leukemia with eosinophilia
Nonspecific esterase (NSE) (α-naphthylacetate)	Variably strong staining of monocytic cells (diffuse) and megakaryoblasts (punctate) Sodium fluoride inhibition of monocytic esterase Weak reaction may be found in granulocytic elements Reports of moderate positivity in some APL cases that are purely granulocytic by all other features
Nonspecific esterase (α-naphthylbutyrate)	Diffuse positivity of monocytic cells (reaction weak to strong) May be weakly positive in granulocytic precursors but generally negative
Periodic acid–Schiff (PAS)	Large granules and globules of PAS-positive material (glycogen or glycoprotein) in leukemic lymphoblasts and erythroblasts; diffuse cytoplasmic positivity in more mature neoplastic erythrocytic elements Diffuse or globular positivity also found in megakaryoblasts Weak diffuse positivity common in granulocytic and monocytic precursors
Toluidine blue	Positive in both mast cells and basophils Mast cells also CAE positive
Ultrastructural myeloperoxidase and platelet peroxidase	Possible detection of myeloperoxidase in very early granulocytic precursors by electron microscopy, in contrast to light microscopy Platelet peroxidase detectable by electron microscopy in endoplasmic reticulum and perinuclear cisternae of megakaryoblasts (not detectable by light microscopy)
Acid phosphatase	Focal, paranuclear positivity originally noted in T-ALL, later found in other immunologic subtypes of ALL
Oil red O	Vacuoles in Burkitt or L3 leukemia/lymphoma cells positive

†Note: Abbreviation: APL, acute promyelocytic leukemia. Blasts in ALL, in contrast to those in several other leukemias, do not have a specific cytochemical profile.

consisting of numerical abnormalities or reciprocal translocations are detected in the majority of AMLs and ALLs by standard cytogenetic analyses (Tables 4–8 and 4–9). Genes at the site of most of the common reciprocal translocations have been cloned and sequenced, providing critical information about the genetic events that produce acute leukemia and facilitating development of specific probes for leukemogenic events (Caligiuri et al 1997; Greaves, 1997; Rubnitz & Look, 1998; Russell, 1997; Sawyers, 1997; Zeleznik-Le et al, 1995). Rapid polymerase chain reaction (PCR) analyses for selected fusion gene products may be used in initial diagnostic screening of new cases of acute leukemia. In most cases, standard cytogenetic analysis is needed to determine the complete genotypic profile of a leukemic case, since molecular analyses probe only highly restricted genetic loci and do not detect additional abnormalities.

In addition to the utility of genotypic analyses in defining specific leukemogenic events, these studies also distinguish biologic subsets of leukemia with varying optimal therapy and prognosis. In AML, genotypic studies may broadly separate cases into chemotherapy-sensitive and chemotherapy-resistant groups, whereas genotypic studies in ALL are crucial for assigning low-, intermediate-, and high-risk status.

Clonal cytogenetic abnormalities are identified in the majority of cases of AML (Casasnovas et al, 1998; Dastugue et al, 1995; Martinez-Climent, 1995b; Rubnitz & Look, 1998; Walker et al, 1994) (see Table 4–8). In AML, numerical abnormalities such as −5/5q − and −7 are linked to prior alkylating agent chemotherapy, multidrug resistance of the leukemic clone, and background dysplastic features of mature hematopoietic elements. Cases of AML demonstrating these numerical abnormalities are much more common in elderly patients. The incidence of this biologic type of AML in pediatric patients is low. The structural abnormalities delineated in Table 4–8 are more commonly encountered in children and young adults with AML. These patients generally respond to standard chemotherapy and may experience long-term remission.

With current cytogenetic and molecular techniques, clonal abnormalities are detected in approximately 90% of cases of ALL (Heerema et al, 1992; Kaspers et al, 1995; Kersey, 1997; Martinez-Climent, 1997; Pui et al, 1990; Raimondi et al, 1991; Rubnitz & Look, 1998) (see Table 4–9). The most frequent chromosomal abnormality in ALL is hyperdiploidy, identified in over 40% of B cell precursor ALL (B-ALL) cases. The prognostic significance of hyperdiploidy has been established in ALL patients in whom a good prognosis is associated with a chromosome number ≥50 or a DNA content index ≥1.16. A minority of ALL cases (usually T-ALL) demonstrate a normal karyotype. Hypodiploidy is a very uncommon karyotypic abnormality in ALL that is linked to poor prognosis. (See Hyperdiploid ALL section.)

Approximately 40% of pediatric cases of ALL and >50% of adult ALL cases demonstrate clonal structural chromosomal abnormalities by routine cytogenetic studies (see Table 4–9). The two most frequent translocations so detected, t(1;19) and t(9;22), occur in <10% of cases of ALL in children and are

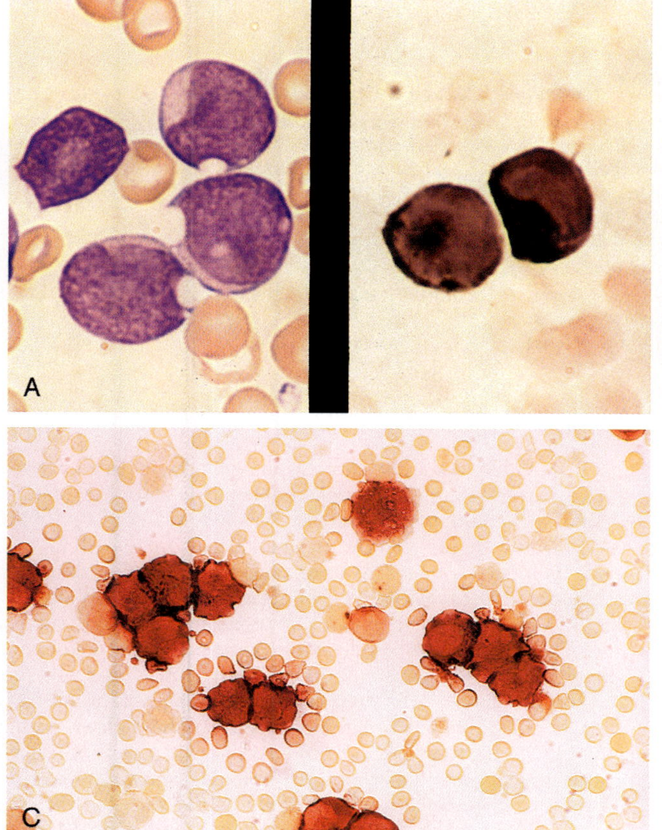

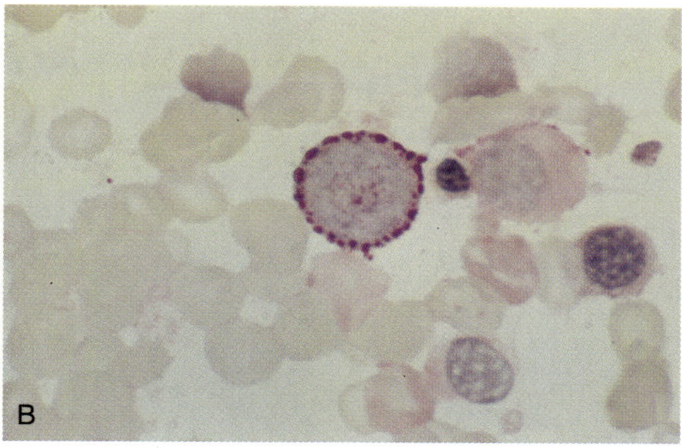

Figure 4–18

AML, cytochemistry. *A*. Myeloblasts are strongly Sudan black B positive (right panel). *B*. Globular PAS positivity is observed in erythroblasts. *C*. Diffuse nonspecific esterase positivity occurs in monoblasts.

much more prevalent in adult patients. Cryptic t(12;21)(p13;q22) has been identified in ALL and linked to good outcome (see ALL with cryptic t(12;21) section). Molecular techniques have been used to identify fusion genes and fusion gene products in ALL as well as to assess immunoglobulin heavy-chain and light-chain and T cell receptor (TCR) gene rearrangements (Table 4–10). As predicted, immunoglobulin heavy-chain gene rearrangement is identified in the majority of cases exhibiting a B lineage immunophenotypic profile, whereas T lineage antigens and TCR gene rearrangement are demonstrated in T-ALL (Beishuizen et al, 1994; Felix & Poplack, 1991; Foucar, 1995a; Tien et al, 1991). Many cases of B-ALL demonstrate TCR gene rearrangement, and a few cases of T-ALL demonstrate immunoglobulin heavy-chain or light-chain gene rearrangements (see Table 4–10).

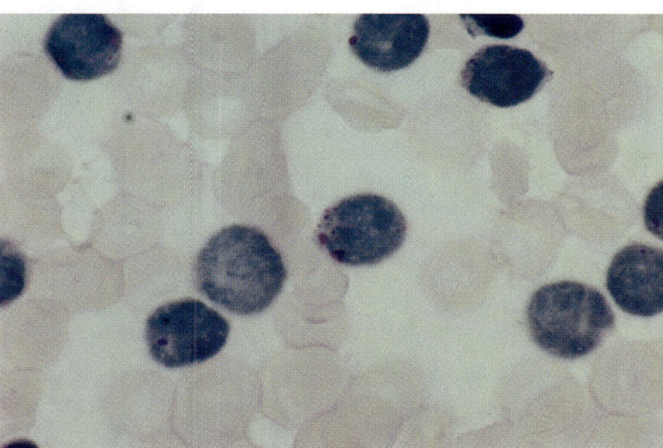

Figure 4–19

ALL. A lymphoblast containing blocks of PAS positivity is illustrated.

APPROACH TO THE DIAGNOSIS AND CLASSIFICATION OF ACUTE LEUKEMIAS

The initial basic decisions in a case of possible acute leukemia involve analysis of morphologic and hematologic parameters to determine whether the process is benign or malignant, acute or chronic, and lymphocytic or myelocytic. The latter two decisions are facilitated by cytochemical and immunophenotypic studies. Ideally, additional information relevant to treatment, prognosis, and identification of specific biologic subsets of acute leukemia should be provided to clinicians at the time of diagnosis. Consequently, a biologically relevant classification system of acute leukemia blends the traditional analysis and information from more sophisticated characterization of the phenotypic and genotypic profiles of leukemic cells.

To be biologically relevant, a classification system should relate the predominant cells in leukemic cases to stages of differentiation of normal hematopoietic elements as well as offer insights into pathogenetic mechanisms. Basic assumptions in such a classification are that cases of acute leukemia will be accurately and reproducibly identified as to lineage and stage of maturation by the readily available methods of morphologic study, cytochemical analysis, and imunophenotyping and that unique features of individual cases will be determined by specialized cytogenetic and/or genotypic techniques. To be maximally useful clinically, classification terminology should

Table 4–4
Flow Cytometric Analyses Useful in Leukemias

Technique	Utility
Multicolor immunophenotyping	Determine lineage and stage of maturation of leukemia Determine clonality of mature B lymphocytic disorders Assess surface, cytoplasmic, and nuclear antigen profile at diagnosis Evaluate for minimal residual disease
DNA content analysis	Determine whether ALL is diploid, hypodiploid, or hyperdiploid
Multidrug resistance assays	Assess for expression of multidrug resistance–associated proteins Assess efflux properties of leukemic cells

incorporate multidrug resistance features and thereby facilitate selection of therapy and development of new treatments.

The most widely accepted current classification system for acute leukemias was initially proposed by the FAB Cooperative Group in 1976 (Bennett et al, 1976) (Table 4–11). Subsequent revisions of this FAB classification system improved diagnostic concordance and provided criteria for newly recognized acute leukemia subtypes (Bennett et al, 1991, 1985a, 1985b, 1981). The FAB criteria are generally useful in classifying cases of acute leukemia, but this lineage-based system does not consistently define many important subsets of acute leukemia that have clinical and biologic importance. Consequently, new classification strategies have been proposed, especially for AML (Pui et al, 1995), including separating cases of AML into two broad "biologic" groups, de novo AML and myelodysplasia-related AML (Head, 1996) (Table 4–12). The prototypic features of de novo AML include a reciprocal cytogenetic translocation, a stable lifetime incidence rate that does not vary by patient age, a lack of background dysplasia and antecedent hematologic disorders, and, in general, a chemotherapy sensitivity. Myelodysplasia-related AML predominates in the elderly, is dramatically increased in incidence with age, is linked to prior oncogenic "hits," is associated with numerical chromosomal aberrations and background dyspoiesis, and is linked to multidrug resistance and poor survival time. This approach to myelogenous leukemias incorporates important clinical and genotypic information, but it does not provide specific diagnostic criteria and is not applicable to all cases of AML, since significant minority of AML patients have normal cytogenetics. Further investigations of leukemogenesis will likely provide insights relevant to optimal acute leukemia classification. Most cases of acute leukemia in children fall into the de novo category. Some of the specific types of AML and ALL described in the next section are unique to children. Diagnostic criteria for each include multiparameter data.

Table 4–5
Immunophenotypic Profile of Immature Myelocytes and Lymphocytes

Cell Type	Characteristic Immunophenotypic Features and Comments
Myeloblast	CD34, HLA-DR, CD13, CD33, CD15, antimyeloperoxidase, CD11±
Promyelocyte	CD13, CD33, CD15, CD11 Loss of HLA-DR and acquisition of strong CD15 and CD11 associated with maturation Gradual loss of CD33 in successive maturation stages
Monoblast	CD34±, HLA-DR, CD13, CD33, CD14, CD4, CD15±, CD11
Promonocyte	HLA-DR, CD13, CD33 ±, CD14, CD4, CD15 ±, CD11
Erythroblast	Glycophorin A, hemoglobin A
Megakaryoblast	HLA-DR, CD34±, CD41,[a] CD13±, CD33±, CD61+ Progressive maturation characterized by loss of CD34 and acquisition of CD42 and von Willebrand factor
B lymphocyte[b]	
CALLA (CD10) negative	HLA-DR, TdT, CD34, CD19 (usually), cCD22[c]
"Common"	HLA-DR, TdT, variable CD34, CD19, CD10, cCD22, variable CD20[c]
Pre-B	HLA-DR, variable TdT, CD19, CD10, CD20, CD22, cytoplasmic μ[c]
B	HLA-DR, CD19, variable CD10, CD20, CD22, SIg[c]
T Lymphocyte[b]	
Early T precursor	CD7, TdT, CD34[c]
Immature thymocyte	CD7, TdT, CD34, CD5, CD38, CD2, cCD3[c]
Common thymocyte	CD7, variable TdT, CD5, CD38, CD2, CD1, CD3, CD4, CD8[c]
Mature thymocyte	CD7, CD5, CD38, CD2, CD3, CD4 or CD8[c]

Abbreviations before CD: c, cytoplasmic.

[a] False-positive CD41 expression by flow cytometric analysis may be secondary to platelet adherence to blasts.

[b] Majority of ALL of B lineage; 15–25% of ALL of T lineage.

[c] Numerous aberrations of antigen profile described in ALL. Majority of cases do *not* fit currently recognized patterns of antigen expression of normal B and T precursors.

Table 4–6
Three-Color Flow Cytometric Immunophenotyping in Acute Leukemia

Value in Diagnosis	Detector 1	Detector 2	Detector 3
"Core" panel for acute leukemia diagnosis[a]	K	Λ	CD19
	CD34	CD33	CD45
	HLA-DR	CD13	CD45
	CD10	CD19	CD45
	CD5	CD22	CD45
	CD7	CD3	CD45
Additional markers for T-lineage ALL	CD8	CD4	CD45
	CD1	CD2	CD45
	cMPO	cCD3	
	TdT		
Additional markers for B-lineage ALL	CD20	CD34	CD45
	TdT		
	DNA content		
Additional markers for AML	cMPO	cCD3	
	CD14	CD56	CD45

Abbreviations: c, cytoplasmic; MPO, myeloperoxidase.

[a] Gating by CD45 or side scatter.

SPECIFIC BIOLOGIC SUBSETS OF AML AND ALL

Congenital Leukemia with t(v;11)(v;q23) or t(1;22)(p12–13;q13)

Cases of AML and ALL are rare in neonates. Cases occurring within the first month of life are termed congenital leukemia. These leukemias occur at a rate of 1 in 5 million births (Pui et al, 1995b). Most cases of congenital leukemia, either AML or ALL, are associated with translocations involving 11q23 and various partner chromosomes (Behm et al, 1996; Heerema et al, 1994; Martinez-Climent et al, 1995a; McCoy & Overton, 1995; Rubnitz et al, 1996; Rubnitz & Look, 1998; Taki et al, 1996). The commonest translocations involving 11q23 in ALL are the t(4;11) and t(11;19), whereas in de novo AML the t(9;11), t(6;11), and t(11;19) appear most frequent. In addition to these commonly detected translocations, 11q23 rearrangements may also be detected at a molecular level in AML patients with apparently normal cytogenetics (Caligiuri et al, 1997). In particular, 11q23 rearrangement may be found in up to 80% of infant acute leukemia cases if molecular methods are used (Chen et al, 1993; Cimino et al, 1993; Martinez-Climent et al, 1995a).

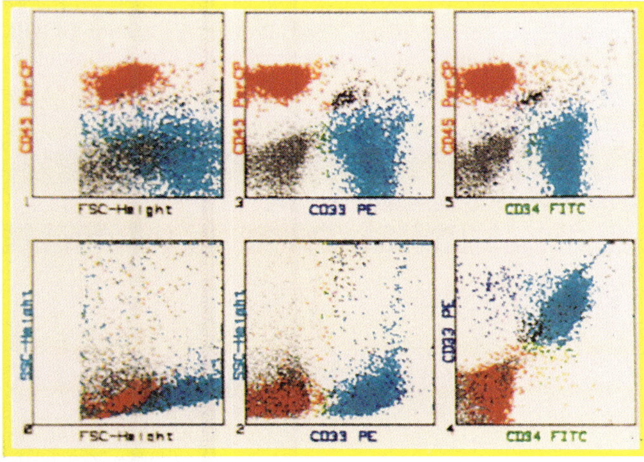

Figure 4–20

AML, flow cytometry. This flow cytometric histogram composite illustrates typical patterns of reactivity for CD13, CD33, and CD34 as well as weak CD45 reactivity.

These 11q23-associated congenital leukemias represent a distinctive biologic group characterized by marked hepatosplenomegaly, profound leukocytosis, severe anemia, and severe thrombocytopenia (Fig. 4–22). Monocytic leukemias (either FAB M5 or FAB M4) constitute the majority of 11q23-associated congenital AML cases, whereas the cases of congenital ALL are generally FAB L1 or L2 morphologic subtypes. A characteristic immunophenotypic profile (CD10−, CD15+) is found in congenital B cell precursor ALL with 11q23 translocation.

The gene involved in all 11q23 translocations has been named the *MLL, ALL1, HRX*, or *HTRX1* gene by the various research groups that independently cloned the gene (Djabali et al, 1992; Gu et al, 1992; Tkachuk et al, 1992; Ziemin-van der Poel et al, 1991). The *MLL* gene encodes a protein that is involved in positive transcriptional regulation of homeotic genes critical in normal hematopoiesis. Rearrangement of MLL results in disruption of the normal regulation of other genes involved in hematopoiesis (Caligiuri et al, 1997). Abnormalities of 11q23 are identified best by molecular techniques (Poirel et al, 1996; Rubnitz et al, 1996). Southern blotting detects all 11q23 rearrangements (the partner chromosomes need not be known), and reverse transcriptase pdymerase chain reaction (RT-PCR) techniques detect about 90% of cases. The latter technique is much more sensitive in detecting 11q23 abnormalities at a minimal residual disease level (Rubnitz 1996).

A much less common subset of congenital leukemia is associated with t(1;22)(p12–13;q13) and megakaryoblastic morphologic features (Lion et al, 1992; Martinez-Climent, 1997; Rubnitz & Look, 1998). In contrast to neonates with 11q23-associated congenital leukemia, those with acute megakaryoblastic t(1;22)-associated leukemia have a reduced WBC count along with severe anemia and thrombocytopenia. Marrow fibrosis and hepatosplenomegaly may be striking in these infants. Prognosis is dismal for patients with all types of congenital leukemia.

Table 4–7
Immunoperoxidase Techniques in Acute Leukemia

Marker Available	Utility[a]
CD34	Identification and localization of immature cells
TdT	Delineation and localization of immature lymphocytes (both leukemic cells and hematogones)
Myeloperoxidase, CD43	Delineation and localization of immature granulocytic elements
CD20, CD45RO, CD43, CD3, CD79a	Delineation and localization of B and T cell populations
CD68, lysozyme, CD43	Identification of monocytic elements
Hemoglobin A	Identification of erythrocyte precursors
Factor VIII, glycoprotein 1	Identification of megakaryocytic elements
Tryptase	Identification of mast cells

[a] For marrow biopsy and clot sections; some antibody stains do not work on decalcified specimens, depending on technique used.

Acute Leukemia in Down Syndrome Patients (AML, ALL)

As described earlier, there is a striking association between Down syndrome and childhood AML and ALL (Creutzig et al, 1996; Horwitz, 1997; Lange et al, 1998; Lanza et al, 1997a; Robison, 1992). Neonates with Down syndrome may also present with a transient, spontaneously regressing myeloproliferative disorder that mimics AML (see Chap. 9). Most cases of overt acute leukemia in children with Down syndrome occur after 6 months of age. For infants and toddlers, acute megakaryoblastic leukemias predominate (Fig. 4–23), whereas ALL is much more common in children with Down syndrome who are over 4 years of age. In both acute megakaryoblastic leukemia and ALL in Down syndrome patients, there may be cytogenetic abnormalities in addition to the constitutional trisomy 21. The marrow architecture is effaced by blasts in these patients, although some marrow fibrosis is common in acute megakaryoblastic leukemia. The acute leukemias in patients with Down syndrome are similar morphologically to analogous acute leukemias in constitutionally normal patients, but studies document a more favorable response to therapy in the Down syndrome patients with AML (Lange et al, 1998).

The basis for the association between constitutional trisomy 21 and the development of leukemia is uncertain. Clearly, trisomy 21 is a predisposing factor for hematologic malignancies, but specific leukemogenic mechanisms and secondary events involving chromosome 21 have not yet been clearly delineated. An interstitial deletion on the long arm of chromosome 21 that was restricted to the leukemic clone in five Down syndrome patients with leukemia suggests that a gene or genes on chromosome 21 play a role in leukemogenesis (Kempski et al, 1997).

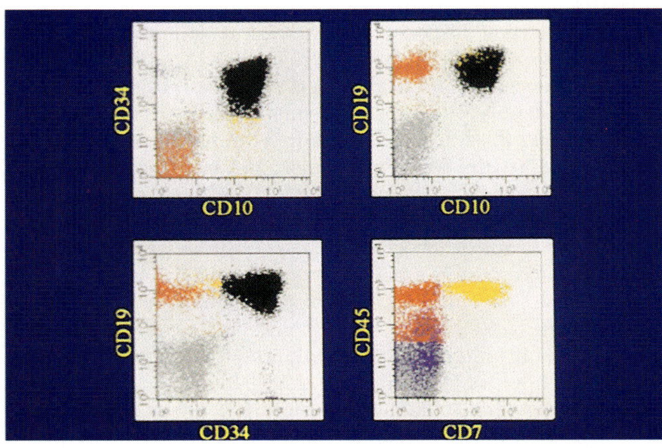

Figure 4–21

ALL, B cell precursor, flow cytometry. This composite histogram demonstrates weak CD45 positivity in lymphoblasts that coexpress CD19, CD10, and CD34.

Biologic Subsets of AML

Acute Promyelocytic Leukemia: t(15;17)(q22;q21)

APL (AML-M3) is one of the best characterized subtypes of AML, making up 7–15% of all pediatric AML cases. The frequency may be significantly higher among Latino patients (Douer et al, 1996; Martinez-Climent, 1997; Rubnitz & Look, 1998). The vast majority of APL cases are characterized by distinctive morphologic characteristics and an underlying cytogenetic event: the t(15;17)(q22;q21) (Table 4–13). Both features have become required for diagnosis in APL. APL patients also have unique clinical features. They often have life-threatening DIC at presentation or during tumor lysis from induction chemotherapy. In addition, the leukemic blasts in patients with APL are uniquely responsive to the differentiating agent all-transretinoic acid. Treatment with this agent in conjunction with conventional chemotherapy has led to a high cure rate (Fenaux et al, 1997; Tallman, 1996). Prompt recognition of APL at diagnosis is thus essential for optimal patient management.

Table 4–8
Cytogenetic Abnormalities in AML

Numerical Abnormalities	Structural Abnormalities
−5/5q−	t(8;21)(q22;q22)
−7	inv(16)(p13;q22)
+8	t(15;17)(q21;q21)
20q−	t(v;11)(v;q23)
16q−	t(3;v)(q26;v)
	t(3;5)(q35;q35)
	t(6;9)(p23;q34)
	t(1;22)(p12-13;q13)

Source: Martinez-Climent JA: Molecular cytogenetics of childhood hematological malignancies. Leukemia 11:1999, 1997; Rubnitz JE, Look AT: Molecular genetics of childhood leukemias. J Pediatr Hematol Oncol 20:1, 1998.

Table 4–9
Cytogenetic Abnormalities in ALL

Numerical Abnormalities	Structural Abnormalities
Hypodiploid	Cryptic t(12;21)(p13;q22)
Hyperdiploid (47–49 chromosomes)	t(1;19)(q23;p13) t(4;11)(q21;q23)
Hyperdiploid (≥50 chromosomes)	t(v;11)(v;q23) t(7;v)(q34;v)
Near triploidy	t(9;22)(q34;q11)
Near tetraploid	t(8;14)(q24;q32) t(5;14)(q31;q32) t(11;14)(p15;q11) t(10;14)(q24;q11) t(1;14)(p32;q11)

Source: Martinez-Climent JA: Molecular cytogenetics of childhood hematological malignancies. Leukemia 11:1999, 1997; Rubnitz JE, Look AT: Molecular genetics of childhood leukemias. J Pediatr Hematol Oncol 2:1, 1998.

Table 4–10
Percentages of "Appropriate" and "Inappropriate" Gene Rearrangement in ALL

B-Lineage ALL	T-Lineage ALL
IgH: 98%	IgH: 20–30%
IgK: 30%	IgK: 10%
TCRγ: 60–80%	TCRγ: 96%
TCRβ: 30%	TCRβ: 97%

APL has two distinct morphologic subtypes in the FAB classification scheme: the classic hypergranular form and the microgranular variant (Bennett et al, 1976; Castoldi et al, 1994). The classic form of APL shows a preponderance of promyelocytes in the marrow, cells with numerous azurophilic granules that often blur the nuclear outline (Fig. 4–24). Auer rods are common and may form small stacks (so-called faggot cells). The leukemic cells in the peripheral blood are often inconspicuous. The WBC count is frequently low, and the circulating cells may have less prominent granulation than do corresponding marrow cells. In the microgranular variant of APL, the leukemia cells generally resemble the blasts of monocytic leukemia and have bilobed or reniform nuclei and moderately abundant cytoplasm (Fig. 4–25). Granules are sparse and indistinct, with variable numbers of cells containing Auer rods. In contrast to the classic form, the WBC count may be significantly elevated in these cases. The marrow in these patients may contain more classic APL features.

The leukemic promyelocyte of APL (both classic and microgranular forms) invariably shows intense staining with Sudan black B, myeloperoxidase, and specific esterase. The staining is sufficiently intense in most cells to obscure the nucleus (Fig. 4–26). Some cases show staining with nonspecific esterase, a feature that should not distract the interpreting physician from a diagnosis of APL. Promyelocytes have a characteristic phenotype, expressing myelocyte antigens CD13 and CD33 and lacking expression of the stem cell antigen CD34 and HLA-DR. Absence of HLA-DR expression is a clue that a leukemia may be APL but is not diagnostic per se. The blasts in the microgranular variant may also express CD2 (Biondi et al, 1995; Tallman, 1996).

The underlying t(15;17)(q21;q21) is a reciprocal translocation that involves the promyelocytic leukemia (*PML*) gene on chromosome 15 and the retinoic acid receptor (*RARα*) gene on chromosome 17. Two fusion genes are formed: *PML/RARα* on 15q+ and *RARα*/PML on 17q−. The *RARα* gene is critical in normal myelocytic differentiation. The PML/RARα fusion protein blocks this *RARα*-induced differentiation, resulting in the accumulation of cells at the promyelocyte stage. Pharmacologic doses of all-transretinoic acid reverse this differentiation blockade and result in differentiation of the leukemic promyelocytes to mature granulocytes. The PML/RARα fusion protein may also have leukemogenic effects by disrupting the normal nuclear localization of the wild-type PML protein, which appears to encode for a DNA-binding protein (Grignani et al, 1994; Lavau & Dejean, 1994).

Classic cytogenetic analysis will not detect the t(15;17) in all APL cases. However, RT-PCR molecular techniques show that the vast majority of t(15;17)-negative cases of APL harbor the *PML/RARα* fusion transcript, and this technique is recommended in all suspected APL cases.

AML with t(8;21)(q22;q22)

A t(8;21) is found in about 10–15% of children with AML (Martinez-Climent, 1997; Rubnitz & Look, 1998). Morphologically this translocation may be suspected on the basis of a distinctive constellation of abnormalities (see Table 4–13) (Nucifora et al, 1994; Swirsky et al, 1984). Characteristically the leukemia cells show some maturation (FAB M2). In some cases the blast percentage is <30%, causing confusion with high-grade myelodysplasia (MDS) (Chan et al, 1997; Taj et al, 1995; Xue et al, 1994). The blasts often contain finely tapered Auer rods and may also exhibit cytoplasmic vacuoles. Salmon-pink cytoplasmic granules surrounded by a basophilic rim as well as intracytoplasmic pink globules are seen in promyelocytes and myelocytes (Fig. 4–27). Marrow eosinophilia is also common (see Table 4–13). Cytochemical and immunophenotypic clues to the presence of a t(8;21) include strong Sudan black and myeloperoxidase positivity in the blasts, coexpression of CD19 or CD56 by blasts, and strong CD34 expression (Hurwitz et al, 1992; Porwit-MacDonald et al, 1996).

The genes involved in the t(8;21) are two transcription factors: the *AML1* gene at 21q22 and *ETO* (for *eight twenty-one*) at 8q22 (Nucifora & Rowley, 1995; Tanaka et al, 1998). The translocation produces a novel chimeric *AML1/ETO* gene. The normal AML1 protein is part of the "master switch" that controls many genes expressed in myelocytic development. The chimeric *AML1/ETO* transcript may induce leukemia through an altered interaction with genes normally controlled by AML1 (Nucifora & Rowley, 1995).

As with other fusion genes, the chimeric *AML1/ETO* transcript may be detected by RT-PCR. This method has demonstrated the fusion transcript in a proportion of AML cases with typical t(8;21) morphologic features that lack the cytogenetic translocation (Nucifora et al, 1994). Since these patients have a prognosis similar to that of patients with cytogenetically detectable t(8;21), molecular analysis is warranted in cases morphologically suspicious for t(8;21) if cytogenetic study results are negative. Molecular studies are also very useful in separating t(8;21) AML with a low blast count from high-grade MDS.

The prognostic significance of the t(8;21) in childhood AML is not entirely clear. In contrast to the favorable prognosis in adults, children with t(8;21) AML have a high rate of relapse and poor survival time despite frequent initial remission (Martinez-Climent et al, 1995b; Pearson et al, 1996). Their poor survival may result from an unusually high frequency of expression of the multidrug resistance gene or functional drug

Table 4–11
FAB Classification of AML and ALL

Subtype	Definition[a]
AML-M0	30% blasts (type 1) <3% Sudan black B or myeloperoxidase positivity Myeloid antigen expression by immunophenotyping or myeloperoxidase expression by electron microscopy
AML-M1	30% blasts (types 1, 2, and rarely 3) 3% Sudan black B or myeloperoxidase positivity in blasts <10% cells exhibiting maturation beyond blast stage
AML-M2	30% blasts (types 1, 2, and 3) 3% Sudan black B or myeloperoxidase positivity in blasts >10% granulocytic cells exhibiting maturation beyond blast stage <20% monocytic cells
AML-M3	30% blasts (types 1, 2, and 3) + hypergranular promyelocytes[b] Intense myeloperoxidase or Sudan black B reaction in virtually all cells
AML-M3m	Same criteria, except that granules within most promyelocytes very inconspicuous and nuclei highly grooved and reniform
AML-M4	Monocytosis (5000/μl); increased lysozyme 30% myeloblasts + monoblasts + promonocytes >20% Sudan black B–myeloperoxidase-positive cells >20% nonspecific esterase–positive cells
AML-M4eos	Same criteria as AML-M4 plus abnormal eosinophils in marrow
AML-M5a,b	30% myeloblasts + monoblasts + promonocytes <20% Sudan black B–or myeloperoxidase-positive cells >80% nonspecific esterase–positive cells Monoblasts predominate in M5a Promonocytes predominate in M5b
AML-M6a,b	30% of cells, other than erythrocyte precursors, myeloblasts (types 1, 2, and 3) >50% erythrocyte precursors Erythroblasts predominate (provisional in AML-M6b category)
AML-M7	30% blasts (myeloblasts + megakaryoblasts) >30% megakaryocytic elements defined by immunophenotyping or electron microscopy
ALL-L1	High nuclear-cytoplasmic ratio Nuclei with inconspicuous nucleoli Blasts variable in size but often small
ALL-L2	Moderate to abundant amounts of cytoplasm Nuclei with one or more distinct, prominent nucleoli Blasts medium to large
ALL-L3	Scant to abundant amounts of deeply basophilic cytoplasm containing abundant distinct vacuoles Nuclear chromatin homogeneous with one or more generally indistinct nucleoli Blasts medium to large

[a] National Cancer Institute recommends classification as acute leukemia when blood blasts exceed 30% regardless of marrow blast percentage. (See "AML with t(8;21)(q22;q22)" and "AML with Myelodysplastic Features" for our approach to distinction between leukemia and myelodysplasia.)

[b] Promyelocytes usually predominate in AML-M3.

efflux activity found in pediatric but not adult patients with t(8;21) AML (Pearson et al, 1996).

AML with inv(16)(p13q22)

The inv(16)(p13q22) and the related but less commonly identified t(16;16) are recurring chromosomal translocations in AML associated with unique morphologic features. These two cytogenetic abnormalities are seen in 10–12% of pediatric AML cases (Martinez-Climent, 1997; Rubnitz & Look, 1998). This entity is important, since it is associated with a particularly favorable prognosis, being highly amenable to cure by chemotherapy alone. Most patients enjoy prolonged disease-free survival periods (Le Beau et al, 1983; Marlton et al, 1995).

In almost all cases of inv(16)-associated AML, the marrow is infiltrated by a myelomonocytic blast population and a variable percentage of dysplastic eosinophils (see Table 4–13). These unique features were first recognized in the early 1980s, prompting subsequent modification of the FAB classification scheme to AML-M4eos (Arthur & Bloomfield, 1983; Bennett et al, 1985b; Le Beau et al, 1983). This constellation of features predicts the presence of an inv(16) or t(16;16). The reverse is not true: inv(16) or molecular evidence of inv(16) is found in a minority of patients with other FAB morphologic features, including cases lacking marrow eosinophilia (Langabeer et al, 1997; Tobal et al, 1995).

The eosinophils of AML-M4eo constitute about 2–10% of marrow cells and are dysplastic, with abnormal basophil cyto-

Table 4–12
Criteria That Identify "Biologic" Subgroups of AML

Feature	MDS-Related AML	De novo AML
Age	Predominates in elderly	All ages
Incidence	Increased in elderly	Stable rate by age
Morphologic features	Background MDS features	No MDS features
Cytogenetic features	Numerical abnormalities	Translocations
Multidrug resistance	Present	Absent
Prognosis	Poor risk	Good risk

Abbreviation: MDS, myelodysplasia.

Source: Head DR: Revised classification of acute myeloid leukemia. Leukemia 10:1826, 1996.

plasmic granules and abnormal cytochemical staining characteristics (Fig. 4–28 and Table 4–13). Similar dysplastic eosinophils may be found in the peripheral blood of most patients but are usually inconspicuous. These abnormal eosinophils are part of the neoplastic clone and contain the inv(16) (Haferlach et al, 1996).

In AML with inv(16), the underlying molecular event is rearrangement of the *CBFβ* gene (a mouse transcription factor also called *PEBP2B*) on 16q into the smooth-muscle myosin heavy-chain gene, *MYH11*, on 16p with formation of a *CBFβ*/MYH11 chimeric gene and fusion protein (Liu et al, 1995). *CBFβ* encodes a protein that, along with the AML1 protein, makes up a "master switch" regulating many genes specifically expressed in myelocytic development. The chimeric CBFβ/MYH11 protein presumably induces leukemia through disruption of this "master switch," with resultant loss of the normal regulation of the downstream target genes (Liu et al, 1995).

Detection of the inv(16) by classic cytogenetic analysis is often difficult because of poor metaphase resolution, but RT-PCR techniques sensitively detect chimeric *CBFβ*/MYH11 mRNA (Claxton et al, 1994). The *CBFβ*/MYH11 fusion transcript may be found in about 10% of de novo AML cases (Langabeer et al, 1997). A third of these cases lacked the inv(16) and classic AML-M4eo morphologic features, suggesting that the inv(16) may be underdiagnosed. If patients with a cryptic *CBFβ*/MYH11 fusion share the same excellent prognosis as those inv(16) patients with classic AML-M4eo, then RT-PCR at diagnosis to look for the fusion product appears mandatory for optimal patient care (Langabeer et al, 1997). Flow cytometric techniques utilizing an antibody to the fusion protein may be a useful method for rapid detection of cases of inv(16) and t(16;16) (Viswanatha et al, 1998).

AML with Myelodysplastic Features

Some cases of AML have marked background dyspoiesis of the more mature marrow hematopoietic elements, including hypogranular neutrophils with nuclear segmentation defects, large hypogranular platelets, and anisopoikilocytosis of erythrocytes (Brito-Babapulle et al, 1987; Goasguen et al, 1992; Kuriyama et al, 1994), a distinct morphologic picture that indicates the AML has arisen from an antecedent MDS. In other cases these changes are present in apparently de novo disease. Due to the lack of uniform criteria to define such MDS-type features, the frequency of background dysplasia varies among studies but appears to increase with patient age (Hast & Widell, 1992). The clinical outcome is worse in patients whose marrows show background dysplasia than in patients who lack such changes (Gahn et al, 1996). Furthermore, dysplastic features in AML of the elderly have been linked to other indicators of poor prognosis, such as expression of the multidrug resistance gene and unfavorable karyotype (Gahn et al, 1996; Leith & Willman, 1996). Thus, assessment of MDS changes is likely to be of value clinically. The presence of dysplastic features should trigger a search for morphologic evidence of a t(8;21), since this AML subtype

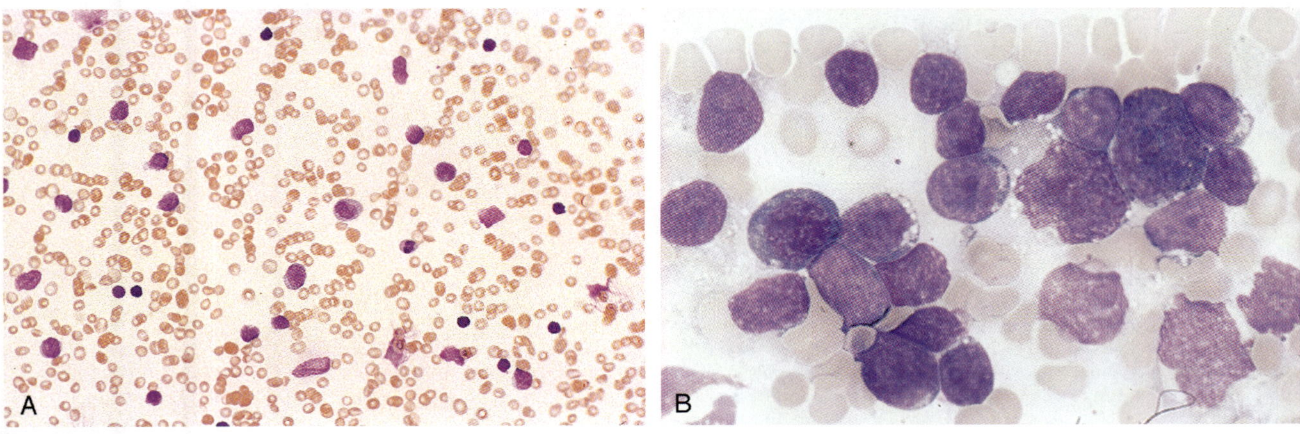

Figure 4–22

Congenital leukemia. *A*. A peripheral blood film from a 2-week-old infant with congenital leukemia shows leukocytosis (WBC $>150{,}000/\mu l$). *B*. Marrow is packed, containing immature myelomonocytic elements. Wright stain.

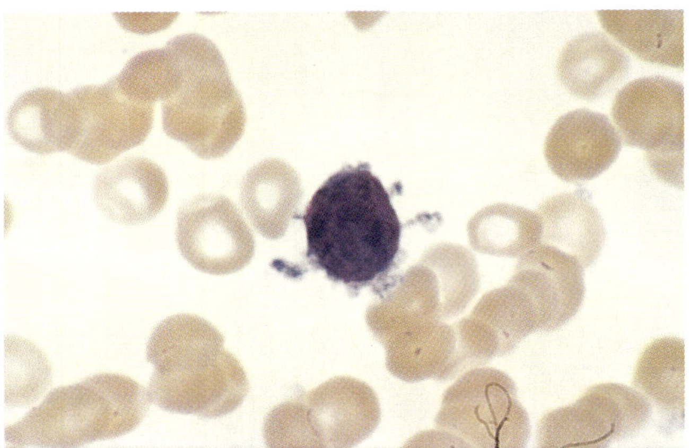

Figure 4–23

Acute megakaryoblastic leukemia, Down syndrome, peripheral blood. A circulating megakaryoblast is evident in this 3-year-old child with Down syndrome. Wright stain.

may show single or even multilineage dysplasia while biologically behaving as de novo disease.

The frequency of background MDS in AML in elderly adults is quite high, but no specific studies have determined their frequency in younger adults or pediatric patients. Since MDS changes mirror the frequency of multidrug resistance gene 1 expression and MDS-type cytogenetic features, the frequency of multilineage dysplasia in AML in childhood is probably low. Nevertheless, identification of such dysplastic changes indicates cytogenetic abnormalities that are associated with a poor clinical response.

AML in Patients with Monosomy 7 Syndrome

Monosomy 7 is detected in several pediatric hematologic disorders that may be broadly categorized as MDS or AML and then subcategorized as primary, secondary to antecedent chemotherapy or radiotherapy, and occurring in patients with various constitutional disorders (Johnson & Cotter, 1997; Luna-Fineman et al, 1995). Monosomy 7 is also rarely found in lymphocytic malignancies (Russo et al, 1991).

Monosomy 7 is found in about 40–50% of pediatric MDS cases, frequently as the sole abnormality, and in about 7% of pediatric AML cases (Johnson & Cotter, 1997; Luna-Fineman et al, 1995; Passmore et al, 1995). Pediatric MDS cases may be broadly subcategorized into MDS, monosomy 7 syndrome, and juvenile chronic myelomonocytic leukemia (Johnson & Cotter, 1997; Luna-Fineman et al, 1995). Children with monosomy 7 syndrome are usually boys who present in infancy or early childhood (6 months to 2 years of age) with pallor, bleeding, and hepatosplenomegaly. The marrow shows marked dyspoiesis and increased numbers of blasts, often with a prominent monocytic component. In many cases the process transforms

Table 4–13
Genotypic Subtypes of AML

Genotype	Morphologic Features	Morphologic Caveats	Cytochemical Features	IP	Molecular Features
t(15;17)	Classic APL: hypergranular blasts and numerous promyelocytes, many with Auer rod bundles Microgranular variant: folded nuclei and moderately abundant cytoplasm resembling immature monocytes	Only rare circulating blasts may be present in classic form.	Intense SBB positivity	HLA-DR–; CD34–; M3v (variant); CD2+	PML/RAR fusion transcript; more sensitive than cytogenetic studies
t(8;21)	Significant myelocytic maturation (generally M2); prominent tapered Auer rods; salmon-pink granules surrounded by basophilic rim in myelocytes and metamyelocytes; may show dyspoiteic features, especially in myelocytic elements	Blast percentage maybe <30%, leading to mistaken diagnosis of MDS.	Many SBB- or MPO-positive cells; less uniform intensity than APL	CD34+; may be CD19+, CD56+	*AML/ETO* detected by RT-PCR
inv(16)	Myelomonocytic blasts; dysplastic eosinophils with characteristic mixed eosinophilic or basophilic granules in cytoplasm in marrow	Very low percentage of abnormal eosinophils may be seen in AML with deletions of chromosome 16 and other abnormalities.	Eosinophils: PAS positive, chloroacetate esterase positive	CD13+; blast subsets are CD34+ or CD14+; CD2+	*CBFβ/MYH11* transcript detected by RT-PCR; other cytogenetic abnormalities in 40% of cases (particularly +22, +8, +21)

Abbreviations: APL, acute promyelocytic leukemia; IP, immunophenotype; MDS, myelodysplastic syndrome; MPO, myeloperodixase; SBB, Sudan black B.

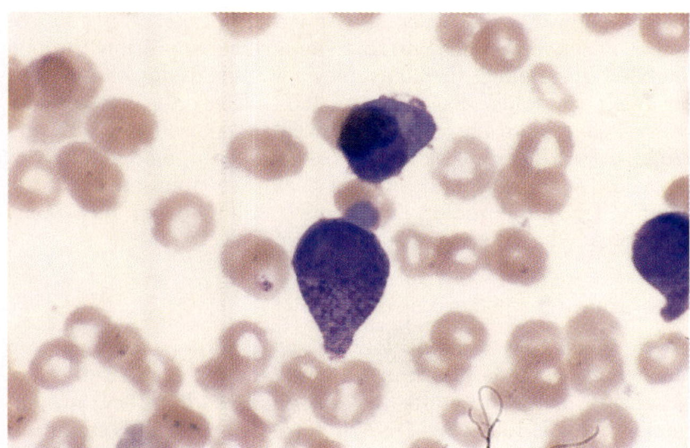

Figure 4–24

Acute promyelocytic leukemia. Hypergranular cells of the common type of promyelocytic leukemia are illustrated in this photomicrograph. Wright stain.

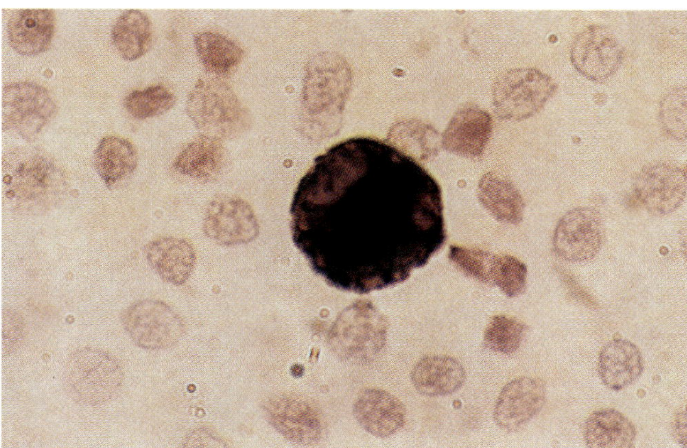

Figure 4–26

Acute promyelocytic leukemia. Intense positivity characteristically obscures the nucleus. Sudan black B.

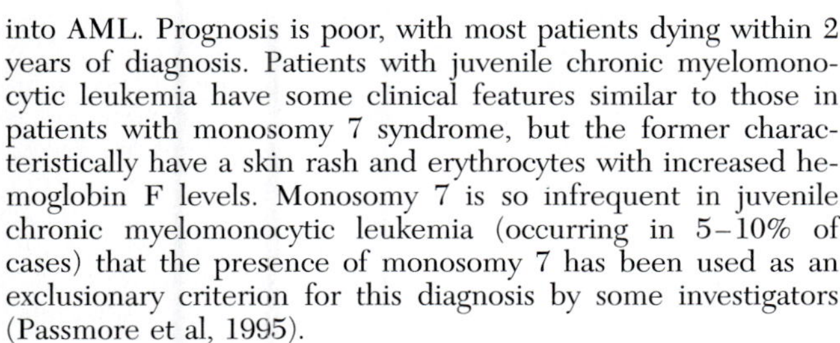

into AML. Prognosis is poor, with most patients dying within 2 years of diagnosis. Patients with juvenile chronic myelomonocytic leukemia have some clinical features similar to those in patients with monosomy 7 syndrome, but the former characteristically have a skin rash and erythrocytes with increased hemoglobin F levels. Monosomy 7 is so infrequent in juvenile chronic myelomonocytic leukemia (occurring in 5–10% of cases) that the presence of monosomy 7 has been used as an exclusionary criterion for this diagnosis by some investigators (Passmore et al, 1995).

About 7% of *de novo* pediatric AML cases exhibit monosomy 7. As in adults, AML patients with monosomy 7 have a very poor prognosis. Marrow transplant appears to offer the only chance for cure in these patients.

Secondary MDS or AML occurs in 1–2% of children treated with cancer chemotherapy. Monosomy 7 is found in 60% of such cases and is particularly associated with antecedent alkylating agent therapy. The incidence of secondary MDS or AML following alkylating therapy peaks 3 to 7 years post treatment.

MDS or AML also occurs in patients treated for severe aplastic anemia. In these patients, monosomy 7 is found very infrequently (about 1% of cases) at diagnosis but is detected in >50% of cases of MDS or AML arising in treated patients (Kalra et al, 1995; Ohara et al, 1997). The complications of MDS or AML may be associated with specific therapies, such as recombinant granulocyte-macrophage colony-stimulating factor (GM-CSF) or immunosuppressive agents. Alternatively, MDS or AML may represent a natural history of the underlying disease, apparent due to longer survival times of patients with severe aplastic anemia.

MDS and AML have markedly increased frequency in children with a variety of constitutional disorders, including Kostmann syndrome, Schwachman syndrome, Fanconi anemia, and neurofibromatosis type 1 (Fischer et al, 1997; Johnson & Cotter, 1997; Kalra et al, 1995). A significant proportion of these MDS and AML cases harbor monosomy 7, but the pathogenetic mechanisms involved are not entirely clear. In neurofibromatosis 1, deregulation of the *RAS* gene appears to be important. For unknown reasons, the high risk of MDS or AML is found only in affected children under 5 years of age.

In addition to these constitutional abnormalities underlying MDS or AML, a familial monosomy 7 syndrome has been reported in about 10 families. These patients also develop

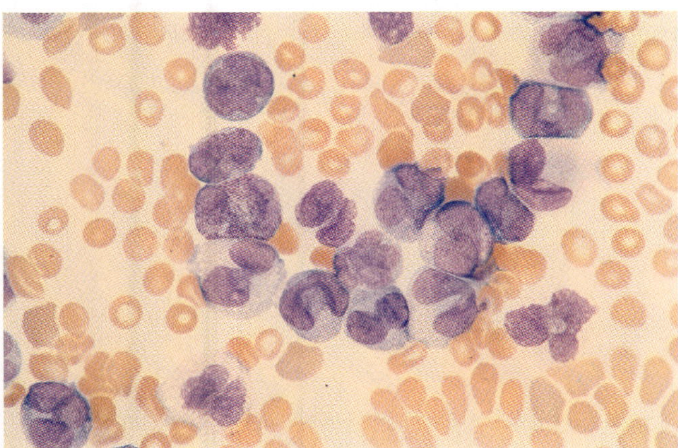

Figure 4–25

Acute promyelocytic leukemia, microgranular. This photomicrograph illustrates the striking nuclear folding and sparsely granular cytoplasm typical of the microgranular form. Wright stain.

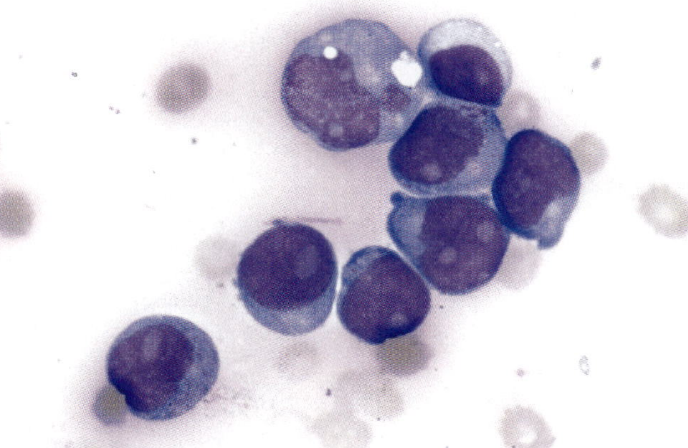

Figure 4–27

AML. In this patient with t(8;21), poor cytoplasmic granulation and a rim of basophilia are evident. Wright stain.

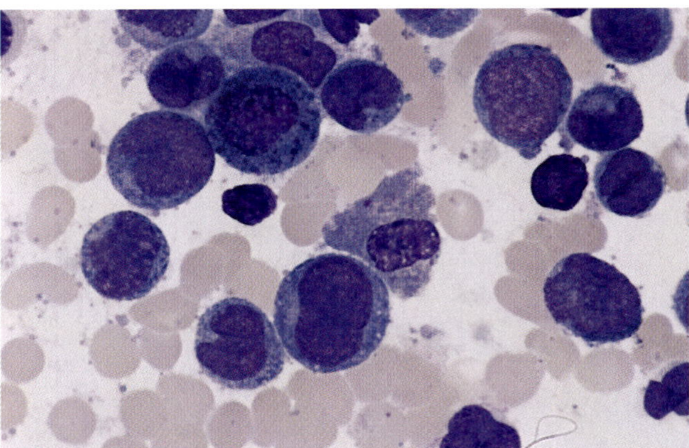

Figure 4–28

AML M4eos, marrow aspirate. This photomicrograph illustrates increased eosinophils with abnormal granulation in a patient with eosinophilia and inv(16). Wright stain.

MDS or AML but at an older age than do patients with monosomy 7 syndrome (Johnson & Cotter, 1997). The inheritance pattern in this disorder is not established. There is no evidence of inheritance of an abnormal tumor suppressor gene on chromosome 7 as in the retinoblastoma model. Abnormal loci on other chromosomes may be inherited that predispose to development of monosomy 7. Monosomy 7 is rarely detected in lymphocytic malignancies; a small subset of ALL patients with t(9;22) also show a monosomy 7. The prognosis for these patients is extremely poor (Russo et al, 1991).

Data suggest that monosomy 7 is likely a secondary event in AML. Monosomy 7 appears to contribute to leukemic transformation, but other genetic events, such as changes in RAS signaling pathways are likely also important. Loss of a gene or genes on 7q may contribute to leukemogenesis, possibly through a gene dosage effect (haploinsufficiency leads to decreased levels of critical proteins) (Savage et al, 1994). The critical regions involved in monosomy 7/7q− are well recognized at 7q22 and 7q32–34. Although several genes have been mapped to this area, no single gene is deleted in each case (Johnson & Cotter, 1996). Thus, the molecular events resulting from monosomy 7/7q− may be heterogeneous (Fischer et al, 1997).

Therapy-Related Leukemias

Acute leukemias and myelodysplastic disorders secondary to alkylating agent or radiation therapy have been the subject of extensive investigation for several decades, but the development of AML following DNA topoisomerase II inhibitor therapy has only been identified since 1991 (Devereux, 1991; Karp & Smith, 1997; Pedersen-Bjergaard et al, 1995; Pedersen-Bjergaard et al, 1993; Pui et al, 1995c; Sandoval et al, 1993; Super et al, 1993). The clinical and pathologic features of these two types of therapy-related AML are detailed in Table 4–14. Although mechanisms vary, both treatments induce permanent DNA damage, the presumed first step in leukemogenesis. The interval from initiation of therapy to onset of therapy-related leukemia ranges between 1 and 11 years and is characteristically shorter in patients with topoisomerase II inhibitor–related leukemia. A greater risk of leukemia and a shorter latent period before leukemia development are linked to a higher cumulative dose of alkylating agents. Prior myelodysplastic phases and multilineage dyspoiesis characterize alkylating agent–related AML. Leukemias linked to topoisomerase II inhibitor therapy generally have a more abrupt onset and usually demonstrate a striking monoblastic component (Fig. 4–29).

Clonal cytogenetic abnormalities are identified in at least 90% of patients developing therapy-related leukemias. For

Table 4–14
Comparison of Clinicopathologic Features of Two Types of Therapy-Related AML

	Secondary to Alkylating Agent Therapy	Secondary to Topoisomerase II Inhibitor Therapy
Therapy	Alkylating agents or radiotherapy induce permanent genetic abnormalities	Epipodophyllotoxins and related agents target DNA–topoisomerase II
Latent period	2–11 years; shorter for patients with higher cumulative alkylating agent dose	<1–3 years
Blood	Myelodysplastic phase characterized by severe cytopenias, marked trilineage dyspoiesis, and basophilia	Abrupt onset of AML Usually lack myelodysplastic phase or exhibit very brief phase
Marrow	Usually hypercellular, but may be hypocellular Fibrosis common Multilineage dyspoiesis present Blasts undifferentiated, with high CD34 expression, weak cytochemical reactions, and few Auer rods Most common types: AML-M2, AML-M4, AML-M6	Hypercellular, with prominent monoblastic component (AML-M5a or AML-M4)
Cytogenetics	−5/5q−, −7/7q− Complex karyotypic abnormalities frequent Rare translocations (of type found in de novo AML)	11q23 translocations in most cases
Response to therapy	Poor response to conventional antileukemic therapy Expression of multidrug resistance–associated proteins and drug efflux	Good response to induction chemotherapy but high rate of relapse
Survival	Poor	Variable; may be improved with marrow transplantation

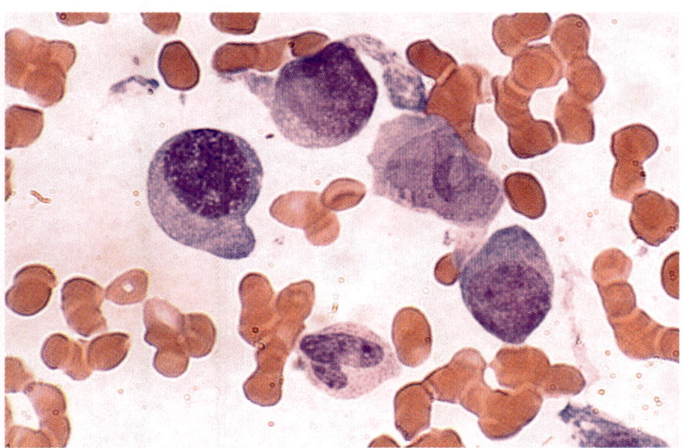

Figure 4–29

Acute monocytic leukemia, marrow aspirate. This film shows a sheet of monoblasts in a patient who developed acute monocytic leukemia following topoisomerase II inhibitor therapy. Wright stain.

alkylating agent–related lesions, loss of all or part of chromosomes 5 and/or 7 is characteristic. Complex karyotypic abnormalities are common in patients with alkylating agent–related AML, but the types of translocations typically found in cases of de novo AML are rare. In contrast, translocations involving 11q23 typify topoisomerase II inhibitor–related leukemias.

Multidrug-Resistant AML

AML patients frequently achieve remission with current induction therapies, but a large proportion of these patients subsequently experience relapse and die. Expression of multidrug-resistant protein 1 (MDR1, or p-glycoprotein) is a mechanism important in the resistance of AML to chemotherapy (Dalton, 1997; Del Poeta et al, 1996; Leith et al, 1997b; List, 1996; Marie et al, 1997; Willman, 1997). MDR1 confers multidrug resistance through the ATP-dependent efflux from the cell of a wide variety of compounds, including drugs, such as daunomycin, that are key to AML therapy. Thus, MDR1+ AML blasts are inherently more resistant to daunomycin-induced cell death than MDR1− cells. The frequency of MDR1 expression in AML increases sharply with patient age (Leith 1997a, Leith 1997b), an expected finding, since AML in the elderly more closely resembles secondary AML (frequently MDR1+) than de novo AML. The few studies of multidrug resistance in pediatric AML have shown a frequency of MDR1 expression of 8–20%, similar to that in younger adults (Ivy et al, 1996). One study revealed an association between MDR1 expression and drug efflux with the t(8;21) (Pearson et al, 1996). This preliminary finding may explain the poor prognosis this translocation carries in pediatric AML (Martinez-Climent, 1997).

Biologic Subsets of ALL

Hyperdiploid ALL

Hyperdiploidy (a numerical increase in the chromosome number) is the most frequently identified cytogenetic abnormality in ALL. Over 40% of pediatric ALL cases are hyperdiploid. About 15% of ALL cases have 47 to 50 chromosomes, and 27% have over 50 chromosomes (Martinez-Climent, 1997; Pui et al, 1990). Those hyperdiploid ALL (Fig. 4–30) patients with over 50 chromosomes or a DNA index over 1.16 are associated with other favorable features at presentation and demonstrate a particularly favorable response to antimetabolite-based therapy (Pui et al, 1989; Pui et al, 1994; Trueworthy et al, 1992). Patients with chromosome numbers of 47 to 50 appear to have a prognosis intermediate between those over 50 hyperdiploidy and diploid or pseudodiploid patients. A DNA index over 1.16 remains an important independent prognostic indicator of outcome, even after accounting for the other favorable features found in these patients at presentation. The good prognosis of this group has been attributed to increased sensitivity of the blasts to antimetabolites, increased spontaneous apoptosis, and lower tumor burden (Kaspers et al, 1995; Kumagai et al, 1996; Pui et al, 1989). The presence of an additional chromosome 4 or 10 identifies a subset of hyperdiploid ALL cases with a particularly favorable response (Harris et al, 1992).

Triploid or tetraploid states (more than 65 chromosomes) are seen in about 1% of cases and are associated with poor outcome (Pui et al, 1994).

ALL with Cryptic t(12;21)(p13;q22)

The t(12;21) is the commonest genetic translocation in pediatric ALL (Romana et al, 1995b; Rubnitz & Look, 1998). The

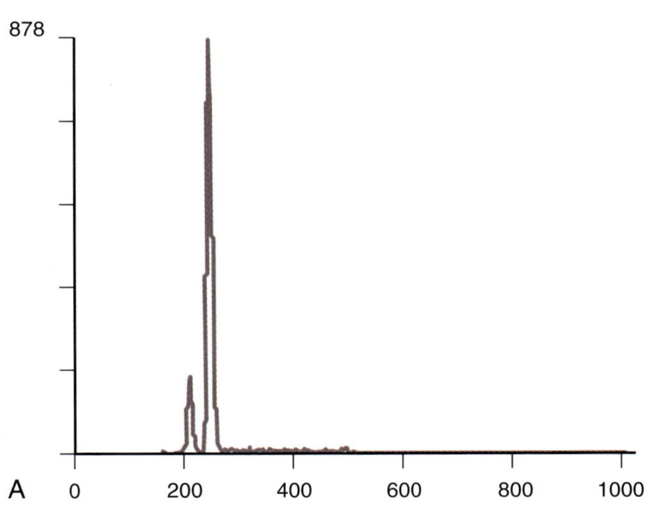

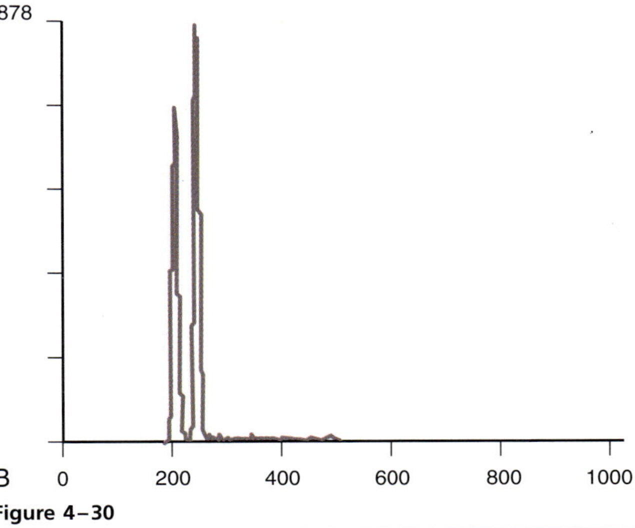

Figure 4–30

ALL, hyperdiploid type. *A*. The hyperdiploid peak of the leukemic population is demonstrated. *B*. There is an equal mixture of leukemic and normal cells, with an increase in the normal diploid spike.

high prevalence of this translocation has been established. The translocation is usually cryptic, being detected by classic cytogenetic analysis in <0.5% of ALL cases. The incidence of t(12;21) in 20–25% of cases of B precursor pediatric ALL was established only after the genes involved were identified and molecular methods were developed to detect the resultant fusion transcript (McClean et al, 1996; Raynaud et al, 1996; Romana et al, 1995b; Rubnitz & Look, 1998; Shih et al, 1996; Shurtleff et al, 1995).

The t(12;21) results in formation of a fusion transcript between the *TEL* gene on chromosome 12p13 and the *AML1* gene on 21q22. *TEL* is a member of a family of genes that presumably act as transcriptional modulators, whereas the *AML1* gene acts as a transcriptional regulator. The *TEL/AML1* fusion transcript resulting from the t(12;21) causes transcription factor deregulation, a critical event in leukemogenesis (Romana et al, 1995b).

Reports are conflicting, but most evidence indicates that patients with the t(12;21) usually have a favorable prognosis, similar to that of patients with hyperdiploid ALL (Borkhardt et al, 1997; Lanza et al, 1997b; Rubnitz & Look, 1998; Seeger et al, 1998). If the t(12;21) is shown to be a favorable prognostic factor in pediatric ALL in larger trials, molecular screening for the translocation should become standard practice for improving the management of such patients.

Pre-B ALL with t(1;19) or Variants

The t(1;19)(q23;p13) translocation is another abnormality in pediatric ALL, identified by cytogenetic study in about 5% of cases (Martinez-Climent, 1997; Rubnitz & Look, 1998). These patients do poorly on standard chemotherapeutic regimens, with a high risk of relapse and death. However, they do well on more intensive regimens. Thus, identification of patients with a t(1;19) ensures that they receive appropriately intensive chemotherapy (Crist et al, 1990).

Patients with t(1;19) ALL have features of high-risk disease at presentation. They often have high peripheral WBC counts and increased frequency of CNS disease. Even in the context of such high-risk features, the t(1;19) is an independent prognostic factor for poor outcome (Crist et al, 1990). Morphologically, blasts in t(1;19) ALL are indistinguishable from those in other ALL types. However, the immunophenotype is characteristic, since the vast majority (>90%) of cases show a pre–B cell phenotype (cytoplasmic immunoglobulin positive). Only a small percentage of t(1;19) ALLs have a more immature B precursor phenotype. The blasts generally lack CD34 expression and show heterogeneous CD20 expression, with some blasts CD20 − (Borowitz et al, 1993b). DNA content is usually pseudodiploid (Pui et al, 1994). The presence of the t(1;19), found in 20–25% of pre–B cell ALLs, explains the poor prognosis previously associated with this phenotype. Thus, analysis for the t(1;19) translocation is clinically much more valuable than assessment of cytoplasmic immunoglobulin expression (Crist et al, 1990; Crist et al, 1989; Hunger, 1996).

The t(1;19) involves the *E2A* gene on chromosome 19 and the pre–B cell leukemia transcription factor 1 (*PBX1*) gene on chromosome 1 (Hunger et al, 1991). *E2A* acts as a transcriptional activator important in normal regulation of B cell development, whereas *PBX1* may have a role in growth cycle regulation (Hunger, 1996; Hunger et al, 1991). The E2A/PBX1 fusion protein formed by the t(1;19) has properties of a chimeric transcription factor and has been shown experimentally to act as a potent oncogene.

Molecular studies have shown that 25–50% of t(1;19) translocations may be missed by classic cytogenetic analysis (Hunger, 1996; Izraeli et al, 1993; Borowitz et al, 1993). Since patients with t(1;19) ALL have a greatly improved prognosis if intensive therapy is given, RT-PCR analysis to look for a cryptic t(1;19) is particularly important in children who would otherwise be given standard therapy.

Philadelphia Chromosome–Positive ALL: t(9;22)(q34;q11)

The Philadelphia chromosome (Ph^1) is present in 3–5% of pediatric ALL cases (Rubnitz & Look, 1998; Schlieben et al, 1996). Earlier studies suggested that children with Ph^1 ALL had poor prognostic features, such as older age and higher WBC count, at presentation, but subsequent studies show no significant differences between Ph^1-positive and Ph^1-negative ALL with regard to clinical features at presentation (Ribeiro et al, 1987; Schlieben et al, 1996). In addition, Ph^1 ALL cases have a phenotype similar to that of the common pediatric ALL (early B cell precursor). Most of the remainder have a pre–B cell phenotype. A T cell phenotype is rare (Schlieben et al, 1996). CD34 is expressed in most cases of either common ALL or pre-B phenotype (Schlieben et al, 1996), and expression of myeloid antigens such as CD13 or CD33 may be seen. Since such antigens are also commonly present on other ALL subtypes, the diagnosis of Ph^1 ALL rests on cytogenetic and molecular analysis.

Classic cytogenetic analysis has been the standard for detection of the Ph^1 chromosome. In most cases the Ph^1 results from the classic t(9;22)(q34;q11), whereas in a minority classic cytogenetics detects a complex "variant" Ph^1 translocation.

Cases of Ph^1 ALL may be missed by cytogenetic analysis because of technical problems. Occasionally, cases with negative cytogenetic study results are shown to have breakpoint cluster region–Abelson leukemia virus (*BCR/ABL*) fusion by RT-PCR analysis (Beyermann et al, 1996; Devaraj et al, 1995). RT-PCR techniques are useful adjuncts to routine cytogenetic studies in detecting cases with an occult Ph^1 chromosome. Secondary cytogenetic abnormalities are well described in Ph^1 ALL, including a monosomy 7 associated with a particularly poor prognosis (Rieder et al, 1996). Thus, cytogenetic analysis remains a part of the standard diagnostic work-up in ALL.

The t(9;22)(q34;q11) juxtaposes the *ABL* gene on chromosome 9 with the *BCR* gene on chromosome 22. The chimeric *BCR/ABL* transcript encodes for a protein with enhanced tyrosine kinase activity. In chronic myelogenous leukemia, the chimeric *BCR/ABL* transcript produces a 210-kD (p210) protein, while a 190-kD (p190) protein is produced in most pediatric ALL cases. The p190 protein is possibly more leukemogenic than the p210 protein (resulting in acute rather than chronic leukemia), but there is no convincing evidence that leukemic type is dependent on which protein is produced.

Ph^1 ALL is associated with a poor response to therapy, and patients may be candidates for alternative therapies, such as allogeneic marrow transplantation, in first remission. Duration of the first complete remission is often short, and many patients relapse on therapy. The likelihood of a second complete remission and of event-free survival is much lower among Ph^1 ALL patients (Beyermann et al, 1997; Beyermann et al, 1996).

Burkitt Lymphoma/ALL-L3: t(8;14)(q24;q32)

ALL-L3 is a leukemic phase of small noncleaved cell lymphoma (Burkitt lymphoma) but is by convention considered a leukemia, rather than a lymphoma in FAB classification (Martinez-Climent, 1997; Rubnitz & Look, 1998). These cases constitute about 2% of childhood "ALL" cases. Recognition of ALL-L3 is important, since patients should receive Burkitt lymphoma treatment. Morphologically, L3 blasts are large, with fine chromatin, multiple distinct nucleoli, and vacuolated ba-

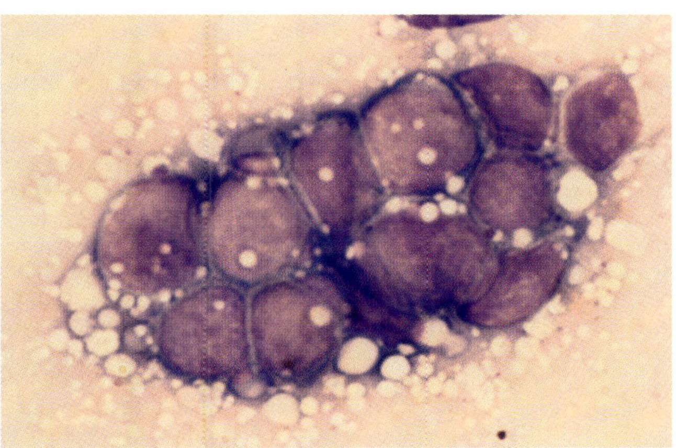

Figure 4–31

Burkitt lymphoma, marrow aspirate. Numerous L3 lymphoblasts are evident. Note the basophilic cytoplasm and prominent vacuolization. Wright stain.

sophilic cytoplasm (see Figs. 4–16 and 4–31). Phenotypically, these blasts have a mature B cell phenotype, with surface immunoglobulin expression and light-chain restriction. Rarely, cases have cytoplasmic immunoglobulin without surface light chains. TdT positivity has also been rarely reported (Magrath et al, 1992).

The hallmark of ALL-L3 is a cytogenetic abnormality, t(8;14)(q24;q32), juxtaposing a myelocytomatosis (*MYC*) protooncogene and the immunoglobulin promoter region. Constitutive overexpression of *MYC* and excessive cell proliferation result. ALL-L3 is less commonly associated with the t(2;8) or the t(8;22), in which case the juxtaposition of *MYC* and the promoter region of the immunoglobulin light-chain genes leads to the same net effect of uncontrolled *MYC* expression.

T-ALL

Ten to 15% of all pediatric ALL cases have a T cell phenotype (Martinez-Climent 1997; Rubnitz & Look, 1998). Most children with T cell ALL are male and are 7 to 8 years of age or older at presentation. Patients typically present with very high WBC, counts (>100,000/mm^3), lymphadenopathy, and organomegaly. Many have an anterior mediastinal mass (Uckun et al, 1998), a finding highly predictive of a T cell phenotype. T-ALL is the leukemic counterpart of T lymphoblastic lymphoma, which is characteristically seen as an anterior mediastinal mass in adolescent males. Distinction between these two diseases is arbitrary, with ALL diagnosed when leukemic blasts constitute >25% of marrow cells (Foucar, 1995a).

The lymphoblasts of T-ALL recapitulate, although often not precisely, the phenotype of immature T cells at one of the stages of thymic development. T-ALL lymphoblasts therefore generally express surface CD7/CD2 and quite often CD5. Some cases express CD1 and may coexpress CD4/CD8. T-ALL cells (and normal immature T cells) may express intracytoplasmic but not surface CD3. T-ALL lymphoblasts routinely express TdT but are usually HLA-DR negative. Some T-ALL cases may coexpress myeloid antigens. Differentiation of T-ALL from AML requires a battery of immunophenotypic markers, since many AMLs express the "T cell" antigens—CD7, CD4, and CD2—and may also express dim TdT (Borowitz, 1992). The marker most useful in differentiating T-ALL from AML is expression of cytoplasmic CD3. This marker is very sensitive and highly specific for T-ALL. In addition, AML cases usually express HLA-DR and have characteristic cytochemical profiles.

No single cytogenetic abnormality is characteristic of T-ALL, although 40% of cases show chromosomal translocations. About half of these have breakpoints involving the TCR genes at 14q11 (Tα/δ), 7q35 (Tβ), or 7p15 (Tγ) (Martinez-Climent, 1997; Pui et al, 1990; Rubnitz & Look, 1998). Various other chromosomes are partners in these translocations involving the TCR genes. One of the commonest is seen in about 10% of T-ALL in children: the t(11;14)(p15;q11), involving the *TCRα/δ* gene and the *TTG2* gene on chromosome 11. Other genes that may be involved include the *MYC* gene on chromosome 8q24 and the *TAL1* gene on chromosome 1p32 [t(1;14)(p32–p34;q11)]. Cytogenetic translocations involving *TAL1* on 1p32 are found in only about 3% of T-ALL cases, but molecular studies have found that about 25% of patients with T-ALL harbor *TAL1* gene rearrangements that are not detected cytogenetically. Most T-ALL lymphoblasts produce TAL1 mRNA and protein, even in the absence of *TAL1* rearrangement (Bash et al, 1995; Bash et al, 1993; Chetty et al, 1995; Kikuchi et al, 1993). Ectopic expression of this gene (not normally expressed by T cells during their development) may be one mechanism of leukemogenesis in this disease (Bash et al, 1995).

Homozygous deletions or, much less commonly, mutations of the tumor suppressor genes *P16^{INK4A}/MTS1* and *P15^{INK4B}/MTS2* on chromosome 9p have been found in up to 80% of T-ALL cases (Hebert et al, 1994; Ohnishi et al, 1995; Okuda et al, 1995). These genes encode proteins that are important regulators of the cell cycle, and thus their deletion presumably results in uncontrolled cell growth and leukemogenesis. Deletions of p16 and p15 appear characteristic of T-ALL and are observed infrequently (<5%) in B lineage ALL (Hebert et al, 1994). Molecular analysis is necessary to detect these deletions in most cases, since only about 10% of cases exhibit abnormalities of 9p detected by classic cytogenetic analysis.

ALL with Eosinophilia and t(5;14)(q31;q32)

A striking blood, marrow, and tissue eosinophilia is identified in rare ALL patients and is associated with t(5;14)(q31;q32)(Meeker 1990, Rubnitz 1998). Lymphoblasts usually have L1 or L2 morphologic features. Compared to other ALL patients, those with associated eosinophilia tend to be older; exhibit a greater male predominance, striking organomegaly, and cardiovascular abnormalities; and experience an aggressive disease course. The eosinophilia may precede, occur simultaneously with, or follow the development of ALL. This eosinophilia is the presumed consequence of the fusion of the *IL3* gene into the immunoglobulin heavy-chain gene locus, resulting in a sustained stimulus for eosinophil production (Meeker et al, 1990). The eosinophils may exhibit striking nuclear and cytoplasmic dysplasia, including hypogranular cytoplasm, cytoplasmic vacuoles, and nuclear hypersegmentation (Fig. 4–32). Persistent eosinophilia may result in extensive tissue damage, especially cardiovascular and neural, and thereby result in substantial rates of morbidity and mortality in these patients.

Granular ALL

Approximately 2–7% of cases of ALL in children demonstrate distinct cytoplasmic granules, mimicking AML (Cerezo et al, 1991), in which >5% of the lymphoblasts contain scattered azurophilic granules (Fig. 4–33). These blasts also often demonstrate L2 morphologic features, causing further confusion with AML. Ultrastructural studies show that these granules are either mitochondria or lysosomes. On cytochemical staining, the granules are acid phosphatase or α-naphthylacetate esterase positive, weakly PAS positive, Sudan black B positive (occa-

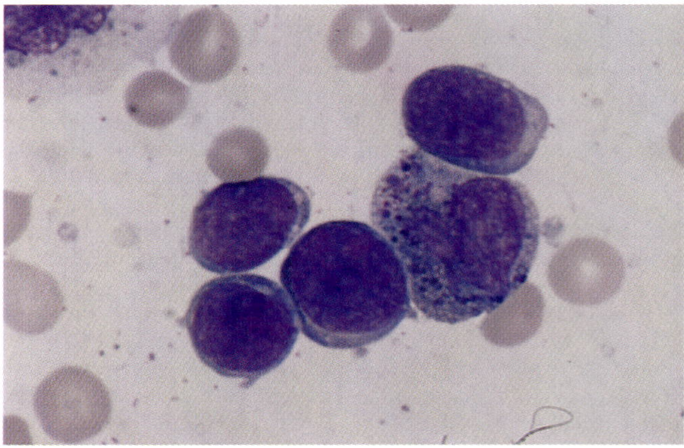

Figure 4–32

Acute lymphoblastic leukemia with t(5:14), marrow aspirate. This film shows a striking predominance of lymphoblasts with admixed dyspoietic eosinophils. Wright stain.

sional cases), and myeloperoxidase negative. Immunophenotypic profiles are straightforward precursor B cell ALL in type (Cerezo et al, 1991). Patients with granular ALL have a worse prognosis than do other pediatric ALL patients.

"Mixed Lineage" Acute Leukemia

Coexpression of antigens of more than one lineage is frequently encountered in acute leukemia, generally as expression of lymphocytic antigens in AML or myelocytic antigens in ALL. Such phenotypes were initially often described as of "mixed lineage" and were considered to be phenotypic aberrations. It has been recognized that many antigens are not lineage specific. For example, dim CD4 expression is found on normal monocytes and is also frequently found in AML, particularly, though not exclusively, on the monocytic subtypes (Larson & McCurley et al, 1995; Pui et al, 1993). Small subpopulations of normal marrow progenitor cells expressing antigens of more than one lineage have been identified. For example, CD2 expression is found on some normal B lymphocyte progenitors. Leukemias with "aberrant" phenotypes may be derived from such progenitor cells (Pui et al, 1993).

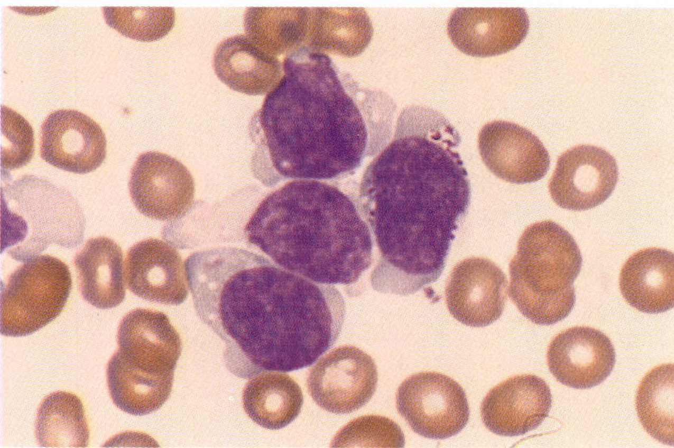

Figure 4–33

ALL, L2 with granules, marrow aspirate. This film shows scattered cytoplasmic granules within blasts. Wright stain.

The importance of "mixed lineage" phenotypes has been difficult to determine because of varying immunophenotypic criteria in identification of cases and poorly standardized methods of detecting antigen expression. Taking these limitations into consideration, investigators have reported that myeloid antigen expression apparently does not affect the response of ALL to current treatment regimens. A similar conclusion may be reached about cases of AML with lymphoid antigens once other prognostic factors, such as cytogenetic, features, have been considered (Drexler et al, 1993; Leith & Willman, 1996; Smith et al, 1992). One exception to this conclusion is a rarely described AML that is clearly Sudan black B and myeloperoxidase positive and yet is characterized by blasts that coexpress T cell antigens, including cytoplasmic CD3. Children with this disease are older, have lymphadenopathy, and tend to have higher WBC counts. Responses to ALL therapy subsequent to failure with AML therapy are reported in this group (Cross et al, 1988). These cases may be best described as lineage indeterminant.

From a practical standpoint, correct diagnosis of ALL (T or B cell types) or AML is problematic in cases in which the leukemic blasts coexpress antigens from multiple lineages. Studies have found that at least 25% of ALL cases coexpress myeloid antigens such as CD13 or CD33, whereas up to 60% of pediatric AML cases coexpress lymphoid-associated antigens, including CD2, CD4, and CD19. A fairly comprehensive immunophenotyping panel is essential and should include several markers for each lineage (Davis et al, 1997). The use of markers highly sensitive for the lineage (e.g., CD7 for T cells) as well as those that are lineage specific (e.g., cytoplasmic CD3) is helpful. Interpretation of the results of immunophenotyping in cases in which the leukemic blasts coexpress antigens from multiple lineages requires knowledge of the relative lineage specificity of each antigen used.

Extramedullary Disease

Although acute leukemias are marrow-derived neoplasms, extramedullary manifestations are relatively common. Leukemias, especially ALL, typically involve extramedullary sites, such as liver, spleen, and nodes, at presentation. However, some patients have tumorous infiltrates that precede or follow the diagnosis of acute leukemia as well as occur simultaneously. The term extramedullary myeloid cell tumor has generally replaced the earlier terms granulocytic or monoblastic sarcoma and chloroma (Byrd et al, 1995; Quintanilla-Martinez et al, 1995; Roth et al, 1995; Traweek et al, 1993). Associations between specific types of AML and the development of extramedullary tumors have been established. For example, these tumors are much commoner in cases of AML in which either t(8;21) or inv(16) is detected and in AML FAB subtypes M2, M4, and M5 (Figs. 4–34 and 4–35) (Byrd, 1995). Extramedullary manifestations are consistently seen in patients with monocytic leukemia (Fig. 4–36). In particular, cutaneous monoblastic lesions commonly occur in neonates with acute monocytic leukemia and t(4;11). Coexpression of CD56, CD2, CD4, and CD1 in cases of AML is also linked to a greater likelihood of extramedullary tumors.

The temporal association of extramedullary tumors with the marrow picture of AML is clinically significant. Extramedullary tumors occurring along with marrow involvement at presentation or relapse of AML are generally of no clinical significance, although recent reports suggest an adverse outcome for those patients with t(8;21) (Byrd et al, 1997; Traweek et al, 1993). In contrast, extramedullary tumors in patients with underlying chronic myeloproliferative disorders represent blast crises that are often difficult to control. If extramedullary tu-

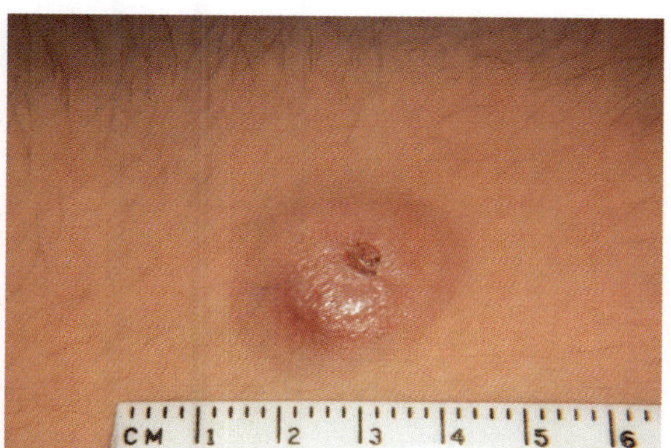

Figure 4–34

Acute monocytic leukemia. This photograph shows a single lesion in a young adult with multiple cutaneous masses. (Courtesy Dr. J. Saiki.)

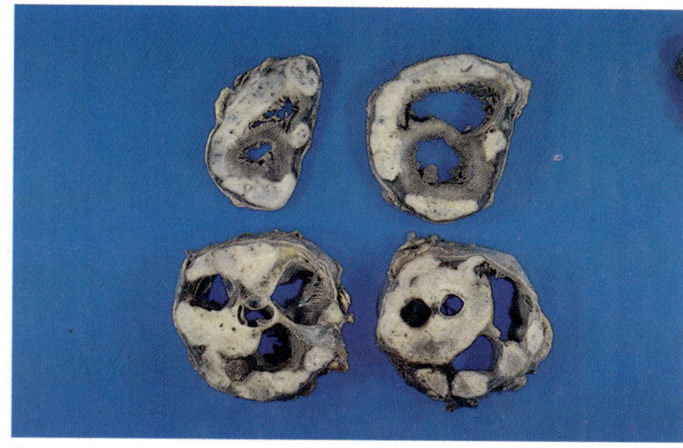

Figure 4–35

Acute myelomonocytic leukemia. Death occurred suddenly in this young man with acute heart failure from massive cardiac involvement by leukemia.

mors precede marrow disease in untreated patients, overt marrow involvement by AML generally occurs within 1 to 2 years. Consequently, treatment currently recommended for isolated extramedullary tumor is AML-type induction therapy to prevent eventual marrow disease (Byrd et al, 1995).

Extramedullary tumors are often misdiagnosed. Their morphologic appearance is variable and overlaps substantially with B and T cell lymphomas and undifferentiated nonhematopoietic malignant tumors (Fig. 4–37). Recognition of extramedullary tumors preceding AML is often dependent on paraffin immunoperoxidase techniques, since electron microscopy is usually not available and appropriate samples for flow cytometric immunophenotyping or frozen-section immunoperoxidase studies may not be obtained. The actual paraffin immunoperoxidase profile of extramedullary tumors lacks specificity (Table 4–15). One of its most sensitive markers (CD43 expression) is present in most T cell processes, including T-ALL and T lymphoblastic lymphoma. Additional potential problems include the frequent failure of extramedullary tumors to express either CD34 or CD45 (common leukocyte

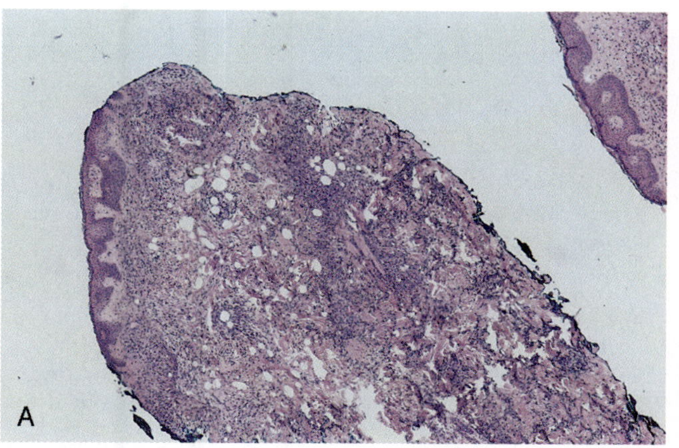

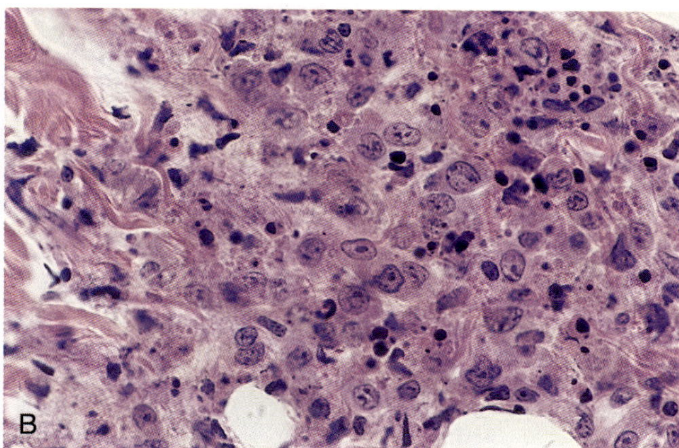

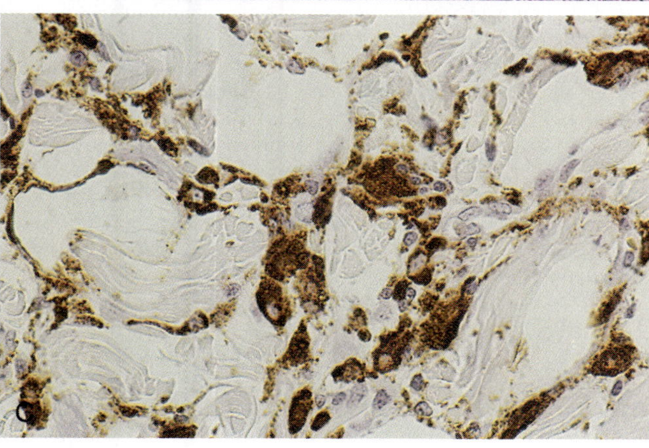

Figure 4–36

Acute monocytic leukemia, skin. *A*. This low-magnification photomicrograph illustrates a pattern of involvement often seen in leukemic infiltrates, with extensive permeation of the dermis and subcutaneous tissue. *B*. This high-magnification photomicrograph shows blasts with distinct nucleoli and slight nuclear folding. Monocytic infiltrates often show more folding than in this case. *C*. Immunoperoxidase procedures may facilitate recognition of monocytic infiltrates. In this instance the antimicrophagic antibody HAM56 was used.

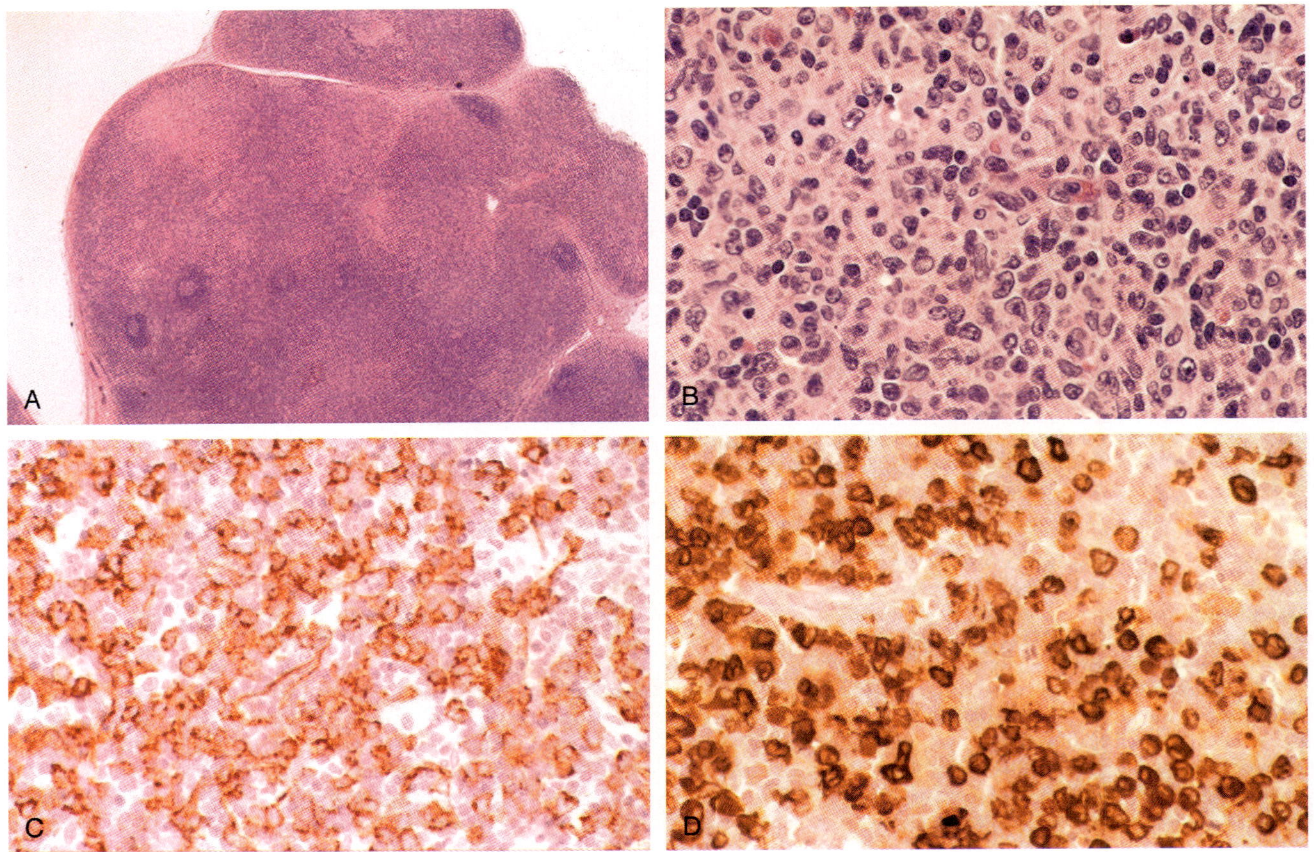

Figure 4–37

Acute leukemia, lymph node. *A*. This low-magnification photomicrograph illustrates striking nodal effacement by an extensive infiltrate of blasts in a 1-year-old infant. *B*. This high-magnification photomicrograph illustrates a spectrum of immature cells that have no apparent differentiation by hematoxylin-eosin staining. *C*. Immunoperoxidase staining facilitates the identification of leukemic infiltrates in extramedullary sites. Immunoperoxidase for CD34. *D*. Strong myeloperoxidase positivity is evident in this immunoperoxidase preparation.

antigen) in paraffin immunoperoxidase studies. The most sensitive and specific marker in these cases is antimyeloperoxidase (Fig. 4–37*D*), and CD68 and lysozyme studies may also be useful.

Extramedullary infiltrates of immature T or B cells are "diagnosed" as to lymphomatous or leukemic origin by arbitrary criteria, with cases in which lymphoblasts exceed 25% of marrow elements designated as ALL. Infiltrates in lymph node, spleen, liver, and mediastinum (Fig. 4–38) are common manifestations of ALL, whereas relapses often involve the CNS and testes. In general, T cell lymphoblastic infiltrates predominate in extramedullary sites (Fig. 4–39), and the paraffin immunoperoxidase profile of these tumors includes the consistent expression of cytoplasmic CD3, CD43, and CD45 and the variable expression of markers of immaturity, such as TdT and CD34. In contrast, the diagnosis of B cell precursor ALL or B lymphoblastic lymphoma by paraffin immunoperoxidase studies is more difficult, since CD45 and CD20 expression is frequently not detected in these malignancies. CD79a may be useful in these cases. TdT and CD34 may be expressed in extramedullary precursor B-ALL or B lymphoblastic lymphoma but are not uniformly identified. The differential diagnosis for extramedullary infiltrate of lymphoblasts includes the look-alikes of AML, "small blue-cell tumors" in pediatric patients, and the B T cell lymphomas (see Table 4–15). The approach to the diagnosis of extramedullary acute leukemic infiltrates includes correlation with the blood and marrow picture, a high index of suspicion, and a comprehensive immunoperoxidase panel (see Table 4–15) if cell suspensions or electron microscopy is not available.

MINIMAL RESIDUAL DISEASE

Following antileukemic therapy, most patients with AML or ALL enter a morphologic and hematologic complete remission. However, by more sensitive techniques, small numbers of residual neoplastic cells may often be detected in the marrow. The techniques used to detect minimal residual disease and their relative sensitivities in recognizing neoplastic cells admixed with normal marrow may be found in Table 4–16. In general, PCR-based molecular techniques are the most sensitive and specific for detecting minimal residual disease. The sensitivity of cytogenetic studies for this purpose may be enhanced by fluorescence in situ hybridization methods, while immunophenotypic marker analyses are dependent upon a unique leukemia-specific antigen profile utilizing multicolor coexpression analyses.

The clinical significance of minimal residual disease is controversial and apparently depends on factors that vary for each type of leukemia (Brisco et al, 1996). Two major variables are the sensitivity of the methods used to detect residual disease and the time during therapy when the residual disease is detected (El-Rifai et al, 1997; Jacquy et al, 1997; Kaspryzk &

Table 4–15

Paraffin Immunoperoxidase Studies in Extramedullary Myelogenous and Lymphoblastic Tumors

Antibodies	Comments and Caveats
Myeloid	
CD43	Highly sensitive for myelocytic tumors but *not* specific Also detected in T cells, some B cells, and erythrocytic precursors; rare reports in nonhematopoietic neoplasms
Antimyeloperoxidase	Highly sensitive and specific marker for myelocytic elements
Antilysozyme	Sensitive but not entirely specific for immature myelocytic infiltrates
CD68, CD15	Moderate sensitivity; more often detected on more differentiated granulocytic (CD15) and monocytic (CD68) processes
CD45 (CLA)	Detected in only about half of extramedullary myelocytic tumors
CD34	Valuable indicator of immaturity of cells but detected in less than half of extramedullary myelocytic tumors
Lymphoid	
CD3	Highly sensitive and specific for T cell neoplasms; cytoplasmic reaction common in immature T cell tumors
CD43	Sensitive but not specific for T cell tumors (see above)
CD45 (CLA)	Expressed on most immature T cell infiltrates of T-ALL or T-LL but often *negative* on precursor B-ALL or B-LL
TdT, CD34	Useful markers of immaturity but not expressed in all cases of blastic T or B cell neoplasms (ALL or LL); also expressed on a minority of myelocytic tumors
CD20	Specific for B cell tumors although not expressed on very immature precursor B-ALL or B-LL; rare reports of CD20 expression on myelocytic tumors
CD79a	Useful marker for B cells in tissue; greater sensitivity for immature B cells than CD20; also expressed in some AML cases and rare T-LL/T-ALL
CD99	Often expressed in B and T cell blastic tumors (ALL or LL)

Abbreviations: ALL, acute lymphoblastic leukemia; LL, lymphoblastic lymphoma.

Secker-Walker, 1997; Knechtli et al, 1995; Owen et al, 1997). In t(8;21) AML patients, the *AML1/ETO* fusion gene may be detected in patients who experience prolonged relapse-free survival, suggesting that molecular evidence of disease is not linked to clinical outcome in this situation (Nucifora et al, 1993). The significance of PCR-detected minimal residual disease is controversial and varies by disease type (Hunger et al, 1998). In contrast, the detection of residual disease by less sensitive parameters (standard cytogenetics or morphologic or cytochemical characteristics) is much more closely associated with eventual overt relapse.

RELAPSE OF ACUTE LEUKEMIA

Approximately one-half of AML patients and one-third of ALL patients suffer a relapse, generally manifested in the marrow as >5% marrow blasts unattributable to another cause (Cheson et al, 1990). If the percentage of marrow blasts is low and the diagnosis of overt relapse is inconclusive, a repeat marrow examination in 1 week is warranted. In most cases of relapse, the number of marrow blasts unambiguously exceeds 5%, and these blasts generally resemble the original leukemic cells morphologically and cytochemically. Foci of blasts may be evident on clot and biopsy sections, while other areas of the marrow are unaffected (Fig. 4–40). The use of CD34 and TdT immunoperoxidase stains on marrow sections is very helpful in detecting ALL relapse (Rimsza et al, 1998).

Relapse may also be confirmed in extramedullary sites either as an isolated focus or in conjunction with marrow relapse. Numerous sites may be involved in extramedullary relapse in AML, whereas CNS and testicular relapse is typical of ALL.

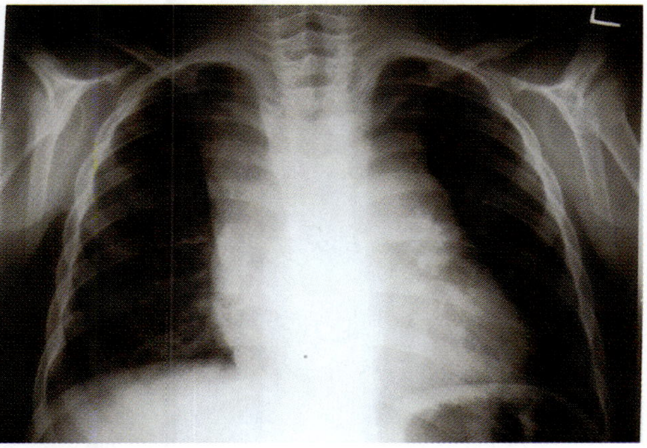

Figure 4–38

A prominent mediastinal mass is evident in this 11-year-old boy with T-ALL.

DIFFERENTIAL DIAGNOSIS OF ACUTE LEUKEMIA

Myelodysplastic syndromes are the primary differential diagnostic consideration in adult patients with AML (see Chap. 7) but are rarely a consideration in children. By FAB criteria, a diagnosis of AML arbitrarily requires that blasts represent at least 30% of either all marrow elements or at least 30% of elements other than erythrocyte precursors when the latter exceeds 50% on differential cell counts (Bennett et al, 1985). This arbitrary definition of acute leukemia has been challenged, and some propose a category of "low blast count" AML (i.e., cases with <30% marrow blasts), especially in patients with t(8;21)-associated AML (Chan et al, 1997).

In ALL, the primary marrow differential diagnostic consideration is increased benign lymphocyte precursor cells, so-called hematogones (Foucar, 1995d; Longacre et al, 1989). Hematogones are commonly encountered in marrow specimens from children, especially young infants, in whom they may be sufficiently numerous in response to a variety of marrow insults

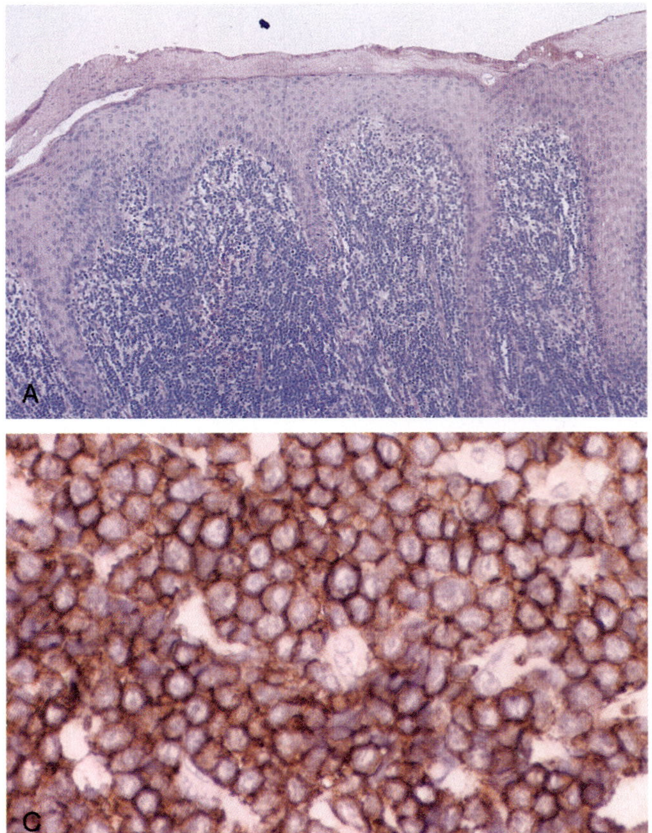

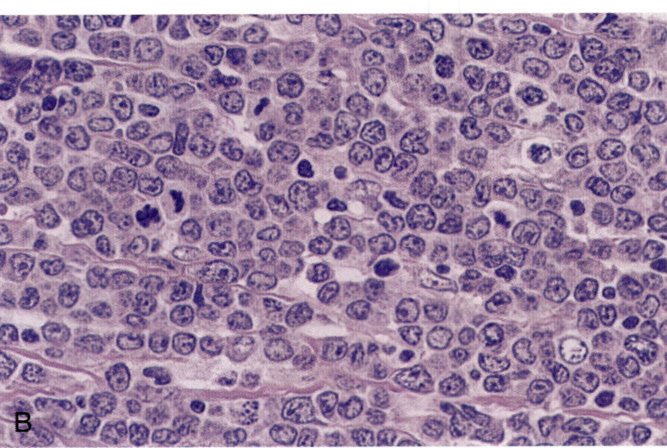

Figure 4–39

T-ALL, skin. *A.* This low-magnification photomicrograph illustrates a dense dermal infiltrate. *B.* This high-magnification photomicrograph shows scant cytoplasm and prominent mitotic activity. *C.* Strong CD43 positivity facilitates identification as a T cell neoplasm confirmed by flow cytometric immunophenotyping. Immunoperoxidase for CD43.

to cause confusion with ALL. Conditions associated with increased marrow hematogones are listed in Table 4–17 and consist of single or multilineage cytopenias as well as marrow suppression from therapy. The association of increased marrow hematogones in staging specimens from children with solid tumors likely reflects the young age of many of these patients.

Hematogones are characterized by a dense homogeneous nuclear chromatin pattern without nucleoli. Nuclear contours are round to irregular, while cytoplasm is scant. These cells are the size of normal lymphocytes or moderately larger (Fig. 4–41) (Foucar, 1995; Longacre et al, 1989; Rimsza et al, 1998). Marrow clot or biopsy sections may show a diffuse increase in lymphocytes, particularly in patients with numerous hematogones on aspirate films. On sections, these benign cells do not exhibit the convoluted nuclei and dispersed chromatin typical of lymphoblasts (Fig. 4–42). By flow cytometric immunophenotyping, a spectrum of immature and polyclonal mature B lymphocytes is detected. The immature cells mimic the lymphoblasts of ALL by expressing TdT and CD34, but generous numbers of admixed, mature, polyclonal B cells are also evident (Longacre et al, 1989). On tissue sections, CD34+ hematogones are individually scattered throughout the marrow, in contrast to sections in ALL, characterized by clusters of blasts (Rimsza et al, 1998). Hematogones exhibit a diploid DNA content and normal cytogenetic karyotype and are nonclonal by molecular analyses (Longacre et al, 1989). The cor-

Table 4–16

Methods of Detecting Minimal Residual Leukemia in Marrow or Blood

Technique	Approximate Sensitivity (%)	Comments
Morphologic or cytochemical	<5–10	Variable sensitivity, dependent on unique features, e.g., Auer rods
Cytogenetics	5–10	Cells must undergo mitosis
Immunophenotyping	1–5	Greater sensitivity if unique leukemia-specific profile defined by multicolor analysis
FISH	2–5	Applicable only if appropriate probe available; must exceed background levels of false positivity
PCR	<0.01	Applicable only if appropriate probe available; may be utilized for gene rearrangement studies and assessment for specific translocations

Abbreviations: FISH, fluorescence in situ hybridization; PCR, polymerase chain reaction.

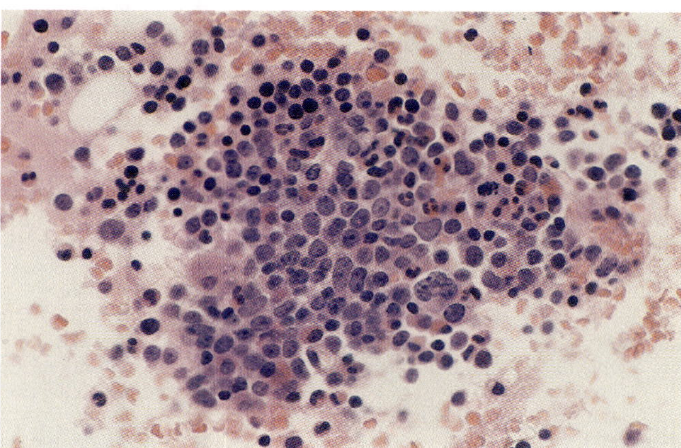

Figure 4–40

T-ALL, marrow section, early relapse. A focus of blasts is evident, indicating early relapse.

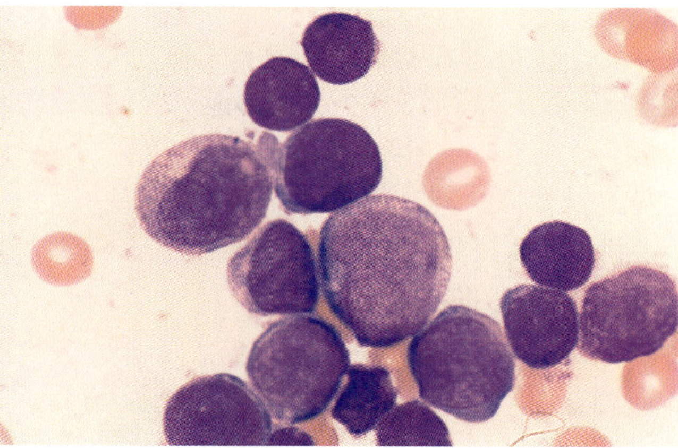

Figure 4–41

Hematogones, marrow aspirate. The cytologic features of hematogones are illustrated in this photomicrograph from a 1-year-old child with retinoblastoma. The finely dispersed chromatin of the myeloblast in the center of the photomicrograph should be compared to the condensed chromatin of the hematogones. Wright stain.

rect identification of hematogones depends upon recognition of their distinctive morphologic and immunophenotypic features as well as understanding the clinical circumstances in which these benign precursor cells in marrow are typically encountered. These immature and mature B cells likely function in both immune and hematopoietic recovery following diverse marrow insults. Evolution to ALL has not been described in these patients.

PROGNOSTIC FACTORS IN ACUTE LEUKEMIA

Many studies have analyzed prognostic markers in AML, but it is often difficult to evaluate the significance of these findings because studies are often limited by patient cohort size or lack of uniform patient treatment. In addition, since most studies have been performed on adult patients, the results may not be able to be extrapolated to children with AML. Two readily determined laboratory measurements are associated with poor prognosis in pediatric AML: prognosis is significantly poorer with high WBC counts at presentation and if there is CNS disease (as detected by cell counts >5 WBCs/mm^3 and blasts in cerebrospinal fluid) (Smith, 1995; Woods et al, 1993).

Cytogenetic characteristics are a second important prognostic indicator in AML (Dastugue et al, 1995). Data on pediatric AML are more limited than in adults, but clinical outcome is correlated with cytogenetic features. As in adults, AML with inv(16) is associated with a favorable outcome. The t(15;17) is also associated with a favorable response if the patient achieves a complete remission. The data on the prognostic relevance of the t(8;21) are less clear. Some studies show that pediatric patients with the t(8;21) have a favorable response similar to that in adults, but others show that such patients have a high rate of relapse (Creutzig et al, 1995; Martinez-Climent, 1997; Pearson et al, 1996).

Other predictors of response are likely to be uncovered. An intriguing finding is the association of B cell leukemia/lymphoma 2 (BCL2) gene overexpression with fewer complete remissions and increased relapse rates in univariate analysis in adult AML, presumably due to the antiapoptotic effects of BCL2 (Reed, 1997). Larger groups of patients must be studied to determine whether BCL2 overexpression is an independent predictor of outcome in pediatric AML.

With current treatments, about 70% of pediatric ALL patients experience a prolonged disease-free survival, and a

Table 4–17

Conditions Associated with Increased Marrow Hematogones

Fanconi anemia
Diamond-Blackfan anemia
Transient erythroblastopenia of childhood
Congenital or acquired neutropenia
Immune thrombocytopenic purpura
Staging for various childhood tumors
Following chemotherapy
Following marrow transplantation
Congenital amegakaryocytosis

Note: Young patients have a greater proportion of hematogones. For further details, see Chap. 9.

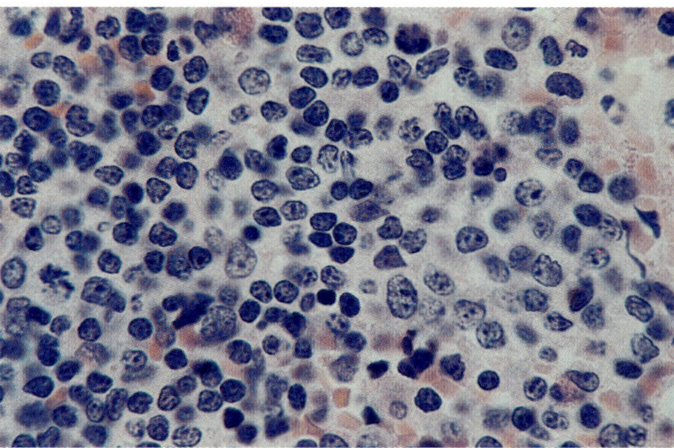

Figure 4–42

Hematogones, marrow section. This marrow clot section from a patient with constitutional red cell aplasia and increased hematogones illustrates the morphologic features of hematogones on clot section. Note the paucity of mitotic figures and the condensed chromatin.

Table 4–18
Prognostic Variables in ALL

Age
Gender
WBC count
Ploidy
Structural chromosome abnormalities
Race
Response to therapy
Type of therapy

substantial portion of these children are likely cured (Reiter et al, 1994). Various factors predict good, intermediate, or poor risk status in these patients. The accepted prognostic variables in ALL are listed in Table 4–18 and range from hematologic parameters to type of therapy (Behm et al, 1996; Chessells et al, 1995; Gajjar et al, 1995; Heerema et al, 1994; Lilleyman et al, 1997; Rubnitz & Look, 1998; Secker-Walker, 1997; Seeger et al, 1998). With progressively improving treatment options for pediatric ALL patients, these prognostic variables will likely change. For example, T cell phenotype was initially a poor prognostic factor in children with ALL, but, with improved high-risk treatment protocols, this variable no longer has independent prognostic significance. Those variables currently linked to good outcome include age over 1 year but less than 10 years, low WBC count, female sex, DNA content greater than 1.16, and rapid complete response to induction therapy. Adverse outcome is linked to age under 1 year and over 10 years, high WBC count, male sex, diploid DNA content, reciprocal translocations [notably t(9;22), t(4;11), and t(1;19)], and delayed response to therapy.

CONCLUSION

This chapter has presented a broad overview of acute leukemias, with emphasis on the various methods used to characterize these neoplastic cells, ranging from standard morphologic classification to sophisticated molecular analyses. Each of these methods contributes to either the phenotypic or the genotypic characterization of the leukemic clone. By the integration of clinical, morphologic, and genetic findings, many leukemias may be classified into biologic subtypes that are of critical importance in determining prognosis and optimal therapy. In other cases this biologic categorization is not clear-cut, and further investigations are necessary to understand specific leukemogenic events. Such understanding will likely contribute to improved classification, prognostication, and treatment of acute leukemia.

REFERENCES

Adriaansen HJ, te Boekhorst AW, Hagemeijer AM, et al: Acute myeloid leukemia M4 with bone marrow eosinophilia (M4Eo) and inv(16)(p13q22) exhibits a specific immunophenotype with CD2 expression. Blood 81:3043, 1993.

Arber DA, Jenkins KA, Slovak ML: CD79a expression in acute myeloid leukemia: high frequency of expression in acute promyelocytic leukemia. Am J Pathol 149:1105, 1996.

Arthur DC, Bloomfield CD: Partial deletion of the long arm of chromosome 16 and bone marrow eosinophilia in acute non-lymphocytic leukemia: a new association. Blood 61:994, 1983.

Barnard DR, Kalousek DK, Wiersma SR, et al: Morphologic, immunologic, and cytogenetic classification of acute myeloid leukemia and myelodysplastic syndrome in childhood: a report from the Childrens Cancer Group. Leukemia 10:5, 1996.

Bash RO, Crist WM, Shuster JJ, et al: Clinical features and outcomes of T-cell acute lymphoblastic leukemia in childhood with respect to alterations at the TAL1 locus: a Pediatric Oncology Group study. Blood 81:2110, 1993.

Bash RO, Hall S, Timmons CF, et al: Does activation of the TAL1 gene occur in a majority of patients with T-cell acute lymphoblastic leukemia? A Pediatric Oncology Group study. Blood 86:666, 1995.

Behm FG, Raimondi SC, Frestedt JL, et al: Rearrangement of the MLL gene confers a poor prognosis in childhood acute lymphoblastic leukemia, regardless of presenting age. Blood 87:2870, 1996.

Beishuizen A, Verhoeven M-AJ, van Wering ER, et al: Analysis of Ig and T-cell receptor genes in 40 childhood acute lymphoblastic leukemias at diagnosis and subsequent relapse: implications for the detection of minimal residual disease by polymerase chain reaction analysis. Blood 83:2238, 1994.

Bennett JM, Catovsky D, Daniel M-T, et al: Criteria for the diagnosis of acute leukemia of megakaryocyte lineage (M7): a report of the French-American-British Cooperative Group. Ann Intern Med 103:460, 1985a.

Bennett JM, Catovsky D, Daniel MT, et al: The morphological classification of acute lymphoblastic leukaemia: concordance among observers and clinical correlations. Br J Haematol 47:553, 1981.

Bennett JM, Catovsky D, Daniel M-T, et al: Proposal for the recognition of minimally differentiated acute myeloid leukaemia (AML-MO). Br J Haematol 78:325, 1991.

Bennett JM, Catovsky D, Daniel M-T, et al: Proposals for the classification of the acute leukaemias. Br J Haematol 33:451, 1976.

Bennett JM, Catovsky D, Daniel MT, et al: Proposed revised criteria for the classification of acute myeloid leukemia: a report of the French-American-British Cooperative Group. Ann Intern Med 103:620, 1985b.

Beyermann B, Adams H-P, Henze G, for the Berlin-Frankfurt-Münster Study Group: Philadelphia chromosome in relapsed childhood acute lymphoblastic leukemia: a matched-pair analysis. J Clin Oncol 15:2231, 1997.

Beyermann B, Agthe AG, Adams H-P, et al: Clinical features and outcome of children with first marrow relapse of acute lymphoblastic leukemia expressing BCR-ABL fusion transcripts. Blood 87:1532, 1996.

Bhatia S, Neglia JP: Epidemiology of childhood acute myelogenous leukemia. J Pediatr Hematol Oncol 17:94, 1995.

Biondi A, Luciano A, Bassan R, et al: CD2 expression in acute promyelocytic leukemia is associated with microgranular morphology (FAB M3v) but not with any PML gene breakpoint. Leukemia 9:1461, 1995.

Bitter MA, Le Beau MM, Larson RA, et al: A morphologic and cytochemical study of acute myelomonocytic leukemia with abnormal marrow eosinophils associated with inv(16)(p13q22). Am J Clin Pathol 81:733, 1984.

Borkhardt A, Cazzaniga G, Viehmann S, et al: Incidence and clinical relevance of TEL/AML1 fusion genes in children with acute lymphoblastic leukemia enrolled in the German and Italian Multicenter Therapy Trials. Blood 90:571, 1997.

Borowitz MJ: Acute lymphoblastic leukemia. In: Knowles DM (ed): Neoplastic Hematopathology. Williams & Wilkins, Baltimore, p 1295, 1992.

Borowitz MJ, Guenther L, Shults KE, et al: Immunophenotyping of acute leukemia by flow cytometric analysis: use of CD45 and right-angle light scatter to gate on leukemic blasts in three-color analysis. Am J Clin Pathol 100:534, 1993a.

Borowitz MJ, Hunger SP, Carroll AJ, et al: Predictability of the t(1;19)(q23;p13) from surface antigen phenotype: implications for screening cases of childhood ALL for molecular analysis, a Pediatric Oncology Group study. Blood 82:1086, 1993b.

Brisco MJ, Hughes E, Neoh SH, et al: Relationship between minimal residual disease and outcome in adult acute lymphoblastic leukemia. Blood 87:5251, 1996.

Brito-Babapulle F, Catovsky D, Galton DAG: Clinical and laboratory features of de novo acute myeloid leukaemia with trilineage myelodysplasia. Br J Haematol 66:445, 1987.

Byrd JC, Edenfield WJ, Shields DJ, et al: Extramedullary myeloid cell tumors in acute nonlymphocytic leukemia: a clinical review. J Clin Oncol 13:1800, 1995.

Byrd JC, Weiss RB, Arthur DC, et al: Extramedullary leukemia adversely affects hematologic complete remission rate and overall survival in patients with t(8;21)(q22;q22): results from Cancer and Leukemia Group B 8461. J Clin Oncol 15:466, 1997.

Caligiuri MA, Strout MP, Gilliland DG: Molecular biology of acute myeloid leukemia. Semin Oncol 24:32, 1997.

Casasnovas RO, Campos L, Mugneret F, et al: Immunophenotypic patterns and cytogenetic anomalies in acute non-lymphoblastic leukemia subtypes: a prospective study of 432 patients. Leukemia 12:34, 1998.

Cascavilla N, Musto P, D'Arena G, et al: Adult and childhood acute lymphoblastic leukemia: clinicobiological differences based on CD34 antigen expression. Haematologica 82:31, 1997.

Castoldi GL, Liso V, Specchia G, et al: Acute promyelocytic leukemia: morphological aspects. Leukemia 8:1441, 1994.

Cavenagh JD, Richardson DS, Gibson RA, et al: Fanconi's anaemia presenting as acute myeloid leukaemia in adulthood. Br J Haematol 94:126, 1996.

Cerezo L, Shuster JJ, Pullen J, et al: Laboratory correlates and prognostic significance of granular acute lymphoblastic leukemia in children: a Pediatric Oncology Group study. Am J Clin Pathol 95:526, 1991.

Chan GCF, Wang WC, Raimondi SC, et al: Myelodysplastic syndrome in children: differentiation from acute myeloid leukemia with a low blast count. Leukemia 11:206, 1997.

Chen C-S, Sorensen PHB, Domer PH, et al: Molecular rearrangements on chromosome 11q23 predominate in infant acute lymphoblastic leukemia and are associated with specific biologic variables and poor outcome. Blood 81:2386, 1993.

Cheson BD, Cassileth PA, Head DR, et al: Report of the National Cancer Institute–sponsored workshop on definitions of diagnosis and response in acute myeloid leukemia. J Clin Oncol 8:813, 1990.

Chessells JM, Richards SM, Bailey CC, et al: Gender and treatment outcome in childhood lymphoblastic leukaemia: report from the MRC UKALL trials. Br J Haematol 89:364, 1995.

Chetty R, Pulford K, Jones M, et al: SCL/Tal-1 expression in T-acute lymphoblastic leukemia: an immunohistochemical and genotypic study. Hum Pathol 26:994, 1995.

Cimino G, Lo Coco F, Biondi A, et al: ALL-1 gene at chromosome 11q23 is consistently altered in acute leukemia of early infancy. Blood 82:544, 1993.

Cimino G, Rapanotti MC, Elia L, et al: ALL-1 gene rearrangements in acute myeloid leukemia: association with M4-M5 French-American-British classification subtypes and young age. Cancer Res 55:1625, 1995.

Claxton DF, Liu P, Hsu HB, et al: Detection of fusion transcripts generated by the inversion 16 chromosome in acute myelogenous leukemia. Blood 83:1750, 1994.

Creutzig U, Harbott J, Sperling C, et al: Clinical significance of surface antigen expression in children with acute myeloid leukemia: results of study AML-BFM-87. Blood 86:3097, 1995.

Creutzig U, Ritter J, Vormoor J, et al: Myelodysplasia and acute myelogenous leukemia in Down's syndrome: a report of 40 children of the AML-BFM Study Group. Leukemia 10:1677, 1996.

Crist W, Boyett J, Jackson J, et al: Prognostic importance of the pre–B-cell immunophenotype and other presenting features in B-lineage childhood acute lymphoblastic leukemia: a Pediatric Oncology Group study. Blood 74:1252, 1989.

Crist WM, Carroll AJ, Shuster JJ, et al: Poor prognosis of children with pre-B acute lymphoblastic leukemia is associated with the t(1;19)(q23;p13): a Pediatric Oncology Group study. Blood 76:117, 1990.

Cross AH, Goorlha RM, Nuss R, et al: Acute myeloid leukemia with T-lymphoid features: a distinct biologic and clinical entity. Blood 72:579, 1988.

Dalton WS: Mechanisms of drug resistance in hematologic malignancies. Semin Hematol 34:3, 1997.

Dastugue N, Payen C, Lafage-Pochitaloff M, et al: Prognostic significance of karyotype in *de novo* adult acute myeloid leukemia. Leukemia 9:1491, 1995.

Davey DD, Patil SR, Echternacht H, et al: 8;21 translocation in acute nonlymphocytic leukemia: occurrence in M1 and M2 FAB subtypes. Am J Clin Pathol 92:172, 1989.

Davis BH, Foucar K, Szczarkowski W, et al: U.S.–Canadian consensus recommendations on the immunophenotypic analysis of hematologic neoplasia by flow cytometry: medical indications. Cytometry 30:249, 1997.

Dayton VD, Arthur DC, Gajl-Peczalska KJ, et al: L3 acute lymphoblastic leukemia: comparison with small noncleaved cell lymphoma involving the bone marrow. Am J Clin Pathol 101:130, 1994.

Dehner LP, Price RA: Cytochemical profiles in acute lymphoblastic leukemia. Am J Pediatr Hematol Oncol 1:263, 1979.

Del Poeta G, Stasi R, Aronica G, et al: Clinical relevance of P-glycoprotein expression in de novo acute myeloid leukemia. Blood 87:1997, 1996.

Devaraj PE, Foroni L, Kitra-Roussos V, et al: Detection of BCR-ABL and E2A-PBX1 fusion genes by RT-PCR in acute lymphoblastic leukaemia with failed or normal cytogenetics. Br J Haematol 89:349, 1995.

Devereux S: Therapy associated leukaemia. Blood Rev 5:138, 1991.

Djabali M, Selleri L, Parry P, et al: A trithorax-like gene is interrupted by chromosome 11q23 translocations in acute leukaemias. Nat Genet 2:113, 1992.

Douer D, Preston-Martin S, Chang E, et al: High frequency of acute promyelocytic leukemia among Latinos with acute myeloid leukemia. Blood 87:308, 1996.

Drexler HG, Thiel E, Ludwig W-D: Acute myeloid leukemias expressing lymphoid-associated antigens: diagnostic incidence and prognostic significance. Leukemia 7:489, 1993.

El-Rifai W, Ruutu T, Elonen E, et al: Prognostic value of metaphase-fluorescence in situ hybridization in follow-up of patients with acute myeloid leukemia in remission. Blood 89:3330, 1997.

Evans PAS, Short MA, Jack AS, et al: Detection and quantitation of the CBF/MYH11 transcripts associated with the inv(16) in presentation and follow-up samples from patients with AML. Leukemia 11:364, 1997.

Felix CA, Hosler MR, Winick NJ, et al: ALL-1 gene rearrangements in DNA topoisomerase II inhibitor-related leukemia in children. Blood 85:3250, 1995.

Felix CA, Poplack DG: Characterization of acute lymphoblastic leukemia of childhood by immunoglobulin and T-cell receptor gene patterns. Leukemia 5:1015, 1991.

Fenaux P, Chomienne C, Degos L: Acute promyelocytic leukemia: biology and treatment. Semin Oncol 24:92, 1997.

Fischer K, Frohling S, Scherer SW, et al: Molecular cytogenetic delineation of deletions and translocations involving chromosome band 7q22 in myeloid leukemias. Blood 89:2036, 1997.

Foucar K: Acute lymphoblastic leukemia. In: Bone Marrow Pathology. ASCP Press, Chicago, p 379, 1995a.

Foucar K: Acute myelogenous leukemia. In: Bone Marrow Pathology. ASCP Press, Chicago, p 189, 1995b.

Foucar K: Effects of therapy and transplantation, and detection of minimal residual disease. In: Bone Marrow Pathology. ASCP Press, Chicago, p 531, 1995c.

Foucar K: Reactive lymphoid proliferations in blood and bone marrow. In: Bone Marrow Pathology. ASCP Press, Chicago, p 255, 1995d.

Gahn B, Haase D, Unterhalt M, et al: De novo AML with displastic hematopoiesis: cytogenetic and prognostic significance. Leukemia 10:946, 1996.

Gajjar A, Ribeiro R, Hancock MH, et al: Persistence of circulating blasts after 1 week of multiagent chemotherapy confers a poor prognosis in childhood acute lymphoblastic leukemia. Blood 86:1292, 1995.

Gale RE, Linch DC: Clonality studies in acute myeloid leukemia. Leukemia 12:117, 1998.

Gardie B, Cayuela J-M, Martini S, et al: Genomic alterations of the $p19^{ARF}$ encoding exons in T-cell acute lymphoblastic leukemia. Blood 91:1016, 1998.

Goasguen JE, Matsuo T, Cox C, et al: Evaluation of the dysmyelopoiesis in 336 patients with de novo acute myeloid leukemia: major importance of dysgranulopoiesis for remission and survival. Leukemia 6:520, 1992.

Greaves MF: Aetiology of acute leukaemia. Lancet 349:344, 1997.

Grignani F, Fagioli M, Alcalay M, et al: Acute promyelocytic leukemia: from genetics to treatment. Blood 83:10, 1994.

Gu Y, Nakamura T, Alder H, et al: The t(4;11) chromosome translocation of human acute leukemias fuses the ALL-1 gene, related to *Drosophila trithorax*, to the AF-4 gene. Cell 71:701, 1992.

Guglielmi C, Cordone I, Boecklin F, et al: Immunophenotype of adult and childhood acute lymphoblastic leukemia: changes at first relapse and clinico-prognostic implications. Leukemia 11:1501, 1997.

Gurney JG, Ross JA, Wall DA, et al: Infant cancer in the U.S.: histology-specific incidence and trends, 1973 to 1992. J Pediatr Hematol Oncol 19:428, 1997.

Haferlach T, Winkemann M, Loffler H, et al: The abnormal eosinophils are part of the leukemic cell population in acute myelomonocytic leukemia with abnormal eosinophils (AML M4Eo) and carry the pericentric inversion 16: a combination of May-Grunwald-Giemsa staining and fluorescence *in situ* hybridization. Blood 87:2459, 1996.

Harris MB, Shuster JJ, Carroll A, et al: Trisomy of leukemic cell chromosomes 4 and 10 identifies children with B-progenitor cell acute lymphoblastic leukemia with a very low risk of treatment failure: a Pediatric Oncology Group study. Blood 79:3316, 1992.

Hast R, Widell S: Dysplastic peripheral blood polymorphs link acute myeloblastic leukaemia in elderly to the myelodysplastic syndromes. Eur J Haematol 48:163, 1992.

Hayhoe FGJ: Cytochemistry of the acute leukaemias. Histochem J 16:1051, 1984.

Head DR: Revised classification of acute myeloid leukemia. Leukemia 10:1826, 1996.

Hebert J, Cayuela JM, Barkeley J, et al: Candidate tumor-suppressor genes MTS1 (p16INK4A) and MTS2 (p15INK4B) display frequent homozygous deletions in primary cells from T- but not from B-cell lineage acute lymphoblastic leukemias. Blood 84:4038, 1994.

Heerema NA, Arthur DC, Sather H, et al: Cytogenetic features of infants less than 12 months of age at diagnosis of acute lymphoblastic leukemia: impact of the 11q23 breakpoint on outcome, a report of the Children's Cancer Group. Blood 83:2274, 1994.

Heerema NA, Palmer CG, Weetman R, et al: Cytogenetic analysis in relapsed childhood acute lymphoblastic leukemia. Leukemia 6:185, 1992.

Henderson ES: History of leukemia. In: Henderson ES, Lister TA, Greaves MF (eds): Leukemia. 6th ed. W.B. Saunders Co, Philadelphia, p 1, 1996.

Horwitz M: The genetics of familial leukemia. Leukemia 11:1347, 1997.

Hunger SP: Chromosomal translocations involving the E2A gene in acute lymphoblastic leukemia: clinical features and molecular pathogenesis. Blood 87:1211, 1996.

Hunger SP, Fall M, Camitta BM, et al: E2A-PBX1 chimeric transcript status at end of consolidation is not predictive of treatment outcome in childhood acute lymphoblastic leukemias with a t(1;19)(q23;p13): a pediatric oncology group study. Blood 91:1021, 1998.

Hunger SP, Galili N, Carroll AI, et al: The t(1;19)(q23;p13) results in consistent fusion of E2A and PBX1 coding sequences in acute lymphoblastic leukemias. Blood 77:687, 1991.

Hurwitz CA, Raimondi SC, Head D, et al: Distinctive immunophenotypic features of t(8;21)(q22;q22) acute myeloblastic leukemia in children. Blood 80:3182, 1992.

Ioachim HL, Pambuccian S, Giancotti F, et al: Reactivity of lung tumors with lung-derived and non-lung-derived monoclonal antibodies. Int J Cancer 8:132, 1994.

Ivy SP, Olshefski RS, Taylor BJ, et al: Correlation of P-glycoprotein expression and function in childhood acute leukemia: a Children's Cancer Group study. Blood 88:309, 1996.

Izraeli S, Janssen WSG, Haas OA, et al: Detection and clinical relevance of genetic abnormalities in pediatric acute lymphoblastic leukemia: a comparison between cytogenetic and polymerase chain reaction analyses. Leukemia 7:671, 1993.

Jacquy C, Delepaut B, van Daele S, et al: A prospective study of minimal residual disease in childhood B-lineage acute lymphoblastic leukaemia: MRD level at the end of induction is a strong predictive factor of relapse. Br J Haematol 98:140, 1997.

Jennings CD, Foon KA: Flow cytometry: recent advances in diagnosis and monitoring of leukemia. Cancer Invest 15:384, 1997.

Johnson E, Cotter FE: Monosomy 7 and 7q−-associated with myeloid malignancy. Blood Rev 11:46, 1997.

Kalra R, Dale D, Freedman M, et al: Monosomy 7 and activating RAS mutations accompany malignant transformation in patients with congenital neutropenia. Blood 86:4579, 1995.

Karp JE, Smith MA: The molecular pathogenesis of treatment-induced (secondary) leukemias: foundations for treatment and prevention. Semin Oncol 24:103, 1997.

Kaspers GJL, Smets LA, Pieters R, et al: Favorable prognosis of hyperdiploid common acute lymphoblastic leukemia may be explained by sensitivity to antimetabolites and other drugs: results of an in vitro study. Blood 85:751, 1995.

Kasprzyk A, Secker-Walker LM: Increased sensitivity of minimal residual disease detection by interphase FISH in acute lymphoblastic leukemia with hyperdiploidy. Leukemia 11:429, 1997.

Keifer J, Abromowitch M, Stass SA: Chloroacetate esterase positivity in acute lymphoblastic leukemia. Am J Clin Pathol 83:647, 1985.

Kempski HM, Chessells JM, Reeves BR: Deletions of chromosome 21 restricted to the leukemic cells of children with Down syndrome and leukemia. Leukemia 11:1973, 1997.

Kersey JH: Fifty years of studies of the biology and therapy of childhood leukemia. Blood 90:4243, 1997.

Khalidi HS, Medeiros LJ, Chang KL, et al: The immunophenotype of adult acute myeloid leukemia: high frequency of lymphoid antigen expression and comparison of immunophenotype, French-American-British classification, and karyotypic abnormalities. Am J Clin Pathol 109:211, 1998.

Kikuchi A, Hayashi Y, Kobayashi S, et al: Clinical significance of TAL1 gene alteration in childhood T-cell acute lymphoblastic leukemia and lymphoma. Leukemia 7:933, 1993.

Knechtli CJC, Goulden NJ, Langlands K, et al: The study of minimal residual disease in acute lymphoblastic leukaemia. J Clin Pathol Mol Pathol 48:M65, 1995.

Kumagai M, Manabe A, Pui C-H, et al: Stroma-supported culture of childhood B-lineage acute lymphoblastic leukemia cells predicts treatment outcome. J Clin Invest 97:755, 1996.

Kuriyama K, Tomonaga M, Matsuo T, et al: Poor response to intensive chemotherapy in de novo acute myeloid leukaemia with trilineage myelodysplasia. Br J Haematol 86:767, 1994.

Lacombe F, Durrieu F, Briais A, et al: Flow cytometry CD45 gating for immunophenotyping of acute myeloid leukemia. Leukemia 11:1878, 1997.

Langabeer SE, Walker H, Gale RE, et al: Frequency of CBF/MYH11 fusion transcripts in patients entered into the U.K. MRC AML trials. Br J Haematol 96:736, 1997.

Lange B: Editorial overview: progress in acute myelogenous leukemia: the one hundred years' war. J Pediatr Hematol Oncol 17:91, 1995.

Lange BJ, Kobrinsky N, Barnard DR, et al: Distinctive demography, biology, and outcome of acute myeloid leukemia and myelodysplastic syndrome in children with Down syndrome: Children's Cancer Group studies 2861 and 2891. Blood 91:608, 1998.

Lanza C, Volpe G, Basso G, et al: The common TEL/AML1 rearrangement does not represent a frequent event in acute lymphoblastic leukaemia occurring in children with Down syndrome. Leukemia 11:820, 1997a.

Lanza C, Volpe G, Basso G, et al: Outcome and lineage involvement in t(12;21) childhood acute lymphoblastic leukaemia. Br J Haematol 97:460, 1997b.

Larson RS, McCurley TL: CD4 predicts nonlymphocytic lineage in acute leukemia: insights from analysis of 125 cases using two-color flow cytometry. Am J Clin Pathol 104 204, 1995.

Lavau C, Dejean A: The t(15;17) translocation in acute promyelocytic leukemia. Leukemia 8:1615, 1994.

Le Beau MM, Larson RA, Bitter MA, et al: Association of an inversion of chromosome 16 with abnormal marrow eosinophils in acute myelomonocytic leukemia. N Engl J Med 309:630, 1983.

Leith CP, Kopecky KJ, Chen I-M, et al: Frequency and clinical significance of expression of the multidrug resistance proteins, MDR1, MRP1 and LRP in acute myeloid leukemia patients less than 65 years old: a Southwest Oncology Group study. Blood 90:389a, 1997a.

Leith CP, Kopecky KJ, Godwin J, et al: Acute myeloid leukemia in the elderly: assessment of multidrug resistance (MDR1) and cytogenetics distinguishes biologic subgroups with remarkably distinct responses to standard chemotherapy, a Southweset Oncology Group study. Blood 89:3323, 1997b.

Leith CP, Willman CL: Prognostic markers in acute leukemia. Curr Opin Hematol 3:329, 1996.

Li C-Y, Yam LT: Cytochemical characterization of leukemic cells with numerous cytoplasmic granules. Mayo Clin Proc 62:978, 1987.

Lilleyman JS, Gibson BES, Stevens RF, et al: Clearance of marrow infiltration after 1 week of therapy for childhood lymphoblastic leukaemia: clinical importance and the effect of daunorubicin. Br J Haematol 97:603, 1997.

Lion T, Hass OA, Harbott J, et al: The translocation t(1;22)(p13;q13) is a nonrandom marker specifically associated with acute megakaryocytic leukemia in young children. Blood 79:3325, 1992.

List AF: Role of multidrug resistance and its pharmacological modulation in acute myeloid leukemia. Leukemia 10:937, 1996.

Liu PP, Hajra A, Wijmenga C, et al: Molecular pathogenesis of the chromosome 16 inversion of the M4Eo subtype of acute myeloid leukemia. Blood 85:2289, 1995.

Longacre TA, Foucar K, Crago S, et al: Hematogones: a multiparameter analysis of bone marrow precursor cells. Blood 73:543, 1989.

Luna-Fineman S, Shannon KM, Lange BJ: Childhood monosomy 7: epidemiology, biology, and mechanistic implications. Blood 85:1985, 1995.

Magrath IT, Jain V, Jaffe ES: Small noncleaved cell lymphoma in neoplastic hematopathology. In: Knowles DK (ed): Neoplastic Hematopathology. Williams & Wilkins, Baltimore, p 749, 1992.

Marie J-P, Legrand O, Perrot J-Y, et al: Measuring multidrug resistance expression in human malignancies: Elaboration of consensus recommendations. Semin Hematol 34:63, 1997.

Marlton P, Keating M, Kantarjian H, et al: Cytogenetic and clinical correlates in AML patients with abnormalities of chromosome 16. Leukemia 9:965, 1995.

Martinez-Climent JA: Molecular cytogenetics of childhood hematological malignancies. Leukemia 11:1999, 1997.

Martinez-Climent JA, Espinosa R, Thirman MJ, et al: Abnormalities of chromosome band 11q23 and the MLL gene in pediatric myelomonocytic and monoblastic leukemias. Identification of the t(9;11) as an indicator of long survival. J Pediatr Hematol Oncol 17:277, 1995a.

Martinez-Climent JA, Lane NJ, Rubin CM, et al: Clinical and prognostic significance of chromosomal abnormalities in childhood acute myeloid leukemia *de novo*. Leukemia 9:95, 1995b.

Martinez-Climent JA, Thirman MJ, Espinosa R, et al: Detection of 11q23/MLL rearrangements in infant leukemias with fluorescence *in situ* hybridization and molecular analysis. Leukemia 9:1299, 1995c.

McCoy JP, Overton WR: Immunophenotyping of congenital leukemia. Cytometry 22:85, 1995.

McKenna RW, Brynes RK, Nesbit ME, et al: Cytochemical profiles in acute lymphoblastic leukemia. Am J Pediatr Hematol Oncol 1:263, 1979.

McLean TW, Ringold S, Neuberg D, et al: TEL/AML-1 dimerizes and is associated with a favorable outcome in childhood acute lymphoblastic leukemia. Blood 88:4252, 1996.

Meeker TC, Hardy D, Willman C, et al: Activation of the interleukin-3 gene by chromosome translocation in acute lymphocytic leukemia with eosinophilia. Blood 76:285, 1990.

Muto A, Mori S, Matsushita H, et al: Serial quantification of minimal residual disease of t(8;21) acute myelogenous leukaemia with RT-competitive PCR assay. Br J Haematol 95:85, 1996.

Nucifora G, Dickstein JI, Torbenson V, et al: Correlation between cell morphology and expression of the AML1/ETO chimeric transcript in patients with acute myeloid leukemia without the t(8;21). Leukemia 8:1533, 1994.

Nucifora G, Larson RA, Rowley JD: Persistence of the 8;21 translocation in patients with acute myeloid leukemia type M2 in long-term remission. Blood 82:712, 1993.

Nucifora G, Rowley JD: AML1 and the 8;21 and 3;21 translocations in acute and chronic myeloid leukemia. Blood 86:1, 1995.

Ohara A, Kojima S, Hamajima N, et al: Myelodysplastic syndrome and acute myelogenous leukemia as a late clonal complication in children with acquired aplastic anemia. Blood 90:1009, 1997.

Ohnishi H, Kawamura M, Ida K, et al: Homozygous deletions of p16/MTS1 gene are frequent but mutations are infrequent in childhood T-cell acute lymphoblastic leukemia. Blood 86:1269, 1995.

Okuda T, Shurtleff SA, Valentine MB, et al: Frequent deletion of $p16^{INK4a}$/MTS1 and $p15^{INK4b}$/MTS2 in pediatric acute lymphoblastic leukemia. Blood 85:2321, 1995.

Owen RG, Goulden NJ, Oakhill A, et al: Comparison of fluorescent consensus IgH PCR and allele-specific oligonucleotide probing in the detection of minimal residual disease in childhood ALL. Br J Haematol 97:457, 1997.

Pasqualetti P, Festuccia V, Acitelli P, et al: Tobacco smoking and risk of haematological malignancies in adults: a case-control study. Br J Haematol 97:659, 1997.

Passmore SJ, Hann IM, Stiller CA, et al: Pediatric myelodysplasia: a study of 68 children and a new prognostic scoring system. Blood 85:1742, 1995.

Pearson L, Leith CP, Duncan MH, et al: Multidrug resistance-1 (MDR1) expression and functional dye/drug efflux is highly correlated with the t(8;21) chromosomal translocation in pediatric acute myeloid leukemia. Leukemia 10:1274, 1996.

Pedersen-Bjergaard J, Pedersen M, Roulston D et al: Different genetic pathways in leukemogenesis for patients presenting with therapy-related myelodysplasia and therapy-related acute myeloid leukemia. Blood 86:3542, 1995.

Pedersen-Bjergaard J, Philip P, Larsen SO, et al: Therapy-related myelodysplasia and acute myeloid leukemia: cytogenetic characteristics of 115 consecutive cases and risk in seven cohorts of patients treated intensively for malignant diseases in the Copenhagen series. Leukemia 7:1975, 1993.

Piller G: The history of leukemia: a personal perspective. Blood Cells 19:521, 1993.

Poirel H, Rack K, Delabesse E, et al: Incidence and characterization of MLL gene (11q23) rearrangements in acute myeloid leukemia M1 and M5. Blood 87:2496, 1996.

Porwit-MacDonald A, Janossy G, Ivory K, et al: Leukemia-associated changes identified by quantitative flow cytometry: IV CD34 overexpression in acute myelogenous leukemia M2 with t(8;21). Blood 87:1162, 1996.

Pui C-H, Behm FG, Crist WM: Clinical and biologic relevance of immunologic marker studies in childhood acute lymphoblastic leukemia. Blood 82:343, 1993.

Pui C-H, Campana D, Crist WM: Toward a clinically useful classification of the acute leukemias. Leukemia 9:2154, 1995a.

Pui C-H, Crist WM: Biology and treatment of acute lymphoblastic leukemia. J Pediatr 124:491, 1994.

Pui C-H, Crist WM, Look AT: Biology and clinical significance of cytogenetic abnormalities in childhood acute lymphoblastic leukemia. Blood 76:1449, 1990.

Pui C-H, Kane JR, Crist WM: Biology and treatment of infant leukemias. Leukemia 9:762, 1995b.

Pui C-H, Raimondi SC, Dodge RK, et al: Prognostic importance of structural chromosomal abnormalities in children with hyperdiploid (>50 chromosomes) acute lymphoblastic leukemia. Blood 73:1963, 1989.

Pui C-H, Raimondi SC, Hancock ML, et al: Immunologic, cytogenetic, and clinical characterization of childhood acute lymphoblastic leukemia with the t(1;19)(q23;p13) or its derivative. J Clin Oncol 12:2601, 1994.

Pui C-H, Relling MV, Rivera GK, et al: Epipodophyllotoxin-related acute myeloid leukemia: a study of 35 cases. Leukemia 9:1990, 1995c.

Quintanilla-Martinez L, Zukerberg LR, Ferry JA, et al: Extramedullary tumors of lymphoid or myeloid blasts: the role of immunohistology in diagnosis and classification. Am J Clin Pathol 104:431, 1995.

Raimondi SC, Privitera E, Williams DL, et al: New recurring chromosomal translocations in childhood acute lymphoblastic leukemia. Blood 77:2016, 1991.

Raimondi SC, Pui C-H, Hancock ML, et al: Heterogeneity of hyperdiploid (51–67) childhood acute lymphoblastic leukemia. Leukemia 10:213, 1996.

Raynaud S, Cavé H, Baens M, et al: The 12;21 translocation involving *TEL* and depletion of the other *TEL* allele: two frequently associated alterations found in childhood acute lymphoblastic leukemia. Blood 87:2891, 1996.

Raynaud S, Mauvieux L, Cayuela JM, et al: TEL/AML1 fusion gene is a rare event in adult acute lymphoblastic leukemia. Leukemia 10:1529, 1996.

Reed JC: Bcl-2 family proteins: regulators of apoptosis and chemoresistance in hematologic malignancies. Semin Hematol 34:9, 1997.

Reiter A, Schrappe M, Ludwig W-D, et al: Chemotherapy in 998 unselected childhood acute lymphoblastic leukemia patients: results and conclusions of the multicenter trial ALL-BFM86. Blood 84:3122, 1994.

Rieder H, Ludwig WD, Gassmann W, et al: Prognostic significance of additional chromosome abnormalities in adult patients with Philadelphia chromosome positive acute lymphoblastic leukaemia. Br J Haematol 95:678, 1996.

Ribeiro RC, Abromowitch M, Raimondi SC, et al: Clinical and biological hallmarks of the Philadelphia chromosome in childhood acute lymphoblastic leukemia. Blood 70:948, 1987.

Ribeiro RC, Pui C-H, Schell MJ: Vertebral compression fracture as a presenting feature of acute lymphoblastic leukemia in children. Cancer 61:589, 1988.

Rimsza LM, Viswanatha DS, Winter SS, et al: The presence of CD34+ cell clusters predicts impending relapse in children with acute lymphoblastic leukemia receiving maintenance chemotherapy. Am J Clin Pathol 110:313, 1998.

Robison LL: Down syndrome and leukemia. Leukemia 6:5, 1992.

Romana SP, Mauchauffé M, Le Coniat M, et al: The t(12;21) of acute lymphoblastic leukemia results in a tel-AML1 gene fusion. Blood 85:3662, 1995a.

Romana SP, Poirel H, Leconiat M, et al: High frequency of t(12;21) in childhood B-lineage acute lymphoblastic leukemia. Blood 86: 4263, 1995b.

Roth MJ, Medeiros LJ, Elenitoba-Johnson K, et al: Extramedullary myeloid cell tumors: an immunohistochemical study of 29 cases using routinely fixed and processed paraffin-embedded tissue sections. Arch Pathol Lab Med 119:790, 1995.

Rothe G, Schmitz G: Consensus protocol for the flow cytometric immunophenotyping of hematopoietic malignancies. Leukemia 10:877, 1996.

Rubnitz JE, Behm FG, Downing JR: 11q23 rearrangements in acute leukemia. Leukemia 10:74, 1996.

Rubnitz JE, Downing JR, Pui C-H, et al: TEL gene rearrangement in acute lymphoblastic leukemia: a new genetic marker with prognostic significance. J Clin Oncol 15:1150, 1997.

Rubnitz JE, Look AT: Molecular genetics of childhood leukemias. J Pediatr Hematol Oncol 20:1, 1998.

Rubnitz JE, Shuster JJ, Land VJ, et al: Case-control study suggests a favorable impact of TEL rearrangement in patients with B-lineage acute lymphoblastic leukemia treated with antimetabolite-based therapy: a Pediatric Oncology Group study. Blood 89:1143, 1997.

Russell NH: Biology of acute leukaemia. Lancet 349:118, 1997.

Russo C, Carroll A, Kohler S, et al: Philadelphia chromosome and monosomy 7 in childhood acute lymphoblastic leukemia: a Pediatric Oncology Group study. Blood 77:1050, 1991.

Sandoval C, Pui C-H, Bowman LC, et al: Secondary acute myeloid leukemia in children previously treated with alkylating agents, intercalating topoisomerase II inhibitors, and irradiation. J Clin Oncol 11:1039, 1993.

Savage P, Frenck R, Paderanga D, et al: Parental origins of chromosome 7 loss in childhood monosomy 7 syndrome. Leukemia 8:485, 1994.

Sawyers CL: Molecular genetics of acute leukaemia. Lancet 349:196, 1997.

Schlieben S, Borkhardt A, Reinisch J, et al: Incidence and clinical outcome of children with BCR/ABL-positive acute lymphoblastic leukemia (ALL): a prospective RT-PCR study based on 673 patients enrolled in the German pediatric multicenter therapy trials ALL-BFM-90 and CoALL-05-92. Leukemia 10:957, 1996.

Secker-Walker LM, Craig JM: Prognostic implications of breakpoint and lineage heterogeneity in Philadelphia-positive acute lymphoblastic leukemia: a review. Leukemia 7:147, 1993.

Secker-Walker LM, Prentice HG, Durrant J, et al: Cytogenetics adds independent prognostic information in adults with acute lymphoblastic leukaemia on MRC trial UKALL XA. Br J Haematol 96:601, 1997.

Seeger K, Adams H-P, Buchwald D, et al: TEL-AML1 fusion transcript in relapsed childhood acute lymphoblastic leukemia. Blood 91:1716, 1998.

Shih L-Y, Chou T-B, Liang D-C, et al: Lack of TEL-AML1 fusion transcript resulting from a cryptic t(12;21) in adult B lineage acute lymphoblastic leukemia in Taiwan. Leukemia 10:1456, 1996.

Shurtleff SA, Buijs A, Behm FG, et al: TEL/AML1 fusion resulting from a cryptic t(12;21) is the most common genetic lesion in pediatric ALL and defines a subgroup of patients with an excellent prognosis. Leukemia 9:1985, 1995.

Smith FO: Prognostic factors in leukemia and lymphoma. Curr Opin Hematol 2:322, 1995.

Smith FO, Lampkin B, Dinndorf PA, et al: Lymphoid-associated cell surface antigens on childhood acute myeloid leukemia lack prognostic significance. Blood 79:2415, 1992.

Sorahan T, Prior P, Lancashire RJ, et al: Childhood cancer and parental use of tobacco: deaths from 1971 to 1976. Br J Cancer 76:1525, 1997.

Soslow RA, Bhargava V, Warnke RA: MIC2, TdT, bcl-2, and CD34 expression in paraffin-embedded high-grade lymphoma/acute lymphoblastic leukemia distinguishes between distinct clinicopathologic entities. Hum Pathol 28:1158, 1997.

Sperling C, Büchner T, Creutzig U, et al: Clinical, morphologic, cytogenetic and prognostic implications of CD34 expression in childhood and adult *de novo* AML. Leuk Lymphoma 17:417, 1995.

Stewart CC, Behm FG, Carey JL, et al: U.S.–Canadian consensus recommendations on the immunophenotypic analysis of hematologic neoplasia by flow cytometry: selection of antibody combinations. Cytometry 30:231, 1997.

Super HJG, McCabe NR, Thirman MJ, et al: Rearrangements of the MLL gene in therapy-related acute myeloid leukemia in patients previously treated with agents targeting DNA-topoisomerase II. Blood 82:3705, 1993.

Swirsky DM, Li YS, Matthews JG, et al: 8;21 translocation in acute granulocytic leukemia: cytological, cytochemical, and clinical features. Br J Haematol 56:199, 1984.

Taj AS, Ross FM, Vickers M, et al: t(8;21) myelodysplasia, an early presentation of M2 AML. Br J Haematol 89:890, 1995.

Taki T, Ida K, Bessho F, et al: Frequency and clinical significance of the MLL gene rearrangements in infant acute leukemia. Leukemia 10:1303, 1996.

Tallman MS: Differentiating therapy with all-trans retinoic acid in acute myeloid leukemia. Leukemia 10(suppl 1):S12, 1996.

Tanaka K, Tanaka T, Kurokawa M, et al: The AML1/ETO(MTG8) and AML1/Evi-1 leukemia-associated chimeric oncoproteins accumulate PEBP2 (CBF) in the nucleus more efficiently than wild-type AML1. Blood 91:1688, 1998.

Taylor CG, Stasi R, Bastianellic, et al: Diagnosis and classification of the acute leukemias: recent advances and controversial issues. Hematopathol Mol Hematol 10:1, 1996.

Tien H-F, Wang C-H, Su I-J, et al: Immunoglobulin and T-cell receptor gene rearrangements in acute lymphoblastic leukemia: a higher incidence of double rearrangements in patients with myeloid antigen expression. Leuk Res 15:91, 1991.

Tkachuk DC, Kohler S, Cleary ML: Involvement of a homolog on *Drosophila trithorax* by 11q23 chromosomal translocations in acute leukemias. Cell 71:691, 1992.

Tobal K, Johnson PRE, Saunders MJ, et al: Detection of CBFB/MYH11 transcripts in patients with inversion and other abnormalities of chromosome 16 at presentation and remission. Br J Haematol 91:104, 1995.

Tobal K, Liu Yin JA: Monitoring of minimal residual disease by quantitative reverse transcriptase-polymerase chain reaction for AML1-MTG8 transcripts in AML-M2 with t(8;21). Blood 88:3704, 1996.

Traweek ST: Immunophenotypic analysis of acute leukemia. Am J Clin Pathol 99:504, 1993.

Traweek ST, Arber DA, Rappaport H, et al: Extramedullary myeloid cell tumors: an immunohistochemical and morphologic study of 28 cases. Am J Surg Pathol 17:1011, 1993.

Trueworthy R, Shuster J, Look T, et al: Ploidy of lymphoblasts is the strongest predictor of treatment outcome in B-progenitor cell acute lymphoblastic leukemia of childhood: a Pediatric Oncology Group study. J Clin Oncol 10:606, 1992.

Uckun FM, Sather HN, Gaynon PS, et al: Clinical features and treatment outcome of children with myeloid antigen positive acute lymphoblastic leukemia: a report from the Children's Cancer Group. Blood 90:28, 1997.

Uckun FM, Sensel MG, Sun L, et al: Biology and treatment of childhood T-lineage acute lymphoblastic leukemia. Blood 91:735, 1998.

van Dongen JJM, Adriaansen HJ: Immunobiology of leukemia. In: Henderson ES, Lister TA, Greaves MF (eds): Leukemia 6th ed. W.B. Saunders Co. Philadelphia, p 83, 1996.

Viswanatha DS, Chen I-M, Liu PP, et al: Characterization and use of an antibody detecting the CBF-SMMHC fusion protein in inv(16)/t(16;16)-associated acute myeloid leukemias. Blood 91:1882, 1998.

Walker H, Smith FJ, Betts DR: Cytogenetics in acute myeloid leukaemia. Blood Rev 8:30, 1994.

Wallis JP, Reid MM: Bone marrow fibrosis in childhood acute lymphoblastic leukaemia. J Clin Pathol 42:1253, 1989.

Wang JCY, Beauregard P, Soamboonsrup P, et al: Monoclonal antibodies in the management of acute leukemia. Am J Hematol 50:188, 1995.

Weinstein HJ: Acute myelogenous leukemia in infants and children. In: Henderson ES, Lister TA, Greaves MF (eds): Leukemia. 6th ed. W.B. Saunders Co, Philadelphia, p 509, 1996.

Willman CL: The prognostic significance of the expression and function of multidrug resistance transporter proteins in acute myeloid leukemia: studies of the Southwest Oncology Group Leukemia Research Program. Semin Hematol 34:25, 1997.

Woods WG, Kobrinsky N, Buckley J, et al: Intensively timed induction therapy followed by autologous or allogeneic bone marrow transplantation for children with acute myeloid leukemia or myelodysplastic syndrome: a Children's Cancer Group pilot study. J Clin Oncol 11:1448, 1993.

Xue Y, Yu F, Zhou Z, et al: Translocation (8;21) in oligoblastic leukemia: Is this a true myelodysplastic syndrome? Leuk Res 18:761, 1994.

Zack M, Adami H-O, Ericson A: Maternal and perinatal risk factors for childhood leukemia. Cancer Res 51:3696, 1991.

Zeleznik-Le NJ, Nucifora G, Rowley JD: The molecular biology of myeloproliferative disorders as revealed by chromosomal abnormalities. Semin Hematol 32:201, 1995.

Ziemin-van der Poel S, McCabe NR, Gill HJ, et al: Identification of a gene, MLL, that spans the breakpoint in 11q23 translocations associated with human leukemias. Proc Natl Acad Sci USA 88:10735, 1991.

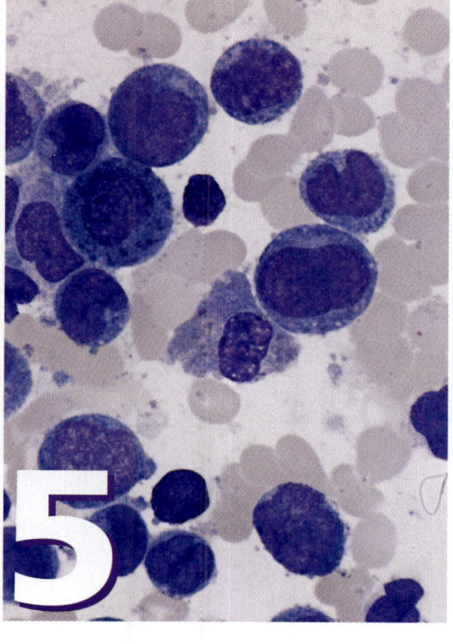

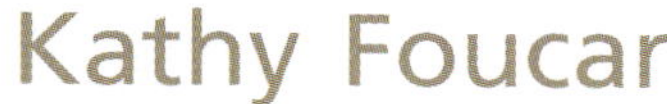

Kathy Foucar

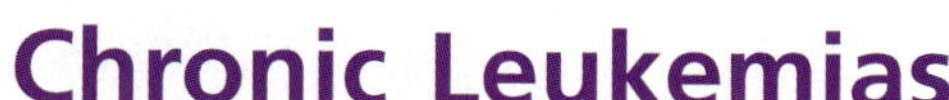

5 Chronic Leukemias

The diagnosis of chronic leukemia is rarely made in children. Only two such disorders occur in children—chronic myelogenous leukemia (CML) and so-called juvenile chronic myelogenous leukemia (juvenile myelomonocytic leukemia, JMML). CML and JMML are biologically distinct and are discussed separately in this chapter, although they are compared in the discussion of differential diagnosis. CML is a well-characterized neoplasm that makes up only 2–5% of childhood leukemias and is much more frequent in adults (Melo, 1996b; Vardiman, 1992). JMML is a controversial entity whose existence as a distinct pathologic disorder has been challenged. A rare disorder, JMML is similar to chronic myelomonocytic leukemia except for elevated hemoglobin F levels, prompting investigators to propose the designation *juvenile myelomonocytic leukemia* (Arico et al, 1997). Chronic myelomonocytic leukemia is also controversial: it is categorized as a myelodysplastic syndrome by the French-American-British (FAB) work group, but many assert that it is intermediate between chronic myeloproliferative disorders and myelodysplastic syndromes (Bennett et al, 1982; Rosati et al, 1996). JMML is included here because it currently bears the designation *leukemia*. (See Chap. 7 for a discussion of all types of chronic myeloproliferative disorders and myelodysplastic syndromes.)

CHRONIC MYELOGENOUS LEUKEMIA

CML is a clonal stem cell neoplasm in which there is excess production of one or more mature granulated white blood cells (WBCs). CML has a unique and defining cytogenetic molecular feature: the [t(9;22)(q34;q11)], known as the Philadelphia chromosome. The resultant *BCR/ABL* fusion gene results in a leukemia in which there are initially a striking neutrophilia of blood and granulocytic hyperplasia of marrow. The disease course of CML generally consists of three phases: an initial chronic phase; an intermediate accelerated phase; and, finally, a "blast crisis," with acute leukemia. All are described below.

The incidence of CML is much greater in adults than in children. Most patients are in their fourth through sixth decades, whereas about 9% of cases of CML occur in children (Savage et al, 1997). CML has occasionally been diagnosed in children younger than 5 years of age, but adolescents are usually affected. A clear association with prior radiation exposure has been established, and rare cases of CML are thought to arise from prior chemotherapy (Kamada & Uchino, 1978).

Patients with CML may present with nonspecific symptoms, such as fatigue, bleeding, malaise, and weight loss, or they may have symptoms from splenomegaly, a feature present at diagnosis in 80% of patients (Savage et al, 1997; Vardiman, 1992) (Fig. 5–1). The WBC counts in children with CML are often higher than adult counts, and symptoms from hyperleukocytosis are more common in pediatric patients (Vardiman, 1992). Hepatomegaly is noted in about 20% of patients, whereas lymphadenopathy is uncommon. CML is an incidental finding in about 20% of patients (Savage et al, 1997).

Blood and Bone Marrow Findings

A constellation of peripheral blood abnormalities is characteristic in CML, including pronounced leukocytosis often exceeding 100,000/µl (Foucar, 1995; Savage et al, 1997; Vardiman, 1992) (Table 5–1). Mature, seemingly normal neutrophils clearly predominate in stable-phase CML, but there is a left shift with a "bulge" of myelocytes and usually 1–3% circulating myeloblasts (Fig. 5–2*A*). Absolute basophilia is a hallmark of CML, even though the basophils usually constitute only 1–3% of cells on differential counts (Fig. 5–2*B*). Because of the pronounced leukocytosis, there is a striking absolute basophilia greatly exceeding normal ranges. Eosinophilia is also usually evident, while circulating erythroblasts, although typical, are infrequent. The platelet count in CML is usually increased and is sometimes so strikingly elevated that a diagnosis of essential thrombocythemia is entertained (Fig. 5–2*C*). Circulating megakaryocytes and megakaryocyte fragments may be noted. Aside from large atypical platelets, dyspoiesis of blood elements is not prominent in the chronic, stable phase of CML.

The marrow is characteristically packed by granulocytes (Fig. 5–3, Table 5–1). Immature granulocytes surround bony trabeculae and blood vessels to form a distinct cuff or collar, and more mature elements fill the intertrabecular spaces (Fig. 5–4). Megakaryocytes are abundant and often clustered. Megakaryocyte size is quite variable, but in some cases small mononuclear megakaryocytes are prominent (see Fig. 5–3). Such megakaryocytes may be useful in distinguishing CML from other chronic myeloproliferative disorders, which consistently have enlarged, hyperlobulated megakaryocytes (Foucar, 1995).

Cytogenetic Molecular Features

The hallmark of CML is demonstration of the Philadelphia chromosome, a reciprocal translocation between chromosomes 9 and 22, by cytogenetic analysis or the *BCR/ABL* fusion gene–gene product by molecular techniques (Gordon &

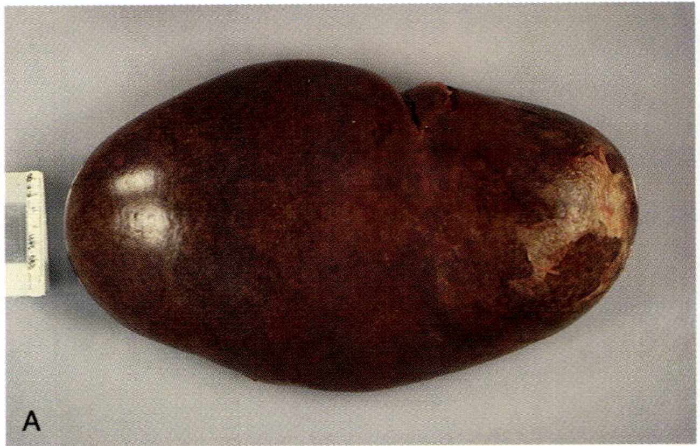

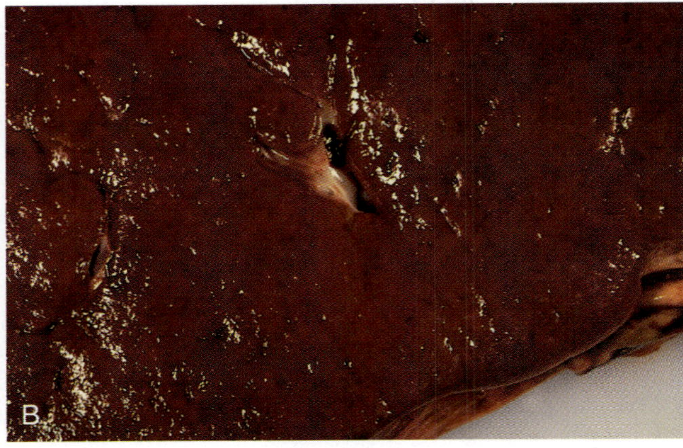

Figure 5–1

Chronic myelogenous leukemia, spleen. These gross photographs illustrate the massive splenomegaly that may occur in patients with CML. *A*. Note the area of infarction. *B*. On cut sections, the spleen has a uniform, beefy, red appearance secondary to red pulp infiltration by leukemia.

Goldman, 1996; Melo, 1996a; Savage et al, 1997) (Fig. 5–5). Routine cytogenetic studies identify the Philadelphia chromosome in >95% of cases, whereas the remaining Philadelphia chromosome–negative cases exhibit *BCR/ABL* gene rearrangement (Gordon & Goldman, 1996; Savage et al, 1997). This chimeric gene encodes a novel mRNA that is translated into a tyrosine kinase protein (Sawyers, 1997). The unregulated production of this protein presumably drives cell growth in CML by activating mitogenic signaling pathways (Sawyers, 1997). However, this fusion gene may not be the initial cytogenetic lesion in CML, since there is evidence that an initial cytogenetic event results in clonal hematopoiesis that precedes the reciprocal translocation between chromosomes 9 and 22 (Gordon & Goldman, 1996). Various breakpoints in the two fused genes are linked to features at presentation, duration of the chronic phase, and type of blast crisis (Cervantes et al, 1996; Melo, 1996a; Urbano-Ispizua et al, 1993). The *BCR/ABL* fusion gene has been documented in all hematopoietic elements as well as some T and B lymphocytes, validating the stem cell nature of this disorder (Tefferi et al, 1995).

Table 5–1

Chronic Myelogenous Leukemia: Blood and Marrow Features

Blood

- Pronounced leukocytosis with a predominance of mature neutrophils
- Left shift with a myelocyte "bulge"
- Myeloblasts usually <3%
- Absolute basophilia; variable eosinophilia
- Variable, possibly pronounced, thrombocytosis
- Occasional erythroblasts; erythrocytes unremarkable

Marrow

- Marked hypercellularity (usually 100% cellular) with granulocytic hyperplasia; maturation intact
- Megakaryocytic hyperplasia with clustering; small forms may predominate
- Pseudo-Gaucher cells and sea-blue histiocytes present (secondary to increased cell turnover)

Source: Foucar K: Chronic myeloproliferative disorders. In: Foucar K (ed): Bone Marrow Pathology. ASCP Press, Chicago, p 121, 1995. Vardiman JW: Chronic myelogenous leukemia and the myeloproliferative disorders. In: Knowles DK (ed): Neoplastic Hematopathology. Williams & Wilkins, Baltimore, p 1405, 1992.

Disease Course

Most patients with CML have an initial indolent disease course (so-called chronic phase). In the vast majority, an aggressive phase eventually develops and is characterized by a progressive increase in blasts usually within the marrow but also in extramedullary sites, progressive dyspoiesis of cells, and cytopenias (Arlin et al, 1990; Foucar, 1995; Kantarjian et al, 1988; Vardiman, 1992) (Fig. 5–6 and Table 5–2). The period between the chronic phase and the overt acute leukemia phase has been designated the accelerated phase (Kantarjian et al, 1988), perhaps best viewed as the harbinger of blast crisis (Anastasi et al, 1995; Nanjangud et al, 1994) (Fig. 5–7). Karyotypic evolution accompanies the progressive increase in blasts, progressive cytologic dyspoiesis, progressive cytopenias, and refractoriness to therapy. In addition to the determination of differential cell counts on marrow aspirate smears (Orazi et al, 1994), evaluation for CD34 expression by paraffin immunoperoxidase techniques is a practical method of assessing disease progression in CML. Occasionally, blast crises are first detected in extramedullary sites but usually the marrow shows a progressive increase in blasts as well (Arlin et al, 1990) (Figs. 5–8 and 5–9). Blast crises of CML may be indistinguishable from de novo acute myelogenous leukemia or acute lymphoblastic leukemia (see Fig. 5–7*B*), although residual dyspoietic mature components may be intermixed with the acute leukemia. The blast crisis in CML may contain virtually any hematopoietic or lymphocytic cell, and multilineage blast crises are common, further evidence of the stem cell nature of this disease (Akashi et al, 1993; Derderian et al, 1993; Hernandez et al, 1991; Rosenthal et al, 1995; Urbano-Ispizua et al, 1993; Warzynski et al, 1989).

Types of blast crises of CML are listed in Table 5–3. The morphologic appearance varies among the types of blast crisis, depending on the lineage involved and the degree of maturation. Clues to antecedent CML include a residual basophilic or eosinophilic component as well as residual small mononuclear megakaryocytes typical of chronic-phase CML. In most pa-

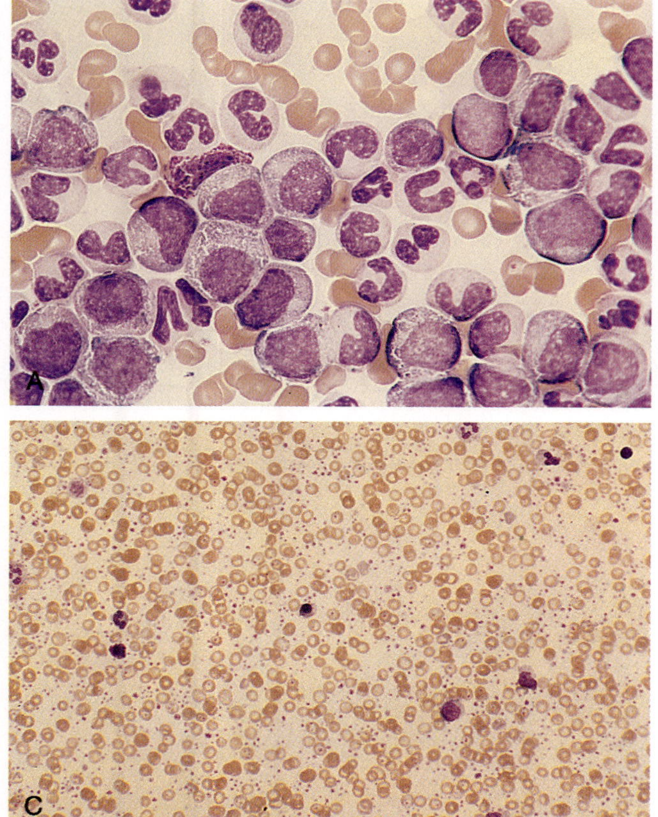

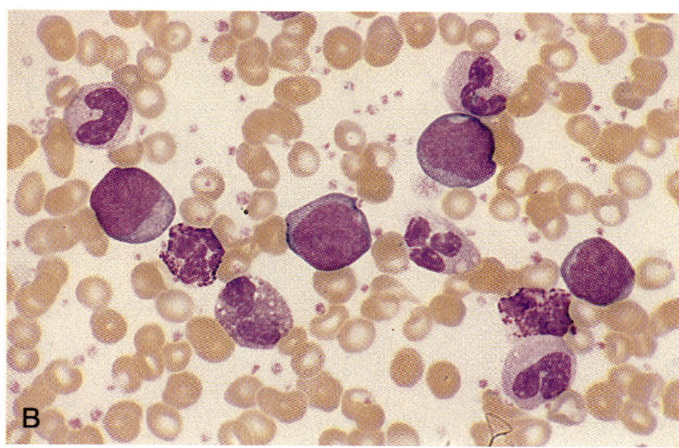

Figure 5–2

Chronic myelogenous leukemia, peripheral blood. *A*. Note the predominance of mature neutrophils, myelocyte bulge, and occasional myeloblasts. *B*. Prominent basophilia is evident in another patient with CML. Wright stain. *C*. Striking thrombocytosis is noted in another patient with CML. Wright stain.

tients detection of underlying evidence of CML is moot, since the prior chronic phase of CML has been well documented and the cytogenetic studies at blast crisis demonstrate the Philadelphia chromosome and additional cytogenetic abnormalities compatible with clonal evolution. Response to therapy is generally poor for patients with all types of blast crisis of CML.

Differential Diagnosis of CML

The differential diagnosis of CML may be challenging, since it includes reactive neutrophilias, other chronic myeloproliferative disorders, and myelodysplastic syndromes. The first step in establishing a diagnosis of CML is to rule out a reactive neutrophilia. Various clinical and laboratory parameters are useful

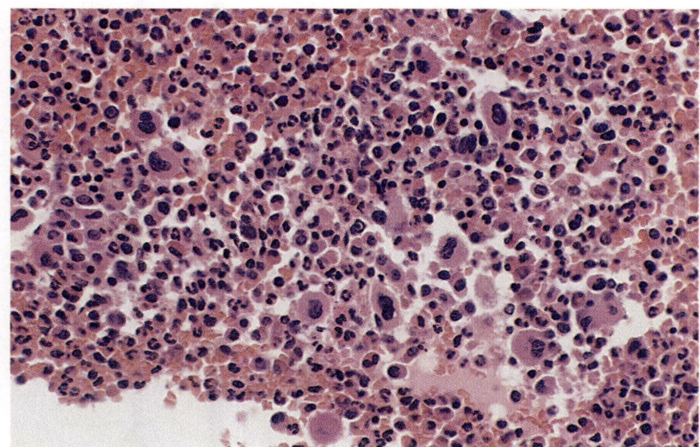

Figure 5–3

Chronic myelogenous leukemia, marrow particle section. A particle with 100% cellularity is shown. Note granulocytic and megakaryocytic hyperplasia. Many mononuclear megakaryocytes are evident.

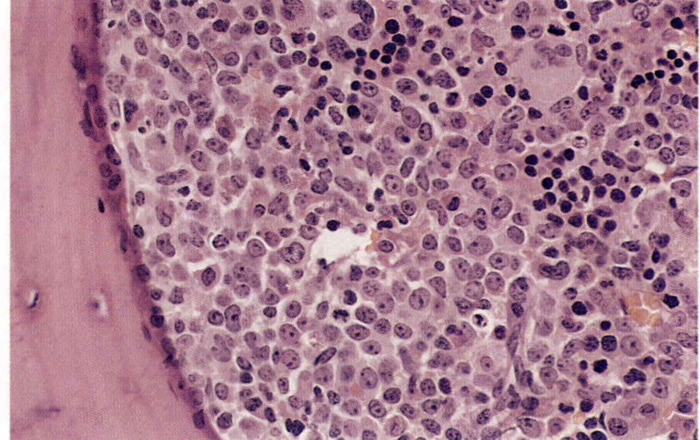

Figure 5–4

Chronic myelogenous leukemia, marrow biopsy. At high magnification there is a prominent paratrabecular collar of immature granulocytic elements.

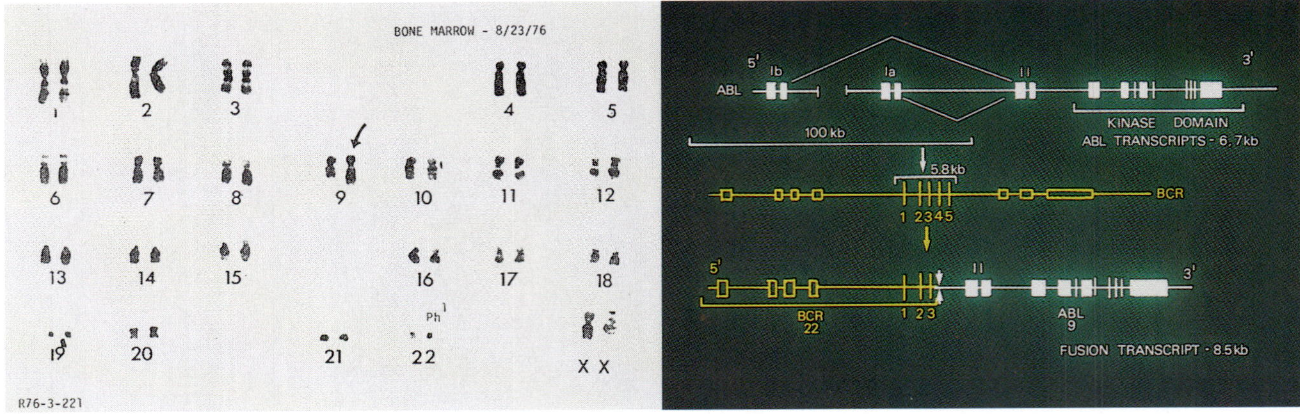

Figure 5–5

Chronic myelogenous leukemia, cytogenetic and molecular genetic features. *A*. The Philadelphia chromosome is shown by classic cytogenetic techniques. *B*. The *BCR/ABL* fusion gene is shown in this sketch. (Courtesy Dr. C. Willman.)

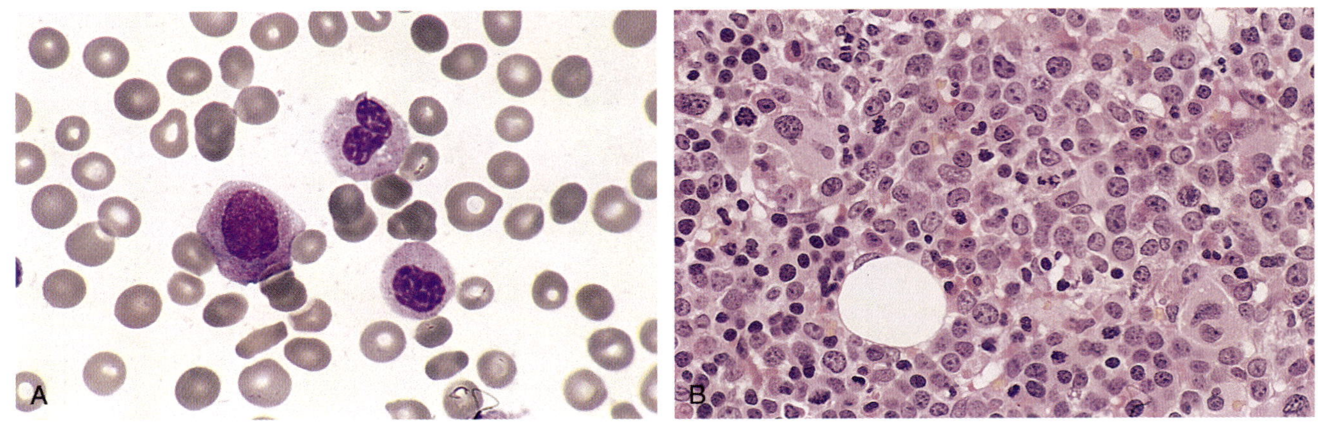

Figure 5–6

Chronic myelogenous leukemia, accelerated phase, blood and marrow. *A*. This peripheral blood film illustrates progressive dyspoiesis with a pseudo–Pelger-Huet change in neutrophils, hypogranular cytoplasm, and increased blasts. Wright stain. *B*. A marrow biopsy section demonstrates a prominent parenchymal focus of blasts; the blast count on this marrow was 22%.

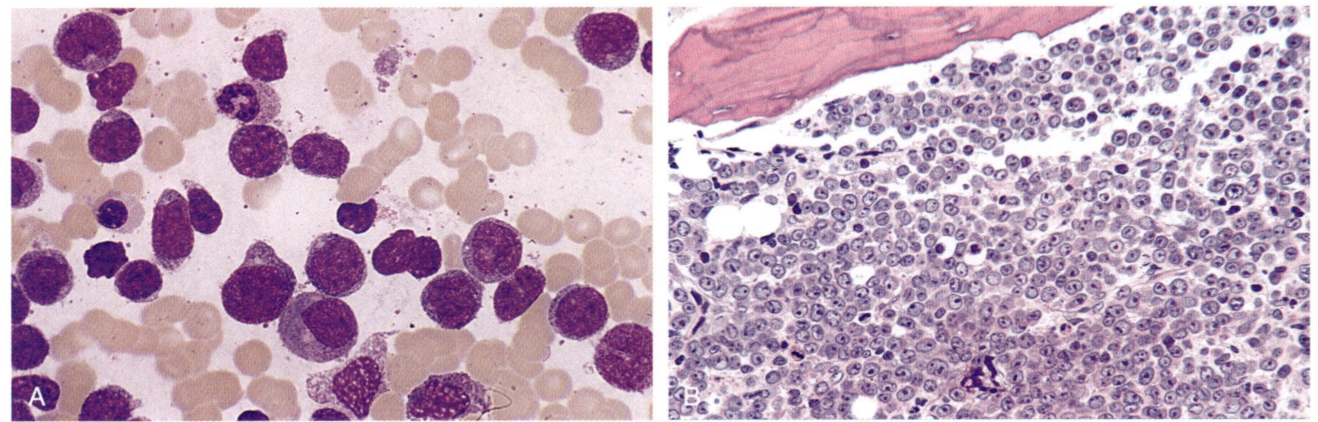

Figure 5–7

Chronic myelogenous leukemia, blast crisis, marrow. *A*. This marrow aspirate film demonstrates a predominance of blasts. Wright stain. *B*. A marrow biopsy section shows complete effacement by blasts.

Table 5–2
Chronic Myelogenous Leukemia: Disease Phases

Chronic (stable) phase	Blood and marrow blasts <5% Clinically stable for several years
Accelerated phase	Poorly defined intermediate phase characterized by increasing blood and marrow blast counts (<30%) and cytopenias May also demonstrate progressive dyspoiesis, rising absolute basophil count, progressive marrow fibrosis, or refractoriness to therapy Clonal karyotypic evolution common
Blast crisis	Blasts exceed 30% (20% for lymphocytic blast crisis) in blood or marrow *or* extra- or intramedullary focus of blasts Similar but progressive dyspoiesis; cytopenias; rising basophilia; progressive clinical symptoms, as noted in accelerated phase but more pronouced Clonal karyotypic evolution

in making this distinction (Table 5–4). In general, the causes of a reactive neutrophilia are usually clinically apparent, and the neutrophils demonstrate toxic changes, such as toxic granulation, Dohle bodies, and cytoplasmic vacuoles. Left shift may be present in reactive processes, but circulating myeloblasts are generally not observed, except in septic infants. Many cases of reactive neutrophilia are secondary to infection and therefore accompanied by fever, whereas most patients with CML are afebrile. Splenomegaly is almost universal in CML but is not evident in most patients with reactive neutrophilia. Documentation of the Philadelphia chromosome or *BCR/ABL* confirms the diagnosis of CML and excludes reactive processes.

CML must also be distinguished from other chronic myeloproliferative disorders, such as essential thrombocythemia, chronic idiopathic myelofibrosis, and polycythemia vera. Such disorders are discussed in detail in Chap. 7. All are exceedingly rare in pediatric patients. In general, these disorders are characterized by a more prolonged indolent disease course, and affected patients rarely develop an acute leukemia phase. Distinction between CML and myelodysplastic syndromes is also clinically important. The myelodysplastic syndromes are characterized by low, rather than high, cell counts in the blood, and mature cells have prominent dyspoietic features. Cytogenetic studies distinguish CML from other myeloid neoplasms, which may exhibit a variety of karyotypic aberrations, but lack the Philadelphia chromosome.

JUVENILE MYELOMONOCYTIC LEUKEMIA

Approximately 2% of childhood leukemias are designated JMML, a disorder that principally affects young children. Despite the nosologic similarity to CML, JMML is a distinct disorder characterized by moderate leukocytosis with prominent monocytosis, leukoerythroblastosis, erythrocyte abnormalities, hepatosplenomegaly, lymphadenopathy, skin lesions, and increased fetal hemoglobin levels (Table 5–5) (Busque et al, 1995; Hess et al, 1996; Vardiman, 1992). Furthermore, neither the Philadelphia chromosome nor the *BCR/ABL* fusion gene is present, clearly distinguishing this type of leukemia from CML. JMML is virtually indistinguishable from chronic myelomonocytic leukemia except for increased hemoglobin F levels (Arico et al, 1997; Hess et al, 1996; Niemeyer et al, 1997; Passmore et al, 1995; Vardiman, 1992). Overlap exists between JMML and another childhood entity, termed infantile monosomy 7 syndrome. One proposal suggests that these two disorders are part of a disease spectrum (Hess et al, 1996; Luna-Fineman et al, 1995; Hasle, 1999; Luna-Fineman, 1999). The salient features of JMML are presented here, and childhood myelodysplastic syndromes are presented in Chap. 7.

Clinical Features

Children with JMML typically are <4 years old and present with malaise, bleeding, fever, and skin rash. JMML is associated with neurofibromatosis, which may dominate the cuta-

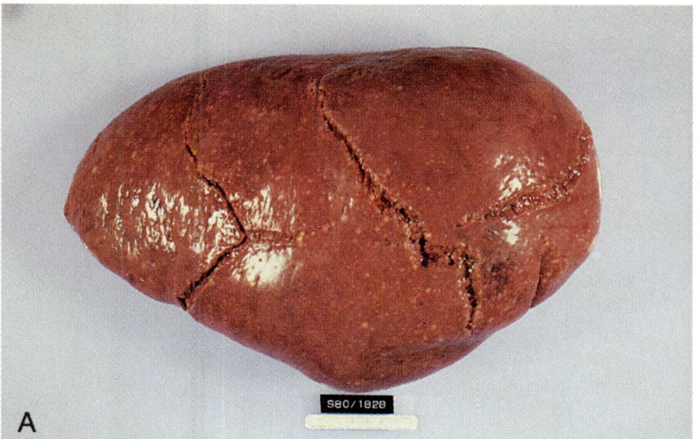

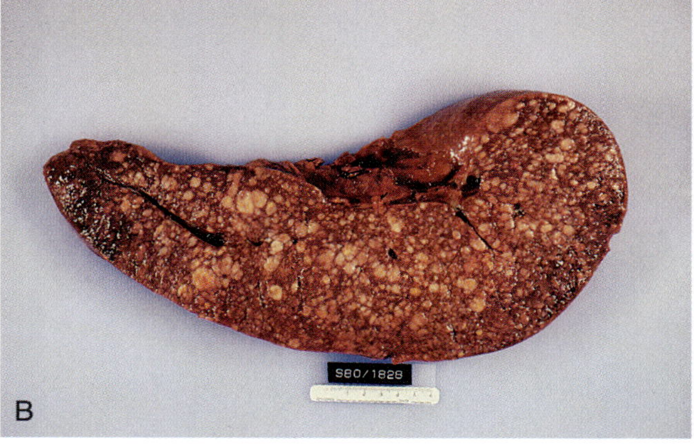

Figure 5–8

Chronic myelogenous leukemia, blast crisis, spleen. This patient with extramedullary blast crisis of CML (compare to Fig. 5–1*A* and *B*) had spontaneous rupture of the spleen secondary to extensive infiltration of blasts. The (*A*) external and (*B*) cut surfaces of the spleen are shown.

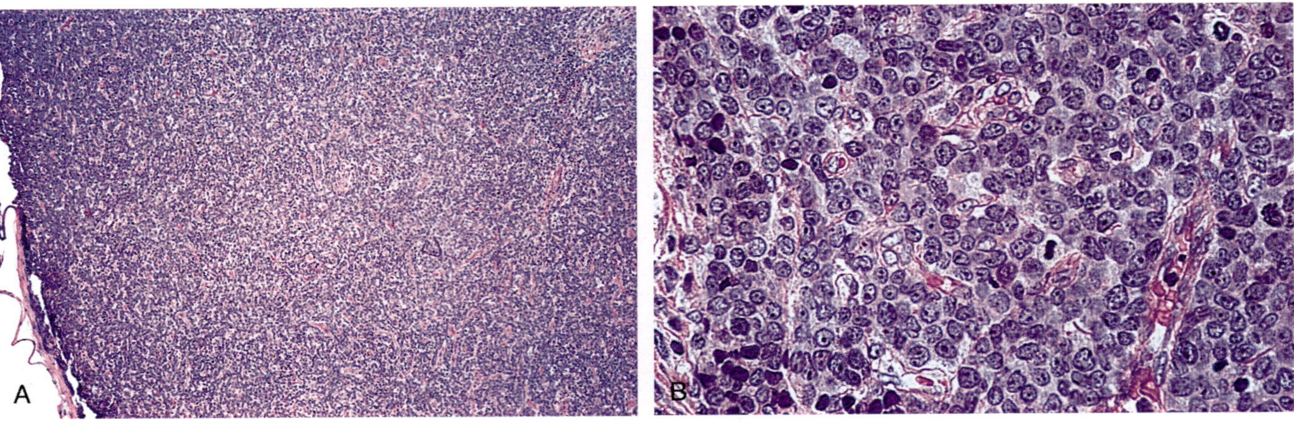

Figure 5–9

Chronic myelogenous leukemia, blast crisis, lymph node. (*A*) Low- and (*B*) high-magnification photomicrographs demonstrate a lymphocytic blast crisis in a patient with known CML.

neous picture at presentation. The WBC count is characteristically elevated (usually $< 100{,}000/\mu l$) with an absolute monocytosis, left-shifted granulocytosis with mild dysplastic features, $<5\%$ blasts, frequent nucleated red blood cells, anemia, and thrombocytopenia (Fig. 5–10). The fetal hemoglobin level is consistently increased, and fetal hemoglobin uniformly distributed within erythrocytes (Niemeyer et al, 1997). The marrow in these children is characterized by hypercellularity, with moderately increased numbers of myeloblasts (5–20%), atypical monocytosis, and mild multilineage dysplasia (Fig. 5–11).

Table 5–3
Chronic Myelogenous Leukemia: Blast Crisis

Lineage	Comments
Myelocytic	Most common type of blast crisis May be granulocytic or myelomonocytic Usual types of clonal evolution: duplicate Philadelphia chromosome, trisomies of 8, 19, 20, or 21, and i(17q) Occasional cases demonstrate t(8;21), inv(16), or t(15;17)
Multilineage	Variable patterns: mixed myelocytic, erythrocytic, megakaryoblastic, and lymphocytic Blasts may coexpress antigens characteristic of different lineages (mixed lineage), or two or more distinct cell populations may be noted (bilineage)
Lymphocytic	B, T, and natural killer cell blast crises noted Often extramedullary May be mixed B and T
Erythrocytic	Rare in pure form
Megakaryoblastic	Rare in pure form Frequent component of multilineage blast crisis Linked to chromosome 3 abnormalities
Promyelocytic	May mimic acute promyelocytic leukemia Associated with t(15;17) or i(17q)
Mast cell	Very rare; cells exhibit admixed basophil and mast cell granules

In approximately one third of patients, the disease is rapidly progressive, with survival times of under 2 years. Other patients experience a more indolent, prolonged disease course (Arico et al, 1997). A rapidly progressive terminal phase may occur in a substantial proportion of the latter group (Arico et al, 1997). Factors linked to better outcome include a high hemoglobin F level, platelet count $>40{,}000/mm^3$, and normal cytogenetic analysis (Passmore et al, 1995).

Cytogenetic Features

Cytogenetic findings vary in cases of JMML, depending on the diagnostic criteria utilized. According to some investigators, the identification of monosomy 7 precludes a diagnosis of JMML. Other investigators include cases with this cytogenetic feature if other findings are supportive. The controversy is related to whether JMML and infantile monosomy 7 syndrome are a single disease (Luna-Fineman et al, 1995). In one series that included both JMML and infantile monosomy 7 syndrome in a single diagnostic group termed childhood chronic myelomonocytic leukemia, 65% of cases had a normal karyotype, 25% demonstrated monosomy 7, and 10% had cytogenetic abnor-

Table 5–4
Features Differentiating Chronic Myelogenous Leukemia from Reactive Neutrophilia

Feature	CML	Reactive Neutrophilia
Fever	Absent	Present
Splenomegaly	Present	Absent (usually)
Toxic neutrophils	Absent	Present
Basophilia	Present	Absent
Myeloblasts in blood	Present	Absent
Erythroblasts in blood	Present	Absent
Thrombocytosis	Present	Absent (usually)
Uric acid	Increased	Normal
Neutrophil alkaline phosphatase	Decreased	Increased
Philadelphia chromosome	Present	Absent
BCR/ABL fusion gene	Present	Absent

Table 5–5

Comparison of Clinical, Hematologic, and Cytogenetic Features of Juvenile Myelomonocytic Leukemia and Chronic Myelogenous Leukemia

Feature	JMML	CML
Age, sex	<4 years, usually male	>4 years, usually young adult
Skin lesions	Present	Absent
Splenomegaly	Present	Present
Lymphadenopathy	Present	Absent
Recurrent infections, hemorrhage	Common	Infrequent
Leukocytosis	<100,000/μl	>100,000/μl (usually)
Dyspoiesis	Mild	Absent (usually)
Monocytosis	Present	Absent
Basophilia	Absent	Present
Platelets	Decreased	Increased (usually)
Anemia	Present	Absent (usually)
Hemoglobin F	Increased	Absent
Neutrophil alkaline phosphatase	Variable	Decreased
Percent blasts in marrow	<25%	<5%
Cell types, blood and marrow	Monocytosis, neutrophilia	Neutrophilia, basophilia
Philadelphia chromosome	Absent	Present
BCR/ABL fusion gene	Absent	Present
Blast crisis	Variable	Common

malities other than monosomy 7 (Niemeyer et al, 1997). Similar cytogenetic results have been reported for cases designated juvenile myelomonocytic leukemia (Arico et al, 1997). The current recommendation is to view JMML and infantile monosomy 7 syndrome as a single disease entity (Hasle, 1999; Luna-Fineman, 1999).

Differential Diagnosis of JMML

The differential diagnosis of JMML includes reactive processes, especially chronic Epstein-Barr virus (EBV) infection, childhood myelodysplasias, and CML. In children, especially immunosuppressed patients, chronic EBV infection may be

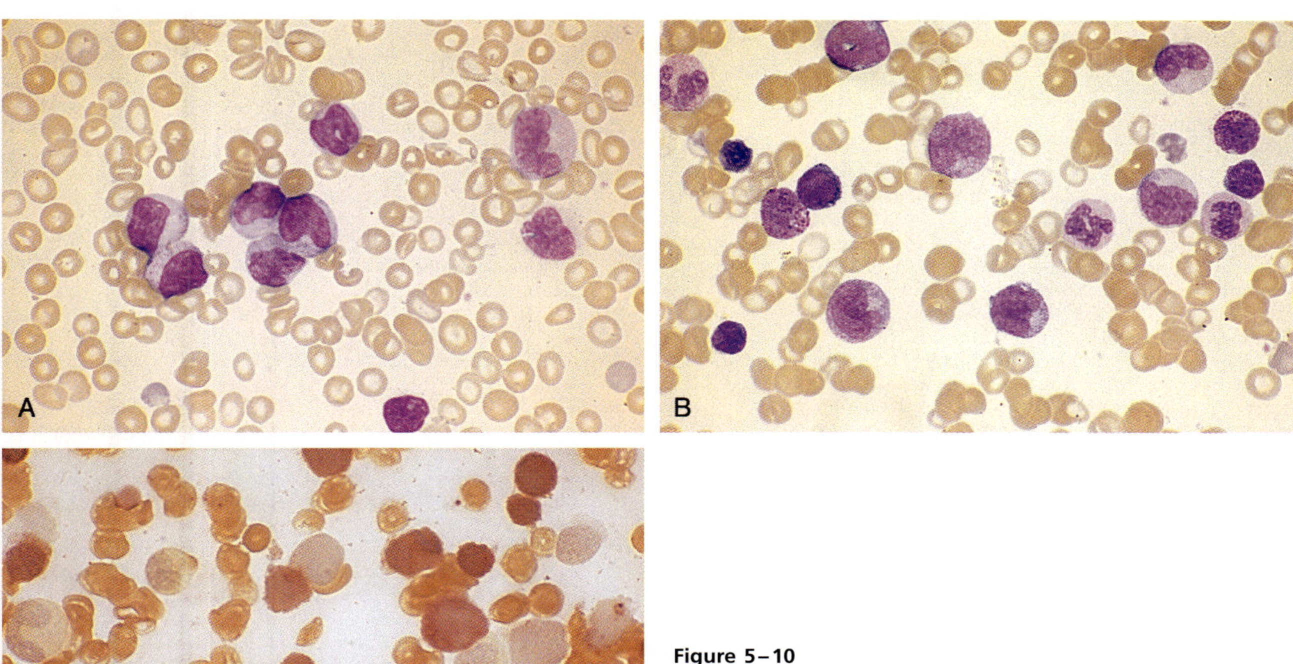

Figure 5–10

Juvenile myelomonocytic leukemia, peripheral blood. *A*. This peripheral blood film illustrates the monocytosis with left shift and moderate leukocytosis that characterize this disease. Wright-Giemsa stain. *B*. Immature granulocytic elements, basophilia, monocytosis, and an occasional nucleated red blood cell are present in another patient. Wright-Giemsa Stain. (Courtesy Dr. R. Brynes.) *C*. Nonspecific esterase stain highlights the monocytic component.

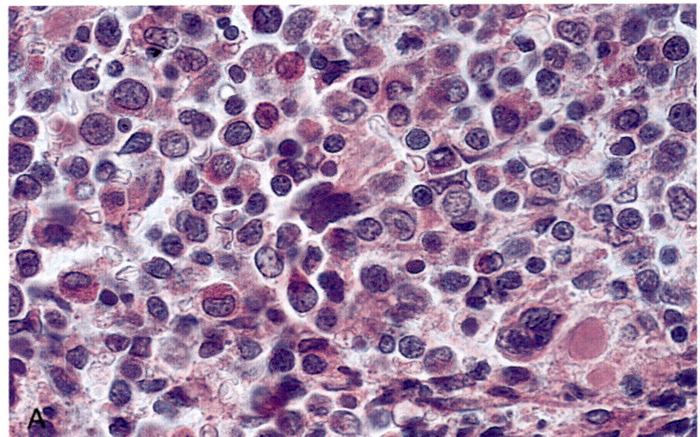

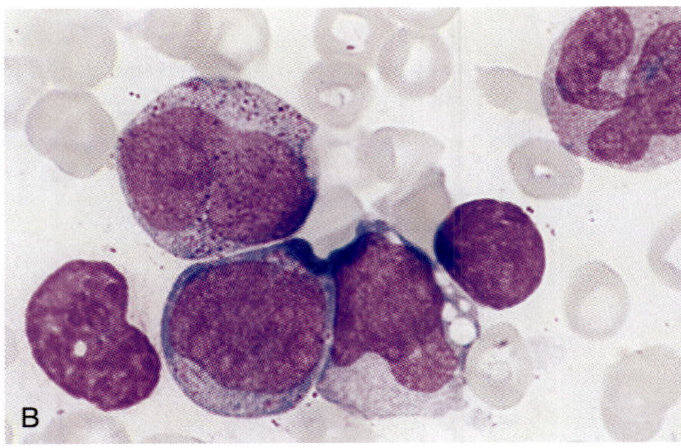

Figure 5–11

Juvenile myelomonocytic leukemia, marrow. *A*. A high-magnification photomicrograph of a biopsy section demonstrates hypercellularity, left-shifted granulopoiesis, and megakaryocyte atypia. Hematoxylin-eosin stain. (Courtesy Dr. R. Brynes.) *B*. This aspirate film demonstrates left-shifted granulopoiesis with increased monocytes. Wright-Giemsa stain.

associated with hepatosplenomegaly, leukocytosis with an absolute monocytosis, anemia, and thrombocytopenia, closely mimicking JMML. Serologic studies for evidence of acute and persistent EBV infection are essential to identifying this group of patients (Herrod et al, 1983). The distinction between JMML and childhood myelodysplastic disorders, including infantile monosomy 7 syndrome, is largely semantic. Most current data support the proposal that these various diagnostic labels have been used for parts of a single disease. JMML must also be distinguished from CML (see Table 5–5). In general, a constellation of clinical and hematologic parameters readily distinguishes these biologically discrete disorders. Cytogenetic and molecular studies may be used to establish the diagnosis of CML.

REFERENCES

Akashi K, Mizuno S, Harada M, et al: T lymphoid/myeloid bilineal crisis in chronic myelogenous leukemia. Exp Hematol 21:743, 1993.

Anastasi J, Feng J, Le Beau MM, et al: The relationship between secondary chromosomal abnormalities and blast transformation in chronic myelogenous leukemia. Leukemia 9:628, 1995.

Arico M, Biondi A, Pui C-H: Juvenile myelomonocytic leukemia. Blood 90:479, 1997.

Arlin ZA, Silver RT, Bennett JM: Blastic phase of chronic myeloid leukemia (blCML): a proposal for standardization of diagnostic and response criteria. Leukemia 4:755, 1990.

Bennett JM, Catovsky D, Daniel MT, et al: Proposals for the classification of the myelodysplastic syndromes. Br J Haematol 51:189, 1982.

Busque L, Gilliland DG, Prchal JT, et al: Clonality in juvenile chronic myelogenous leukemia. Blood 85:21, 1995.

Cervantes F, Colomer D, Vives-Corrons JL, et al: Chronic myeloid leukemia of thrombocythemic onset: a CML subtype with distinct hematological and molecular features? Leukemia 10:1241, 1996.

Derderian PM, Kantarjian HM, Talpaz M, et al: Chronic myelogenous leukemia in the lymphoid blastic phase: characteristics, treatment response, and prognosis. Am J Med 94:69, 1993.

Ferro MT, Steegman JL, Escribano L, et al: Ph-positive chronic myeloid leukemia with t(8;21)(q22;q22) in blastic crisis. Cancer Genet Cytogenet 58:96, 1992.

Foucar K: Chronic myeloproliferative disorders. In: Foucar K (ed): *Bone Marrow Pathology*. ASCP Press, Chicago, p 121, 1995.

Gordon MY, Goldman JM: Cellular and molecular mechanisms in chronic myeloid leukaemia: biology and treatment. Br J Haematol 95:10, 1996.

Hasle H, Arico M, Basso G, et al: Myelodysplastic syndrome, juvenile myelomonocytic leukemia, and acute myeloid leukemia associated with complete or partial monosomy 7. European Working Group on MDS in Childhood (EWOG-MDS). Leukemia 13:376, 1999.

Hernandez JM, Gonzalez-Sarmiento R, Martin C, et al: Immunophenotypic, genomic and clinical characteristics of blast crisis of chronic myelogenous leukaemia. Br J Haematol 79:408, 1991.

Herrod HG, Dow LW, Sullivan JL. Persistent Epstein-Barr virus infection mimicking juvenile chronic myelogenous leukemia: immunologic and hematologic studies. Blood 61:1098, 1983.

Hess JL, Zutter MM, Castleberry RP, et al: Juvenile chronic myelogenous leukemia. Am J Clin Pathol 105:238, 1996.

Kamada N, Uchino H: Chronologic sequence in appearance of clinical and laboratory findings characteristic of chronic myelocytic leukemia. Blood 51:843, 1978.

Kantarjian HM, Dixon D, Keating MJ, et al: Characteristics of accelerated disease in chronic myelogenous leukemia. Cancer 61:1441, 1988.

Luna-Fineman S, Shannon KM, Lange BJ: Childhood monosomy 7: epidemiology, biology, and mechanistic implications. Blood 85: 1985, 1995.

Luna-Fineman S, Shannon KM, Atwater SK, et al: Myelodysplastic and myeloproliferative disorders of childhood: A study of 167 patients. Blood 93:459, 1999.

Melo JV: The diversity of BCR-ABL fusion proteins and their relationship to leukemia phenotype. Blood 88:2375, 1996a.

Melo JV: The molecular biology of chronic myeloid leukaemia. Leukemia 10:751, 1996b.

Nanjangud G, Kadam PR, Saikia T, et al: Karyotypic findings as an independent prognostic marker in chronic myeloid leukaemia blast crisis. Leuk Res 18:385, 1994.

Niemeyer CM, Arico M, Basso G, et al: Chronic myelomonocytic leukemia in childhood: a retrospective analysis of 110 cases. Blood 89:3534, 1997.

Orazi A, Neiman RS, Cualing H, et al: CD34 immunostaining of bone marrow biopsy specimens is a reliable way to classify the phases of chronic myeloid leukemia. Am J Clin Pathol 101:426, 1994.

Passmore SJ, Hann IM, Stiller CA, et al: Pediatric myelodysplasia: a study of 68 children and a new prognostic scoring system. Blood 85:1742, 1995.

Rosati S, Anastasi J, Vardiman J: Recurring diagnostic problems in the pathology of the myelodysplastic syndromes. Semin Hematol 33:111, 1996.

Rosenthal NS, Knapp D, Farhi DC: Promyelocytic blast crisis of chronic myelogenous leukemia: a rare subtype associated with disseminated intravascular coagulation. Am J Clin Pathol 103:185, 1995.

Savage DG, Szydlo RM, Goldman JM: Clinical features at diagnosis in 430 patients with chronic myeloid leukaemia seen at a referral centre over a 16-year period. Br J Haematol 96:111, 1997.

Sawyers CL: Molecular genetics of acute leukaemia. Lancet 349:196, 1997.

Tefferi A, Schad CR, Pruthi RK, et al: Fluorescent in situ hybridization studies of lymphocytes and neutrophils in chronic granulocytic leukemia. Cancer Genet Cytogenet 83:61, 1995.

Urbano-Ispizua A, Cervantes F, Matutes E, et al: Immunophenotypic characteristics of blast crisis of chronic myeloid leukaemia: correlations with clinico-biological features and survival. Leukemia 7:1349, 1993.

Vardiman JW: Chronic myelogenous leukemia and the myeloproliferative disorders. In: Knowles DK (ed): *Neoplastic Hematopathology*. Williams & Wilkins, Baltimore, p 1405, 1992.

Warzynski MJ, White C, Golightly MG, et al: Natural killer lymphocyte blast crisis of chronic myelogenous leukemia. Am J Hematol 32:279, 1989.

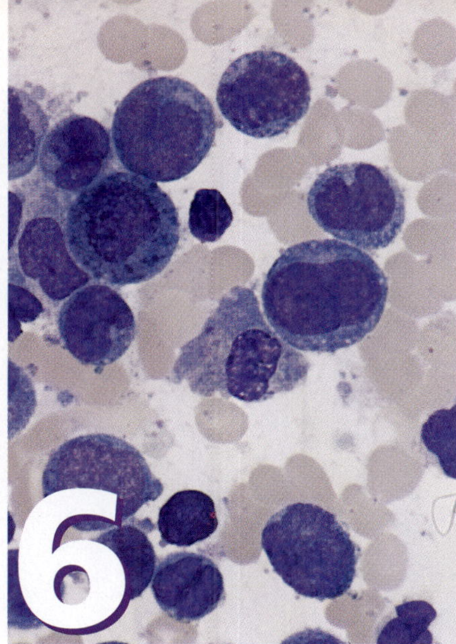

Sherrie Perkins

Disorders of Hematopoiesis

INHERITED ANEMIAS: HEMOGLOBINOPATHIES

Sickle Cell Disease

Sickle cell anemia (SS) and the less severe heterozygous sickle cell trait (SA) are common hemoglobinopathies characterized by an autosomally dominant mutation in the β-globin gene in which a valine residue replaces a glutamic acid in the number 6 position to form hemoglobin S (HgS) (Ingram, 1957). HgS is a common mutant in central Africa and is also found in the Near East, Mediterranean and parts of India. This geographic distribution parallels the incidence of *falciparum malaria*. The sickling may protect against malarial infection by impeding infection of the cell by increasing membrane rigidity, by providing a hostile intracellular environment for the parasite, or by facilitating more rapid removal of infected cells from the circulation (Johnson, 1985).

The HgS mutant may be heterozygous (SA), usually producing no symptoms, or homozygous, producing SS. Mutation induces abnormal polymerization of deoxygenated hemoglobin to form long, fibrillar crystalline arrays that create the characteristic sickle shape (Eaton & Hofrichter, 1987; Rodgers et al, 1987). Hemoglobin polymerization is usually seen physiologically only in the homozygous state because of the relative insolubility of the abnormal hemoglobin molecules. Polymerization and associated red blood cell shape changes are usually reversed by oxygenation. Sickling is irreversible in a few cells and may be seen on routine peripheral blood films.

Repeated episodes of sickling induce membrane changes in red cells, including loss of normal deformability, changes in lipid orientation, ATP depletion, and abnormalities in ion transport (Ballas & Smith, 1992; Eaton et al, 1979; Lubin et al, 1981). These ultimately cause cellular dehydration by alterations in cellular cation and water concentrations. As individual cells become dehydrated, hemoglobin concentration rises and solubility decreases. Resultant small aggregates of hemoglobin ("micro-Heinz bodies") adhere to the cell membrane and are targeted for removal by the mononuclear phagocytic system (Evans & Mohandas, 1987). All of these changes contribute to the shortened life span of sickle cells and accelerated hemolysis intrinsic to the disease. Sickle cell membranes also interact abnormally with vascular endothelium, contributing to the characteristic vaso-occlusive phenomena (Hebbel & Vercellotti, 1997).

Clinical Features

The clinical manifestations of SS are extremely variable (Powars, 1975). Since the high levels of hemoglobin F (HgF) in the newborn have a protective effect by decreasing hemoglobin solubility, patients are often not anemic and have no symptoms. Later, anemia and compensatory reticulocytosis develop. Hemoglobin levels of 7–10 g/dl and reticulocyte counts of 5–20% are often seen by 4 months of age, although characteristic sickle cells are not usually seen in the peripheral smear (Hayes et al, 1985). By 3 years of age, the decrease in splenic function gives rise to the characteristic blood smear, including irreversibly sickled cells, cellular fragments, spherocytes, target cells, nucleated red cells, and Howell-Jolly bodies. Early diagnosis and comprehensive care improve survival of infants with SS anemia, decreasing mortality rates from 25 to <3%. Because of these results, neonatal screening of all infants at risk for sickle cell disease is advocated (Consensus Conference, 1987). Older patients may be virtually asymptomatic or have frequent painful episodes from vaso-occlusion and infarction (Baum et al, 1987). Vaso-occlusion most commonly involves bone, with spleen, liver, lungs, brain, and penis also frequently affected. Splenic infarction is so common that most children with SS have a completely autoinfarcted spleen by age 7. Hyposplenism increases susceptibility to bacterial infections, in particular from *Pneumococcus* and *Haemophilus influenzae* (Barrett-Connor, 1971).

Other precipitous hematologic events in patients with SS include acute splenic sequestration and aplastic or hemolytic crises. Acute splenic sequestration occurs in young children (the spleen must be partially intact) with frequent acute upper respiratory infections (Emond et al, 1985). Patients experience severe anemia, hypoxia, and cardiovascular collapse (Seeler & Shwiaki, 1972) from massive splenic trapping of red cells. Aplastic crisis develops when viral or bacterial infections suppress hematopoiesis. This inability to compensate for the increased red cell turnover inherent in SS leads to a precipitous fall in hematocrit. Patients characteristically have no compensatory reticulocytosis. Recovery is evidenced in the peripheral blood by increased numbers of nucleated red cells and brisk reticulocytosis. The period of aplasia is usually short but in some patients is severe and requires transfusion therapy. Parvovirus B19 infection is a common cause of aplastic crisis (Goldstein et al, 1987; Rao et al, 1992) and should be searched for routinely. Folate deficiency, another cause of aplastic crisis, is detected by severe megaloblastic changes in both red and white cells. Hemolytic crises occur in some SS patients and are most often associated with an additional glucose-6-phosphate dehydrogenase (G6PD) deficiency and oxidative stress owing to infection or drug ingestion. Hemolytic crises may occasionally be seen in patients with bacterial infections in the absence of G6PD deficiency (Smits et al, 1969).

Table 6–1
Laboratory Features of Sickle Cell (Hemoglobin SS) Disease

Peripheral blood	
RBCs	Mild to moderate normocytic, normochromic anemia with anisocytosis, poikilocytosis Reticulocytosis; nucleated RBCs may be seen Howell-Jolly bodies and irregular cell shapes consistent with asplenia Sickle cells, fragments
WBCs	Normal to slightly increased; neutrophilia with left shift
Platelets	Normal to increased (up to 1 millionn/μl)
Other	Positive sickle preparation test results Positive sickle solubility test results Hg analysis revealing dominant HgS species Decreased RBC life span
Marrow	Hypercellular, with erythrocyte hyperplasia
Chemistries	Evidence of hemolysis; increased LDH level, elevated direct bilirubin level

Abbreviations: Hg, hemoglobin; LDH, lactate dehydrogenase; RBC, red blood cell, WBC, white blood cell.

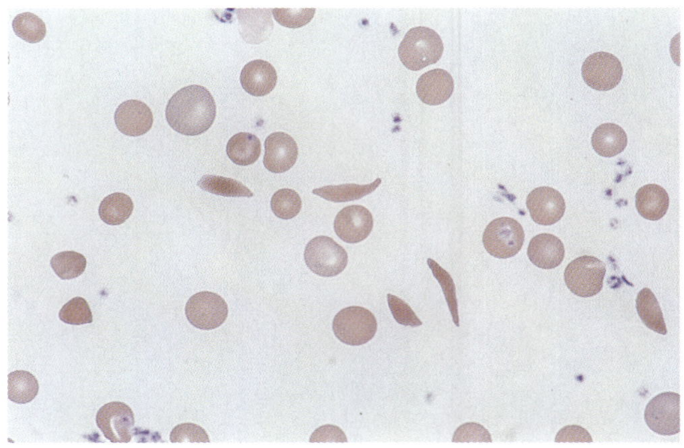

Figure 6–1

Sickle cells, peripheral blood. This film shows prominent sickle cell formation in a patient with hemoglobin SS disease. The nonsickled cells show characteristic increased anisocytosis and poikilocytosis. Wright-Giemsa stain.

Laboratory Features

Laboratory features of SS disease (Table 6–1) include normochromic, normocytic anemia with hemoglobin levels of 5–11 g/dl and reticulocytosis of 5–20%. There may be peripheral neutrophilia with a left shift (Buchanan & Glader, 1978) and thrombocytosis (up to 1 million/μl^3) with numerous large platelets (Freedman & Karpatkin, 1975). Mean corpuscular hemoglobin concentration (MCHC) is usually normal. Hemolysis is evidenced by increased direct bilirubin levels, reticulocytosis, and circulating nucleated red cells. The hematologic parameters among patients with sickle cell disease vary widely, but the values for a single patient tend to remain stable over time (Hayes et al, 1985).

The peripheral blood film in patients with SS (Fig. 6–1) demonstrates marked heterogeneity of red cell shape, size, and hemoglobin density, reflecting the various ages of cells in the film and variations in HgF levels. HgF interferes with polymerization of HgS, and cells with a higher proportion of HgF have a longer life span. Cells with lower levels of HgF show progressive increases in hemoglobin concentration owing to membrane loss, leading eventually to irreversibly sickled cells (Bookchin & Nagel, 1974). Since splenic hypofunction is common, films of peripheral blood show Howell-Jolly bodies, irregularly shaped red cells, spherocytes, cellular fragments, and target cells. Polychromatophilic cells and nucleated red cells may also be seen, reflecting the physiologic response to chronic hemolysis.

The marrow in SS exhibits hypercellularity owing to marked erythrocyte hyperplasia. The rapid turnover of red cells leads to nutritional deficiencies of folate and cobalamin, causing abnormalities in red cell maturation. Chronic hemolysis also leads to increased iron deposition in macrophages of marrow and other organs.

Laboratory tests used to diagnose SA or SS include the sickle preparation test for screening as well as the more definitive hemoglobin analysis for HgS. In the sickle preparation test, a reducing agent (usually sodium metabisulfate) is added to fresh blood, and after 1 h of incubation a wet mount is examined for the presence of sickled cells. Both heterozygotes and homozygotes for HgS exhibit sickled cells. Most screening tests are unreliable in newborns owing to the increased levels of fetal hemoglobin. Thus, in many centers screening is performed by hemoglobin electrophoresis on blood from the umbilical cord or from a heel stick. The levels of HgF decrease over the first 20 weeks of life, with concomitant increases in HgS production. Hemoglobin is analyzed to demonstrate HgS by hemoglobin gel electrophoresis using cellulose acetate at pH 8.4 and citrate agar at pH 6.0–6.2. This two-gel system allows for separation and identification of most of the major

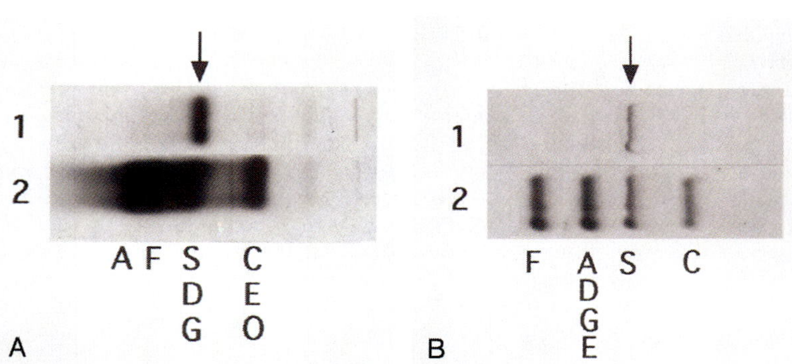

Figure 6–2

Sickle cell disease, hemoglobin electrophoretic pattern. *A.* Cellulose acetate gel (pH 8.4). The patient's sample is in lane 1, and control hemoglobins are in lane 2. An arrow indicates the HgS band. *B.* Citrate agar gel (pH 6.0–6.2). The patient's sample is in lane 1, and control hemoglobins are in lane 2. The arrow indicates the HgS band in the patient's sample.

Table 6–2
Laboratory Features of Homozygous Hemoglobin C Disease

Peripheral blood	
RBCs	Mild normocytic, normochromic anemia Target cells, HgC crystal, spherocytes Reticulocytosis
WBCs	Normal
Platelets	Normal
Other	Hg analysis shows predominant HgC species Negative sickle cell preparation and sickle solubility test results Decreased RBC life span
Marrow	Hypercellular with erythrocyte hyperplasia
Chemistries	Evidence of mild hemolysis, increased LDH level, elevated direct bilirubin level

Abbreviations: Hg, hemoglobin; LDH, lactate dehydrogenase; RBC, red blood cell; WBC, white blood cell.

hemoglobin species and definitive diagnosis of many hemoglobinopathies. The HgS migrates to the same position as hemoglobins D and G on cellulose acetate gel (Fig. 6–2*A*) but separates from these other species on citrate agar gel (Fig. 6–2*B*). Thin-layer isoelectric focusing (Galacteros et al, 1980), high-performance liquid chromatography, mass spectrography, or DNA analysis (Steinberg, 1993) may also be used to identify abnormal hemoglobins.

Sickle Trait

SA is usually a benign condition that affects up to 8% of American blacks and a higher proportion of the population in malarial endemic areas of Africa (Johnson, 1985). Since the blood film appears normal, diagnosis is dependent on the demonstration of both HgS and hemoglobin A (HgA) by hemoglobin electrophoresis (Vichinsky et al, 1988). The levels of HgS are lower than those of HgA owing to decreased efficiency of HgS protein synthesis, and sickling does not occur under most physiologic conditions (an oxygen tension of <15 mmHg is required for sickling). Red cell life span is normal, and hemoglobin levels of affected individuals are often normal. Renal abnormalities that may occur in patients with SA include increased incidence of hematuria, hyposthenuria, and increased incidence of urinary tract infections during pregnancy (Schlitt & Keitel, 1960).

Other Hemoglobinopathies

Several other hemoglobinopathies seen either as pure traits or in combination with the more common thalassemia and sickle traits have an effect on hematologic status. Myriad abnormal hemoglobins have been described, but the following discussion is limited to diseases of hemoglobin C (HgC) and hemoglobin E (HgE), unstable hemoglobins, and some of the more common mixed hemoglobinopathies.

Hemoglobin C

In HgC, a mutation replaces the glutamic acid in the sixth position from the N terminus of the β chain with lysine. Red cells thereby become more rigid (Fabry et al, 1981), with increased red cell fragmentation and spherocytosis. The red cell life span in HgC homozygotes is reduced to approximately 30 to 35 days (Hirsch et al, 1988), and the cells appear to have lower oxygen affinity than do normal red cells (Murphy, 1976). Characteristic intracellular crystals of HgC are seen in peripheral films, especially in splenectomized patients. Cells containing higher levels of HgF form fewer crystals (Hirsch et al, 1988).

HgC may be inherited as a heterozygous trait or as a homozygote (CC disease). The HgC gene is found in 17–28% of West Africans, especially in northern Ghana, whereas the frequency in American blacks is 2–3% (Schneider, 1954). Clinically, patients present with anemia and splenomegaly. The anemia may worsen following infections, but HgC disease is usually mild and does not require specific therapy. Laboratory findings (Table 6–2) include mild chronic hemolytic anemia, with hemoglobins in the range of 8–12 mg/dl, and reticulocytosis of 3–10%. The peripheral blood film shows increased numbers of target cells, spherocytes, and occasional intracellular crystals (Fig. 6–3). Osmotic fragility may be decreased. Diagnosis requires hemoglobin electrophoresis. HgC migrates to the same position as HgA2 and HgE on cellulose acetate gel (Fig. 6–4*A*) but may be separated from those hemoglobins on citrate agar gel (Fig. 6–4*B*).

Mixed Hemoglobinopathies

Mixed hemoglobinopathies with heterozygous expression of HgC and HgS (SC disease) are seen because of the high incidence of the HgC gene in the black population. SC disease is milder clinically than SS disease, with only anemia and few clinical complications in most patients (Ballas et al, 1982). Some patients have a more severe clinical course, with significant sickling, sickle crises, and increased susceptibility to infections (Tuttle & Koch, 1960). Pregnancies may be complicated by crises with massive fat emboli. In contrast to SS disease, splenomegaly is seen in SC disease. The peripheral blood film shows rare sickle cells, HgC crystals, and many poikilocytes that have dense chromatin or abnormal shapes (Bain, 1993). Target cells are usually prominent, whereas polychromasia is modest. Hemoglobin electrophoresis demonstrates the presence of both HgS and HgC.

Hemoglobin E

HgE results from a mutation of the hemoglobin β chain that substitutes lysine for glutamic acid at position 26 (Chernoff et

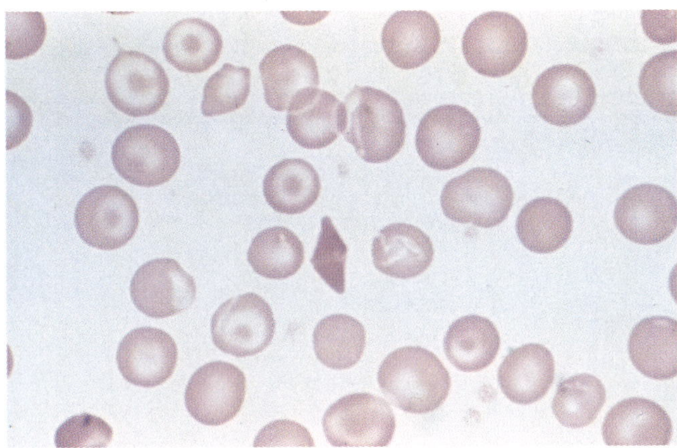

Figure 6–3

Hemoglobin C disease, peripheral blood. This film from a patient shows a crystalline structure with target cells and spherocytes. Wright-Giemsa stain.

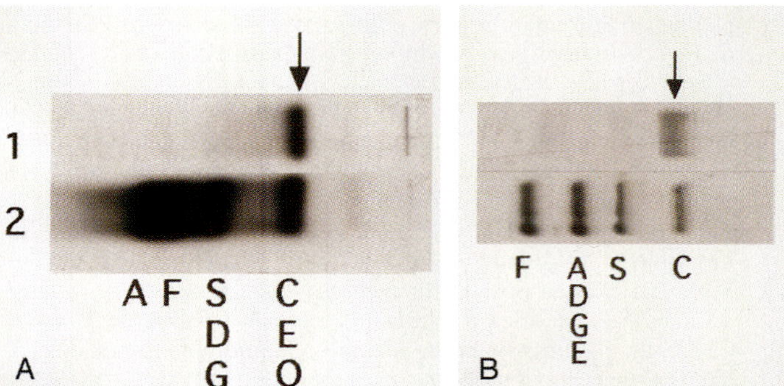

Figure 6–4

Hemoglobin C disease, hemoglobin electrophoretic pattern. *A.* Cellulose acetate gel (pH 8.4). The patient's sample is in lane 1, and control hemoglobins are in lane 2. An arrow indicates the hemoglobin C band. *B.* Citrate agar gel (pH 6.0–6.2). The patient's sample is in lane 1, and control hemoglobins are in lane 2. The arrow indicates the hemoglobin C band in the patient's sample.

al, 1956; Lachant, 1987). This mutation induces hemoglobin instability in the oxidized state and provides a site where alternative splicing of the hemoglobin mRNA may occur (Frischer & Bowman, 1975; Orkin et al, 1982). Relative instability of the hemoglobin molecule gives rise to a thalassemic phenotype. HgE is inherited similarly to the other β-chain mutations, with homozygotes demonstrating the full disease phenotype and heterozygotes the HgE trait. The HgE gene is found principally in Southeast Asia, where the carrier rate may be as high as 30% of the population. Homozygous HgE disease (Table 6–3) is manifested by marked microcytosis, hypochromia, and target cells in the peripheral film without significant anemia (Fig. 6–5), similar to β-thalassemia minor (Fairbanks et al, 1979). Patients often have a hemoglobin level of 10 g/dl or higher, little increase in reticulocytes, and microcytosis (mean corpuscular volume [MCV] 50–66 fl). The red cell life span is normal, and splenomegaly is unusual. Hemoglobin electrophoresis demonstrates a band that comigrates with HgA2 and HgC on cellulose acetate gel (Fig. 6–6*A*) but may be separated on citrate agar gel (Fig. 6–6*B*). There is no apparent adverse effect on red cell life span. The HgE trait is asymptomatic but demonstrates microcytosis of the red cells, with a characteristic MCV value of 74 ± 10.6 fl. Occasionally, target cells are seen in peripheral films. HgE and β-thalassemia heterozygotes have moderate hypochromic, microcytic anemia as well as splenomegaly and a higher morbidity rate than patients with homozygous HgE disease.

Unstable Hemoglobins

Various mutations produce unstable hemoglobins that spontaneously denature and precipitate as insoluble globulins (Williamson, 1993) recognized as Heinz bodies. Heinz bodies impair red cell membrane deformability and increase splenic transit time, leading to premature hemolysis (Jandl et al, 1961). Most unstable hemoglobins are inherited as autosomal dominant traits and affect the α chain of the hemoglobin molecule. Phenotypes within this group of hemoglobin abnormalities range from slight hemolysis to severe hemolysis with associated jaundice, splenomegaly, and anemia. Drugs or other oxidant stresses may precipitate hemolytic episodes (Winterbourn, 1990). Laboratory features also reflect marked clinical heterogeneity, with variable degrees of anemia, hypochromia, poikilocytosis, polychromasia, anisocytosis, and reticulocytosis. Laboratory tests used to demonstrate unstable hemoglobins include the isopropanol stability test (Carrell & Kay, 1972), the heat instability test, and supravital staining with brilliant cresyl blue to demonstrate Heinz bodies (Fig. 6–7). Heinz body numbers are increased in splenectomized patients. Hemoglobin electrophoresis may not reveal any abnormalities. Detection of some abnormal hemoglobins requires demonstration of abnormal oxygen affinities, isoelectric focusing, or DNA sequence analysis. Treatment of these disorders is usually not necessary unless there is severe hemolysis. Patients should avoid oxidative drugs and sulfonamides, which tend to increase the frequency of hemolytic episodes.

Table 6–3
Laboratory Features of Homozygous Hemoglobin E Disease

Peripheral blood	
RBCs	Mild to moderate microcytic, hypochromic anemia (MCV 50–66fl)
	Target cells
	Low reticulocyte count
WBCs	Normal
Platelets	Normal
Other	Hg analysis shows predominant HgE species
	Normal RBC life span
Marrow	Mild erythrocyte hyperplasia
	Normal iron stores
Chemistries	Normal iron study results

Abbreviations: Hg, hemoglobin; MCV, mean corpuscular volume; RBC, red blood cell; WBC, white blood cell.

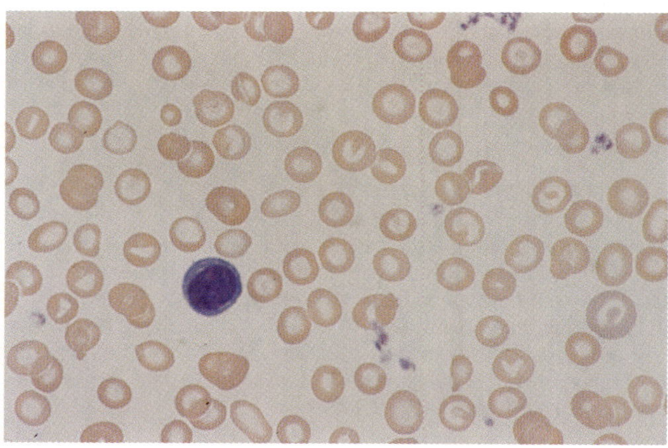

Figure 6–5

HgS disease, peripheral blood. This film from a patient shows microcytosis, hypochromia, and numerous target cells. Wright-Giemsa stain.

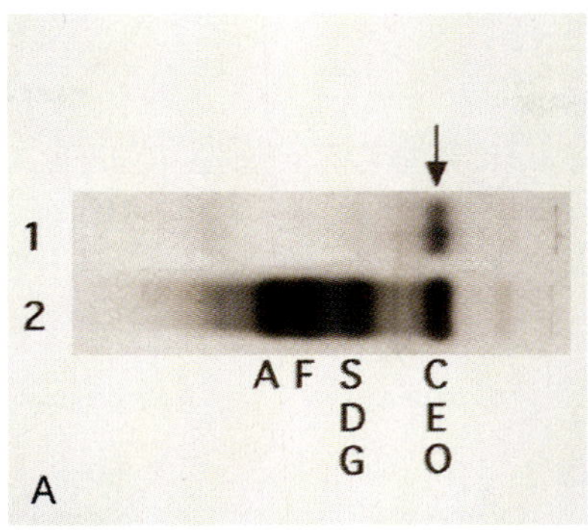

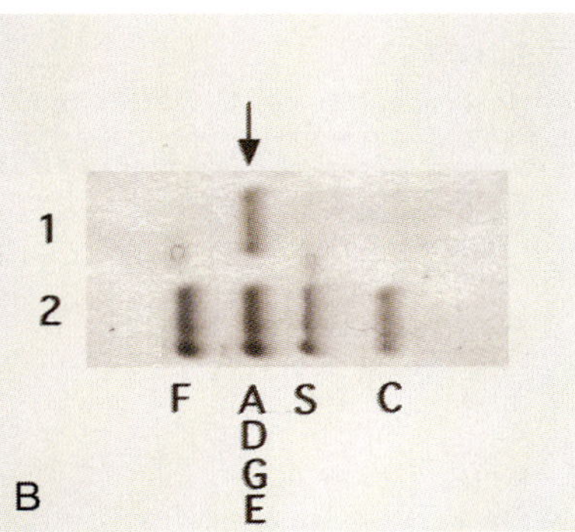

Figure 6–6

Hemoglobin E disease, hemoglobin electrophoretic pattern. *A.* Cellulose acetate gel (pH 8.4). The patient's sample is in lane 1, and control hemoglobins are in lane 2. An arrow indicates the hemoglobin E band. *B.* Citrate agar gel (pH 6.0–6.2). The patient's sample is in lane 1, and control hemoglobins are in lane 2. The arrow indicates the hemoglobin E band in the patient's sample.

OTHER INHERITED ANEMIAS

Spherocytosis and Other Membrane Abnormalities

The life span of circulating red cells is related to membrane properties affecting cell shape and deformability. Alterations in membranes often cause premature hemolysis. The hereditary disorders of spherocytosis, elliptocytosis, stomatocytosis, and xerocytosis involve defects in red cell membranes, with resultant hemolytic anemias.

Red cell membranes are composed of a phospholipid bilayer with intercalated cholesterol and glycolipids as well as protein components. The latter include structural proteins affecting cellular shape and functional proteins that act as cell antigens or receptors and participate in enzymatic reactions and ion and water transport. Structural proteins include spectrin, actin, protein 4.1, protein 4.9, and adducin as the main components, with variable amounts of ankyrin, protein 3, and protein 7 (Goodman et al, 1988; Lux, 1979). Spectrin interacts with actin and ankyrin to form a hexagonal latticework comprising the red cell skeleton (Lui et al, 1978). The characteristic shape and deformability of red cells arise from interaction of the skeleton, other structural membrane components, and lipid bilayers through a network of microfilaments. Red cells must be sufficiently pliant to pass through capillaries and splenic cords without disruption and must have the stamina for the usual life span of 120 days.

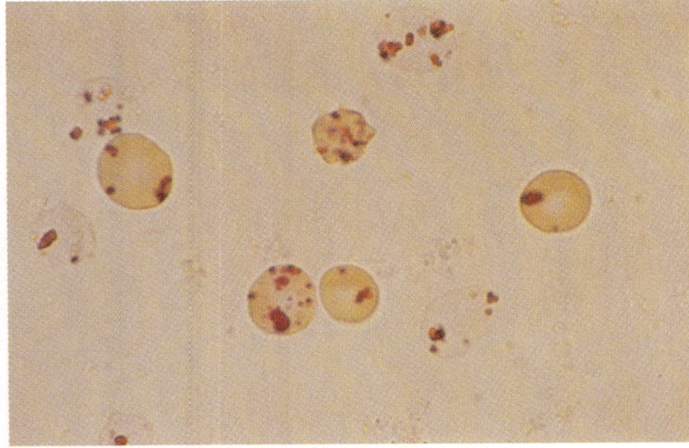

Figure 6–7

Heinz bodies, peripheral blood. Insoluble precipitates of unstable hemoglobin adhere to the red cell membrane as Heinz bodies, shown by supravital staining with brilliant cresyl blue.

Hereditary Spherocytosis

Hereditary spherocytosis (HS) is classic hereditary hemolytic anemia owing to defects in red cell membranes. Patients have mild to severe hemolysis, perhaps reflecting the various biochemical changes involved in membrane instability. Most patients have hemolytic anemia, spherocytes in the peripheral blood film, increased osmotic fragility, and a favorable response to splenectomy. HS is most common in northern Europeans, with an estimated carrier frequency of 1 in 5000 (Morton et al, 1962), a probable underestimation, since there are many asymptomatic or mildly affected individuals. The actual frequency may be closer to the 1% of increased osmotic fragility found in blood donors (Eber et al, 1992; Godal & Heisto, 1981). HS is also described in Japanese and in South African black populations. Molecular analysis has identified several membrane protein defects involving various genetic loci and variable patterns of inheritance (Table 6–4). Most cases of HS are autosomal dominant, although autosomal recessive inheritance and spontaneous mutations exist (Agre et al, 1982; Morton, et al, 1962; Stevens & Evans, 1981). Most patients have partial spectrin deficiency, associated with deficiencies in ankyrin, protein 4.2, or other membrane skeletal proteins. Only about 10% of HS patients have defects in spectrin alone (Agre et al, 1986). One of the most common abnormalities is a combined defect of spectrin and ankyrin, the primary protein linking spectrin to the red cell membrane (Coetzer et al, 1988).

Regardless of the skeletal protein defect implicated, the interactions between cytoskeleton and membrane are weakened in HS. Membranous material is lost through the formation of microvesicles containing membrane material and sometimes skeletal proteins (Hassoun & Palek, 1996). Spherocytes form when cellular surface area decreases from loss of membrane material. Since spherocytes have reduced deformability, their transit times through the spleen are prolonged (Mohandas et al, 1980; Nakashima & Beutler, 1979), leading to further membrane loss, acidosis, and ATP depletion, with premature phagocytosis of the red cell by cordal macrophages (Emerson & Wilkinson, 1966). Splenectomy or partial splenectomy usually reverses the shortened red cell life span observed in HS (Agre et al, 1986; Tchernia et al, 1993).

Clinical Features

Clinically, HS is highly variable, although the classic features are mild to moderate anemia dating from the neonatal period, splenomegaly, jaundice, and a positive family history. Mild jaundice may be the chief clinical feature if anemia is well compensated. Some patients have extremely mild jaundice or are asymptomatic and thereby escape detection until adulthood unless hemolysis is exacerbated by infection. Other patients

Table 6–4
Heterogeneity of Hereditary Spherocytosis

Protein Defect	Hemolysis	Inheritance Pattern	Incidence
Mild to moderate β-spectrin deficiency	Mild to moderate	Autosomal dominant	Common (75% of patients); associated with ankyrin deficiency
Moderate to severe α-spectrin deficiency	Severe	Autosomal recessive	Rare (25% of patients)
Ankyrin deficiency	Mild to moderate	Autosomal dominant	Common; assocated with spectrin deficiency
Protein 4.1 deficiency	Mild	Autosomal dominant	Common in North Africa
Protein 4.2 deficiency	Mild to moderate	Autosomal recessive	Rare in Europeans, commoner in Japanese
Protein 3 deficiency	Mild	Autosomal dominant	Rare (10% of patients)

These are some of the described defects in protein cytoskeletal proteins that give rise to hereditary spherocytosis and its variable clinical and epidemiologic features.

have severe, unremitting hemolysis that requires splenectomy and transfusions. Complications of the disease include crises of various types. Aplastic crises are usually secondary to infection, such as parvovirus infection, megaloblastic crises are due to folate deficiency, and hemolytic crises arise when infections increase the rate of hemolysis. Gallstones and iron overload may occur, as in other hemolytic anemias. Rarely, specific defects are associated with other congenital anomalies. For example, defects in ankyrin give rise to psychomotor retardation and dysmorphism in addition to HS (Chilcote et al, 1987).

Laboratory Features

Variations in laboratory findings in HS (Table 6–5) parallel clinical variability. Hemoglobin levels may be decreased or normal, with a high reticulocyte count, whereas white cell and platelet counts are usually normal. Most older children and adults have relatively normal hemoglobin levels owing to adequate compensation, whereas infants and young children often have more severe anemia (Krueger & Burgert, 1966). Many patients have a lower MCV than expected for the degree of reticulocytosis. Increased MCHC is a sensitive and fairly specific indicator for spherocytosis (Pati et al, 1989). Some patients with hemolysis have increased unconjugated bilirubin and lactate dehydrogenase levels with decreased haptoglobin levels. Blood films show variable numbers of spherocytes, which may be recognized by slightly smaller size, lack of central pallor, and appearance of dense hemoglobinization. Cells artifactually resembling spherocytes may be seen in excessively thin areas of blood films (Fig. 6–8). Polychromasia is often prominent, and circulating nucleated red blood cells may be seen. The marrow often exhibits erythrocyte hyperplasia.

Osmotic fragility testing of red cells is useful in screening for HS (Goda et al, 1979). Spherocytes have a decreased surface-to-volume ratio and are thereby more susceptible to osmotic hemolysis. Aliquots of heparinized blood are placed in solutions of known osmolarity (Table 6–6). After incubation for 1 h at room temperature, the samples are centrifuged, and the amount of hemoglobin released is determined by spectrophotometric absorbance at 540 nm. Fresh blood or blood incubated for 24 h at 37°C (incubated osmotic fragility) may be used. The latter is more sensitive but less specific (Godal & Heisto, 1981; Young et al, 1951). The expected levels of hemolysis are shown in Table 6–6, or results may be presented graphically (Fig. 6–9). The presence of spherocytes is indicated by an increased osmotic lysis. In some patients a population of severely af-

Table 6–5
Laboratory Features of Hereditary Spherocytosis

Peripheral blood	
RBCs	Variable normochromic, normocytic anemia; patients may not be anemic MCV lower than expected for degree of reticulocytosis MCHC increased Reticulocyte count may be increased Spherocytes present
WBCs	Normal
Platelets	Normal
Other	Increased osmotic fragility Abnormal RBC membrane electrophoresis
Marrow	Ranges from normal to hypercellular with erythrocyte hyperplasia
Chemistries	Evidence of hemolysis; increased LDH level, elevated direct bilirubin level

Abbreviations: LDH, lactate dehydrogenase; MCHC, mean corpuscular hemoglobin concentration; MCV, mean corpuscular volume; RBC, red blood cell; WBC, white blood cell.

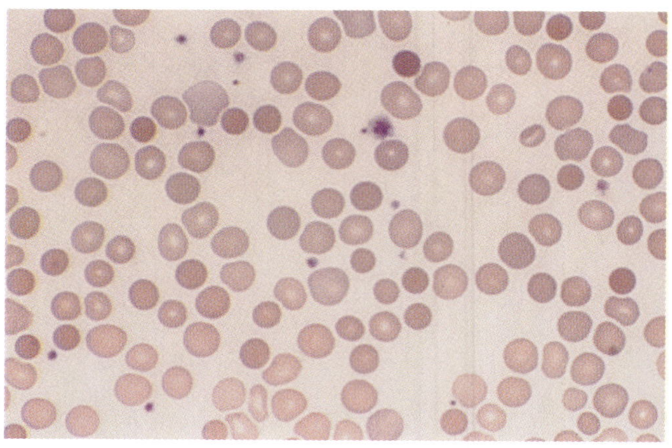

Figure 6–8

Hereditary spherocytosis, peripheral blood. This film shows many spherocytes with small size, dense hemoglobinization, and lack of central pallor. Wright-Giemsa stain.

Table 6–6
Normal Values for Osmotic Fragility Test Results

NaCl(%)	Lysis(%) Fresh	Lysis(%) Incubated
0.20	97–100	95–100
0.30	97–100	85–100
0.35	90–99	75–100
0.40	50–90	65–100
0.45	5–45	55–95
0.50	0–5	40–85
0.55	0	15–70
0.60	0	0–40
0.65	0	0–10
0.70	0	0–5
0.75	0	0

fected, very fragile cells forms a "tail" on the curve, which usually disappears after splenectomy (Young et al, 1951). Increased lysis is also seen in autoimmune hemolytic disease, but conditions that increase the cell surface-to-volume ratio (thalassemia, iron deficiency, and some liver diseases) decrease red cell osmotic fragility. The osmotic fragility test should not be used as a screening test in newborns unless appropriate age-matched control subjects or incubated blood is used (Schroter & Kahsnitz, 1983; Trucco & Brown, 1967).

Hereditary Elliptocytosis

Hereditary elliptocytosis (HE) is another disease resulting from abnormal membrane cytoskeletal proteins and occurs in 250 to 500 per million population in the United States (Wyandt et al, 1941). The defects in HE weaken bonds between proteins and destabilize the cellular skeleton. Cells are thereby unable to return rapidly to a biconcave disk shape after deformation in small vessels and permanently retain an elliptical shape (Palek, 1985; Palek & Lux, 1983). Poikilocytosis, often seen in association with HE, reflects the increased sensitivity of abnormal cells to fragmentation and hemolysis. The several defects described in HE (Table 6–7) fall into four basic categories: (1) defects in spectrin that affect spectrin dimer and tetramer formation, (2) abnormal spectrin and ankyrin association, (3) protein 4.1 defects; and (4) deficiencies in glycophorin C (see Table 6–7) (Palek, 1985; Palek, 1987; Palek & Lux, 1983).

Clinical Features

The clinical manifestations of HE range from none to severe hemolytic anemia. Black patients tend to be affected most often. In mild cases, patients may have a normal red cell life span or well-compensated mild hemolytic anemia, and the defect is discovered incidentally. In such cases, elliptocytes are scattered in the peripheral film. Patients with mild disease are most likely to have spectrin mutations, partial protein 4.1 deficiency, or glycophorin C deficiency. Sporadic increases in hemolysis may occur with infections or nutritional deficiencies. Patients with moderate to severe hemolytic anemia may require splenectomy. These patients have numerous elliptocytes and poikilocytes. Homozygous defects are expected in spectrin or protein 4.1, or combinations of these defects (double heterozygote) may occur. Patients with somewhat round-appearing elliptocytes as well as spherocytes and moderate to severe hemolysis are likely to have protein 4.1 defects inherited in an autosomal dominant fashion (Tchernia et al, 1981).

Laboratory Features

The laboratory work-up of HE begins with examination of the peripheral blood film (Fig. 6–10). Patients with elliptocytosis as the only abnormality have minimal hemolysis, probably reflecting a minor membrane defect. In patients with more severe membrane abnormalities, shear stresses cause red cell fragmentation and poikilocytosis. There is a direct association between the level of poikilocytosis and the degree of hemolysis. Moderate to severe hemolysis and rounder elliptocytes and spherocytes are seen in the spherocytic variant of HE. Osmotic fragility is usually normal unless numerous spherocytes are present. The specific molecular defect may be identified by gel electrophoretic analysis of red cell skeletal proteins or tryptic protein digests to identify abnormal or decreased protein species. In general, the level of hemolysis is inversely related to the amount of spectrin and the percentage of dimeric spectrin, indicative of mutations that affect dimerization (Coetzer et al, 1988; Palek & Lambert, 1990).

The clinical and laboratory manifestations of HE are age related. Elliptocytes are a minor population in affected infants and usually do not reach maximal levels until 3 to 4 months of age. Family histories are useful in suggesting the diagnosis. Elliptocytosis may be acquired in myelofibrosis, myelodysplasia, pyruvate kinase deficiency, thalassemia, congenital dyserythropoiesis syndromes, and iron or folate deficiency. Normal blood films contain <5% elliptocytes (Palek, 1985).

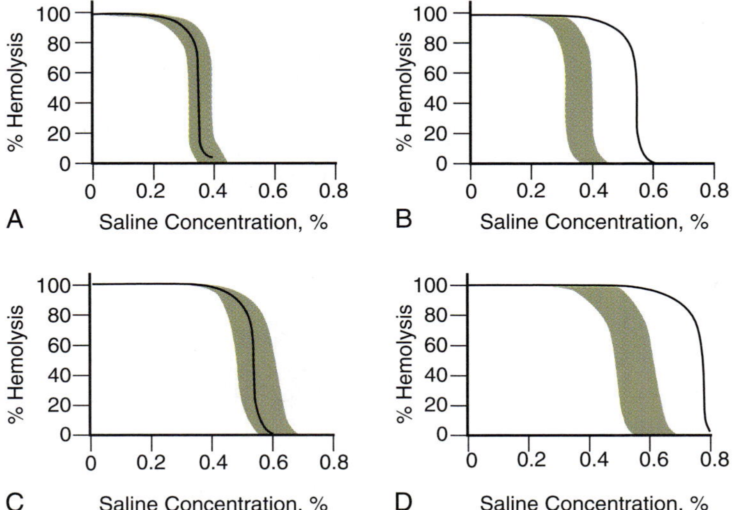

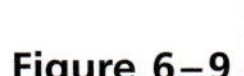

Figure 6–9

Hemolysis curves, osmotic fragility testing. *A.* Control osmotic fragility curves. *B.* Increased osmotic fragility, as evidenced by increased hemolysis in a patient with hereditary spherocytosis. *C.* Control values for osmotic fragility following incubation of the sample for 24 h at 37°C (incubated osmotic fragility test). *D.* Increased osmotic fragility observed in an incubated osmotic fragility test performed on a patient with hereditary spherocytosis.

Table 6–7
Molecular Defects Giving Rise to Hereditary Elliptocytosis

Molecular Defect	Clinical Presentation	Red Cell Morphologic Features	Inheritance
Abnormal spectrin self-association; may have either abnormal α-spectrin or -β spectrin	Commonest type; variable levels of hemolysis from asymptomatic to severe, depending on defect	Elliptocytes; some poikilocytosis or fragmented cells may be seen	Autosomal dominant in most cases; some autosomal recessive defects
Defective spectrin-ankyrin binding	Rare; usually mild hemolysis	Elliptocytes	Autosomal dominant
Protein 4.1 defect	Rare; usually mild hemolysis except severe hemolysis in homozygote	Elliptocytes; may also see rounder elliptocytes with associated spherocytes	Autosomal dominant
Glycophorin C deficiency	Rare; mild or absent hemolysis	Elliptocytes or normal cell shape	Autosomal dominant

Hereditary Pyropoikilocytosis

Hereditary pyropoikilocytosis (HPP) is a rare subtype of HE with severe hemolytic anemia and an autosomal recessive inheritance pattern. Hemoglobin levels are often as low as 4.5–6.5 g/dl. The MCV is decreased due to fragmentation of red cells. The blood film (Fig. 6–11) shows marked poikilocytosis, with many small fragmented cells, elliptocytes, and spherocytes (Palek & Lambert, 1990). The red cells are very sensitive to thermal stress and fragment after heating for 10–15 min at 45°C or after 6 h at lower temperatures. Affected patients usually carry two mutations in spectrin (Coetzer et al, 1990). Blacks tend to have more severe disease than do whites or Arabs.

Stomatocytic HE presents as an asymptomatic trait in 30% of individuals from parts of Papua New Guinea, Southeast Asia, and Indonesia. The elliptocytes have a characteristic spoon shape with a central hemoglobin bar. This variant of HE is due to an abnormality in band 3 protein (Liu et al, 1990) and may convey partial immunity to malarial infection (Hadley et al, 1983; Jones et al, 1990).

Stomatocytes have shapes like a cup or bowl in addition to a centrally placed stoma and are seen in various acquired and uncommon inherited disorders. In the latter, a defect in sodium regulation in the red cell is manifested as a sodium leak, leading to increased sodium concentrations and subsequent overhydration (Mentzer et al, 1975). Sodium permeability may increase by 15 to 40 times normal levels (Zarkowsky et al, 1968). The molecular basis of the disease is not known, and several defects may produce a similar phenotype (Eber et al, 1989; Kanzaki & Yawata, 1992). When inherited as an autosomal dominant trait, stomatocytosis results in moderate to severe hemolytic anemia. There are 10–30% stomatocytes on the peripheral blood film, and osmotic fragility is usually increased. Acquired stomatocytosis is seen in malignancy, cardiovascular disease, hepatobiliary disease, alcoholism, and ingestion of certain drugs (Davidson et al, 1977; Douglass & Twomey, 1970; Neville et al, 1984). Normal blood films may have 3–5% stomatocytes (Douglass & Twomey, 1970).

Hereditary Xerocytosis

Hereditary xerocytosis is a rare disorder inherited as an autosomal dominant trait and characterized by red cell dehydration and decreased red cell osmotic fragility (McGrath et al, 1984; Snyder et al, 1978). Cells have a defect in potassium regulation that causes a net loss of potassium through the cell membrane and a secondary influx of sodium into the cell (Glader et al, 1974; Joiner et al, 1986). Intracellular osmotic pressure is maintained by depletion of intracellular cations and water loss. The molecular basis of the defect is unknown.

Patients have a moderate to severe hemolytic anemia and increased MCHC (Glader et al, 1974). The blood film shows stomatocytes, target cells, and a population of spiculated cells

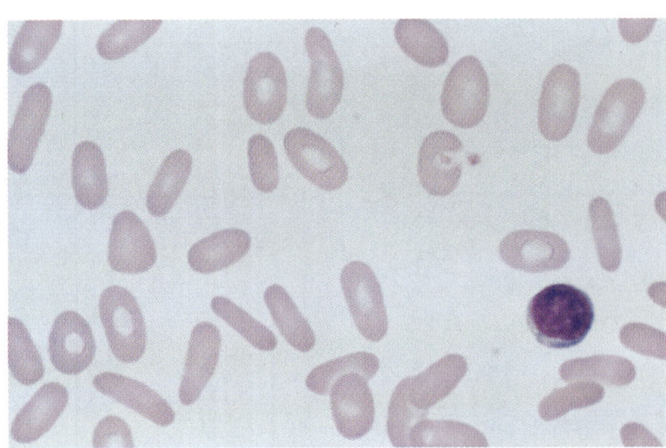

Figure 6–10

Hereditary elliptocytosis, peripheral blood. This film shows numerous elliptocytes in a patient with hereditary elliptocytosis. Wright-Giemsa stain.

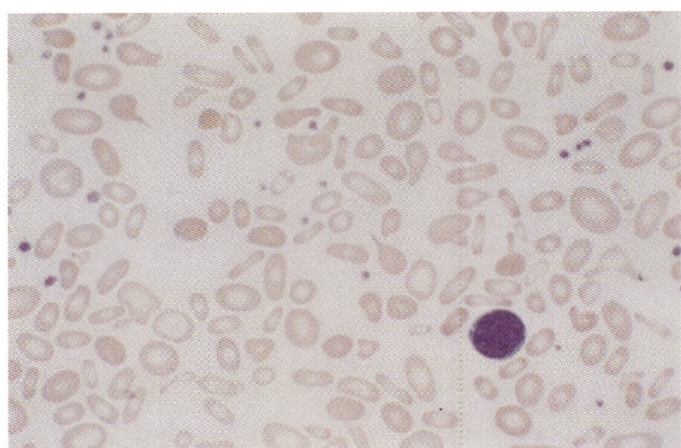

Figure 6–11

Hereditary pyropoikilocytosis, peripheral blood. This film shows marked poikilocytosis with small, fragmented cells, elliptocytes, and spherocytes characteristic of hereditary pyropoikilocytosis. Wright-Giemsa stain.

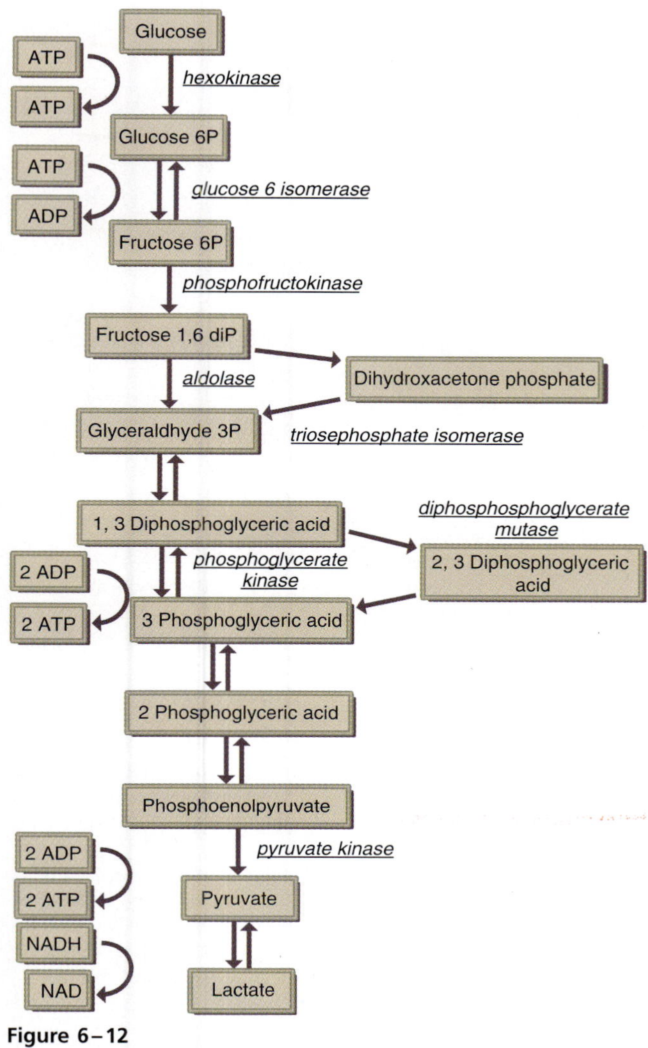

Figure 6–12

The glycolytic pathway. Enzyme deficiencies associated with the development of hemolytic anemia are underlined.

with hemoglobin condensation on the cell periphery. Numerous fragmented cells may be noted, indicating that the cells are sensitive to shear stress (Platt et al, 1981; Snyder et al, 1978). Osmotic fragility is markedly decreased (i.e., cells are resistant to osmotic lysis). Intracellular potassium levels are decreased to 50% of normal values (Glader et al, 1974; Platt et al, 1981).

PYRUVATE KINASE DEFICIENCY AND OTHER RELATED CAUSES OF ANEMIA

The energy requirements of mature red cells are solely dependent on the glycolytic pathway (Fig. 6–12) for production of ATP. Defects or deficiencies in glycolytic pathway enzymes markedly affect red cell metabolism and may produce a congenital nonspherocytic hemolytic anemia (Tanaka & Zerez, 1990; Valentine & Paglia, 1984) (Table 6–8). A defect in glycolysis should be suspected in patients with chronic hemolysis if hemoglobin electrophoresis results and osmotic fragility are normal and there are no significant alterations in red cell morphologic features (Lakomek et al, 1989).

Pyruvate kinase deficiency is the most common glycolytic pathway defect, with approximately 400 known patients, most being of northern European extraction. There is an autosomal recessive inheritance pattern. Pyruvate kinase has three subunits that are produced by two distinct genes. The M, or muscle, type is not found in erythrocytes. An isomer of the L, or liver, form, designated the R form, is found in red cells, and mutations of this isoform give rise to hemolytic disease (Marie et al, 1981).

Hemolysis of pyruvate kinase–deficient red cells principally affects newly formed red cells in the marrow, spleen, and liver (Mentzer et al, 1971). Often splenectomy is followed by a "paradoxical" increase in reticulocyte counts owing to improved survival of newly formed cells. Spleens exhibit large numbers of reticulocytes with prominent erythrophagocytosis and relatively empty sinuses (Bowman & Procopio, 1963).

The peripheral blood film reveals normal red cell morphologic features without spherocytes. In some cases macrocytes and rare, shrunken, spiculated red cells may be seen, particularly in splenectomized patients (Oski et al, 1964). Reticulocyte counts are elevated. White blood cells and platelets are normal in number and morphologic characteristics. Marrow examination usually reveals erythrocytic hyperplasia.

GLUCOSE-6-PHOSPHATE DEHYDROGENASE DEFICIENCY

G6PD is an essential enzyme in the hexose monophoshate shunt (Fig. 6–13), a pathway that is essential for genesis of reduced nicotinamide-adenine dinucleotide phosphate (NADPH). The red cell, by virtue of its role in oxygen transport, is highly susceptible to damage by oxygen radicals and other reactive oxygen species. The reactive oxygen radicals are converted to H_2O_2 by superoxide dismutase, and glutathione reduces H_2O_2 to water. NADPH is required to reoxidize glutathione, thereby ensuring that the pathway remains functional and that oxidative damage to the cell is prevented (Arese & De Flora, 1990; Beutler, 1991). Mutations in G6PD are common, and G6PD deficiency is the commonest red cell enzymatic abnormality. Incidences are 50% in male Kurdish Jews, 11% in West African males, 0.1% in northern Europeans (Heller et al, 1979), 1% in U.S. white populations, and 2.4% in U.S. black populations (Mohrenweiser, 1987).

Since the gene for G6PD is located on the X chromosome, males are either fully deficient or of normal phenotype. Females may exhibit an intermediate expression of the phenotype owing to heterozygous inheritance of one abnormal and

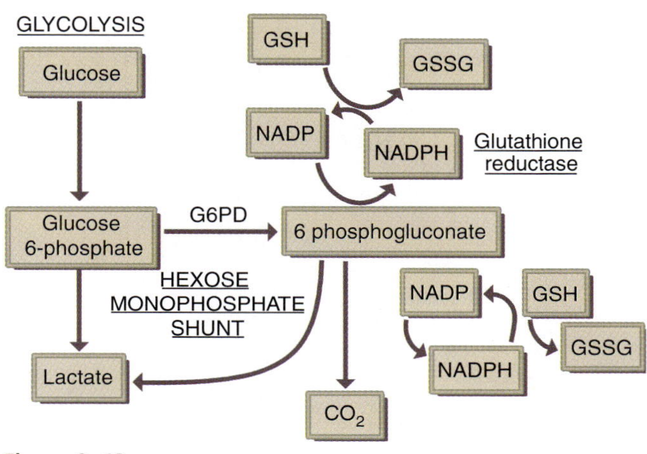

Figure 6–13

G6PD pathway.

Table 6–8
Defects in Glycolysis Associated with Hemolysis

Enzyme	Clinical Presentation	Red Cell Morphologic Features	Inheritance Pattern	Frequency
Hexokinase	CNSHA	Unremarkable	Autosomal recessive	< 100 cases reported
Glucose-6-isomerase	CNSHA	Unremarkable	Autosomal recessive	> 100 casese reported
Phosphofructokinase	CNSHA and/or muscle glycogen storage disorder	Unremarkable	Autosomal recessive	< 100 cases reported
Aldolase	CNSHA and liver glycogen storage abnormality	Unremarkable	Autosomal recessive	< 10 cases reported
Triosephosphate isomerase	CNSHA and severe neuromuscular disease	Unremarkable	Autosomal recessive	< 100 cases reported
Phosphoglycerate kinase	CNSHA, myoglobinuria, behavioral abnormalities	Unremarkable	X-linked	< 100 cases reported
Diphosphoglycerate mutase	CNSHA, polycythemia	Unremarkable	Autosomal recessive	< 100 cases reported
Pyruvate kinase	CNSHA	Usually unremarkable; occasionally echinocytes seen	Autosomal recessive	~ 400 cases reported

Abbrevations: CNSHA, congenital nonspherocytic hemolytic anemia.

Source: Adapted from Beutler E: Glucose-6-phosphate dehydrogenase deficiency and other enzyme abnormalities. In: Beutler E, Lichtman M, Coller BS et al (eds): Williams Hematology, 5th ed. McGraw-Hill, New York, p 565 1995.

one normal gene. Heterozygotes usually have approximately 50% of normal levels of G6PD in their red cells. There may be significant deviation from this level due to X chromosome inactivation, resulting in only one functional X chromosome per cell (Beutler, 1990).

Clinical Features

The clinical expression of G6PD deficiency is varied. Unless they are exposed to oxidative stress from drug ingestion or infection, patients may have no evidence of anemia. Children exposed to an oxidative challenge have, within 6–12 h, an episode of hemolysis associated with mild fever, hemoglobinuria, and jaundice. The numerous agents inducing hemolysis in G6PD-deficient patients are shown in Table 6–9. Other manifestations of G6PD disease include markedly increased neonatal jaundice. Jaundice is usually apparent at 2–3 days after birth and in most cases is more severe than the rather mild anemia. Jaundice may be mild or sufficiently severe to require exchange transfusion. Since not all affected infants develop neonatal jaundice, the inciting factors may involve liver dysfunction as much as a red cell abnormality. A third manifestation of G6PD deficiency is chronic nonspherocytic hemolytic anemia that may be mild or severe. These patients have a baseline hemolytic anemia and are also susceptible to exacerbations of hemolysis following exposure to oxidative stress.

Laboratory Features

Laboratory findings in G6PD deficiency are shown in Table 6–10. Most patients with episodic hemolysis have a normal red cell life span, laboratory values, and blood films between hemolytic episodes, when anemia may become severe. Marked anisopoikilocytosis, shrunken cells with irregular distribution of hemoglobin, and "bite" cells are seen (Fig. 6–14). Numbers of reticulocytes are increased, and the blood film shows polychromatophilia. Supravital staining with methylene blue or crystal violet demonstrates precipitates of denatured hemoglobin or Heinz bodies during a hemolytic episode (see Fig. 6–7). Removal of these deposits by the spleen gives rise to the characteristic "bite" cells seen in the blood film. Heinz bodies disappear as the episode resolves. Hemoglobinuria, suggested by darkness of urine, is an important clinical feature of the disease, since it is seen in a small number of hemolytic episodes (Table 6–11). G6PD deficiency is diagnosed by demonstrating decreased enzymatic activity in red cells. Screening tests (e.g., the fluorescent spot test) are based on the ability of NADPH to fluoresce under ultraviolet light (Beutler & Mitchell, 1968). Heterozygotes or patients with a marked reticulocytosis following a hemolytic episode may have near-normal amounts of enzyme when tested by these assays, and retesting may be needed after reticulocytosis abates. Studies using polymerase

Table 6–9
Causes of Hemolysis in Patients with G6PD Deficiency

Foods
- Fava beans

Antimalarial agents
- Primaquine
- Pamaquine

Sulfonamides
- Sulfanilamide
- Sulfamethoxazole
- Sulfacetamide
- Sulfapyridine

Other antibacterial agents
- Nitrofurantoin
- Nitrofurazone
- Para-aminosalicyclic acid
- Nalidixic acid
- Phenazopyridine

Analgesics
- Acetanilid

Sulfones
- Diaminodiphenyl sulfone
- Thiazosulfone

Miscellaneous agents
- Naphthalene (mothballs)
- Methylene blue
- Trinitrotoluene
- Toludine blue

Table 6–10
Laboratory Features of G6PD Deficiency

Peripheral blood	
RBCs	May be normal unless there is oxidant stress Normochromic, normocytic anemia with oxidant stress Bite cells, cell fragments *without* spherocytes Increased reticulocytes
WBCs	Normal
Platelets	Normal
Other	Increased numbers of Heinz bodies Decreased fluorescent spot test results Decreased G6PD enzymatic activity
Marrow	Varies from normal to hypercellular with erythrocyte hyperplasia
Chemistries	Evidence of hemolysis; increased LDH level, elevated direct bilirubin level Hemoglobinuria

Abbreviations: LDH, lactate dehydrogenase; RBC, red blood cell, WBC, white blood cell.

chain reaction (PCR) may identify the abnormal gene (Beutler et al, 1991) as well as the biochemical abnormality (Beutler, 1992). Prenatal screening using PCR may also be performed in kindreds at risk for inheriting the trait (Beutler et al, 1992).

Clinical criteria are combined with the amount of residual enzymatic activity to classify G6PD deficiency (Table 6–12). The wide spectrum of clinical and laboratory findings in G6PD-deficient patients is probably due to the extensive genetic polymorphism associated with this enzyme. Various mutations alter enzyme synthesis or stability and change enzymatic affinity for substrate and other biochemical parameters (Beutler, 1990). Specific genotypic variants have geographic localization (Table 6–13). The highest incidence of G6PD deficiency occurs in Africa, the Mediterranean, the Middle East, Southeast Asia, India, and Central and South America. As with sickle cell mutations, G6PD deficiency may provide protection against malarial infection, probably by impeding intracellular

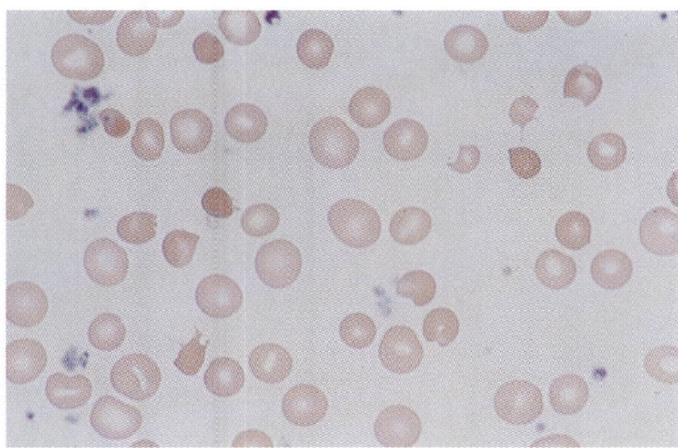

Figure 6–14

G6PD deficiency, peripheral blood. This film shows numerous bite cells with anisocytosis and poikilocytosis in a patient with G6PD deficiency undergoing active hemolysis following an oxidative challenge. Wright-Giemsa stain.

Table 6–11
Diseases Associated with Hemoglobinuria in Children

Disease	Inciting Event
G6PD deficiency	Exposure to oxidative stress
Blackwater fever	Malarial infection
Paroxysmal cold hemoglobinuria	Viral infection
Paroxysmal nocturnal hemoglobinuria	Marrow stem cell abnormality; rare in children
Mismatched blood transfusion	ABO mismatch

development of the parasite (Bienzle et al, 1972). Treatment of the disorder is avoidance of oxidizing agents.

CONGENITAL DYSERYTHROPOIETIC ANEMIAS

Congenital dyserythropoietic anemias (CDAs) are rare inherited anemias characterized by erythrocyte hyperplasia with extensive dyserythropoiesis and ineffective marrow production manifested by inappropriately few reticulocytes. Sufficent numbers of cases have been reported to allow classification into three major subtypes based on the morphologic features of red cells and erythroblasts in addition to other laboratory findings (Table 6–14). The inheritance pattern for type 1 and type 2 CDA is autosomal recessive, whereas type 3 has an autosomal dominant pattern.

CDA should be suspected in infants with mild to severe anemia without appropriate reticulocytosis. It is surprising that many patients are often not identified until later in life. The anemias are macrocytic in most cases, although some cases of CDA type 2 are normocytic. The diagnosis is based on combining analysis of marrow erythroblast morphologic characteristics with results of the acid serum hemolysis (Ham) test and serologic reactions with antibodies against the red cell proteins i and I (anti-i and anti-I).

Type 1 CDA is often not diagnosed until adulthood, since patients may have only a mild to moderate macrocytic anemia (Heimpel et al, 1971; Lewis et al, 1972). Peripheral blood films reveal anisopoikilocytosis, punctate basophilia, occasional Cabot rings, with normal white cells and platelets. There is laboratory evidence of ineffective erythropoiesis, since lactate dehydrogenase and bilirubin levels are elevated despite normal to slightly decreased red cell life span. The serum acid hemolysis test result is negative, and there is only slight reaction with antibodies against i and I (Tamary et al, 1996). The marrow exhibits marked erythrocyte hyperplasia, with 1–2% of erythroblasts manifesting binucleation and nuclear chromatin bridges (Fig. 6–15) (Heimpel et al, 1971). The remaining erythrocyte precursors exhibit megaloblastic maturation and nuclear-cytoplasmic dyssynchrony. Most patients do not require supportive therapy.

Table 6–12
Classification of G6PD Deficiency

Class	Hemolysis	G6PD (% of normal)
I	Severe, chronic	<20
II	Mild, episodic	<10
III	Mild, episodic	10–60
IV	None	100
V	None	>100

Source: Beutler E, Yoshida, A: Genetic variation of glucose-6-phosphate dehydrogenase: a catalog amd future prosects. Medicine 67: 311–334, 1988.

Table 6–13
Common G6PD Variants

Described Variant	Hemolysis	Affected Population
G6PD A	No; normal variant	Blacks
G6PD B	No; normal variant	Blacks, whites, Asians
G6PD A−	Yes; moderate	Blacks
$G6PD^{Med}$	Yes; severe	Whites in Mediterranean basin
$G6PD^{Canton}$	Yes; severe	Asians

Type 2 CDA, or hereditary erythroblastic multinuclearity with a positive acidified serum test (HEMPAS), usually presents with a mild to severe normochromic or macrocytic anemia with hyperbilirubinemia and splenomegaly (Iolascon et al, 1996). Diagnosis may be delayed until the teen years or adulthood. Blood films show anisopoikilocytosis, teardrop cells, and basophilic stippling. Laboratory studies reveal a shortened red cell life span (average 17 days, range 7–31 days) and the characteristic finding of lysis in acidified serum from normal control subjects (Crookston et al, 1972). The sugar water test result is negative, as opposed to results in paroxysmal nocturnal hemoglobinuria. Antibody testing shows strong expression of protein antigens i and I on the red cell membrane (Enquist et al, 1972). Other red cell membrane proteins may also exhibit defective glycosylation (Fukada et al, 1986), and a defect in *N*-aceytlglucosaminoyltransferase II has been proposed (Fukada et al, 1987). This defect in glycosylation may contribute to complement lysis susceptibility, as evidenced by positive acidified serum lysis test results (Tomita & Parker, 1994). Marrow examination reveals erythrocytic hyperplasia, with 10–40% of erythrocyte precursors showing binucleation and multinucleation (Fig. 6–16). Patients with severe anemia may require transfusions, and splenectomy may help by increasing red cell life span.

Type 3 CDA is characterized by a mild macrocytic anemia. Diagnosis may also occur in later life. Red cell life span is slightly decreased. The characteristic finding in this subtype is the presence of multinuclearity in 10–40% of erythroblasts. Some cells have extreme multinuclearity, with up to 12 nuclei (gigantoblasts; Fig. 6–17) (Goudsmit et al, 1972). Transfusions are usually not required. The molecular defect has been mapped to chromosome 15 (Lind et al, 1995). Several other variants of CDA do not fit the foregoing criteria (Boogaerts & Verwilghen, 1982), but the small numbers of cases make their classification difficult.

NUTRITIONAL AND TOXIC ANEMIAS

The nutrients iron, cobalamin (B_{12}), and folate are required for normal red cell proliferation and differentiation. Deficiencies markedly affect red cell production. Futhermore, several compounds, such as lead, are toxic to the marrow and affect erythropoiesis by interfering with normal metabolic pathways.

Iron Deficiency Anemia

Iron is essential for the formation and function of hemoglobin. Since iron is a stable compound in either a reduced or an oxidized form when complexed with protein, the iron in hemoglobin can bind and release oxygen without exposing cells to oxidative damage. Iron balance is tightly regulated, with absorption principally in the upper jejunum. Since iron in an unbound form may be toxic, iron is complexed to the transport protein transferrin for safe passage through the circulation to the tissues. Transferrin binds to a cell surface receptor, releasing iron into the cell, where it may be incorporated into ferritin for storage. Approximately 80% of the iron absorbed daily goes to the marrow for erythropoiesis (Finch & Huebers, 1982). Hemoglobin and marrow storage pools contain about 85% of total body iron (Dallman et al, 1980).

Iron deficiency may arise from inadequate intake, abnormal absorption, or increased losses. Infants or young children

Table 6–14
Congenital Dyserythropoietic Anemias

Characteristic	Type I	Type II (HEMPAS)	Type III
Degree of anemia	Mild to moderate	Mild to severe	Mild
Type of anemia	Macrocytic	Normocytic or macrocytic	Macrocytic
Acidified serum lysis test result	Negative	Positive	Negative
Sugar-water test result	Negative	Negative	Negative
Anti-*i* reactivity	Slight	Strong	Slight
Anti-I reactivity	Slight	Strong	Slight
Marrow features	Megaloblastic maturation; 1–3% binucleated or chromatin bridges in erythrocyte precursors	10–40% binucleated or multinucleated erythrocyte precursors	10–40% multinucleated erythrocyte precursors, including extreme multinucleation
Inheritance	Autosomal recessive	Autosomal recessive	Autosomal dominant

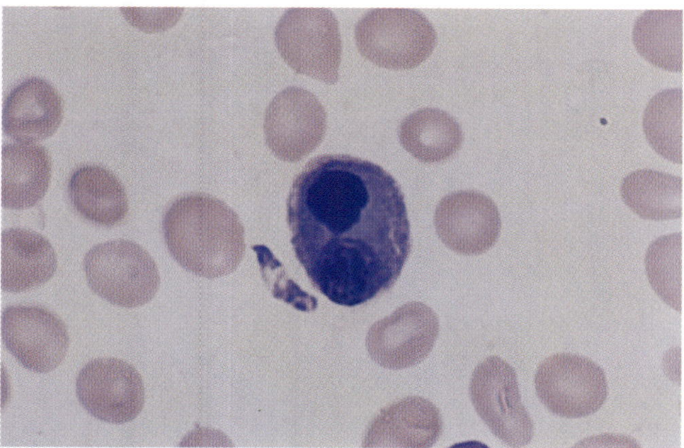

Figure 6–15

Congenital dyserythropoietic anemia, type I, marrow aspirate. Intranuclear bridging in normoblasts is demonstrated. Wright-Giemsa stain.

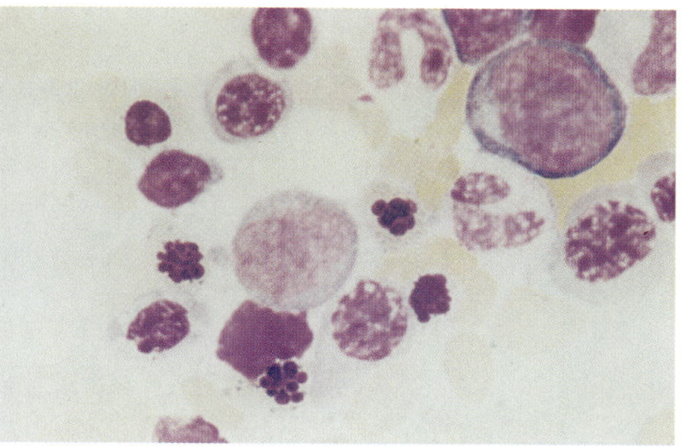

Figure 6–17

Congenital dyserythropoietic anemia, type III, marrow aspirate. Pronormoblasts are illustrated that have extreme multinuclearity (gigantoblasts). Wright-Giemsa stain.

in their rapid growth phase commonly have inadequate intake, and thus iron deficiency is the commonest cause of anemia in children. Certain periods of growth and development are associated with increased risk of iron depletion. At birth, the infant usually has adequate iron stores, but gradual depletion follows birth, particularly if dietary iron intake is low. At about 4 months of age, iron deficiency is common because of the concurrence of increasing iron requirements owing to rapid growth and feeding with cow's milk or non–iron fortified formula (Dallman et al, 1984; McMillan et al, 1977). Some children also have milk intolerance, which may exacerbate iron loss by increasing occult fecal blood losses (Fomon et al, 1981). Iron deficiency affects almost 10% of children between 6 months and 2.5 years of age, although full-blown anemia is much rarer (Yip et al, 1987). Premature infants are at greater risk owing to faster growth rates (Lundstrom et al, 1977). Preschool and school-aged children acquire sufficient iron from dietary sources, but adolescence is another high-risk time for iron deficiency (Dallman et al, 1984).

Anemias owing to iron deficiency are characterized by inadequate hemoglobin synthesis, which inexorably follows depletion of marrow iron stores. If this deficiency persists, the subsequent anemia is distinguished by red cells that are hypochromic and microcytic (Fig. 6–18). Anemias with decreased MCV and MCHC as well as increased red cell distribution width are most likely due to iron deficiency rather than to other causes of microcytosis, such as hemoglobinopathy, infection, or chronic disease (Abshire, 1996; Bessman et al, 1983; Beutler, 1988; Jansson et al, 1986; Lee, 1983). The aforementioned blood parameters, combined with the results of iron studies, differentiate cases of iron deficiency from other microcytic anemias (Table 6–15).

Laboratory Features

Laboratory testing for iron deficiency analyzes marrow iron stores, plasma iron levels, and red cell iron content. Infections and inflammation, in addition to other conditions, interfere with normal iron metabolism and affect iron study results (Table 6–16), discussed later. Iron stores are measured directly by marrow iron stains and indirectly by serum ferritin determinations, which are roughly proportional to storage iron levels (Siimes et al, 1974). Infections and liver disease are often associated with elevated ferritin levels, which may obscure

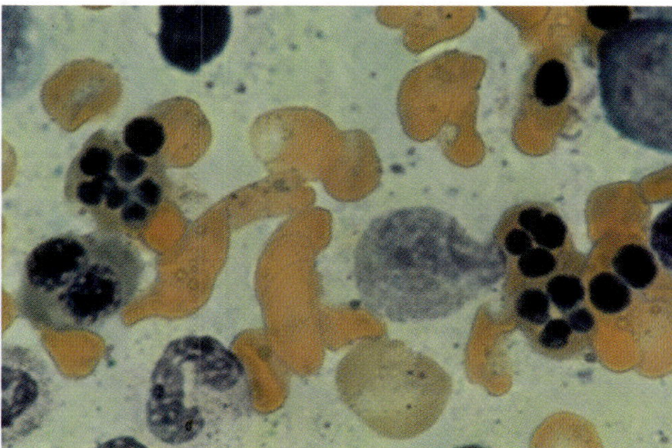

Figure 6–16

Congenital dyserythropoietic anemia, type II, marrow aspirate. There are marked dyserythropoiesis, megaloblastic maturation, and multinuclearity. Wright-Giemsa stain.

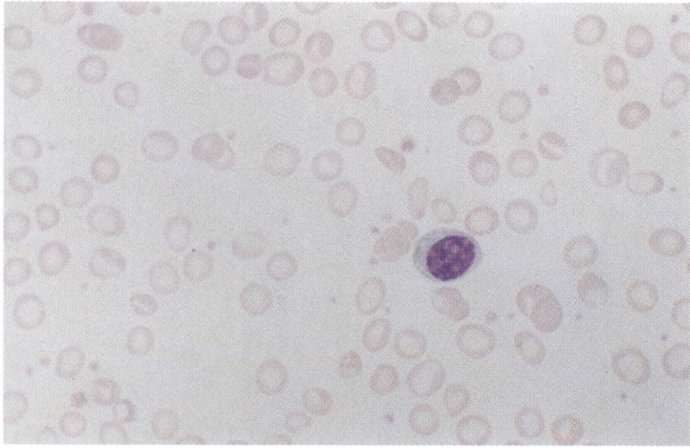

Figure 6–18

Iron deficiency, peripheral blood. This film shows hypochromic, microcytic red cells. Wright-Giemsa stain.

Table 6–15
CBC and Iron Study Parameters Useful in Distinguishing Microcytic, Hypochromic Anemias

Anemia	MCV	RDW	Serum Iron	TIBC	% Solution	Erythrocyte Protoporphyrin	Marrow Storage Iron
Iron deficiency	Decreased	Increased	Decreased	Increased	Decreased	Increased	Decreased
Thalassemia	Decreased	Normal	Increased or normal	Decreased or normal	Increased or normal	Normal	Increased or normal
Sideroblastic anemia	Decreased or normal	Increased	Increased	Decreased or normal	Increased	Increased	Increased
Chronic disease	Decreased or normal	Normal or increased	Decreased	Decreased	Decreased	Increased	Increased
Inflammation	Decreased or normal	Normal or increased	Decreased or normal	Increased	Decreased	Normal	Increased or normal

Abbreviations: RDW, red cell distribution width; TIBC, total iron-binding capacity.

decreased iron stores (Lipschitz et al, 1974; Reeves et al, 1984). Plasma iron levels are measured by total iron-binding capacity (TIBC) and serum iron levels, the latter subject to wide diurnal variations (Dallman, 1984). Samples collected in the morning or early afternoon showing values of <30 μg/dl or <5.4 μmol/l are most indicative of iron deficiency. TIBC increases with iron deficiency. Transferrin saturation (calculated as the ratio between serum iron level and TIBC $\times$ 100) is often more reliable than individual measurements of serum iron or TIBC. A transferrin saturation of $<12\%$ in infants and preschoolers, $<14\%$ in school-aged children, or $<16\%$ in preadolescents and adolescents is highly suggestive of iron deficiency. Transferrin saturation may be decreased in inflammatory disease (Jansson et al, 1986). Red cell iron levels are reflected by erythrocyte protoporphyrin levels, which increase when iron levels are too low for heme formation (Thomas et al, 1977). This measurement assesses iron levels even in the face of recent iron therapy. Erythrocyte protoporphyrin levels are also elevated in lead poisoning, often to a marked degree.

Cases of full-blown anemia (hemoglobin <10 g/dl) with decreased MCV or MCHC, decreased serum ferritin levels, decreased transferrin saturation, or increased transferrin receptor levels are confidently identified as iron deficiency anemia. Iron supplementation should result in reticulocytosis within 1–2 weeks and a gradually increasing hemoglobin level and hematocrit within 2–4 weeks. Such a response to iron therapy confirms the diagnosis, and testing by marrow examination is not required. Milder cases of iron deficiency anemia, with slight decreases in hemoglobin level and hematocrit, may be more difficult to identify but also respond promptly to iron supplementation.

Sideroblastic Anemia

Sideroblastic anemias are a heterogeneous group of hereditary or acquired disorders (Table 6–17) characterized by a dimorphic blood film with varying numbers of microcytic, hypochromic cells and normocytic, normochromic cells (Fig. 6–19). The anemia is hypoproliferative, with low reticulocyte counts a reflection of ineffective erythropoiesis. Ringed sideroblasts are present in the marrow (Bottomley et al, 1992). Disrupted iron metabolism and heme synthesis are reflected by elevated erythrocyte protoporphyrin levels and increased marrow iron stores in some patients (Romslo et al, 1982). Hemolysis may exacerbate the anemia, and some children acquire a form of hemoglobin H disease (Higgs et al, 1983).

Sideroblastic anemias in children are usually congenital. Hereditary sideroblastic anemias affect males more often than females, suggesting an X-linked mode of inheritance. Some patients have a pattern suggestive of autosomal recessive inheritance (Nusbaum, 1991). Many children show defects in heme biosynthesis owing to impairment of δ-aminolevulinic acid synthetase production, the rate-limiting initial reaction in heme biosynthesis (Bottomley et al, 1992; Cotter et al, 1992). Children with the rare Wolfram syndrome (diabetes insipidus,

Table 6–16
Conditions That May Alter Iron Study Results

Test	Elevated Results	Decreased Results
Serum iron	Sample taken late in day (diurnal variation) Recent iron intake	Infections
Serum ferritin	Infection Inflammation Liver disease	Hypothyroidism
Transferrin		Infection Inflammation
Erythrocyte protoporphyrin	Lead poisoning Infection Inflammation Protoporphyria	

Table 6–17
Sideroblastic Anemias

Hereditary
- X-linked
- Autosomal recessive

Acquired
- Idiopathic: myelodysplasia
- Disease associated
  - Inflammatory disease
  - Neoplasms
- Toxic
  - Alcohol
  - Lead
  - Drugs: isoniazid, chloramphenicol
  - Zinc

diabetes mellitus, optic atrophy, and deafness) develop sideroblastic anemias with megaloblastic features from defects in thiamine phosphokinase activity (Borgna-Pignatti et al, 1989). Patients with hereditary sideroblastic anemias may present within a few months of birth or later in life (Cotter et al, 1995). The anemia is usually progressive and requires transfusion therapy.

Sideroblastic anemias may be acquired after exposure to drugs and toxins as well as in association with neoplasms or chronic inflammatory disease. Lead, zinc, alcohol, isoniazid, other antitubercular drugs, and chloramphenicol are the agents usually implicated. Sideroblastic anemias are also caused by alkylating agents in chemotherapuetic regimens. Many drugs inhibit heme biosynthetic enzymes to produce the sideroblastic phenotype. Lead poisoning is covered in detail later (see "Lead- and Toxin-Associated Anemias"). Children may also develop an idiopathic acquired sideroblastic anemia, more commonly seen in adults. Classified in the spectrum of myelodysplastic syndromes, it is discussed in Chap. 7.

Patients with sideroblastic anemia usually present with a microcytic, hypochromic or normocytic, normochromic anemia with a reticulocyte count of 1–2%. Patients may also have leukopenia and thrombocytopenia, and poor platelet and white cell function may be observed, suggesting a stem cell defect (Soslau & Brodsky, 1989). These patients present with infection or bleeding.

Laboratory Features

Laboratory studies usually reveal elevated serum iron and transferrin levels, with elevated lactate dehydrogenase and bilirubin levels with hemolysis. The peripheral film usually reveals hypochromia and microcytosis as well as normochromic, normocytic cells (see Fig. 6–19). In some patients one pattern may predominate. Sideroblastic anemia is diagnosed by demonstrating ringed sideroblasts in the marrow (Fig. 6–20). Iron stains reveal increased macrophage iron levels as well as granules of iron scattered around normoblast nuclei. Electron microscopy studies reveal iron deposits in mitochondria (Goodman & Hall, 1967). In the hereditary form, ringed iron is found in late normoblasts, whereas, in acquired forms, early normoblasts are involved (Buchanan et al, 1980). The marrow often demonstrates erythrocyte hyperplasia, with megaloblastic maturation of erythrocyte precursors or frank dyserythropoiesis. Abnormalities in white cells and megakaryocytes may also be seen. Cytogenetic analysis may reveal chromosomal abnormalities, particularly in idiopathic acquired sideroblastic anemias, including abnormalities of long arms of chromosomes 5 or 7, hypodiploidy, and random loss or breaks of chromosomes (Clark et al, 1986).

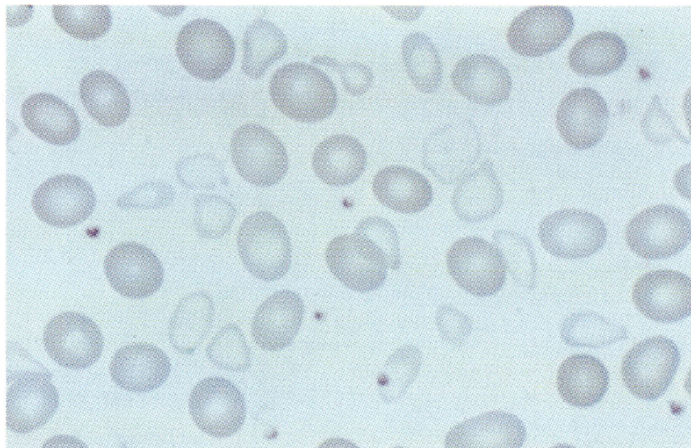

Figure 6–19

Hereditary sideroblastic anemia, peripheral blood. A dimorphic red cell population is demonstrated with hypochromic as well as macrocytic cells. Wright-Giemsa stain.

Treatment of sideroblastic anemia is to some extent dependent on the cause of the disease. Most patients respond at least partially to a trial of vitamin therapy with either oral pyridoxine or pyridoxal-5′-phosphate therapy (Hines, 1976; Mason & Emerson, 1973). Some children with sideroblastic anemia progress to development of acute leukemia. Dependence on transfusion means that iron overload becomes a difficult problem in children. Bone marrow transplantation may provide a therapeutic option (Urban et al, 1992).

Megaloblastic Anemias

Megaloblastic anemias are usually due to deficiencies in either folate or cobalamin (vitamin B_{12}), although rare cases are hereditary or related to drug intake (Table 6–18). All megaloblastic anemias are characterized by ineffective erythropoiesis (Finch et al, 1956) owing to defects in DNA replication. Erythrocyte precursors contain less DNA, more RNA, and more cytoplasm per cell than normal. Since chromatin

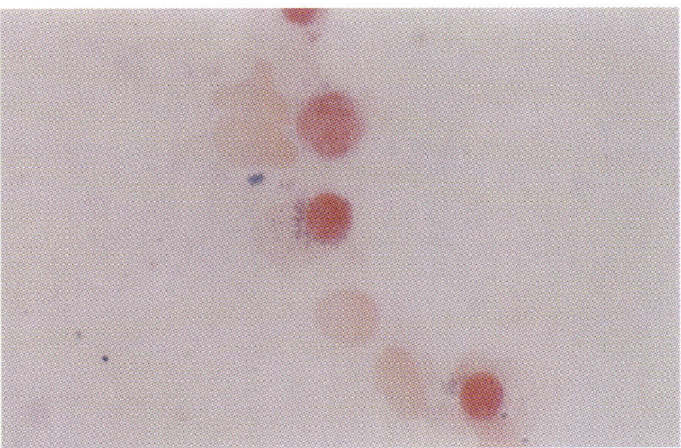

Figure 6–20

Hereditary sideroblastic anemia, marrow aspirate. This iron stain demonstrates iron ringing the nucleus of a sideroblast. Perls stain.

Table 6–18
Factors Associated with Megaloblastic Anemia

Folate Deficiency
- Decreased intake
  - Poor diet
  - Premature infants
  - Goat's milk
  - Hemodialysis
  - Hyperalimentation
- Impaired absorption
  - Small intestinal disease: tropical and nontropical sprue
- Increased requirements
  - Rapid cell turnover: hemolytic anemia, exfoliative dermatitis
  - Pregnancy

Cobalamin (B_{12}) Deficiency
- Decreased intake: vegetarianism
- Impaired absorption
  - Gastric causes: pernicious anemia, gastrectomy
  - Intestinal causes: diseases of the ileum, fish tapeworm, blind loop syndrome
  - Pancreatic insufficiency

Drugs
- Nitrous oxide
- Chemotherapeutic agents: antimetabolites, dihydrofolate reductase inhibitors
- Oral contraceptives
- Anticonvulsants

Hereditary (Rare)
- Enzymatic deficiencies
- Deficiencies in binding proteins

condenses more slowly than normal, large cells with nuclear features more "immature" than cytoplasm are produced (Glazer et al, 1954), a phenomenon termed nuclear-cytoplasmic dyssynchrony (Wickremasinghe & Hoffbrand, 1980). DNA is also more fragile and subject to chromosomal breaks (Das et al, 1986).

Folate is a cofactor for many enzymes involved in DNA synthesis. One of the most important enzymes is dihydrofolate reductase, the target of many chemotherapeutic drugs. Since folate is widely found in foods, the minimum daily requirements of 3.6 μg/kg/day for infants and 3.3 μg/kg/day for children are usually met without exogenous supplementation (Chung et al, 1961). However, cow's and goat's milk contains little folate, and infants receiving these milks are at risk for dietary deficiency (Collins et al, 1951), particularly since infants and young children have higher requirements. Folate is absorbed in the small intestine, and diseases such as sprue and regional enteritis may affect gut absorption. Patients with hemolytic anemias of all types have increased folate requirements due to rapid cell turnover. Oral contraceptives and antiepileptics interfere with folate metabolism. A number of drugs are direct inhibitors of folate, including methotrexate (used in treatment of cancers and autoimmune diseases), pyrimethamine (used to treat malaria), purine analogues (used to treat HIV infection and malignancy), and trimethoprim-based antibiotics.

Vitamin B_{12} is a cofactor for enzymes involved in methionine synthesis and conversion of methylmalonyl CoA to succinyl CoA, reactions that consume and remove potentially harmful homocysteine and methylmalonate as well as maintain methionine levels. B_{12} is found in meat and animal products, and strict vegetarians are at risk for deficiencies. The B_{12} requirement is 0.1 μg/day for infants and 1.0 μg/day for adults (Chung et al, 1961). Because B_{12} occurs at low levels in foods, its absorption by the gut requires multiple steps. B_{12} is released from food in the stomach, and it binds to haptocorrin from the saliva. Haptocorrin is digested by stomach enzymes as the complex enters the intestine, allowing B_{12} binding to intrinsic factor. The intrinsic factor–B_{12} complex binds to ileal cells for uptake.

B_{12} deficiency arises from any defects in the uptake pathway, including rare hereditary defects of intrinsic factor production or function (Qureshi et al, 1994). Megaloblastic anemia in infancy is most often due to an inherited failure of the ileum to absorb the intrinsic factor–cobalamin complex (Imerslund-Grasbeck disease) but is also due to congenital intrinsic factor deficiency (Katz et al, 1972). Immunologic destruction of the gastric parietal cells and associated gastric atrophy (pernicious anemia) are uncommon in children (McIntyre et al, 1965). Transport in the blood is by binding to transcobalamin, and

Table 6–19
Laboratory Features of Megaloblastic Anemia

Peripheral blood	
RBCs	Macrocytic anemia (MCV > 100fl^3) with normal MCHC Oval macrocytes and anisocytosis, schistocytes Basophilic stippling and nucleated RBCs may be seen Reticulocytopenia
WBCs	Hypersegmented neutrophils (>5 lobes/cell); may have neutropenia
Platelets	Usually normal; may be decreased
Other	Decreased RBC life span
Marrow	Hypercellular marrow with erythrocyte hyperplasia Megaloblastic erythrocyte maturation Ineffective erythropoiesis, dyspoiesis Megaloblastic myelocyte maturation with giant bands and metamyelocytes Increased iron stores
Cytogenetics	Normal karyotype
Chemistries	Decreased folate or B_{12} level Increased serum muramidase level Evidence of hemolysis; increased LDH level, elevated direct bilirubin level

Abbreviations: LDH, lactate dehydrogenase; MCHC, mean corpuscular hemoglobin concentration; MCV, mean corpuscular volume; RBC, red blood cells; WBC, white blood cells.

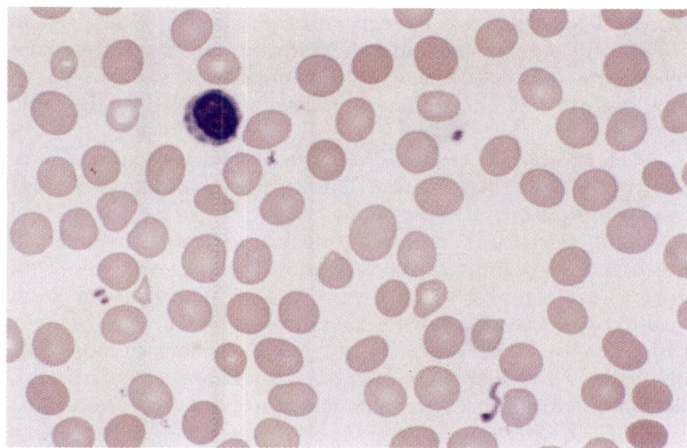

Figure 6–21

Folate deficiency, peripheral blood. This film demonstrates macrocytosis with numerous macroovalocytes in a patient with macrocytic anemia. Wright-Giemsa stain.

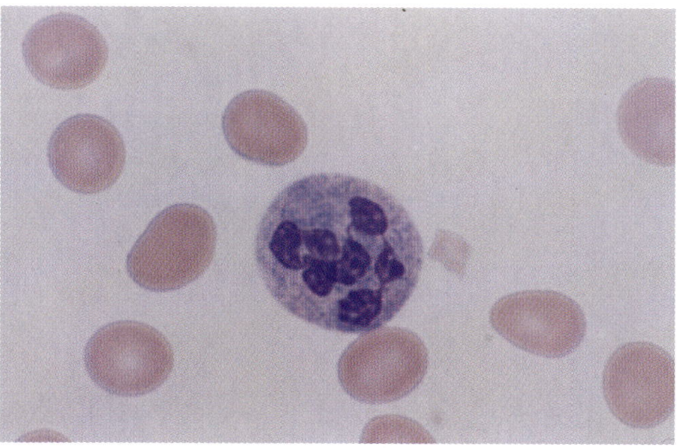

Figure 6–22

Folate deficiency, peripheral blood. A hypersegmented neutrophil is demonstrated in a patient with macrocytic anemia. Wright-Giemsa stain.

hereditary deficiency may cause megaloblastic anemia in children (Monagle & Tauro, 1995). Several disease states that affect either small intestinal absorption sites or the synthesis or binding to transport proteins may give rise to deficiency states. Fish tapeworms may induce a deficiency by causing premature release of B_{12} from intrinsic factor and competition for the factor by the parasite (Nyberg, 1963). Nutritional competition due to bacterial overgrowth in blind intestinal loops may be seen. B_{12} deficiency causes megaloblastic anemia and neurologic disease, the manifestations of which include decreased vibration sense and paresthesias, as well as dementia and depression. Patients with severe cases may develop the rare complication of subacute combined degeneration of the spinal cord.

Laboratory Features

The laboratory findings in megaloblastic anemia from either folate or B_{12} deficiency (Table 6–19) include a macrocytic anemia with marked anisopoikilocytosis. Red cells are enlarged (MCV 100–150 fl) and may have an oval appearance with little central pallor (Fig. 6–21). Reticulocyte counts are low, and nucleated red cells may be seen in peripheral films. Neutrophil nuclei often exhibit hypersegmentation (Fig. 6–22), with many cells having more than five nuclear segments per cell. Normally, $<5\%$ of neutrophils are hypersegmented (Lindenbaum & Nath, 1980). Platelets are often slightly smaller that normal (Bessman et al, 1982). The marrow exhibits marked erythrocytic hyperplasia with megaloblastic maturation and nuclear-cytoplasmic asynchrony (Fig. 6–23). The numbers of pronormoblasts may be so increased as to mimic an acute leukemia. Bilirubin, iron, and ferritin levels are usually increased, and serum lactate dehydrogenase levels are very high, particularly in patients with severe anemia (Emerson & Wilkinson, 1966). Serum erythropoietin levels are also increased (de Klerk et al, 1981). Direct measurements of serum folate levels are highly susceptible to alterations in intake, but the red cell folate level is useful in diagnosis, since it remains fairly stable during the life span of the cell (Hoffbrand et al, 1966). Some patients with B_{12} deficiency have serum levels that are normal or only slightly reduced. Methylmalonuria is seen in significant B_{12} deficiency (Kahn et al, 1965), with elevated serum methylmalonic acid and homocysteine levels (Allen et al, 1990; Lindenbaum et al, 1990). Detection of intrinsic factor deficiency by the Schilling test may provide information about the mechanisms of B_{12} deficiency (Fairbanks et al, 1983).

Megaloblastic anemias are readily treated by replacement therapy of folate (1–5 mg/day) or parenteral B_{12}. Vegetarian or severely malnourished patients and some patients with pernicious anemia are given high-dose oral therapy (Lederle, 1991). Replacement usually achieves a rapid response, with decreases in bilirubin, lactate dehydrogenase, and serum iron levels. Reticulocyte counts rise in 3–5 days, with maximal reticulocytosis at 4–10 days after therapy. Megaloblastic changes in the marrow resolve within 2–3 days. Replacement or transfusion prior to marrow examination may mask megaloblastic changes. The anemia should be corrected within 1–2 months. Hyperlobated neutrophils may persist in the peripheral blood film for up to 2 weeks. Another or coexisting cause for the anemia should be investigated if hematologic parameters are not normalized within 2 months.

Lead- and Toxin-Associated Anemias

Red cells are subject to several environmental hazards. The most significant in children is lead. Lead has a high affinity for

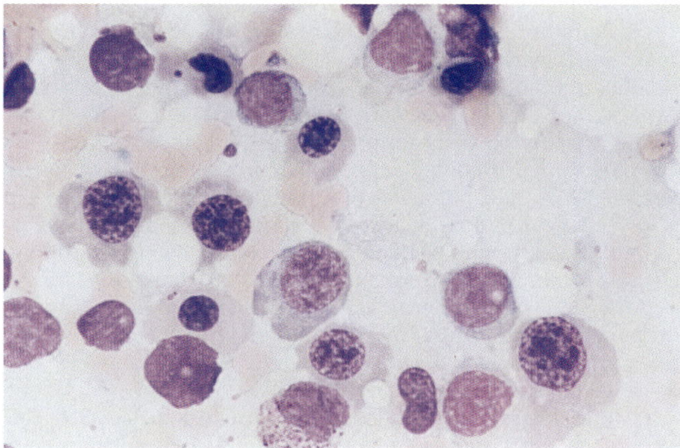

Figure 6–23

Folate deficiency, marrow aspirate. There is marked megaloblastic maturation of red cell precursors. Dispersed nuclear chromatin and early cytoplasmic hemoglobinization are features characteristic of nuclear-cytoplasmic dyssynchrony. Wright-Giemsa stain.

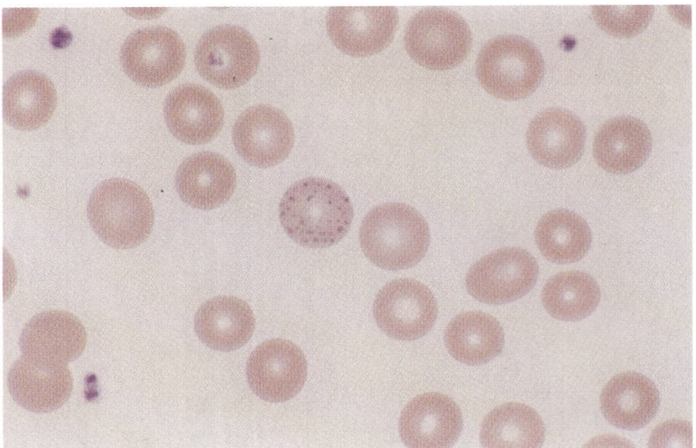

Figure 6–24

Lead poisoning, peripheral blood. This film shows coarse basophilic stippling in red cells, characteristic of lead poisoning. Wright-Giemsa stain.

sulfhydryl groups and affects many cellular enzymatic functions, especially heme synthesis. Children may be exposed to lead from ingestion of paint, inhalation of vapors from gasoline products and smelters, inhalation of contaminated dusts in older houses, and ingestion of canned or contaminated foods. Paint in older homes is the most concentrated source of lead. Exposure may be through direct ingestion by younger children or breathing contaminated dusts. Lead levels in children have fallen since the proscription against leaded gasoline (Annest et al, 1983), but city children remain at great risk from urban pollution and residence in older homes. By promoting lead uptake by the intestine and red cells, iron deficiency, increases the risk of lead poisoning (Kaplan et al, 1975; Six & Goyer, 1972).

Lead accumulates in mitochondria and inhibits their production of reduced nicotinamide-adenine dinucleotide (NADH) (Goyer & Moore, 1974) as well as markedly impairing synthesis of hemoglobin at several points. Specifically, lead inhibits δ-amino-levulinic acid (ALA) synthetase (Nakao et al, 1968) in a dose-dependent manner (Hernberg & Nikkanen, 1970); ferrochelatase, which inserts iron into the porphyrin ring (Gibson & Goldberg, 1970); iron uptake by mitochrondria (Lamola et al, 1975); and pyrimidine-5′-nucleotidase (Paglia et al, 1975).

Laboratory findings in children with lead poisoning include microcytic, hypochromic anemia with prominent basophilic stippling of red cells (Fig. 6–24). Anemia is a late manifestation in children and often follows neurologic abnormalities, such as behavioral changes, cognitive deficits, or encephalopathy. Basophilic stippling represents remnants of ribosomal DNA and mitochondrial fragments that persist owing to inhibition of pyrimidine-5′-nucleotidase (Paglia et al, 1975). Osmotic fragility may be increased, probably owing to poisoning of membrane transport function (Waldron, 1964). Free erythrocyte protoporphyrin levels are increased and may be used as a screening test for lead poisoning (Kaul et al, 1983). Lead levels may be measured directly. Treatment is to decrease lead exposure and remove lead by chelation.

Many compounds (Table 6–20) with toxic effects on the marrow are used in industry and agriculture. Plants, drugs, and other substances may produce toxicity by acting in an idiosyncratic manner. Toxic effects include marrow necrosis, cellular dysplasia, macrophage hyperplasia, and marrow aplasia (Rebar, 1993). Patients often present with one or more cytopenias. Occasionally, peripheral blood findings are normal, with evidence of toxic damage only in marrow samples (Cullen et al, 1983). The outcome of toxic injury to the marrow varies from permanent marrow damage, culminating in aplastic anemia, to total recovery of hematopoiesis following removal of the toxic agent.

Infections may also cause marrow suppression or injury and produce anemia. The best-known infectious cause of marrow suppression is parvovirus infection (see "Red Cell Aplasia"). Parvovirus causes a transient decrease in red cell precursors, cessation of erythropoiesis, and development of anemia (Young, 1988), with few or no symptoms in most healthy patients. However, parvovirus infections in patients with increased red cell turnover, which occurs in hemoglobinopathies and hemolytic anemias, may cause an aplastic crisis. Immunosuppressed patients may also have a severe anemia owing to the inability to clear the virus and chronic infection (Kurtzman et al, 1989). Hepatitis (Hagler et al, 1975), Epstein-Barr virus (Lazarus & Baehner, 1981), and HIV infections (Grau et al, 1989) may also cause marrow supression and toxicity, with effects ranging from mild, transient cytopenia to severe aplastic anemia.

OTHER HEMOLYTIC ANEMIAS

Disorders causing hemolysis by immune mechanisms or peripheral destruction are summarized in Table 6–21. Antibodies producing autoimmune hemolytic anemia usually arise in children after infection, and red cell survival is proportional to the amount of antibody attached to the cells. The most common antibodies are IgG (Pirofsky, 1976), directed against Rh antigen (Vos et al, 1971), and are warm in type. An IgG that is cold-acting follows viral infection (Wolach et al, 1981) and reacts against Donath-Landsteiner antigen. *Mycoplasma pneumoniae* infections occasionally produce cold-acting IgM antibodies (Salama & Mueller-Eckhardt, 1987). Erythrocyte destruction is dependent on the binding of antibody to red cell surfaces and on mediating complement fixation. The latter requires a single IgM molecule, as opposed to two IgG molecules, in close proximity. Cells coated with IgM effectively bind complement and activate C3 component, leading to their removal by the liver. IgG-coated cells are usually removed by the spleen (Schreiber & Frank, 1972).

Hemolysis may cause a rapid fall in hemoglobin levels (Buchanan & Glader, 1978), particularly in children under the age of 5 years (Habibi et al, 1974; Zuelzer et al, 1970). Patients have symptoms of hemolysis, including pallor, jaundice, dark urine, fever, and abdominal pain. Resolution is expected in about 50% of cases in 3–6 months, and a chronic

Table 6–20

Some Drugs and Chemicals Commonly Associated with Marrow Toxicity

Drugs

- Cytotoxic drugs: busulfan, melphalan
- Antimetabolites: nucleotide analogues, methotrexate
- Antimitotics: colchicine, vincristine
- Antibiotics: chloramphenicol, sulfonamides
- Anticonvulsants
- Anti-inflammatories: phenylbutazone

Chemicals

- Organic solvents
- Benzene and associated derivatives
- Insecticides: chlordane, parathion
- Metals: gold, bismuth, mercury, lead

Table 6–21
Causes of Hemolytic Anemia

Hereditary
- Hemoglobinopathies: sickle cell, thalassemia, unstable hemoglobins
- RBC membrane abnormalities: hereditary spherocytosis, hereditary elliptocytosis
- RBC enzyme abnormalities: G6PD deficiency, pyruvate kinase deficiency

Immune Mediated
- Autoimmune
  - Idiopathic
  - Due to underlying disease
    - Infections: viral infection, *Mycoplasma pneumoniae,* EBV
    - Autoimmune disorders: rheumatoid arthritis, SLE
    - Immunodeficiency: HIV
    - Malignancy: lymphomas, ALL, carcinoma
- Alloimmune: hemolytic disease of the newborn
- Drug induced
- Paroxysmal nocturnal hemoglobinuria

Peripheral Destruction
- Thrombotic disorders: HUS, TTP, Kasabach-Merritt syndrome
- Cardiac valve prostheses
- Burns

Abbreviations: ALL, acute lymphoblastic leukemia; EBV, Epstein-Barr virus; HUS, hemolytic uremic syndrome; RBC, red blood cell; SLE, systemic lupus erythematosus; TTP, thrombotic thrombocytopenic purpura.

relapsing and remitting course is seen in the remaining patients (Heisel & Ortega, 1983; Zupanska et al, 1976).

Laboratory findings include anemia, hyperbilirubinemia, reticulocytosis, and demonstration of the autoantibody by the direct antibody test (direct Coombs test). The pattern of cell agglutination facilitates antibody identification (Table 6–22). In general, IgM is commoner in acute cases, IgG in chronic cases. Treatment of autoimmune hemolytic anemia ranges from no therapy in acute, self-limited disease to corticosteroids. Splenectomy may be useful in refractory cases.

Alloimmune hemolytic anemias are due to preformed antibodies and occur particularly in the newborn period when antibodies cross the placenta or are given by blood transfusions. Maternofetal incompatibilities are of two major types: Rh disease and ABO incompatibility. Infants develop evidence of hemolysis, including anemia, jaundice, and hepatosplenomegaly. In severe cases, infants develop hydrops fetalis or bilirubin encephalopathy.

In hemolytic disease of the newborn, hemolysis develops shortly after birth and may continue until the antibody is eliminated, which, in the case of IgG type, may be 3 weeks or longer. Infants may develop hemolysis days to a week after birth. Severe hemolysis prior to birth causes hydrops fetalis. Treatment includes phototherapy for increased bilirubin levels, immunoglobulin administration, plasmapheresis, or exchange transfusion in severe cases.

Hemolytic disease of the newborn is diagnosed by demonstrating anemia and hyperbilirubinemia and by a positive direct antibody test result. Detection of alloantibodies in the mother should lead to testing of cord blood (Judd et al, 1990). The level of antibody in the infant correlates poorly with the degree of anemia and hyperbilirubinemia (Brouwers et al, 1988). Blood films show spherocytosis, polychromatophilia, and nucleated red blood cells. Platelet levels may be decreased owing to increased splenic function.

Hemolytic anemias from drugs involve three main mechanisms (Table 6–23). All give rise to hemolysis associated with a positive direct antiglobulin test result. In the hapten–drug absorption type, a drug bonds to a protein on the red cell membrane. Antibodies to the complex, usually of the IgG type, coat red cells and cause their premature removal by splenic macrophages. Hemolysis may appear after 7–10 days of therapy and continue for days to weeks after the termination of drug use. In the second type, the ternary complex mechanism of hemolysis is attributed to a complex of drug, antibody, and red cell antigen (Habibi, 1985). Hemolysis requires low levels of the drug and appears to be mediated by complement activation. Hemolysis in these patients may be quite severe or life threatening (Garratty et al, 1992). In the third major mechanism of drug-related hemolysis, drugs induce formation of autoantibodies against red cell antigens, usually of the Rh locus (Joseph, 1972). Drugs may bind to and alter red cell antigens, causing autoantibody formation. Antibodies are usually of the IgG class, and no antidrug antibodies are detected. Hemolysis may not appear for 3–6 months after initiation of drug therapy and is mediated by the spleen.

Paroxysmal nocturnal hemoglobinuria (PNH) is an acquired chronic hemolytic anemia in which a clonal abnormality increases sensitivity to complement-mediated lysis. Patients have episodic hemolytic anemia and nocturnal hemoglobinuria, often with visceral thromboses. A few have thrombocytopenia and neutropenia. Therefore, PNH should be considered in patients presenting with pancytopenia as well as hemolytic anemia. In PNH there are defects in the X-linked phosphatidylinositol glycan class A gene that produces a protein-anchoring complement component to red cell membranes (Takeda et al, 1993). Other genetic defects have also been described (Nafa et al, 1995; Nagarajan et al, 1995).

The laboratory features of PNH are summarized in Table 6–24. Several confusing variables alter this picture. Hemolytic episodes occur at irregular intervals, patients may develop iron deficiency from hemoglobinuria, thrombocytopenia and neutropenia are described, and the marrow may be hypercellular or aplastic. There is usually less reticulocytosis than in other hemolytic anemias.

Screening tests used in PNH include the sucrose hemolysis test (Hartmann & Jenkins, 1965). If the sucrose hemolysis test result is positive, it should be followed by a Ham acid hemolysis test to confirm that the defect is due to the patient's cells and that the active component is a heat-sensitive factor present in serum (Ham & Dingle, 1939). Urine may also be screened for hemosiderin. PNH may also be demonstrated by flow cytometric staining with CD59 that binds to the phosphoinositol-binding protein. Analysis of CD59 staining in reticulocytes shows decreased levels of staining in patients with PNH (Ware et al, 1995).

Treatment of PNH is predominantly supportive, with transfusions, antibiotics, and anticoagulants. Marrow transplantation is curative (Kawahara et al, 1992) and is of particular value in children, since their clinical course is often more severe (Ware

Table 6–22
Major Reactions Seen in Direct Antibody Testing

Anti-IgG	Anti-C_3	Interpretation
Positive	Negative	RBCs coated only with IgG
Positive	Positive	RBCs coated with IgG and C_3
Negative	Positive	RBCs coated with C_3, usually IgM antibody

Abbreviations: RBC, red blood cell.

Table 6–23
Drug-Mediated Hemolysis

	Mechanisms		
	Hapten or Drug Absorption	Ternary Complex	Autoantibody
Associated drugs	Penicillin and penicillin-type drugs	Quinine, quinidine, nonsteroidal anti-inflammatory	Alpha methyldopa, procainamide, mefanammic acid
Dose of drug	High	Low	High
Role of drug	Strongly binds to RBC membrane	Weak binding to RBC to form complex	Stimulates formation of cross-reactive antibody
Antibody formed	IgG against drug	IgM or IgG against drug	IgG against RBC
Proteins detected with direct antiglobulin test	IgG; rarely complement	Complement	IgG; rarely complement
Drug needed for hemolysis	Yes	Yes	No
Mechanism of RBC destruction	Splenic sequestration of IgG-coated cells	Complement-mediated lysis and splenic clearance of C_3b-coated cells	Splenic sequestration

Abbreviations: RBC, red blood cell.

et al, 1991). A small number of cases may progress to myelodysplasia or acute myelogenous leukemia (Devine et al, 1987; Graham & Gastineau, 1992).

Hemolysis from mechanical destruction of red cells has been seen in diseases with intravascular coagulation, burns, other traumatic injury, and cardiac abnormalities, including valvular diseases. Many of these processes produce increased numbers of schistocytes and spherocytes in the peripheral film (Fig. 6–25). Patients with heart abnormalities and burns often present with normal platelet counts. There are several diseases associated with hemolysis and thrombocytopenia, including hemolytic uremic syndrome, thrombotic thrombocytopenia purpura, microangiopathic processes, and Kasabach-Merritt syndrome with numerous congenital capillary hemangiomas.

Table 6–24
Laboratory Features of Paroxysmal Nocturnal Hemoglobinuria

Peripheral blood	
RBCs	Mild to severe normochromic, normocytic anemia; may be macrocytic if reticulocyte count high or hypochromic and microcytic if iron deficient; reticulocytosis
WBCs	Usually leukopenic
Platelets	Usually thrombocytopenic
Other	Positive sucrose hemolysis test result Positive acidified serum lysis test (Ham test) result Decreased CD59 expression on reticulocytes by flow cytometric analysis
Marrow	Normocellular to hypocellular marrow Erythrocytic hyperplasia Decreased or absent iron stores
Chemistries	May have increased urine hemoglobin level Hemosiderinuria May have decreased serum iron or ferritin level

Abbreviations: RBC, red blood cell; WBC, white blood cell.

RED CELL APLASIAS

In pure red cell aplasia erythropoiesis fails, whereas granulopoiesis and megakaryocytopoiesis are maintained. Patients have anemia, low reticulocyte counts, and decreased erythro-

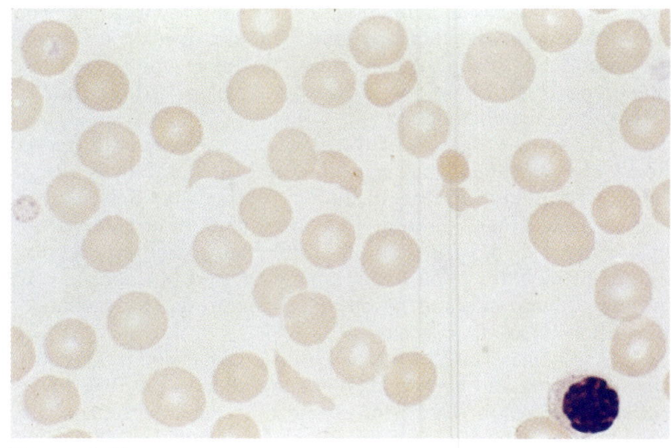

Figure 6–25

Hemolytic uremic syndrome, peripheral blood. Numerous red cell fragments and spherocytes, characteristic of hemolysis, are demonstrated in a patient with hemolytic uremic syndrome. Wright-Giemsa stain.

Table 6–25

Factors Associated with Pure Red Cell Aplasia in Childhood

Hereditary
Diamond-Blackfan anemia

Acquired
Idiopathic
Drugs: chloramphenicol, azothioprine, sulfonamides, antiepileptics, isoniazid
Viral infection: parvovirus B19, hepatitis, Epstein-Barr virus, HIV
Collagen vascular diseases: systemic lupus erythematosus, rheumatoid arthritis, juvenile rheumatoid arthritis
Thymoma
Malignancy: malignant histiocytosis, acute lymphoblastic leukemia
Myelodysplastic syndromes
Myeloproliferative syndromes

cytes in the marrow. Inherited and acquired forms of pure red cell aplasia occur (Table 6–25). There are many causes (Alter, 1980; Alter & Nathan, 1979), but those particularly important in the pediatric population are parvovirus B19 infection, transient erythroblastosis of childhood, and Diamond-Blackfan syndrome.

Parvovirus B19 infection is common in children, causing erythema infectiosum, or fifth disease (Harris, 1992). Parvovirus infects and destroys erythrocyte precusors (Ozawa et al, 1987), as evidenced by the presence of giant pronormoblasts, some of which may contain viral inclusions (Krause et al, 1992) (Fig. 6–26). Normal children are usually asymptomatic despite a transient fall in hematocrit. Children with increased red cell production demands (those with hemoglobinopathies, red cell membrane abnormalities, or enzymatic deficiencies) often develop a transient aplastic crisis (Brown & Young, 1996). An abrupt cessation of erythropoiesis is followed by a rapid fall in hematocrit due to the shortened red cell life span. Red cell production usually resumes in 1–2 weeks. The parvovirus infection may persist and produce a chronic hypoproliferative anemia in some patients with underlying immune deficiency (Kurtzman et al, 1987). Laboratory findings other than giant pronormoblasts (see Fig. 6–26) include anemia, reticulocytopenia, and a rise in IgM titers (Harris, 1992). Viral sequences may be detected by PCR amplification from the marrow (Patou et al, 1993).

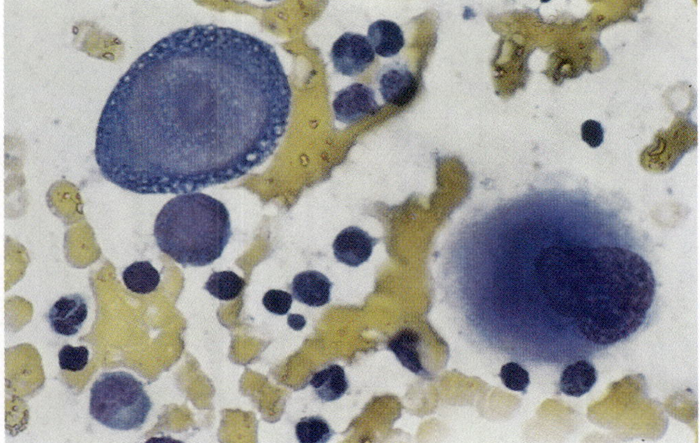

Figure 6–26

Parvovirus infection, marrow aspirate. A giant pronormoblast with a viral inclusion is shown in a marrow aspirate from a patient with parvovirus infection. Wright-Giemsa stain.

In transient erythroblastopenia there is transient cessation in erythropoiesis in children with previously normal hematologic features. Very young children are affected, with the median age of onset at 23 months. A clear viral cause has not been documented for the disease, and results of tests for parvovirus infection have been generally negative (Young et al, 1984). A serum factor, possibly IgG, has been shown to inhibit erythropoiesis (Dessypris et al, 1982; Freedman, 1983; Koenig et al, 1979).

Laboratory findings include moderate to severe normochromic, normocytic anemia with reticulocyte counts $<1\%$. White cell counts are often normal, but neutropenia and thrombocytopenia may be seen (Hanada et al, 1989). The marrow examination reveals a marked decrease in erythrocyte precursors as well as erythrocyte maturational arrest. Lymphocytes may be increased. Erythropoietin levels are high.

Recovery is spontaneous, with resolution of the anemia expected in 1–2 months. A few children take up to 8 months to recover, but relapse or recurrence is extremely rare (Freedman, 1983). Recovery is heralded by a marked reticulocytosis, followed by a rise in hemoglobin level to normal.

Diamond-Blackfan anemia is a congenital pure red cell aplasia that develops in children. The leukocyte and platelet counts are essentially normal, thereby differentiating this process from aplastic anemia. Patients usually present in infancy with severe anemia. The average age at diagnosis is 2 months, and over 90% of cases are detected by 1 year of age (Diamond et al, 1976). An autosomal dominant pattern (Diamond et al, 1976; Falter & Robinson, 1972) and an autosomal recessive pattern have been described (Starling & Fernbach, 1973). Affected infants may have other congenital abnormalities, including short stature and abnormalities of the head, face, upper limb, and eye (Cathie, 1950; Diamond et al, 1961).

Laboratory findings (Table 6–26) include moderate to severe anemia. The blood film shows macrocytosis, anisocytosis, and teardrop cells. Reticulocyte counts are low. Analysis of the

Table 6–26

Laboratory Features of Diamond-Blackfan Anemia

Peripheral blood	
RBCs	Mild to severe macrocytic anemia Decreased reticulocyte count RBC morphology shows macrocytes, teardrop cells, anisocytosis
WBCs	Usually normal; may be decreased
Platelets	Usually normal; may be decreased
Other	Increased fetal hemoglobin level
Marrow	Normocellular marrow Erythrocyte precursors usually aplastic or hypoplastic In rare cases, normal numbers of erythrocyte precursors with maturational arrest Dyserythropoiesis
Cytogenetics	Usually normal karyotype
Chemistries	Increased erythropoietin levels Increased B_{12} and folate levels Increased serum iron and ferritin levels Increased RBC adenosine deaminase levels

Abbreviations: RBC, red blood cell; WBC, white blood cell.

Table 6–27

Comparative Features of Diamond-Blackfan Anemia and Transient Erythroblastopenia of Childhood

Features	Diamond-Blackfan Anemia	Transient Erythroblastopenia of Childhood
Clinical Features		
Average age at diagnosis	5 months (range 0–72)	26 months (range 1–92)
Previous viral infection	No	Yes
Congenital abnormalities	Yes in 30%	No
Laboratory Findings		
RBCs	Macrocytic anemia	Normocytic anemia; may be macrocytic during recovery phase
WBCs	Usually normal; may be decreased	Usually normal; may be decreased
Platelets	Usually normal; may be increased	Usually normal; may be increased
HgF	Increased	Normal; may be increased during recovery phase
i antigen	Increased	Normal; may be increased during recovery phase
RBC adenosine deaminase levels	Increased	Normal

Abbreviations: HgF, hemoglobin F; RBC, red blood cell; WBC, white blood cell.

Source: Adapted from Alter BP: Aplastic anemia. Am J Pediatr Hematol Oncol 2:119–139, 1980.

red cells show increased levels of HgF distributed among cells. Levels of the red cell antigen i, usually seen in fetal hematopoiesis, are also increased, and antigen I levels are near adult levels, a pattern seen in "stress erythropoiesis" following marrow failure (Alter & Nathan, 1979). Adenine deaminase levels are often elevated (Glader et al, 1983). Serum levels of iron, ferritin, folate, cobalamin, and erythropoietin are elevated, indicating that deficiencies are not the cause of the anemia. Marrows are normocellular, with selective erythrocytic hypoplasia or aplasia. Results of chromosomal analysis are usually normal (Alter, 1980).

The main differential diagnostic consideration is transient erythroblastopenia of childhood (Table 6–27) (Alter, 1980). This disorder usually affects older patients, with a mean age of 26 months versus 5 months for Diamond-Blackfan syndrome. There is often an antecedent viral infection. An abrupt onset with a "spontaneous" resolution is characteristic. Adenosine deaminase levels are normal.

The pathophysiologic features of red cell aplasia in Diamond-Blackfan anemia may involve a defect in erythrocyte stem cells (Lipton et al, 1986; Nathan et al, 1978; Tsai et al, 1989). Treatment includes supportive transfusion therapy, corticosteroids, and marrow transplantation, the latter offering the possibility of cure. About 20% of patients have a spontaneous remission, but prognosis is otherwise poor, since many patients die with severe anemia or complications of therapy, such as hemosiderosis. There is an increased risk of development of leukemia or myelodysplasia as well as other malignancies.

APLASTIC ANEMIA

In aplastic anemia all hematopoiesis fails, as evidenced by pancytopenia (Camitta et al, 1979). There are hereditary and acquired forms (Table 6–28). Most cases are idiopathic, although aplastic anemia has developed after exposure to a multitude of environmental hazards, including chemicals, drugs, radiation, and viruses. Particularly notable hazards are benzene (Goldstein et al, 1987; Smith, 1996), chloramphenicol (Smick et al, 1964), and hepatitis (Ajlouni & Doeblin, 1974; Hagler et al, 1975), especially an unusual non–A-, non–B-type virus, possibly hepatitis G (Brown et al, 1997). These various agents must damage either hematopoietic stem cells or marrow stroma that provides the essential microenvironment for hematopoiesis (Juneja & Gardner, 1985; Knospe & Crosby, 1971; Marsh et al, 1991; Scopes et al, 1996).

Among inherited forms of aplastic anemia, Fanconi anemia is the most common, with over 800 cases reported in the literature (Alter, 1992). Inherited as an autosomal recessive trait, Fanconi anemia is associated with short stature, abnormal skin pigmentation, renal anomalies, and abnormal thumbs and radii. Other inherited causes of aplastic anemia are dyskeratosis congenita and Schwachman-Diamond syndrome (pancreatic insufficiency with neutropenia).

Patients with aplastic anemia have fatigue, weakness, petechiae, and bruising as well as an increased incidence of infection. Since the onset may be insidious, some patients

Table 6–28

Factors Associated with Aplastic Anemia

Hereditary
- Fanconi anemia
- Dyskeratosis congenita
- Schwachman syndrome

Acquired
- Idiopathic (65% of cases)
- Chemicals: benzene, insecticides, solvents
- Drugs: chloramphenicol, phenylbutazone, anticonvulsants, gold
- Radiation exposure
- Viruses: non-A, non-B hepatitis; Epstein-Barr virus
- Autoimmune disorders: rheumatoid arthritis, systemic lupus erythematosus
- Pregnancy

Table 6–29

Laboratory Features of Aplastic Anemia

Peripheral blood	
RBCs	Normocytic, normochromic anemia; may be macrocytic
WBCs	Leukopenia Neutropenia Relative lymphocytosis
Platelets	Thrombocytopenia
Marrow	Markedly hypocellular Mild dyspoiesis or megaloblastic maturation
Cytogenetics	Usually normal

Abbreviations: RBC, red blood cell; WBC, white blood cell.

present with marked pancytopenia. Laboratory findings (Table 6–29) include pancytopenia, thrombocytopenia, low reticulocyte counts, and neutropenia with normal or only slightly decreased lymphocyte counts. Occasionally patients present with single cell deficits, but other blood elements fail in days to weeks. Erythropoietin and serum iron levels are high (Adams & Barrett, 1982).

The marrow aspirate reveals marked hypocellularity, with increased amounts of fat. Plasma cells, lymphocytes, mast cells, and macrophages are usually the predominant cellular components, with only rare hematopoietic cells. The biopsy confirms marked hypocellularity (Fig. 6–27) that may be patchy, with small islands of hypercellular residual hematopoiesis. Lymphocyte aggregates and clusters of plasma cells may be seen. Cytogenetic analysis may be difficult due to the paucity of hematopoietic cells, and only a few patients have demonstrated abnormalities (Mikhailova et al, 1996).

Other causes of marrow aplasia and pancytopenia must be excluded before a definitive diagnosis of aplastic anemia is made. PNH should be excluded by normal sucrose hemolysis and Ham tests, acute lymphoblastic leukemia (Reid & Summerfield, 1992) or myelodysplastic syndromes (Tuzuner et al, 1995) by careful marrow examination.

Treatment of aplastic anemia in children usually involves allogeneic marrow transplantation in moderate to severe cases (Doney et al, 1997), whereas occasionally patients with less severe aplasia have spontaneous recovery. Marrow transplantation is curative in up to 89% of patients, with improved survival time seen in patients who had not received transfusions prior to transplant (Bunin et al, 1996; Doney et al, 1997; Margolis et al, 1996). Patients who are not suitable candidates for marrow transplantation may receive immunosuppressive therapy and androgen therapy (Fonseca & Tefferi, 1997). Immunosuppressive therapy is successful in about half of patients, but some develop PNH, myelodysplasia, or acute myelogenous leukemia (Moore & Castro-Malaspina, 1991). Poor prognostic indicators appear to be absolute neutrophil count $<200/\mu l$ and aplastic anemia following hepatitis infection (Bacigalupo et al, 1988; Najean & Pecking, 1979).

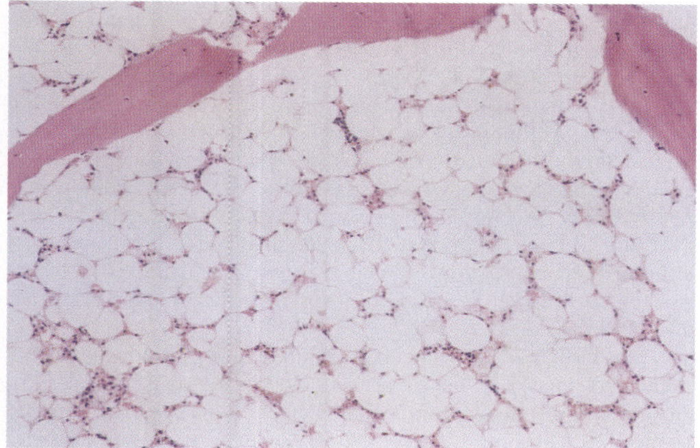

Figure 6–27

Aplastic anemia, marrow biopsy. In a child presenting with pancytopenia, the marrow is characteristically hypocellular, containing only scattered hematopoietic cells, lymphocytes, and plasma cells. Hematoxylin-eosin stain.

DISORDERS OF MYELOCYTES AND MONOCYTES

Children may have hereditary and acquired disorders of neutrophils, monocytes, eosinophils, and basophils. Many of them are associated with significant rates of morbidity and mortality.

Neutrophilic Disorders

Neutrophils differentiate in the marrow for about 7 days and then circulate for about 6.5 h (Athens et al, 1961) before entering a tissue pool. Neutrophil number is affected by age and genetic characteristics. Newborns often have neutrophilia for the first 2 weeks (mean 11,000 cells/μl, range 6,000–28,000 cells/μl). Children between 1 month and 8 years of age have mean counts of 3500–3800 cells/μl (range 1000–9000 cells/μl). Above this age, counts are similar to adult levels.

Neutropenia in children has hereditary and acquired causes (Table 6–30) and is often categorized as transient or chronic. Susceptibility to bacterial infections is a major complication of neutropenia. Work-up requires documentation of the neutrope-

Table 6–30

Factors Associated with Neutropenia

Hereditary
- Infantile genetic agranulocytosis (Kostmann syndrome)
- Chronic congenital neutropenia
  - Cyclic neutropenia
  - Benign chronic neutropenia
- Reticular dysgenesis
- Myelokathexis
- Cartilage-hair hypoplasia
- Dyskeratosis congenita
- Chédiak-Higashi syndrome

Acquired
- Transient
  - Infections: viral, bacterial, tularemia
  - Burns
  - Drugs
  - Hemodialysis
  - Vitamin deficiency: B_{12}, folate
- Chronic
  - Myelophthisic process
  - Hematologic malignancies
  - Myelodysplasia
  - Autoimmune mechanisms
  - Hypersplenism
  - Idiopathic

nia over time, elimination of precipitating causes by history and physical examination, and marrow examination in those children in whom a clear cause is not found (Bernini, 1996).

Infantile genetic agranulocytosis, or Kostmann syndrome, is a rare autosomal recessive hereditary deficiency in neutrophil differentiation that causes extreme neutropenia, severe infections, often beginning in the first month of life, and premature death. Laboratory findings include severe neutropenia (absolute count $<500/\mu l$) or an absolute lack of neutrophils (Welte & Dale, 1996), whereas numbers of eosinophils and monocytes may be increased. Red cells and platelets are usually normal in number. The marrow shows normal cellularity, but there is absent or markedly decreased myelocyte precursors with a maturational arrest at the promyelocyte or myelocyte stage. Granulopoiesis may be stimulated by treatment with granulocyte colony-stimulating (G-CSF) factor (Bonilla et al, 1989) or marrow transplant may be effective (Rappeport et al, 1980). Children often die of infection by 3 years of age, but a few patients have developed acute leukemia (Lui et al, 1978; Rosen & Kang, 1979; Welte & Dale, 1996). Mutations in the receptor for G-CSF identified in some patients may be associated with progression to acute myelogenous leukemia (Dong et al, 1995; Dong et al, 1997). Other hereditary disorders causing neutropenia include reticular dysgenesis (Rosen et al, 1984), myelocathexis (Zuelzer et al, 1970), cartilage-hair hypoplasia (Lux et al, 1970), and dyskeratosis congenita (Dokal 1996; Putterman et al, 1993).

Other chronic congenital neutropenias, also called benign familial neutropenia, form a syndrome presenting with a lesser degree of neutropenia than in the severe congenital neutropenia previously described. The susceptibility of these patients to infection is correlated to the level of neutropenia, and some have mild infections. The marrow often exhibits decreased numbers of myelocyte precursors or maturational arrest. Cyclic neutropenia is included in this group of disorders and is named for the oscillation of neutrophil counts over a 21-day cycle (Dale & Hammond, 1988; Wright et al, 1981). Other blood cells co-oscillate but usually cycle between normal and elevated levels. The marrow often exhibits myelocytic maturational arrest 1 week prior to the neutropenic nadir. There is spontaneous resolution of the neutropenia. Inheritance is variable but fits an autosomal dominant pattern in some families (Palmer et al, 1996). Treatment with hematopoietic growth factors may be useful (Dale, 1995).

Acquired disorders of neutrophil quantities occur in metabolic disturbances, ineffective granulopoiesis due to folate or B_{12} deficiencies, infections, autoimmune destruction, splenic sequestration, and drug-induced neutropenia. Viral infections commonly cause transient neutropenia in children, particularly infections with Epstein-Barr virus, hepatitis A or B, respiratory syncytial virus, influenza A and B, rubella, rubeola, and varicella (Murdoch & Smith, 1972). Neutropenia develops in the first 24–48 h of infection and may persist for 3–6 days. This neutropenia results from neutrophil infiltration of virally affected tissues and splenic sequestration. Epstein-Barr virus infection also induces antineutrophil antibodies that accelerate neutrophil destruction (Schooley et al, 1984). The marrow often exhibits normal or increased granulopoiesis. Patients with processes that infiltrate the bone marrow, such as metastatic tumor, hematologic malignancies, granulomatous disorders, or fibrosis may present with neutropenia or pancytopenia.

Neutrophilia usually represents reactions to stress, infection, or chronic inflammation. Some drugs, particularly lithium and corticosteroids, produce neutrophilia. Chronic causes of neutrophilia include myeloproliferative syndromes (see Chap. 7), chronic infections, and hyposplenism.

Several qualitative abnormalities of neutrophils have been described. Most are rare hereditary disorders in which dysfunction is due to abnormalities of degranulation, leukocyte adhesion, and microbial killing (Table 6–31). Chédiak-Higashi syndrome, chronic granulomatous disease, and myeloperoxidase deficiency are particularly important and are discussed below.

Table 6–31
Qualitative Defects in Neutrophil Function

Degranulation Abnormalities
Chédiak-Higashi syndrome
Specific granule deficiency
Neutrophil Adheshion Abnormalities
Leukocyte adhesion deficiency
Abnormalities in Chemotaxis
IgG deficiency
C3 deficiency
Neonatal defects in chemotaxis
Immune complex disorder
Defects in Microbial Killing
Chronic granulomatous disease
Myeloperoxidase deficiency
Severe G6PD deficiency
Glutathione reductase deficiency
Glutathione synthetase deficiency

Chédiak-Higashi is a rare autosomal recessive disorder in which neutrophils, monocytes, and lymphocytes contain giant intracytoplasmic granules that include coalesced lysosomes (Fig. 6–28). The genetic defect has been mapped to chromosome 1 and appears to cause defects in protein sorting into cytoplasmic organelles (Nagle et al, 1996), with ineffective myelopoiesis and microorganism killing capacity (Boxer & Blackwood, 1996). Patients are characteristically hypopigmented, lack natural killer cells, and have bleeding tendencies and frequent infections. Older children enter a life-threatening accelerated phase (see also Chap. 8), with development of extensive lymphohistiocytic infiltrates that are not cytologically malignant involving spleen, liver, and lymph nodes (Rubin et al, 1985). Most patients die in childhood of progressive pancytopenia. Marrow transplantation has been used to correct the defect and treat the accelerated phase (Haddad et al, 1995).

In chronic granulomatous disease, neutrophils and monocytes are unable to generate superoxide and thereby kill phagocytized organisms that are catalase positive. Chronic granulomatous disease is caused by mutations in one of the four subunits of NADPH oxidase (Roos et al, 1996). In all forms the characteristic laboratory finding is decreased production of superoxide or hydrogen peroxide following neutrophil stimulation (Ottonello et al, 1995). The patterns of inheritance are X-linked and autosomal recessive. Pneumonitis, dermatitis, and lymphadenitis are the common resultant infections. Patients may present as infants, or presentation may be delayed until late childhood. Patients are treated supportively with antibiotics and γ-interferon (Forrest et al, 1988), but marrow transplantation provides the opportunity for cure (Calvino et al, 1996).

Myeloperoxidase deficiency, either inherited or acquired in myelodysplasia, is characterized by a functional, cytochemical, and immunohistochemical absence of myeloperoxidase in neutrophil granules. Myeloperoxidase deficiency appears to arise from a variety of mutations in the myeloperoxidase gene (Selsted et al, 1993). When inherited, the pattern is autosomal recessive, with a frequency of approximately 1:2000–1:4000 (Kizaki et al, 1994). Ingested microorganisms cannot be killed rapidly, although killing by other mechanisms may occur after

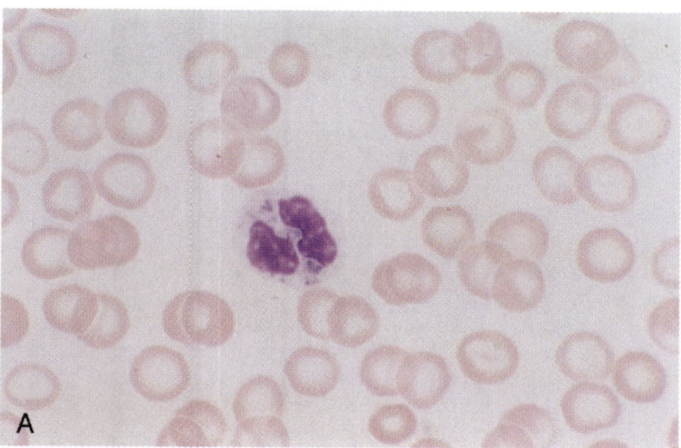

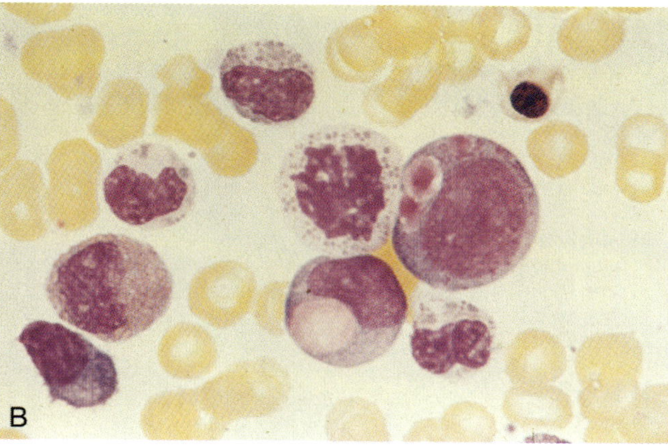

Figure 6–28

Chédiak-Higashi disease, peripheral blood and marrow. *A*. A peripheral blood neutrophil with large, fused granules is characteristic of Chédiak-Higashi disease. *B*. The marrow aspirate from the same patient demonstrates the abnormal granulation throughout myelocyte maturation. Wright-Giemsa stain.

a longer period of time (Nauseef, 1988). The neutrophils in this disease are incapable of killing yeast. An important clinical manifestation is susceptibility of diabetic patients to infections with *Candida albicans*. The frequency of bacterial infections is usually not increased.

Eosinophilic Disorders

The quantitation of eosinophils in peripheral blood is clinically important as an indicator of underlying disease. Excess production of eosinophils in the hypereosinophilic syndromes is very rare in children (Table 6–32).

Reactive eosinophilia is seen in asthma, hay fever, acute allergic reactions, reactions to drugs, parasitic infections, and lymphomas, particularly Hodgkin disease and T cell lymphoblastic lymphoma. Hypereosinophilic syndromes vary in severity and outcome, ranging from fairly benign to fatal proliferations (Hardy & Anderson, 1968). In hypereosinophilic syndromes there are numerous circulating eosinophils (Fig. 6–29) as well as tissue infiltration, with resultant damage from inflammatory mediators. Hepatosplenomegaly, cardiac damage or fibrosis, pulmonary fibrosis, central nervous system disease, anemia, fever, and weight loss may be seen. Cardiac fibrosis is the most common cause of death. Very high eosinophil counts (>100,000 cells/ml), abnormal cytogenetic, features, and decreased leukocyte alkaline phosphatase scores are associated with a poor outcome (Flaum et al, 1981).

Basophilic Disorders

Basophilic granules contain inflammatory mediators, especially those involved in hypersensitivity reactions, and marrow and peripheral basophilia are seen in a number of hypersensitivity and inflammatory reactions (Table 6–33) (Mitchell, 1957). Basophilia is frequently associated with myelodysplastic syndromes and myeloproliferative disorders (see Chap. 7).

Monocytic Disorders

Relatively little information is available on monocyte and macrophage subpopulations and their involvement in childhood diseases. Monocytosis is common in the period of marrow recovery, when it is absolute and more striking because of neu-

Table 6–32
Causes of Eosinophilia

Hereditary
Hereditary eosinophilia

Acquired
Reactive causes
- Allergic disorders: asthma, hay fever, atopic dermatitis
- Drug reaction
- Skin diseases: pemphigoid
- Parasitic infections: nematodes, trematodes
- Tumors: brain tumors, lymphomas

Primary marrow disorders
- Hypereosinophilic syndromes
- Eosinophilic leukemia

Other
- Loeffler syndrome (pulmonary eosinophilia)
- Polyarteritis nodosa

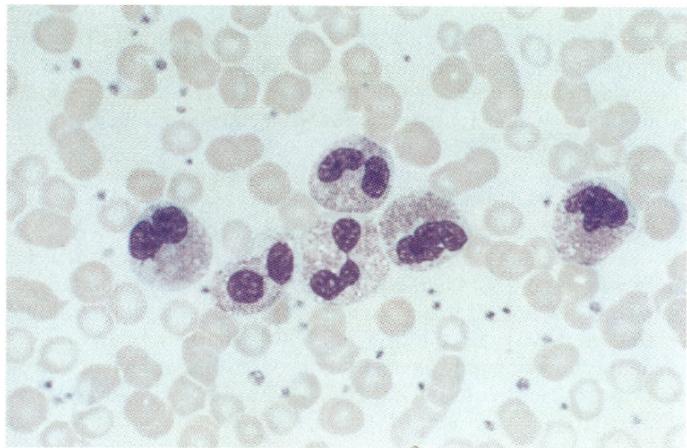

Figure 6–29

Hypereosinophilic syndrome, peripheral blood. This film from a patient with hypereosinophilic syndrome shows marked eosinophilia with minimal dysplastic features. Wright-Giemsa stain.

Table 6–33
Causes of Basophilia

Hypersensitivity reactions
Urticaria
Drug allergy
Food allergy
Inflammation or infection
Influenza
Varicella infection
Tuberculosis
Rheumatoid arthritis
Ulcerative colitis
Myeloproliferative disorders
Myelodysplastic disorders
Acute myelogenous leukemias

tropenia; in granulomatous disease; and in various hematologic disorders (Table 6–34). Monocytic leukemias are covered in Chap. 4. Monocyte and macrophage proliferation is an important part of infection-associated hemophagocytic syndrome, covered in Chap. 16.

MAST CELL DISEASE

Mast cells, derived from CD34 positive marrow stem cells, share morphologic and functional properties with basophils. Mast cells do not circulate in appreciable numbers, but remain in connective tissues in the skin, mucosal sites, lymph nodes, liver, spleen, and marrow. Mast cells are also often found in association with nerves, blood vessels, and mucosal surfaces. The mast cell has many high affinity surface IgE receptors and participates in both immediate and cutaneous hypersensitivity reactions. Cellular degranulation may be induced by localized trauma or response to IgE binding and receptor cross-linking. Mast cell granules contain many mitogenic and inflammatory cytokines (interleukins 1, 3, 4, 5, and 6; tumor necrosis factor alpha; and granulocyte-macrophage colony stimulating factor) as well as histamine and heparin-like substances (Longley et al, 1995; Marone et al, 1995; Weber et al, 1995). Release of these substances causes many of the symptoms associated with mast cell disease, including pruritus, flushing, urticaria, diarrhea, nausea, cramping, headaches, and palpitations, or full-blown anaphylactic symptoms. Serum histamine or urinary histamine metabolite levels may be increased, whereas serum seratonin and hyaluronic acid levels are decreased (Bateman et al, 1995).

Mast cell disease in children and adults includes a spectrum of disorders, ranging from localized skin disease to full-blown mast cell leukemia (Golkar & Bernhard, 1997). Most children have indolent or localized forms of disease that are characterized by large numbers of mast cells in the skin or gastrointestinal tract mucosa (Kettelhut & Metcalfe, 1994). Skin disease is the most common manifestation of mast cell disease in children, and is characterized by dermal accumulation of mast cells. Clinically this may give rise to a solitary nodule (mast cell nevus) or multiple nodules, or the more common presentation of patchy involvement as in urticaria pigmentosa (Golkar & Bernhard, 1997; Longley et al, 1995; Marone et al, 1995). Urticaria pigmentosa appears before the age of 2 years in 55% of cases, and an additional 10% of cases develop before the age of 15 years (Kettelhut & Metcalfe, 1994).

Children have brownish papules that are symmetrically distributed over the trunk and other sites. Upon minor trauma, the mast cells degranulate, causing urticarial lesions, dermatographism, and blistering. Many patients also experience intense pruritus. Biopsy samples of the skin show nodules of bland-appearing mast cells with varying degrees of degranulation in the dermis (Fig. 6–30*A*). Mast cells may be identified as spindle-shaped cells with oval nuclei (Kettelhut & Metcalfe, 1994; Marone et al, 1995). The cytoplasm contains granules that do not stain well with hematoxylin and eosin, but do stain well with Giemsa/toluidine blue stains and mast cell tryptase (Li et al, 1996) (Fig. 6–30*B*).

Patients with urticaria pigmentosa often have increased numbers or nodular aggregates of mast cells in other sites, including marrow and gut. Marrow involvement in children is usually manifested by eosinophilia with focal perivascular and peritrabecular aggregates of mast cells (Kettelhut et al, 1989) (Fig. 6–31). Adults are more likely to have nodular mast cell nodules or diffuse infiltrates (Horny et al, 1985; Topar et al, 1998). Rarely, cutaneous mast cell disease in children may diffusely infiltrate the skin, which appears normal or has red-brown/yellow coloration with thickening. Yellow papules that resemble xanthomas may occur (i.e., pseudoxanthomatous mastocytosis). There may be diffuse erythroderma. Often, extensive bullae formation occurs in these children, with blisters at birth in some. Diffuse cutaneous mastocytosis frequently resolves spontaneously between the ages of 2 to 5 years, although during the disease course sepsis and gastrointestinal symptoms of diarrhea may be severe and lead to hypotension, shock, and even death (Kettelhut & Metcalfe, 1994; Marone et al, 1995).

Most cases of urticaria pigmentosa subside at puberty, but a small proportion persist into adulthood. Most cases of mast cell disease in adults do not remain localized to the skin, but develop into either a benign or an aggressive systemic form that involves spleen, liver, lymph nodes, gut, and marrow (Kors et al, 1996; Travis et al, 1988a). Onset of the aggressive systemic form is usually associated with progressive anemia, thrombocytopenia, leukopenia, and hepatosplenomegaly in addition to the characteristic skin disease (Golkar & Bernhard,

Table 6–34
Causes of Monocytosis

Newborn state
Infections
Bacterial: recovery phase, mycobacteria, subacute bacterial endocarditis
Rickettsia: Rocky Mountain spotted fever
Protozoa: malaria
Postsplenectomy
Hematologic disorders
Myeloproliferative disorders: CML, JMML, CMML
Acute myelogenous leukemia: AML-M4, AML-M5
Myelodysplastic syndromes: infantile monosomy 7 syndrome
Chronic neutropenia
Cyclic neutropenia
Malignant histiocytosis
Hodgkin disease
Collagen vascular diseases
Rheumatoid arthritis
Systemic lupus erythematosus
Gastrointestinal diseases
Sprue
Inflammatory bowel disease
Sarcoidosis

Abbreviations: AML, acute myelogenous leukemia; CML, chronic myelogenous leukemia; CMML, chronic myelomonocytic leukemia; JMML, juvenile myelomonocytic leukemia.

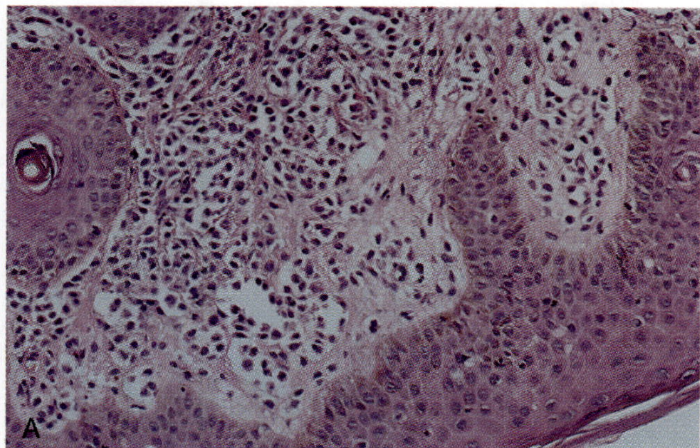

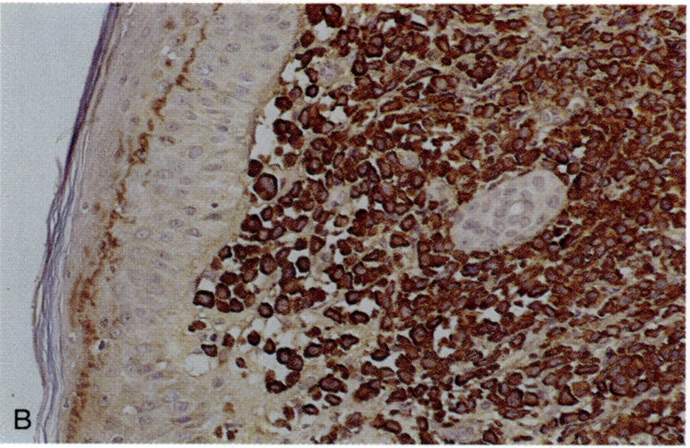

Figure 6–30

Skin, mast cell disease (urticaria pigmentosa). *A.* A skin biopsy from a 3-year-old with brown plaques and itching showed dermal infiltrate of spindled mast cells. *B.* Immunohistochemical stain for mast cell tryptase demonstrated strong positivity of the spindle cells.

1997). Up to 15% of patients with aggressive systemic mast cell disease may develop a frank mast cell leukemia (Travis et al, 1986). Adults may also present with aggressive mast cell disease without preexistent indolent disease (Golkar & Bernhard, 1997; Longley et al, 1995). Children rarely develop aggressive systemic forms of mast cell disease (Kettelhut & Metcalfe, 1994).

Mast cell proliferations have been seen in children and adults in association with other hematologic disorders, in particular myeloproliferative disorders, malignant lymphomas, and acute leukemias (Travis et al, 1988b). Concurrent association of mast cell disease with another hematologic disorder is usually seen with a more aggressive course. Treatment of the underlying disorder often causes regression of the mast cell disease (Hutchinson, 1992; Travis et al, 1988b).

Controversy exists as to whether mast cell disease represents reactive disorders or malignancies (Krober et al, 1997; Longley, 1994). Clonality studies in females suggest that localized skin disease and benign systemic skin forms of disease are reactive polyclonal proliferations of mast cells, whereas the more aggressive systemic disorders and mast cell leukemia represent clonal disorders (Krober et al, 1997). Most patients experience disease progression from localized or benign systemic disease to aggressive disease, although a small proportion of patients experience de novo aggressive systemic disease.

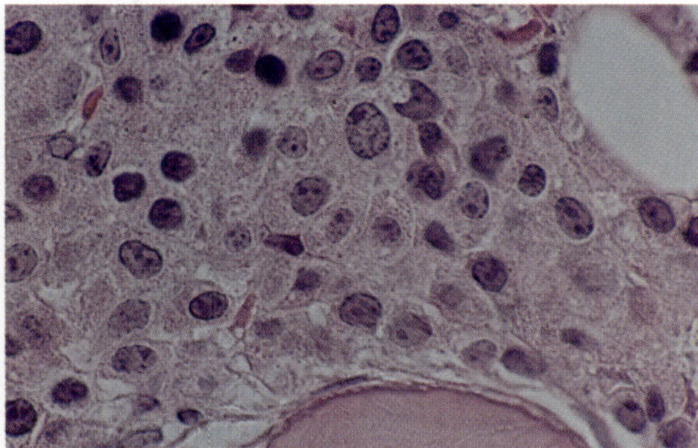

Figure 6–31

Marrow, mast cell disease.
The marrow in this child with urticaria pigmentosa demonstrated a paratrabecular collection of mast cells.

Treatment of localized mast cell disease is usually excision. Benign systemic forms are often treated with agents to block degranulation and mediator release. Histamine antagonists to block histamine effects and other drugs to ameliorate symptoms of itching, diarrhea, flushing, and urticaria may also be used. The aggressive mast cell disorders are treated with chemotherapeutic agents, although results are generally disappointing (Golkar & Bernhard, 1997; Marone et al, 1995). Marrow transplant has also been utilized in aggressive or malignant mast cell disease with some success (Przepiorka et al, 1998).

MEGAKARYOCYTIC OR PLATELET DISORDERS

Platelet counts represent the balance between platelet production and platelet removal or utilization. Most cases of thrombocytopenia in children are associated with excess removal or destruction. Failures of megakaryocytopoiesis are uncommon and are often associated with general marrow failure, as in aplastic anemia or leukemia. Pure failures in megakaryocytopoiesis are very rare and may be acquired or hereditary (Table 6–35).

Acquired megakaryocytopenia is very rare, with fewer than 50 patients reported (Manoharan et al, 1989). The patients had both thrombocytopenia and markedly reduced megakaryocytes. Autoimmune, infectious, and myelodysplastic

Table 6–35

Causes of Thrombocytopenia (Associated with Decreased Marrow Megakaryocytes)

Hereditary
Thrombocytopenia with absent radii syndrome
Hereditary amegakaryocytic thrombocytopenia
Acquired
Myelodysplasia
Viral infections
Autoimmune disorders

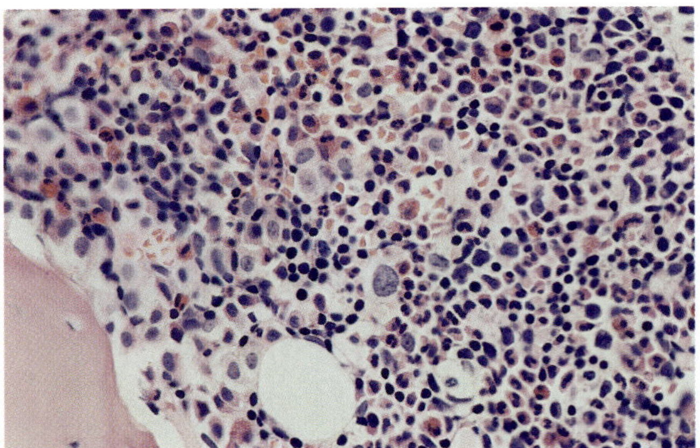

Figure 6–32

Thrombocytopenia with absent radii syndrome, marrow aspirate. A clot section from an affected infant shows decreased numbers of megakaryocytes as well as the characteristic mononuclear and hypolobated forms. Hematoxylin-eosin stain.

disorders may cause megakaryocytopenia by affecting the marrow precursor cell or its response to thrombopoietin (Gewirtz et al, 1986; Hoffman et al, 1982). Viral infections have been associated with transient thrombocytopenia. The mechanisms may involve decreasing the numbers of megakaryocytes as well as increasing splenic removal of platelets.

Hereditary thrombocytopenia is associated with absent radii (Hedberg & Lipton, 1988). Patients are usually identified at birth by lack of radii, presence of thumbs, and thrombocytopenia. Inheritance is autosomal recessive, and all racial groups are affected. In addition to thrombocytopenia, patients have anemia if significant bleeding has occurred. Reticulocytosis after anemia differentiates this syndrome from Fanconi anemia. The levels of white cells are often elevated at birth but usually return to normal over time. White counts $>100{,}000/\mu l$ have been reported. The marrow exhibits normal myelopoiesis and erythropoiesis, and megakaryocytes are decreased or absent. The megakaryocytes are often small or immature appearing (Fig. 6–32). Cytogenetic testing reveals normal chromosomal breakage and karyotype. Platelet transfusions may be used to help control bleeding in infancy but are usually not required in older children. There is no association with development of leukemia or other hematologic complications in later life.

Thrombocytosis in children and adults is often secondary. Malignancy, inflammatory disorders, blood loss, iron deficiency, splenectomy, or exercise (Davis & Ross, 1973) may elevate platelet counts. Infants with vitamin E deficiency also may have increased platelet counts (Lundstrom, 1979; Ritchie et al, 1968). This thrombocytosis is occasionally complicated by thrombosis (Buss et al, 1985). The myeloproliferative disorders (see Chap. 7) may cause thrombocytosis.

Platelets may function abnormally in inherited or acquired disorders. Acquired abnormalities in platelet function are seen with many drugs, hematologic diseases, uremia, and other systemic diseases. The hereditary disorders are often detected in childhood and are associated with specific defects that affect platelet function. Three of the more important disorders are Glanzmann thrombasthenia, Bernard-Soulier syndrome, and Wiskott-Aldrich syndrome.

Glanzmann thrombasthenia is a congenital bleeding disorder in which platelets fail to aggregate in response to ADP, epinepherine, collagen, and thrombin (Coller et al, 1994; George et al, 1990). Patients have normal platelet counts and morphologic features, prolonged bleeding times, abnormal clot retraction times, and abnormal platelet aggregation with all agonists except ristocetin. Analysis of glycoprotein IIb/IIIa levels shows variation among patients, with levels ranging from $<5\%$ in most patients to 50% of normal (George et al, 1990). Molecular analysis of the defects associated with Glanzmann thrombasthenia has shown a wide variety of defects in the glycoprotein IIb and IIIa coding regions (Bray, 1994; Seligsohn & Peretz, 1994). The glycoproteins act as platelet receptors for fibrinogen (Phillips et al, 1988). Treatment is by prevention of bleeding and avoidance of aspirin and other platelet inactivators. Platelet transfusions or desmopressin may be needed when serious bleeding occurs. The overall prognosis is good. Allogeneic bone marrow transplantation has been used in patients with severe bleeding (Johnson et al, 1994).

Bernard-Soulier syndrome is characterized by thrombocytopenia and giant platelets that fail to participate in interactions with von Willebrand factor and thrombin (Howard et al, 1973; Jantunen, 1994) due to deficiencies in glycoproteins Ib, V, and IX (Degos et al, 1977; Sae-Tung et al, 1996). This rare disease is usually inherited as an autosomal recessive trait. Patients of varying age present with epistaxis or ecchymoses of varying severity. The blood film shows thrombocytopenia and characteristic large platelets, some larger than lymphocytes (Fig. 6–33). Platelet function tests show failure to aggregate with ristocetin due to the glycoprotein Ib defect, with normal or enhanced aggregation with ADP, collagen, and epinephrine (Bithell et al, 1972). Flow cytometric analysis shows decreased glycoprotein Ibα expression on platelets, allowing for rapid diagnosis (Cohn et al, 1997). PCR analysis may also be used to demonstrate specific defects in glycoproteins Ib and IX (Bray, 1994). Patients are treated with platelet transfusions and desmopressin during severe bleeding episodes.

Wiskott-Aldrich syndrome is an X-linked disorder characterized by thrombocytopenia, small platelets, recurrent infections, eczema, and a predisposition to the development of malignancy (Sullivan et al, 1994). There are abnormalities in T cell immunity as well as deficiencies in platelet, lymphocyte, and monocyte expression of the surface glycoprotein CD43 (Parkman et al, 1981). Platelets have decreased survival times, and many patients show qualitative defects in storage pool adenine nucleotides (Baldini, 1972). The blood film shows varying thrombocytopenia and very small platelets. Bleeding times are usually increased, and platelet aggregation tests have variable results. Thrombocytopenia improves with splenectomy. Marrow

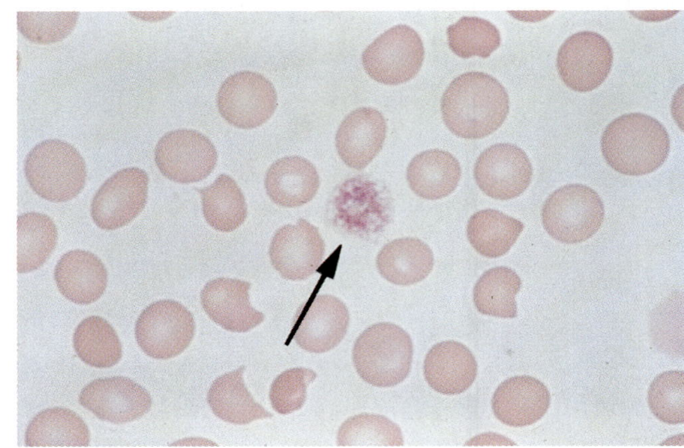

Figure 6–33

Bernard-Soulier disease, peripheral blood. This film shows a giant platelet. Wright-Giemsa stain.

transplantation is curative, particularly if performed early in the course of the disease before significant immunodeficiency evolves (Mullen et al, 1993).

SUGGESTED READINGS

Sickle Cell Disease

Eaton WA, Hofrichter J: Hemoglobin S gelation and sickle cell disease. Blood 70:1245–1266, 1987.

Hayes RJ, Beckford M, Grandison Y, et al: The haemotology of steady state homozygous sickle cell disease: frequency distributions, variation with age and sex, longitudinal observations. Br J Haematol 59:369–382, 1985.

Johnson CS: Sickle cell anemia. JAMA 254:1958–1963, 1985.

Lane PA: Sickle cell disease. Pediatr Hematol 43:639–664, 1996.

Powars DR: Natural history of sickle cell disease: the first ten years. Semin Hematol 12:267–285, 1975.

Other Hemoglobinopathies

Ballas SK, Lewis CN, Noone AM, et al: Clinical, hematological, and biochemical features of Hb SC disease. Am J Hematol 13:37–51, 1982.

Glader BE, Look KA: Hematologic disorders in children from southeast Asia. Pediatr Hematol 43:665–681, 1996.

Lachant NA: Hemoglobin E: an emerging hemoglobinopathy in the United States. Am J Hematol 25:449–462, 1987.

Tuttle AH, Koch B: Clinical and hematological manifestations of hemoglobin CS disease in children. J Pediatr 56:331–342, 1960.

Willamson D: The unstable hemoglobins. Blood Rev 7:146–163, 1993.

Hereditary Spherocytosis and Other Membrane Abnormalities

Cynober T, Mohandas N, Tchernia G: Red cell abnormalities in hereditary spherocytosis: relevance to diagnosis and understanding of the variable expression of clinical severity. J Lab Clin Med 128:259–269, 1996.

Lusher JM, Barnhart MI: The spleen as related to hematologic disorders of childhood, continued: the role of the spleen in the pathophysiology of hereditary spherocytosis and hereditary elliptocytosis. Am J Pediatr Hematol Oncol 2:31–39, 1980.

Palek J: Hereditary elliptocytosis, spherocytosis and related disorders: consequences of a deficiency or a mutation of membrane skeletal proteins. Blood Rev 1:147–168, 1987.

Palek J, Jarolim P: Clinical expression and laboratory detection of red blood cell membrane protein mutations. Semin Hematol 30:249–283, 1993.

Pyruvate Kinase and Other Red Cell Enzyme Deficiencies

Tanaka KR, Zerez CR: Red cell enzymopathies of the glycolytic pathway. Semin Hematol 27:165–185, 1990.

Valentine WN, Paglia DE: Erythrocyte enzymopathies, hemolytic anemia, and multisystem disease: an annotated review. Blood 64:583–591, 1984.

G6PD Deficiency

Arese P, De Flora A: Pathophysiology of hemolysis in glucose-6-phosphate dehydrogenase deficiency. Semin Hematol 27:1–40, 1990.

Beutler E: The genetics of glucose-6-phosphate dehydrogenase deficiency. Semin Hematol 27:137–164, 1990.

Beutler E: Glucose-6-phosphate dehydrogenase deficiency. N Engl J Med 324:169–174, 1991.

Iron Deficiency

Beutler E: The common anemias. JAMA 259:2433–2437, 1988.

Bothwell TH: Overview and mechanisms of iron regulation. Nutr Rev 53:237–245, 1995.

Dallman PR: Diagnosis of anemia and iron deficiency: analytic and biological variations of laboratory tests. Am J Clin Nutr 39:937–941, 1984.

Dallman PR, Siimes MA, Stekel A: Iron deficiency in infancy and childhood. Am J Clin Nutr 33:86–118, 1980.

Hastka J, Lasserre J, Schwarzbeck A, et al: Laboratory tests of iron status: correlation or common sense? Clin Chem 42:718–724, 1996.

Sideroblastic Anemia

Nusbaum NJ: Genetic bases for sideroblastic anemia. Am J Hematol 37:41–44, 1991.

Megaloblastic Anemia

Allen RH, Stabler SP, Savage DG, et al: Diagnosis of cobalamin deficiency I: usefulness of serum methylmalonic acid and total homocysteine concentrations. Am J Hematol 34:90–98, 1992.

Beutler E: The common anemias. JAMA 259:2433–2437, 1988.

Chung ASM, Pearson WN, Darby WJ, et al: Folic acid, vitamin B_6, pantothenic acid and vitamin B_{12} in human dietaries. Am J Clin Nutr 9:573–582, 1961.

Lindenbaum J, Savage DG, Stabler SP, et al: Diagnosis of cobalamin deficiency: II. Relative sensitivities of serum cobalamin, methylmalonic acid, and total homocysteine concentrations. Am J Hematol 34:99–107, 1990.

McIntyre OR, Sullivan LW, Jefries GH, et al: Pernicious anemia in childhood. N Engl J Med 272:981–986, 1965.

Lead and Toxins

Kaul B, Slavin G, Davidow B: Free erythrocyte protoporphyrin and zinc protoporphyrin measurements compared as primary screening methods for detection of lead poisoning. Clin Chem 29:1467–1470, 1983.

Paglia DE, Valentine WN, Dahlgren JG: Effects of low-level lead exposure on pyrimidine 5′-nucleotidase and other erythrocyte enzymes. J Clin Invest 56:1164–1169, 1975.

Hemolytic Anemias

Habibi B, Homberg J, Schaison G, et al: Autoimmune hemolytic anemia in children. Am J Med 56:61–69, 1974.

Judd WJ, Luban NLC, Ness PM, et al: Pernatal and perinatal immunohematology: recommendations for serologic management of the fetus, newborn infant and obstetric patient. Transfusion 30:175–183, 1990.

Parker CJ: Molecular basis of paroxysmal nocturnal hemoglobinuria. Stem Cells 14:396–411, 1996.

Pirofsky B: Clinical aspects of autoimmune hemolytic anemia. Semin Hematol 13:251–265, 1976.

Whittle MJ: Rhesus haemolytic disease. Arch Dis Child 67:65–68, 1992.

Red Cell Aplasia

Alter BP, Nathan DG: Red cell aplasia in children. Arch Dis Child 54:263–267, 1979.

Brown KE, Young NS: Parvoviruses and bone marrow failure. Stem Cells 14:151–163, 1996.

Freedman MH, Saunder EF: Transient erythroblastopenia of childhood: varied pathogenesis. Am J Hematol 14:247–254, 1983.

Freedman MH: Pure red cell aplasia in childhood and adolescence: pathogenesis and approaches to diagnosis. Br J Haematol 85:246–253, 1993.

Aplastic Anemia

Alter BP: Aplastic anemia. Am J Pediatr Hematol Oncol 2:119–139, 1980.

Fonseca R, Tefferi A: Practical aspects in the diagnosis and management of aplastic anemia. Am J Med Sci 313:159–169, 1997.

Myelomonocytic Disorders

Bain BJ: Eosinophilic leukaemias and the idiopathic hypereosinophilic syndrome. Br J Haematol 95:2–9, 1996.

Bernini JC: Diagnosis and management of chronic neutropenia during childhood. Pediatr Clin North Am 43:773–792, 1996.

Boxer LA, Blackwood A: Leukocyte disorders: quantitative and qualitative disorders of the neutrophil, part 2. Pediatr Rev 17:47–50, 1996.

Forrest CB, Forehand JR, Axtell RA, et al: Clinical features and current management of chronic granulomatous disease. Hematol Oncol Clin North Am 2:253–266, 1988.

Maldonado JE, Hanlon DG: Monocytosis: a current appraisal. Mayo Clin Proc 40:248–259, 1965.

Nauseef WM: Myeloperoxidase deficiency. Hematol Oncol Clin North Am 2:135–158, 1988.

Palmer SE, Stephens K, Dale DC: Genetics, phenotype and natural history of autosomal dominant cyclic hematopoiesis. Am J Med Genet 66:413–422, 1996.

Weller PF, Bubley GJ: The idiopathic hypereosinophilic syndrome. Blood 83:2759–2779, 1994.
Welte K, Dale D: Pathophysiology and treatment of severe chronic neutropenia. Ann Hematol 72:158–165, 1996.

Mast Cell Disorders

Golkar L, Bernhard JD: Mastocytosis. Lancet 349:1379–1385, 1997.
Horny HP, Parawaresch MR, Lennert K: Bone marrow findings in systemic mastocytosis. Hum Pathol 16:808–814, 1985.
Kettelhut BV, Metcalfe DD: Pediatric mastocytosis. Ann Allergy 73: 197–202, 1994.
Kettelhut BV, Parker RI, Travis WD, Metcalfe DD: Hematopathology of the bone marrow in pediatric cutaneous mastocytosis. Am J Clin Pathol 91:558–562, 1989.
Marone G, Spadero G, Genovese A: Biology, diagnosis and therapy of mastocytosis. Chem Immunol 62:1–21, 1995.
Travis WD, Li C-Y, Yam LT, et al: Significance of systemic mast cell disease with associated hematologic disorders. Cancer 62:965–972, 1988b.

Megakaryocytic and Platelet Disorders

George JN, Caen JP, Nurden AT: Glanzmann's thrombasthenia: the spectrum of clinical disease. Blood 75:1383–1395, 1990.
Hedberg VA, Lipton JM: Thrombocytopenia with absent radii: a review of 100 cases. Am J Pediatr Hematol Oncol 10:51–64, 1988.
Jantunen E: Inherited giant platelet disorders. Eur J Haematol 53:191–196, 1994.
Seligsohn U, Peretz H: Molecular genetics aspects of factor XI deficiency and Glanzmann thrombasthenia. Haemostasis 24:81–85, 1994.
Sullivan KE, Mullen CA, Blaese RM, et al: A multiinstitutional survey of the Wiskott-Aldrich syndrome. J Pediatr 125:876–885, 1994.

REFERENCES

Abshire TC: The anemia of inflammation: a common cause of childhood anemia. Pediatr Hematol 43:623–637, 1996.
Adams JA, Barrett AJ: Haematopoietic stimulators in the serum of patients with severe aplastic anaemia. Br J Haematol 52:327–335, 1982.
Agre P, Asimos A, Casella JF, et al: Inheritance pattern and clinical response to splenectomy as a reflection of erythrocyte spectrin deficiency in hereditary spherocytosis. N Engl J Med 315: 1579–1583, 1986.
Agre P, Orringer EP, Bennett V: Deficient red-cell spectrin in severe, recessively inherited spherocytosis. N Engl J Med 306: 1155–1161, 1982.
Ajlouni K, Doeblin TD: The syndrome of hepatitis and aplastic anemia. Br J Haematol 27:345–355, 1974.
Allen RH, Stabler SP, Savage DG, et al: Diagnosis of cobalamin deficiency I: usefulness of serum methylmalonic acid and total homocysteine concentrations. Am J Hematol 34:90–98, 1990.
Alter BP: Aplastic anemia. Am J Pediatr Hematol Oncol 2:119–139, 1980.
Alter BP: Fanconi's anemia. Am J Pediatr Hematol Oncol 14: 170–176, 1992.
Alter BP, Nathan DG: Red cell aplasia in children. Arch Dis Child 54:263–267, 1979.
Annest JL, Pirkle JL, Makuc D, et al: Chronological trend in blood lead levels between 1976 and 1980. N Engl J Med 308: 1373–1377, 1983.
Arese P, De Flora A: Pathophysiology of hemolysis in glucose-6-phosphate dehydrogenase deficiency. Semin Hematol 27:1–40, 1990.
Athens JW, Haab OP, Raab SO, et al: Leukokinetic studies: IV. The total blood, circulating and marginal granulocyte pools and the granulocyte turnover rate in normal subjects. J Clin Invest 40:989–995, 1961.
Bacigalupo A, Hows J, Gluckman E, et al: Bone marrow transplantation (BMT) versus immunosuppression for the treatment of severe aplastic anaemia (SAA): a report of the EBMT SAA Working Party. Br J Haematol 70:177–182, 1988.
Bain BJ: Blood film features of sickle cell-haemoglobin C disease. Br J Haematol 83:516–518, 1993.
Baldini MG: Nature of the platelet defect in the Wiskott-Aldrich syndrome. Ann NY Acad Sci 301:437–444, 1972.
Ballas SK, Lewis CN, Noone AM, et al: Clinical, hematological, and biochemical features of Hb SC disease. Am J Hematol 13:37–51, 1982.
Ballas SK, Smith ED: Red blood cell changes during the evolution of the sickle cell painful crisis. Blood 79:2154–2163, 1992.
Baronciani L, Beutler E: Analysis of pyruvate kinase–deficiency mutations that produce nonspherocytic hemolytic anemia. Proc Natl Acad Sci USA 90:4324–4327, 1993.
Barrett-Connor E: Bacterial infection and sickle cell anemia. Medicine 50:97–112, 1971.
Bateman HE, Scroff V, Centeno LV, et al: Systemic mastocytosis: a diagnostic challenge. Ann Allergy, Asthma, Immunol 74:379–386, 1995.
Baum KF, Dunn DT, Maude GH, et al: The painful crisis of homozygous sickle cell disease. Arch Intern Med 147:1231–1234, 1987.
Bernini JC: Diagnosis and management of chronic neutropenia during childhood. Pediatr Clin North Am 43:773–792, 1996.
Bessman JD, Gilmer PR, Gardner FH: Improved classification of anemias by MCV and RDW. Am J Clin Pathol 80:322–326, 1983.
Bessman JD, Williams LJ, Gilmer PR: Platelet size in health and hematologic disease. Am J Clin Pathol 78:150–153, 1982.
Beutler E: The common anemias. JAMA 259:2433–2437, 1988.
Beutler E: The genetics of glucose-6-phosphate dehydrogenase deficiency. Semin Hematol 27:137–164, 1990.
Beutler E: Glucose-6-phosphate dehydrogenase deficiency. N Engl J Med 324:169–174, 1991.
Beutler E: The molecular biology of G6PD variants and other red cell enzyme defects. Ann Rev Med 43:47–59, 1992.
Beutler E: Why has the autohemolysis test not gone the way of the cephalin flocculation test? Blood 51:109–110, 1978.
Beutler E, Baranko PV, Feagler J, et al: Hemolytic anemia due to pyrimidine-5′-nucleotidase deficiency: report of eight cases in six families. Blood 56:251–255, 1980.
Beutler E, Blume KG, Kaplan JC, et al: International Committee for Standardization in Haematology: recommended methods for red-cell enzyme analysis. Br J Haematol 35:331–340, 1977.
Beutler E, Blume KG, Kaplan JC, et al: International Committee for Standardization in Haematology: recommended screening test for glucose-6-phosphate dehydrogenase (G-6-PD) deficiency. Br J Haematol 43:469–477, 1979.
Beutler E, Kuhl W, Fox M, et al: Prenatal diagnosis of glucose-6-phosphate-dehydrogenase deficiency. Acta Haematol 87:103–104, 1992.
Beutler E, Kuhl W, Gelbart T, et al: DNA sequence abnormalities of human glucose-6-phosphate dehydrogenase variants. J Biol Chem 266:4145–4150, 1991.
Beutler E, Mitchell M: Special modifications of the fluorescent screening method for glucose-6-phosphate dehydrogenase deficiency. Blood 32:816–818, 1968.
Bienzle U, Lucas AO, Ayeni O, et al: Glucose-6-phosphate dehydrogenase and malaria: greater resistance of females heterozygous for enzyme deficiency and of males with nondeficient variant. Lancet 1:107–110, 1972.
Bithell TC, Parekh SJ, Strong RR: Platelet-function studies in the Bernard-Soulier syndrome. Ann NY Acad Sci 201:145–160, 1972.
Boivin P, Galand C, Hakim J, et al: Acquired erythroenzymopathies in blood disorders: study of 200 cases. Br J Haematol 31:531–543, 1975.
Bonilla MA, Gillio AP, Ruggeiro M, et al: Effects of recombinant human granulocyte colony-stimulating factor on neutropenia in patients with congenital agranulocytosis. N Engl J Med 320:1574–1580, 1989.
Boogaerts MA, Verwilghen RL: Variants of congenital dyserythropoietic anaemia: an update. Haematologia 15:211–219, 1982.
Bookchin RM, Nagel RL: Interaction between human hemoglobins: sickling and related phenomena. Semin Hematol 11:577–595, 1974.
Borgna-Pignatti C, Marradi P, Pinelli L, et al: Thiamine-responsive anemia in DIDMOAD syndrome. J Pediatr 114:405–410, 1989.
Bottomley SS, Healy HM, Brandenburg MA, et al: 5-aminolevulinate synthase in sideroblastic anemias: mRNA enzyme activity levels in bone marrow cells. Am J Hematol 41:76–83, 1992.
Bowman HS, Procopio F: Hereditary non-spherocytic hemolytic anemia of the pyruvate-kinase deficient type. Ann Intern Med 58:567–591, 1963.

Bowman JM, Pollock JM, Manning FA, et al: Maternal K blood group alloimmunization. Obstet Gynecol 79:239–244, 1992.

Boxer LA, Blackwood A: Leukocyte disorders: quantitative and qualitative disorders of the neutrophil, part 2. Pediatr Rev 17:47–50, 1996.

Bray PF: Inherited diseases of platelet glycoproteins: considerations for rapid molecular characterization. Thromb Haemost 72:492–502, 1994.

Brouwers HAA, van Ertbruggen I, Alsbach GPJ, et al: What is the best predictor of the severity of ABO-haemolytic disease of the newborn? Lancet 335:641–644, 1988.

Brown KE, Tisdale J, Barrett AJ, et al: Hepatitis-associated aplastic anemia. N Engl J Med 336:1059–1064, 1997.

Brown KE, Young NS: Parvoviruses and bone marrow failure. Stem Cells 14:151–163, 1996.

Buchanan GR, Bottomley SS, Nitschke R: Bone marrow delta-aminolaevulinate synthase deficiency in a female with congenital sideroblastic anemia. Blood 55:109–115, 1980.

Buchanan GR, Glader BE: Leukocyte counts in children with sickle cell disease. Am J Dis Child 132:396–398, 1978.

Bunin N, Leahey A, Kamani N, et al: Bone marrow transplantation in pediatric patients with severe aplastic anemia: cyclophosphamide and anti-thymocyte globulin conditioning followed by recombinant human granulocyte-macrophage colony stimulating factor. J Pediatr Hematol Oncol 18:68–71, 1996.

Buss DH, Stuart JJ, Lipscomb GE: The incidence of thrombotic and hemorrhagic disorders in association with extreme thrombocytosis: an analysis of 129 cases. Am J Hematol 20:365–372, 1985.

Calvino MC, Maldonado MS, Otheo E, et al: Bone marrow transplantation in chronic granulomatous disease. Eur J Pediatr 155:877–879, 1996.

Camitta BM, Thomas ED, Nathan DG, et al: A prospective study of androgens and bone marrow transplantation for treatment of severe aplastic anemia. Blood 53:504–514, 1979.

Carrell RW, Kay R: A simple method for the detection of unstable haemoglobins. Br J Haemotol 23:615–619, 1972.

Cathie IAB: Erythrogenesis imperfecta. Arch Dis Child 25:313–324, 1950.

Cazzola M, Barosi G, Bergamaschi G, et al: Iron loading in congenital dyserythropoietic anaemias and congenital sideroblastic anaemias. Br J Haematol 54:649–654, 1983.

Chernoff AI, Minnich V, Na-Nakorn S, et al: The clinical, hematologic, and genetic characteristics of the hemoglobin E syndromes. J Lab Clin Med 47:455–489, 1956.

Chilcote RR, Le Beau MM, Dampier C, et al: Association of red cell spherocytosis with deletion of the short arm of chromosome 8. Blood 69:156–159, 1987.

Chung ASM, Pearson WN, Darby WJ, et al: Folic acid, vitamin B_6, pantothenic acid and vitamin B_{12} in human dietaries. Am J Clin Nutr 9:573–582, 1961.

Clark R, Peters S, Hoy T, et al: Prognostic importance of hypodiploid hemopoietic precursors in myelodysplastic syndromes. N Engl J Med 314:1472–1475, 1986.

Coetzer TL, Lawler J, Liu SC, et al: Partial ankyrin and spectrin deficiency in severe, atypical hereditary spherocytosis. N Engl J Med 318:230–234, 1988.

Coetzer T, Palek J, Lawler J, et al: Structural and functional heterogeneity of α spectrin mutations involving the spectrin heterodimer self-association site: relationships to hematologic expression of homozygous hereditary elliptocytosis and hereditary pyropoikilocytosis. Blood 75:2235–2244, 1990.

Cohn RJ, Sherman GG, Glencross DK: Flow cytometric analysis of platelet surface glycoproteins in the diagnosis of Bernard-Soulier syndrome. Pediatr Hematol Oncol 14:43–50, 1997.

Coller BS, Seligsohn U, Peretz H, et al: Glanzmann thrombasthenia: new insights from an historical perspective. Semin Hematol 31:301–311, 1994.

Collins RA, Harper AE, Schreiber M, et al: The folic acid and vitamin B_{12} content of the milk of various species. J Nutr 43:313–321, 1951.

Consensus Conference: Newborn screening for sickle cell disease and other hemoglobinopathies. JAMA 258:1205–1208, 1987.

Cotter PD, Baumann M, Bishop DF: Enzymatic defect in "X-linked" sideroblastic anemia: molecular evidence for erythroid δ-aminolevulinate synthase deficiency. Proc Natl Acad Sci USA 89: 4028–4032, 1992.

Cotter PD, May A, Fitzsimons EJ, et al: Late-onset X-linked sideroblastic anemia: missense mutations in the erythroid δ-aminolevulinate synthase *(ALAS2)* gene in two pyridoxine-responsive patients initially diagnosed with acquired refractory anemia and ringed sideroblasts. J Clin Invest 96:2090–2096, 1995.

Croft JD, Swisher SN, Gilliland BG, et al: Coombs'-test positivity induced by drugs. Ann Intern Med 68:176–187, 1968.

Crookston JH, Crookston MC, Rosse WF: Red-cell abnormalities in HEMPAS (hereditary erythroblastic multinuclearity with a positive acidified-serum test). B J Haematol 23:83–91, 1972.

Cullen MR, Rado T, Waldron JA, et al: Bone marrow injury in lithographers exposed to glycol ethers and organic solvents used in multicolor offset and ultraviolet curing printing processes. Arch Environ Health 38:347–354, 1983.

Dale DC: Hematopoietic growth factors for the treatment of severe chronic neutropenia. Stem Cells 13:94–100, 1995.

Dale DC, Hammond WP: Cyclic neutropenia: a clinical review. Blood Rev 2:178–185, 1988.

Dallman PR: Diagnosis of anemia and iron deficiency: analytic and biological variations of laboratory tests. Am J Clin Nutr 39: 937–941, 1984.

Dallman PR, Siimes MA, Stekel A: Iron deficiency in infancy and childhood. Am J Clin Nutr 33:86–118, 1980.

Dallman PR, Yip R, Johnson C: Prevalence and causes of anemia in the United States, 1976 to 1980. Am J Clin Nutr 39:437–445, 1984.

Das KC, Mohanty D, Garewal G: Cytogenetics in nutritional megaloblastic anaemia: prolonged persistence of chromosomal abnormalities in lymphocytes after remission. Acta Haematol 76: 146–154, 1986.

Davidson RJ, How J, Lessels S: Acquired stomatocytosis: its prevalence and significance in routine haematology. Scand J Haematol 19:47–53, 1977.

Davis WM, Ross AOM: Thrombocytosis and thrombocythemia: the laboratory and clinical significance of an elevated platelet count. Am J Clin Pathol 59:243–247, 1973.

Degos L, Tobelem G, Lethielleux P, et al: Molecular defect in platelets from patients with Bernard-Soulier syndrome. Blood 50:899–903, 1977.

de Klerk G, Rosengarten CJ, Vet RJWM, et al: Serum erythropoietin (ESF) titers in anemia. Blood 58:1164–1170, 1981.

Dessypris EN, Krantz SB, Roloff JS, et al: Mode of action of the IgG inhibitor of erythropoiesis in transient erythroblastopenia of childhood. Blood 59:114–123, 1982.

Devine DV, Gluck WL, Rosse WF, et al: Acute myeloblastic leukemia in paroxysmal nocturnal hemoglobinuria. J Clin Invest 79: 314–317, 1987.

Diamond LK, Allen, M, Magill FB: Congenital (erythroid) hypoplastic anemia. Am J Dis Child 102:403–415, 1961.

Diamond LK, Wang WC, Alter BP: Congenital hypoplastic anemia. Adv Pediatr 22:349–378, 1976.

Dokal I: Dyskeratosis congenita: an inherited bone marrow failure syndrome. Br J Haematol 92:775–779, 1996.

Doney K, Leisenring W, Storb R, et al: Primary treatment of acquired aplastic anemia: outcomes with bone marrow transplantation and immmunosuppressive therapy. Ann Intern Med 126:107–115, 1997.

Dong F, Brynes RK, Tidow N, et al: Mutations in the gene for the granulocyte colony-stimulating-factor receptor in patients with acute myeloid leukemia preceeded by severe congenital neutropenia. N Engl J Med 333:487–493, 1995.

Dong F, Dale DC, Bonilla MA, et al: Mutations in the granulocyte colony-stimulating factor receptor gene in patients with severe congenital neutropenia. Leukemia 11:120–125, 1997.

Douglass CC, Twomey JJ: Transient stomatocytosis with hemolysis: a previously unrecognized complication of alcoholism. Ann Intern Med 72:159–164, 1970.

Eaton JW, Jacob HS, White JG: Membrane abnormalities of irreversibly sickled cells. Semin Hematol 16:52–64, 1979.

Eaton WA, Hofrichter J: Hemoglobin S gelation and sickle cell disease. Blood 70:1245–1266, 1987.

Eber SW, Lande WM, Iarocci TA, et al: Hereditary stomatocytosis: consistent association with an integral membrane protein deficiency. Br J Haematol 72:452–455, 1989.

Eber SW, Pekrun A, Neufeldt A, et al: Prevalence of increased osmotic fragility of erythrocytes in German blood donors: screening using a modified glycerol lysis test. Ann Hematol 64:88–92, 1992.

Emerson PM, Wilkinson JH: Lactate dehydrogenase in the diagnosis and assessment of response to treatment of megaloblastic anaemia. Br J Haematol 12:678–688, 1966.

Emond AM, Collis R, Darvill D, et al: Acute splenic sequestration in homozygous sickle cell disease: natural history and management. J Pediatr 107:201–206, 1985.

Enquist RW, Gockerman JP, Jenis EH, et al: Type II congenital dyserythropoietic anemia. Ann Intern Med 77:371–376, 1972.

Evans EA, Mohandas N: Membrane-associated sickle hemoglobin: a major determinant of sickle erythrocyte rigidity. Blood 70: 1443–1449, 1987.

Fabry ME, Kaul DK, Raventos C, et al: Some aspects of the pathophysiology of homozygous Hb CC erythrocytes. J Clin Invest 67: 1284–1291, 1981.

Fairbanks VF, Beutler E: A simple method for detection of erythrocyte glucose-6-phosphate dehydrogenase deficiency (G-6-PD spot test). Blood 20:591–601, 1962.

Fairbanks VF, Gilchrist GS, Brimhall B, et al: Hemoglobin E trait reexamined: a cause of microcytosis and erythrocytosis. Blood 53: 109–115, 1979.

Fairbanks VF, Wahner HW, Phyliky RL: Tests for pernicious anemia: the "Schilling test." Mayo Clin Proc 58:541–544, 1983.

Falter MI, Robinson MG: Autosomal dominant inheritance and amino aciduria in Blackfan-Diamond anaemia. J Med Genet 9:64–66, 1972.

Finch CA, Coleman DH, Motulsky AG, et al: Erythrokinetics in pernicious anemia. Blood 11:807–820, 1956.

Finch CA, Huebers H: Perspectives in iron metabolism. N Engl J Med 306:1520–1528, 1982.

Flaum MA, Schoole RT, Fauci AS, et al: A clinicopathologic correlation of the idiopathic hypereosinophilic syndrome: I. hematologic manifestations. Blood 58:1012–1020, 1981.

Fomon SJ, Ziegler EE, Nelson SE, et al: Cow milk feeding in infancy: gastrointestinal blood loss and iron nutritional status. J Pediatr 98:540–545, 1981.

Fonseca R, Tefferi A: Practical aspects in the diagnosis and management of aplastic anemia. Am J Med Sci 313:159–169, 1997.

Forrest CB, Forehand JR, Axtell RA, et al: Clinical features and current management of chronic granulomatous disease. Hematol Oncol Clin North Am 2:253–266, 1988.

Freedman MH: "Recurrent" erythroblastopenia of childhood. Am J Dis Child 137:458–460, 1983.

Freedman ML, Karpatkin S: Short communication: elevated platelet count and megathrombocyte number in sickle cell anemia. Blood 46:579–582, 1975.

Frischer H, Bowman J: Hemoglobin E, and oxidatively unstable mutation. J Lab Clin Med 85:531–539, 1975.

Fukada MN, Dell A, Scartezzini P: Primary defect of congenital dyserythropoietic anemia type II. J Biol Chem 262:7195–7206, 1987.

Fukada MN, Klier G, Yu J, et al: Anomalous clustering of underglycosylated band 3 in erythrocytes and their precursor cells in congenital dyserythropoietic anemia type II. Blood 68:521–529, 1986.

Galacteros F, Kleman K, Caburi-Martin J, et al: Cord blood screening for hemoglobin abnormalities by thin layer isoelectric focusing. Blood 56:1068–1071, 1980.

Garratty G, Nance S, Lloyd M, et al: Fatal immune hemolytic anemia due to cefotetan. Transfusion 32:269–271, 1992.

George JN, Caen JP, Nurden AT: Glanzmann's thrombasthenia: the spectrum of clinical disease. Blood 75:1383–1395, 1990.

Gewirtz AM, Sacchetti MK, Bien R, et al: Cell-mediated suppression of megakaryocytopoiesis in acquired amegakaryocytic thrombocytopenic purpura. Blood 68:619–626, 1986.

Gibble JW, Ness PM: Maternal immunity to red cell antigens and fetal transfusion. Clin Lab Med 12:553–576, 1992.

Gibson SLM, Goldberg A: Defects in haem synthesis in mammalian tissues in experimental lead poisoning and experimental porphyria. Clin Sci 38:63–72, 1970.

Gilliland BC: Coombs-negative immune hemolytic anemia. Semin Hematol 13:267–275, 1976.

Glader BE, Backer K, Diamond LK: Elevated erythrocyte adenosine deaminase activity in congenital hypoplastic anemia. N Engl J Med 309:1486–1490, 1983.

Glader BE, Fortier N, Albala MM, et al: Congenital hemolytic anemia associated with dehydrated erythrocytes and increased potassium loss. N Engl J Med 291:491–496, 1974.

Glazer HS, Muelle JF, Jarrold T, et al: The effect of vitamin B_{12} and folic acid on nucleic acid composition of the bone marrow of patients with megaloblastic anemia. J Lab Clin Med 43:905–913, 1954.

Godal HC, Heisto H: High prevalence of increased osmotic fragility of red blood cells among Norwegian blood donors. Scand J Haematol 27:30–34, 1981.

Godal HC, Nyvold N, Rustad A: The osmotic fragility of red blood cells: a re-evaluation of technical conditions. Scand J Haematol 23:55–58, 1979.

Goldstein AR, Anderson MJ, Serjeant GR: Parvovirus associated aplastic crisis in homozygous sickle cell disease. Arch Dis Child 62:585–588, 1987.

Golkar L, Bernhard JD: Mastocytosis. Lancet 349:1379–1385, 1997.

Goodman JR, Hall SG: Accumulation of iron in mitochondria of erythroblasts. Br J Haematol 13:335–340, 1967.

Goodman SR, Krebs KE, Whitfield CF, et al: Spectrin and related molecules. CRC Crit Rev Biochem 23:171–234, 1988.

Goudsmit R, Beckers D, de Bruijne JI, et al: Congenital dyserythropoietic anaemia, type II. Br J Haematol 23:97–105, 1972.

Goyer RA, Moore JF: Cellular effects of lead. Adv Exp Med Biol 48:447–462, 1974.

Graham DL, Gastineau DA: Paroxysmal nocturnal hemoglobinuria as a marker for clonal myelopathy. Am J Med 93:671–674, 1992.

Grau JM, Bosch X, Salgado AC, et al: Human immunodeficiency virus (HIV) and aplastic anemia. Ann Intern Med 110:576–577, 1989.

Habibi B: Drug induced red blood cell autoantibodies co-developed with drug specific antibodies causing haemolytic anaemias. Br J Haematol 61:139–143, 1985.

Habibi B, Homberg J, Schaison G, et al: Autoimmune hemolytic anemia in children. Am J Med 56:61–69, 1974.

Haddad E, Le Deist F, Blanche S, et al: Treatment of Chédiak-Higashi syndrome by allogenic bone marrow transplantation: report of 10 cases. Blood 85:3328–3333, 1995.

Hadley T, Saul A, Lamont G, et al: Resistance of Melanesian elliptocytes (ovalocytes) to invasion by *Plasmodium knowlesi* and *Plasmodium falciparum* malaria parasites in vitro. J Clin Invest 71:780–782, 1983.

Hagler L, Pastore RA, Bergin JJ: Aplastic anemia following viral hepatitis: report of two fatal cases and literature review. Medicine 54:139–164, 1975.

Ham TH, Dingle JH: Studies on destruction of red blood cells: chronic hemolytic anemia with paroxysmal nocturnal hemoglobinuria: certain immunological aspects of the hemolytic mechanism with special reference to serum complement. J Clin Invest 18: 657–672, 1939.

Hanada T, Koike K, Hirano C, et al: Childhood transient erythroblastopenia complicated by thrombocytopenia and neutropenia. Eur J Haematol 42:77–80, 1989.

Hardy WR, Anderson RE: The hypereosinophilic syndromes. Ann Intern Med 68:1220–1229, 1968.

Harris JW: Parvovirus B19 for the hematologist. Am J Hematol 39:119–130, 1992.

Hartmann RC, Jenkins DE: The "sugar-water" test for paroxysmal nocturnal hemoglobinuria. N Engl J Med 275:155–157, 1965.

Hassoun H, Palek J: Hereditary spherocytosis: a review of the clinical and molecular aspects of the disease. Blood Rev 10:129–147, 1996.

Hayes RJ, Beckford M, Grandison Y, et al: The haemotology of steady state homozygous sickle cell disease: frequency distributions, variation with age and sex, longitudinal observations. Br J Haematol 59:369–382, 1985.

Hebbel RP, Vercellotti GM: The endothelial biology of sickle cell disease. J Lab Clin Med 129:288–293, 1997.

Hedberg VA, Lipton JM: Thrombocytopenia with absent radii: a review of 100 cases. Am J Pediatr Hematol Oncol 10:51–64, 1988.

Heimpel H, Forteza-Vila J, Queisser W, et al: Electron and light microscopic study. Blood 37:299–310, 1971.

Heisel MA, Ortega JA: Factors influencing prognosis in childhood autoimmune hemolytic anemia. Am J Pediatr Hematol Oncol 5:147–152, 1983.

Heller P, Best WR, Nelson RB, et al: Clinical implications of sickle-cell trait and glucose-6-phosphate dehydrogenase deficiency in hospitalized black male patients. N Engl J Med 300:1001–1005, 1979.

Table 6–36
Comparison of Major Subtypes of α- and β-Thalassemias Based on Clinical Severity

α-Thalassemia	β-Thalassemia	Clinical Features
Hydrops fetalis with Hg Bart	Thalassemia major	Severe anemia (<7 g/dl) α: fetal or neonatal death β: growth retardation, splenomegaly, bony deformities
HgH	Thalassemia intermedia	Chronic hemolytic anemia (7–10 g/dl)
α-Thalassemia trait	Thalassemia minor (trait)	Little or no anemia (>10 g/dl)

Constant Spring, Hg Lepore, and HgE (Lukens, 1999; Weatherall, 1995).

The clinical features of thalassemic patients vary among the types of thalassemia. The type reflects specific defects of globin genes and their expression (Lukens, 1999; Weatherall, 1995) (see "Pathogenesis"). Alpha- and β-thalassemias are divided into three subtypes by clinical severity (Table 6–36). The salient clinical features in thalassemia include anemia, jaundice, hepatosplenomegaly, skeletal abnormalities, extramedullary hematopoiesis, and delayed growth and sexual development.

Hydrops fetalis with Hg Bart is the most severe form of thalassemia and is frequently observed in Southeast Asian populations. The affected die in utero or shortly after birth. Owing to the total lack of α-globin chain and the high oxygen affinity of Hg Bart (γ-globin chain tetramer), the fetus develops cardiopulmonary failure and a grossly hydropic appearance indistinguishable from hydrops fetalis in isoimmune hemolytic diseases (Lie-Injo et al, 1968). β-Thalassemia major, or Cooley anemia, is the most severe form of β-thalassemia and is characterized by progressive anemia and splenomegaly after the first few months of life; hepatomegaly and mild jaundice; skeletal changes, especially craniofacial deformities resulting in the "thalassemic facies;" osteopenia predisposing to pathologic fractures of long bones and vertebrae; growth retardation; and delayed development of secondary sexual characteristics. After the first decade, many patients have such complications as sterile pericarditis, myocardial hemosiderosis, small airway obstruction, and hyperinflation or restrictive lung disease (Engle, 1964; Hoyt et al, 1986). Hypersplenism may produce thrombocytopenia and leukopenia in addition to progressive anemia, for which transfusions are usually given (Weatherall, 1995).

Patients with thalassemia intermedia do not require transfusions except during intercurrent illnesses. The disease is generally less severe than thalassemia major, and survival into adulthood is expected. HgH disease varies in clinical severity, but most cases are comparable to β-thalassemia intermedia. Approximately one third of patients have skeletal changes, and mental retardation has been noted rarely. Anemia is accentuated during infections and after exposure to oxidant drugs. The traits α-thalassemia and β-thalassemia minor may produce slight anemia or no clinical symptoms. Silent carriers have neither anemia nor abnormal red cell morphologic features.

The prognosis of thalassemia major was grim before the advent of hypertransfusion therapy. Most patients died in the first decade from severe anemia and intercurrent infections or in the second or third decade from cardiopulmonary complications. The majority now develop normally into the second decade with transfusions, but then complications of iron overload and transfusion-related illnesses, such as hepatitis, develop (Lukens 1999; Weatherall, 1995).

Laboratory Features

Patients with all forms of thalassemia have altered red cell morphologic features, including microcytosis, hypochromia, anisocytosis, and poikilocytosis (Fig. 6–34). Target cells, ovalocytes, and fragmented red cells may be seen, along with

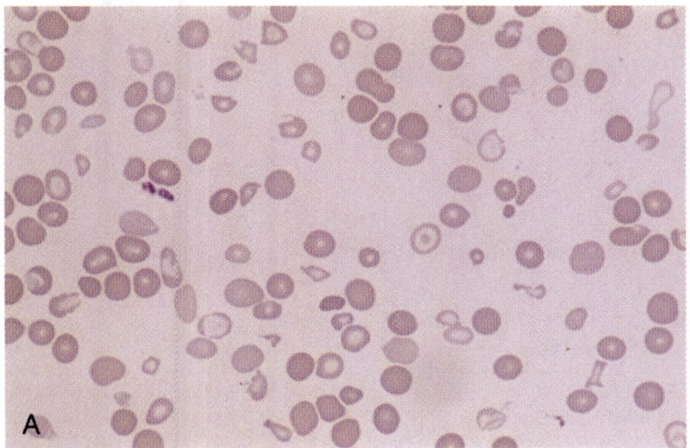

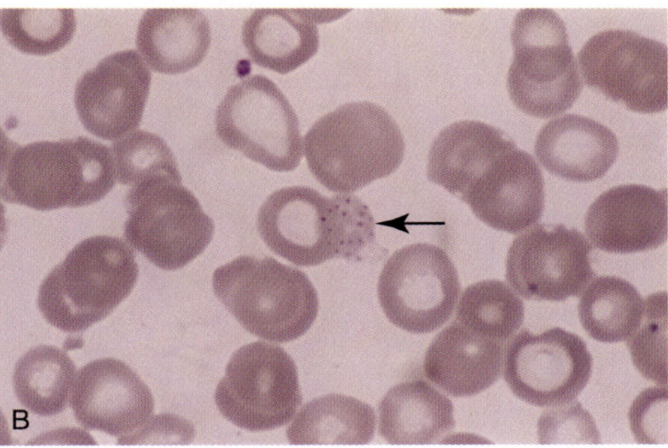

Figure 6–34

Thalassemia, peripheral blood changes. *A.* Anisocytosis and poikilocytosis are demonstrated. Hypochromia is not prominent due to previous blood transfusion. Polychromasia is also noted. *B.* β-Thalassemia major after hypertransfusion therapy. Abnormal red cell morphologic characteristics are less obvious. However, basophilic stippling (*arrow*) is detectable in this case. Wright stain.

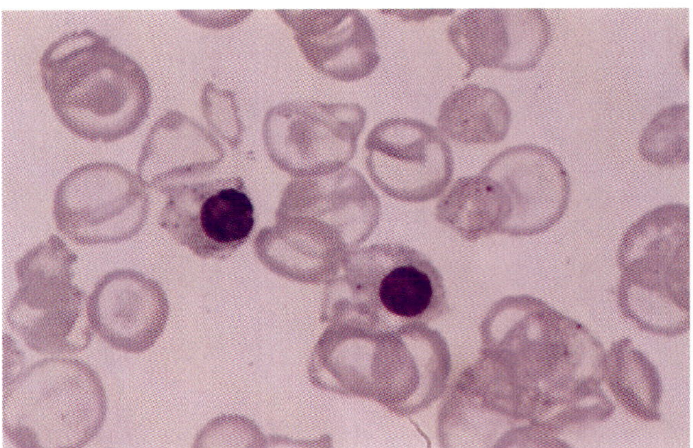

Figure 6–35

Thalassemia, postsplenectomy, peripheral blood. Basophilic stippling and inclusions are more discernible, along with nucleated erythrocytes. Wright stain.

basophilic stippling. Red cell features vary with the severity of thalassemia as well as the presence of the spleen (Lukens, 1999; Weatherall, 1995). Stippling and inclusions are more discernible after splenectomy (Fig. 6–35). Reticulocyte counts are elevated (5–15%) but lower than expected from the degree of anemia owing to ineffective erythropoiesis. The mean cell volume (MCV) (50–70 fl) and mean cell hemoglobin (MCH) are low (20–22 pg).

Erythrocyte hyperplasia is variably present in thalassemia (Sonakul et al, 1989; Weatherall & Clegg, 1981; Whipple & Bradford, 1936) (Fig. 6–36), the degree varying with the severity of tissue hypoxia. Unpaired α-globin chains in β-thalassemia form insoluble inclusion bodies in the earliest hemoglobinized erythrocyte precursors that may be demonstrated by both light and electron microscopy (Polliack & Rachimelewitz, 1973). Supravital stains, including methyl violet, are required to demonstrate these inclusions, which appear in late normoblasts as large irregular structures that are usually single and closely adherent to the nucleus (Fessas, 1963). Ineffective erythropoiesis in the marrow is the result. Gaucher-like histiocytes may be seen because of high cell turnover (Zaino et al, 1971). The unpaired γ-globin chains and β-globin chains in α-thalassemia form soluble tetramers that do not precipitate in the marrow. Therefore, erythropoiesis is less affected in α-thalassemia (Weatherall, 1995). β_4 tetramers precipitate as red cells age, forming HgH inclusions and leading to sequestration in the splenic microvasculature (Fessas & Yataghanas, 1968).

In addition to erythrocyte hyperplasia in the marrow, important pathologic findings encountered in other organs and tissues are extramedullary hematopoiesis (EMH), hemosiderosis, and mononuclear phagocyte system (MPS) hyperplasia (Sonakul, 1989; Weatherall & Clegg, 1981; Whipple & Bradford, 1936). EMH is typically present in the spleen and liver, but it may be found in unusual sites, such as paraspinal soft tissue. Hemosiderosis is seen in thalassemia mostly after the second decade and is responsible for cardiomegaly, pigmentary cirrhosis, and endocrinopathologic disorders including diabetes mellitus, adrenal insufficiency, and infertility (Fig. 6–37).

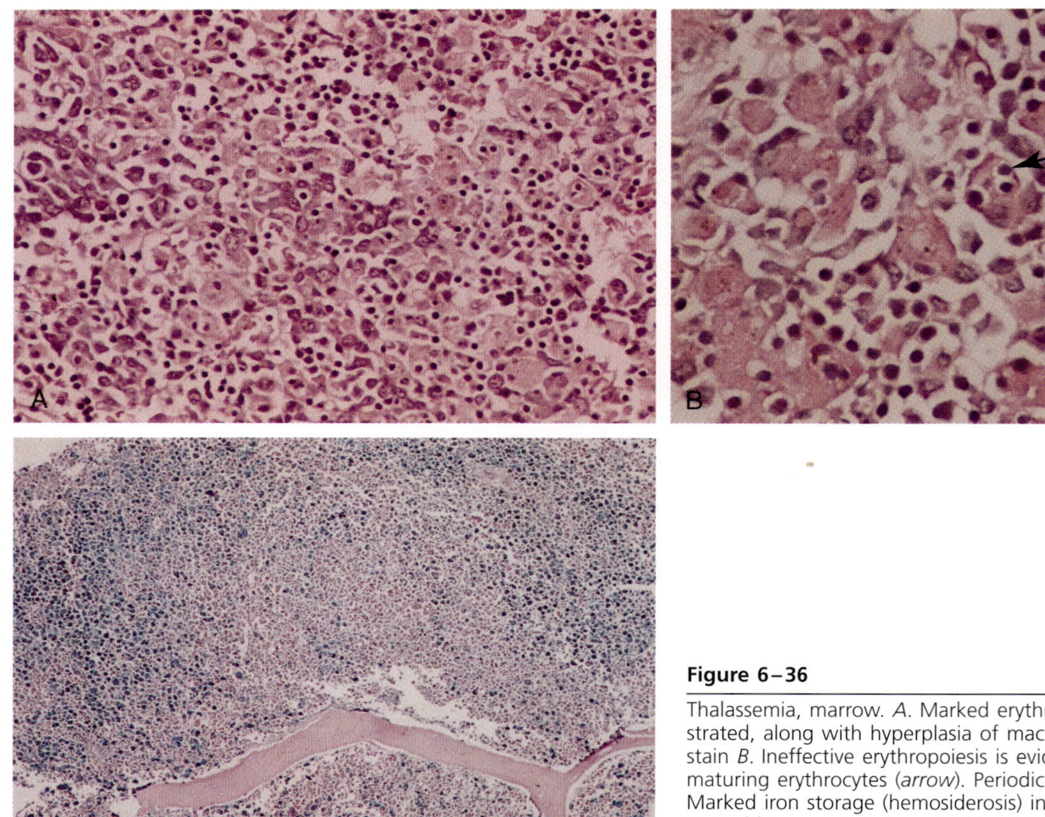

Figure 6–36

Thalassemia, marrow. *A*. Marked erythrocyte hyperplasia is demonstrated, along with hyperplasia of macrophages. Hematoxylin-eosin stain *B*. Ineffective erythropoiesis is evidenced by phagocytosis of maturing erythrocytes (*arrow*). Periodic acid–Schiff stain. *C*. Marked iron storage (hemosiderosis) in the marrow, as demonstrated by numerous Prussian blue–stained hemosiderin-laden macrophages. Perls Prussian blue.

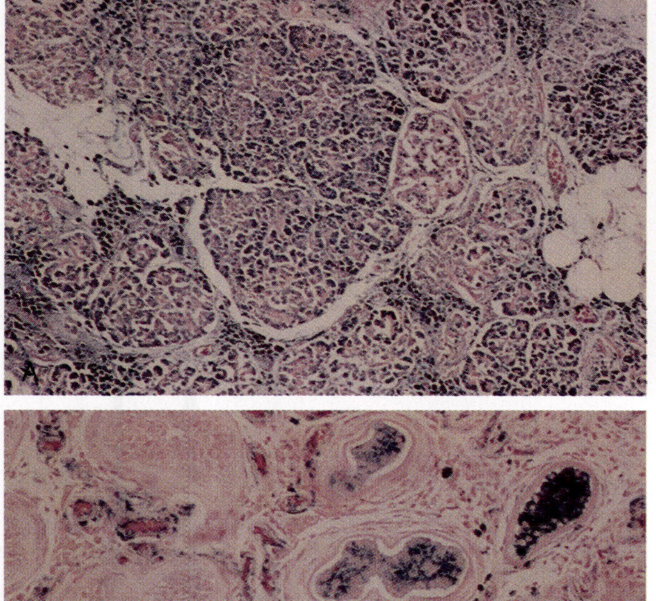

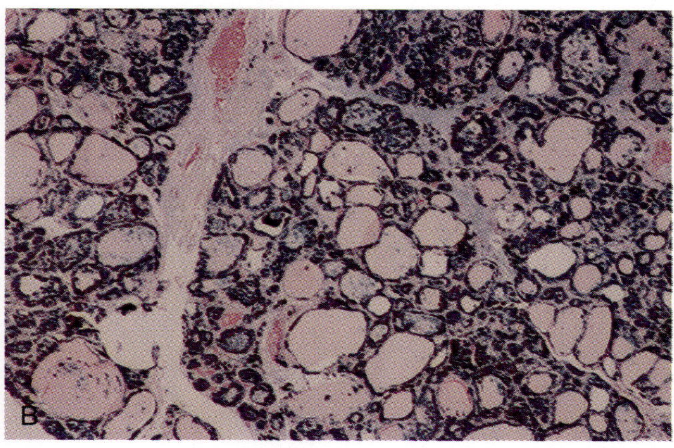

Figure 6–37

Thalassemia with hemosiderosis, various sites. *A*. In the pancreas both endocrine (islets of Langerhans) and exocrine (pancreatic acini) tissues are affected. *B*. In the thyroid gland, the follicular epithelium is affected. *C*. In the testis, cells in seminiferous tubules and blood vessels contain hemosiderin. Perls Prussian blue.

Splenomegaly is attributed to hyperplasia of the MPS from destruction of erythrocytes containing precipitated globin chains and sequestration (Sonakul, 1989). Pulmonary arterial thromboembolism is a noteworthy albeit uncommon complication in β-thalassemia/HgE disease (Sonakul et al, 1980).

Red Cell Inclusions

Inclusions alone are not diagnostic for thalassemia. HgH inclusions in α-thalassemia and α-chain inclusions in β-thalassemia resemble Heinz bodies found in unstable hemoglobin diseases, chemical poisoning, drug intoxication, and glucose-6-phosphate dehydrogenase (G6PD) deficiency. HgH inclusions appear as multiple pale-staining green-blue dots or spherical bodies of varying size that are easily distinguished from the darker-staining reticulofilamentous material of reticulocytes (Fig. 6–38). Heinz bodies vary from 1 to 3 μm and stain intensely purple. One or more may be present in a single cell. Precipitated α-chain inclusions have been inappropriately described as Heinz bodies. Certain staining techniques facilitate recognition of specific red cell inclusions. One percent brilliant cresyl blue and new methylene blue are excellent stains for HgH inclusions, whereas methyl violet stains Heinz bodies and precipitated α chains (Brozovic & Henthorn, 1995).

Hemoglobin Electrophoresis

Cellulose acetate electrophoresis at pH 8.4–8.6 is simple, rapid, and sensitive in detecting most common hemoglobin variants (see Chap. 6). Even though Hg electrophoresis is helpful in characterizing symptomatic thalassemia, α-thalassemia trait may be difficult to diagnose because there is no characteristic elevation in HgA_2 or HgF, and HgH inclusions are not always demonstrable (Weatherall, 1995).

Globin Biosynthesis Ratio

The α- and β-globin chains are isolated by ion exchange chromatography after incubating the blood for 2 h with ^{14}C-leucine.

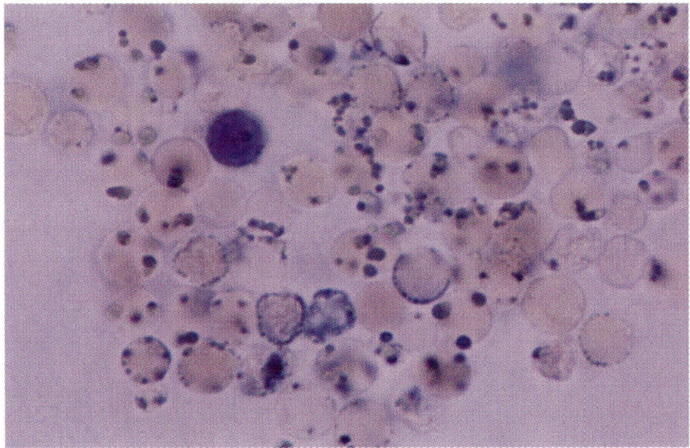

Figure 6–38

HgH inclusions, peripheral blood. Inclusions ranging from multiple greenish-blue dots to spherical bodies are noted in many erythrocytes. One percent brilliant cresyl violet.

Table 6–37

Common Genotypes of α- and β-Thalassemias

α-Thalassemia	β-Thalassemia
Hydrops fetalis with Hg Bart $--/--$	Thalassemia major β^0/β^0, β^+/β^+, β^0/β^+, $\beta^0/(\delta\beta)^{\text{Lepore}}$, β^0/β^{E}
HgH disease $--/-\alpha$, $--/\alpha^{\text{CS}}\alpha$, $--/\alpha\alpha^{\text{T}}$, $\alpha\alpha^{\text{T}}/\alpha\alpha^{\text{T}}$	Thalassemia intermedia β^+/β^+, β^0/β, β^0/β^{E}, $\beta^0/(\delta\beta)^{\text{Lepore}}$, $\beta^+/(\delta\beta)^{\text{Lepore}}$
α-Thalassemia trait $-\alpha/-\alpha$ (Asian, African, Mediterranean), $--/\alpha\alpha$ (Asian), $-\alpha/\alpha\alpha^{\text{T}}$	Thalassemia minor β^0/β, β^+/β, β^+/β^{E}
Silent carrier $-\alpha/\alpha\alpha$	Silent carrier $\beta^{\text{silent}}/\beta$
Normal $\alpha\alpha/\alpha\alpha$	Normal β/β

Symbols: $--$, deletion of both loci of α-globin gene; $-\alpha$, deletion of one locus of α-globin gene; $\alpha^{\text{CS}}\alpha$, α-globin gene for Hg Constant Spring; $\alpha\alpha^{\text{T}}$, nondeletion α-thalassemia gene; β^0, β^0-thalassemia haplotype; β^+, β^+-thalassemia haplotype; β^{E}, β-globin gene for HgE; $(\delta\beta)^{\text{Lepore}}$, $\delta\beta$ gene for Hg Lepore; β^{silent}, silent β-thalassemic gene.

The specific activity of the globin chains and the ratio of their radioactivities are then determined (Nathan, 1972). The globin biosynthesis ratio is helpful in problematic diagnoses, especially in cases of thalassemia minor.

Molecular Pathology

Molecular diagnostic techniques, such as Southern blotting of DNA using either restriction fragment length polymorphism (RFLP) linkage analysis or hybridization techniques and polymerase chain reaction (PCR) techniques, greatly facilitate identification of thalassemia mutations and are very useful in prenatal diagnosis (Kazazian, 1990). The common genotypes of α- and β-thalassemias are summarized in Table 6–37. The cause of α-thalassemia is mainly deletion of one or more loci of α-globin gene, but nondeletional forms account for almost 20% of all cases (Weatherall, 1995). The doubly heterozygous state for the α^0-thalassemia haplotype ($--$) and Hg Constant Spring are manifested clinically as HgH disease. β-Thalassemias that totally lack β-globin chain production in the homozygous state are called β^0-thalassemias, and those that have a deficient synthesis of β-globin chain are called β^+-thalassemias. Most of the β-thalassemias result from mutations, and over 100 have been identified. Details of these mutations and their effects on β-globin chain synthesis may be found in specialized monographs (Lukens, 1999; Weatherall, 1995). The doubly heterozygous state for β-thalassemia and Hg Lepore is manifested clinically primarily as thalassemia intermedia. The doubly heterozygous state for β-thalassemia and HgE may be characterized clinically as thalassemia major or intermedia (Lukens, 1999; Weatherall, 1995).

Diagnostic Criteria

Thalassemia is diagnosed in patients who have (1) a history of hereditary anemia; (2) hypochromic microcytic anemia with anisocytosis, poikilocytosis, basophilic stippling, and target cells; (3) Hg electrophoretic abnormalities in some thalassemia syndromes, including decreased or absent HgA plus Hg Bart in hydrops fetalis with Hg Bart, HgH in HgH diseases, and variably elevated HgA or HgF levels in β-thalassemias. HgH inclusions are useful in recognizing HgH disease. α-Chain synthesis is reduced in reticulocytes in α-thalassemia syndrome and β-chain synthesis reduced in β-thalassemia syndrome (globin biosynthesis ratio).

In order to provide complete genetic counseling, the homozygous or compound heterozygous state for various forms of thalassemia should be determined. Generally, there is no requirement for marrow examination in thalassemia except for evaluation of diseases simulating thalassemia.

Differential Diagnosis

Overt cases of thalassemia, such as homozygous β-thalassemia and HgH disease, are easily diagnosed. In thalassemia intermedia or minor, the following conditions should be excluded:

- ☐ Iron deficiency anemia. Minimal anisocytosis and poikilocytosis are noted. Basophilic stippling and target cells are rarely seen. Determination of serum ferritin and serum iron concentration, determination of the globin biosynthesis ratio, and molecular genetic analysis may be required to distinguish between α-thalassemia trait and iron deficiency anemia (Weatherall, 1995).
- ☐ Hemoglobinopathy. Complete Hg electrophoresis, determination of the globin biosynthesis ratio, and molecular genetic studies are required to distinguish between thalassemia and hemoglobinopathy (Weatherall, 1995).
- ☐ Hereditary sideroblastic anemia. Patients may have splenomegaly as well as microcytic, hypochromic red cells with anisocytosis and poikilocytosis. Their marrow has numerous sideroblasts (Beutler, 1995).
- ☐ Congenital dyserythropoietic anemia. Patients may have marked aniso- and poikilocytosis, hypochromia, and evidence of ineffective erythropoiesis. Marrow examination reveals characteristic abnormal erythrocytes, such as multinucleated erythroblasts (Beutler, 1995).

Pathogenesis

The pathogenesis of thalassemia is related to defective globin-chain synthesis because of a mutation in the corresponding globin gene (Lukens, 1999; Weatherall, 1995). The main effects of deficiency of one or more globin chains are decreased hemoglobin synthesis and an excess of unpaired globin chains. The former results in hypochromic, microcytic anemia, whereas the latter causes many pathologic consequences in thalassemia. Because of their high oxygen affinity, Hg Bart (γ_4) and HgH (β_4) in α-thalassemia cause tissue hypoxia, whereas precipitated α-globin chains in β-thalassemia are insoluble, resulting in ineffective erythropoiesis and splenic sequestration of the defective erythrocytes. Hyperplasia of the mononuclear phagocyte system is pronounced.

Active erythropoiesis secondary to tissue hypoxia then causes marrow expansion and bony deformities. In severe forms of thalassemia, extramedullary hematopoiesis can occur. Iron overload results not only from ineffective erythropoiesis and splenic sequestration but also from iron absorption from the gastrointestinal tract and blood transfusions. This secondary hemosiderosis adversely affects many organs, particulary the heart, the liver, and the endocrine system.

Thalassemic erythrocytes are abnormal as a result of pitting of inclusions by macrophages in the spleen, oxidative damage to the cell membrane from excess globin chains, decreased cell deformability from polymerization of membrane components secondary to lipid peroxidation, and interaction of the excess globin chains with membrane cytoskeletons (McDonagh & Nienhuis, 1993).

REFERENCES

Beutler E: The congenital dyserythropoietic anemias. In: Beutler E, Lichtman MA, Coller BS, et al (eds): Williams Hematology, 5th ed. McGraw-Hill, New York, pp 467–470, 1995.

Beutler E: Hereditary and acquired sideroblastic anemias. In: Beutler E, Lichtman MA, Coller BS, et al (eds): Williams Hematology, 5th ed. McGraw-Hill, New York, pp 747–750, 1995.

Brozovic M, Henthorn J: Investigation of abnormal haemoglobins and thalassaemia. In: Dacie JV, Lewis SM (eds): Practical Haematology, 8th ed. Churchill Livingstone, Edinburgh, pp 249–286, 1995.

Cooley TB, Lee P: A series of cases of splenomegaly in children with anemia and peculiar bone change. Trans Am Pediatr Soc 37:29–30, 1925.

Engle MA: Cardiac involvement in Cooley's anemia. Ann NY Acad Sci 119:694–702, 1964.

Fessas P: Inclusions of hemoglobin in erythroblasts and erythrocytes of thalassemia. Blood 21:21–32, 1963.

Fessas P, Yataghanas X: Intraerythroblastic instability of hemoglobin β_4 (Hgb H). Blood 31:323–331, 1968.

Hoyt RW, Scarpa N, Wilmott RW, et al: Pulmonary function abnormalities in homozygous β-thalassemia. J Pediatr 109:452–455, 1986.

Kazazian HH Jr: The thalassemia syndromes: molecular basis and prenatal diagnosis in 1990. Semin Hematol 27:209–228, 1990.

Lie-Injo LE, Lopez CG, Dutt AK: Pathological findings in hydrops foetalis due to alpha-thalassaemia: a review of 32 cases. Trans R Soc Trop Med Hyg 62:874–879, 1968.

Lukens JN: The thalassemias and related disorders: quantitative disorders of hemoglobin synthesis. In: Lee GR, Foerster J, Lukens JN, et al (eds): Wintrobe's Clinical Hematology, 10th ed. Lippincott Williams & Wilkins, Philadelphia, pp 1405–1448, 1999.

McDonagh KT, Nienhuis AW: The thalassemias. In: Nathan DG, Oski FA (eds): Hematology of Infancy and Childhood, 4th ed. W.B. Saunders, Philadelphia, pp 783–879, 1993.

Nathan DG: Thalassemia. N Engl J Med 286:586–594, 1972.

Polliack A, Rachmilewitz EA: Ultrastructural studies in β-thalassemia major. Br J Haematol 24:319–326, 1973.

Sonakul D: Pathology of Thalassaemic Diseases. Amarin Printing Group, Bangkok, 1989.

Sonakul D, Pacharee P, Laohapand T, et al: Pulmonary artery obstruction in thalassaemia. Southeast Asian J Trop Med Pub Hlth 11:516–523, 1980.

Weatherall DJ: The thalassemias. In: Beutler E, Lichtman MA, Coller BS, et al (eds): Williams Hematology, 5th ed. McGraw-Hill, New York, pp 581–615, 1995.

Weatherall DJ, Clegg JB: The Thalassaemia Syndromes, 3rd ed. Blackwell Scientific, Oxford, 1981.

Whipple GH, Bradford WL: Mediterranean disease—thalassemia (erythroblastic anemia of Cooley). Associated pigment abnormalities simulating hemochromatosis. J Pediatr 9:279–311, 1936.

Zaino EC, Rossi MB, Pham TD, et al: Gaucher's cells in thalassemia. Blood 38:457–462, 1971.

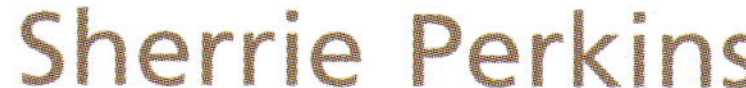
Sherrie Perkins

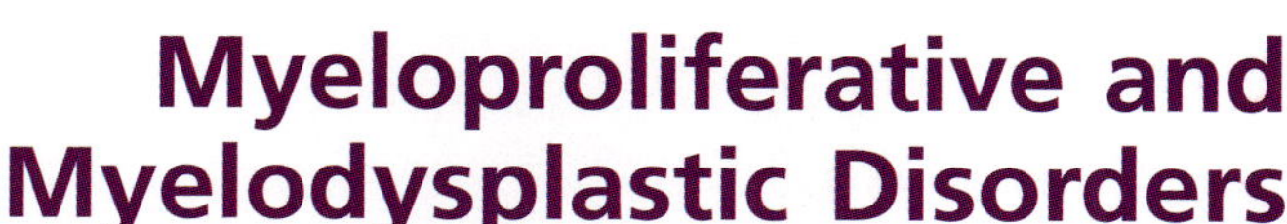

7 Myeloproliferative and Myelodysplastic Disorders

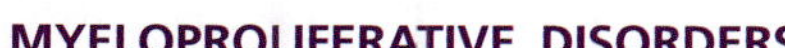

MYELOPROLIFERATIVE DISORDERS

The myeloproliferative disorders—polycythemia vera (PV), essential thrombocythemia (ET), and myelofibrosis or agnogenic myeloid metaplasia (AMM)—are typically seen in adults and are very rare in children (Table 7–1). These processes have in common a clonal proliferation of an abnormal stem cell and the tendency for overproduction of one or more cell lines, leading to polycythemia, leukocytosis, or thrombocytosis. All may progress to an acute leukemia. Two other diseases apparently unique to children are often classified as myeloproliferative disorders: juvenile myelomonocytic leukemia (JMML) and a transient myeloproliferative disorder of newborns, particularly those with trisomy 21. The latter is covered in Chap. 9. JMML and standard chronic myelogenous leukemia are covered in Chap. 5.

Polycythemia Vera

PV, characterized by an increase in erythrocyte mass, is extremely rare in children (Berlin, 1975). There are only a few pediatric cases (Danish et al, 1980), including a familial polycythemic syndrome (Adamson, 1975; Prchal et al, 1985). As a clonal disorder, PV has abnormal pluripotential stem cells that are extremely sensitive to the growth and differentiation effects of erythropoietin (Adamson et al, 1976; Casadevall et al, 1982). All hematopoietic cell lines may show increased sensitivity to other hematopoietic cytokines (Dai et al, 1992). The criteria defining PV (Table 7–2) were developed by the Polycythemia Vera Study Group (Berlin, 1975). Secondary or reactive polycythemia must be excluded by ruling out cardiac disease, lung disease, and abnormal hemoglobins with increased oxygen affinities.

Presenting symptoms in PV reflect the increased blood volume and include headaches, dizziness, flushing, and increased blood pressure. Splenomegaly is common, while abnormal bleeding or thrombosis may also occur. Laboratory findings (Table 7–3) include increased red cell mass with normal to decreased erythropoietin levels (de Klerk et al, 1981), leukocytosis in two thirds of patients, thrombocytosis in half of patients (Berlin, 1975), and basophilia in many. The leukocyte alkaline phosphatase (LAP) score is often elevated. Platelets exhibit an abnormal primary wave of aggregation in response to epinephrine (Yamamoto et al, 1984). Serum B_{12} levels are increased. The marrow is hypercellular, often with panhyperplasia, and iron stores are usually decreased. Cytogenetic studies may reveal a clonal abnormality in a minority of patients (Testa et al, 1981).

Patients are often treated with phlebotomy to decrease red cell mass, and iron supplementation is usually required. Treatment for leukocytosis and thrombocytosis may be associated with increased incidence of acute leukemia (Berk et al, 1981) and may be inappropriate for children. PV may proceed to a spent phase, characterized by increasing marrow fibrosis, splenomegaly, cytopenias, and transformation to acute leukemia (Silverstein, 1976).

Essential Thrombocythemia

The thrombocytosis in ET is due to increased responsiveness of a marrow clone to thrombopoietin or other factors favoring the differentiation of megakaryocytes and formation of platelets (Fialkow et al, 1981). Other causes of thrombocytosis in children (Chan et al, 1989; Heath & Pearson, 1989) must be excluded (Table 7–4). Some patients are asymptomatic, whereas other have thrombosis or bleeding. Laboratory findings (Table 7–5) include a normal red cell mass or evidence of mild anemia, platelet counts $>600{,}000/\mu l$ or higher, and a mild leukocytosis in some. The platelets are often large and hypogranulated (Fig. 7–1), and megakaryocytic fragments may be seen in peripheral blood films. Platelet aggregation studies show loss of the aggregation response to epinephrine as well as other variable defects in aggregation or hyperaggregability (Cortelazzo et al, 1980; Hehlmann et al, 1988). The marrow biopsy is hypercellular, with increased numbers of megakaryocytes that are often in clusters and have increased numbers of nuclei (Fig. 7–2). Large megakaryocytes, increased numbers of platelets, and platelet debris may be present in aspirate films (Burkhardt et al, 1986). Reticulin fibrosis is usually absent or mild. Cytogenetic studies are usually normal, although a small group of patients have *BCR-ABL* translocation and follow a clinical course like that of chronic myelogenous leukemia, including an eventual blast crisis (Aurer, 1991).

Treatment of ET is usually directed at bleeding or thrombotic events, although cytoreduction may be attempted with hydroxyurea. A newer agent, anagrelide, reduces platelet counts without significant toxic effects (Chintagumpala et al, 1995). Aspirin therapy may be useful in patients with thrombotic complications. Progression to acute leukemia is infrequent (Geller & Shapiro, 1982), except in the small subset with *BCR-ABL* translocation.

Table 7–1
Myeloproliferative Disorders in Children

Disorder	Incidence in Children	Postulated Defect
Polycythemia vera	Very rare	Increased sensitivity to erythropoietin and other cytokines
Essential thrombocythemia	Very rare	Increased sensitivity to thrombopoietin or other cytokines
Myelofibrosis or agnogenic myeloid metaplasia	Very rare	Increased production of growth factors by megakaryocytes that induce fibrosis, cell proliferation

Note: Standard and juvenile myelomonocytic leukemias are considered myeloproliferative disorders by some. They are covered in Chap. 5.

Agnogenic Myeloid Metaplasia

AMM in children is usually reported in the first year of life (Boxer et al, 1975; Cohn et al, 1991), and some cases appear to be familial (Mallouh & Sa'di, 1992). AMM in adults and children is characterized by marrow fibrosis, leukoerythroblastosis in the peripheral blood, teardrop cells, and extramedullary hematopoiesis causing splenomegaly. Laboratory findings (Table 7–6) include a normochromic, normocytic anemia with teardrop cells, a leukoerythroblastosis with immature white cells (Fig. 7–3), leukocytosis, and basophilia. Neutrophils may show nuclear abnormalities and atypical granulation. The LAP score is variable. Platelets are increased in one third of patients and decreased in another third and demonstrate abnormal epinephrine-induced aggregation patterns (Yamamoto et al, 1984). A few patients present with pancytopenia secondary to ineffective hematopoiesis and hypersplenism (Hasselbalch, 1990).

The marrow in AMM is often difficult to aspirate owing to varying degrees of reticulin fibrosis (Fig. 7–4*A*), highlighted by silver staining (Fig. 7–4*B*). Osteosclerosis may be prominent. Some cases exhibit dense marrow fibrosis and megakaryocytes interspersed with a few other hematopoietic cells. Megakaryocytes are usually increased in number and abnormal, with increased size, hyperlobation, hypolobation, or naked megakaryocytic nuclei. Cytogenetic abnormalities are common although difficult to demonstrate owing to scant marrow aspirates (Greenberg et al, 1987). The clonal disorder in AMM involves a hematopoietic stem cell (Jacobson et al, 1978), whereas the marrow fibrosis may result from elaboration of growth factors by megakaryocytes. Extramedullary hematopoiesis is often an important cause of clinical symptoms. In addition to the characteristic splenomegaly, patients may have lymphadenopathy or tumorous masses of hematopoietic tissue.

Differential diagnosis of marrow fibrosis in children includes metastatic tumors, metabolic diseases, and inflammatory disorders (Table 7–7), which must be excluded before a diagnosis of AMM is made. Treatment of AMM may be symptomatic, although marrow transplantation may be curative (Dokal et al, 1989; Rossbach et al, 1996). Complications include bleeding, infection, and transformation to acute leukemia (Hernandez et al, 1992).

MYELODYSPLASTIC SYNDROMES

Myelodysplastic syndromes (MDSs) are clonal disorders of multipotential hematopoietic stem cells characterized by peripheral cytopenias, marrow hypercellularity, and ineffective

Table 7–2
Diagnostic Criteria for Polycythemia Vera

Major Criteria
- Increased red cell mass adjusted for age and sex
- Oxygen saturation ≥92%
- Splenomegaly

Minor Criteria
- Thrombocytosis (>400,000 platelets/l)
- Leukocytosis (>12,000 cells)
- Elevated leukocyte alkaline phosphatase score
- Increased levels of vitamin B_{12} (>900 pg/ml) or increased unsaturated B_{12} binding capacity (>2200 pg/ml)

Note: For diagnosis of polycythemia vera, all three major criteria or increased red cell mass and oxygen saturation plus two minor criteria must be met.

Source: Adapted from Berlin NI: Diagnosis and classification of the polycythemias. Semin Hematol 12:339–351, 1975.

Table 7–3
Laboratory Features of Polycythemia Vera

Peripheral Blood	
RBCs	Increased RBC count, hematocrit, hemoglobin level
WBCs	Increased; usually neutrophilia
Platelets	Normal to increased numbers
Other	Abnormal platelet aggregation with epinephrine
	Arterial oxygen saturation >92%
	Leukocyte alkaline phosphatase score often increased; may be normal
Marrow	Panhyperplasia
	Iron stores often low
Cytogenetics	Usually normal; may have karyotypic abnormalities in 10–25% of cases
Chemistry	Serum vitamin B_{12} levels increased (>900 pg/ml)
	Unsaturated vitamin B_{12} binding capacity increased (>2200 pg/ml)
	Erythropoietin levels normal to decreased

Abbreviations: RBC, red blood cell; WBC, white blood cell.

Table 7–4
Causes of Thrombocytosis in Children

Reactive
- Trauma: surgery, fracture, hemorrhage
- Inflammatory diseases: collagen vascular disease, inflammatory bowel disease, sarcoid
- Infections: viral, bacterial
- Nutritional: iron deficiency, B_{12} or folate deficiency
- Drugs: corticosteroids
- Splenectomy

Neoplastic
- Myeloproliferative disorders
- Lymphoma
- Hepatoblastoma
- Neuroblastoma

Adapted from Chan KW, Kaikov Y, Wadsworth LD: Thrombocytosis in childhood: a survey of 94 patients. Pediatrics 84:1064–1067, 1989.

Heath HW, Pearson HA: Thrombocytosis in pediatric outpatients. Clin Lab Observ 114:805–807, 1989.

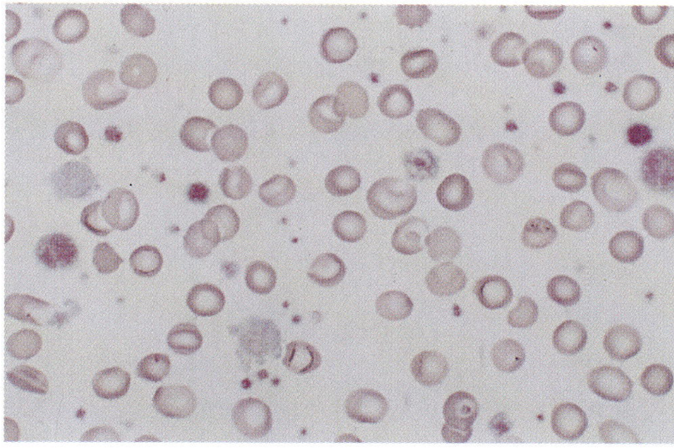

Figure 7–1

ET, peripheral blood. The characteristic thrombocytosis, numerous large platelets, and atypical platelet granulation patterns are present. Wright-Giemsa stain.

hematopoiesis. MDSs have also been termed preleukemia because of their frequency of transformation into acute leukemia. MDSs are much less common in children than in adults, and children may have unique forms of myelodysplasia, such as the monosomy 7 syndrome. In addition, MDSs are associated with a number of congenital abnormalities, including trisomy 21, Schwachman syndrome, Fanconi anemia, neurofibromatosis type 1, and other, less well-defined congenital abnormalities. Finally, MDSs develop after toxin exposure or tumor therapy, especially if alkylating agents are used (Cronkite, 1987; de Gramont et al, 1986).

The most widely accepted classification of MDS is by the French-American-British (FAB) group (Bennett et al, 1982) (Table 7–8). This classification is more applicable to adults than to children. The latter rarely have refractory anemia or refractory anemia with ringed sideroblasts. Many patients diagnosed with monosomy 7 syndrome are not included in the FAB classification (Locatelli et al, 1994; Passmore et al, 1995). By FAB criteria, most children with MDS have refractory anemia with excess blasts, refractory anemia with excess blasts in transformation, or an unclassifiable MDS (Passmore et al, 1995).

MDSs are clonal abnormalities of hematopoietic stem cells, although the defect is not well understood. The progeny of this clone have abnormal morphologic features and function, manifested by abnormal proliferation and disordered differentiation. The susceptibility of the myelodysplastic clone to additional genetic damage leads to transformation to an acute leukemia (Bartram, 1992; Raskind et al, 1984).

Several morphologic features of MDS allow for identification of the dysplastic process (Table 7–9). Abnormalities of all hematopoietic cells are found in both the peripheral blood and the marrow. Peripheral cytopenias in the presence of a normocellular or hypercellular marrow are presumed to reflect the ineffective hematopoiesis characteristic of this disorder. Dyserythropoiesis is often one of the earliest manifestations of MDS. The resultant anemia is often normochromic and normocytic but may be microcytic or megaloblastic. Increased numbers of oval macrocytes or a dimorphic population may be

Table 7–5
Laboratory Features of Essential Thrombocythemia

Peripheral blood	
RBCs	Hemoglobin level < 13 g/dl or normal red cell mass
WBCs	Usually normal
Platelets	Increased > 600,000 platelets/μl Large platelets with hypogranular forms
Other	Platelet aggregation abnormalities Variable qualitative platelet defects May have prolonged bleeding time
Marrow	Hypercellular marrow with megakaryocytic hyperplasia, megakaryocytic clustering Variable to absent reticulin fibrosis Normal iron stores
Cytogenetics	Usually normal karyotype

Abbreviations: RBC, red blood cell, WBC, white blood cell.

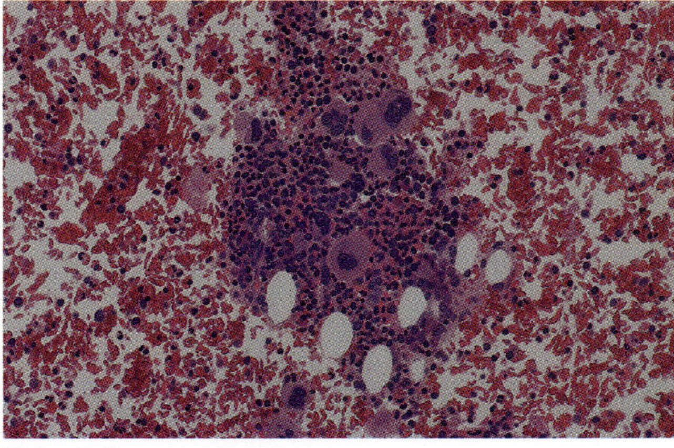

Figure 7–2

ET, marrow biopsy. Megakaryocytic hyperplasia is demonstrated, with clustering of megakaryocytes within the marrow. Many of the megakaryocytes show hyperlobation. Hematoxylin-eosin stain.

Table 7–6

Laboratory Features of Myelofibrosis or Agnogenic Myeloid Metaplasia

Peripheral blood	
RBCs	Normochromic, normocytic anemia Numerous teardrop cells Anisopoikilocytosis
WBCs	Usually increased ($<$ 40,000/μl) with left shift
Platelets	May be elevated, normal, or decreased
Other	Prominent leukoerythroblastotic reaction with nucleated RBCs; left shift in myelocytes
Marrow	Variable cellularity with increased numbers of megakaryocytes Increased reticulin fibrosis or sclerosis Osteosclerosis
Cytogenetics	Abnormal in 50%; variable

Abbreviations: RBC, red blood cell; WBC, white blood cell.

seen. Since anemia is often due to ineffective erythropoiesis, the reticulocyte count is low. The marrow shows abnormal erythrocyte maturation, with nuclear-cytoplasmic maturation dyssynchrony (megaloblastic maturation) and abnormal nuclear features, such as nuclear budding, karyorrhexis, and multinuclearity (Fig. 7–5), findings similar to those in severe B_{12} or folate deficiency. Dysmyelopoiesis is manifested in the peripheral blood as abnormal segmentation and granulation of granulocytes. Hypersegmentation, hyposegmentation with formation of bilobed psuedo–Pelger-Huët cells (Fig. 7–6*A*), and ringed nuclei may be seen. Cytoplasmic granulation is often decreased (Fig. 7–6*B*), or abnormal granules may be seen. Numbers of basophils and mast cells are often increased. The marrow shows abnormal maturation of myelocytes. The stage of maturation may be obscured by abnormalities in nuclear and cytoplasmic features. Numbers of immature cells and blasts are increased and located in clusters away from bony trabeculae, a process termed atypical localization of immature precursors. Myelocytes may also have abnormal cytochemical characteristics, including decreased myeloperoxidase activity or decreased leukocyte alkaline phosphatase staining. Flow cytometric analysis may reveal abnormal patterns of myelocyte antigen expression. Dysmegakaryopoiesis results in thrombocytopenia and platelets that are functionally abnormal. The peripheral blood platelets are often large or bizarrely shaped, with abnormal granulation, including increased, decreased, or large granules. The marrow often shows small mononuclear megakaryocytes

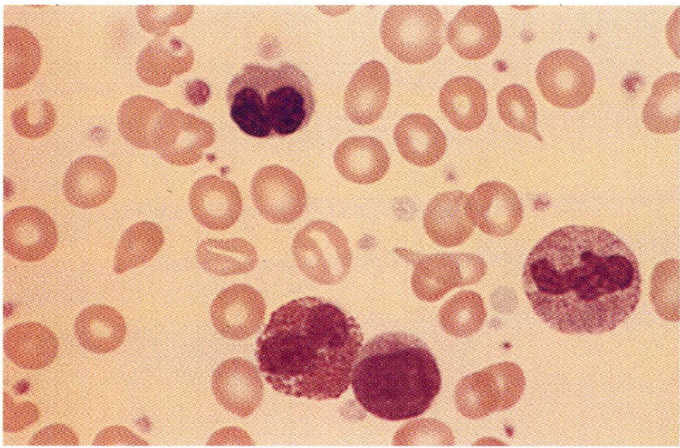

Figure 7–3

AMM, peripheral blood. Numerous teardrop-shaped red blood cells and a circulating binucleated red blood cell are revealed. Wright-Giemsa stain.

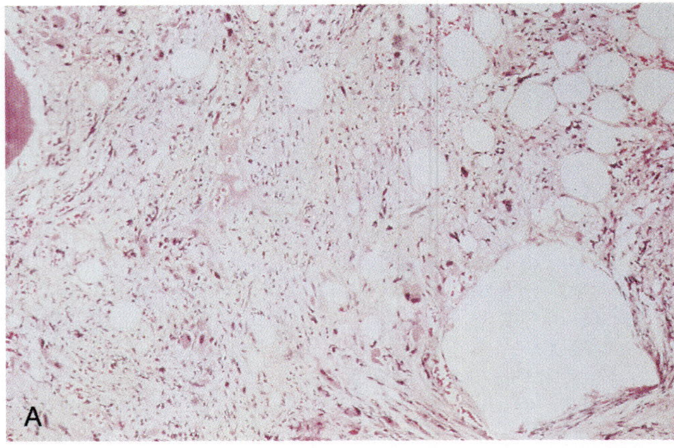

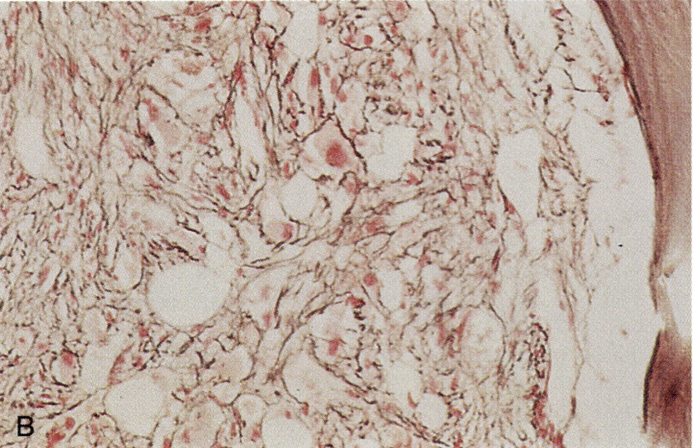

Figure 7–4

AMM, marrow biopsy. *A*, This section demonstrates increased fibrosis within the marrow and distortion of the normal architecture. Megakaryocytes are prominent. Hematoxylin-eosin stain. *B*, A silver stain highlights the reticulin fibrosis. Gordon and Sweet silver stain.

Table 7–7

Conditions Associated with Marrow Fibrosis in Children

Metastatic tumors Neuroblastoma Hodgkin disease B and T cell lymphomas	Metabolic diseases Chronic renal failure Hypoparathyroidism
Hematologic disorders Myeloproliferative disorders Acute leukemias, particularly megakaryocytic leukemia Myelodysplasia	Granulomatous diseases Sarcoidosis Infections
Bone diseases Osteopetrosis Osteomyelitis	Collagen vascular diseases

Table 7–8
Laboratory Features of Myelodysplastic Syndromes by the FAB Criteria

	RA	RARS	RAEB	RAEBIT
Peripheral blood				
Anemia	+	+	+	+
Neutropenia	−/+	−/+	+	+
Monocytosis (>1000/l)	−	−	−	−
Peripheral blood blasts	≤1%	≤1%	<5%	May be >5%
Marrow				
Erythrocyte dysplasia	+	+	+	+
Trilineage dysplasia	−/+	−/+	+	+
Ringed sideroblasts (>15%)	−	+	−	−
Marrow blasts	<5%	<5%	5–20%	21–30%
Marrow monocytes and promonocytes				

Abbreviations: RA, refractory anemia; RAEB, refractory anemia with excess blasts; RAEBIT, refractory anemia with excess blasts in transformation; RARS, refractory anemia with ringed sideroblasts.

Source: Derived from Bennett JM, Catovsky D, Daniel MT, et al: Proposals for the classification of myelodysplastic syndromes. Br J Haematol 51:189–199, 1982.

(Fig. 7–7) or very large megakaryocytes with increased numbers of nuclei or bizarre segmentation. Other nonspecific findings of MDS in the marrow include increased iron stores and increased reticulin fibrosis.

In the FAB classification for MDS, most children fall into the refractory anemia with excess blasts or refractory anemia with excess blasts in transformation categories, with refractory anemia less frequent (Passmore et al, 1995). Refractory anemia with ringed sideroblasts is extremely rare in children, and an alternative diagnosis of hereditary sideroblastic anemia or toxic exposure should always be considered (Passmore & Hann, 1996) (see Chap. 6). Patients with refractory anemia present with anemia, decreased reticulocyte response, and evidence of dyserythropoiesis. Blast numbers are usually not significantly increased in the marrow. Dysplasia of the myelocytic and megakaryocytic lines is minimal to absent (Bennett et al, 1982).

Table 7–9
Morphologic Features of Myelodysplasia

Cell Line	Peripheral Blood	Marrow
Erythrocytes	Anemia: normocytic or macrocytic; dual population of red cells Anisocytosis Poikilocytosis Oval macrocytes Polychromasia Basophilic stippling Nucleated red blood cells with abnormal features	Erythrocyte hyperplasia or hypoplasia Partial maturation arrest Dyssnchrony of nuclear and cytoplasmic maturation Nuclear abnormalities Megaloblastic maturation Nuclear budding Multinuclearity Karyorrhexis Nuclear bridging Abnormal mitotic figures Cytoplasmic abnormalities Ringed sideroblasts Cytoplasmic vacuolation Impaired hemoglobinization
Granulocytes	Neutropenia Monocytosis Hypogranular neutrophils Abnormal segmentation (hypo- or hypersegmentation) Immature granulocytes Basophilia	Myelocyte hyperplasia or hypoplasia Partial maturational arrest Decreased secondary granules or abnormal granulation Abnormal segmentation Irregular cytoplasmic basophilia Increased blasts Increased monocytes Atypical localization of immature precursors Abnormal mitotic figures
Platelets	Thrombocytopenia Large, atypical platelets Abnormal granulation of platelets	Megakaryocytic hyperplasia or hypoplasia Micromegakaryocytes Mononuclear megakaryocytes Abnormal nuclear segmentation Macromegakaryocytes

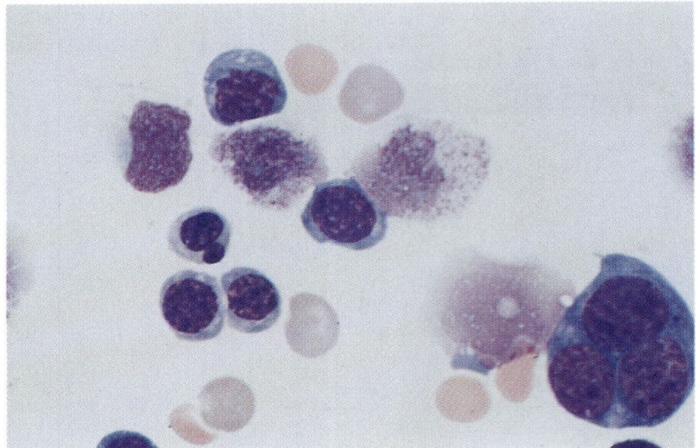

Figure 7–5

MDS, marrow aspirate. Dysplasia of the erythrocyte precursors, including binucleation, nuclear budding, and nuclear-cytoplasmic dyssynchrony, is similar to that seen in severe B_{12} or folate deficiency. Wright-Giemsa stain.

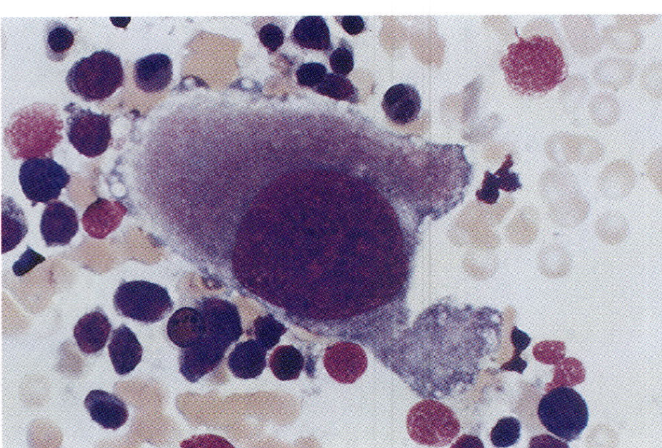

Figure 7–7

MDS, marrow aspirate. A dysplastic mononuclear megakaryocyte is shown. Wright-Giemsa stain.

Refractory anemia is often difficult to diagnose unless associated with cytogenetic abnormalities. It is often a diagnosis of exclusion in children, made after ruling out congenital dyserythropoietic anemia or abnormalities in folate metabolism (Passmore et al, 1995; Passmore & Hann, 1996).

Patients with refractory anemia with excess blasts present with anemia, but pancytopenia is common. Transient monocytosis has been described. Dysplastic nucleated red cells and circulating blasts may be seen. The platelets are often abnormal in size, shape, and granulation. The marrow is usually hypercellular and shows trilineage dysplasia with abnormalities in morphologic features and maturation. Myeloblasts compose 5–20% of the nucleated cells. Refractory anemia with excess blasts in transformation has similar findings, although the blast percentage is increased to >20%. Patients have a rapid progression to acute myelogenous leukemia. Many institutions now consider refractory anemia with excess blasts as a type of acute myelogenous leukemia. It is also anticipated that the myelodysplastic category will be eliminated when the WHO classification of hematologic malignancies is published, since it uses myeloid blast counts of 20% or more as a criterion of acute myeloid leukemia.

An MDS unique to children is infantile monosomy 7 (Table 7–10). This disorder occurs in infants less than 2 years of age with hepatosplenomegaly, recurrent infections, anemia, leukocytosis, and thrombocytopenia. The marrow is hypercellular due to erythrocytic and/or myelocytic hyperplasia and mild to moderate dysplastic features. The defining cytogenetic finding of monosomy 7 is seen in the marrow cells. Most patients exhibit a rapid progression to acute leukemia (Evans et al, 1988; Sieff et al, 1981). An increased incidence of infantile monosomy 7 is noted in patients with neurofibromatosis type 1 (Niemeyer et al, 1997; Shannon et al, 1992). Since monosomy 7 may be seen as a cytogenetic abnormality in other MDSs and has a particular association with secondary myelodysplasia, the diagnosis of infantile monosomy 7 requires correlation of cytogenetic, laboratory, and clinical findings (Sieff et al, 1981). Clearly, there is extensive overlap in clinical and laboratory findings among chronic myelogenous leukemia, juvenile myelomonocytic leukemia, and infantile monosomy 7. The lit-

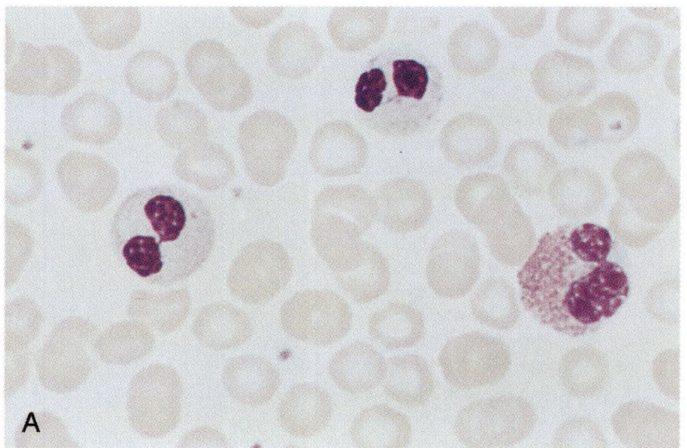

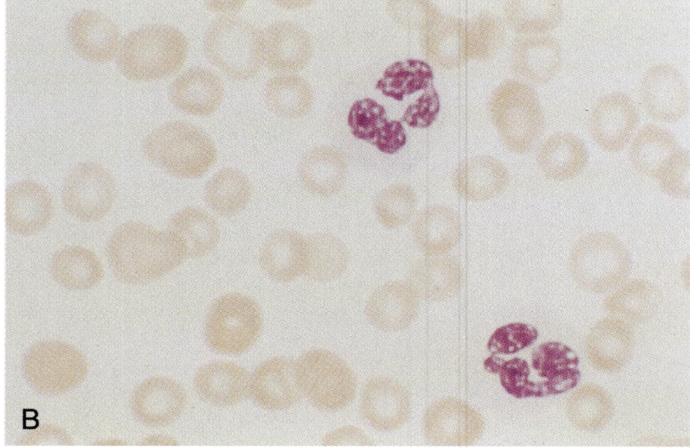

Figure 7–6

MDS, peripheral blood. *A*, This dysplastic neutrophil has a pseudo–Pelger-Huët bilobed nucleus. *B*, Dysplastic neutrophils characterized by markedly decreased cytoplasmic granulation are shown. Wright-Giemsa stain.

Table 7–10
Laboratory Features of Infantile Monosomy 7 Syndrome

Peripheral blood	
RBCs	Normochromic, normocytic anemia
WBCs	Leukocytosis with myeloid left shift, monocytosis
Platelets	Decreased
Fetal hemoglobin	Normal to slightly increased
Marrow	Hypercellular with myeloid or erythroid hyperplasia
Cytogenetics	Monosomy 7

Abbreviations: RBC, red blood cell, WBC, white blood cell.

erature is contentious as to whether these entities are spectra of a single disease or unique diseases (Butcher et al, 1995; Niemeyer et al, 1997; Passmore et al, 1995). For further discussion see Chap. 5.

MDS is more likely in children with certain genetic disorders. Children with trisomy 21 are very likely to develop acute leukemia, particularly acute megakaryoblastic leukemia (Zipursky et al, 1994a). Leukemia is often preceded by a period of myelodysplasia with thrombocytopenia, occasional circulating blasts, and variable anemia. Marrow examination reveals abnormal megakaryopoiesis, as evidenced by small, mononuclear megakaryocytes that may contain nucleoli. Numbers of megakaryoblasts are increased and may constitute <30% of total nucleated cells. There is increased marrow reticulin fibrosis in about half of cases. Cytogenetic analysis reveals frequent acquisition of additional karyotypic abnormalities, the most common being trisomy 8 (Zipursky et al, 1994a). Neurofibromatosis type 1 is associated with increased incidence of MDS, often with monosomy 7. Patients are usually older than expected in the infantile monosomy 7 syndrome (Maris et al, 1997). MDS is also significant in the evolution of Fanconi anemia, in which susceptibility to chromosomal damage apparently affects hematopoiesis and eventually results in development of acute leukemia (Auerbach & Allen, 1991). Patients with Schwachman-Diamond syndrome (exocrine pancreatic insufficiency, marrow hypoplasia, and neutropenia) are prone to myelodysplasia. Anemia and thrombocytopenia in these cases often herald progression to acute leukemia (Schwachman et al, 1964).

Secondary myelodysplasia or dysplasia following treatment with alkylating agents or exposure to toxins is also seen in children (Hawkins et al, 1992) and is frequently associated with acquisition of monosomy 7, monosomy 5, or other cytogenetic abnormalities (Le Beau et al, 1986). Studies of the tumor suppressor gene *P53* have failed to demonstrate increased mutations in pediatric patients with therapy-related myelodysplasia (Felix et al, 1996). Increases in cytogenetic abnormalities, myelodysplasia, and acute leukemia have also been described in patients with Kostmann syndrome (severe congenital neutropenia) treated with long-term granulocyte-monocyte colony-stimulating factor therapy (Bonilla et al, 1994; Smith et al, 1995).

The clinical course of MDS in children is progressive, often culminating in development of acute leukemia (Blank & Lange, 1981; Gadner & Haas, 1992). Marrow transplantation is the definitive treatment for children, with the possible exceptions of patients with refractory anemia with normal cytogenetic features, and any patient in whom the diagnosis is not certain (Passmore et al, 1995). A prognostic scoring system that incorporates diagnosis, platelet count, cytogenetic complexity, and hemoglobin F level may identify patients most at risk for death and may aid in the timing of transplantation (Passmore et al, 1995). Both related and unrelated donors have been used for pediatric MDS patients, with long-term disease-free survival periods in about 50% of patients (Davies et al, 1997). Some patients respond briefly to a course of chemotherapy but usually develop progressive disease or acute leukemia (Passmore & Hann, 1996).

SELECTED READINGS

Myeloproliferative Disorders

Burkhardt R, Bartl R, Jager K, et al: Working classification of chronic myeloproliferative disorders based on histological, haematological, and clinical findings. J Clin Pathol 39:237–252, 1986.

Castro-Malaspina H, Schaison G, Briere J, et al: Philadelphia chromosome–positive chronic myelocytic leukemia in children. Cancer 52:721–727, 1983.

Chan KW, Kaikov Y, Wadsworth LD: Thrombocytosis in childhood: a survey of 94 patients. Pediatrics 84:1064–1067, 1989.

Myelodysplastic Disorders

Bennett JM, Catovsky D, Daniel MT, et al: Proposals for the classification of the myelodysplastic syndromes. Br J Haematol 51: 189–199, 1982.

Evans JPM, Czepulkowski B, Gibbons B, et al: Childhood monosomy 7 revisited. Br J Haematol 69:41–45, 1988.

Locatelli F, Zecca M, Pession A, et al: Myelodysplastic syndromes: the pediatric point of view. Haematologica 80:268–279, 1995.

Niemeyer CM, Arico M, Basso G, et al: Chronic myelomonocytic leukemia in childhood: a retrospective analysis of 110 cases. Blood 89:3534–3543, 1997.

Passmore SJ, Hann IM: Paediatric myelodysplasia. Br Med Bull 52: 778–786, 1996.

Passmore SJ, Hann IM, Stiller CA, et al: Pediatric myelodysplasia: a study of 68 children and a new prognostic scoring system. Blood 85:1742–1750, 1995.

REFERENCES

Adamson JW: Familial polycythemia. Semin Hematol 12:383–396, 1975.

Adamson JW, Fialkow PJ, Murphy S, et al: Polycythemia vera: stem-cell and probable clonal origin of the disease. N Engl J Med 295:913–916, 1976.

Auerbach AD, Allen RG: Leukemia and preleukemia in Fanconi anemia patients. Cancer Genet Cytogenet 51:1–12, 1991.

Aurer I, Butturini A, Gale RP: *BCR-ABL* rearrangements in children with Philadelphia chromosome-positive chronic myelogenous leukemia. Blood 78:2407–2410, 1991.

Bartram CR: Molecular genetic aspects of myelodysplastic syndromes. Hematol Oncol Clin North Am 6:557–570, 1992.

Bennett JM, Catovsky D, Daniel MT, et al: Proposals for the classification of the myelodysplastic syndromes. Br J Haematol 51: 189–199, 1982.

Berk PD, Goldberg JD, Silverstein MN, et al: Increased incidence of acute leukemia in polycythemia vera associated with chlorambucil therapy. N Engl J Med 304:441–447, 1981.

Berlin NI: Diagnosis and classification of the polycythemias. Semin Hematol 12:339–351, 1975.

Bizzozero OJ, Johnson KG, Ciocco A, et al: Radiation-related leukemia in Hiroshima and Nagasaki 1946–1964. Ann Intern Med 66: 522–530, 1967.

Blank J, Lange B: Preleukemia in children. J Pediatr 98:565–568, 1981.

Bonilla MA, Dale D, Zeidler C, et al: Long-term safety of treatment with recombinant human granulocyte colony-stimulating factor (r-metHuG-CSF) in patients with severe congenital neutropenias. Br J Haematol 88:723–730, 1994.

Boxer LA, Camitta BM, Berenberg W, et al: Myelofibrosis-myeloid metaplasia in childhood. Pediatrics 55:861–865, 1975.

Brodeur GM, Dow LW, Williams DL: Cytogenetic features of juvenile chronic myelogenous leukemia. Blood 53:812–819, 1979.

Burkhardt R, Bartl R, Jager K, et al: Working classification of chronic myeloproliferative disorders based on histological, haematological, and clinical findings. J Clin Pathol 39:237–252, 1986.

Busque L, Gilliland DG, Prchal JT, et al: Clonality in juvenile chronic myelogenous leukemia. Blood 85:21–30, 1995.

Butcher M, Frenck R, Emperor J, et al: Molecular evidence that childhood monosomy 7 syndrome is distinct from juvenile chronic myelogenous leukemia and other childhood myeloproliferative disorders. Gene Chromosome Cancer 12:50–57, 1995.

Casadevall N, Vainchenker W, Lacombe C, et al: Erythroid progenitors in polycythemia vera: demonstration of their hypersensitivity to erythropoietin using serum free cultures. Blood 59:447–451, 1982.

Castro-Malaspina H, Schaison G, Briere J, et al: Philadelphia chromosome–positive chronic myelocytic leukemia in children. Cancer 52:721–727, 1983.

Castro-Malaspina H, Schaison G, Passe S, et al: Subacute and chronic myelomonocytic leukemia in children (juvenile CML). Cancer 54:675–686, 1984.

Chan KW, Kaikov Y, Wadsworth LD: Thrombocytosis in childhood: a survey of 94 patients. Pediatrics 84:1064–1067, 1989.

Chintagumpala MM, Kennedy LL, Steuber CP: Treatment of essential thromocythemia with anagrelide. J Pediatr 127:495–498, 1995.

Cohn SL, Cohn RA, Chou P, et al: Infantile myelofibrosis with nephromegaly secondary to myeloid metaplasia. Clin Pediatr 30: 59–61, 1991.

Cortelazzo S, Barbui T, Bassan R, et al: Abnormal aggregation and increased size of platelets in myeloproliferative disorders. Thromb Haemost 43:127–130, 1980.

Coulombel I, Derycke M, Villeval JL, et al: Characterization of the blast cell population in two neonates with Down's syndrome and transient myeloproliferative disorder. Br J Haematol 66:69–76, 1987.

Cronkite EP: Chemical leukemogenesis: benzene as a model. Semin Hematol 24:2–11, 1987.

Dai CH, Krantz SB, Dessypris EN, et al: Polycythemia vera: II. Hypersensitivity of bone marrow erythroid, granulocyte-macrophage, and megakaryocyte progenitor cells to interleukin-3 and granulocyte-macrophage colony-stimulating factor. Blood 80: 891–899, 1992.

Danish EH, Rasch CA, Harris JW: Polycythemia vera in childhood: case report and review of the literature. Am J Hematol 9:421–428, 1980.

Davies SM, Wagner JE, Defor T, et al: Unrelated donor bone marrow transplantation for children and adolescents with aplastic anemia or myelodysplasia. Br J Haematol 96:749–756, 1997.

de Alarcon PA, Patil S, Golberg J, et al: Infants with Down's syndrome: use of cytogenetic studies and *in vitro* colony assay for granulocyte progenitor to distinguish acute nonlymphocytic leukemia from a transient myeloproliferative disorder. Cancer 60:987–993, 1987.

de Gramont A, Louvet C, Krulik M, et al: Preleukemic changes in cases of nonlymphocytic leukemia secondary to cytotoxic therapy. Cancer 58:630–634, 1986.

de Klerk G, Rosengarten CJ, Vet RJWM, et al: Serum erythropoietin (ESF) titers in anemia. Blood 58:1170–1174, 1981.

Dekmezian R, Kantarjian HM, Keating MJ, et al: The relevance of reticulin stain–measured fibrosis at diagnosis in chronic myelogenous leukemia. Cancer 59:1739–1743, 1987.

Denegri JF, Rogers PCJ, Chan KW, et al: In vitro cell growth in neonates with Down's syndrome and transient myeloproliferative disorder. Blood 58:675–677, 1981.

Dokal I, Jones L, Deenmamode M, et al: Allogeneic bone marrow transplantation for primary myelofibrosis. Br J Haematol 71:158–160, 1989.

Dosik H, Rosner F, Sawitsky A: Acquired lipidosis: Gaucher-like cells and "blue cells" in chronic granulocytic leukemia. Semin Hematol 9:309–316, 1972.

Emanuel PD, Bates LJ, Zhu S-W, et al: The role of monocyte-derived hemopoietic growth factors in the regulation of myeloproliferation in juvenile chronic myelogenous leukemia. Exp Hematol 19:1017–1024, 1991.

Estrov Z, Grunberger T, Chan HSL, et al: Juvenile chronic myelogenous leukemia: characterization of the disease using cell cultures. Blood 67:1382–1387, 1986.

Evans JP, Czepulkowski B, Gibbons B, et al: Childhood monosomy 7 revisited. Br J Haematol 69:41–45, 1988.

Fauser AA, Kanz L, Bross KJ, et al: T cells and probably B cells arise from the malignant clone in chronic myelogenous leukemia. J Clin Invest 75:1080–1082, 1985.

Felix CA, Hosler MR, Provisor D, et al: The p53 gene in pediatric therapy-related leukemia and myelodysplasia. Blood 87: 4376–4381, 1996.

Fialkow PJ, Faguet GB, Jacobson RJ, et al: Evidence that essential thrombocythemia is a clonal disorder with origin in a multipotent stem cell. Blood 58:916–919, 1981.

Fialkow PJ, Jacobson RJ, Papayannopoulou T: Chronic myelocytic leukemia: clonal origin in a stem cell common to the granulocyte, erythrocyte, platelet and monocyte/macrophage. Am J Med 63: 125–130, 1977.

Foucar K, Friedman K, Llewellyn A, et al: Prenatal diagnosis of transient myeloproliferative disorder via percutaneous umbilical blood sampling. Am J Clin Pathol 97:584–590, 1992.

Freedman MH, Estrov Z, Chan HSL: Juvenile chronic myelogenous leukemia. Am J Pediatr Hematol Oncol 10:261–267, 1988.

Gadner H, Haas OA: Experience in pediatric myelodysplastic syndromes. Hematol Oncol Clin North Am 6:655–672, 1992.

Geller SA, Shapiro E: Acute leukemia as a natural sequel to primary thrombocythemia. Am J Clin Pathol 77:353–356, 1982.

Greenberg BR, Woo L, Veomett IC, et al: Cytogenetics of bone marrow fibroblastic cells in idiopathic chronic myelofibrosis. Br J Haematol 66:487–490, 1987.

Griffin JD, Todd III RF, Ritz J, et al: Differentiation patterns in the blastic phase of chronic myeloid leukemia. Blood 61:85–91, 1983.

Gualtieri RJ, Emanuel PD, Zuckerman KS, et al: Granulocyte-macrophage colony-stimulating factor is an endogenous regulator of cell proliferation in juvenile chronic myelogenous leukemia. Blood 74:2360–2367, 1989.

Guinan EC, Tarbell NJ, Tantravahi R, et al: Bone marrow transplantation for children with myelodysplastic syndromes. Blood 73: 619–622, 1989.

Hasselbalch H: Idiopathic myelofibrosis: a clinical study of 80 patients. Am J Hematol 34:291–300, 1990.

Hawkins MM, Kinnier Wilson LM, Stovall MA, et al: Epipodophyllotoxins, alkylating agents, and radiation and risk of secondary leukaemia after childhood cancer. Br Med J 304: 951–958, 1992.

Hayashi Y, Eguchi M, Sugita K, et al: Cytogenetic findings and clinical features in acute leukemia and transient myeloproliferative disorder in Down's syndrome. Blood 72:15–23, 1988.

Heath HW, Pearson HA: Thrombocytosis in pediatric outpatients. Clin Lab Observ 114:805–807, 1989.

Hehlmann R, Jahn M, Baumann B, et al: Clinical characteristics and course of 61 cases: essential thrombocythemia. Cancer 61: 2487–2496, 1988.

Heisterkamp N, Stephenson JR, Groffen J, et al: Localization of the *c-abl* oncogene adjacent to a translocation break point in chronic myelocytic leukaemia. Nature 306:239–242, 1983.

Hernandez JM, San Miguel JF, Gonzalez M, et al: Development of acute leukaemia after idiopathic myelofibrosis. J Clin Pathol 45: 427–430, 1992.

Herrod HG, Dow LW, Sullivan JL: Persistent Epstein-Barr virus infection mimicking juvenile chronic myelogenous leukemia: immunologic and hematologic studies. Blood 61:1098–1104, 1983.

Hess JL, Zutter MM, Castelberry RP, et al: Juvenile chronic myelogenous leukemia. Am J Clin Pathol 105:238–248, 1996.

Jacobson RJ, Salo A, Fialkow PJ: Agnogenic myeloid metaplasia: a clonal proliferation of hematopoietic stem cells with secondary myelofibrosis. Blood 51:189–194, 1978.

Janossy G, Woodruff RK, Pippard MJ, et al: Relation of "lymphoid" phenotype and response to chemotherapy incorporating vincristine-prednisolone in the acute phase of Ph^1 positive leukemia. Cancer 43:426–434, 1979.

Kirby M, Weitzman S, Freedman MH: Juvenile chronic myelogenous leukemia: differentiation from infantile cytomegalovirus infection. Am J Pediatr Hematol Oncol 12:292–296, 1990.

Krilov LR, Jacobson M, Shende A: Acute febrile neutrophilic dermatosis (Sweet's syndrome) presenting as facial cellulitis in a child with juvenile chronic myelogenous leukemia. Pediatr Infect Dis 6:77–79, 1987.

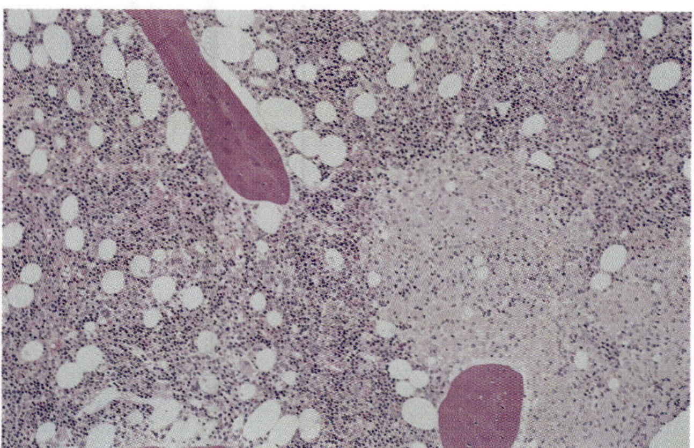

Figure 8–3

Granulomatous inflammation, marrow section. Granulomas usually form discrete nodules in the marrow and may contain areas of necrosis as well as giant cells. Hematoxylin-eosin stain.

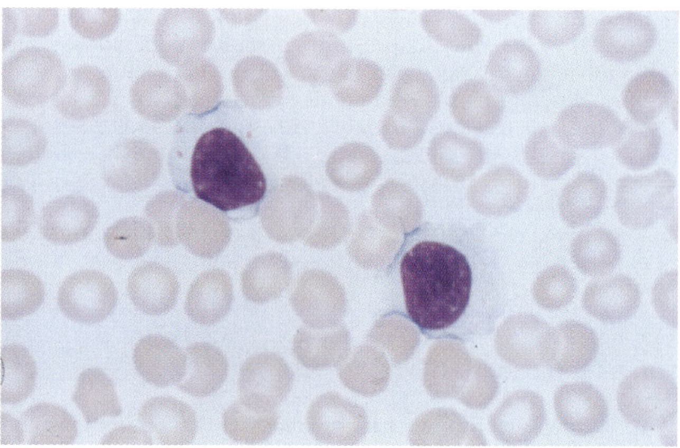

Figure 8–5

Activated lymphocyte, peripheral blood. Lymphocyte from a patient with infectious mononucleosis shows the characteristic fine chromatin and abundant cytoplasm that envelops surrounding red blood cells ("ballerina skirt"). Wright-Giemsa stain.

normal to increased numbers of megakaryocytes and red cell precursors.

Infectious mononucleosis or EBV infection is most frequent in adolescents and young adults and is manifested by malaise, fatigue, sore throat, fever, and lymphadenoapthy. Younger children may only have symptoms of an upper respiratory infection. The blood film reveals a lymphocytosis composed of lymphocytes of varying sizes, including large transformed lymphocytes. These cells were called atypical before it was understood that lymphocytes could change in appearance from small round cells. Now such "atypical" cells are deemed characteristic of EBV and other viral infections, highlighting the difficulties of nomenclature as knowledge evolves. Their nuclei tend to be large and eccentric and have distinct, coarse chromatin and occasional nucleoli. The cytoplasm is abundant and often basophilic. In some cells the cytoplasm appears to flow around adjacent red cells, resulting in a scalloped appearance (Fig. 8–5). Immunophenotyping shows that most of these large lymphocytes are T cells and represent an immune reaction against EBV infection (Enberg et al, 1974). Neutropenia is common during the acute phase of the infection, and a minority of patients

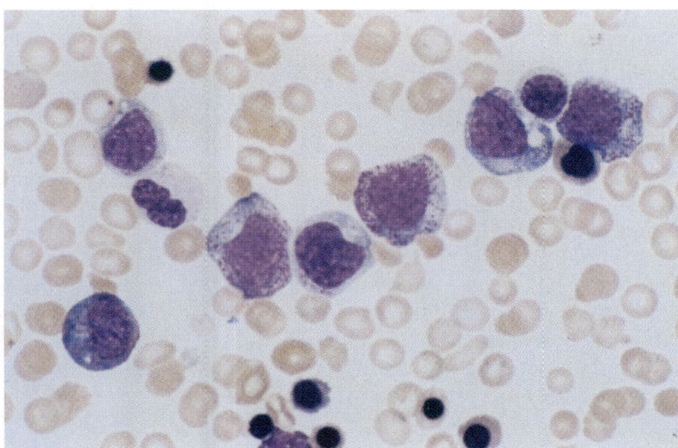

Figure 8–4

Myelophthisic pattern, peripheral blood. Nucleated red blood cells, teardrop-shaped red blood cells, and immature myelocytes are present. Wright-Giemsa stain.

develop anemia or thrombocytopenia. The anemia is often an immune-mediated hemolytic anemia associated with reactivity against the i antigen (Jenkins et al, 1965). Rare cases exhibit decreased red cell precursors or bone marrow aplasia (Baranski et al, 1988). The discussion of X-linked lymphoproliferative disease in Chap. 3 includes details about the response of these children to EBV infection. Thrombocytopenia, usually mild in degree, is caused by immune-mediated mechanisms (Radel & Schorr, 1963). The diagnosis of EBV infection may be confirmed by a positive heterophile antibody test result or by more detailed serologic evidence.

HIV infection also has profound hematologic effects either from direct viral injury or from multiple infections and therapeutic drugs. Peripheral cytopenias are very common, and most HIV patients have some degree of anemia and granulocytopenia. Most cytopenias in HIV patients are attributed to ineffective hematopoiesis as well as increased peripheral destruction.

HIV patients usually have normochromic, normocytic anemia that increases in severity with progression of the disease. Reticulocyte counts are often low, and there may be moderate to severe anisocytosis and poikilocytosis. Up to 40% of HIV patients have a positive direct antibody test result, although severe hemolysis is infrequent (Mayer, 1990). Up to 75% of patients on zidovudine (AZT) therapy develop macrocytosis, which in the initial stages of therapy is not always associated with anemia (Snower & Weil, 1993). AZT therapy has also been associated with marrow suppression, as evidenced by granulocytopenia and reticulocytopenia (Richman et al, 1987). Thrombocytopenia has been attributed to both antiplatelet antibodies and nonspecific antibody coating of platelets commonly observed in these patients. Immune-mediated platelet destruction or idiopathic thrombocytopenic purpura is seen in 5–12% of patients (Walsh & Karpatkin, 1990).

The marrow in HIV infections is usually hypercellular, with adequate hematopoiesis, normal to increased numbers of megakaryocytes, and nonparatrabecular lymphocyte aggregates with increased numbers of plasma cells and histiocytes. Fine reticulin fibrosis is seen in about 50% of patients, and patients in the later stages of disease develop serous fat atrophy. Stainable iron levels are usually increased, but sideroblastic iron levels are decreased, which is consistent with the pattern of anemia of chronic disease. Dysplastic features are common, including megaloblastic maturation, abnormal neutrophil segmentation, decreased granulation of myelocyte precursors, and increased immature precursors (Castella et al, 1985; Shenoy & Lin, 1986). Marrow biopsies or particle preparations may exhibit evidence of opportunistic mycobacterial or fungal infection in the form of granulomas or numerous histiocytes. Organisms are usually abundant, with single or multiple infectious agents (Nichols et al, 1991). HIV-associated lymphomas may be seen in marrow biopsies and are usually of large-cell or small noncleaved subtypes.

Another viral infection, dengue fever, is discussed later (see "Dengue Hemorrhagic Fever and Dengue Shock Syndrome").

Fungal Infections

Fungal infections are usually a complication of immunosuppression from chemotherapy or HIV infection. There is usually a peripheral monocytosis, and the neutrophil count may be increased, normal, or decreased. Marrow biopsy specimens may exhibit granulomas. Extensive marrow infiltration by granulomas may result in myelophthisis, with circulating nucleated red blood cells, teardrop cells, and immature myelocytes. Special stains readily demonstrate the causative organism or organisms.

Parasitic Infections

The most common hematologic manifestation of parasitic infection in children is peripheral and marrow eosinophilia. Other effects vary with the agent. For example, malaria is associated with hemolytic anemia and intestinal parasitization by hookworms with iron deficiency anemia.

Hemophagocytic Syndrome

Infection-associated hemophagocytic syndrome (IAHS) is a rare, potentially fatal complication of systemic infections in immunocompromised patients that is characterized by fevers, hepatosplenomegaly, cytopenias involving at least two cell lines, and coagulopathy (Risdall et al, 1979). Skin rashes, lymphadenopathy, and pulmonary infiltrates are seen in some patients. Infectious agents implicated in IAHS include EBV, herpesvirus, and adenovirus as well as some bacterial, fungal, and parasitic infections. The disease is characterized by a widespread proliferation of benign histiocytes, particularly in the marrow. Histiocytes contain ingested red cells, red cell precursors, and other hematopoietic agents (Fig. 8–6). In addition to hemophagocytosis, the marrow often exhibits normal or decreased numbers of myelocyte and erythrocyte precursors as well as normal or increased numbers of megakaryocytes. The most common cause of hemophagocytosis is IAHS, but the differential diagnosis includes malignant histiocytoses and familial hemophagocytic lymphohistiocytosis syndrome. Children with IAHS may have "atypical" mononuclear cells similar to those in infectious mononucleosis in the peripheral blood and marrow (Wong et al, 1994). The pathogenesis of IAHS is unclear, although abnormal activation or regulation of the immune response, with resultant overexpression of inflammatory and macrophage-activating cytokines, has been proposed (Ohga et al, 1993). Patients may recover spontaneously, but many die from complications of IAHS or their underlying diseases.

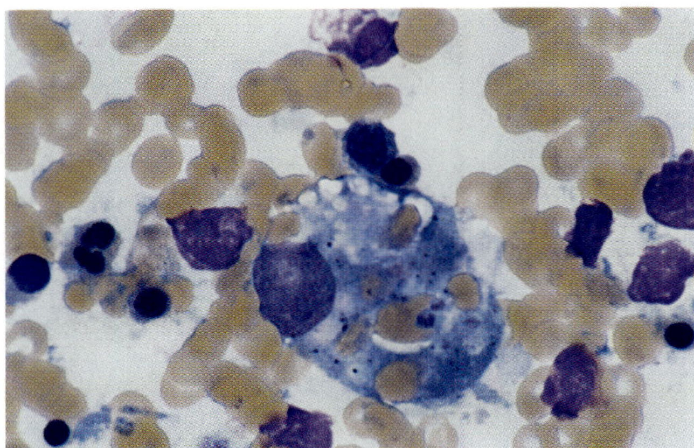

Figure 8–6

Hemophagocytosis of red blood cells, marrow aspirate. Marrow macrophages in a patient with infectious hemophagocytic syndrome exhibit prominent phagocytosis of red cells. Wright-Giemsa stain.

MANIFESTATIONS OF SYSTEMIC DISEASE

Individual systemic diseases are associated with relatively specific hematologic and marrow findings, as discussed later. Anemia is seen in many systemic diseases. The term *anemia of chronic disease* may be applied if anemia is of moderate severity and if there are low serum iron levels, low iron-binding capacity, increased iron tissue stores, and decreased sideroblastic iron levels (Richer, 1997), all leading to decreased red cell production. The red cell life span also appears to be slightly shortened (Dinant & de Maat, 1978). Anemia of chronic disease may be due to macrophage activation and resultant increases in cytokine production. Together these may enhance removal of red cells by mononuclear phagocytes, suppress erythropoietin secretion by the kidneys, or affect erythropoietin action on red cell precursors (Means & Krantz, 1992). Iron metabolism is also deranged in anemia of chronic disease. Low serum iron levels with adequate tissue iron stores are attributed to impaired macrophage release of iron.

Patients usually have a mild to moderate anemia, with hemoglobin levels of 7–11 g/dl. The anemia is usually normochromic and normocytic, although blood films may reveal many hypochromic cells, and some patients have mildly microcytic indexes. Reticulocyte counts are usually normal to slightly elevated. There are decreased levels of serum iron, with normal or decreased serum iron-binding capacity, making iron deficiency anemia unlikely (Table 8–2). Serum ferritin levels are usually normal or slightly increased.

The marrow aspirate usually exhibits normal cellularity and myelocyte-to-erythrocyte (M/E) ratios, with no evidence of compensatory erythrocyte hyperplasia. The diagnosis of anemia of chronic disease may be confirmed by the characteristic iron staining pattern in the marrow, indicating increased storage iron in marrow macrophages and decreased sideroblastic iron. Usually one third of nucleated red blood cells are termed sideroblasts, since they contain one or more iron granules. In anemia of chronic disease, the number of sideroblasts is markedly reduced despite the increased macrophage iron stores (Cartwright & Deiss, 1975). In contrast, in iron deficiency anemia both macrophage storage iron and sideroblastic iron levels are decreased. Anemia of chronic disease is a common manifestation of many diseases. In addition, many childhood diseases have other noteworthy hematologic manifestations or associations, and they are presented in the following sections.

Cardiac Disease

Children with cyanotic congenital heart disease have intact erythropoietin responses and thus often demonstrate compensatory polycythemia and increased oxygen saturation (Tyndall

Table 8–2
Tests Helpful in Distinguishing Anemia of Chronic Disease from Iron Deficiency

Test	Anemia of Chronic Disease	Iron Deficiency
RBC size	Normocytic to slightly microcytic	Microcytic
RBC hemoglobin	Normochromic to hypochromic	Hypochromic
Serum iron level	Decreased	Decreased
Total iron-binding capacity	Decreased	Increased
Transferrin saturation	Decreased	Decreased
Serum ferritin level	Normal to slightly increased	Decreased
Marrow iron stains		
Reticuloendothelial	Increased	Absent
Sideroblastic	Decreased	Absent

et al, 1987). The resultant nutritional demands place infants at risk for development of iron, folate, or vitamin B_{12} deficiency (Olcay et al, 1996), and hyperviscosity may cause coagulation defects and thrombocytopenia. Qualitative platelet defects have also been described in this setting (Maurer, 1972).

Prosthetic valves may induce microangiopathic hemolytic anemia from traumatic fragmentation of red cells as they pass through the valve and the surrounding distorted vascular surfaces (Nevaril et al, 1968). The blood film often reveals red cell fragments and helmet cells, with accompanying polychromasia and reticulocytosis (Fig. 8–7). Hemoglobinuria, hemoglobinemia, and increased red cell lactate dehydrogenase levels reflect the degree of hemolysis, and the marrow shows compensatory erythrocyte hyperplasia.

Liver Disease

Liver dysfunction causes anemia and coagulation defects, the latter from dyssynthesis of clotting factors. These clotting abnormalities rarely produce severe bleeding unless there is fulminant hepatic failure (O'Grady et al, 1986). Commonly altered clotting factors are the vitamin K–dependent factors (factors II, VII, IX, and X), factor V, plasminogen, and antithrombin III. Levels of these factors fall as the extent of hepatocellular damage increases. Effects on clotting factor levels may not be apparent in diseases such as obstructive jaundice or biliary cirrhosis. Factor VII levels are sensitive indicators of liver cell function and may be used as a monitor of liver status by direct assays or prothrombin time measurements (Lechner et al, 1977).

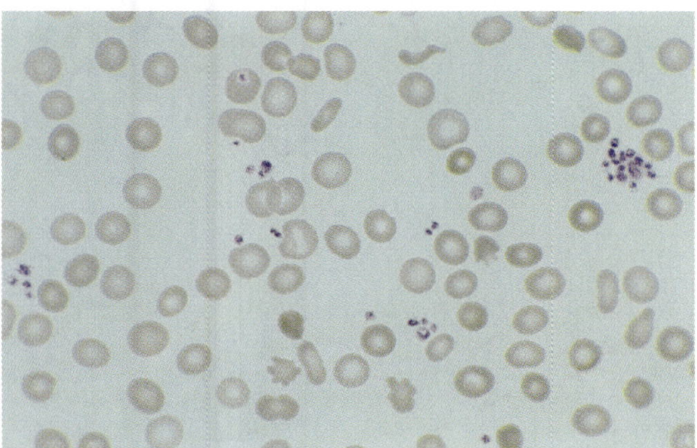

Figure 8–7

Microangiopathic changes, peripheral blood. Red cells in this patient with a heart valve prosthesis show characteristic microangiopathic changes, with numerous red blood cell fragments and polychromasia. Platelets are present in normal numbers. Wright-Giemsa stain.

Anemia is common in liver disease and has several causes. Most patients have macrocytic anemia (mean corpuscular volume 100–110 fl), with increased numbers of target cells, acanthocytes, and spur cells, attributed to alterations in red cell membrane cholesterol and phospholipid content that increase cell membrane surface area (Cooper et al, 1972). Red cell survival may also decrease in hepatic disease, and formation of Heinz bodies probably reflects oxidant stresses (Cooper, 1980).

Gastrointestinal Diseases

Hematologic abnormalities are seen in many diseases of the gastrointestinal tract, usually from inadequate gastrointestinal absorption of essential nutrients or from blood loss. Iron deficiency anemia strongly indicates blood loss, which has a multitude of causes, including esophageal webs, reflux, gastric ulcers, gastritis, regional enteritis, celiac disease, and ulcerative colitis.

Impaired absorption of folate and vitamin B_{12} follows gastritis or gastric resection, leading to decreased levels of intrinsic factor and impaired B_{12} absorption (McIntyre et al, 1965). Celiac disease may cause malabsorption of both folate and B_{12}, partly owing to impaired absorption and also to bacterial overgrowth (Katz & Falchuk, 1975).

Anemia is common in inflammatory bowel disease (Grand et al, 1995), in part from blood loss through the ulcerated intestinal mucosa with iron deficiency. Patients may also develop immune-mediated hemolytic anemia (Gumaste et al, 1989) or anemia of chronic disease. The peripheral blood has microcytic or normocytic indexes in most cases. Neutrophilia or monocytosis may be present, reflecting the underlying inflammation (Mee et al, 1980).

Renal Disease

Anemia is very common in renal diseases and may be attributed to various causes, including anemia of chronic disease. Decreased red cell production follows a decrease in erythropoietin levels and marrow toxicity from uremia. Decreased red cell survival and nutritional deficiencies from dialysis may contribute to but are probably not the major factors in anemia (Zachee et al, 1994). The anemia in renal disease is usually normochromic and normocytic, with no specific morphologic abnormalities. The marrow is often normal, although levels of erythrocyte progenitors may be increased owing to ineffective erythropoiesis (Barak et al, 1994). Since erythropoietin levels are often subnormal, most patients respond vigorously to erythropoietin (Hanna et al, 1996; Hutchinson & Jones, 1997). Macrocytosis, occasionally seen in peripheral and marrow red cells, is usually attributable to folate deficiency from poor intake and dialysis losses.

White cell counts are usually normal in uremic patients. Mild thrombocytopenia found in 25% of patients with acute renal failure and 10% of patients with chronic renal failure has been attributed to decreased platelet production and increased platelet consumption (George et al, 1974). Many patients acquire platelet function defects that affect adhesion, aggregation, or degranulation (Gordge et al, 1988). These defects are due in part to anemia and are correctable by transfusion (Moia et al, 1987) or are from toxic substances that may be removed by dialysis (Livio et al, 1985).

Pulmonary Disease

Patients with severe pulmonary disorders usually compensate for poor oxygenation and cyanosis with polycythemia and shifting of the oxygen desaturation curve. Despite chronic lung disease, patients with cystic fibrosis usually do not develop compensatory polycythemia because of overriding anemia of chronic disease or iron deficiency (Vichinsky et al, 1984). Superimposed infections in patients with cystic fibrosis may lead to neutrophilia with a left shift. Idiopathic pulmonary hemosiderosis is characterized by an iron deficiency anemia due to recurrent pulmonary hemorrhages.

Collagen Vascular Diseases

Collagen vascular disorders with prolonged inflammation and/or autoimmunity as prominent features are often associated with anemia of chronic disease (Means & Krantz, 1992). Iron deficiency or autoimmune hemolytic anemia may also be present. The altered immune function and inflammatory episodes in many of these patients may produce leukocytosis and neutrophilia. Treatment with anti-inflammatory agents, such as steroids, may cause a relative lymphopenia and reactive neutrophilia. Antimetabolites used in severe cases may cause cytopenia by marrow suppression. Platelet counts are often normal or increased, except in systemic lupus erythematosus. Some patients with this disorder develop immune-mediated thrombocytopenia (Karpatkin et al, 1972).

Rheumatoid arthritis, neutropenia, and splenomegaly constitute the triad of Felty syndrome. The neutropenia may be secondary to a decrease in hematopoietic growth factors (Rosenstein & Kramer, 1991), resulting in decreased granulopoiesis in the marrow. Neutropenia often responds to therapy with granulocyte colony-stimulating (G-CSF) factor over prolonged periods (Choi et al, 1994). Another disorder, termed pseudo-Felty syndrome, exhibits a proliferation of large granular lymphocytes and neutropenia. It is uncertain whether this is a lymphoproliferative disorder or a reaction to prolonged inflammation (Rosenstein & Kramer, 1991).

INVOLVEMENT BY TUMORS

In childhood, marrow metastases are commonest from neuroblastoma, rhabdomyosarcoma, synovial sarcoma, peripheral neuroectodermal tumor, Ewing sarcoma, and lymphomas, whereas metastases from Wilms tumors, hepatoblastoma, retinoblastoma, and other sarcomas are less common. Neuroblastoma ranks second only to acute lymphoblastic leukemia as a cause of marrow infiltration in children (Reid & Hamilton, 1988). (For a discussion of leukemias, see Chaps. 4 and 5.) The presence of marrow involvement places a tumor into an unfavorable group, since the patient's prognosis is tied to the tumor stage. Rarely, metastatic tumor is first detected when marrow is examined to evaluate cytopenia.

Metastatic tumor in the marrow is often associated with mild to moderate cytopenia and a myelophthisic pattern in the blood (Papac, 1994). Patients often have mild to moderate normochromic, normocytic anemia. Peripheral blood film shows schistocytes, teardrop cells, moderate anisocytosis, and poikilocytosis. Nucleated red blood cells and immature myelocytes may be seen, a process termed a leukoerythroblastic reaction.

Marrow biopsy and aspiration are extremely useful in documenting metastatic involvement. That random biopsies at presentation show tumor indicates the widespread nature of some malignancies (de Wolf-Peeters, 1991). Marrow aspirations may produce clumps of tumor cells (Fig. 8–8A). There is often failure to obtain a bone marrow aspirate ("dry tap") since many metastatic tumors associated with fibrosis or venous spaces are obliterated by extensive tumor deposits. In such cases, touch imprints from the marrow biopsy specimen facilitate identification of tumor cells. Tumor cells are usually identified by their large size and anaplasia as well as by their clumping or molding, in contrast to the dispersed pattern of hematopoietic cells. Marrow biopsies are more reliable than

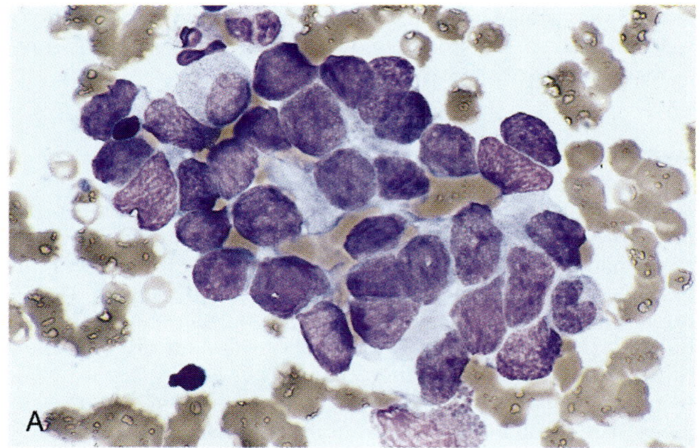

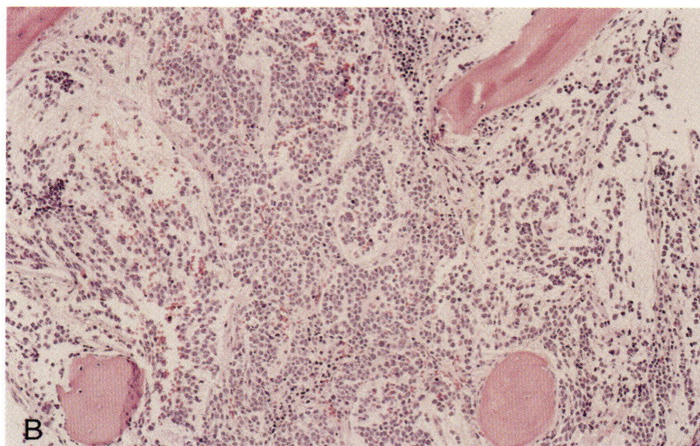

Figure 8–8

Metastatic neuroblastoma, marrow. *A*, Marrow aspirate contains clumps of cells with nuclear molding and cytologic features indicating malignancy. Wright-Giemsa stain. *B*, A marrow biopsy specimen from the same patient demonstrates extensive replacement of the marrow by metastatic neuroblastoma and fibrosis. Hematoxylin-eosin stain.

Table 8–3
Immunophenotypic Analysis of Metastatic Tumors in Marrow in Children

Tumor	Reactivity Expected with Immunohistochemical Preparations
Lymphoblastic lymphoma[a]	CD3, CD43
B cell lymphoma	CD20
Anaplastic large-cell lymphoma	CD3, UCHL1, CD30
Hodgkin disease	CD15, CD30
Neuroblastoma	Synaptophysin, neuron-specific enolase
Rhabdomyosarcoma	Myo D1, myogenin, desmin, muscle-specific actin
Ewing sarcoma, PNET[b]	O13 (CD99), variable staining with neuron-specific enolase, synaptophysin
Synovial sarcoma	Vimentin, keratin

[a] More than 90% of cases are TdT positive.

[b] PAS cytoplasmic positivity is usually manifested as small globules.

Abbreviations: PAS, periodic acid–Schiff; PNET, peripheral neuroectodermal tumor; TdT, terminal deoxytidyltransferase.

aspirations for demonstrating metastatic tumor, although their value is somewhat limited by the size of the sample (Westerman, 1981). At least 0.5 cm of well-preserved marrow should be obtained (Reid & Roald, 1996). Positive biopsy results reveal varying degrees of marrow infiltration by tumor and fibrosis (Fig. 8–8*B*). When primary tumors are unknown, morphologic patterns and immunohistochemical profiles (Table 8–3) are often definitive (Papac, 1994).

Lymphomas may involve the marrow in advanced stage disease, as covered in more detail in Chaps. 14 and 15. Hodgkin disease is associated with a fibrotic response in the marrow, and a leukoerythroblastic reaction may be seen (Doll et al, 1989). In contrast, most B and T cell lymphomas are not associated with fibrosis and do not cause leukoerythroblastosis. Lymphoma cells are not adherent and may be dispersed among normal hematopoietic precursor cells in the aspirate film. The pattern of marrow involvement varies from an interstitial infiltrate to replacement by tumor. The common B and T cell lymphomas of children are intermediate to high grade and are easily distinguished by morphologic features from normal components in the marrow, although special studies may be useful in some cases (Schwonzen et al, 1992). In particular, some cases of anaplastic large-cell lymphoma have a subtle interstitial pattern of marrow involvement that may be overlooked (Fraga et al, 1995) unless CD30 (Ki-1 or BerH2) immunostaining on the biopsy specimen is used to highlight tumor involvement. Circulating tumor cells may be seen in the peripheral films of patients with extensive marrow involvement.

THERAPY-RELATED CHANGES

Chemotherapy

Antimetabolites and other agents used to treat childhood cancers have profound effects on the marrow and hematologic status of the patient, since currently used drugs do not discriminate between tumor and rapidly proliferating hematopoietic cells. Marrow toxicity is a significant complication of many cancer treatment regimens. The marrow injury and recovery following treatment are reflected in blood counts as well as marrow appearance.

Myeloablative therapy for acute leukemia is particularly toxic to the marrow, which initially exhibits extensive necrosis, followed by marked hypocellularity that persists for 1–2 weeks. Repopulation of hematopoietic cells occurs 1–3 weeks after injury. The stage of hypocellularity is characterized by edema, dilated sinuses, multiloculated fat cells, and eosinophilic degeneration of the stromal cells (Fig. 8–9). Macrophages are often prominent, and mild reticulin fibrosis may develop (Islam et al, 1980; Wittels, 1980). Clusters or colonies of regenerating cells then develop, often surrounding loculated fat cells. Regeneration is well under way but still occurs in patches by the third to fifth week after therapy. Myelocyte and erythrocyte regeneration usually occurs before megakaryocytes proliferate (Islam et al, 1980). Dyspoiesis may be seen in regenerating marrow cells, accompanied by decreases in reticulin and adipose cells (Wittels, 1980). Marrow status at 1–4 weeks is critical, since patients have significantly better chances of remission if marrow at that time contains no residual blasts (Cheson et al, 1990; Potter, 1992). However, some patients have vigorous regeneration 2–3 weeks after therapy, with numerous blasts and promyelocytes that are difficult to distinguish from residual acute myelogenous leukemia (Dick et al, 1995). In these patients repeat biopsy after another 1–2 weeks may be required to determine remission or relapse status.

The marrow, but not the peripheral blood, of children contains small to medium-sized benign lymphocytes called

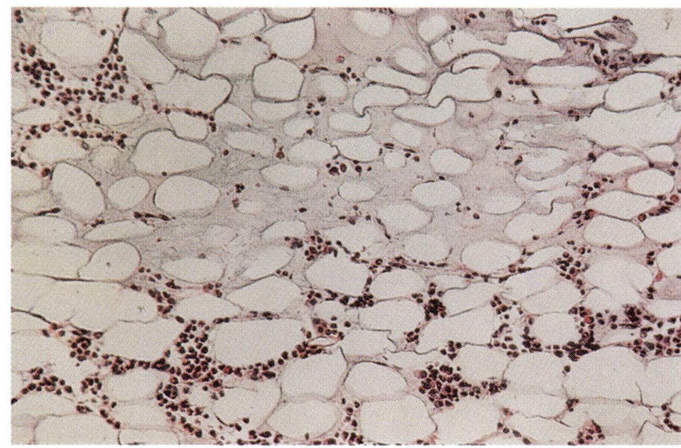

Figure 8–9

Marrow depletion from myeloablative chemotherapy, marrow biopsy. Marked depletion with eosinophilic stromal degeneration 5 days following myeloablative chemotherapy is demonstrated. Scattered residual lymphocytes and plasma cells are admixed with rare regenerating marrow elements. Hematoxylin-eosin stain.

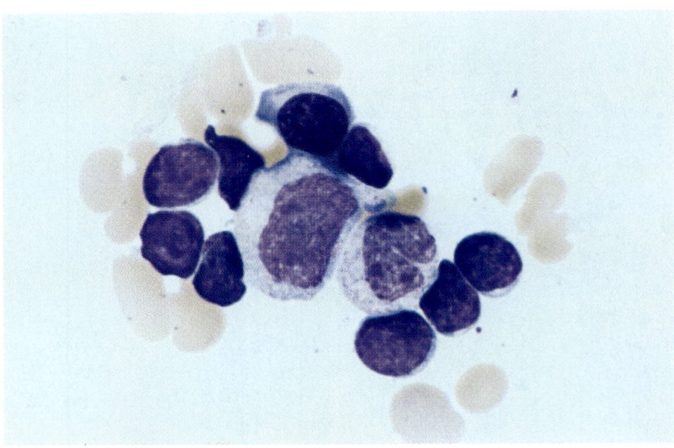

Figure 8–10

Hematogones in marrow after myeloablative chemotherapy. A marrow aspirate exhibits numerous hematogones in a child recovering from myeloablative chemotherapy. The hematogones are medium to large in size, with hyperchromatic chromatin; chromatin is dispersed but not as fine as that seen in leukemic blasts. Nucleoli are usually not seen. Wright-Giemsa stain.

hematogones, cells with agranular cytoplasm and compact hyperchromatic nuclei. Nuclear chromatin is smooth, homogeneous, and without nucleoli (Fig. 8–10). Children under the age of 5 years may have >30% hematogones in normal marrow, whereas these cells are much rarer in older children and adults (Caldwell et al, 1991). Hematogones are precursors of B lymphocytes; have an immature B cell phenotype, with coexpression of CD19 and CD10 and terminal deoxynucleotidyltransferase and CD34 positivity; and thereby resemble blasts of common acute lymphoblastic leukemia (Ryan et al, 1987). Hematogones make up >50% of the marrow cells after chemotherapy (Longacre et al, 1989) and may be confused with residual blasts (Muehleck et al, 1983). Features helpful in distinguishing hematogones from lymphoblasts may be found in Table 8–4 (Longacre et al, 1989) (also see Chap. 9). The absence of cytogenetic abnormalities in hematogones may be particularly helpful. Occasionally, sequential marrow examinations are required to exclude acute lymphoblastic leukemia. Periodic acid–Schiff stains may also help by showing blocklike positivity in lymphoblasts, whereas negative reactions are the rule in hematogones.

Chemotherapy or radiotherapy for neoplasms other than acute leukemias also affect the marrow. Radiation therapy usually suppresses all hematopoietic cell lines and may lead to irreversible depletion of marrow stem cells (Dritschilo & Sherman, 1981). Many drugs used in treating other tumors cause a "nonspecific" inhibition of DNA synthesis that results in dyspoietic marrow cell maturation, especially in the red cell line. Morphologically, there are nuclear-cytoplasmic dyssynchrony, megaloblastic maturation, and nuclear abnormalities (Hoagland, 1982). Neutropenia and thrombocytopenia may also be seen.

Marrow Transplantation

Bone marrow transplantation (BMT) is increasingly favored in treatment of tumors in children, particularly for poor-risk acute leukemias, relapsed or nonresponsive lymphomas, and some solid tumors (Amylon, 1997; Shen et al, 1997). The rationale of BMT is to give very high doses of therapy, which in other circumstances would be lethal owing to the effects on the marrow. Patients are rescued by transplantation of marrow elements in the hope of reconstituting the hematopoietic system. In patients with solid tumors, stem cells may be harvested from marrow or peripheral blood and infused as an autologous transplant (Shen et al, 1997). In tumors such as leukemias, marrow stem cells of the patient may carry the karyotypic abnormality in the tumor. Therefore, these patients are usually given an infusion of marrow or stem cells from an HLA-

Table 8–4
Features Helpful in Distinguishing Hematogones from Lymphoblasts

Features	Hematogones	Lymphoblasts
Morphologic features		
Size (compared to small lymphocyte)	Smaller	Usually larger
Nuclear features	Dense, homogenous chromatin, round to notched contours, nucleoli usually absent	Dispersed fine chromatin, may have convoluted nuclear contours, nucleoli often present
Cytoplasmic features	Scant, lacks vacuoles or granules	Scant to moderate, may have granules or vacuolization
Mitoses	Absent	Present
Cytochemical staining		
TdT	Positive	Positive
PAS	Negative in majority, occasional granular staining	Positive, blocklike pattern
Clinical features	Not seen in peripheral blood May be associated with solid tumors, marrow recovery, immune-mediated disease	Often seen in peripheral blood Associated with cytopenias
Flow cytometric analysis	See spectrum of CD19, CD20, CD10, cytoplasmic immunoglobulin, TdT, CD34, HLA-DR positivity suggesting maturational spectrum	Often one peak correlating to neoplastic clone
Cytogenetic analysis	Normal karyotype	May exhibit abnormal karyotype
DNA content	Diploid	May be aneuploid
Gene rearrangements	Not clonal	Clonal

Source: Derived from Longacre TA, Foucar K, Crago S, et al: Hematogones: a multiparameter analysis of bone marrow precursor cells. Blood 73: 543–552, 1989.

matched donor. This allogeneic transplant carries additional risks over autologous transplant because of possible immunologic mismatches. Allogenic marrow transplantation is also used in children for treatment of life-threatening conditions other than cancers, such as aplastic anemia, sickle cell anemia, or thalassemia major (Davies & Roberts, 1996; Vellodi et al, 1994). The rationale of treatment is to ablate the abnormal stem cells in the recipient's marrow and to reconstitute hematopoiesis with normal cells from an autologous donor.

The morphologic findings immediately following BMT are similar to those following myeloablative chemotherapy and include edema, eosinophilic stromal degeneration, increased reticulin fibrosis, and small, nonspecific granulomas (Sale & Buckner, 1988). Reconstitution of the marrow occurs in a stepwise fashion. The patient's marrow stromal cells may have varying degrees of damage, depending on the conditioning regimen for marrow ablation. Since stromal cells provide the microenvironment necessary for hematopoiesis, recovery of stromal cells for 14 days is often required before the marrow engrafts (Sale & Buckner, 1988; van den Berg et al, 1990).

Immediately following the transplant, the infused marrow may be found in other sites, such as the liver. Dispersed colonies of monomorphic (i.e., erythrocytic or myelocytic) cells may then appear in the marrow, eventually progressing to patchy regeneration (van den Berg et al, 1990). Erythrocytes usually appear first, followed by myelocytes and then by megakaryocytes. The blood counts after engraftment reflect this sequence, with pancytopenia followed by increasing red cell counts; then by increasing white cell counts, which usually normalize by day 21 after transplant; and finally by increasing platelet counts, which usually normalize by days 25–30 after transplant (Sale & Buckner, 1988). Autologous transplant patients tend to engraft earlier than do allogeneic transplant patients. Evidence of engraftment may be found in marrow biopsy specimens as early as 7 days following transplant (Naeim et al, 1978; Neiman et al, 1974), with recovery to half normal cellularity by about 21 days in many cases (Sale & Buckner, 1988; van den Berg et al, 1990). The recovery of normal marrow cellularity shows marked variability, ranging from weeks to a year. Hematogone levels are often increased following BMT, suggesting recurrent acute lymphoblastic leukemia (Kobayashi et al, 1991; Leitenberg et al, 1994). Extensive transfusion therapy in these patients may increase storage iron levels and result in ringed sideroblasts (Macon et al, 1995).

Several complications may occur after BMT during the period of pancytopenia. The marked leukopenia may lead to a widespread infection involving the marrow. Occasionally, the transplanted marrow will not engraft or may engraft briefly and then fail. Graft failure or rejection is evidenced by worsening pancytopenia, increasing transfusion requirements, and decreasing marrow cellularity (Champlin et al, 1989). In these circumstances the marrow aspirate or biopsy specimen reveals decreased numbers of hematopoietic cells and increased numbers of stromal cells, lymphocytes, and plasma cells (Rosenthal & Farhi, 1994). Stromal damage, marrow necrosis, hemorrhage, and "nonspecific" granulomas may be seen (Naeim et al, 1978). Rarely, only a single lineage, such as megakaryocytes, fails. Finally, marrows may reveal recurrence of the primary disorder.

Most patients are given cytokine therapy in the immediate posttransplant period to minimize the neutropenic interval. Cytokines are beneficial clinically but may cause dramatic changes in the peripheral blood and marrow. In some patients these changes increase the difficulty of identifying early infection and/or relapse of acute leukemia. (See "Cytokines".)

Most patients after BMT are on protocols that require marrow sampling at specific intervals, usually after 100 days and after 1 year, to assess the adequacy of engraftment by evaluation of the marrow cellularity and cellular composition. In heavily treated patients who have received autologous transplants, the marrow is also evaluated for possible treatment-associated dysplasia. Additional marrow examinations may be performed to rule out marrow relapse, to assess the possibility of infection, and to identify possible causes for prolonged or worsening cytopenias.

Cytokines

Hematopoietic cytokines are now used widely to stimulate marrow recovery following myelotoxic chemotherapy, radiation therapy, or BMT as well as to treat neutropenia of other causes (Lieschke & Burgess, 1992b). The most commonly used cytokines are G-CSF and granulocyte-macrophage colony-stimulating factor (GM-CSF), which act to stimulate predominantly myelocyte proliferation and differentiation.

G-CSF and GM-CSF cause specific morphologic alterations in the blood and marrow myelocyte precursors (Table 8–5). GM-CSF and G-CSF have similar effects, although G-CSF appears more effective than GM-CSF in stimulating granulocyte precursors. GM-CSF causes peripheral monocytosis and eosinophilia, changes infrequently seen with G-CSF. GM-CSF in particular may cause a transient fall in platelet count (Lieschke & Burgess, 1992a). These cytokines have profound effects on the myelocyte series, as manifested by peripheral blood neutrophilia (left shift) that may include blasts. The neutrophils and their precursors have increased azurophilic granulation and Döhle bodies, with multiple Döhle bodies or coalescent Döhle bodies in a single cell (Fig. 8–11). Occasional cells may show segmentation abnormalities, including hypolobation, hyperlobation, or ringed nuclei, as well as cytoplasmic vacuolization (Schmitz et al, 1994b). Giant neutrophils, or macropolycytes, representing tetraploid neutrophils are commonly seen in the peripheral blood films or by automated hematologic analyzers (Campbell et al, 1992). Leukoerythroblastosis may be seen in $<50\%$ of patients. Leukocyte alkaline phosphatase scores are increased (Schmitz et al, 1994a).

The marrow following G-CSF or GM-CSF therapy becomes hypercellular, particularly from an increase in promyelocytes and myelocytes. Promyelocytes may constitute 14–22% (mean 19%) of marrow cells and myelocytes 18–52% (mean 30%). These cells are larger than normal, with occasional binucleation and prominent azurophilic granulation similar to that seen in the peripheral blood. Later in therapy, the M/E ratio normalizes, and there is a shift in maturation to myelocytes and band forms (Schmitz, et al, 1994b). GM-CSF is associated with eosinophilic (Ryder et al, 1992) and histiocytic (Wilson et al, 1993) hyperplasia. Some patients on growth factor therapy develop foci of extramedullary hematopoiesis (EMH) in lymph nodes or spleen, which may be confused with leukemic infiltrates or granulocytic sarcoma (Litam et al, 1993). A small percentage of patients with aplasia or marrows replaced by tumor do not respond to growth factor therapy (Schmitz et al, 1994a). Following the cessation of cytokine therapy, marrow cellularity and the M/E ratio return to normal within 4–8 weeks (Schmitz et al, 1994b), whereas peripheral white blood cell counts and absolute neutrophil counts tend to be maintained (Ryder et al, 1992).

The use of G-CSF and GM-CSF therapy causes a difficult differential diagnostic problem: the detection of early relapse of acute myelogenous leukemia (Table 8–6). Blasts may be seen in the peripheral blood with cytokine therapy, but in general the peripheral blood and marrow blast count does not exceed 3%. In addition, the blasts are seen in the context of a myelocyte surge with evidence of maturation, whereas relapsed leukemia often has higher peripheral blast counts, Auer rods, and little evidence of myelocyte maturation. Certainly, blast counts over 3% or persistence of blasts after cessation of cytokine therapy may suggest leukemic relapse, and evaluations

Table 8–5
Changes Associated with G-CSF and GM-CSF Therapy

Changes	G-CSF and GM-CSF	Unique to G-CSF	Unique to GM-CSF
Peripheral blood			
WBC count	Increased neutrophil count with left shift, including blasts and promyelocytes	Monocytosis at high doses	Eosinophilia, monocytosis
WBC morphologic features	Prominent granulation, Döhle bodies, vacuolization, nuclear segmentation abnormalities, nuclear-cytoplasmic assynchrony	Macropolycytes	
Platelets	Enlarged	Mild, transient decrease	Transient decrease
Leukoerythroblastotic findings	Seen in 50% of cases		
LAP score	Increased		
Marrow			
Cellularity	Hypocellular to hypercellular		
M/E ratio	Increased		
Morphologic features	Cytoplasmic basophilia, increased granulation, enlarged promyelocytes and myelocytes		
Neutrophil production rate	Increased	9.4-fold	1.5-fold

Abbreviations: G-CSF, granulocyte colony-stimulating factor; GM-CSF, granulocyte-macrophage colony-stimulating factor; LAP, leukocyte alkaline phosphatase; M/E, myelocyte-to-erythrocyte; WBC, white blood cell.

Source: Modified from Lieshke GJ, Burgess AW: Granulocyte colony-stimulating factor and granulocyte-macrophage colony-stimulating factor: 1 and 2. N Engl J Med 327: 28–34, 327: 99–106, 1992.

of the blood films for 1–2 weeks may be required to differentiate growth factor effect from early relapse (Schmitz et al, 1994a). Similarly, the marrow aspirate may be difficult to interpret owing to the marked left shift, especially in cases of acute myelogenous leukemia. Diffusely distributed granulation, perinuclear cytoplasmic clearing, and higher numbers of promyelocytes than blasts are features suggesting response to cytokines (Harris et al, 1994). The presence of Auer rods, irregularly distributed cytoplasmic granules, extensive dysplasia, or high numbers of blasts may help identify leukemic relapse. If the marrow findings are indeterminant, repeated biopsy 1–2 weeks after cessation of growth factor therapy often clarifies the diagnosis (Schmitz et al, 1994a).

Cytokine therapy also obscures early changes of infection, particularly bacterial infection. Prominent azurophilic granulation, Döhle bodies, and a left shift are hallmarks of infection as well as cytokine effects. It is important that cytokine status is known when films are reviewed for evidence of infection.

Other cytokines, such as stem cell factor, have been used occasionally to stimulate trilineage hematopoiesis following chemotherapy. These cytokines have doubled very early progenitor cells (CD34+ cells) and increased peripheral neutrophil and reticulocyte counts (Orazi et al, 1995).

Erythropoietin administration to patients with end-stage renal disease after 4 months selectively increases erythrocyte mass, normalizes the maturational sequence of erythrocyte precursors,

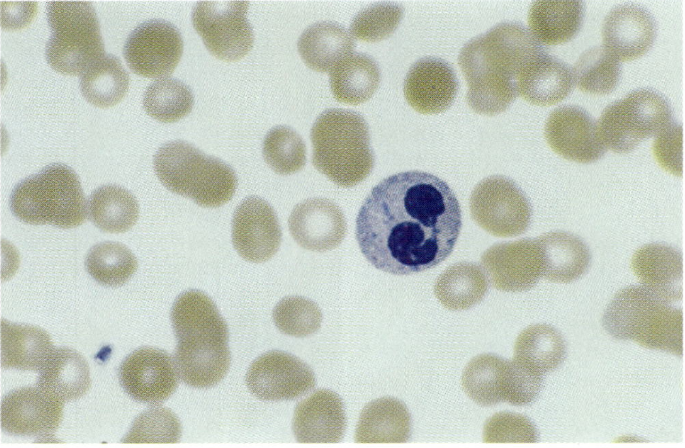

Figure 8–11

Myelocytes after cytokine therapy, peripheral blood. The characteristic changes of cytokine therapy with granulocyte colony-stimulating factor are demonstrated. The myelocyte has abnormal nuclear segmentation, prominent azurophilic granules, and multiple, coalescent Döhle bodies. Wright-Giemsa stain.

Table 8–6
Features Helpful in Distinguishing Leukemic Relapse from Cytokine Effects

Features	Growth Factor	Leukemic Relapse
Blood		
Blasts	0–3%	0–100%
Dysplastic features	Absent	Present
Neutrophilia	Marked	Variable, may be absent
Marrow		
Left shift	Present	Present
Increased blasts	Absent	Present
Auer rods	Absent	Present
Dysplastic features of myelocytic and other cell lines	Absent	Present

Source: Modified from Schmitz LL, Litz CE, Brunning RD: Morphologic and quantitative alterations in hematopoietic cells associated with growth factor therapy: review of the literature. Hematol Pathol 8: 55–73, 1994.

and notably increases the number of megakaryocytes. The increase in red cell mass in the marrow is accompanied by increased red cell counts and hemoglobin levels after 26 months of erythropoietin therapy. Platelet counts increase by an average of 30,000 platelets/μl over 26 months (Horina et al, 1991).

Thrombopoietin is a cytokine that specifically promotes megakaryocytopoiesis. In an initial study, thrombopoietin caused a dose-dependent increase in platelet counts up to 200% and marrow megakaryocytes up to fourfold. Morphologic evaluation and platelet aggregation study results were normal. There was also a marked expansion of other marrow hematopoietic cells, with increased red and white cell counts in the peripheral blood (Vadhan-Raj et al, 1997).

SELECTED READINGS

Inflammation and Infection

Abshire TC: The anemia of inflammation: a common cause of childhood anemia. Pediatr Hematol 43:623–637, 1996.

Murdoch JM, Smith CC: Infection. Clin Haematol 1:619–644, 1972.

Shenoy CM, Lin JH: Bone marrow findings in acquired immunodeficiency syndrome (AIDS). Am J Med Sci 292:372–375, 1986.

Manifestations of Systemic Diseases

Maurer HM: Hematologic effects of cardiac disease. Pediatr Clin North Am 19:1083–1093, 1972.

Means RT, Krantz SB: Progress in understanding the pathogenesis of the anemia of chronic disease. Blood 80:1639–1647, 1992.

Bone Marrow Involvement by Tumors

de Wolf-Peeters C: Bone marrow trephine interpretation: diagnostic utility and potential pitfalls. Histopathology 18:489–493, 1991.

Doll DC, Ringenberg QS, Anderson SP, et al: Bone marrow biopsy in the initial staging of Hodgkin's disease. Med Pediatr Oncol 17:1–5, 1989.

Papac RJ: Bone marrow metastases. Cancer 74:2403–2413, 1994.

Schwonzen M, Pohl C, Steinmetz T, et al: Bone marrow involvement in non-Hodgkin's lymphoma: increased diagnostic sensitivity by combination of immunocytology, cytomorphology and trephine histology. Br J Haematol 81:362–369, 1992.

Therapy-Related Changes

Dick FR, Burns CP, Weiner GJ, et al: Bone marrow morphology during induction phase of therapy for acute myeloid leukemia (AML). Hematol Pathol 9:95–106, 1995.

Islam A, Catovsky D, Galton DAG: Histological study of bone marrow regeneration following chemotherapy for acute myeloid leukaemia and chronic granulocytic leukaemia in blast transformation. Br J Haematol 45:535–540, 1980.

Lieschke GJ, Burgess AW: Granulocyte colony-stimulating factor and granulocyte-macrophage colony-stimulating factor: 1. N Engl J Med 327:28–34, 1992.

Longacre TA, Foucar K, Crago S, et al: Hematogones: a multiparameter analysis of bone marrow precursor cells. Blood 73:543–552, 1989.

Sale GE, Buckner D: Pathology of bone marrow in transplant recipients. Hematol Oncol Clin North Am 2:735–756, 1988.

Schmitz LL, Litz CE, Brunning RD: Morphologic and quantitative alterations in hematopoietic cells associated with growth factor therapy: review of the literature. Hematol Pathol 8:55–73, 1994.

REFERENCES

Abshire TC: The anemia of inflammation: a common cause of childhood anemia. Pediatr Hematol 43:623–637, 1996.

Amylon MD: Allogeneic bone marrow transplant in pediatric patients with high-risk hematopoietic malignancies early in the course of their disease. J Pediatr Hematol Oncol 19:54–61, 1997.

Arnez M, Cizman M, Jazbec J, et al: Acute infectious lymphocytosis caused by coxsackie virus B2. Pediatr Infect Dis J 15:1127–1128, 1996.

Bagby GC, Gilbert DN: Suppression of granulopoiesis by T-lymphocytes in two patients with disseminated mycobacterial infection. Ann Intern Med 94:478–481, 1981.

Barak Y, Sinai-Treiman L, Karov Y, et al: Hematopoietic progenitors in children with end-stage renal disease. Pediatr Hematol Oncol 11:633–639, 1994.

Baranski B, Armstrong G, Truman JT, et al: Epstein-Barr virus in the bone marrow of patients with aplastic anemia. Ann Intern Med 109:695–704, 1988.

Brown KE, Young NS: Parvovirus B19 infection and hematopoiesis. Blood Rev 9:176–182, 1995.

Caldwell CW, Poje E, Helikson MA: B-cell precursors in normal pediatric bone marrow. Am J Clin Pathol 95:816–823, 1991.

Campbell LJ, Maher DW, Tay DLM, et al: Marrow proliferation and the appearance of giant neutrophils in response to recombinant human granulocyte colony stimulating factor (rhG-CSF). Br J Haematol 80:298–304, 1992.

Cartwright GE, Deiss A: Sideroblasts, siderocytes, and sideroblastic anemia. N Engl J Med 292:185–193, 1975.

Castella A, Croxson TS, Mildvan D, et al: The bone marrow in AIDS. Am J Clin Pathol 84:425–432, 1985.

Champlin RE, Horowitz MM, van Bekkum DW, et al: Graft failure following bone marrow transplantation for severe aplastic anemia: risk factors and treatment results. Blood 73:606–613, 1989.

Cheson BD, Cassileth PA, Head DR, et al: Report of the National Cancer Institute–sponsored workshop on definitions and response in acute myelogenous leukemia. J Clin Oncol 8:812–819, 1990.

Choi MFV, Mant MJ, Turner AR, et al: Successful reversal of neutropenia in Felty's syndrome with recombinant granulocyte colony stimulating factor. Br J Haematol 86:663–664, 1994.

Christensen RD, Rothstein G: Exhaustion of mature marrow neutrophils in neonates with sepsis. J Pediatr 96:316–320, 1980.

Cooper RA: Hemolytic syndromes and red cell membrane abnormalities in liver disease. Semin Hematol 17:103–112, 1980.

Cooper RA, Diloy-Puray M, Lando P, et al: An analysis of lipoproteins, bile acids, and red cell membranes associated with target cells and spur cells in patients with liver disease. J Clin Invest 51: 3182–3192, 1972.

Corrigan JJ: Thrombocytopenia: a laboratory sign of septicemia in infants and children. J Pediatr 85:219–221, 1974.

Corrigan JJ, Ray WL, May N: Changes in the blood coagulation system associated with septicemia. N Engl J Med 279:851–856, 1968.

Davies SC, Roberts IAG: Bone marrow transplant for sickle cell disease: an update. Arch Dis Child 75:3–6, 1996.

de Wolf-Peeters C: Bone marrow trephine interpretation: diagnostic utility and potential pitfalls. Histopathology 18:489–493, 1991.

Dick FR, Burns CP, Weiner GJ, et al: Bone marrow morphology during induction phase of therapy for acute myeloid leukemia (AML). Hematol Pathol 9:95–106, 1995.

Dinant HJ, de Maat CEM: Erythropoiesis and mean red-cell lifespan in normal subjects and in patients with the anaemia of active rheumatoid arthritis. Br J Haematol 329:437–444, 1978.

Doll DC, Ringenberg QS, Anderson SP, et al: Bone marrow biopsy in the initial staging of Hodgkin's disease. Med Pediatr Oncol 17: 1–5, 1989.

Dritschilo A, Sherman DS: Radiation and chemical injury in the bone marrow. Environ Health Perspect 39:59–64, 1981.

Enberg RN, Eberle BJ, Williams RC: T- and B-cells in peripheral blood during infectious mononucleosis. J Infect Dis 130:104–111, 1974.

Fraga M, Brousset P, Schlaifer D, et al: Bone marrow involvement in anaplastic large cell lymphoma. Am J Clin Pathol 103:82–89, 1995.

George CRP, Slighter SJ, Quadracci LJ, et al: A kinetic evaluation of hemostasis in renal disease. N Engl J Med 291:1111–1115, 1974.

Glasser RM, Walker RI, Herion JC: The significance of hematologic abnormalities in patients with tuberculosis. Arch Intern Med 125: 691–695, 1970.

Gordge MP, Faint RW, Rylance PB, et al: Platelet function and the bleeding time in progressive renal failure. Thromb Haemost 60: 83–87, 1988.

Grand RJ, Ramakrishna J, Calenda KA: Inflammatory bowel disease in the pediatric patient. Gastroenterol Clin North Am 24:613–632, 1995.

Gumaste V, Greenstein AJ, Meyers R, et al: Coombs-positive autoimmune hemolytic anemia in ulcerative colitis. Dig Dis Sci 34: 1457–1461, 1989.

Hanna JD, Krieg RJ, Scheinman JI, et al: Effects of uremia on growth in children. Semin Nephrol 16:230–241, 1996.

Harris AC, Todd WA, Hackney MH, et al: Bone marrow changes associated with recombinant granulocyte-macrophage and granulocyte colony-stimulating factors. Arch Pathol Lab Med 118:624–629, 1994.

Harris JW: Parvovirus B19 for the hematologist. Am J Hematol 39: 119–130, 1992.

Hoagland HC: Hematologic complications of cancer chemotherapy. Semin Oncol 9:95–102, 1982.

Horina JH, Schmid CR, Roob JM, et al: Bone marrow changes following treatment of renal anemia with erythropoietin. Kidney Int 40: 917–922, 1991.

Hutchinson FN, Jones WJ: A cost-effective analysis of anemia screening before erythropoietin in patients with end-stage renal disease. Am J Kidney Dis 29:651–657, 1997.

Islam A, Catovsky D, Galton DAG: Histological study of bone marrow regeneration following chemotherapy for acute myeloid leukaemia and chronic granulocytic leukaemia in blast transformation. Br J Haematol 45:535–540, 1980.

Jenkins WJ, Koster HG, Marsh WL, et al: Infectious mononucleosis: an unsuspected source of anti-i. Br J Haematol 11:480–483, 1965.

Karpatkin S, Strick N, Karpatkin MB, et al: Cumulative experience in the detection of antiplatelet antibody in 234 patients with idiopathic thrombocytopenic purpura, systemic lupus erythematosus and other clinical disorders. Am J Med 52:776–785, 1972.

Katz AJ, Falchuk ZM: Current concepts in gluten sensitive enteropathy (celiac sprue). Pediatr Clin North Am 22:767–785, 1975.

Kobayashi SD, Seki K, Suwa N, et al: The transient appearance of small blastoid cells in the marrow after bone marrow transplantation. Am J Clin Pathol 96:191–195, 1991.

Kubic VL, Kubic PT, Brunning RD: The morphologic and immunophenotypic assessment of the lymphocytosis accompanying *Bordetella pertussis* infection. Am J Clin Pathol 95:809–815, 1991.

Laurence J: T-cell subsets in health, infectious disease, and idiopathic CD4+ T lymphocytopenia. Ann Intern Med 119:55–62, 1993.

Lechner K, Niessner H, Thaler E: Coagulation abnormalities in liver disease. Semin Thromb Hemost 4:40–56, 1977.

Leitenberg D, Rappeport JM, Smith BR: B-cell precursor bone marrow reconstitution after bone marrow transplantation. Am J Clin Pathol 102:231–236, 1994.

Lentnek AL, Schreiber AD, MacGregor RR: The induction of augmented granulocyte adherence by inflammation. J Clin Invest 57: 1098–1103, 1976.

Lieschke GJ, Burgess AW: Granulocyte colony-stimulating factor and granulocyte-macrophage colony-stimulating factor: 1. N Engl J Med 327:28–34, 1992a.

Lieschke GJ, Burgess AW: Granulocyte colony-stimulating factor and granulocyte-macrophage colony-stimulating factor: 2. N Engl J Med 327:99–106, 1992b.

Litam PP, Friedman HD, Loughran TP Jr: Splenic extramedullary hematopoiesis in a patient receiving intermittently administered granulocyte colony-stimulating factor. Ann Intern Med 118: 954–955, 1993.

Livio M, Benigni A, Remuzzi G: Coagulation abnormalities in uremia. Semin Nephrol 5:82–90, 1985.

Longacre TA, Foucar K, Crago S, et al: Hematogones: a multiparameter analysis of bone marrow precursor cells. Blood 73:543–552, 1989.

Macon WR, Tham KT, Greer JP, et al: Ringed sideroblasts: a frequent observation after bone marrow transplantation. Mod Pathol 8: 782–785, 1995.

Mahn E, Chile S, Dantuono LM: Postabortal septicotoxemia due to *Clostridium welchii*. Am J Obstet Gynecol 70:604–610, 1955.

Maldonado JE, Hanlon DG: Monocytosis: a current appraisal. Mayo Clin Proc 40:248–259, 1965.

Maurer HM: Hematologic effects of cardiac disease. Pediatr Clin North Am 19:1083–1093, 1972.

Mayer K: Transfusion of the patient with acquired immunodeficiency syndrome. Arch Pathol Lab Med 114:295–297, 1990.

McIntyre OR, Sullivan LW, Jeffries GH, et al: Pernicious anemia in childhood. N Engl J Med 272:981–986, 1965.

Means RT, Krantz SB: Progress in understanding the pathogenesis of the anemia of chronic disease. Blood 80:1639–1647, 1992.

Mee AS, Berney J, Jewell DP: Monocytes in inflammatory bowel disease: absolute monocyte counts. J Clin Pathol 33:917–920, 1980.

Moia M, Vizzotto L, Cattaneo M, et al: Improvement in the haemostatic defect of uraemia after treatment with recombinant human erythropoietin. Lancet 1:1227–1229, 1987.

Muehleck SD, McKenna RW, Gale PF, et al: Terminal deoxynucleotidyl transferase (TdT)-positive cells in bone marrow in the absence of hematologic malignancy. Am J Clin Pathol 79: 277–284, 1983.

Murdoch JM, Smith CC: Infection. Clin Haematol 1:619–644, 1972.

Naeim F, Smith GS, Gale RP: Morphologic aspects of bone marrow transplantation in patients with aplastic anemia. Hum Pathol 9: 295–308, 1978.

Neiman P, Thomas ED, Buckner CD, et al: Marrow transplantation for aplastic anemia and acute leukemia. Annu Rev Med 25: 179–198, 1974.

Nevaril CG, Lynch EC, Alfrey CP, et al: Erythrocyte damage and destruction induced by shearing stress. J Lab Clin Med 71: 784–790, 1968.

Nichols L, Florentine B, Lewis W, et al: Bone marrow examination for the diagnosis of mycobacterial and fungal infections in the acquired immunodeficiency syndrome. Arch Pathol Lab Med 115: 1125–1132, 1991.

O'Grady JG, Langley PG, Isola LM, et al: Coagulopathy of fulminant hepatic failure. Semin Liver Dis 6:159–163, 1986.

Ohga S, Matsuzaki A, Nishizaki M, et al: Inflammatory cytokines in virus-associated hemophagocytic syndrome. Am J Pediatr Hematol Oncol 15:291–298, 1993.

Olcay L, Ozer S, Gurgey A, et al: Parameters of iron deficiency in children with cyanotic congenital heart disease. Pediatr Cardiol 17: 150–154, 1996.

Orazi A, Gordon MS, John K, et al: *In vivo* effects of recombinant human stem cell factor treatment. Am J Clin Pathol 103:177–184, 1995.

Papac RJ: Bone marrow metastases. Cancer 74:2403–2413, 1994.

Person PL, Korngold R, Teuscher C: Pertussis toxin–induced lymphocytosis is associated with alterations in thymocyte subpopulations. J Immunol 148:1506–1511, 1992.

Potter MN: The detection of minimal residual disease in acute lymphoblastic leukemia. Blood Rev 6:68–82, 1992.

Radel EG, Schorr JB: Thrombocytopenic purpura with infectious mononucleosis. J Pediatr 63:46–60, 1963.

Reid MM, Hamilton PJ: Histology of neuroblastoma involving bone marrow: the problem of detecting residual tumor after initiation of chemotherapy. Br J Haematol 69:487–490, 1988.

Reid MM, Roald B: Adequacy of bone marrow trephine biopsy specimens in children. J Clin Pathol 49:226–229, 1996.

Richer S: A practical guide for differentiating between iron deficiency anemia and anemia of chronic disease in children and adults. Nurse Pract 22:82–101, 1997.

Richman DD, Fischl MA, Grieco MH, et al: The toxicity of azidothymidine (AZT) in the treatment of patients with AIDS and AIDS-related complex. N Engl J Med 317:192–197, 1987.

Risdall RJ, McKenna RW, Nesbit ME, et al: Virus-associated hemophagocytic syndrome. Cancer 44:993–1002, 1979.

Rosenstein ED, Kramer N: Felty's and pseudo-Felty's syndromes. Semin Arthritis Rheum 21:129–142, 1991.

Rosenthal NS, Farhi DC: Failure to engraft after bone marrow transplantation: bone marrow morphologic findings. Am J Clin Pathol 102:821–824, 1994.

Ryan DH, Chapple CW, Kossover SA, et al: Phenotypic similarities and differences between CALLA-positive acute lymphoblastic leukemia cells and normal marrow CALLA-positive B-cell precursors. Blood 70:814–821, 1987.

Ryder JW, Lazarus HM, Farhi DC: Bone marrow and blood findings after marrow transplantation and rhGM-CSF therapy. Am J Clin Pathol 97:631–637, 1992.

Sale GE, Buckner D: Pathology of bone marrow in transplant recipients. Hematol Oncol Clin North Am 2:735–756, 1988.

Saulsbury FT: B cell proliferation in acute infectious lymphocytosis. Pediatr Infect Dis J 6:1127–1129, 1987.

Schmitz LL, Litz CE, Brunning RD: Morphologic and quantitative alterations in hematopoietic cells associated with growth factor therapy: review of the literature. Hematol Pathol 8:55–73, 1994a.

Schmitz LL, McClure JS, Litz CE, et al: Morphologic and quantitative changes in blood and marrow cells following growth factor therapy. Am J Clin Pathol 101:67–75, 1994b.

Schwonzen M, Pohl C, Steinmetz T, et al: Bone marrow involvement in non-Hodgkin's lymphoma: increased diagnostic sensitivity by combination of immunocytology, cytomorphology and trephine histology. Br J Haematol 81:362–369, 1992.

Shen V, Woodbury C, Killen R, et al: Collection and use of peripheral blood stem cells in young children with refractory solid tumors. Bone Marrow Transplant 19:197–204, 1997.

Shenoy CM, Lin JH: Bone marrow findings in acquired immunodeficiency syndrome (AIDS). Am J Med Sci 292:372–375, 1986.
Snower DP, Weil SC: Changing etiology of macrocytosis: zidovudine as a frequent causative factor. Am J Clin Pathol 99:57–60, 1993.
Tyndall MR, Teitel DF, Lutin WA, et al: Serum erythropoietin levels in patients with congenital heart disease. J Pediatr 110:538–544, 1987.
Vadhan-Raj S, Murray LJ, Bueso-Ramos C, et al: Stimulation of megakaryocyte and platelet production by a single dose of recombinant human thrombopoietin in patients with cancer. Ann Intern Med 126:673–681, 1997.
van den Berg H, Kluin PM, Vossen JM: Early reconstitution of haematopoiesis after allogeneic bone marrow transplantation: a prospective histopathological study of bone marrow biopsy specimens. J Clin Pathol 43:365–369, 1990.
Vellodi A, Picton S, Downie CJC, et al: Bone marrow transplantation for thalassaemia: experience of two British centres. Bone Marrow Transplant 13:559–562, 1994.
Verschueren H, Dewit J, Van der Wegen A, et al: The lymphocytosis promoting action of pertussis toxin can be mimicked in vitro. J Immunol Methods 144:231–240, 1991.
Vichinsky EP, Pennathur-Das R, Nickerson B, et al: Inadequate erythroid response to hypoxia in cystic fibrosis. J Pediatr 105:15–21, 1984.
Walsh CM, Karpatkin S: Thrombocytopenia and human immunodeficiency virus-1 infection. Semin Oncol 17:367–374, 1990.
Westerman MP: Bone marrow needle biopsy: an evaluation and critique. Semin Hematol 18:293–300, 1981.
Wilson PA, Ayscue LH, Jones GR, et al: Bone marrow histiocytic proliferation association with colony-stimulating factor therapy. Am J Clin Pathol 99:311–313, 1993.
Wittels B: Bone marrow biopsy changes following chemotherapy for acute leukemia. Am J Surg Pathol 4:135–142, 1980.
Wong KF, Chan JKC, Ha SY, et al: Reactive hemophagocytic syndrome in childhood: frequent occurrence of atypical mononuclear cells. Hematol Oncol 12:67–74, 1994.
Zachee P, Vermylen J, Boogaerts MA: Hematologic aspects of end-stage renal failure. Ann Hematol 69:33–40, 1994.
Zipursky A, Palko J, Milner R, et al: The hematology of bacterial infections in premature infants. Pediatrics 57:839–853, 1976.

Sanya Sukpanichnant

Dengue and Malaria

DENGUE HEMORRHAGIC FEVER AND DENGUE SHOCK SYNDROME

Equivalent Terms

Dengue hemorrhagic fever is also known as break-bone fever.

Definition

Dengue hemorrhagic fever and shock syndrome are mosquito-borne viral hemorrhagic fevers caused by dengue virus serotypes 1, 2, 3, and 4 and are characterized by increased vascular permeability and abnormal hemostasis. Prevalent in the tropical and subtropical regions, the principal vector of dengue is the *Aedes aegypti* mosquito (Isaäcson & Hale, 1995).

Clinical Features

Clinical features range from a mild fever to fatal shock syndrome, the latter being more common in older children and adolescents. Shock syndrome is rare in infants, except in those born to dengue-immune mothers. After an incubation period of 3–14 days following the bite of an infected mosquito, there is an abrupt onset of fever, chills, and other constitutional symptoms, including lassitude, headache, anorexia, nausea, vomiting, myalgia, and a morbilliform rash. The second to fifth day is the time of defervescence of classic dengue, but a few patients experience shock and bleeding disorders, such as hematemesis and vaginal bleeding. The mortality rate varies from less than 5% to 50% (Nimmannitya et al, 1969). Cases complicated by hepatic failure or encephalopathy have been documented.

Laboratory Features

Thrombocytopenia in the shock syndrome is due in large part to maturation arrest of megakaryocytes. Aplastic anemia and hemophagocytic syndrome may also occur. Generalized lymphocytic depletion is seen in lymph nodes, spleen, and thymus (Aung-Khin et al, 1975). At autopsy, hemorrhages in multiple organs and serous effusion in the pleural and peritoneal cavities are noted.

Hemoconcentration is an important finding in diagnosing the shock syndrome. Increments of hematocrit by 20% are often observed. Paired serum samples obtained 14 days apart may be used to detect rising antibody titers by complement fixation, hemagglutination inhibition, and neutralization tests. Cross-reactivity among the four dengue serotypes is commonly seen. Viremia may be detected by reverse transcriptase polymerase chain reaction (Brown et al, 1996) or virus demonstrated by in situ hybridization (Killen & O'Sullivan, 1993). Dengue antigens may also be identified in paraffin-embedded tissue by immunohistochemical analysis (Hall et al, 1991).

Diagnostic Criteria

The diagnosis is made on the basis of acute onset of fever, hemorrhagic manifestations, hepatomegaly, shock, thrombocytopenia (≤100,000 platelets/ml), hemoconcentration (hematocrit increased by at least 20%), and a serologic test result indicating a recent dengue infection (World Health Organization, 1986).

Differential Diagnosis

Hemorrhagic diatheses and multiple organ failure are found in yellow fever, malaria, leptospirosis, and other viral hemorrhagic fevers.

Pathogenesis

Dengue viruses replicate in the cells of the mononuclear phagocyte system. If patients are exposed to one serotype of the dengue virus, usually type 2, following exposure to another serotype or if they have passively acquired maternal antibodies, viral replication is apparently enhanced by concomitant enhancing antibodies to heterologous dengue serotypes. The formation of antigen-antibody complexes and subsequent activation of the complement system produce a hemorrhagic diathesis and the increased vascular permeability of the dengue shock syndrome (Halstead, 1989). Dengue viruses also infect the marrow stromal cells. Altered cytokine production by these cells may transiently suppress the marrow (Rothwell et al, 1996).

MALARIA

Definition

Malaria is caused by protozoan parasites of the genus *Plasmodium*, including *P. vivax, P. falciparum, P. ovale*, and *P. malariae*. Malaria is one of the commonest parasitic diseases in the world, with 270 to 450 million new cases developing worldwide each year (Marty & Andersen, 1995).

Clinical Features

Periodic febrile paroxysms, including cold, hot, and perspiration stages, are pathognomonic of malaria, although they are not always present in children. These febrile cycles correspond to red cell lysis and parasitic release (Randall & Seidel, 1985) and were once used to describe the types of malaria. There are no reliable clinical features of malaria in children other than the periodic febrile paroxysms. Anemia and leukopenia are common, but leukemoid reactions may be observed during periods of red cell lysis and release of parasites. In endemic areas splenomegaly is found in >50% and hepatomegaly in >25% of cases. Black water fever is most often associated with *P. falciparum*. Sudden intravascular hemolysis results in a dramatically dark-colored urine. Children are at risk for developing nephrotic syndrome, especially in *P. malariae* infection. Transfusion malaria may occur if the screening techniques for donors are ineffective. Congenital malaria occurs if the mother has parasitemia during pregnancy. Affected infants generally present days or weeks after birth. Malaria is difficult to distinguish from other congenital infections because the fever pattern is generally not synchronized.

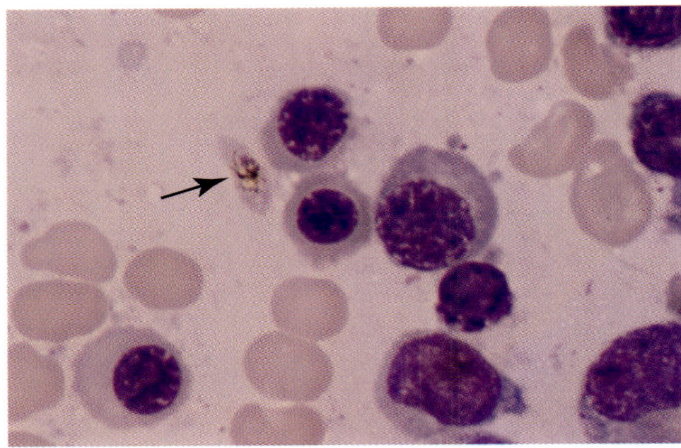

Figure 8–13

Malaria, *Plasmodium falciparum*, marrow. A fusiform gametocyte *(arrow)*, a finding diagnostic of falciparum malaria, is found in this film from a child who had malaria-associated hemophagocytic syndrome (not shown). Wright stain. (Marrow film kindly provided by Dr. Gavivann Veerakul.)

Malaria causes an estimated 1.5 to 2.5 million deaths per year. Most deaths are due to *P. falciparum*–induced cerebral involvement, renal failure, and pulmonary edema. Traumatic or spontaneous splenic rupture may cause death in patients with species other than *P. falciparum*. Recrudescence or relapse occurs, especially in *P. vivax* and *P. ovale* infections (Marty & Andersen, 1995).

Laboratory Features

The presence of asexual and sexual forms of parasites in erythrocytes is pathognomonic of malaria. The asexual forms include the early trophozoites (ring forms), late trophozoites, and schizonts containing merozoites, which are released to enter other erythrocytes (Fig. 8–12). The sexual forms are male and female gametocytes (Fig. 8–13). The diagnostic features of the four species of malarial parasites in Giemsa-stained peripheral blood smears are compared in Table 8–7 (Marty & Andersen, 1995). Dark-brown malarial pigments as well as

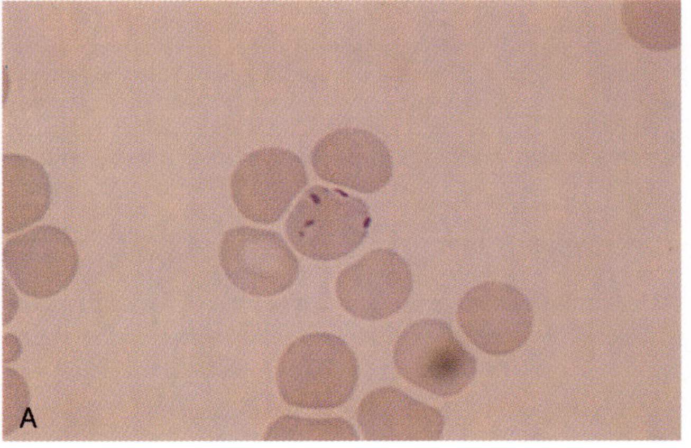

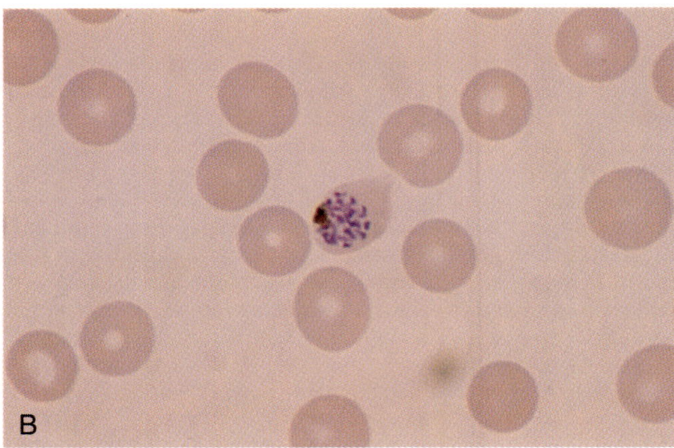

Figure 8–12

Malaria, *Plasmodium falciparum*, peripheral blood. *A*, Multiple ring forms (early trophozoites) in one erythrocyte. Also note the appliqué form at the cytoplasmic membrane of the erythrocyte. *B*, Approximately 20 merozoites in one erythrocyte. Also note the dark-brown malarial pigment. It is rare to see schizont or merozoites in falciparum malaria except in the advanced stage. Wright stain.

Table 8–7

Diagnostic Features of the Four Malarial Parasites in Giemsa-Stained Peripheral Blood Films

Features	P. falciparum	P. vivax	P. ovale	P. malariae
Erythrocyte size	Normal	Enlarged	Enlarged	Normal
Inclusions	Maurer dots (rare)	Schüffner stippling	Schüffner stippling	Ziemans dots (rare)
Multiple parasites per erythrocyte	Frequent	Occasional	Rare	Rare
Double chromatin dot	Frequent	Occasional	Occasional	Rare
Pigment	Brown-black	Yellow-brown	Yellow-brown	Black
Stages detected	Usually only rings and/or gametocytes	All	All	All
Rings	Small, delicate, $\frac{1}{5}$ size of erythrocyte	$\frac{1}{3}$ size of erythrocyte, large chromatin dot	Like *P. vivax*	Small and thick, large chromatin dot
Trophozoites	Small and solid (rare)	Large, very ameboid	Usually compact, dense, and round	Usually like *P. ovale* but smaller
Merozoites per schizont	8–24 (rare)	12–24	4–16	6–12, rosette pattern
Gametocytes	Crescent or banana shaped	Round	Round	Round
Remarks	Frequent appliqué forms in ring stage		Erythrocytes often oval and fimbriated	Trophozoites may form band or basket shape

Source: Marty AM, Andersen EM: Malaria. In Doerr W, Seifert G (eds): Tropical Pathology, 2nd ed. Springer, Berlin, pp 557–596, 1995.

phagocytosed parasitized erythrocytes may be found in monocytes (Fig. 8–14).

Localization of parasites in tissue capillaries depends on the level of parasitemia. In all patients, there is pronounced hyperplasia of cells in the mononuclear phagocyte system, particularly Kupffer cells and sinus histiocytes in the spleen. Malarial pigments are found within these cells (Fig. 8–15). Engorgement of the splenic red pulp is constantly found. Hemorrhage and infarction are occasionally seen, and fibrosis and siderotic nodules are found in chronic malaria. Disseminated intravascular coagulation is sometimes observed. Malaria-associated hemophagocytic syndrome can occur.

In addition to the conventional examination for malarial parasites in erythrocytes with thin and thick films, other methods have been developed for the diagnosis of malaria: (1) quantitative blood technique using acridine orange and fluorescent microscopy (Cabezos & Bada, 1993); (2) a dipstick technique (ParaSight F) to detect the presence of histidine-rich protein II in the serum of patients with *P. falciparum* (Marty & Andersen, 1995); (3) flow cytometric analysis and DNA staining of the parasites (van Vianen et al, 1993); and (4) molecular biology techniques, including detection of *P. falciparum* by DNA probe (Liu et al, 1993) and polymerase chain reaction (Snounou et al, 1993).

Diagnostic Criteria

A history of visiting an endemic area is an important diagnostic clue. Residents of such areas are presumed to be at risk. Periodic fever should trigger a peripheral blood examination for malarial parasites in Giemsa-stained blood films. Malaria with low parasitemia may be difficult to diagnose. Two hundred to 300 oil immersion fields of thin films should be examined before a negative result is reported. Additional methods described earlier may be useful in cases with scant numbers of parasites.

Differential Diagnosis

Babesiosis, a tick-borne disease caused by *Babesia microti*, may mimic malaria. Babesiae appear as pleomorphic ringlike struc-

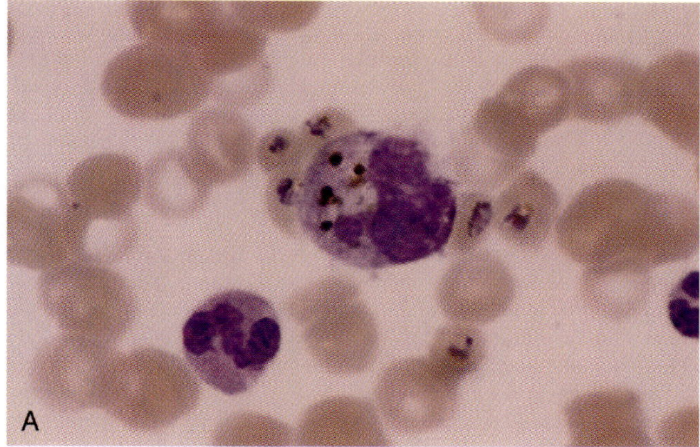

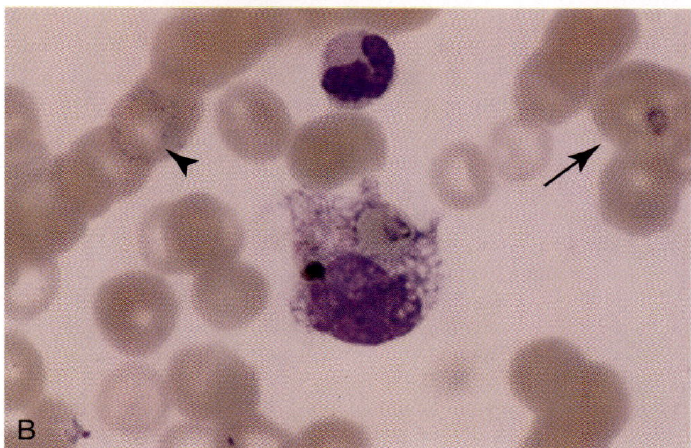

Figure 8–14

Malaria, peripheral blood. *A*, Dark-brown malarial pigment in the cytoplasm of a monocyte. Also note malarial trophozoites in the surrounding erythrocytes. *B*, Dark-brown malarial pigment and a phagocytosed, parasitized erythrocyte in the cytoplasm of a monocyte. Also note a malarial trophozoite in one erythrocyte *(arrow)* and gray-blue–staining Maurer dots in the other erythrocyte *(arrowhead)*. Wright stain.

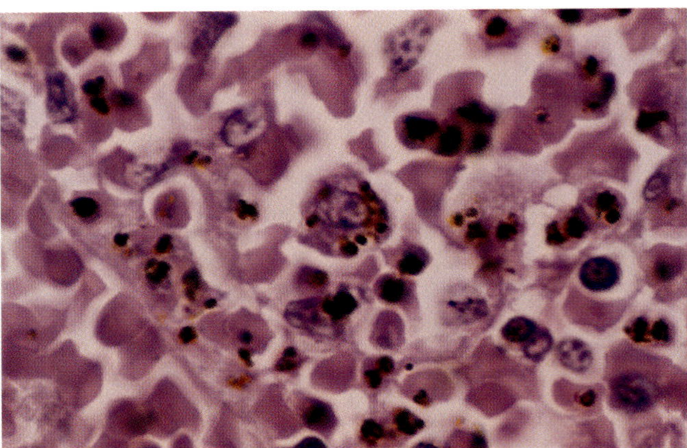

Figure 8–15

Malaria, spleen. Note dark-brown malarial pigments in macrophages and erythrocytes. It is difficult to determine the precise stages of malarial parasites in histologic sections. Hematoxylin-eosin stain.

tures in erythrocytes, resembling the ring forms of *P. falciparum*. Moreover, serologic studies reveal cross-reactivity among various species of *Babesia* and several species of *Plasmodium* (Ruebush et al, 1981). The correct diagnosis may be made based on the presence of tetrads (Maltese crosses), variation in size of the parasites, absence of pigments, and presence of more extracellular parasites in babesiosis.

Pathogenesis

The life cycle of malarial parasites consists of a sexual phase in female anopheline mosquitoes and an asexual phase in humans. As a female *Anopheles* mosquito takes its blood meal, sporozoites are injected into the human host and enter hepatocytes, where they undergo asexual multiplication, a process known as exoerythrocytic schizogony. After several days, tissue schizonts release thousands of merozoites into the circulation, where they enter erythrocytes and begin the second phase of asexual reproduction. In *P. vivax* and *P. ovale*, some sporozoites in hepatocytes lie dormant as hypnozoites and are responsible for the relapses seen in these two types of malaria.

The merozoites enter erythrocytes via a species-specific glycoprotein on the surface of erythrocytes. The erythrocytic stages are separated into asexual and sexual reproductions. After several cycles of asexual reproduction, the sexual forms occur as male and female gametocytes, which enter the mosquito during a blood meal and eventually produce sporozoites to complete the life cycle.

Transfusion malaria occurs by inoculation of blood containing malarial parasites in erythrocytic stages. The incubation period is shorter but there is no relapse because there are no sporozoites to infect the hepatocytes. Parasites have been found in the placentae of mothers whose infants develop congenital malaria. Most of the ill effects of malaria may be attributed to intravascular hemolysis and vaso-occlusion.

Intravascular hemolysis is responsible for anemia, unconjugated hyperbilirubinemia, hyperkalemia, and fever from release of plasmodial antigens and pyrogens. *Plasmodium falciparum* causes erythrocytes to stick to endothelium and thereby occludes microcirculation. Immune responses to malaria produce tropical splenomegaly, glomerulonephritis, and thrombocytopenia. Cytokine production by parasite-reactive T cells as well as alteration of erythrocytes contributes to cerebral malaria in *P. falciparum* infection (Marty & Andersen, 1995).

Anemia in malaria is caused not only by increased destruction of erythrocytes but also by decreased production due to marrow suppression seen in acute infections. Tumor necrosis factor may contribute to dyserythropoiesis and erythrophagocytosis in malaria (Clark & Chaudhri, 1988).

REFERENCES

Dengue Hemorrhagic Fever and Dengue Shock Syndrome

Aung-Khin M, Ma-Ma K, Thant-Zin: Changes in the tissues of the immune system in dengue haemorrhagic fever. J Trop Med Hyg 78: 256–261, 1975.

Brown JL, Wilkinson R, Davidson RN, et al: Rapid diagnosis and determination of duration of viraemia in dengue fever using a reverse transcriptase polymerase chain reaction. Trans R Soc Trop Med Hyg 90:140–143, 1996.

Hall WC, Crowell TP, Watts DM, et al: Demonstration of yellow fever and dengue antigens in formalin-fixed paraffin-embedded human liver by immunohistochemical analysis. Am J Trop Med Hyg 45: 408–417, 1991.

Halstead SB: Antibody, macrophages, dengue virus infection, shock, and hemorrhage: a pathogenetic cascade. Rev Infect Dis 11(suppl 4):S830–S839, 1989.

Isaäcson M, Hale MJ: The viral haemorrhagic fever. In Doerr W, Seifert G (eds): Tropical Pathology, 2nd ed. Springer, Berlin, pp 427–430, 1995.

Killen H, O'Sullivan MA: Detection of dengue virus by in situ hybridization. J Virol Methods 41:135–146, 1993.

Nimmannitya S, Halstead SB, Cohen SN, et al: Dengue and Chikungunya virus infection in man in Thailand, 1962–1964: I. Observations on hospitalized patients with hemorrhagic fever. Am J Trop Med Hyg 18:954–971, 1969.

Rothwell SW, Putnak R, La Russa VF: Dengue-2 virus infection of human bone marrow: characterization of dengue-2 antigen-positive stromal cells. Am J Trop Med Hyg 54:503–510, 1996.

World Health Organization: Dengue haemorrhagic fever: diagnosis, treatment, and control. World Health Organization, Geneva, pp 1–58, 1986.

Malaria

Cabezos J, Bada JL: The diagnosis of malaria by the thick film and the QBC: a comparative study of both technics. Med Clin (Barc) 101: 91–94, 1993.

Clark IA, Chaudhri G: Tumor necrosis factor may contribute to the anemia of malaria by causing dyserythropoiesis and erythrophagocytosis. Br J Haematol 70:99–103, 1988.

Liu KY, Huang BC, Zhang HH, et al: Cloning of a DNA probe and its application in the detection of *Plasmodium falciparum*: a preliminary report. Chin Med J (Engl) 106:31–34, 1993.

Marty AM, Andersen EM: Malaria. In Doerr W, Seifert G (eds): Tropical Pathology, 2nd ed. Springer, Berlin, pp 557–596, 1995.

Randall G, Seidel JS: Malaria. Pediatr Clin North Am 32:893–916, 1985.

Ruebush TK II, Chisholm ES, Sulzer AJ, et al: Development and persistence of antibody in persons infected with *Babesia microti*. Am J Trop Med Hyg 30:291–292, 1981.

Snounou G, Viriyakosol S, Jarra W, et al: Identification of the four human malaria parasite species in field samples by the polymerase chain reaction and detection of a high prevalence of mixed infections. Mol Biochem Parasitol 58:283–292, 1993.

van Vianen PH, van Engen A, Thiathong S, et al: Flow cytometric screening of blood samples for malarial parasites. Cytometry 14:276–280, 1993.

9

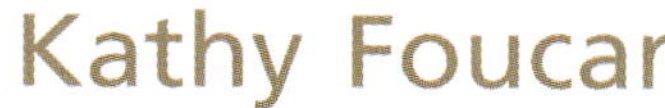

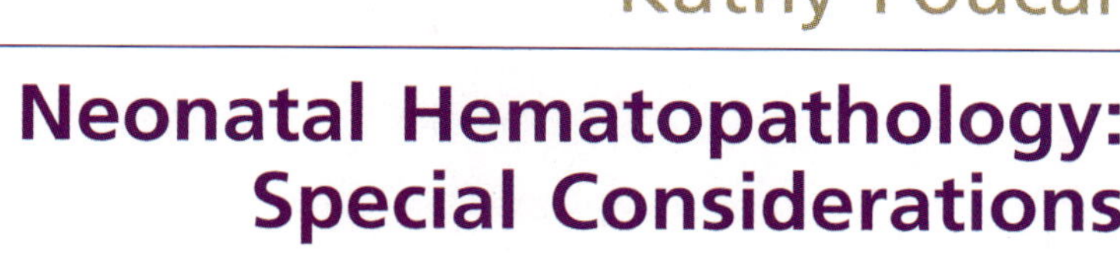

Kathy Foucar

Neonatal Hematopathology: Special Considerations

Remarkable physiologic changes in red blood cells (RBCs) and white blood cells (WBCs) characterize the neonatal blood picture. The unique "hematologic profile" of the neonate must be appreciated in order to recognize the various diseases that may affect these patients (Brugnara, 1998; Foucar, 1995e; Matsunaga & Lubin, 1995; Miller, 1995c; Oski & Naiman, 1982c). This chapter reviews the normal hematologic parameters of term and preterm neonates and discusses RBC, WBC, and platelet disorders that may present at birth or during the first weeks of life. Many of the disorders affecting neonates are discussed in detail in other chapters. These disorders are listed for differential diagnostic considerations, and the reader is referred to the appropriate chapter for a more comprehensive discussion.

Age-related normal values have been established for all hematologic parameters. Normal neonatal hematologic parameters differ substantially from those of older children and adults. Term neonates usually have higher hemoglobin levels, hematocrit levels, RBC counts, WBC counts, absolute neutrophil counts, reticulocyte counts, and mean corpuscular volume (MCV) than normal for patients of any other age (Table 9–1) (Fig. 9–1*A*). Circulating erythrocyte precursors, especially orthochromic normoblasts, are also normally present in neonates (Fig. 9–1*B*). These nucleated RBCs should be rapidly cleared from the blood, and nucleated erythrocytes do not persist beyond 3–4 days of life in normal-term infants. Because of the hypoxic in utero environment, hemoglobin and hematocrit levels of normal-term neonates are typically around 19 g/dl and 58%, respectively (Attias, 1995e; Brugnara, 1998; Miller, 1995). The dominant hemoglobin (hemoglobin F) contributes to this hypoxic environment because of its high oxygen affinity. Erythropoiesis, driven by erythropoietin production, is abundant in utero, as might be anticipated. The marked increase in oxygen availability that follows birth of a normal infant precipitates a marked decrease in serum erythropoietin levels, which in turn is reflected during the first several months of life by gradually decreasing hemoglobin, hematocrit, and RBC counts. Eventually, erythropoietin production resumes, and this "physiologic anemia" gradually resolves.

Preterm infants have hematologic parameters that differ substantially from those of term infants (Table 9–2) (Attias, 1995; Foucar, 1995e; Miller, 1995; Shannon, 1995). Hemoglobin and hematocrit levels are characteristically lower, while MCV, reticulocyte count, and the number of nucleated RBCs are all higher in preterm infants (Fig. 9–2). Likewise, the physiologic postnatal anemia is more exaggerated in preterm infants, resulting in a more rapid decline in hemoglobin levels and a lower hemoglobin level nadir. These effects are attributed to either diminished erythropoietin production or blunted responsiveness to lower hemoglobin levels (Shannon, 1995).

A brisk physiologic neutrophilia with left shift, including occasional circulating myeloblasts, is characteristic at birth in term infants (see Fig. 9–1*A*). The mean WBC count at birth is approximately 20,000/mm^3 but may be substantially greater, especially in infants born at high altitude (Carballo et al, 1991). In healthy neonates, this neutrophilia rapidly resolves, and lymphocytes predominate by approximately 1–2 weeks of age. Even though the mean WBC count is substantially lower in preterm infants, the physiologic changes in absolute neutrophil count and absolute lymphocyte count that occur during the first weeks of life parallel those of term infants (see Table 9–2) (Foucar, 1995e). By 2 weeks of age, lymphocytes predominate in the blood of normal-term and preterm neonates, a pattern that continues throughout early childhood. Some variation in platelet count may occur during the neonatal period, but the mean platelet count parallels adult values throughout this period for healthy term and preterm infants. Likewise, there are no significant variations from adult values in eosinophil or basophil levels during the neonatal period. Although the absolute monocyte count is characteristically higher throughout infancy than in older children and adults, there are no physiologic variations in this lineage during the neonatal period. Since variations in eosinophils, basophils, and monocytes are not typical in the neonatal period, these cell types are not individually discussed in this chapter.

Marrow evaluation is seldom necessary in neonates, but normal ranges for cellularity and cell distribution have been established. Cellularity is typically 100% in neonates, and the only substantial differences in cell distribution between neonatal marrow specimens and those obtained from older patients are in the proportions of erythroid cells and lymphocytes (Foucar, 1995e). The proportion of erythroid cells within the marrow is directly correlated with erythropoietin production, and a decline in erythroid cells parallels the precipitous postnatal drop in serum erythropoietin levels. Erythroid cells may constitute <5% in marrow differential cell counts during the nadir in erythrocyte production. The "physiologic anemia" of infancy is terminated by the resumption of erythropoietin production.

The proportion of lymphocytes within the marrow is characteristically higher in children, particularly in young

Thanks to Drs. Susan Scott and Dale Alverson, both neonatologists, who provided many helpful comments in reviewing this chapter.

Table 9–1
Usual Hematologic Values from Birth to 1 Month in Term Infants

Parameter/Units	Cord Blood	Day 1	Day 3	Week 1	Week 2	Week 4
Hemoglobin (g/dl)[a]	16.5	19	18	17	16	14
Hematocrit (%)	53	58	55	54	52	43
RBC ($\times 10^6/\mu l$)	5.3	5.8	5.6	5.2	4.8	4.0
MCV (μm^3)	110–115	110	105	99	99	96
MCHC (g/dl)	32	32	33	33	33	33
Reticulocytes (% of RBC)	3–7	3–7	1–4	0–1	0	0
Nucleated RBC (per 100 WBC)	500	200	0–5	0	0	0
WBC ($\times 10^3/\mu l$)	20	19	14	12	11	10
Absolute neutrophil count ($\times 10^3/\mu l$)	13	12	8	5	5	4
Absolute lymphocyte count ($\times 10^3/\mu l$)	5	5	5	5	6	6
Platelet count ($\times 10^3/\mu l$)	290	250	250	250	250	250

Note: Mean values given.

[a]Capillary samples have higher hemoglobin concentration than venous specimens.

infants, than in adults. These lymphocytes may express antigens associated with immaturity. Marked physiologic increases in lymphocyte precursors, termed hematogones, may mimic acute lymphocytic leukemia, discussed later.

ASSESSMENT OF HEMATOLOGIC ABNORMALITIES IN NEONATES

Assessments of hematologic abnormalities in neonates are uniquely complicated. Not only are there normal and dramatic physiologic variations during the neonatal period, but various maternal, familial, and obstetrical factors are linked to distinct hematologic aberrations in neonates (Foucar, 1995e; Miller, 1995c). Specific examples of factors that affect fetal and neonatal hematologic parameters are listed in Table 9–3. Any hematologic abnormality in neonates may be due to maternal, familial, or obstetrical events acting singly or in concert. For example, maternal medications, infections, and hypertension are all associated with hematologic aberrations in neonates, and various fetal or neonatal factors, such as in utero transfusions, internal hemorrhage, congenital anomalies, and rare congenital neoplasms, may also produce hematologic abnormalities (see Table 9–3). A broad range of laboratory tests used to diagnose and monitor neonates with hematologic abnormalities is given in Table 9–4.

NEONATAL ANEMIA

Differential diagnostic considerations for neonatal anemia may generally be grouped into the three major categories of blood loss, hemolysis, and reduced RBC production (Table 9–5). As emphasized earlier, determining the cause of neonatal anemia requires integrating obstetrical, familial, and maternal histories; clinical assessment; and laboratory studies, including determinations of RBC parameters (see Tables 9–3 and 9–4). Anemia has varying physiologic effects regardless of its cause (Alverson, 1995).

Most cases of neonatal anemia are from blood loss or hemolysis (see Table 9–5) (Brugnara & Platt, 1998; Miller, 1995a; Newland & Evans, 1997; Tannirandorn & Rodeck, 1991). Acquired anemia in ill neonates is often caused by iatrogenic blood withdrawal for laboratory testing. There are no

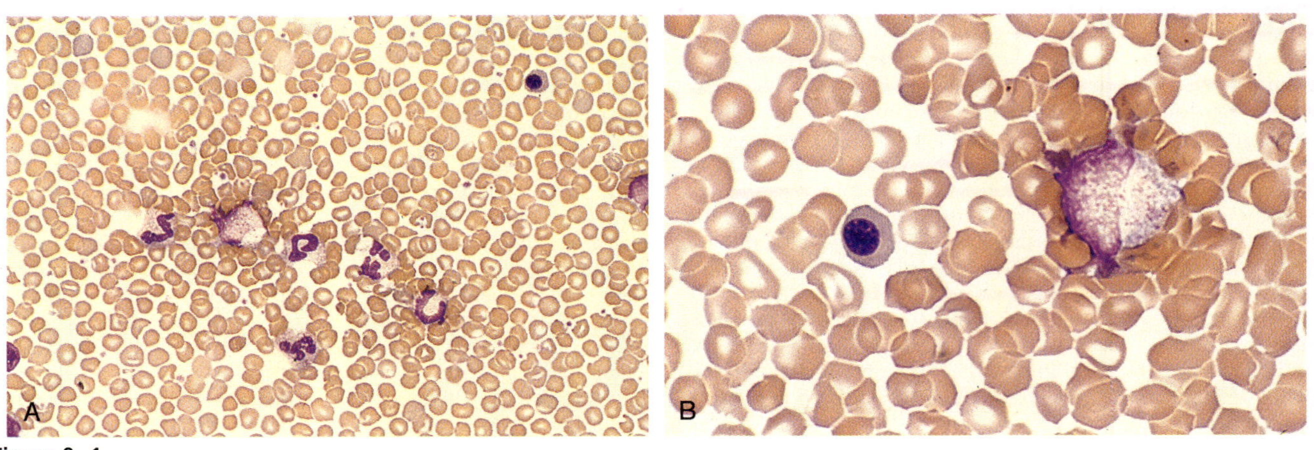

Figure 9–1

Peripheral blood, normal-term infant. *A*, This low-magnification photomicrograph illustrates neutrophilia with left shift and circulating normoblasts that are physiologic for this age. Wright stain. *B*, Higher magnification shows a promyelocyte and a circulating orthochromic normoblast. Wright stain.

Table 9–2

Physiologic Variations in Hematologic Values in Preterm Infants

RBC Parameters
- Lower hemoglobin and hematocrit levels at birth
- Higher MCV, reticulocyte percent, and number of nucleated RBCs at birth
- Shorter RBC survival time (35–50 days vs. 60–80 days for term infant)
- More rapid and more pronounced physiologic anemia; nadir at 1–2 months

WBC Parameters
- WBC count 30–50% lower at birth

Note: All parameters compared to those in term infants.

specific erythrocyte abnormalities in anemias secondary to blood loss, but sustained reticulocytosis and numerous circulating normoblasts are expected. In contrast, a variety of RBC abnormalities characterize the various types of hemolytic anemia that may occur during the neonatal period. Immune-mediated hemolytic anemias, including Rh or ABO incompatibility, are characterized by spherocytosis with striking reticulocytosis and many circulating normoblasts. A microangiopathic blood picture with erythrocytic fragmentation and microspherocytes may be seen in neonates with disseminated intravascular coagulation secondary to bacterial sepsis, various congenital infections, or congenital vascular anomalies. Hereditary RBC membrane or enzyme disorders may also be evident at birth. These disorders include hereditary spherocytosis and glucose-6-phosphate dehydrogenase deficiency.

Reduced erythrocyte production is less commonly responsible for neonatal anemia. Constitutional disorders associated with reduced erythrocyte production include Diamond-Blackfan anemia (RBC aplasia) and very rare constitutional megaloblastic, sideroblastic, and dyserythropoietic anemias, all reviewed in Chap. 6. The only acquired type of red cell aplasia in the neonatal period is secondary to maternal parvovirus infection. As noted earlier reduced erythropoietin production and blunted erythropoietin response are linked to the exaggerated "physiologic anemia" that develops shortly after birth in preterm infants (Alverson, 1995).

NEONATAL POLYCYTHEMIA

Polycythemia, defined as a venous hematocrit exceeding 65%, has several causes, including intrauterine hypoxia from hypoglycemia, cardiomegaly, and central nervous system injury (Brugnara, 1998; Miller, 1995c; Oski, 1993; Werner, 1995). Those cases caused by chronic hypoxia in utero often have increased circulating normoblasts and high reticulocyte counts. Neonatal polycythemia may also be due to increased placental transfusion at the time of delivery or twin-to-twin transfusions (Werner, 1995). Neonatal polycythemia affects approximately 2–4% of infants and is associated with maternal diabetes and infant Down syndrome. In some patients, partial plasma exchange transfusion (isovolumic erythropheresis) may be required to alleviate the neurologic, cardiopulmonary, metabolic, and vascular complications of hyperviscosity syndrome (Miller, 1995; Oski, 1993; Oski & Naiman, 1982; Werner, 1995).

NEUTROPHILIA AND NEUTROPENIA

There are both qualitative and quantitative differences between neutrophils in neonates and those in older individuals. Numerous studies demonstrate reduced adherence, chemotaxis, phagocytosis, and bacterial killing in neonatal neutrophils compared with those in older subjects (Curnette, 1993). Since the neonatal immune system is not fully operational, the increased susceptibility of neonates to life-threatening infections is understandable. The marrow of infants with infections is often unable to sustain neutrophil production and release. Consequently, "marrow exhaustion" may occur in septic neonates, a phenomenon that is more common in fatal cases. However, recent studies suggest that human recombinant granulocyte colony-stimulating factor (G-CSF) therapy may enhance neutrophil production in infected neutropenic neonates (Al-Mulla & Christensen, 1995).

The brisk neutrophilia with left shift that is evident at birth rapidly resolves in the healthy neonate (Baehner & Miller, 1995; Foucar, 1995). Persistence of toxic neutrophilia with left shift suggests ongoing stress, particularly bacterial

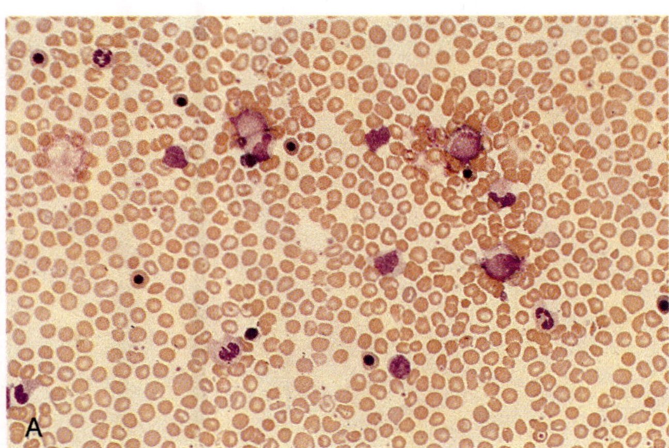

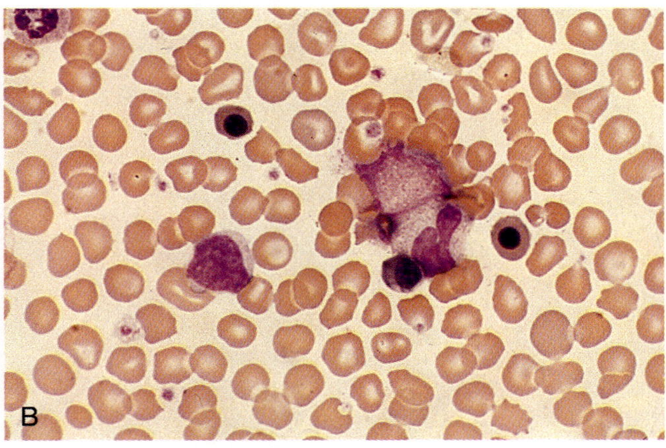

Figure 9–2

Peripheral blood, preterm infant. *A*, This low-magnification photomicrograph demonstrates a prominent left shift of granulocytic elements and numerous circulating normoblasts. Wright stain. *B*, A more prominent left shift and greater numbers of circulating normoblasts are seen. Wright stain.

Table 9–3
Hematologic Abnormalities in Neonates in Relation to Factors Associated with Disease

Factors	Considerations: Examples
Maternal	Medications: Fetal or neonatal hyperbilirubinemia, hemolysis, thrombocytopenia, neutropenia, coagulation defects Exposures or infections: hemolysis, RBC aplasia, thrombocytopenia, lymphocyte abnormalities Obstetrical complications (maternal hypertension): neonatal neutropenia Underlying illness (systemic lupus erythematosus): alloimmune fetal or neonatal thrombocytopenia, hemolytic anemia, neutropenia, other abnormalities
Familial	Rh or ABO incompatibility: variably severe hemolytic anemia secondary to maternal antibody production vs. fetal antigens inherited from father Consanguinity: increased incidence of recessive genetic disorders Constitutional disorders: numerous rare hereditary disorders of hematopoietic cell production, e.g., Diamond-Blackfan anemia (RBC aplasia), thalassemia (hemoglobinopathy), hereditary spherocytosis (RBC membrane defect), Kostmann syndrome (granulocytic aplasia), thrombocytopenia with absent radii (megakaryocyte aplasia)
Obstetrical	Traumatic birth: may cause fetal hemorrhage and neonatal anemia Chorioamnionitis: may cause fetal or neonatal infections linked to WBC abnormalities
Fetal and neonatal	Fetomaternal or twin-to-twin transfusions: neonatal anemia Internal (e.g., intracranial) hemorrhage: anemia in preterm infants Congenital anomalies Various cardiac and vascular anomalies, e.g., Kasabach-Merritt syndrome, linked to macro- or microangiopathic hemolytic anemia with variable thrombocytopenia Down syndrome linked to transient myeloproliferative disorders and other transient hematologic aberrations associated with many qualitative and quantitative abnormalities in the blood of neonates Congenital neoplasms Congenital acute leukemia linked to loss of normal hematopoietic elements and leukocytosis with many circulating blasts Stage IVS neuroblastoma with extensive marrow involvement linked, in rare cases, to neonatal cytopenia

Table 9–4
Laboratory Assessment of Hematologic Disorders in Neonates

Laboratory Test	Useful in Evaluating
Hemoglobin, hematocrit, RBC count	Anemia vs. normal vs. polycythemia
MCV	Gestational age variations
Reticulocyte count	RBC production
Nucleated erythrocyte precursor level	RBC production
Coombs test	Allo- (rarely auto-) erythrocyte antibodies
Maternal antibody titers	Source of alloantibodies
Maternal CBC	Assess for autoantibody-mediated cytopenia
Kleihauer Betke of maternal blood	Fetomaternal transfusion
ABO and Rh typing of neonate and mother	Assess for incompatibility
Bilirubin level	Chronic hemolysis
RBC morphologic features	Evidence of microangiopathic hemolysis or constitutional anemia, e.g., hereditary spherocytosis
DIC work-up	Septic or other type of coagulopathy
TORCH screening	Congenital infections
Cultures	Possibility of infection
Marrow examination	Rarely indicated unless constitutional aplasia, congenital leukemia, or transient myeloproliferative disorder suspected

Abbreviations: DIC, disseminated intravascular coagulation; TORCH antibody screening for toxoplasmosis, rubella, cytomegalovirus, and herpesvirus.

Table 9–5
Neonatal Anemias Grouped by Mechanism

Mechanism	Examples and Comments
Blood Loss	
Occult hemorrhage	Fetomaternal hemorrhage
Blood loss from phlebotomy	Laboratory test monitoring in ill neonate
Obstetrical accidents	Ruptured umbilical cord
Malformations of placenta or cord	Placenta previa
Internal hemorrhage	Intracranial hemorrhage
Hemolysis	
Immune mediated	Rh incompatibility
Infection	Bacterial sepsis, congenital CMV
Macro- or microangiopathic	Cavernous hemangioma, DIC
Hereditary disorders of RBC membrane	Hereditary spherocytosis[a]
Hereditary RBC enzyme deficiencies	G6PD deficiency[a]
	PK deficiency[a]
Thalassemias	Severe forms[a]
Reduced Production	
RBC aplasia	Maternal parvovirus infection, Diamond-Blackfan anemia[a]
Constitutional megaloblastic anemia[a]	Rarely encountered in clinical practice
Constitutional sideroblastic anemia[a]	Rarely encountered in clinical practice
Congenital dyserythropoietic anemia[a]	Rarely encountered in clinical practice

[a]See Chapter 6.
Abbreviations: CMV, cytomegalovirus; DIC, disseminated intravascular coagulation; G6PD, glucose-6-phosphate dehydrogenase; PK, pyruvate kinase.

infection. Except for the transient myeloproliferative disorders in neonates with Down syndrome, discussed later, constitutional disorders linked to sustained mature neutrophilia are exceedingly rare.

In contrast, neonatal neutropenia is a frequently encountered hematologic abnormality. The differential diagnoses in these patients include neonatal infections (the commonest cause); maternal factors, such as hypertension or drug treatments; maternal antibody production resulting in immune-mediated neutrophil destruction; and a variety of rare constitutional disorders characterized by defective neutrophil maturation or production (see Tables 9–3 and 9–6) (Al-Mulla & Christensen, 1995; Baehner & Miller, 1995; Baley et al, 1988; Curnette, 1993; Foucar, 1995a; Koenig & Christensen, 1989; Oski & Naiman, 1982c; Sievers & Dale, 1996; Smith et al, 1996). These constitutional neutrophil disorders are detailed in Chap. 6.

LYMPHOCYTOSIS

Circulating lymphocytes are abundant in the blood of neonates and become the predominant WBC as the transient antepartum neutrophilia subsides. These lymphocytes typically demonstrate finer nuclear chromatin and greater nuclear irregularity than seen in older individuals, presumably reflecting an immature immune system. Neonates with congenital infections often have circulating reactive lymphocytes. T cells predominate within the blood in patients of all ages, but the helper-to-suppressor cell ratio in neonates exceeds that in normal adults (Kotylo et al, 1993). Likewise, B cells are more numerous in neonates and young infants than in older subjects (Kotylo et al, 1993; Motley et al, 1996).

Lymphocytes are abundant within the marrow of children and in some circumstances may morphologically and immunophenotypically mimic acute lymphoblastic leukemia (Caldwell et al, 1991; Foucar, 1995c; Longacre et al, 1989; Mandel et al, 1991). These benign lymphocyte precursor cells, or hematogones, are especially numerous in the marrow of young infants and may be encountered on marrow examination of neonates. Conditions associated with substantially increased numbers of marrow hematogones include a variety of constitutional and acquired hematologic disorders.

Infants and children undergoing tumor staging and children recovering from marrow suppression typically demonstrate an increase in hematogones (Table 9–7). Hematogones characteristically have round to irregular nuclei with dense,

Table 9–6
Neutropenia in Early Infancy: Constitutional Disorders

Disorder	Comments
Cyclic neutropenia	Regulatory defect with intermittent reduction in hematopoietic elements followed by rebound
Kostmann syndrome	Marrow granulocyte production failure
Schwachman-Diamond syndrome	Marrow granulocyte production and/or maturation failure; other lineages possibly affected
Chédiak-Higashi syndrome	Defective granule formation in many lineages; intramedullary cell death
Myelokathexis	Intramedullary death of defective granulocytic elements
T cell and B cell immunodeficiency disorders	Failure of marrow regulation of granulopoiesis

Table 9–7
Increased Marrow Hematogones: Associated Conditions

Conditions	Comments
Cytopenias	Constitutional and acquired anemia, neutropenia, and thrombocytopenia
Nonhematologic neoplasms	Staging for retinoblastoma, neuroblastoma (including stage IVS), and Wilms tumor
Marrow suppression	Following aggressive multiagent chemotherapy for hematologic or nonhematologic disorders Following viral infections that cause significant suppression of hematopoiesis Following marrow transplantation

homogeneously condensed chromatin, inconspicuous nucleoli, and a very high nuclear-cytoplasmic ratio (Fig. 9–3). Immunophenotyping studies on marrow samples from children with numerous hematogones reveal increased numbers of lymphocytes expressing an immature phenotype as well as abundant, mature polyclonal B cells (Fig. 9–4). Although their immunophenotypic profile suggests acute lymphoblastic leukemia, these lymphocyte precursors are shown to be nonclonal by cytogenetic and molecular studies. Evolution to acute lymphoblastic leukemia has not been described in these patients (Longacre et al, 1989). In all likelihood, these abundant hematogones represent an exaggerated normal B cell constitution that is particularly apparent in recovery or regeneration following various marrow insults.

DISORDERS OF PLATELETS AND MEGAKARYOCYTES

Thrombocytopenia is common in distressed neonates but occurs in <1% of healthy term infants (Dreyfus et al, 1997; Newland & Evans, 1997). Neonatal thrombocytopenia has numerous causes, including maternal drug ingestion; maternal illnesses, such as systemic lupus erythematosus or infections; maternal alloimmunization against fetal platelet antigens; fetal or neonatal infections; fetal chromosomal abnormalities, such as trisomy 13, 18, or 21; and various therapeutic measures (see Table 9–3) (Alter & Young, 1993; Burrows & Kelton, 1995; Bussel & Corrigan, 1995; Dreyfus et al, 1997; Hohlfeld et al, 1994; Oski & Naiman, 1982b; Panzer et al, 1995; Udom-Rice & Bussel, 1995). In all these disorders, bone marrow megakaryocytes are abundant, and circulating megakaryocytes may be evident on blood smear review or by specialized elutriation studies (Levine et al, 1996). Only very rare constitutional disorders, such as thrombocytopenia with absent radii and X-linked amegakaryocytic thrombocytopenia, are associated with decreased numbers of bone marrow megakaryocytes in neonates (Alter & Young, 1993; Beardsley, 1993; Bussel & Corrigan, 1995; Foucar, 1995d; Oski & Naiman, 1982b; Newland & Evans, 1997; Udom-Rice & Bussel, 1995). The most dramatic platelet and megakaryocyte abnormalities in the blood and bone marrow of neonates are those associated with Down syndrome, which are described in detail in the next section.

HEMATOLOGIC ABNORMALITIES IN NEONATES WITH DOWN SYNDROME

Neonates and even fetuses studied in utero with Down syndrome (DS) may have various striking but transient blood and marrow aberrations (Table 9–8) (Doyle et al, 1995; Foucar et al, 1992; Litz et al, 1995; Kempski et al, 1997; Horwitz, 1997). Rarely, phenotypically normal neonates with mosaic DS may also develop these transient disorders (Doyle et al, 1995). Polycythemia with a venous hematocrit >65% is a common abnormality in neonatal DS patients and may require aggressive medical management to ameliorate the hyperviscosity. The other hematologic aberrations described in DS neonates include transient myeloproliferative disorders, normoblastosis, and, rarely, thrombocytosis. These idiopathic transient leukocytoses and normoblastoses eventually spontaneously remit, but they must be distinguished from overt neoplastic processes, such as congenital leukemia.

The most commonly encountered "pseudoleukemia" in neonates with DS is usually called transient myeloproliferative

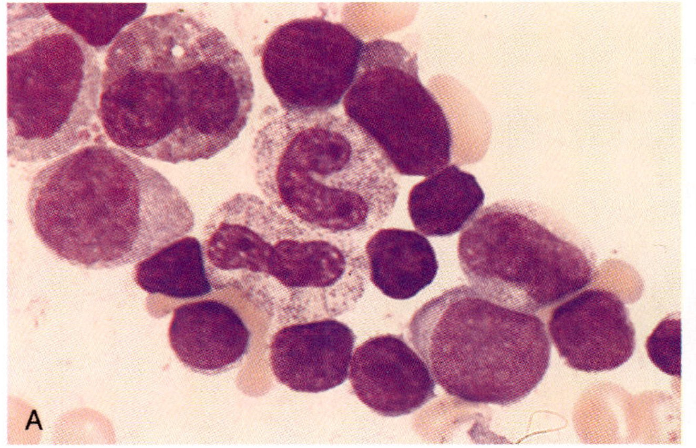

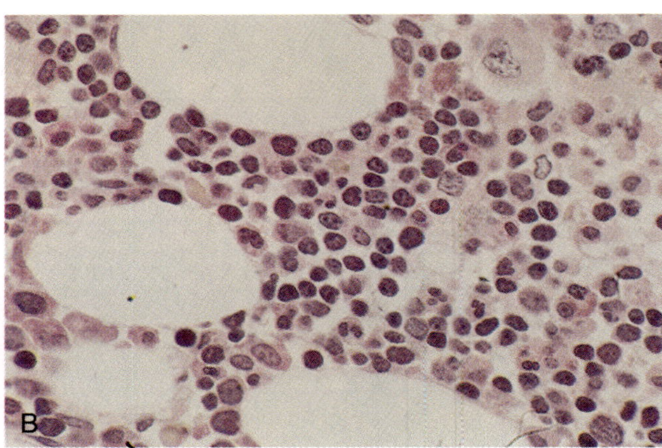

Figure 9–3

Increased hematogones, marrow from infant. *A*, This aspirate film obtained for staging in a patient with retinoblastoma demonstrates a striking increase in hematogones, causing concern for acute lymphoblastic leukemia. Compare the highly condensed nuclear chromatin of these hematogones with the myeloblasts in the lower right-hand corner. Wright stain. *B*, The marrow biopsy section shows a diffuse lymphocytosis; these lymphocytes lack the dusty chromatin and convoluted nuclear configuration of typical lymphoblasts.

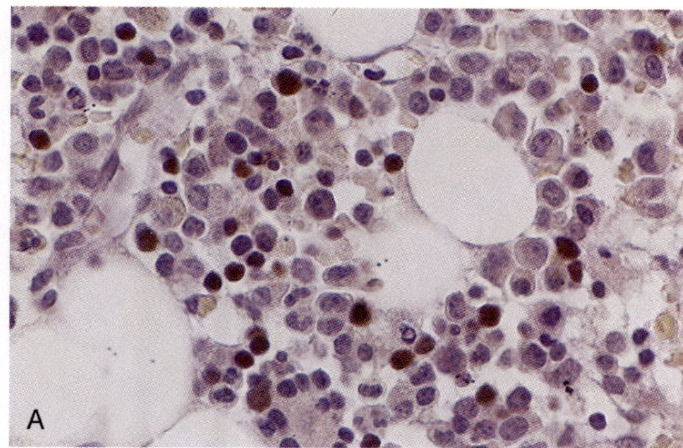

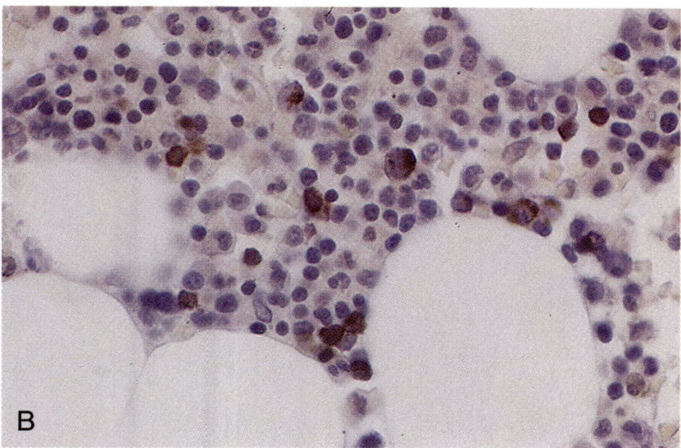

Figure 9–4

Increased hematogones, marrow from infant. *A*, A TdT stain of the marrow clot section shows a diffuse increase in terminal deoxynucleotidyltransferase (TdT)–positive cells, without clustering. TdT by immunoperoxidase. *B*, A diffuse increase in CD34-positive blasts is noted on this marrow clot section. No clustering is evident. CD34 by immunoperoxidase.

disorder (TMD). Other designations are *transient abnormal myelopoiesis* and *transient leukemia.* Affected neonates with DS often have hepatomegaly but appear healthy otherwise. The complete blood count is remarkably abnormal, with a WBC that may exceed 50,000/mm^3 (Fig. 9–5) (Avet-Loiseau et al, 1995; Foucar et al, 1992; Litz et al, 1995). There is maturation, and neutrophils are morphologically normal (Fig. 9–5*B*). However, up to 50% of circulating cells may be blasts, with a predominance of megakaryoblasts and erythroblasts (Fig. 9–5*C*). Massively enlarged platelets may be seen, along with circulating megakaryocytes showing cytoplasmic blebbing (Fig. 9–6*A* and *B*). Auer rods have not been described in myeloblasts in these patients. Hemoglobin levels and platelet counts are variable but are usually normal. Thrombocytopenia and anemia have been described in some patients. The percentage of blasts within the marrow is characteristically lower than that in the blood, and marrow fibrosis has not been described.

In these TMDs, spontaneous resolution of all blood and marrow aberrations occurs within 1–2 months (Fig. 9–6*C*). Chromosome X inactivation techniques have documented the clonal nature of these transient disorders (Kurahashi et al, 1991; Kwong, 1994). All hematopoietic and even lymphocytic elements demonstrate a clonal pattern of X chromosome inactivation. In general, cytogenetic assessment documents only the constitutional trisomy 21, although there are rare reports of additional transient cytogenetic abnormalities (Doyle et al, 1995). The mechanism of this transient event is not known, but these DS neonates are clearly at increased risk for subsequent overt leukemia. Several studies report acute myelogenous leukemia, usually megakaryoblastic anemia, within 6 months to 3 years of the TMD in a substantial proportion of patients (Avet-Loiseau et al, 1995; Doyle et al, 1995; Kempski et al, 1997; Liang et al, 1993) (see Chap. 7). Likewise, the incidence of both acute myelogenous leukemia, usually AML-M7, and acute lymphoblastic leukemia is markedly increased in DS patients, even in those children without antecedent transient myeloproliferative disorders (Avet-Loiseau et al, 1995; Creutzig et al, 1996; Litz et al, 1995; Tchernia et al, 1996; Zipursky et al, 1994) (see Chap. 7). Acute megakaryoblastic leukemia, often with an admixed erythrocytic component, predominates in young children with DS (<3 years of age), whereas acute lymphoblastic leukemia predominates in older patients (>3 years of age, Table 9–9) (Tchernia et al, 1996).

CONGENITAL LEUKEMIA

Acute leukemia is described, albeit rarely, throughout the first year of life. This discussion is restricted to those cases manifested at birth until 1 month of age, an event that occurs

Table 9–8

Neonates with Down Syndrome: Hematologic Abnormalities

Abnormality	Comments
Polycythemia	Venous hematocrit >65%
Transient myeloproliferative disorder	Leukocytosis with increased neutrophil count and sizable proportion of heterogeneous blasts, including many megakaryoblasts; variable hematocrit and platelet count Clonal by molecular studies Spontaneous remission in 2–3 months
Transient normoblastosis	Striking predominance of normoblasts at various stages of development; no associated leukocytosis; no increase in blast numbers Spontaneous resolution in 1–2 weeks
Transient thrombocytosis	Very rare descriptions of striking thrombocytosis without associated WBC abnormalities Spontaneous resolution in 1–2 weeks

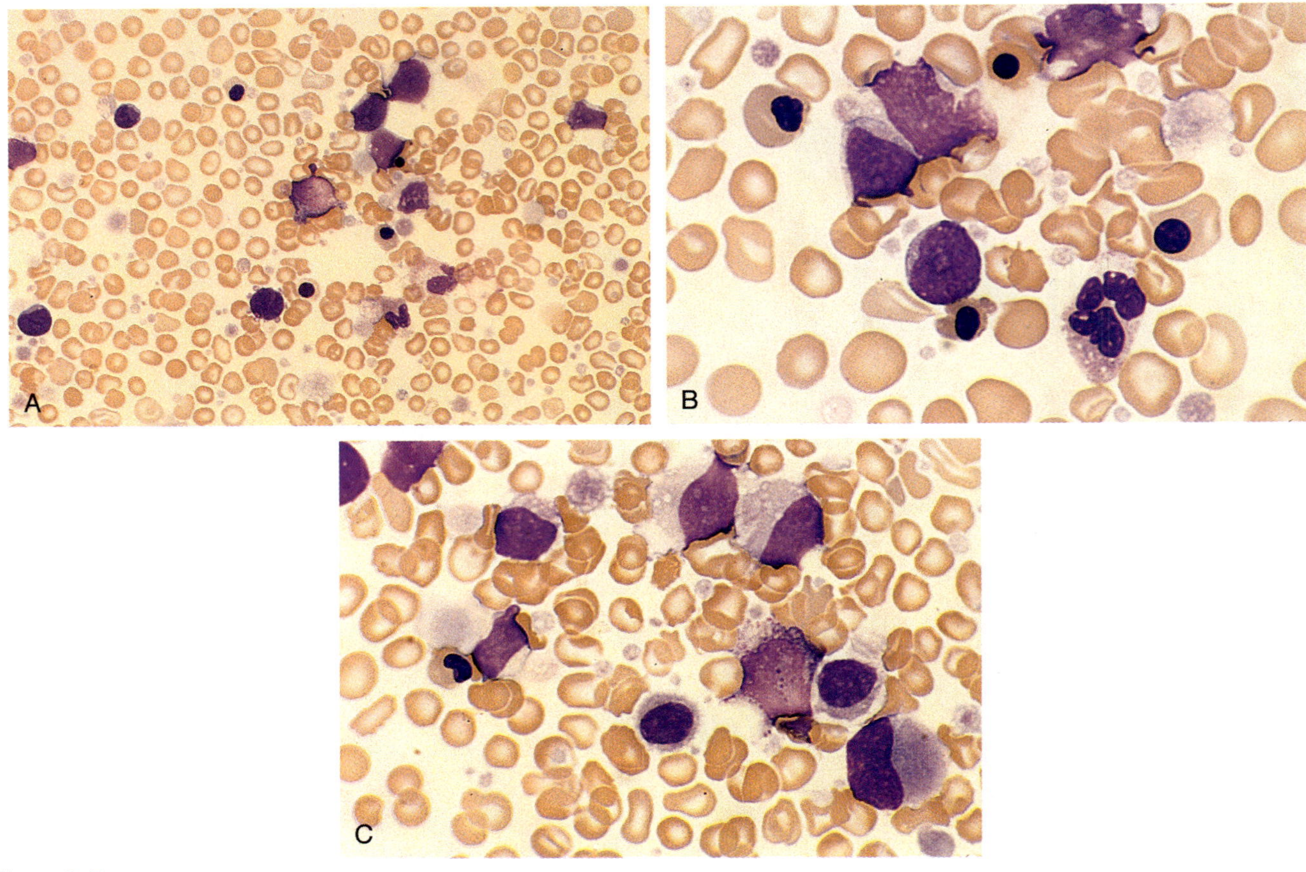

Figure 9–5

Newborn with Down syndrome and transient myeloproliferative disorder, peripheral blood. *A*, This low-magnification photomicrograph illustrates a leukocytosis (WBC count >50,000/μl) with numerous circulating blasts characteristic of transient myeloproliferative disorders. Wright stain. *B*, On high magnification, a spectrum of blasts is seen, along with normal neutrophils and giant platelets. Wright stain. *C*, Myeloblasts, erythroblasts, and megakaryoblasts are evident. Wright stain. (Courtesy Dr. C. Sever.)

Table 9–9

Down Syndrome: Characteristics of Transient Myeloproliferative Disorders and Acute Leukemias

Characteristics	Transient Myeloproliferative Disorder	Acute Leukemias
Onset	Neonatal period; described even in utero	Throughout childhood; usually after 6 months of age
Morphologic features	Spectrum of blasts including myelocytic, megakaryocytic, and erythrocytic blasts Megakaryoblasts abundant Occasionally erythrocytic precursors predominant	Acute megakaryoblastic leukemia (AML-M7) predominant in young children (<3 years) Acute lymphoblastic leukemia commoner in older children (>3 years)
Marrow	Lower percentage of blasts than in blood	Replacement by blasts
Immunophenotype	Heterogeneity of blasts	Blasts more phenotypically uniform
Cytogenetics	Sole abnormality usually constitutional trisomy 21 Rare transient disorders with additional clonal chromosomal abnormality Rare reports of phenotypically normal baby with disorder with trisomy 21 limited to hematopoietic cells	Trisomy 21 plus additional cytogenetic abnormalities frequent
Molecular analysis	Clonal	Clonal
Course	Spontaneous resolution in 2–3 months May later develop acute leukemia	Requires antileukemic therapy for survival

Source: Foucar K: Special considerations for bone marrow evaluation in children. In Bone Marrow Pathology. ASCP Press, Chicago, p 475, 1995e.

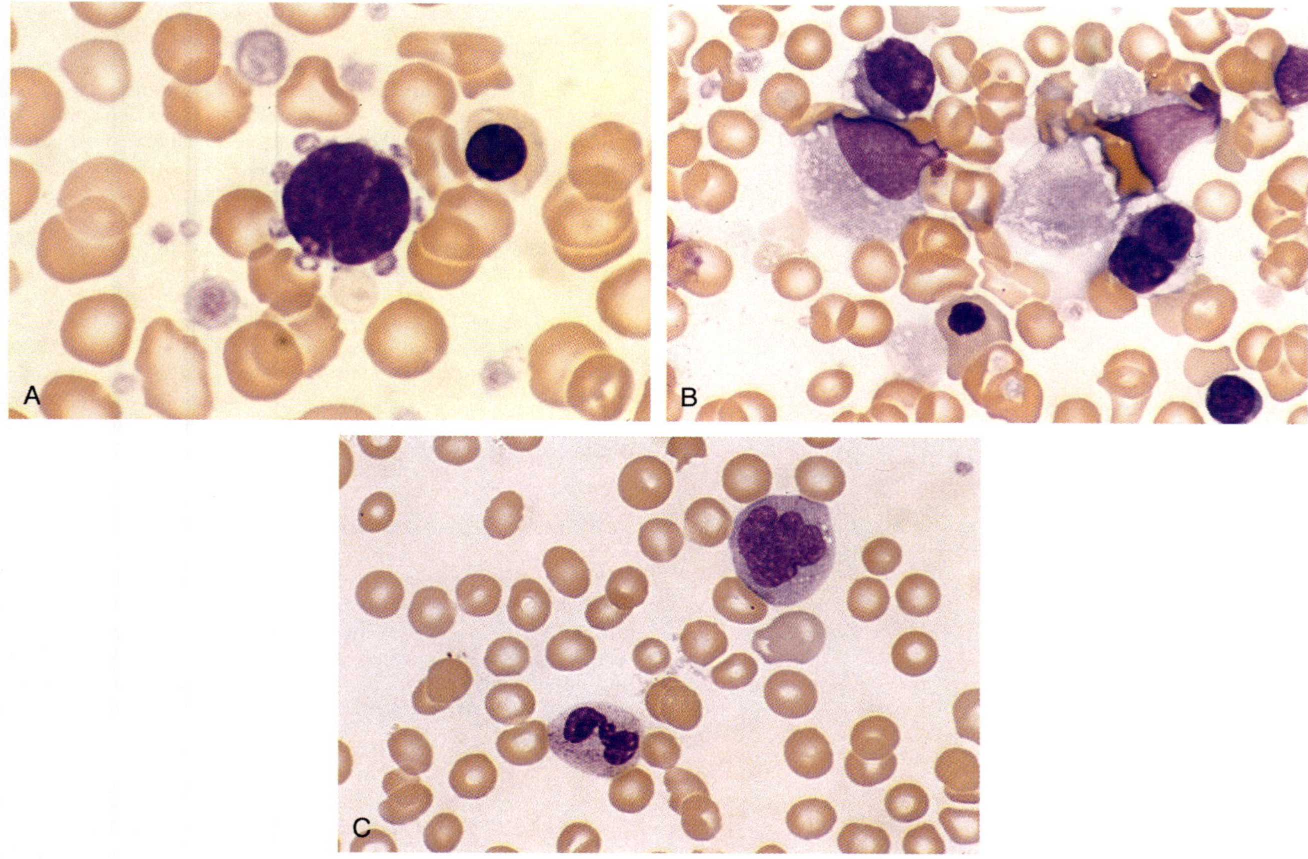

Figure 9–6

Newborn with Down syndrome and transient myeloproliferative disorder, peripheral blood. *A*, Cytoplasmic blebbing is very prominent on this circulating immature megakaryocyte. Wright stain. *B*, Note the massively enlarged platelet and circulating megakaryocytic elements that were evident at birth. Wright stain. *C*, Spontaneous resolution occurred within 1 month. This blood film from that time appears normal. Wright stain. These films are from the same patient as Fig. 9–5. (Courtesy Dr. C. Sever.)

at a rate of 1 per 5 million births (Pui et al, 1995). These congenital leukemias originate in utero and may be linked to parental mutagen exposure (Pui et al, 1995).

There are two distinct biologic subsets of congenital leukemias: those linked to 11q23 translocations and those associated with t(1;22)(p13;q13) (Table 9–10) (Carroll et al, 1991; Cimino et al, 1995; Foucar, 1995e; Greaves, 1996; Lion et al, 1992; McCoy & Overton, 1995; Pui et al, 1995; Pui et al, 1996). The *MLL* gene involved in the 11q23 translocation has been sequenced and cloned, and the genes involved in t(1;22) are unknown. In neonates, *MLL* gene rearrangements are usually linked to acute myelogenous leukemia, especially

Table 9–10

Congenital Leukemia: Characteristics of Biologic Subtypes

Characteristics	*MLL* Gene Rearrangement 11q23	t(1;22)(p13;q13)
WBC count	Very high	Low
Anemia	Severe	Severe
Thrombocytopenia	Severe	Severe
Subtype of leukemia	AML-M5, -M4; ALL-L2, -L1	AML-M7
Marrow fibrosis	No	Yes
Immunophenotype	ALL often coexpresses myelocyte antigens; CD10−	Megakaryocytic antigens present
Hepatosplenomegaly	Marked	Marked
Skin nodules	Frequent (AML-M5)	No
CNS involvement	Yes (ALL)	No
Prognosis	Poor	Poor

Note: Acute leukemia in neonates up to 1 month of age.

Abbreviations: ALL, acute lymphoblastic leukemia; AML, acute myelogenous leukemia; CNS, central nervous system; WBC, white blood cell.

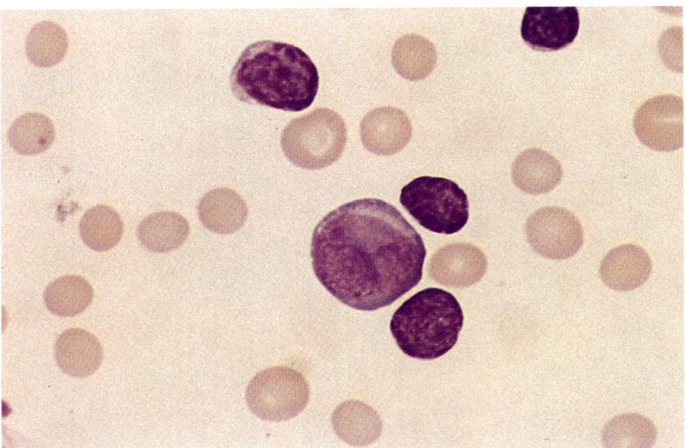

Figure 9–7

Congenital leukemia, peripheral blood. This 4-week-old girl has a striking leukocytosis (WBC count >150,000/μl), severe anemia, and thrombocytopenia. Note the variable appearance of blasts, some resembling lymphoblasts and some myeloblasts. Wright stain.

monocytic subtypes, or, less frequently, to CD10− acute lymphoblastic leukemia (Figs. 9–7 and 9–8). In 11q23-associated leukemia, the neonates present with striking leukocytosis and organomegaly. Skin involvement is common in patients with acute monoblastic leukemia, and central nervous system involvement is common in acute lymphoblastic leukemia (see Table 9–10).

The biologic subtype of congenital leukemia linked to t(1;22) has only recently been identified. These leukemias are consistently megakaryoblastic and have a clinical presentation that mimics a solid tumor. Both marrow and extramedullary infiltrates may be extensively fibrotic, with only isolated nests of leukemic cells (Carroll et al, 1991; Lion et al, 1992). Documentation of megakaryocytic antigen expression is critical in establishing this diagnosis.

The key differential diagnostic considerations for 11q23-associated acute leukemias in neonates include TMD in DS patients and congenital infections. The distinction of t(1;22)-associated acute megakaryoblastic leukemia from solid tumors is a diagnostic challenge in which immunophenotypic investigations may be required. All types of acute leukemia that appear within the first month entail a poor prognosis.

MISCELLANEOUS NEONATAL MARROW DISORDERS

Two very rare disorders, osteopetrosis and stage IV neuroblastoma, may be associated with hematologic and/or marrow abnormalities in neonates. Infantile osteopetrosis, an autosomal recessive disorder, is manifested at birth by macrocytic anemia, prominent reticulocytosis, teardrop erythrocytes, increased numbers of erythroblasts, and leukocytosis with immature

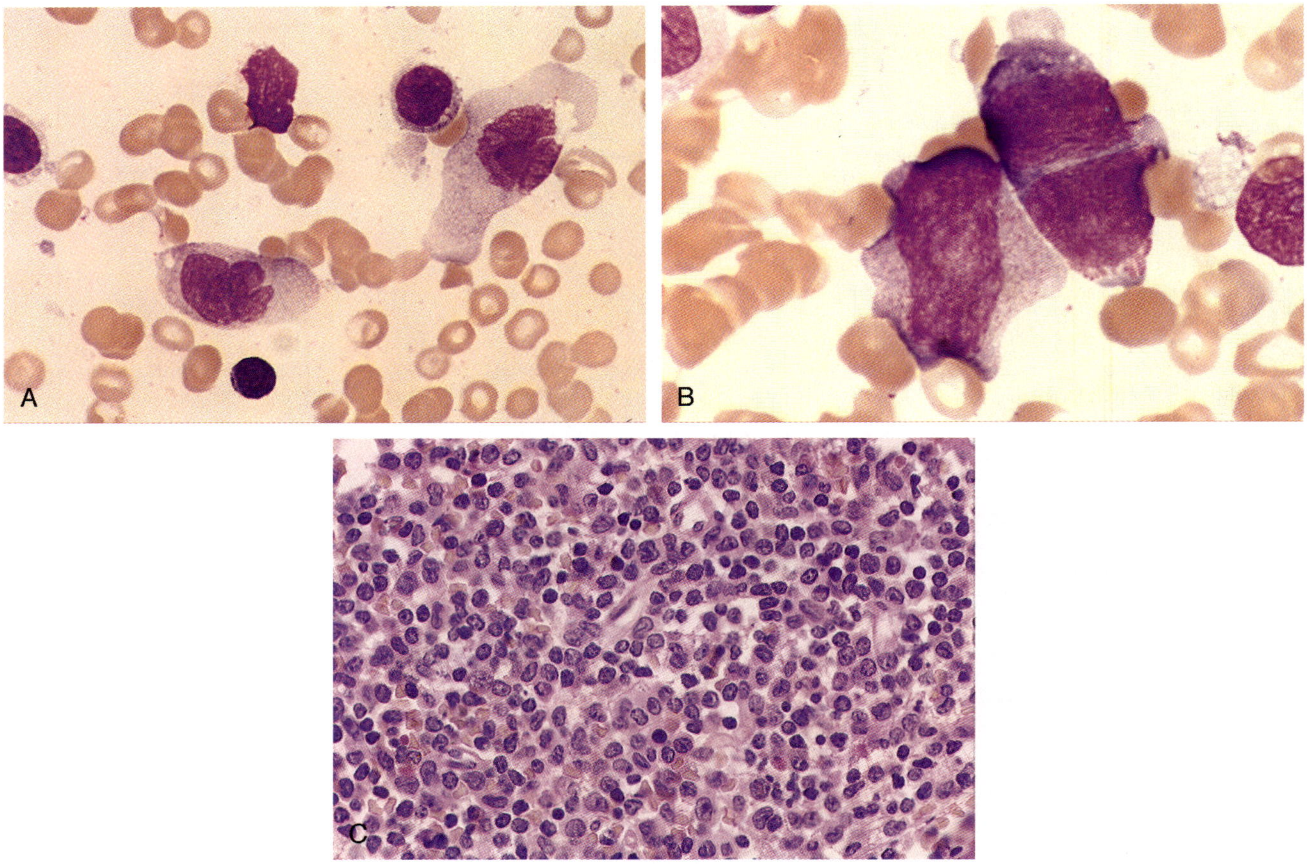

Figure 9–8

Congenital leukemia, marrow. *A*, *B*, These aspirate films from a 4-week-old infant with 11q23-associated congenital leukemia illustrate numerous blasts with a mixture of myeloblasts, monoblasts, and lymphoblasts. Wright stain. *C*, This marrow biopsy section shows effacement of architecture by sheets of blasts.

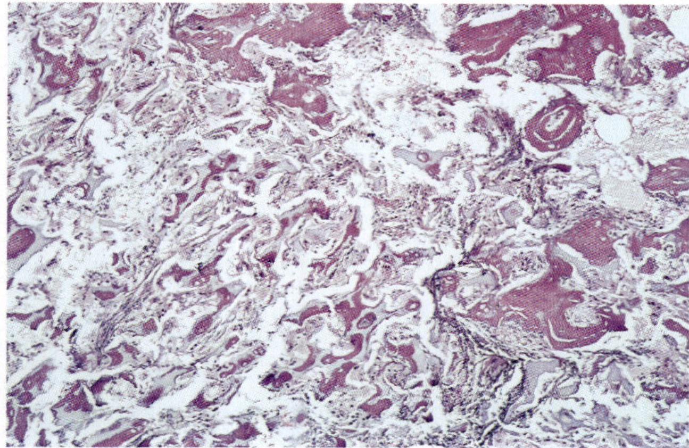

Figure 9–9

Congenital osteopetrosis, marrow. This low-magnification photomicrograph from a child with congenital osteopetrosis demonstrates effacement of all hematopoietic space by fibrous tissue and aberrant bone formation.

myelocytes (Alter & Young, 1993; Solh et al, 1995). Most circulating hematopoietic elements are produced within the massively enlarged spleen and liver, and the marrow has strikingly increased bone and cartilage density with associated fibrosis and is almost devoid of hematopoietic elements. Osteoclast function is defective in these patients, resulting in abnormal bone remodeling (Fig. 9–9). Failure of B and T cells to produce stimulatory enzymes may be linked to functional defects of both osteoclasts and macrophages, suggesting that an underlying immunodeficiency may cause osteopetrosis (Yamamoto et al, 1996).

Patients with stage IVS neuroblastoma may present at birth or during the first year of life with localized primary tumor in conjunction with metastatic disease in liver, skin, and/or marrow (Fig. 9–10) (Hachitanda & Hata, 1996). This incidence of marrow metastasis is 40% in large series. Despite widely metastatic disease, the prognosis is excellent, especially in patients whose tumors exhibit favorable histologic features and lack *MYC* amplification (Hachitanda & Hata, 1996).

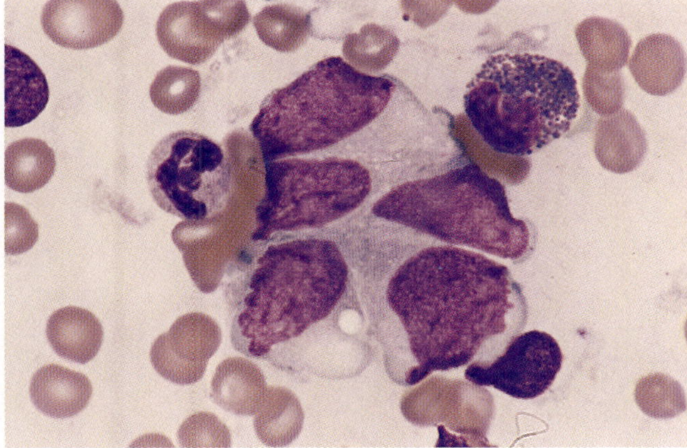

Figure 9–10

Neuroblastoma, marrow aspirate. This film from a neonate shows cohesive clusters of metastatic neuroblastoma cells. Wright stain.

REFERENCES

Alter BP: Arms and the man or hands and the child: congenital anomalies and hematologic syndromes. J Pediatr Hematol/Oncol 19:287, 1997.

Alter BP, Young NS: The bone marrow failure syndromes. In Nathan DG, Oski FA (eds): Hematology of Infancy and Childhood. W.B. Saunders Company, Philadelphia, p 216, 1993.

Al-Mulla ZS, Christensen RD: Neutropenia in the neonate. Clin Perinatol 22:711, 1995.

Alverson DC: The physiologic impact of anemia in the neonate. Clin Perinatol 22:609, 1995.

Attias D: Pathophysiology and treatment of the anemia of prematurity. J Pediatr Hematol Oncol 17:13, 1995.

Avet-Loiseau H, Mechinaud F, Harousseau J-L: Clonal hematologic disorders in Down syndrome: a review. J Pediatr Hematol Oncol 17:19, 1995.

Baehner RL, Miller DR: Disorders of granulopoiesis. In Miller DR, Baehner RL (eds): Blood Disease of Infancy and Childhood. Mosby, St. Louis, p 555, 1995.

Baley JE, Stork EK, Warkentin PI, et al: Neonatal neutropenia: clinical manifestations, cause, and outcome. Am J Dis Child 142:1161, 1988.

Beardsley DS: Platelet abnormalities in infancy and childhood. In Nathan DG, Oski FA (eds): Hematology of Infancy and Childhood. W.B. Saunders Company, Philadelphia, p 1561, 1993.

Brugnara C, Platt OS: The neonatal erythrocyte and its disorders. In Nathan DG, Oski FA (eds): Hematology of Infancy and Childhood. W.B. Saunders Company, Philadelphia, p 19, 1998.

Burrows RF, Kelton JG: Perinatal thrombocytopenia. Clin Perinatol 22:779, 1995.

Bussel JB, Corrigan JJ: Platelet and vascular disorders. In Miller DR, Baehner RL (eds): Blood Disease of Infancy and Childhood. Mosby, St. Louis, p 866, 1995.

Caldwell CW, Poje E, Helikson MA: B-cell precursors in normal pediatric bone marrow. Am J Clin Pathol 95:816, 1991.

Carballo C, Foucar K, Swanson P, et al: Effect of high altitude on neutrophil counts in newborn infants. J Pediatr 119:464, 1991.

Carroll A, Civin C, Schneider N, et al: The t(1;22)(p13;q13) is nonrandom and restricted to infants with acute megakaryoblastic leukemia: a Pediatric Oncology Group study. Blood 78:748, 1991.

Cimino G, Rapanotti MC, Rivolta A, et al: Prognostic relevance of ALL-1 gene rearrangement in infant acute leukemias. Leukemia 9:391, 1995.

Creutzig U, Ritter J, Vormoor J, et al: Myelodysplasia and acute myelogenous leukemia in Down's syndrome: a report of 40 children of the AML-BFM study group. Leukemia 10:1677, 1996.

Curnutte JT: Disorders of granulocyte function and granulopoiesis. In Nathan DG, Oski FA (eds): Hematology of Infancy and Childhood. W.B. Saunders Company, Philadelphia, p 904, 1993.

Dianzani I, Garelli E, Ramenghi U: Diamond-Blackfan anemia: a congenital defect in erythropoiesis. Haematologica 81:560, 1996.

Doyle JJ, Thorner P, Poon A, et al: Transient leukemia followed by megakaryoblastic leukemia in a child with mosaic Down syndrome. Leuk Lymphoma 17:345, 1995.

Dreyfus M, Kaplan C, Verdy E, et al: Frequency of immune thrombocytopenia in newborns: a prospective study. Blood 89:4402, 1997.

Foucar K: Constitutional and reactive myeloid disorders. In Bone Marrow Pathology. ASCP Press, Chicago, p 99, 1995a.

Foucar K: Hematopoiesis. In Bone Marrow Pathology. ASCP Press, Chicago, p 1, 1995b.

Foucar K: Reactive lymphoid proliferations in blood and bone marrow. In Bone Marrow Pathology. ASCP Press, Chicago, p 255, 1995c.

Foucar K: Reactive and neoplastic disorders of megakaryocytes. In Bone Marrow Pathology. ASCP Press, Chicago, p 237, 1995d.

Foucar K: Special considerations for bone marrow evaluation in children. In Bone Marrow Pathology. ASCP Press, Chicago, p 475, 1995e.

Foucar K, Friedman K, Llewellyn A, et al: Prenatal diagnosis of transient myeloproliferative disorder via percutaneous umbilical blood sampling: report of two cases in fetuses affected by Down's syndrome. Am J Clin Pathol 97:584, 1992.

Greaves MF: Infant leukemia biology, etiology and treatment. Leukemia 10:372, 1996.

Hachitanda Y, Hata J-I: Stage IVS neuroblastoma: a clinical, histological, and biological analysis of 45 cases. Hum Pathol 27:1135, 1996.

Hohlfeld P, Forestier F, Kaplan C, et al: Fetal thrombocytopenia: a retrospective survey of 5,194 fetal blood samplings. Blood 84: 1851, 1994.

Horwitz M: The genetics of familial leukemia. Leukemia 11:1347, 1997.

Kempski HM, Chessells JM, Reeves BR: Deletions of chromosome 21 restricted to the leukemic cells of children with Down syndrome and leukemia. Leukemia 11:1973, 1997.

Koenig JM, Christensen RD: Incidence, neutrophil kinetics, and natural history of neonatal neutropenia associated with maternal hypertension. N Engl J Med 321:557, 1989.

Kotylo PK, Fineberg NS, Freeman KS, et al: Reference ranges for lymphocyte subsets in pediatric patients. Am J Clin Pathol 100: 111, 1993.

Kurahashi H, Hara J, Yumura-Yagi K, et al: Monoclonal nature of transient abnormal myelopoiesis in Down's syndrome. Blood 77:1161, 1991.

Kwong YL: Transient abnormal myelopoiesis in Down's syndrome neonates. Am J Pediatr Hematol Oncol 16:387, 1994.

Levine RF, Olson TA, Shoff PK, et al: Mature micromegakaryocytes: an unusual developmental pattern in term infants. Br J Haematol 94:391, 1996.

Liang D-C, Ma S-W, Lu T-H, et al: Transient myeloproliferative disorder and acute myeloid leukemia: study of six neonatal cases with long-term follow-up. Leukemia 7:1521, 1993.

Lion T, Haas OA, Harbott J, et al: The translocation t(1;22)(p13;q13) is a nonrandom marker specifically associated with acute megakaryocytic leukemia in young children. Blood 79:3325, 1992.

Litz CE, Davies S, Brunning RD, et al: Acute leukemia and the transient myeloproliferative disorder associated with Down syndrome: morphologic, immunophenotypic and cytogenetic manifestations. Leukemia 9:1432, 1995.

Longacre TA, Foucar K, Crago S, et al: Hematogones: a multiparameter analysis of bone marrow precursor cells. Blood 73:543, 1989.

Lubin BH: Appendix: reference values in infancy and childhood. In Nathan DG, Oski FA (eds): Hematology of Infancy and Childhood. W.B. Saunders Company, Philadelphia, p i, 1993.

Mandel M, Rechavi G, Neumann Y, et al: Bone marrow cell populations mimicking common acute lymphoblastic leukemia in infants with stage IV-S neuroblastoma. Acta Haematol 86:86, 1991.

Matsunaga AT, Lubin BH: Hemolytic anemia in the newborn. Clin Perinatol 22:803, 1995.

McCoy JP, Overton WR: Immunophenotyping of congenital leukemia. Cytometry 22:85, 1995.

Miller DR: Anemias: general considerations. In Miller DR, Baehner RL (eds): Blood Disease of Infancy and Childhood. Mosby, St. Louis, p 111, 1995a.

Miller DR: Erythropoiesis, hypoplastic anemias, and disorders of heme synthesis. In Miller DR, Baehner RL (eds): Blood Disease of Infancy and Childhood. Mosby, St. Louis, p 140, 1995b.

Miller DR: Origin and development of blood cells and coagulation factors: maternal-fetal interactions. In Miller DR, Baehner RL (eds): Blood Disease of Infancy and Childhood. Mosby, St. Louis, p 3, 1995c.

Motley D, Meyer MP, King RA, et al: Determination of lymphocyte immunophenotypic values for normal full-term cord blood. Am J Clin Pathol 105:38, 1996.

Newland AC, Evans TG: ABC of clinical haematology. Haematologic disorders at the extremes of life. Br Med J 314: 1262, 1997.

Oski FA, Naiman JL: Anemia in the neonatal period. In Hematologic Problems in the Newborn. W.B. Saunders Company, Philadelphia, p 56, 1982a.

Oski FA, Naiman JL: The hematologic aspects of the maternal-fetal relationship. In Hematologic Problems in the Newborn. W.B. Saunders Company, Philadelphia, p 32, 1982b.

Oski FA, Naiman JL: Normal blood values in the newborn period. In Hematologic Problems in the Newborn. W.B. Saunders Company, Philadelphia, p 1, 1982c.

Oski FA, Naiman JL: Polycythemia and hyperviscosity in the neonatal period. In Hematologic Problems in the Newborn. W.B. Saunders Company, Philadelphia, p 87, 1982d.

Panzer S, Auerbach L, Cechova E, et al: Maternal alloimmunization against fetal platelet antigens: a prospective study. Br J Haematol 90:655, 1995.

Pui C-H, Kane JR, Crist WM: Biology and treatment of infant leukemias. Leukemia 9:762, 1995.

Pui C-H, Ribeiro RC, Campana D, et al: Prognostic factors in the acute lymphoid and myeloid leukemias of infants. Leukemia 10:952, 1996.

Shannon K: Recombinant human erythropoietin in neonatal anemia. Clin Perinatol 22:627, 1995.

Sievers EL, Dale DC: Non-malignant neutropenia. Blood Rev 10:95, 1996.

Smith OP, Hann IM, Chessells JM, et al: Haematological abnormalities in Schwachman-Diamond syndrome. Br J Haematol 94:279, 1996.

Solh H, Martins Da Cunha A, Giri N, et al: Bone marrow transplantation for infantile malignant osteopetrosis. J Pediatr Hematol Oncol 17:350, 1995.

Tannirandorn Y, Rodeck CH: Management of immune haemolytic disease in the fetus. Blood Rev 5:1, 1991.

Tchernia G, Lejeune F, Boccara J-F, et al: Erythroblastic and/or megakaryoblastic leukemia in Down syndrome: treatment with low-dose arabinosyl cytosine. J Pediatr Hematol Oncol 18:59, 1996.

Udom-Rice I, Bussel JB: Fetal and neonatal thrombocytopenia. Blood Rev 9:57, 1995.

Werner EJ: Neonatal polycythemia and hyperviscosity. Clin Perinatol 22:693, 1995.

Yamamoto N, Naraparaju VR, Orchard PJ: Defective lymphocyte glycosidases in the macrophage activation cascade of juvenile osteopetrosis. Blood 88:1473, 1996.

Zipursky A, Thorner P, De Harven E, et al: Myelodysplasia and acute megakaryoblastic leukemia in Down's syndrome. Leuk Res 18: 163, 1994.

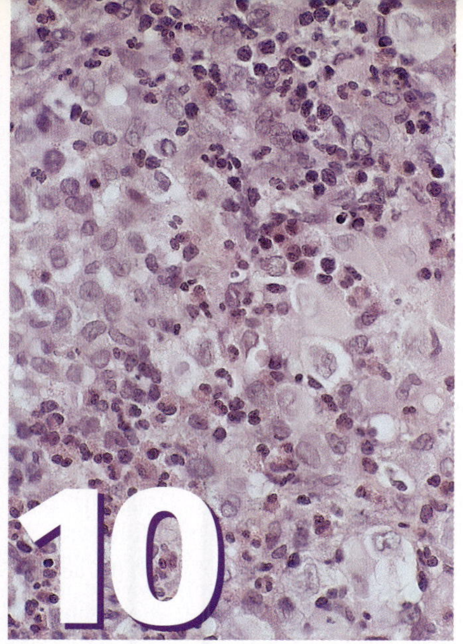

Steven H. Swerdlow
Kevin Salhany
Robert D. Collins

Histiocytoses

Proliferations and neoplasms of histiocytes have been difficult to recognize and classify. Some, especially histiocytic malignancies, are exceedingly rare. Only about 1500 cases of all types were collected worldwide over 10 years to provide the basis for a contemporary classification of histiocytic disorders (Favara et al, 1997). Factors other than rarity that have contributed to slow progress in this area are misdiagnoses of large-cell lymphomas as histiocytic neoplasms, confusion of reactive histiocytoses with neoplasms, limited techniques for establishing the presence of clonality in histiocytoses, and imprecise understanding of the biology of the histiocytic system (Foucar & Foucar, 1990). The classification promulgated by the World Health Organization (WHO) committee on histiocytic and reticulum cell proliferations and the Reclassification Working Group of the Histiocyte Society (Favara et al, 1997) provides a stable framework for improved classification of these diseases. Based partly on biology and partly on clinical behavior, this classification parallels the WHO approach to lymphoma classification. Both give inadequate attention to the organ of origin, but that deficit will be minimized as techniques evolve for recognizing specific subpopulations of histiocytes or lymphocytes that may be programmed for specific functions in individual organs. Both classifications attempt to predict clinical behavior, a useful guide in some cases and in others a gross oversimplification of the potential clinical diversity of individual neoplasms (Table 10–1).

The continued use of the term *histiocytes* is espoused for various macrophages, predominantly antigen-*processing* cells, and dendritic cells, predominantly antigen-*presenting* cells. Favara et al (1997) do not endorse the term *malignant histiocytosis,* even though it parallels the accepted term *malignant lymphoma.* Their choice of *histiocytic sarcoma* by their own admission seems somewhat antiquated. *True histiocytic lymphoma* should be discarded on two counts: *true* is nonsensical in a diagnostic term, and *lymphoma* is a neoplasm of lymphocytes, not histiocytes. *Malignant histiocytosis* is used here because the words are precise. Failure to use them precisely in the past has tarnished their image, but perhaps they are salvageable if used correctly. This approach basically follows that enunciated by Wood and Haber (1993).

Many, if not all, histiocyte populations are derived from a marrow-based progenitor cell, but the neoplastic transformation in many cases seems to be localized to an extramarrow site, as in many lymphomas. Also as in malignant lymphomas, several subtypes of malignant histiocytosis are characterized by having a predominant cell that resembles the presumed normal counterpart. There are too few cases to establish the clinical or therapeutic significance of these categories, much less their natural history. For example, it is not known whether such neoplasms as follicular dendritic histiocytosis are distinct from macrophage-related histiocytoses in natural history or response to treatment.

Regardless of the terms used, the principles of classification should follow those of cancers in general and lymphomas specifically (Lukes & Collins, 1992). The organ of origin should be specified or implied, as in the term *leukemia,* the cell of origin given, and the predominant cell designated. The latter is often predictive of clinical behavior and is reflected in the appearance of the neoplasm. Other features important in classification include the nature of the reactive component and the pathogenetic factors that contribute to development of neoplasia. Specific genotypic abnormalities have been recognized in many neoplasms. They may have significance in classification, as may acquisition of drug resistance genes or susceptibility to growth promoters or inhibitors.

CRITERIA FOR DIAGNOSIS OF MALIGNANCY: MONOCYTIC LEUKEMIA OR MALIGNANT HISTIOCYTOSES

The diagnosis of acute monocytic leukemia in children as well as in adults is straightforward when the patient presents with marrow insufficiency or failure rather than an extramarrow tumor. A tentative diagnosis may usually be made by examining Wright-stained peripheral blood films, and the marrow is generally packed at presentation with monoblasts and partially differentiated monocytes. Since massive necrosis rarely complicates this type of acute leukemia, marrow examinations are not thereby distorted. In addition, we have not found monocytic leukemias in children complicating or confused with myelodysplastic syndromes. Confirmation of the diagnosis of monocytic leukemia is readily accomplished by esterase cytochemical preparations and flow cytometric analysis (see Chap. 4). Skin lesions may precede or be concurrent with the detection of marrow involvement. Even if ideally fixed, such skin lesions may be misinterpreted as containing lymphoma or reactive lymphocytes, diagnoses that are particularly likely unless there is overt involvement of the peripheral blood by abnormal monocytes. Biopsies of second lesions and cytochemical analysis of touch preparations, immunoperoxidase preparations, or electron microscopy may be required to establish the correct diagnosis in cases with minimal blood involvement.

Malignant histiocytoses are diagnosed correctly once or twice a year in most major referral hematopathology laboratories (Lauritzen & Ralfkiaer, 1995) and are therefore about

Table 10–1

Classification of Histiocytic Neoplasms and Proliferations

Malignancies
Leukemias[a]
Acute monocytic leukemia (FAB M5A, M5B)
Acute myelomoncytic leukemia (FAB M4)
Chronic myelomonocytic leukemia
Malignant Histiocytoses[b]
Dendritic type
Follicular, Langerhans cell, indeterminate cell of dermis, interdigitating
Macrophage type

Histocytoses of Varied Biologic Behavior[c]
Dendritic type
Langerhans cell histiocytosis
Juvenile xanthogranuloma
Macrophage type
Solitary histiocytoma with macrophage phenotype

Reactive Histiocytoses[d]
Dendritic proliferations associated with lymphomas, certain infections
Primary hemophagocytic histiocytoses
Secondary hemophagocytic syndromes
Rosai-Dorfman disease (sinus histiocytosis with massive lymphadenopathy)

[a]Presumably marrow based, even when presenting as extramedullary mass.

[b]Cell of origin is probably a multipotential stem cell in some or all cases.

[c]Most cases in this group are localized or indolent in behavior. Langerhans cell histiocytosis is a clonal disorder (Willman et al 1994), and other processes in this group are expected to be.

[d]These reactive histiocytoses are presumably not clonal. Rosai-Dorfman disease has been proven to be polyclonal (Paulli et al, 1995).

0.5–1/1000 as frequent as malignant lymphomas. The reason for the rarity of histiocytic malignancies is not known. Intuitively we assume that all frequently dividing cells, such as histiocytes, are equally subject to malignancy. Tissues often involved by malignant histiocytoses range from skin and soft tissue to any lymphatic tissue (node, spleen, tonsil, thymus) and the gastrointestinal tract. In addition, bone, breast, kidney, and salivary gland have been involved (Kamel et al, 1995). Many large-cell neoplasms previously diagnosed as histiocytic in type have been shown using antibodies to CD30 (Stein et al, 1985) to be anaplastic large-cell lymphomas (Bucsky et al, 1994; Mongkonsritragoon et al, 1998; Wilson et al, 1990). Reports of histiocytoses are therefore suspect if this antibody was not used, even when diagnoses were based on cytochemical preparations (e.g., antilysozyme) and electron microscopy. Incorrect diagnoses may still be made using current sophisticated techniques unless histiocytes are clearly proven to be the neoplastic cell. Activated histiocytes are common in malignant lymphomas and may thereby be confused with the neoplastic lymphocytic component.

How should the diagnosis of malignant histiocytosis then be established? First, a tumorous mass or masses with sheet-like growth should be evident (Figs. 10–1 to 10–4). Proliferations of histiocytes that distort architecture but do not produce mass lesions are almost certainly reactive, even when associated with life-threatening illness or death. Second, there should be morphologic evidence of malignancy in the form of cytologic dysplasia with numerous mitoses (Fig. 10–2), although rare cases accepted as malignant have contained histiocytes judged cytologically benign (Ben-Ezra at al, 1991). Third, dysplastic (or predominant) cells must be identified as histiocytic in type by immunocytochemical techniques and electron microscopy (Fig. 10–3). All cases diagnosed as malignant histiocytoses that have CD30 positivity or T cell gene rearrangement are automatically suspect. The diagnosis of malignancy is confirmed by the demonstration of tumor metastases (Fig. 10–4).

These criteria are perhaps excessively stringent, but stringency is justified in view of the rarity of malignant histiocytoses and the past record of incorrect diagnoses. Most incorrect diagnoses of malignant histiocytoses have been made when malignant lymphomas have an inconspicuous or overlooked, small lymphocytic component and numerous reacting histiocytes, by assuming that sinus infiltrates were more likely histiocytic than lymphocytic (CD30+ anaplastic large-cell lymphomas make up most of these cases), or by assuming that life-threatening illnesses associated with widespread proliferation of histiocytes were malignant histiocytoses (most, if not all, of these cases are infection-associated hemophagocytic syndromes).

The next advances anticipated in this area involve technical developments for more precise delineation of macrophage subpopulations and their attendant neoplasms as well as development of universal techniques to determine histiocyte clonality. Even with these advances, progress will be slow due to the rarity of malignant histiocytoses.

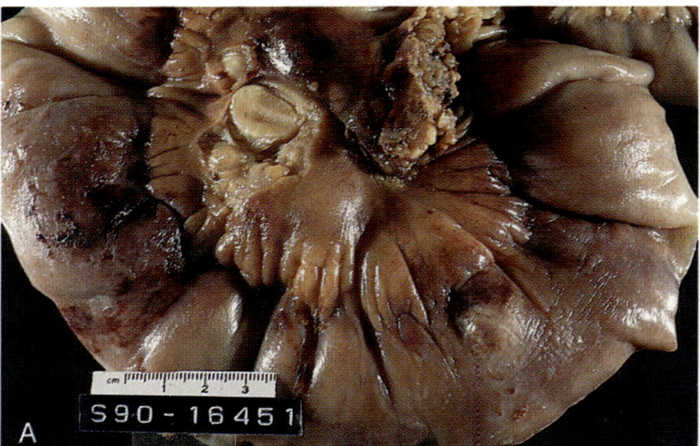

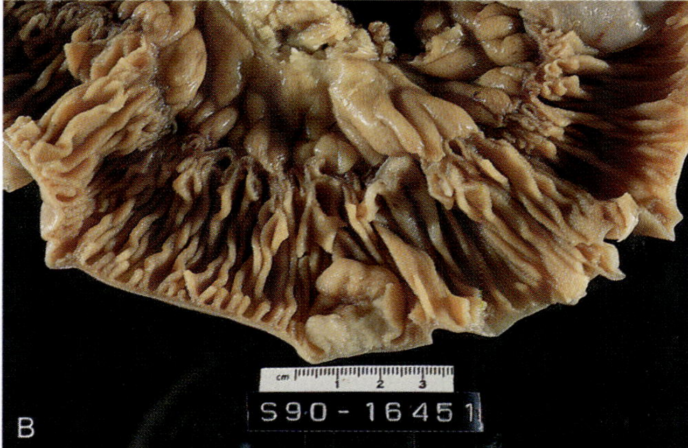

Figure 10–1

Malignant histiocytosis, bowel. In this case there were tumorous masses in the small intestine and adjacent nodes, producing intestinal obstruction. *A,* Photograph of the external surface of the bowel shows a mass in the wall and adjacent adenopathy. *B,* The cut section reveals a distinct mass involving the mucosa with ulceration. Adjacent nodes were enlarged, firm, and pale.

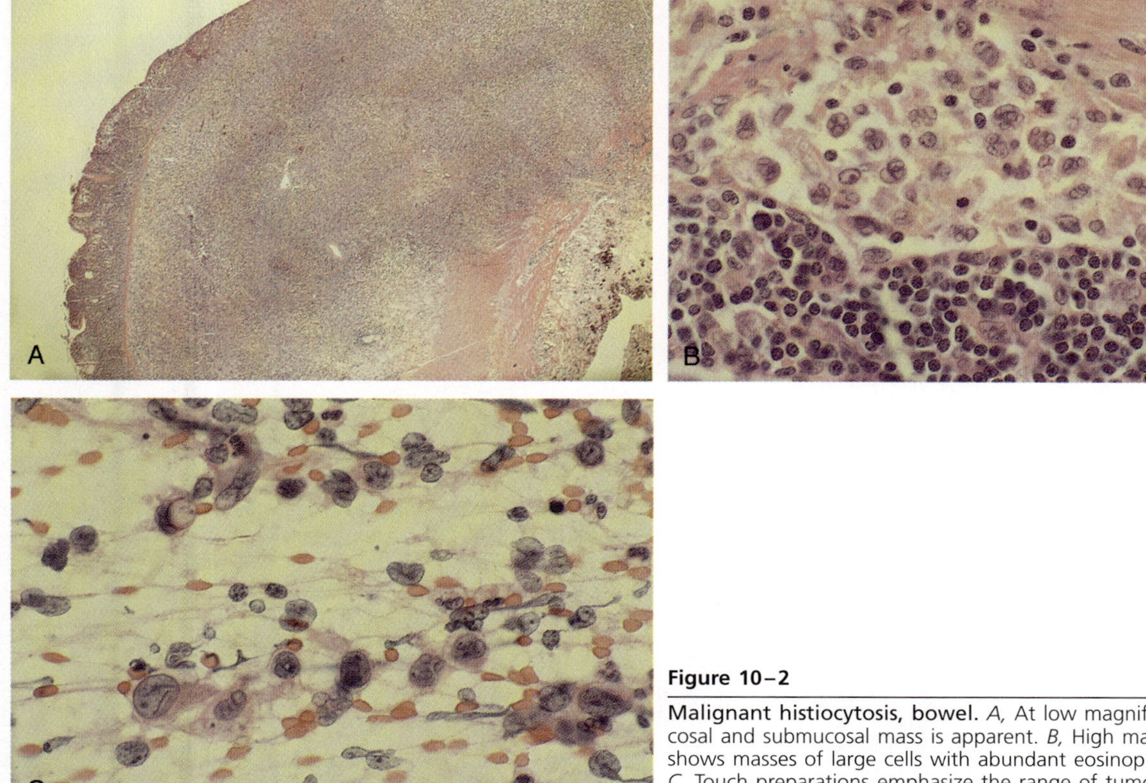

Figure 10–2

Malignant histiocytosis, bowel. *A,* At low magnification a mucosal and submucosal mass is apparent. *B,* High magnification shows masses of large cells with abundant eosinophilic cytoplasm. *C,* Touch preparations emphasize the range of tumor size; some cells have large amounts of cytoplasm.

HISTIOCYTOSES OF CHILDHOOD

The introduction above applies to adults and children, but several recent reports focus on malignant histiocytoses seen in children (Bucsky et al, 1998; Bucsky et al 1994; Malone, 1991). Accepting only cases diagnosed by stringent criteria, including Ki-1 negativity, and based in particular on two series (Ben-Ezra et al, 1991; Lauritzen & Ralfkiaer, 1995), there are fewer than 25 cases of malignant histiocytosis in children worldwide. Malignant histiocytosis of Langerhans cells has been described in a newborn (Ben-Ezra et al, 1991). Two other children in this series are also noteworthy. One, a 3-year-old boy, had multifocal proliferation of Langerhans cells (in the liver, spleen, heart, thymus, marrow, and retroperitoneal area) and died in 1 month despite treatment. The cytologic findings in this case were benign despite the aggressive nature of the process. Another child in the same series, a 4-year-old girl, had bone involvement with malignant cytologic features. There was no evidence of disease 18 years after surgical treatment, indicating cure by local removal. These cases show that "malignant" cytologic features may not be associated with dissemination, even in histiocytoses. They also indicate that benign cytologic features may rarely be seen in clinically aggressive neoplasms. In review of their experience and reported cases, investigators (Lauritzen & Ralfkiaer, 1995) found no cases of follicular dendritic neoplasms in patients under 29 years of age, one case of interdigitating dendritic neoplasm in a 17-year-old (with the other 12 in older patients), several cases of Langerhans cell malignancy [chiefly those referred to earlier (Ben-Ezra et al, 1991)], and 29 cases of macrophage-type malignant histiocytoses. In the latter group there were a few childhood cases, since the age range was 2 months to 75 years, with a mean of 27.5 years. Appropriately studied cases thus reveal that malignant histiocytoses in children are even rarer than in adults and are limited to the Langerhans cell and macrophage types.

MALIGNANT HISTIOCYTOSES

Langerhans Cell Type

Cases from the literature classified as Langerhans cell type (Table 10–2) are those with Langerhans morphologic features and Birbeck granules revealed by electron microscopic study as well as an aggressive clinical course including production of tumorous nodules or cases with local disease and histopathologic features typical of a malignant neoplasm, including cytologic dysplasia, abnormal nuclear shape or chromatin pattern, and abnormal mitoses. It should be noted that Birbeck granules, presumably an indicator of differentiation, have been found in a minority of malignant-appearing tumor cells in children and adults with this type of malignant histiocytosis. The criteria for acceptance of these cases is somewhat at variance with those of the working group of the Histiocyte Society (Favara at al, 1997). In addition, some of the cases listed in Table 10–2 were considered by their investigators to be of uncertain malignant potential despite their aggressive clinical course (Ben-Ezra et al, 1991). Their inclusion in Table 10–2 is based on descriptions of poor clinical outcome or morphologic atypia indicating neoplasia.

Table 10–2
Malignant Histiocytoses of Langerhans Cell Type: Literature Review

Age (years), Sex	Symptoms	Organs Involved	Treatment	Status, Length of Follow-up	Reference
Congenital, M	Skin lesions, respiratory distress	Lymph nodes, lung, muscles, thymus, liver, spleen, blood	Chemotherapy	Dead, 8 days	Ben-Ezra et al, 1991
3,M	Rash, anemia, lymphadenopathy	Liver, spleen, heart, thymus, marrow	Surgery, chemotherapy	Dead, 1 month	Ben-Ezra et al, 1991
4,F	Fever	Bone	Surgery	No evidence of lesion, 18 years	Ben-Ezra et al, 1991
11,F	Pathologic fracture, soft tissue involvement	Clavicle	Surgery	No recurrence, 8 months	Salam et al, 1990
16,M	Unknown	Marrow, thymus, lung	Surgery	Unknown	Ben-Erza et al, 1991[a]

[a]This case (number 1D in the Ben-Ezra et al series) is included because the diagnosis of malignant histiocytosis was indicated by the presence of dysplastic tumor cells as well as disease in marrow, thymus, and lung. Unfortunately, clinical presentation and outcome were not known.

Clinical Features

Speculations rather than conclusions may be drawn from such a small group of cases (see Table 10–2). The age range in this group was 0 to 11 years. It is of particular interest that two of the patients had disease limited to bone (and adjacent soft tissue in the case reported by Salam et al, 1990). One patient was apparently cured by surgery, and the other had no evidence of recurrence at 8 months. The other three patients (see Table 10–2) had widespread disease, including skin lesions as well as involvement of several organs, and died shortly.

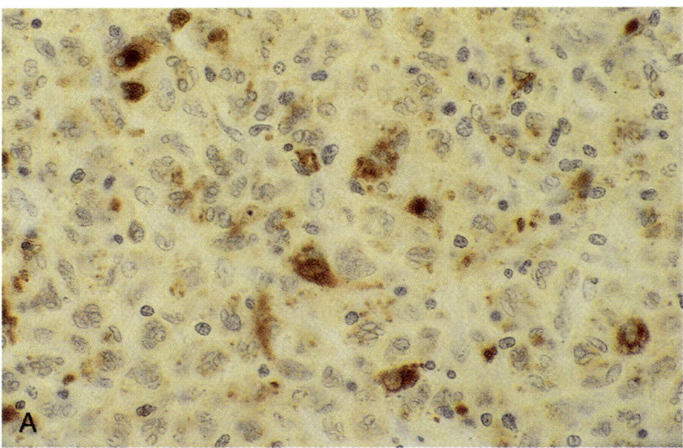

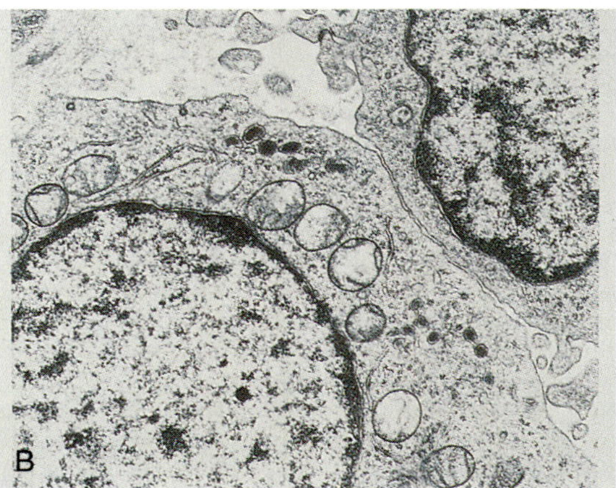

Figure 10–3

Malignant histiocytosis, bowel. *A,* An immunoperoxidase preparation with antibody to CD68 (KP-1) shows marking of many tumor cells. *B,* On ultrastructural examination, dysplastic cells contained haloed granules, a feature that may be taken as evidence of histiocytic differentiation (Collins RD, Bennett B, Glick AD: Neoplasms of the mononuclear phagocyte system. In Herberman RB, Friedman H (eds): The Reticuloendothelial System, Vol. 5. Plenum, New York, 1983).

Histopathologic Findings

The range of histopathologic findings in this type of malignant histiocytosis is best described in the Ben-Ezra et al series from 1991. Some of their patients had infiltrates of typical Langerhans cells exhibiting the expected longitudinal groove and coffee bean appearance. These cells are described as having benign cytologic features. Eosinophils and multinucleated cells were present.

Cases at the opposite pole in terms of appearance had dysplastic, malignant cytologic features, with increased nuclear size, nuclear pleomorphism, and prominent nucleoli. Prominent nuclear grooving was still observed. Some cases had atypical dysplastic cells in some organ infiltrates, whereas other lesions contained typical Langerhans cells. For example, in case 5D of Ben-Ezra et al (1991) (see Table 10–2), typical Langerhans cells were seen in lymph nodes, lung, spleen, liver (discrete tumor nodules were found only in the liver), and muscle, whereas dysplastic cells were identified only in the thymus. Similar variations in histologic appearance were noted in another adult case from the same series. Thus, neoplastic histiocytes may vary in appearance from site to site at a given point in time, as in malignant lymphoma. Sheetlike growth of tumor cells was present, as were extensive eosinophilic infiltrates.

Macrophage Type

Several reports on macrophage-type histiocytosis are restricted to childhood cases (Bucsky et al, 1994; Burgdorf & Zelger, 1996; Malone, 1991). In one, no specific cases are cited (Burdgorf & Zelger, 1996), or it is difficult to be certain the cases cited represent malignant histiocytoses of the macrophage type. In yet another report, a 3-year-old girl with groin adenopathy is reported to have had histopathologic and immunophenotypic features in a tumor, indicating macrophage differentiation (Copie-Bergman et al, 1998). Several general treatments of "true" histiocytic lymphoma and histiocytic sarcomas contain childhood cases, but the data from these cases do

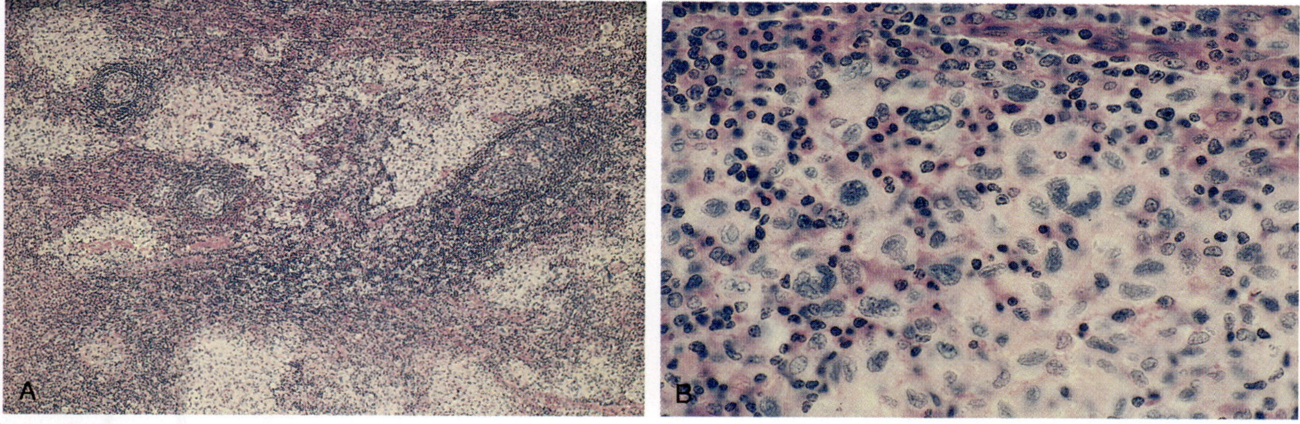

Figure 10–4

Malignant histiocytosis, node. *A,* Low magnification shows nodules of tumor in node sinuses. *B,* At high magnification the tumor cells have indistinct borders and abundant cytoplasm. Figures 10–1 through 10–4 are from the same case.

not seem conclusive for several reasons. For example, evidence of histiocytic differentiation was not cited for a stomach lesion (case 12 of Kamel et al, 1995) in a 9-year-old girl. In another case (case 2 of Soria et al, 1992), multiple skin nodules had immunocytochemical features of monocytes or macrophages. The authors were apparently concerned that this was a case of monocytic leukemia presenting as skin lesions, but the results of pre- and posttreatment marrow examinations were negative. The age and distribution of the disease (skin, liver, spleen, and gastric wall) are more suggestive of leukemia than of malignant histiocytosis.

Malignant histiocytoses of the macrophage type must be exceedingly rare in all patients and especially in children. A decade may pass before sufficient cases accumulate to allow reasonable conclusions as to their presentations, morphologic features, and response to treatment. Assuming it is reasonable to extrapolate from adult cases, children with malignant histiocytoses are most likely to present with nodal and spleen or skin lesions. With dissemination, involvement of marrow, lung, and liver is to be expected (Franchino et al, 1988; Kamel et al 1995; Lauritzen & Ralfkiaer, 1995; Ralfkiaer et al, 1990).

HISTIOCYTOSES OF VARIED BIOLOGIC POTENTIAL

Langerhans Cell Histiocytoses

Formerly known as histiocytosis X, Langerhans cell histiocytosis (LCH) includes proliferations of Langerhans cells that may be localized or widespread, that may spontaneously resolve or progress to death, and that may be congenital or present in adulthood. In addition to cases in which only skin lesions occur, classic clinicopathologic presentations include eosinophilic granuloma (of bones, lung, and nodes), Hand-Schüller-Christian disease (multiple organ involvement, particularly with skull defects, diabetes, insipidus, and exopthalmos), and Letterer-Siwe disease (cutaneous, nodal, visceral, and marrow lesions). Clinical and pathologic descriptions are more voluminous than reports on the basic nature of these various disorders, with certain notable exceptions:

1. Nezelof demonstrated in 1979 that eosinophilic granuloma, Hand-Schüller-Christian disease, and Letterer-Siwe disease have a common histogenesis involving Langerhans cells, as identified by the presence of Birbeck granules.
2. Willman et al (1994) demonstrated the clonal nature of LCH.
3. Prognosis is apparently related more to extent of disease than age of onset, site of disease, or histopathologic features (Nezelof et al, 1979). Spontaneous healing occurs in certain disseminated forms (see "Congenital Self-Healing Reticulohistiocytosis") and is the rule in localized disease.
4. Relatively specific immunocytochemical markers of Langerhans cells are available in addition to the ultrastructural demonstration of Birbeck granules, but most diagnoses of LCH may be made with assurance on morphologic grounds (Favara & Jaffe, 1994; Nezelof et al, 1979); or based on fine-needle aspirate studies in correlation with clinical and radiographic features (Kilpatrick, 1995).

It is still not known whether there is a single population of Langerhans cells and therefore not known whether the diseases outlined here are different manifestations of a single disease or several diseases arising from different subpopulations. Such insights await greater understanding of the biology of the Langerhans cell system, briefly described in the next section, and detection of specific karyotypic abnormalities responsible for clonal proliferations.

Biology of Langerhans Cells

Langerhans cells are a type of dendritic cell. As such, they have antigen-presenting capabilities. Langerhans cells are defined in the dendritic hierarchy as containing Birbeck granules. The relationship of Langerhans cells to other dendritic cells is not clear, but it is known that Langerhans cells may modulate or differentiate in tissue culture to an indeterminate form in which the cultured cells lack Birbeck granules but otherwise resemble Langerhans cells. Similar changes may also occur in vivo, since many, or even most, lesional cells in some cases of eosinophilic granuloma apparently lack Birbeck granules. Uniformity in terms of the presence of Birbeck granules might be expected in such clonal processes. Possibly this distinctive cytologic feature is lost by modulation or differentiation of Langehans cells. These observations imply that Langerhans cells and indeterminate dendritic cells (discussed later) are closely related.

Dendritic cells are derived from the bone marrow, circulate in the peripheral blood, where they constitute $<0.1\%$ of circulating elements, and migrate to various peripheral organs.

The epidermal Langerhans cells trap and process foreign protein antigen and then migrate to regional nodes, where they stimulate antigen-specific T cells. Langerhans cells are apparently highly specialized to initiate primary immune responses through mechanisms that have been conceptualized into three broad groups (Steinman, 1991). As sentinels, Langerhans cells may process and present antigen, then may contact antigen-specific T cells after migration to regional nodes, and finally may function as adjuvant to bind and activate resting T cells.

Clinical Features of Langerhans Cell Histiocytosis

Skin lesions may be present at birth or develop afterward (Esterly et al, 1995). Lesions may be localized in the form of papules, nodules, or vesicopustules. Widespread skin lesions may be manifested as eczematous lesions, often in the scalp and diaper area, or as hemorrhagic rashes. Combinations of lesion types may be noted synchronously or over time. Lesions may resolve or scar. Fluctuation and drainage are apparently unusual. Mucosal lesions, except for gingival lesions (often associated with loose teeth), are also unusual. Some patients present with chronic aural discharge.

Bone involvement is usually solitary rather than multifocal (McCullough, 1980) and may be diagnosed as early as 2 months of age (Kilpatrick et al, 1995). The commonest sites are skull, pelvis, long bones, and vertebrae, in the order given. Mandibular involvement is more likely than maxillary involvement. Bone lesions are signaled by pain that is often worse at night, soft tissue swelling, loose teeth, exopthalmos, deafness, and diabetes insipidus. Radiologic features include irregular lytic areas, often with endosteal erosion and periosteal reaction. Healed lesions may exhibit normalization of trabecular patterns or sclerosis (Sartoris & Parker, 1984).

Other organs are involved much less frequently than skin and bone. They include lung, nodes, liver, spleen, thymus, and the gastrointestinal tract. Lung disease occurs more frequently as an isolated phenomenon than as a manifestation of multisystem disease. In a review of 320 patients with LCH in the lung (Colby & Lombard, 1983), there were 23 under 21 years of age, most of them less than 15 years of age. Patients may be asymptomatic or have dyspnea, shortness of breath, cough, or pneumothorax. Systemic complaints and clubbing are infrequent. Radiographs are usually abnormal, revealing bilateral reticular or reticulonodular infiltrates that are often symmetric. Cavities or honeycombing may be demonstrated (see Chap. 20).

Nodal lesions (see Chap. 16) have been described in a large series of 30 cases (Motoi et al, 1980). Nine patients (30% of cases) were children, including five girls younger than 1 year. The sinuses were involved in all cases, in some nodes to the point of effacing the architecture. Hepatosplenomegaly is seen only in patients with widespread disease. Thymic and gastrointestinal involvement are very rare.

Histopathologic Features

There are criteria by which the diagnosis of LCH may be made with varying degrees of certainty (Favara et al, 1997), with "definitive" diagnosis requiring demonstration of Birbeck granules by electron microscopic studies or demonstration of CD1a antigen in paraffin-embedded specimens. However, careful histopathologic and cytologic examination in correlation with clinical and radiologic data may suffice in most cases (Kilpatrick, 1995), particularly if fixation and processing are optimal (Fig. 10–5). Generally, early lesions are more cellular and have more easily recognized aggregates of Langerhans cells (Malone, 1991). Langerhans cells have homogeneous pink cytoplasm and nuclei distinguished by lobation and a longitudinal nuclear groove. Mitoses are infrequent (Schmitz & Favara, 1998), and phagocytosis is not evident. Eosinophils are more prominent in early lesions, whereas in senescent lesions both eosinophils and Langerhans cells may be difficult to find (Favara & Jaffe, 1994; Munn & Chu, 1998). Areas of necrosis are often evident when the lesion is rich in eosinophils (Fig. 10–6). The term *eosinophilic abscess* is often applied in this circumstance. Cytoplasmic disruption in these areas obscures typical eosinophil morphologic features, although free eosinophil granules are easily detected around the edges of necrotic foci. A carefully studied case of Letterer-Siwe disease showed that Langerhans cells were not homogenous in morphologic features and antigenic properties (Ruco et al, 1988). Thus, careful attention must be paid to the possibility of sampling bias when such cases are diagnosed.

Congenital Self-Healing Reticulohistiocytosis (Hashimoto-Pritzker Disease)

Congenital self-healing reticulohistiocytosis is a rare form of LCH that is significant because it should be distinguished from the aggressive types of LCH (i.e., Letterer-Siwe disease) that it resembles in age of onset, distribution, and histologic features.

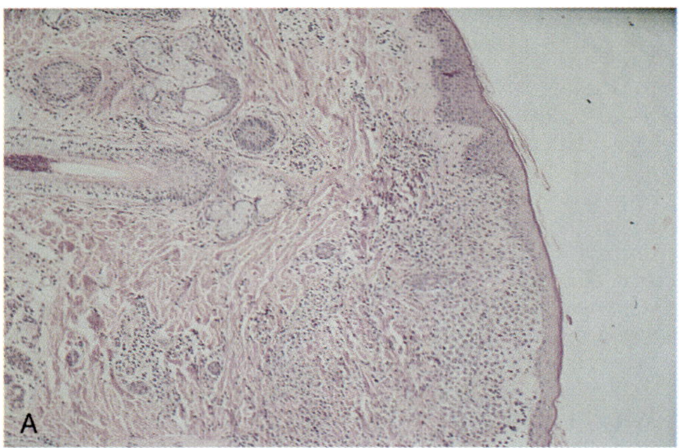

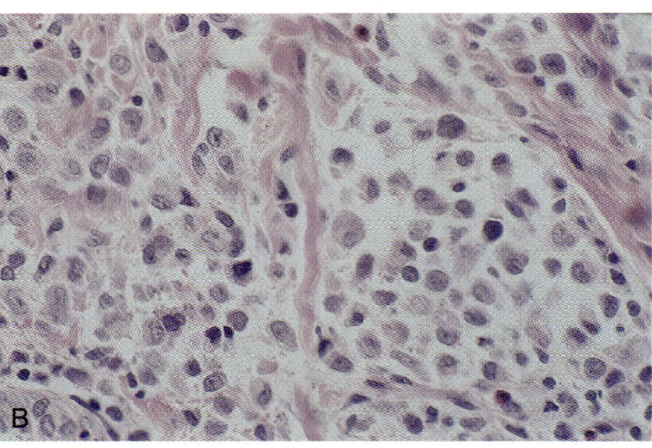

Figure 10–5

Langerhans histiocytosis, skin. *A,* The border between lesion and normal skin is shown. There is a dense infiltrate in the upper dermis. *B,* Large cells with abundant cytoplasm are present. Nuclear grooves are seen in some cells, but fixation with B5 rather than formalin, as was the case here, may be required to enhance nuclear morphologic features.

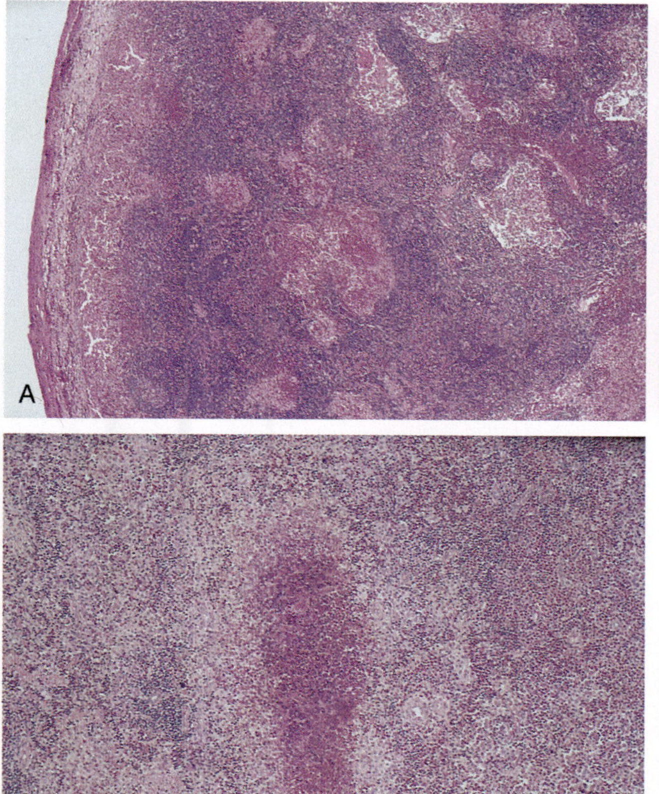

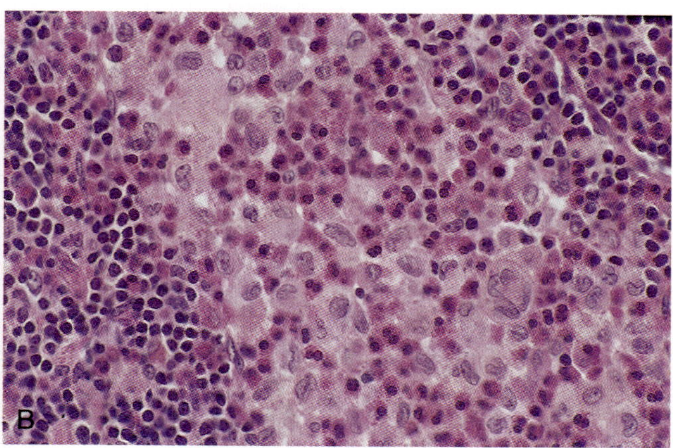

Figure 10–6

Eosinophilic granuloma, node. *A,* A low-magnification photomicrograph shows distortion of nodal architecture by a process localized to sinuses. *B,* At high magnification there are numerous eosinophils, Langerhans cells with nuclear grooves, and rare multinucleated cells, an appearance typical of eosinophilic granuloma wherever located. *C,* Necrosis often occurs, as demonstrated in this photomicrograph from a different case; foci of necrosis are often present in eosinophilic granuloma and almost always involve the sinus infiltrate.

It is characterized by multiple or solitary reddish-brown nodules that are not found on mucous membranes (Divaris et al, 1991) and that spontaneously rapidly regress. Since confirmation of the diagnosis is best obtained by electron microscopic study, glutaraldehyde-fixed material should be set aside at initial biopsy in suspect cases. Microscopic sections exhibit a dense dermal infiltrate of eosinophils, macrophages, and Langerhans cells (Fig. 10–7). Areas of necrosis may be present, as may scattered giant cells. The ultrastructural findings reveal Birbeck granules in a minority of cells, whereas numerous laminated dense bodies are observed (Divaris et al, 1991). Extensive sectioning may reveal Birbeck granules and laminated dense bodies in the same cell, a finding supposedly pathognomonic of the self-healing variant (Hashimoto & Pritzker, 1973).

Lesions typically begin to regress shortly after birth, and complete resolution may be expected between 4 and 8 months. The pathogenesis and biologic significance of this interesting disease are uncertain, although it is presumably a benign clonal proliferation. Careful immunoelectron microscopic studies (Schaumburg-Lever et al, 1994) indicate that the Birbeck granules are present in such low numbers owing to their degradation to laminated dense bodies.

Indeterminate-Cell Histiocytosis

Indeterminate-cell histiocytosis is mentioned for the sake of completion, although a review in 1995 listed only three cases, in a total of nine, that occurred in children (Sidoroff et al, 1996). Its importance may relate more to biologic significance than clinical relevance. Although clinically suggestive of eruptive histiocytomas (Zelger et al, 1996), proliferating cells test positive for S100 protein and CD1. Birbeck granules are notably absent. These data have been interpreted as indicating that indeterminate cells are members of the Langerhans dendritic system on their way from skin to regional nodes (Romani & Schüler, 1992).

Studies of the proliferating cell in indeterminate-cell histiocytosis and self-healing reticulohistiocytosis (discussed earlier) indicate that Langerhans cells lose their Birbeck granules in certain diseases as well as in natural circumstances when they migrate to nodes. In the latter disease the loss is partial, whereas in the former immunocytochemical reactivity (S100 and CD1a positivity) persists even though Birbeck granules have disappeared.

Xanthogranulomas

Xanthogranulomas vary considerably in age of onset, distribution, and morphologic appearance. These variations, particularly in morphologic features, apparently represent maturation of lesions over time (Marrogi et al, 1992), since coordinated histochemical and immunocytochemical studies of variants indicate a common histogenesis for lesions that vary in appearance and distribution (Zelger et al, 1994). The cell of origin for xanthogranuloma is the dermal dendrocyte (Favara et al, 1997), a dermal element of unknown function that is recognizable by its immunoreactivity with factor XIIIa, CD45, and CD68 and negative reactions with S100 and CD1a as well as absent Birbeck granules. Dermal dendrocytes are the predominant cell, and are therefore the presumed cell of origin, for xanthogranulomas

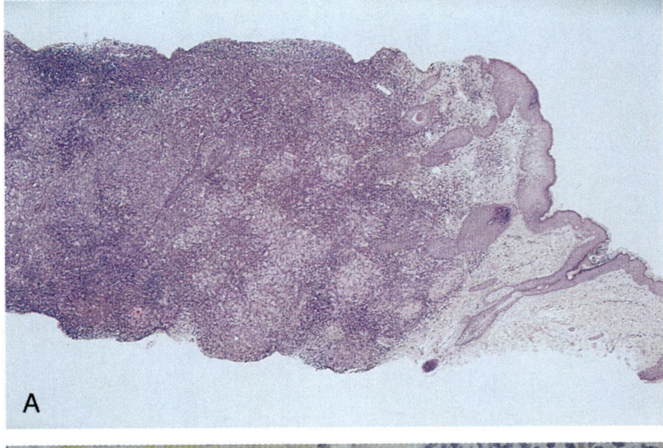

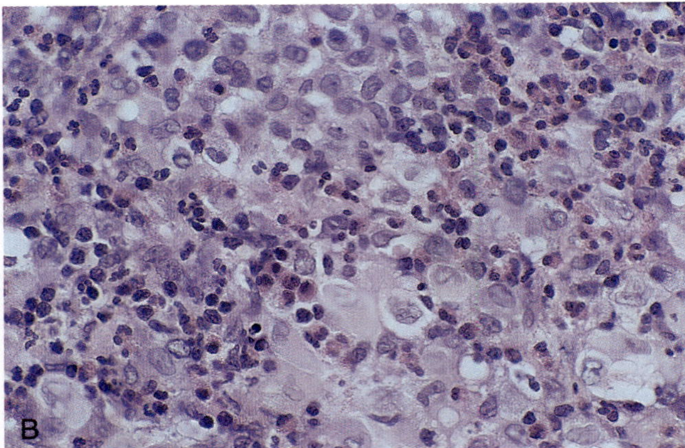

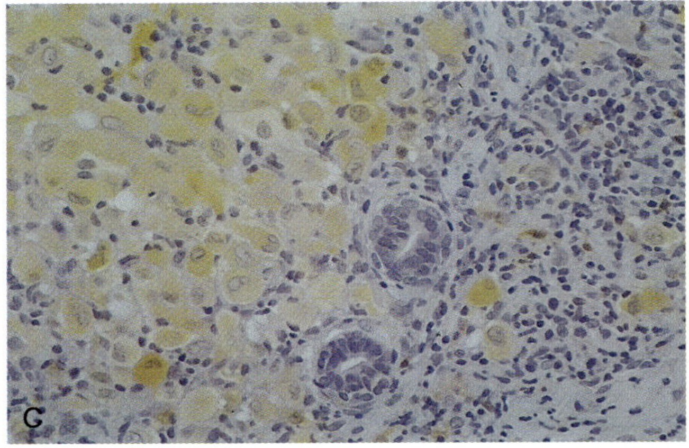

Figure 10–7

Congenital self-healing reticulohistiocytosis, skin. *A,* At low magnification this punch biopsy specimen shows a dense dermal infiltrate under preserved epithelium. *B,* High magnification shows the morphologic features of the Langerhans cell, with grooved nuclei in the group of cells below and a cluster of macrophages above. Numerous inflammatory cells are present, particularly lymphocytes and eosinophils. *C,* An immunoperoxidase preparation with antibody to S-100 protein shows numerous positively stained cells. The skin appendage is not stained, as expected. (Courtesy Dr. Alan Boyd, Associate Professor of Medicine/Dermatology, Vanderbilt University Medical Center, Nashville, TN.)

as well as for xanthoma disseminatum, benign cephalic histiocytosis, and generalized eruptive histiocytosis (Favara et al, 1997). Of these disorders, xanthogranuloma is the commonest, ranking above LCH in frequency and clinical significance. This disorder is thus well known to pediatric dermatologists and pathologists, and its salient features may be summarized as follows:

1. Xanthogranulomas are rarely present at birth but usually arise early in infancy and may be seen in adults.
2. Lesions are often single but may be numerous, with preferential distribution in the head, neck, and shoulder area. Skin lesions are usually described as yellow, pinkish, or lightly pigmented papules or nodules. Rarely, masses measuring several centimeters are produced.
3. Infrequently there are masses in deep soft tissues or involvement of the epibulbar area (leading to glaucoma) or pulmonary or pericardial infiltration. The largest review of cases with systemic involvement is that of Freyer et al (1996), in which 36 patients are described. In addition to skin and subcutaneous lesions, seen in most cases, some patients have hepatosplenomegaly, lung involvement, kidney lesions, abdominal or paravertebral masses, or central nervous system disease. Nineteen of the 36 did not have obvious skin lesions.
4. All but the rarest lesions involute spontaneously (Favara et al, 1997).
5. Multiple xanthogranulomas may be seen in conjunction with neurofibromatous type 1 and chronic myelogenous leukemia.

Histopathologic Features

The histopathologic features of xanthogranulomas vary considerably, reflecting differences from case to case in the shape and cytoplasmic characteristics of the predominant cell as well as the presence and type of giant cells, number of lymphocytes, and amount of connective tissue. These variations in appearance may be due to the age of the lesion alone (Marrogi et al, 1992) or to the age of the lesion as well as the age of the patient and the underlying internal disease (Zelger et al, 1996). These are reasonable possibilities, since there is no evidence of the alternative: that dermal dendrocytes have subpopulations capable of differentiation along various morphologic paths.

The literature on the appearance of xanthogranulomas is considerable, and efforts have been made to correlate variations in appearance with clinical features, such as distribution and recurrence. Histiocytes make up the bulk of the lesion in all cases. Variations in appearance may be attributed to the cytoplasmic appearance of the histiocytes, including whether they exhibit vacuolization or xanthomatization; to the shape of the histiocytic component; to the number and type of giant cells; and to the amount and distribution of collagen. Descriptions of these variations by Malone (1991) and Marrogi et al (1992) seem adequate for the general pathologist attempting to conceptualize the range of histopathologic features. The prototypic form contains vacuolated mononuclear cells and Touton giant cells (Fig. 10–8) that may be scattered or aggregated, whereas the xanthomatous type has foamy histiocytes, with rare or absent Touton giant cells. Fibrohistiocytic types contain spindly or fusiform cells and exhibit collagen deposition. Some xanthogranulomas have a homogenous appearance in all areas, whereas others exhibit intralesional varations in the various components described earlier. Epithelium is intact over xanthogranulomas. The xanthomatous type is the most superficial, whereas other types penetrate the reticular dermis. Lymphocytes may be interspersed throughout, but eosinophils and neutrophils are scant.

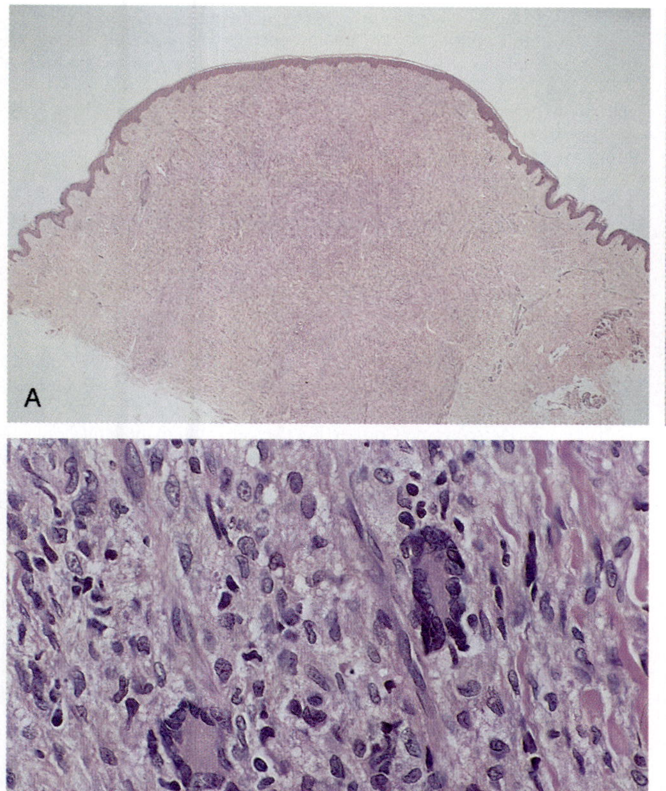

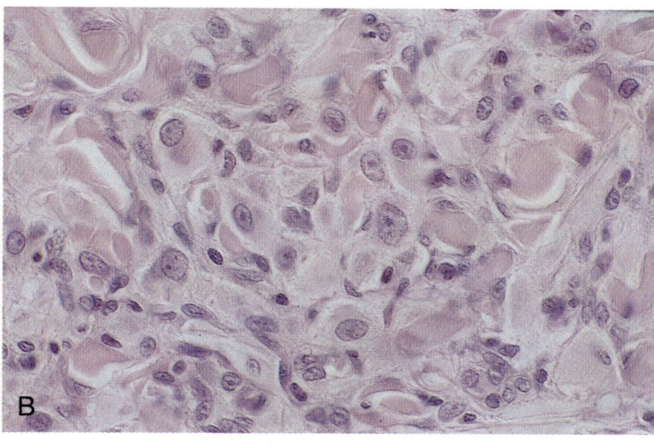

Figure 10–8

Juvenile xanthogranuloma, skin. *A,* Low magnification shows a dome-shaped dermal infiltrate with minimal inflammation. *B,* At high magnification the predominant type of cell has abundant eosinophilic cytoplasm. (*A* and *B* courtesy Dr. Paul Googe, Knoxville Dermatopathology Laboratory, Knoxville, TN.) *C,* A section from another case shows two giant cells of the Touton type. Such cells are often present in early-stage xanthogranulomas. (Courtesy Dr. Alan Boyd, Associate Professor of Medicine/Dermatology, Vanderbilt University Medical Center, Nashville, TN.)

Other Benign Cutaneous Disorders of Childhood Arising from Dermal Dendrocytes

The various terms used for other benign cutaneous disorders of childhood arising from dermal dendrocytes reflect their distribution and expected behavior. Benign cephalic histiocytosis and eruptive histiocytosis produce small red-brown papules, usually on the midface, and recurrent showers of papules, respectively. Both contain bland histiocytes (Fig. 10–9), fade over time, and require no treatment. Progressive nodular histiocytosis produces local disease, whereas xanthoma disseminatum has systemic involvement. Nodular histiocytosis is probably a variant of juvenile xanthogranuloma. Xanthoma disseminatum may have coalescence of lesions as plaques that involve the axilla, neck, or groin. Some of these children have diabetes insipidus or central nervous system or ocular findings. The infiltrates may contain Touton giant cells and may regress, but the prognosis in this disorder is more guarded, with

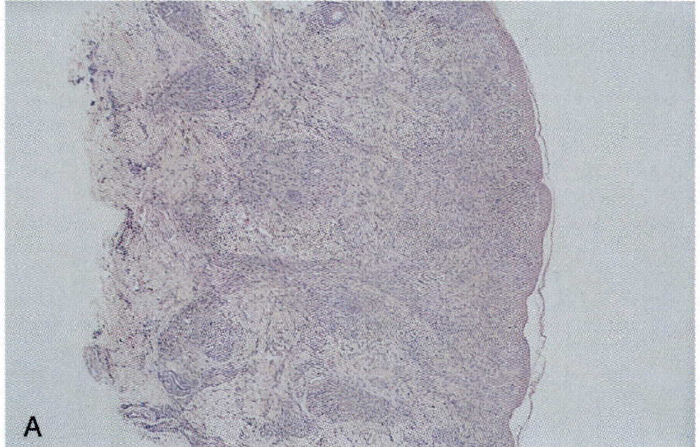

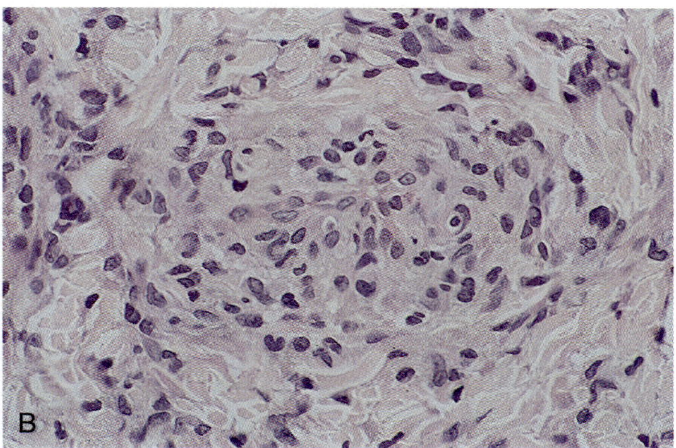

Figure 10–9

Cephalic histiocytosis, skin. *A,* Low magnification shows distortion of the dermal architecture by clusters and aggregates of eosinophilic cells. *B,* At high magnification the histiocytes have bland morphologic features, and there is scant inflammation. Clusters of histiocytes are interspersed among collagen fibers. (Courtesy Dr. Alan Boyd, Associate Professor of Medicine/Dermatology, Vanderbilt University Medical Center, Nashville, TN.)

requirements for both chemotherapy and radiation. For a summary of these rare histiocytic disorders in children, see Table 22–9 in the report of Schachner and Hansen (1995).

REFERENCES

Ben-Ezra J, Bailey A, Azumi N, et al: Malignant histiocytosis X: a distinct clinicopathologic entity. Cancer 68:1050–1060, 1991.

Bucsky P, Egeler RM: Malignant histiocytic disorders in children: clinical and therapeutic approaches with a nosologic discussion. Hematol Oncol Clin North Am 12:465–471, 1998.

Bucsky P, Favara B, Feller AC, et al: Malignant histiocytosis and large cell anaplastic (Ki-1) lymphoma in childhood: guidelines for differential diagnosis, report of the Histiocyte Society. Med Pediatr Oncol 22:200–203, 1994.

Burgdorf WHC, Zelger B: The non-Langerhans' cell histiocytoses in childhood. Pediatr Dermatol 58:201–207, 1996.

Colby TV, Lombard C: Histiocytosis X in the lung. Hum Pathol 14:847–856, 1983.

Collins RD, Bennett B, Glick AD: Neoplasms of the mononuclear phagocyte system. In Herberman RB, Friedman H (eds): The Reticuloendothelial System, Vol. 5. Plenum, New York, 1983.

Copie-Bergman C, Wotherspoon AC, Norton AJ, et al: True histiocytic lymphoma: a morphologic, immunohistiochemical, and molecular genetic study of 13 cases. Am J Surg Pathol 22:1386–1392, 1998.

Divaris DXG, Ling FCK, Prentice RSA: Congenital self-healing histiocytosis: report of two cases with histochemical and ultrastructural studies. Am J Dermatopathol 13:481–487, 1991.

Esterly NB, Maurer HS, Gonzalez-Crussi F: Histiocytosis X: a seven-year experience at a children's hospital. J Am Acad Dermatol 13:481–496, 1995.

Favara BE, Feller AC, Pauli M, et al: Contemporary classification of histiocytic disorders. Med Pediatr Oncol 29:157–166, 1997.

Favara BE, Jaffe R: The histopathology of Langerhans cell histiocytosis. Br J Cancer 70(suppl 23):S17–S23, 1994.

Foucar K, Foucar E: The mononuclear phagocyte and immunoregulatory effector (M-Pire) system: evolving concepts. Semin Diagn Pathol 7:4–18, 1990.

Franchino C, Reich C, Distenfield A, et al: A clinicopathologically distinctive primary splenic histiocytic neoplasm: demonstration of its histiocytic derivation by immunophenotypic and molecular genetic analysis. Am J Surg Pathol 12:398–404, 1988.

Freyer DR, Kennedy R, Bostrom BC, et al: Juvenile xanthogranuloma: forms of systemic disease and their clinical implications. J Pediatr 129:227–237, 1996.

Goerdt S, Kolde G, Bonsmann G, et al: Immunohistochemical comparison of cutaneous histiocytoses and related skin disorders: diagnostic and histogenetic relevance of MS-1 high molecular weight protein expression. J Pathol 170:421–427, 1993.

Hashimoto K, Pritzker MS. Electron microscopic study of reticulohistiocytoma: an unusual case of congenital, self-healing reticulohistiocytosis. Arch Dermatol 107:263–270, 1973.

Kamel OW, Gocke CD, Kell DL, et al: True histiocytic lymphoma: a study of 12 cases based on current definition. Leuk Lymphoma 18:81–86, 1995.

Kilpatrick SE, Wenger DE, Gilchrist GS, et al: Langerhans cell histiocytosis (histiocytosis X) of bone: a clinicopathologic analysis of 263 pediatric and adult cases. Cancer 76:2471–2484, 1995.

Lauritzen AF, Ralfkiaer E: Histiocytic sarcomas. Leuk Lymph 18:73–80, 1995.

Lukes RJ, Collins RD: Tumors of the hematopoietic system. In Hartman WH (ed): Atlas of Tumor Pathology, 2nd series, fascicle 28. Armed Forces Institute of Pathology, Washington DC, 1992.

Malone M: The histiocytoses of childhood. Histopathology 19:105–119, 1991.

Marrogi AJ, Dehner LP, Coffin CM, et al: Benign cutaneous histiocytic tumors in childhood and adolescence, excluding Langerhans' cell proliferations: a clinicopathologic and immunohistochemical analysis. Am J Dermatopathol 14:8–18, 1992.

McCullough CJ: Eosinophilic granuloma of bone. Acta Orthop Scand 51:389–398, 1980.

Mongkonsritragoon W, Li CY, Phytiky RL: True malignant histiocytosis. Mayo Clin Proc 73:520–528, 1998.

Motoi M, Helbron D, Kaiserling E, et al: Eosinophilic granuloma of lymph nodes: a variant of histiocytosis X. Histopathology 4:585–606, 1980.

Munn S, Chu AC: Langerhans cell histiocytosis of the skin. Hematol Oncol Clin North Am 12:269–286, 1998.

Nezelof C: Histiocytosis X: A histological and histogenetic study. Perspect Pediatr Pathol 5:153–178, 1979.

Nezelof C, Frileux-Herbet F, Cronier-Sachot J: Disseminated histiocytosis X: analysis of prognostic factors based on a retrospective study of 50 cases. Cancer 44:1824–1838, 1979.

Ralfkiaer E, Delsol G, O'Conner NTJ, et al: Malignant lymphomas of true histiocytic origin: a clinical histological, immunophenotypic and genotypic study. J Pathol 160:9–17, 1990.

Romani N, Schüler G: The immunologic properties of epidermal Langerhans cells as a part of the dendritic cell system. Springer Semin Immunopathol 13:265–279, 1992.

Ruco LP, Remotti D, Monardo F, et al: Letterer-Siwe disease: immunohistochemical evidence for a proliferative disorder involving immature cells of Langerhans lineage. Virchows Arch A Pathol Anat Histopathol 413:239–247, 1988.

Salam M, Eyres K, Cleary J: Malignant Langerhans' cell histiocytosis of the clavicle: a rare pathological fracture. Br J Clin Pract 44:652–654, 1990.

Sartoris DJ, Parker BR: Histiocytosis X: rate and pattern of resolution of osseous lesions. Radiology 152:679–684, 1984.

Schachner LA, Hansen RC: Benign neoplasms, premalignant conditions and malignancy. Pediatr Dermatol 2:1024–1041, 1995.

Schaumburg-Lever G, Rechowicz E, Fehrenvacher B, et al: Congenital self-healing reticulohistiocytosis: a benign Langerhans cell disease. J Cutan Pathol 59–66, 1994.

Schmitz L, Favara BE: Nosology and pathology of Langerhans cell histiocytosis. Hematol Oncol Clin North Am 12:221–246, 1998.

Sidoroff A, Zelger B, Steiner H, et al: Indeterminate cell histiocytosis: a clinicopathological entity with features of both X- and non-X histiocytosis. Br J Dermatopathol 134:525–532, 1996.

Soria C, Orradre JL, Garcia-Almagro D, et al: True histiocytic lymphoma (monocytic sarcoma). Am J Dermatopathol 14:511–517, 1992.

Stein H, Mason DY, Gerdes J, et al: The expression of the Hodgkin's disease associated antigen Ki-1 in reactive and neoplastic lymphoid tissue: evidence that Reed-Sternberg cells and histiocytic malignancies are derived from activated lymphoid cells. Blood 66:848–858, 1985.

Steinman RM: The dendritic cell system and its role in immunogenicity. Annu Rev Immunol 9:271–296, 1991.

The Writing Group of the Histiocyte Society: Histiocytosis syndromes in children. Lancet 1:208–209, 1987.

Willman CL, Busque L, Griffith BB, et al: Langerhans'-cell histiocytosis (histiocytosis X): a clonal proliferative disease. N Engl J Med 331:154–160, 1994.

Wilson MD, Weiss LM, Gatter KC, et al: Malignant histiocytosis: a reassessment of cases previously reported in 1975 based on paraffin section immunophenotyping studies. Cancer 66:530–536, 1990.

Wood GS, Haber RS: Novel histiocytoses considered in the context of histiocyte subset differentiation. Arch Dermatol 129:210–214, 1993.

Zelger B, Cerio R, Orchard G, et al: Juvenile and adult xanthogranuloma: a histological and immunohistochemical comparison. Am J Surg Pathol 18:126–135, 1994.

Zelger BWH, Sidoroff A, Orchard G, et al: Non-Langerhans cell histiocytoses: a new unifying concept. Am J Dermatopathol 18:490–504, 1996.

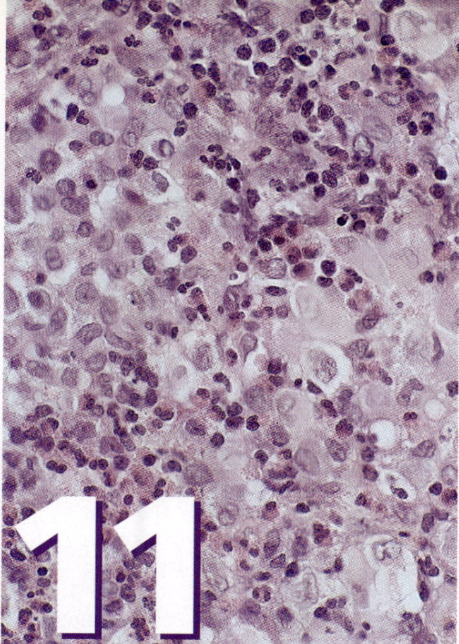

Robert D. Collins

Diagnosis and Classification of Lymphomas

Tissue and fluid samples are usually submitted to a pathology laboratory for diagnosis after a fairly complicated process triggered by patient or family awareness of a health problem, culminating in clinical evaluation and sampling of one or more sites. The intralaboratory component of this process often involves gross examination as well as selection of portions of tissue for microscopic examination, culturing, karyotyping, flow cytometric analysis, and possible storage in a tissue bank. Pathologists should welcome this opportunity to play a central role in patient management. In general, pathologists are held accountable for the successful outcome of the entire process in terms of reaching a diagnosis at minimal cost regardless of the rarity of the lymphoma, the difficulty of the diagnosis, or the adequacy of the sampled tissue.

This chapter discusses

1. Establishing a diagnosis that is appropriate for the clinical setting, that is timely and holds up over time, and that is supportable by consultant review.
2. Optimizing tissue processing. The sophisticated studies available, including expert evaluation of microscopic sections, require sophisticated initial selection of tissue samples based on clinical features, gross examination, or examination of touch preparations or frozen sections. The pathologist must ensure that adequate samples are available for consultant review and future studies.
3. Maintaining a collegial and professional relationship with clinicians and staff.

The most important of these three goals is optimal tissue processing, which is the cornerstone of diagnosis and clinical interaction. If samples are appropriately processed initially, correct diagnoses may usually be made by local pathologists. Approximately seven types of lymphomas are so frequent and have such clearly defined diagnostic criteria that general pathologists should feel comfortable in rendering a specific diagnosis. These lymphomas are listed in Table 11–1. Other lymphomas in Table 11–1 are rare but require early diagnosis because of their aggressive clinical course. The diagnosis in such cases should perhaps be confirmed by consultants because of subtle histologic features coupled with their rarity. Proper handling of tissue samples, diagnosis of lymphomas, and collegial interaction with clinicians and oncologists are greatly facilitated by understanding current concepts about the development and appearance of lymphomas as well as the conceptual framework for their classification.

GENERAL FEATURES OF LYMPHOMA

Lymphomas are derived from precursor lymphocytes by oncogenic genomic changes causing dysregulation of growth factors. Most lymphomas become clinically apparent late in their own life, after about 35 population doublings have produced masses of 10–20 g. Five more doublings result in masses that are usually lethal. Lymphomas are clonal, and the original neoplastic clone is prone to further genetic changes. Subclones, if they survive, may be more aggressive and resistant to treatment. Rapidly proliferating or chronically stimulated lymphocytes are most susceptible to oncogenic genomic changes. In such circumstances, some lymphocyte clones apparently acquire genomic changes that produce a growth advantage. Such abnormal persistent clones may accumulate genomic changes that ultimately lead to neoplasia. Epithelial neoplasms have been shown to acquire sets of abnormalities associated with oncogene activation and loss of growth suppressors. It is not clear whether lymphocytes may become neoplastic with a single change, such as the t8;14, seen in Burkitt lymphoma, or whether comparable sets of genomic abnormalities are required.

Clonal neoplastic expansions are often apparent as discrete masses, although in some cases organomegaly or organ dysfunction may be the presenting manifestation. The intrinsic ability of lymphocytes to circulate is probably responsible for their occasional failure to produce mass lesions. In these cases small lymphocytes with an infiltrative pattern predominate. As a group they are the most challenging for general and special pathologists to recognize as lymphomas. Often confused with infections, many of these lymphomas are diagnosed only after several biopsies in the face of unexplained continued organomegaly and failure to respond to antibiotic treatment.

RELATIONSHIP OF KEY CLINICAL FEATURES TO DIAGNOSIS

Clinical features, including the patient's age and sex, the site of the lesion, and its rate of growth, are often predictive of final diagnosis (Table 11–2) and are therefore very useful in planning optimal work-up of biopsy or fluid samples as well as in establishing the most likely differential diagnosis. Certain lymphomas occur in certain sites in predictable clinical settings. This information provides an important framework, establishing probabilities that usually translate into accurate, reproducible diagnoses sustained by clinical outcome.

Table 11–1

Common Lymphomas in Children with Clearly Defined Diagnostic Criteria and Rare Lymphomas in Which Early Recognition Is Important

Common Lymphomas
Lymphoblastic (convoluted) lymphoma
Large-cell lymphomas in the mediastinum
Small noncleaved (transformed) cell (Burkitt)
Hodgkin disease
  Nodular sclerosing
  Mixed cellularity
  Nodular lymphocyte predominant
Anaplastic large-cell lymphoma, CD30+

Rare Lymphomas[a]
Small-cell variant, anaplastic large-cell lymphoma, CD30+
Hepatosplenic, natural killer–like T cell lymphomas

[a]These lymphomas are important to recognize because of their aggressive course.

CLASSIFICATION OF LYMPHOMAS

Clinicians and pathologists require classifications that are applicable in a community or specialized hospital, have biologic relevance, and are reproducible. The development of a lymphoma classification satisfying these criteria has been hindered by the inherent biologic complexity of lymphomas, their rarity and hence their unfamiliarity to most pathologists, the evolution of clinical protocols that group lymphomas by grade rather than biologic features, and by underlying concerns for turfdom and scientific priority. The approach to lymphoma classification (Table 11–3) taken in this book is based on the following guidelines:

1. Lymphomas should be classified on the same basis as other neoplasms, that is, by site and cell of origin. Grading should be predicated on estimates of the growth potential of the predominant cell. The diagnostic precision inherent in this approach fosters recognition of clinicopathologic entities with attendant specific pathogenetic, prognostic, and therapeutic implications. The framework for this approach is in effect a classification of lymphomas by their B and T cell origin (Lennert, 1973; Lennert et al, 1983; Lukes & Collins, 1974). Current terminology is not fully compliant, but at least lymphomas are now categorized by B or T cell origin and to a certain extent by site of origin. It should be recognized that, for the near future, certain diagnoses may require translation (e.g., in estimating clinical grade) for purposes of treatment protocols.
2. Hodgkin disease is a malignant lymphoma that requires special consideration. First, it is more than one disease in children and adults. Second, the cell or cells of origin are not fully known, although the Reed-Sternberg cell in virtually all cases is a dysplastic, transformed lymphocyte. The site of origin is usually lymph nodes or thymus. Third, the immunologic battle between the injurious agent and the host is apparent microscopically and may dominate the histopathologic picture. The currently recognized subtypes of Hodgkin disease reflect variations in immunologic warfare and perhaps cell of origin. These variations suggest that different pathogenetic factors, different cell types, and different host responses may be involved. One of the types frequent in children, the lymphocyte-predominant type, has been shown to have a B cell origin and probably arises in follicular centers. There is some evidence that Reed-Sternberg cells in other types are B cells, but it is possible that several lymphocyte subpopulations may be induced to neoplasia by pathogenic factors capable of evoking host reactions of the various Hodgkin

Table 11–2

Relationship of Clinical Features to Diagnosis for Common Pediatric Lymphomas

Clinical Features	Diagnosis	Comment
Mediastinum		
Child or teen-ager, male, rapid growth	Lymphoblastic (convoluted) T lymphoma	May have respiratory failure, pleural or pericardial effusion, superior vena caval syndrome, rapid response to steroids
Teen-ager or young adult, female, rapid growth	Large B cell lymphoma	May have compression symptoms
Teen-ager or young adult, female, slow growth	Hodgkin disease, nodular sclerosing type	May have superior vena caval obstruction, tracheal compression, parasternal mass
Abdomen, gastrointestinal tract, ovary		
Child or young adult, rapid growth	Small transformed (noncleaved) lymphoma, Burkitt type	Nonendemic form
Nodes, cervical or axillary		
Child or teen-ager, slow growth	Hodgkin disease, lymphocyte-predominant type	
Child or teen-ager, rapid growth	Anaplastic large-cell lymphoma, CD30+	May present with small-cell variant with clinical features suggesting infection
Bone		
Child, rapid growth	Small transformed (noncleaved) lymphoma, Burkitt type	Endemic form

Table 11–3
Classification of Pediatric Lymphomas

Type	Presenting Sites
T Cell Lymphomas	
Lymphoblastic (convoluted)	Thymus or anterior mediastinum
Anaplastic large-cell, CD30+, small-cell variant	Nodes (cervical, axillary, and skin)
Natural killer–like T cell	Hepatosplenic (intestinal?)
Mycosis fungoides	Skin
B Cell Lymphomas	
Large transformed (noncleaved) cell	Nodes, anterior mediastinum
Small transformed (noncleaved), Burkitt type	Ileum, elsewhere in abdomen, gonads, bone
Follicular center cell, nodular, small cleaved	Nodes, superficial
Immunoblastic lymphoma	Nodes, soft tissue
Lymphoblastic	Mediastinum (?), skin
Hodgkin Diseases	
Lymphocytic and histiocytic, nodular	Node, high cervical, and axillary
Nodular sclerosis	Anterior mediastinal mass, cervical nodes
Mixed cellularity	Superficial nodes

types. Thus, the group of Hodgkin diseases is considered separately in the lymphoma classification, even though some Reed-Sternberg cells are B cells.

3. Light microscopic examination is the cornerstone of lymphoma classification. Many lymphomas may be classified and their behavior predicted by light microscopic study alone. The factors affecting their appearance are therefore of special importance to pathologists. These factors include growth pattern; the mixture of reacting and neoplastic cells; the percentages of neoplastic cells that are dividing, dormant, or differentiated; the inherent cytologic features of the neoplastic clone; and, perhaps most important, the quality of the tissue sections. These factors are described briefly.

Factors Affecting Lymphoma Appearance

The growth patterns of childhood lymphomas are far less complicated than those in adults. This is a mixed blessing, since the growth pattern in adults is often diagnostic of the lymphoma subtype. There are very few lymphomas in children with follicular nodulation. Most childhood lymphomas grow diffusely in sheets and aggregates. Most CD30+ lymphomas have a prominent infiltration of sinuses. Growth patterns in the Hodgkin diseases is also of great help in classifying these processes. In particular, nodular lymphocyte-predominant Hodgkin disease has a virtually diagnostic appearance at low magnification, as does nodular sclerosing Hodgkin disease. As noted earlier, the infiltrative processes composed of small lymphocytes are difficult to recognize as lymphomas and do not have currently recognized characteristic growth features.

In most pediatric lymphomas, clonal expansion of a population results in aggregates, sheets, or masses of neoplastic cells resembling one another in appearance and functional characteristics. Reacting cells usually include macrophages, neutrophils, and eosinophils as well as fibrovascular elements. In some lymphomas, particularly Hodgkin disease, neoplastic cells are in the minority. The reactive component in Hodgkin disease is distinctive and almost specific for purposes of recognition and classification of subtypes.

In pediatric lymphoma cases, the dividing component is usually large, but the percentage of cells in division may vary in individual patients from one part of the tumor to another or at different times. The number of dormant (small) lymphocytes may also vary, as may morphologic or immunophenotypic evidence of differentiation. However, overt plasmacytic differentiation is unusual in pediatric B cell lymphomas, and morphologic criteria for T cell differentiation are not reliable.

Identification of neoplastic cells by cytologic features is part science and part dependence on the eye of the beholder. The difficulties are exemplified by the Reed-Sternberg cell, an extreme example of dysplasia in transformed lymphocytes. No absolutely specific cytologic (or immunophenotypic) markers of these cells have been identified despite the interest in this lymphoma for decades. Recognition of differentiation of neoplastic T cells is even more problematic, although some T cell lymphomas contain specific granules. Identification of neoplastic cells by cytologic features requires high-quality sections, sophistication in microscopy, and some experience. More reliable indicators of cell type are clinical features, growth pattern, and immunophenotypic characteristics. Nevertheless, it is certainly possible for general pathologists to differentiate clearly transformed (noncleaved) cell lymphomas from lymphoblastic processes and to suspect leukemic infiltrates on the basis of growth pattern.

Various explanations have been given to explain the failure to obtain high-quality tissue preparations consistently from lymphatic tissue and marrow. Marrow preparations are subject to crush or aspiration artifact. Nodes are often removed late in the day or week by less experienced surgeons. Specimens not dropped intact into formalin may be submitted for a frozen section for reasons that are often obscure. Proper tissue handling is necessary to obtain accurate diagnoses. Pathologists should become involved in the process before procedures are performed and should select samples on the basis of clinical information supplemented by touch preparations rather than frozen sections. With touch preparations, it is often easier to ensure that diagnostic material has been obtained. They have the additional advantages of speed, avoidance of cryostat contamination, and the ability to be preserved for routine sections, flow cytometric analysis, and cytogenetic study.

ROLE OF FLOW CYTOMETRIC ANALYSIS

Flow cytometric analysis or its equivalent, rapid immunoalkaline phosphatase on air-dried preparations, is necessary for categorization of leukemias and is useful in classifying many lymphomas. However, the common lymphomas in Table 11–1 may all be diagnosed satisfactorily by routine histologic examination and paraffin immunoperoxidase staining. Flow cytometric analysis has the aura of precision, but is subject, as all test results are, to sampling and interpretive errors. Clearly, it should not be performed on all samples. For example, it is not useful in reactive states and Hodgkin disease. Flow cytometric analysis should not be used to compensate for inadequately processed tissue samples. Poor sections coupled with misinterpreted cytometric data may compound diagnostic difficulties.

ROLE OF CLONALITY DEMONSTRATION IN DIAGNOSIS OF LYMPHOMAS

All lymphomas are clonal, but all clonal lymphocytic proliferations are not lymphomas (Collins, 1997). In fact, lymphocytes physiologically respond to antigenic stimulation by clonal expansion. The significance of clonality is particularly problematic in the "pseudolymphomas" that plague adult hematopathologists. Children with clonal proliferations such as eosinophilic granuloma and lymphomatoid papulosis have been shown to have a good prognosis. Thus, clonality alone is not proof of malignancy. Some clonal processes actually producing masses in children with posttransplant lymphoproliferative disorder may resolve with reduction of immunosuppression. Until criteria are established that reliably predict when clonal processes will exhibit malignant behavior, light microscopic study will continue to be the cornerstone of the diagnostic process, with the caveat that clonal tumorous processes may resolve if immunosuppression is reduced after transplantation.

KARYOTYPIC STUDIES

Cancers, including lymphomas, result from genomic aberrations that promote cell proliferation, inhibit suppressors of cell growth, or both. Specific genomic abnormalities are likely to cause specific lymphomas. Karyotypic studies are particularly useful in diagnosing certain leukemias and poorly differentiated neoplasms, such as the "small blue cell" processes. It is likely that, in the future, karyotypic studies will facilitate diagnosis of all lymphomas. At present, it is clear that recognition of the 2;5 translocation has been useful for biologic as well as diagnostic reasons in anaplastic large-cell CD30+ lymphomas. Single karyotypic abnormalities may be sufficient inducers of lymphomas in children, although a clonal evolutionary process would seem to be needed to produce first a sustainable clone and then a malignant lymphoma.

DIFFERENTIAL DIAGNOSIS

Most lymphomas in children are readily apparent as bulky masses containing sheets of rapidly dividing cells. In contrast to adults, there are few, if any, low-grade lymphomas. With rare exceptions known at this time, the predominant cell in childhood lymphomas may be characterized cytologically as a transformed or noncleaved lymphocyte or lymphoblast. One exception is the small-cell variant of anaplastic large-cell lymphoma. This lymphoma requires special attention because of its unusual morphologic features, rarity, and aggressive clinical course.

Lymphomas may be confused with other neoplasms, including rhabdomyosarcomas, small blue cell tumors of various types, and Ewing sarcoma. Presentation of leukemia as skin or node lesions is a particularly difficult problem, but the correct diagnosis in all of the foregoing examples may usually be made by paraffin immunoperoxidase staining, marrow examination with or without flow cytometric analysis, and, rarely, electron microscopic examination.

The distinction of reactive conditions from lymphoma in children may be extraordinarily difficult if the reaction is particularly florid, biopsy specimens are limited, and little clinical information is provided. Infectious mononucleosis is well known for producing alarming nodal or tonsillar immunoblastic proliferations. A greater test of the pathologist's judgment and experience is posed by the spectrum of lymphoproliferative disorders seen in patients with congenital or acquired immunodeficiencies, specifically, posttransplant lymphoproliferative disorders. The difficulty of the problem is illustrated by the lymphoproliferations in X-linked immunodeficiency and after transplantation. In the former, patients may develop polyclonal, florid, fatal, and widespread immunoblastic proliferations from Epstein-Barr virus infection or may present with clonal, more localized lymphomatous masses. Posttransplant lymphoproliferative disorders include a continuum of Epstein-Barr virus–related lymphocytic proliferations following organ transplantation and the associated immunosuppression. The cases range from polymorphic proliferations with B cells at all stages of differentiation and transformation to monomorphic growth of immunoblasts. Rarely, these lymphomas have T cell features or have been diagnosed as Hodgkin disease. Phenotyping has shown polyclonal, oligoclonal, and monoclonal B cell processes. Prognosis is extremely variable and difficult to make, but most of the nonclonal and almost half of the clonal cases respond to reduction in immunosuppression and surgery.

REFERENCES

Collins RD: Is clonality equivalent to malignancy: specifically, is immunoglobulin gene rearrangement diagnostic of malignant lymphoma? Hum Pathol 28:757–759, 1997.

Lennert K: Pathologisch-histologische: Klassifizierung der malignen Lymphome. In Stacher A (ed): Leukämien und maligne Lymphome. Urban and Schwarzenberg, Munich, pp 181–194, 1973.

Lennert K, Collins RD, Lukes RJ: Concordance of the Kiel and Lukes-Collins classifications of non-Hodgkin's lymphomas. Histopathology 7:549–559, 1983.

Lukes RJ, Collins RD: Immunologic characterization of human malignant lymphomas. Cancer 34:1488–1503, 1974.

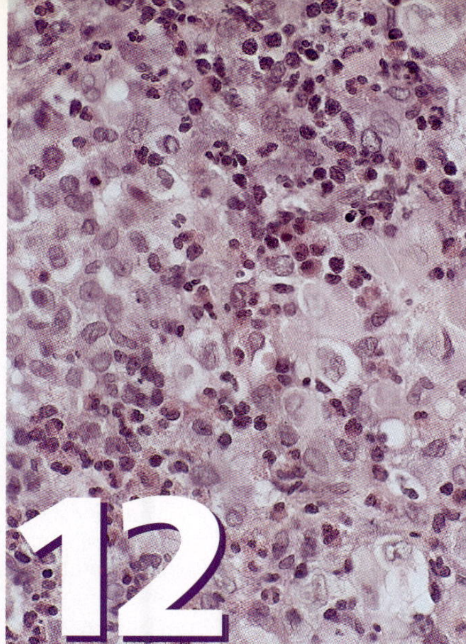

Steven H. Swerdlow

12 Lymphomas: Epidemiologic, Biologic, and Pathogenetic Features

This chapter addresses some of the issues related to the epidemiology of lymphomas in children, the molecular mechanisms involved in oncogenesis, and the pathogenetic factors playing a role in lymphoma development. For some lymphomas there is detailed information on all of these topics, while in others information is sketchy and superficial. Some lymphomas develop in children who have an inherited or acquired immunodeficiency, while others, such as Burkitt lymphoma, apparently result from a viral infection complicated by coexistent infection with malaria. In contrast to adults, children almost never have low-grade lymphomas. Their high-grade lymphomas—lymphoblastic T cell, Burkitt, and anaplastic large-cell Ki-1+—are similar to those in adults with respect to histopathologic features and immunophenotype but differ in some cases in pathogenesis. There are significant differences in Hodgkin disease (HD) between the two age groups with respect to epidemiology and perhaps pathogenesis.

EPIDEMIOLOGY

In order of descending frequency, leukemia, brain tumors, and lymphomas are the most common cancers in children and adolescents in the United States (Bleyer, 1990; Sandlund et al, 1996; Young et al, 1986). About 13% of newly diagnosed pediatric malignant neoplasms are lymphomas. Pediatric lymphomas, particularly those other than HD, increased in frequency during the 1970s and 1980s (Bunin et al, 1996), although more recently there may have been a slight decrease in the group under 20 years of age (Bunin et al, 1996; Chen et al, 1997; Sandlund et al, 1996). The incidence of HD has apparently remained unchanged (Glaser & Swartz, 1990; MacMahon, 1957). Lymphomas in certain areas, such as Zambia, have not followed the same trends (Chintu et al, 1995). There, Burkitt lymphoma is less frequent, whereas B and T cell lymphomas are increasing in incidence overall.

The incidence of pediatric lymphomas varies with geography, race, and gender. Lymphomas, along with leukemias, are the most common childhood cancers in Asia, Africa, and South America (Macharia, 1996; Murphy, 1980; Roguin et al, 1995). In equatorial Africa and Papua, New Guinea, 90% of childhood malignancies are Burkitt lymphoma (Chapman et al, 1995; de Thé, 1993; van den Bosch et al, 1993; and Wright, 1967). Burkitt lymphoma is also very common in northeastern Brazil. In contrast, pediatric B and T cell lymphomas are rare in Japan (Sandlund et al, 1996). The incidence of HD varies widely, with high rates in many underdeveloped countries. Asian children, including those in the United States, have a low incidence (Macfarlane et al, 1995).

In Western developed countries, 60% of childhood lymphomas are B and T cell lymphomas and the remainder HD (Sandlund et al, 1996). Thirty to 50% of B and T cell lymphomas are Burkitt lymphomas, 20–40% T lymphoblastic lymphomas, and 15–30% "large-cell" lymphomas (Link & Donaldson, 1998; Perkins et al, 1995; Sandlund et al, 1996; Wright et al, 1997), with anaplastic large-cell lymphoma (ALCL) the major subset of pediatric large-cell lymphomas. B cell lymphomas make up 90% of all adult lymphomas, but almost half of childhood lymphomas are of T cell origin. These lymphomas include the lymphoblastic T cell lymphomas; the less frequent peripheral T cell lymphomas, most of which are of ALCL type (Agnarsson & Kadin, 1995); and lymphomas resembling adult T cell leukemia or lymphoma, angiocentric immunoproliferative lesions, immunoblastic adenopathy-like T cell lymphoma hepatosplenic T cell lymphoma, and cutaneous T cell lymphomas. Most B cell lymphomas in children are Burkitt in type. B lymphoblastic lymphomas are very rare. More than 33% of pediatric large-cell lymphomas are of B cell origin (Link & Donaldson, 1998). Follicular lymphomas are exceedingly rare in children, and almost half are large cell in type (Pinto et al, 1990). Low-grade B cell lymphomas have been rarely reported (Elenitoba-Johnson et al, 1997).

The subtypes of HD are similar to those in adults. Nodular sclerosis is the most common type, and the lymphocyte-depleted type is very rare. Lymphocyte predominance is frequently seen in developed countries, and mixed cellularity is more common in Latin American children (Razzouk et al, 1997). Children under 10 years of age have incidences of nodular sclerosis and mixed cellularity nearly equal to those in the United States (Jarrett et al, 1996; Medeiros & Greiner, 1995).

In the United States, the 10- to 14-year-old group has the highest incidence of lymphoma (Young et al, 1986), with very few cases in those under 5 years old (Link & Donaldson, 1998). In endemic areas, 50% of Burkitt lymphoma cases occur in 5- to 9-year-olds. Burkitt lymphoma is uncommon in children under 2 years of age (Wright, 1967) and occurs in older individuals outside endemic areas. The median age for pediatric ALCL is 9 years (Massimino et al, 1995). HD is very rare in children under 5 years of age, with the highest incidence among the oldest children (Glaser & Swartz, 1990; Medeiros & Greiner, 1995). However, in developing countries, there may be a peak in children 6 to 12 years old (Armstrong et al, 1993; Chintu et al, 1995), whereas in Hong Kong a peak intermediate between that of underdeveloped countries and that of Western populations was shown (Chan et al, 1995).

Pediatric B and T cell lymphomas, particularly Burkitt lymphoma, have a male predominance of about 2–3:1 (Bunin et al, 1996; Sandlund et al, 1996; Wright et al, 1997). In HD, there is a striking male predominance for those under 10 years of age, a similar sex incidence for those 10 to 14, and a female predominance for those 15 to 19 (Andriko et al, 1997; Bunin et al, 1996; Glaser & Jarrett, 1996; Glaser & Swartz, 1990). B and T cell lymphomas are approximately twice as common in white than in black children (Sandlund et al, 1996). The incidence of HD, particularly the nodular sclerosis type, is higher in black and Hispanic than in white children (Bunin et al, 1996; Cozen et al, 1992; Glaser & Jarrett, 1996; Medeiros & Greiner, 1995).

Inheritance is not known to be a factor in B and T cell lymphomas, although a set of identical twins developing a T lymphoblastic malignancy at 9 and 11 years of age had the same T cell receptor rearrangement (Ford et al, 1997). Familial clustering of Burkitt lymphoma may be related to common environmental factors (Brubaker et al, 1980). Whether low-level ionizing or electromagnetic field radiation is a risk factor in pediatric lymphomas is controversial or of doubtful importance (Kwak & Longo, 1996; Washburn et al, 1994).

The possible causative role of an infectious agent in HD is discussed later in this chapter. An inherited predisposition has been postulated for HD in adults, since monozygotic twins have a high risk of developing coincident disease (Mack et al, 1995). Familial aggregates of HD and parental consanguinity have been reported (Abramson et al, 1978; Glaser & Jarrett, 1996). Some studies suggest that HD is associated with an underlying immune abnormality or, weakly, with certain HLA haplotypes (Mack et al, 1995; Taylor et al, 1996).

GENOTYPIC AND KARYOTYPIC ISSUES

The vast majority of B cell and T cell pediatric lymphomas demonstrate clonal rearrangement of their immunoglobulin and T cell receptor genes, respectively, revealed by Southern blot or polymerase chain reaction (PCR) techniques. This section concentrates on the molecular abnormalities in the neoplastic cells of the major pediatric lymphomas and those that help characterize the precise cell type involved (Table 12–1). Detailed immunophenotypic characterization of these neoplasms is discussed in Chaps. 14 and 15.

Burkitt Lymphoma

Sporadic and endemic Burkitt lymphomas contain clonal B cells with somatically mutated immunoglobulin genes (Chapman et al, 1995; Klein et al, 1995; Tamaru et al, 1995). The frequency of mutation appears lower than in follicular lymphomas. Ongoing mutation, as often seen in follicular lymphomas, does not generally occur. These findings apparently indicate that Burkitt lymphoma cells resemble either early transformed follicular center cells "arrested in a mutation-silent phase" or follicular center cells that have modulated toward IgM+, IgD− memory B cells (Tamaru et al, 1995). CD10 expression by Burkitt lymphomas supports this interpretation. Burkitt lymphoma cells do not morphologically resemble typical memory-type B cells, but *MYC* overexpression might cause their transformation (discussed later). It has also been proposed that Burkitt lymphoma represents a "high-grade MALT lymphoma" [mucosa-associated lymphoid tissue type] (Magrath & Bhatia, 1997).

A critical genotypic abnormality occurs in about 80% of Burkitt lymphomas: the translocation of the *MYC* gene on chromosome 8q24 to the immunoglobulin heavy-chain gene on chromosome 14q32 (Dalla-Favera et al, 1982; Magrath & Bhatia, 1997; Sandlund et al, 1996). Essentially all of the remaining cases demonstrate a "variant" *MYC* translocation to the κ light-chain gene on 2p11 or the λ light-chain gene on 22q11 (Sandlund et al, 1996; Shiramizu et al, 1991). The pathogenesis of the endemic form is different from that of the sporadic type. Most (74–100%) endemic Burkitt lymphomas have breakpoints far upstream from the actual *MYC* gene, whereas most (89–91%) sporadic types have breakpoints within or close to the gene in a region that includes the first intron, exon, and 5′ flanking sequences (Pelicci et al, 1986; Shiramizu et al, 1991). The latter rearrangements lead to varied structural changes in the *MYC* gene (Magrath & Bhatia, 1997). Most of the variant Burkitt lymphoma translocations demonstrate chromosome 8 breakpoints 3′ to the *MYC* locus (Zeidler et al, 1994). The immunoglobulin rearrangements are mostly (73%) outside the switch region, with involvement of the switch region demonstrating an association with sporadic Burkitt lymphoma (Shiramizu et al, 1991). The vast majority (87%) of those with breakpoints in the switch region have a rearranged *MYC* gene.

MYC is a short-lived nuclear phosphoprotein transcription factor that alters the expression of key cellular genes and promotes cell cycle progression from the G1 to the S phase (Packham & Cleveland, 1995; Sandlund et al, 1996; Smith-Sørensen et al, 1996). MYC forms "transcription-activating" heterodimers with the related MAX protein (a zipper protein that forms a DNA-binding complex with MYC), itself, or other proteins. However, the biologic activity of MYC is not completely dependent on MAX (Packham & Cleveland, 1995; Sandlund et al, 1996). MYC also inhibits differentiation and induces apoptosis. The 8q24 translocations in Burkitt lymphoma, together with other molecular abnormalities described later, lead to the constituitive expression of the translocated *MYC*, whereas normal *MYC* is expressed at low levels or not at all (Hörtnagel et al, 1995). This *MYC* dysregulation causes rapid cycling of Burkitt lymphoma cells.

MYC dysregulation is important in the pathogenesis of Burkitt lymphoma but is not sufficient for neoplastic transformation (Chapman et al, 1995; Mautner et al, 1996; Sandlund et al, 1996; Shiramizu et al, 1991; Wolf et al, 1990). Increased *MYC* expression driven by immunoglobulin enhancers in transgenic mice does lead to pre–B and B cell lymphomas after a latent period of months. *MYC* expression is initially in polyclonal cells, and development of monoclonality in these lymphomas infers that an additional oncogenic event or events occur in one of the many B cells overexpressing *MYC* (Adams et al, 1985).

Other abnormalities of importance in the pathogenesis of Burkitt lymphoma are the *MYC* mutations in many or all cases, even when *MYC* translocation occurs far upstream from the *MYC* gene (Bhatia et al, 1995; Chapman et al, 1995; Magrath & Bhatia, 1997). Mutations, present in cases in which much of the *MYC* regulatory region remains, affect the region encompassing the regulatory first exon or first exon-intron boundary (Cesarman et al, 1987; Chapman et al, 1995; Hörtnagel et al, 1995). These mutations may play a part in the promoter switch and release from transcriptional pausing and RNA elongation at the 3′ end of the first exon, which is characteristic of *MYC* expression in Burkitt lymphoma, particularly the endemic type. This loss of transcriptional attenuation resulting from exon 1 mutations may be related to loss of a nuclear MYC inhibitory factor protein–binding site (Smith-Sørensen et al, 1996). The characteristic promoter switch reflects preferential use of the P1 promoter for transcription initiation, in contrast to normal *MYC* in which 80–90% of total *MYC* RNA is derived from the P2 promoter (Hörtnagel et al, 1995). Because many sporadic and a minority of endemic Burkitt lymphomas have *MYC* breakpoints downstream from the P1 and P2 promoters, the

Table 12–1

Cell of Origin, Major Genotypic and Karyotypic Abnormalities, and EBV Association in the Major Types of Pediatric Lymphomas

Diagnosis	Cell Type and Other Important Cellular Constituents	Major Genotypic or Karyotypic Abnormalities	EBV Association
Burkitt lymphoma	B cell similar to those in follicular center or transformed memory–type B cell	*MYC* rearrangement from 8q24 to immunoglobulin heavy-chain (14q32) or, less often, to κ(2p11) or λ(22q11); *MYC* mutations	Endemic: almost all EBV+ Sporadic: 10–40% EBV+
T lymphoblastic lymphoma[a]	Thymic-type T lymphoblast	Translocations involving T cell receptor (α,β,γ, or δ chains on 14q11, 7q32, 14q11, or 7p15, respectively) and protooncogenes (mostly transcription factors)	None
Anaplastic large-cell (Ki-1+) lymphoma	Cytotoxic T cell; less often, "null" (indeterminate) cell	t(2;5)(p23;q35) involving nucleophosmin gene (5) and anaplastic lymphoma kinase gene (2) with *NPM/ALK* fusion product ("p80")	Usually none
HD, nodular lymphocyte predominance	Follicular center B cell ("L and H" Reed-Sternberg variants)	No consistent abnormality in these clonal B cells	None
HD, nodular sclerosis and mixed cellularity types	Reed-Sternberg cells in some cases resemble follicular center cells but do not show immunoglobulin gene expression; some cases of T cell origin; others undefined Reactive cellular elements that, like Reed-Sternberg cells, are important in cytokine secretion	No consistent abnormality but typically aneuploid	>50% EBV+, with highest proportion in children <10 years old

Abbreviations: EBV, Epstein-Barr virus; HD, Hodgkin disease.

[a]Data derived mostly from T cell acute lymphoblastic leukemia studies.

transcription in these cases is initiated within the first intron, possibly because of the juxtaposed immunoglobulin gene enhancer elements (Shiramizu et al, 1991).

Mutations also occur in almost all Burkitt cases in the protein-coding regions that affect the *MYC* transactivating domain. This domain is important for *MYC* function and is a site for phosphorylation (Raffeld et al, 1995). These mutations may resist suppression of *MYC* transactivation by the retinoblastoma-related protein p107 (Bhatia et al, 1995; Raffeld et al, 1995; Smith-Sørensen et al, 1996) and may occur in follicular center cells that already have an *MYC* translocation. The translocated *MYC* may be susceptible to mutations similar to the immunoglobulin V gene region hypermutation that occurs normally in follicular centers (Chapman et al, 1995; Raffeld et al, 1995). This susceptibility to mutations might explain why chronic infections, such as malaria and HIV, that promote follicular hyperplasia might be associated with an increased incidence of Burkitt lymphoma (Chapman et al, 1995).

Other abnormalities of potential importance in Burkitt lymphoma include *BCL6* mutations that affect DNA sequences lying in proximity to gene regulatory sequences and possibly fostering *BCL6* gene dysregulation (Capello et al, 1997). These mutations are seen in 28.6% of sporadic cases and 50% of endemic cases. *BCL6* gene mutations, like the *MYC* mutations, may result from an "ectopic" immunoglobulin variable gene hypermutation mechanism (Capello et al, 1997). *P53* mutations occur inconsistently in Burkitt lymphoma, with maximal incidences of 35–45% of cases (Imamura et al, 1994; Maestro et al, 1997; Preudhomme & Fenaux, 1997). They occur independently of geographic origin, breakpoint location, and presence of Epstein-Barr virus (EBV) (Bhatia et al, 1992; Preudhomme et al, 1995). Burkitt lymphomas also lack CD18 mRNA, leading to a lack of the β_2 integrin CD11a/CD18 on their cell surfaces (Neira et al, 1997). This loss, combined with low expression of other adhesion molecules, may explain the absence of nodal involvement in many cases and provide a possible reason that Burkitt lymphomas apparently escape immunosurveillance.

Lymphoblastic Lymphoma

Most lymphoblastic lymphomas are of T cell origin and have demonstrable clonal T cell receptor gene rearrangements. T cell acute lymphoblastic leukemia is a similar neoplasm morphologically and immunophenotypically, distinguished only by arbitrary criteria. Our understanding of the biology of these neoplasms is based largely on studies of T cell acute lymphoblastic leukemia. The major genotypic abnormalities described in T cell acute lymphoblastic leukemia involve translocations between the regulatory sequences of the T cell antigen receptor genes on chromosomes 7 (β chain, 7q32; δ chain, 7p15) or 14 (α and γ chain, 14q11) and protooncogenes (Sandlund et al, 1996; Uckun et al, 1998). Most involve transcription factor genes, specifically *TAL1* (a genetic locus involved in T cell oncogenesis). In increased levels, the TAL1 protein probably forms complexes with the E2A protein and causes abnormal activation of target genes. Other types of oncogenes and sometimes non–T cell receptor loci are also involved in T cell acute lymphoblastic leukemia translocations (Uckun et al, 1998; Xia et al, 1991). Pediatric T lymphoblastic neoplasms rarely have p53 mutations (Wada et al, 1992), and p53 mutations are more common in T cell acute lymphoblastic leukemia at relapse (Preudhomme & Fenaux, 1997).

Anaplastic Large-Cell Lymphoma

A major karyotypic abnormality associated with ALCL is t(2;5)(p23;q35), which leads to a fusion of the amino-terminal portion of the nucleophosmin gene (*NPM*) from chromosome 5 and the catalytic domain of the anaplastic lymphoma kinase gene (*ALK*) from chromosome 2 (Bischof et al, 1997; Morris et al, 1994). This fusion leads to deregulated expression of a "p80" 75-kD NPM/ALK chimeric protein derived from the fused chromosomes on the derivative chromosome 5.

ALK is a receptor tyrosine kinase of the insulin receptor subfamily that is normally expressed in neural tissues, the testis, and the small intestine (Morris et al, 1994; Sandlund et al, 1996). NPM is a ubiquitously expressed RNA-binding nucleolar phosphoprotein that shuttles ribonucleoproteins from the nucleolus to the ribosomes. In contrast to normal NPM, the fusion protein is present in the cytoplasm, where expression of the truncated ALK may lead to malignant transformation with inappropriate substrate phosphorylation and an unregulated mitogenic signal (Bischof et al, 1997; Fujimoto et al, 1996; Morris et al, 1994; Sandlund et al, 1996). The fusion protein may also be present in the nucleus and nucleolus because of the shuttling activity of NPM, but its presence in cytoplasm is required for oncogenesis (Bischof et al, 1997). NPM is critical because it facilitates NPM/ALK homodimerization, leading to intermolecular cross-phosphorylation and constitutive activation of ALK phosphotransferase activity (Bischof et al, 1997; Kuefer et al, 1997). The neoplastic transforming capabilities of NPM/ALK expression have been demonstrated in NIH 3T3 cells, in a murine retroviral gene transfer model, and in rodent fibroblasts (Bischof et al, 1997; Fujimoto et al, 1996; Kuefer et al, 1997). "Paradoxically," the mice developed large B cell lymphomas.

The t(2;5) translocation is reported in 33–50% of pediatric "large-cell" lymphomas. This translocation and/or the resultant fusion protein is present in many (84–88%) pediatric ALCLs of the T, and less often the null cell type and is much less commonly (18–60%) found in adult ALCLs (Elmberger et al, 1995; Lamant et al, 1996; Nakagawa et al, 1997; Pittaluga et al, 1997; Shiota et al, 1995). One report states that only 58% of childhood ALCLs are NPM/ALK+ (Wellman et al, 1995). Some feel that ALK positivity should be used as a criterion of ALCL, since the histopathologic features are quite variable (Benharroch et al, 1998). The translocation was found in pediatric cases previously diagnosed as malignant histiocytosis (Simonitsch et al, 1996), cases now generally assumed to be ALCL. The translocation is also found in pediatric lymphomas generally of T cell type that have a less obvious CD30+ large-cell population (Weisenburger et al, 1996). These cases are diploid or near diploid, in contrast to classic ALCL, which has a more complex karyotype (Weisenburger et al, 1996). Most of the ALCLs have cytotoxic cell antigenic features that do not correlate with *NPM/ALK* fusion transcript expression (Krenacs et al, 1997). The t(2;5) is also reported in a small number of adult B cell lymphomas. In one study, the *NPM/ALK* fusion RNA was not demonstrable by reverse transcriptase PCR (RT-PCR) (Weisenburger et al, 1996). This translocation is not found in HD, and it is not usually a feature of primary cutaneous or HIV-associated ALCL (DeCoteau et al, 1996; Elmberger et al, 1995; Ladanyi et al, 1994; Lamant et al, 1996; Sarris et al, 1996; Wellman et al, 1995; Wood et al, 1996).

Rare ALCLs are described that have ALK or p80 expression and variant translocations involving 2p23 and a chromosome other than 5 (Lamant et al, 1996; Pittaluga et al, 1997; Pulford et al, 1997), suggesting that genes other than *NPM* can activate ALK (e.g., at 2q35, 1q25) (Lamant et al, 1996; Pittaluga et al, 1997; Touriol et al, 2000).

In contrast to other T cell lymphomas, 45% of CD30+ ALCLs (T or null cell type) express BCL6 (Carbone et al, 1997a). CD30+, BCL6+ cells are normally found in nodal interfollicular areas. This pattern of immunoreactivity and location suggests that they may be the normal cells from which the neoplastic cells in ALCL arise. P53 positivity is common in ALCL (including childhood T and null cell types). No other known oncogene abnormalities characterize t(2;5)-positive ALCL. *MYC* rearrangements or mutations have been reported in six ALCLs. However, five were of B cell origin and therefore different from the usual ALCL (Inghirami et al, 1994a). The genes for CD30 (a member of the tumor necrosis factor receptor superfamily) and for CD30L (a type 2 transmembrane protein that induces numerous biologic effects on CD30+ cells) are not involved in the characteristic ALCL chromosomal translocation. These genes are located on chromosomes 1p36 and 9q33, respectively (Falini et al, 1995), and their importance in the biologic characterization of ALCL is uncertain. The high expression of the cell-cell adhesion cadherin molecule may contribute to the morphologic appearance of ALCLs and their cohesive growth pattern (Ashton-Key et al, 1996). Another cell adhesion protein associated with ALCL is clusterin (Wellmann et al, 1998).

Hodgkin Disease

The nature of HD has fascinated pathologists for many decades. Our poor understanding of this disease is illustrated by the fact that, until recently, HD was considered by some to be an infectious disorder. Malignant clinical and pathologic features have been apparent since the first description of HD. Now the clonality of all types of HD has been shown using various techniques, including many that demonstrate monoclonal Reed-Sternberg (RS) cells. Traditional cytogenetic studies, DNA content studies, genotypic studies, and in situ hybridization studies for immunoglobulin light-chain expression (in some cases of nodular lymphocyte-predominant HD) have all revealed clonality. Another biologic feature of RS cells is their relatively high proliferative fraction, with at least 50% of RS cells often positive for the cell cycle–associated Ki-67 antigen (Elenitoba-Johnson et al, 1996; Gerdes et al, 1987).

Cytogenetic studies have been difficult in HD. When the studies are successful, abnormal results typically show aneuploidy with a predominance of hyperdiploid or near-triploid karyotypes and highly complex structural rearrangements (Döhner et al, 1992; Kwak & Longo, 1996; Tilly et al, 1991). There are no specific cytogenetic abnormalities or recurring translocations, although there are some recurring losses from certain chromosomes. Most report the absence of a t(2;5) translocation. Even when conventional cytogenetic study results are normal, fluorescence in-situ hybridization (FISH) or fluorescent immunophenotyping and interphase cytogenetic analysis (FICTION) studies demonstrate nonuniform numerical chromosome abnormalities with hyperdiploidy in most CD30+ RS cells and variants (Haber et al, 1992; Inghirami et al, 1994b; Weber-Matthiesen et al, 1995). DNA content studies have shown that the same clone of RS cells is present in more than one tissue sample (Inghirami et al, 1994b). The small lymphocytes in HD do not demonstrate chromosomal abnormalities (Pringle et al, 1997).

In nodular lymphocyte-predominant HD, the RS cell variants are B cells. Single-cell genotypic studies have established that these variants are monoclonal B cells that have productive immunoglobulin gene rearrangements (Braeuninger et al,

by reactive T lymphocytes in Hodgkin's disease. Hum Pathol 24: 249–255, 1993.

Hutchison RE, Pui C-H, Murphy SB, et al: Non-Hodgkin's lymphoma in children younger than 3 years. Cancer 62:1371–1373, 1988.

Imai S, Sugiura M, Mizuno F, et al: African Burkitt's lymphoma: a plant, *Euphorbia tirucalli*, reduces Epstein-Barr virus–specific cellular immunity. Anticancer Res 14:933–936, 1994.

Imamura J, Miyoshi I, Koeffler HP: p53 in hematologic malignancies. Blood 84:2412–2421, 1994.

Inghirami G, Macri L, Cesarman E, et al: Molecular characterization of CD30+ anaplastic large-cell lymphoma: high frequency of *c-myc* proto-oncogene activation. Blood 83:3581–3590, 1994a.

Inghirami G, Macri L, Rosati S, et al: The Reed-Sternberg cells of Hodgkin's disease are clonal. Proc Natl Acad Sci USA 91:9842–9846, 1994b.

Jarrett AF, Armstrong AA, Alexander E: Epidemiology of EBV and Hodgkin's lymphoma. Ann Oncol 7:S5–S10, 1996.

Jarrett RF, Gallagher A, Jones DB, et al: Detection of Epstein-Barr virus genomes in Hodgkin's disease: relation to age. J Clin Pathol 44:844–848, 1991.

Jones JF, Shurin S, Abramowsky, C et al: T-cell lymphomas containing Epstein-Barr viral DNA in patients with chronic Epstein-Barr virus infections. N Engl J Med 318:733–741, 1988.

Joske DJL, Emery-Goodman A, Bachmann E, et al: Epstein-Barr virus burden in Hodgkin's disease is related to latent membrane protein gene expression but not to active viral replication. Blood 80:2610–2613, 1992.

Kadin M, Butmarc J, Elovic A, et al: Eosinophils are the major source of transforming growth factor-β_1 in nodular sclerosing Hodgkin's disease. Am J Pathol 142:11–16, 1993.

Kadin ME, Muramoto L, Said J: Expression of T-cell antigens on Reed-Sternberg cells in a subset of patients with nodular sclerosing and mixed cellularity Hodgkin's disease. Am J Pathol 130: 345–353, 1988.

Kamel OW, Chang PP, Hsu FJ, et al: Clonal VDJ recombination of the immunoglobulin heavy chain gene by PCR in classical Hodgkin's disease. Am J Clin Pathol 104:419–423, 1995.

Kamel OW, Gelb AB, Shibuya RB, et al: Leu 7 (CD57) reactivity distinguishes nodular lymphocyte predominance Hodgkin's disease from nodular sclerosing Hodgkin's disease, T-cell–rich B-cell lymphoma and follicular lymphoma. Am J Pathol 142:541–546, 1993.

Kanegane H, Wado T, Nunogami K, et al: Chronic persistent Epstein-Barr virus infection of natural killer cells and B cells associated with granular lymphocytes expansion. Br J Haematol 95:116–122, 1996.

Kanzler H, Küppers R, Hansmann M-L, et al: Hodgkin and Reed-Sternberg cells in Hodgkin's disease represent the outgrowth of a dominant tumor clone derived from (crippled) germinal center B cells. J Exp Med 184:1495–1505, 1996.

Khan G, Gupta RK, Coates PJ, et al: Epstein-Barr virus infection and *bcl-2* proto-oncogene expression: separate events in the pathogenesis of Hodgkin's disease? Am J Pathol 143:1270–1274, 1993.

Khanim F, Yao Q-Y, Niedobitek G, et al: Analysis of Epstein-Barr virus gene polymorphisms in normal donors and in virus-associated tumors from different geographic locations. Blood 88:3491–3501, 1996.

Klein U, Klein G, Ehlin-Henriksson B, et al: Burkitt's lymphoma is a malignancy of mature B cells expressing somatically mutated V region genes. Mol Med 1:495–505, 1995.

Korkolopoulou P, Cordell J, Jones M, et al: The expression of the B-cell marker mb-1 (CD79a) in Hodgkin's disease. Histopathology 24:511–515, 1994.

Krenacs L, Wellmann A, Sorbara L, et al: Cytotoxic cell antigen expression in anaplastic large cell lymphomas of T- and null-cell type and Hodgkin's disease: evidence for distinct cellular origin. Blood 89:980–989, 1997.

Kuefer MU, Look AT, Pulford K, et al: Retrovirus-mediated gene transfer of *NPM-ALK* causes lymphoid malignancy in mice. Blood 90:2901–2910, 1997.

Küppers R, Rajewsky K, Zhao M, et al: Hodgkin disease: Hodgkin and Reed-Sternberg cells picked from histological sections show clonal immunoglobulin gene rearrangements and appear to be derived from B cells at various stages of development. Proc Natl Acad Sci USA 91:10962–10966, 1994.

Kwak LW, Longo DL: Lymphomas. In Pinedo HM, Longo DL, Chabner BA (eds): Elsevier Science, Amsterdam, pp 376–440, 1996.

Ladanyi M, Cavalchire G, Morris SW, et al: Reverse transcriptase polymerase chain reaction for the Ki-1 anaplastic large cell lymphoma-associated t(2;5) translocation in Hodgkin's disease. Am J Pathol 145:1296–1300, 1994.

Lam KMC, Syed N, Whittle H, et al: Circulating Epstein-Barr virus–carrying B cells in acute malaria. Lancet 337:876–878, 1991.

Lamant L, Meggetto F, Saati TA, et al: High incidence of the t(2;5)(p23;q35) translocation in anaplastic large cell lymphoma and its lack of detection in Hodgkin's disease: comparison of cytogenetic analysis, reverse transcriptase-polymerase chain reaction, and P-80 immunostaining. Blood 87:284–291, 1996.

Link MP, Donaldson SS: The lymphomas and lymphadenopathy. In Nathan DG, Orkin SH (eds): W.B. Saunders Company, Philadelphia, pp 1323–1358, 1998.

Macfarlane GJ, Evstifeeva T, Boyle P, et al: International patterns in the occurrence of Hodgkin's disease in children and young adult males. Int J Cancer 61:165–169, 1995.

Macharia WM: Highlight on childhood lymphomas. East Afr Med J 73:341–342, 1996.

Mack TM, Cozen W, Shibata DK, et al: Concordance for Hodgkin's disease in identical twins suggesting genetic susceptibility to the young-adult form of the disease. N Engl J Med 332:413–418, 1995.

MacMahon B: Epidemiological evidence on the nature of Hodgkin's disease. Cancer 10:1045–1054, 1957.

Maestro R, Gloghini A, Doglioni C, et al: Human non-Hodgkin's lymphomas overexpress a wild-type form of p53 which is a functional transcriptional activator of the cyclin-dependent kinase inhibitor p21. Blood 89:2523–2528, 1997.

Magrath IT, Bhatia K: Pathogenesis of small noncleaved cell lymphomas (Burkitt's lymphoma). In Magrath I (ed): The Non-Hodgkin's Lymphomas, 2nd ed. Arnold, London, and Oxford University Press, New York, pp 385–409, 1997.

Marafioti T, Hummel M, Anagnostopoulos I, et al: Origin of nodular lymphocyte-predominant Hodgkin's disease from a clonal expansion of highly mutated germinal-center B cells. N Engl J Med 337:453–458, 1997.

Marafioti T, Hummel M, Foss HD, et al: Hodgkin and Reed-Sternberg cells represent an expansion of a single clone originating from a germinal center B-cell with functional immunoglobulin gene rearrangements but defective immunoglobulin transcription. Blood 95:1443–1450, 2000.

Massimino M, Gasparini M, Giardini R: Ki-1 (CD30) anaplastic large-cell lymphoma in children. Ann Oncol 6:915–920, 1995.

Mautner J, Behrends U, Hörtnagel K, et al: *c-myc* expression is activated by the immunoglobulin k-enhancers from a distance of at least 30 kb, not by elements located within 50 kb of the unaltered *c-myc* locus in *vivo*. Oncogene 12:1299–1307, 1996.

Medeiros LJ, Greiner TC: Hodgkin's disease. Cancer 75:357–369, 1995.

Morris SW, Kirstein MN, Valentine MB, et al: Fusion of a kinase gene, *ALK*, to a nucleolar protein gene, *NPM*, in non-Hodgkin's lymphoma. Science 263:1281–1284, 1994.

Mukherjee S, Trivedi P, Dorfman DM, et al: Murine cytotoxic T lymphocytes recognize an epitope in an EBNA-1 fragment, but fail to lyse EBNA-1–expressing mouse cells. J Exp Med 187: 445–450, 1998.

Munro JM, Freedman AS, Aster JC, et al: In vivo expression of the B7 costimulatory molecule by subsets of antigen presenting cells and the malignant cells of Hodgkin's disease. Blood 83:793–798, 1994.

Murphy EL, Hanchard B, Figueroa JP, et al: Modelling the risk of adult T-cell leukemia/lymphoma in persons infected with human T-lymphotropic virus type I. Int J Cancer 43:250–253, 1989.

Murphy SB: Classification, staging and end results of treatment of childhood non-Hodgkin's lymphomas: dissimilarities from lymphomas in adults. Semin Oncol 7:332–339, 1980.

Murray PG, Oates J, Reynolds GM, et al: Expression of B7 (CD80) and CD40 antigens and the CD40 ligand in Hodgkin's disease is independent of latent Epstein-Barr virus infection. J Clin Pathol Mol Pathol 48:M105–M108, 1995.

Nakagawa A, Nakamura S, Ito M, et al: CD30-positive anaplastic large cell lymphoma in childhood: expression of $p80^{npm/alk}$ and absence of Epstein-Barr virus. Mod Pathol 10:210–215, 1997.

Naresh KN, O'Conor GT, Soman CS, et al: A study of p53 protein, proliferating cell nuclear antigen, and p21 in Hodgkin's disease at presentation and relapse. Hum Pathol 28:549–555, 1996.

Neilly IJ, Dawson AA, Bennett B, et al: Evidence for a seasonal variation in the presentation of Hodgkin's disease. Leuk Lymphoma 18:325–328, 1995.

Neira M, Rincon J, Arias H, et al: Adhesion molecule CD11a/CD18-deficient Burkitt's lymphoma cells lack the transcript for the β, but not the α, integrin subunit. Eur J Haematol 58:32–39, 1997.

Niedobitek G, Kremmer E, Herbst H, et al: Immunohistochemical detection of the Epstein-Barr virus–encoded latent membrane protein 2A in Hodgkin's disease and infectious mononucleosis. Blood 90:1664–1672, 1997.

Ohno T, Stribley JA, Wu G, et al: Clonality in nodular lymphocyte-predominant Hodgkin's disease. N Engl J Med 337:459–465, 1997.

Orazi A, Jiang B, Lee C-H, et al: Correlation between presence of clonal rearrangements of immunoglobulin heavy chain genes and B-cell antigen expression in Hodgkin's disease. Am J Clin Pathol 104:413–418, 1995.

Oudejans JJ, Kummer JA, Jiwa M, et al: Granzyme B expression in Reed-Sternberg cells of Hodgkin's disease. Am J Pathol 148: 233–240, 1996.

Packham G, Cleveland JL: c-Myc and apoptosis. Biochim Biophysi Acta 1242:11–28, 1995.

Pallesen G, Hamilton-Dutoit SJ, Rowe M, et al: Expression of Epstein-Barr virus latent gene products in tumour cells of Hodgkin's disease. Lancet 337:320–322, 1991.

Pelicci P-G, Knowles DM, Magrath I, et al: Chromosomal breakpoints and structural alterations of the *c-myc* locus differ in endemic and sporadic forms of Burkitt lymphoma. Proc Natl Acad Sci USA 83:2984–2988, 1986.

Perkins SL, Segal GH, Kjeldsberg CR: Classification of non-Hodgkin's lymphomas in children. Semin Diagn Pathol 12:303–313, 1995.

Pinkus GS, Lones M, Shintaku IP, et al: Immunohistochemical detection of Epstein-Barr virus–encoded latent membrane protein in Reed-Sternberg cells and variants of Hodgkin's disease. Mod Pathol 7:454–461, 1994.

Pinto A, Hutchison RE, Grant LH, et al: Follicular lymphomas in pediatric patients. Mod Pathol 3:308–313, 1990.

Pittaluga S, Wlodarska I, Pulford K, et al: The monoclonal antibody ALK1 identifies a distinct morphological subtype of anaplastic large cell lymphoma associated with 2p23/*ALK* rearrangements. Am J Pathol 151:343–351, 1997.

Pombo de Oliveira MS, Matutes E, Famadas LC, et al: Adult T-cell leukaemia/lymphoma in Brazil and its relation to HTLV-1. Lancet 336:987–990, 1990.

Preudhomme C, Dervite I, Wattel E, et al: Clinical significance of p53 mutations in newly diagnosed Burkitt's lymphoma and acute lymphoblastic leukemia: a report of 48 cases. J Clin Oncol 13: 812–820, 1995.

Preudhomme C, Fenaux P: The clinical significance of mutations of the p53 tumour suppressor gene in haematological malignancies. Br J Haematol 98:502–511, 1997.

Pringle JH, Shaw JA, Gillies A, et al: Numerical chromosomal aberrations in Hodgkin's disease detected by in situ hybridisation on routine paraffin sections. J Clin Pathol 50:553–558, 1997.

Pulford K, Lamant L, Morris SW, et al: Detection of anaplastic lymphoma kinase (ALK) and nucleolar protein nucleophosmin (NPM)-ALK proteins in normal and neoplastic cells with the monoclonal antibody ALK1. Blood 89:1394–1404, 1997.

Quintanilla-Martinez L, Lome-Maldonado C, Ott G, et al: Primary non-Hodgkin's lymphoma of the intestine: high prevalence of Epstein-Barr virus in Mexican lymphomas as compared with European cases. Blood 89:644–651, 1997.

Raffeld M, Yano T, Hoang AT, et al: Clustered mutations in the transcriptional activation domain of *myc* in 8q24 translocated lymphomas and their functional consequences. Curr Top Microbiol Immunol 194:265–272, 1995.

Razzouk BI, Gan YJ, Mendonça C, et al: Epstein-Barr virus in pediatric Hodgkin disease: age and histiotype are more predictive than geographic region. Med Pediatr Oncol 28:248–254, 1997.

Razzouk BI, Srinivas S, Sample CE, et al: Epstein-Barr virus DNA recombination and loss in sporadic Burkitt's lymphoma. J Infect Dis 173:529–535, 1996.

Renner C, Ohnesorge S, Held G, et al: T cells from patients with Hodgkin's disease have a defective T-cell receptor ζ chain expression that is reversible by T-cell stimulation with CD3 and CD28. Blood 88:236–241, 1996.

Rickinson AB, Moss DJ: Human cytotoxic T lymphocyte responses to Epstein-Barr virus infection. Ann Rev Immunol 15:405–431, 1997.

Roguin A, Ben-Arush MW, Dale J: Incidence of childhood lymphoma in Northern Israel, 1973–1990. Pediatr Hematol Oncol 12: 447–454, 1995.

Rooney CM, Smith CA, Heslop HE: Control of virus-induced lymphoproliferation: Epstein-Barr virus–induced lymphoproliferation and host immunity. Mol Med 3:23–30, 1997.

Sandlund JT, Downing JR, Crist WM: Non-Hodgkin's lymphoma in childhood. N Engl J Med 334:1238–1248, 1996.

Sarris AH, Luthra R, Papadimitracopoulou V, et al: Amplification of genomic DNA demonstrates the presence of the t(2;5)(p23;q35) in anaplastic large cell lymphoma, but not in other non-Hodgkin's lymphomas, Hodgkin's disease, or lymphomatoid papulosis. Blood 88:1771–1779, 1996.

Schlaifer D, March M, Krajewski S, et al: High expression of the bcl-x gene in Reed-Sternberg cells of Hodgkin's disease. Blood 85: 2671–2674, 1995.

Schmid C, Pan L, Diss T, et al: Expression of B-cell antigens by Hodgkin's and Reed-Sternberg cells. Am J Pathol 139:701–707, 1991a.

Schmid C, Sargent C, Isaacson PG: L and H cells of nodular lymphocyte predominant Hodgkin's disease show immunoglobulin light-chain restriction. Am J Pathol 139:1281–1289, 1991b.

Shimakage M, Nakamine H, Tamura S, et al: Detection of Epstein-Barr virus transcripts in anaplastic large-cell lymphomas by mRNA in *situ* hybridization. Hum Pathol 28:1415–1419, 1997.

Shiota M, Nakamura S, Ichinohasama R, et al: Anaplastic large cell lymphomas expressing the novel chimeric protein $p80^{NPM/ALK}$: a distinct clinicopathologic entity. Blood 86:1954–1960, 1995.

Shiramizu B, Barriga F, Neequaye J, et al: Patterns of chromosomal breakpoint locations in Burkitt's lymphoma: relevance to geography and Epstein-Barr virus association. Blood 77:1516–1526, 1991.

Simonitsch I, Panzer-Gruemayer ER, Ghali DW, et al: NPM/ALK gene fusion transcripts identify a distinct subgroup of null type Ki-1 positive anaplastic large cell lymphomas. Br J Haematol 92: 866–871, 1996.

Smith-Sørensen B, Hijmans EM, Beijersbergen RL, et al: Functional analysis of Burkitt's lymphoma mutant c-myc proteins. J Biol Chem 271:5513–5518, 1996.

Su I-J, Hsieh H-C, Lin K-H, et al: Aggressive peripheral T-cell lymphomas containing Epstein-Barr viral DNA: a clinicopathologic and molecular analysis. Blood 77:799–808, 1991.

Su I-J, Lin K-H, Chen C-J, et al: Epstein-Barr virus–associated peripheral T-cell lymphoma of activated CD8 phenotype. Cancer 66:2557–2562, 1990.

Tajima K, T- and B-Cell Malignancy Study Group: The 4th nationwide study of adult T-cell leukemia/lymphoma (ATL) in Japan: estimates of risk of ATL and its geographical and clinical features. Int J Cancer 45:237–243, 1990.

Tamaru J-I, Hummel M, Marafioti T, et al: Burkitt's lymphomas express V_H genes with a moderate number of antigen-selected somatic mutations. Am J Pathol 147:1398–1407, 1995.

Tanaka Y, Sasaki Y, Kurozumi H, et al: Angiocentric immunoproliferative lesion associated with chronic active Epstein-Barr virus infection in an 11-year-old boy. Am J Surg Pathol 18:623–631, 1994.

Tao Q, Robertson KD, Manns A, et al: Epstein-Barr virus (EBV) in endemic Burkitt's lymphoma: molecular analysis of primary tumor tissue. Blood 91:1373–1381, 1998.

Taylor GM, Gokhale DA, Crowther D, et al: Increased frequency of HLA-DPB1°0301 in Hodgkin's disease suggests that susceptibility is HVR-sequence and subtype-associated. Leukemia 10: 854–859, 1996.

Tilly H, Bastard C, Delastre T, et al: Cytogenetic studies in untreated Hodgkin's disease. Blood 77:1298–1304, 1991.

Toren A, Ben-Bassat I, Rechavi G: Infectious agents and environmental factors in lymphoid malignancies. Blood Rev 10:89–94, 1996.

Touriol C, Greenland C, Lamant L, et al: Further demonstration of the diversity of chromosomal changes involving 2p23 in ALK-positive lymphoma: 2 cases expressing ALK kinase fused to CLTCL (clathrin chain polypeptide-like). Blood 95:3204–3207, 2000.

Uckun FM, Sensel MG, Sun L, et al: Biology and treatment of childhood T-lineage acute lymphoblastic leukemia. Blood 91:735–746, 1998.

van den Bosch C, Griffin BE, Kazembe P, et al: Are plant factors a missing link in the evolution of endemic Burkitt's lymphoma. Br J Cancer 68:1232–1235, 1993.

Van Gool SW, Delabie J, Vanderberghe P, et al: Expression of B7-2 (CD86) molecules by Reed-Sternberg cells of Hodgkin's disease. Leukemia 11:846–851, 1997.

Wada M, Bartram C, Nakamura H, et al: Analysis of p53 mutations in a large series of lymphoid hematologic malignancies of childhood. Blood 82:3163–3169, 1992.

Washburn EP, Orza MJ, Berlin JA, et al: Residential proximity to electricity transmission and distribution equipment and risk of childhood leukemia, childhood lymphoma, and childhood nervous system tumors: systematic review, evaluation, and meta-analysis. Cancer Causes Control 5:299–309, 1994.

Weber-Matthiesen K, Deerberg J, Poetsch M, et al: Numerical chromosome aberrations are present within the CD30+ Hodgkin and Reed-Sternberg cells in 100% of analyzed cases of Hodgkin's disease. Blood 86:1464–1468, 1995.

Weidanz WP: Malaria and alterations in immune reactivity. Br Med Bull 38:167–172, 1982.

Weisenburger DD, Gordon BG, Vose JM, et al: Occurrence of the t(2;5)(p23;q35) in non-Hodgkin's lymphoma. Blood 87: 3860–3868, 1996.

Weiss LM, Chang KL: Association of the Epstein-Barr virus with hematolymphoid neoplasia. Adv Anat Pathol 3:1–15, 1996.

Weiss LM, Movahed LA, Warnke RA, et al: Detection of Epstein-Barr viral genomes in Reed-Sternberg cells of Hodgkin's disease. N Engl J Med 320:502–506, 1989.

Weiss LM, Strickler JG, Hu E, et al: Immunoglobulin gene rearrangements in Hodgkin's disease. Hum Pathol 17:1009–1014, 1986.

Wellman A, Otsuki T, Vogelbruch M, et al: Analysis of the t(2;5)(p23;q35) translocation by reverse transcription-polymerase chain reaction in CD30+ anaplastic large-cell lymphomas, in other non-Hodgkin's lymphomas of T-cell phenotype, and in Hodgkin's disease. Blood 86:2321–2328, 1995.

Wellmann A, Thieblemont C, Sakai A, et al: Detection of differentially expressed genes in lymphomas using c-DNA array filters: Identification of a diagnostic marker for anaplastic large cell lymphoma. Blood 92:1290, 1998.

Whittle HC, Brown J, Marsh K, et al: T-cell control of Epstein-Barr virus–infected B cells is lost during *P. falciparum* malria. Nature 312:449–450, 1984.

Wilson JB, Levine AJ: The oncogenic potential of Epstein-Barr virus nucear antigen 1 in transgenic mice. Curr Top Microbiol Immunol 182:375–384, 1992.

Wolf J, Pawlita M, Bullerdiek J, et al: Suppression of the malignant phenotype in somatic cell hybrids between Burkitt's lymphoma cells and Epstein-Barr virus–immortalized lymphoblastoid cells despite deregulated c-*myc* expression. Cancer Res 50:3095–3100, 1990.

Wood GS, Hardman DL, Boni R, et al: Lack of the t(2;5) or other mutations resulting in expression of anaplastic lymphoma kinase catalytic domain in CD30+ primary cutaneous lymphoproliferative disorders and Hodgkin's disease. Blood 88:1765–1770, 1996.

Wright DH: Epidemiology of Burkitt's tumor. Cancer Res 27: 2424–2438, 1967.

Wright D, McKeever P, Carter R: Childhood non-Hodgkin lymphomas in the United Kingdom: findings from the UK Children's Cancer Study Group. J Clin Pathol 50:128–134, 1997.

Xia Y, Brown L, Yang CY-C, et al: *TAL2*, a helix-loop-helix gene activated by the (7;9)(q34;q32) translocation in human T-cell leukemia. Proc Natl Acad Sci USA 88:11416–11420, 1991.

Yatabe Y, Mori N, Oka K, et al: Fatal Epstein-Barr virus–associated lymphoproliferative disorder in childhood. Arch Pathol Lab Med 119:409–417, 1995.

Yatabe Y, Oka K, Asai J, et al: Poor correlation between clonal immunoglobulin gene rearrangement and immunoglobulin gene transcription in Hodgkin's disease. Am J Pathol 149:1351–1361, 1996.

Young JL, Ries LG, Silverberg E, et al: Cancer incidence, survival, and mortality of children younger than age 15 years. Cancer 58: 598–602, 1986.

Zeidler R, Joos S, Delecluse H-J, et al: Breakpoints of Burkitt's lymphoma t(8;22) translocations map within a distance of 300 kb downstream of *MYC*. Genes Chromosomes Cancer 9:282–287, 1994.

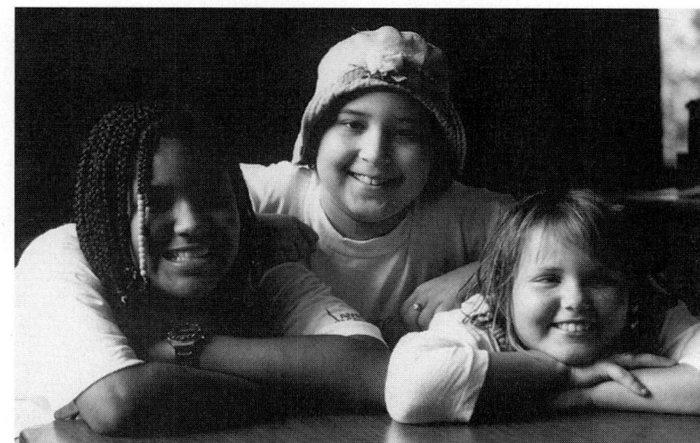

Camp Horizon, near Nashville. From left to right, these girls had Wilms tumor, acute lymphocytic leukemia (currently being treated), and acute lymphocytic leukemia. All were in remission at the time of this writing. (Courtesy of Greg Kinney.)

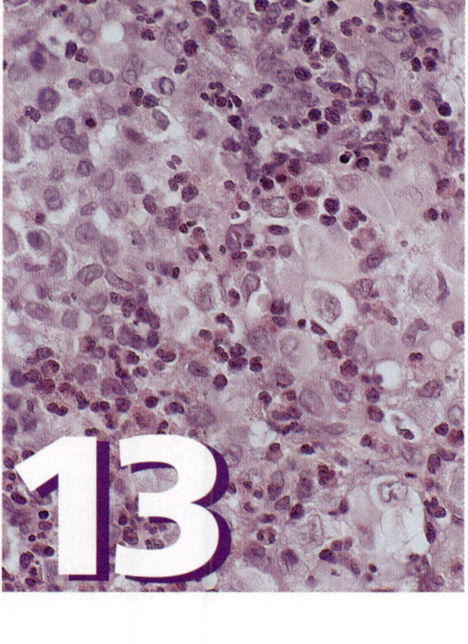

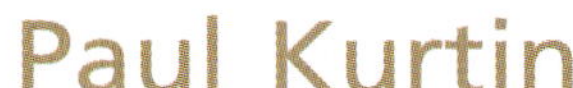

Paul Kurtin

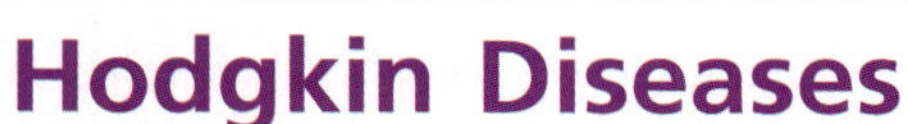

Hodgkin Diseases

In many ways, it is difficult to define precisely the Hodgkin diseases (HDs) because uncertainty remains about the nature of the neoplastic cell itself, explaining why the eponym has been retained 165 years after the disease was first described by Thomas Hodgkin. In simplest terms, HDs are neoplasms of Reed-Sternberg (RS) cells and their variants, often collectively termed Hodgkin cells. The neoplastic cells characteristically are associated with a host immune response that often dominates the histologic picture and is composed of varying numbers of small lymphocytes, plasma cells, eosinophils, neutrophils, and macrophages.

EPIDEMIOLOGY

HD accounts for 15–20% of malignant lymphomas in the United States and has an annual incidence of 3 to 4 cases per 100,000 population (Parker et al, 1996). HD has a bimodal age distribution. It is rare in children under the age of 5 years, and only occasional cases occur in the 5- to 14-year age group. Age-specific incidence increases from ages 10 to 14, peaks at ages 20 to 24, and decreases by ages 40 to 44. After the nadir in the forties, the age-specific incidence rises progressively with age. Nodular sclerosing HD (NSHD) has a unimodal age distribution and is almost solely responsible for the first age-specific incidence peak. Mixed cellularity HD (MCHD) and lymphocyte-predominant HD (LPHD) gradually increase in incidence beginning at ages 10 to 14 years. Lymphocyte-depletion HD is rare under age 40 and then increases in frequency with age (Medeiros & Greiner, 1995).

Overall, more males have HD than do females (1.5:1 male-female ratio). NSHD has an equal gender incidence, but LPHD occurs more often in males than in females (2.6:1 male-female ratio).

Different types of HD vary in frequency in different geographic areas (Macfarlane et al, 1995). The United States and parts of Europe have a high incidence of HD, whereas the disease is rare in Asia. In addition, the bimodal age peak due to NSHD is characteristically seen only in developed countries. In underdeveloped countries, HD occurs at an earlier age, and MCHD is the most frequent type.

Socioeconomic factors appear to affect the risks for the various types of HD and the age distributions of HD. For example, in children under 15 years of age, increased risk of MCHD is associated with large family size, late birth order, multiple-family dwellings, more childhood playmates, low maternal educational level, and lower paternal socioeconomic status. These features, characteristically encountered in underdeveloped countries, may increase exposure to infectious agents at an early age and predispose individuals to develop HD (Correa & O'Connor, 1971). Epstein-Barr virus (EBV) has been implicated as one infectious agent. RS cells in cases of MCHD harbor EBV more frequently than do other histologic types. Children are exposed to EBV at an earlier median age in underdeveloped countries, and these countries have a higher frequency of EBV-related MCHD (Glaser et al, 1997). By contrast, in the 15- to 34-year-old group, an increased risk of NSHD (Medeiros & Greiner, 1995) is correlated with small family size, early birth order, single-family dwellings, fewer neighborhood playmates, higher maternal education, and higher paternal socioeconomic class (Gutensohn, 1982; Gutensohn & Cole, 1981). These are the same factors that were associated with an increased risk for paralytic poliomyelitis, suggesting that an infectious cause may also play a role in the pathogenesis of NSHD. However, the postulated infectious agent or agents remain unidentified. Although serologic evidence of past EBV infection is often present in patients with NSHD, this virus is infrequently demonstrated in the RS cells and lacunar variants from these patients (Gulley et al, 1994; Weiss et al, 1987). Therefore, EBV is not thought to play a major etiologic role in NSHD in developed countries, in contrast to the situation with MCHD.

Some cases of HD cluster in families, perhaps from shared exposure to a common infectious agent, but spouses of affected individuals do not have an increased risk of HD. Clustering of HD cases in families may also be due to a genetic predisposition, a possibility supported by weak links of HD to HLA types A1, B5, B8, and B18 (Prazak & Hermanska, 1989). In addition, a comparison of levels of concordance for HD in pairs of monozygotic and dizygotic twins also suggests a role for heredity. Monozygotic twins of patients with HD have a greatly increased risk of HD compared with dizygotic twins, in whom there is no increased risk (Mack et al, 1995).

CLINICAL FEATURES

Lymphadenopathy is the presenting symptom in 90% of patients (Colby et al, 1982; Lukes et al, 1966), although almost any organ may be involved by HD during its course. A cervical or supraclavicular mass brings most patients (80%) to medical attention, whereas axillary nodes are involved in 10–20% and inguinal nodes in 10%. Adenopathy is often painless, but tenderness does not exclude the diagnosis of HD. In adults, pain after ingestion of alcohol may call the patient's attention to enlarged lymph nodes. The rate of growth of lymph nodes is variable. A few patients seem to have rapid growth, but in most cases lymph node enlargement progresses slowly over several weeks to months. In a small number of individuals with HD, lymphadenopathy waxes and wanes or "spontaneously" remits, only to recur later. Some patients with extensive mediastinal HD and inapparent peripheral adenopathy present with cough, chest pain, or tightness and may have superior vena cava syndrome. HD is usually lymph node based, but lymph nodes in certain locations, particularly the mesenteric and epitrochlear lymph nodes, are very rarely involved at the time of initial diagnosis. Organs with abundant lymphocytic tissue that are rarely involved are the tonsils and Waldeyer ring. HD usually involves the skin, breast, gastrointestinal tract, and thyroid only by contiguous spread from adjacent affected lymph nodes.

HD spreads in a predictable manner (Kaplan, 1980), as shown by studies of many patients carefully staged at diagnosis by lymphangiography and laparotomy and by relapse patterns in patients with limited-stage disease treated with radiation. For example, the spread of HD is usually from one lymph node group to the contiguous lymph node chain directly through connecting lymphatics. The spread through lymphatics may be antegrade or retrograde. Thus, patients with low cervical and mediastinal lymph node involvement usually also have supraclavicular lymph node involvement. Certain patterns of involvement of various organs by HD are predictable. For example, celiac, para-aortic, and/or splenic hilar lymph nodes are usually involved prior to splenic involvement. The liver and marrow very rarely contain HD before the spleen is involved. Pulmonary and pleural HD usually follow extensive mediastinal or pulmonary hilar lymph node involvement, although well-documented cases of primary lung HD have rarely been described.

Lymphadenopathy is accompanied by systemic symptoms and signs at diagnosis in approximately 30% of patients with HD. Enlarged peripheral lymph nodes are associated with fever in about 25% of patients, usually heralding widespread intrathoracic or intra-abdominal disease (Colby et al, 1982). However, a subset of patients with lymphocyte-depletion HD (LDHD) may present with fever of unknown origin and lymphopenia. Lacking superficial adenopathy, they have advanced intra-abdominal nodal, splenic, hepatic, and marrow disease (Bearman et al, 1978; Greer et al, 1986; Neiman et al, 1973). The dramatic diurnal Pel-Ebstein fever rarely seen now was characteristically associated with extensive HD. Weight loss and night sweats, sometimes drenching, have long been associated with HD.

HD has also been associated with various paraneoplastic dermatologic manifestations, the most common being generalized pruritus. Fifteen percent of patients with HD at diagnosis have pruritus, which is so severe in some patients that their skin is excoriated. Severe pruritus is occasionally the major manifestation of HD. When the pruritus is unexplained, these patients often present to dermatologists. Other dermatologic manifestations seen in a few patients with HD include erythema multiforme, erythema nodosum, eczematoid or psoriasiform dermatitis, erythroderma, and bullous pemphigoid.

Patients with HD may exhibit immunologic deficits, particularly if they have widespread disease. Lymphopenia owing to decreased levels of CD4+ T cells is associated with functional impairment of cellular immunity. Consequently, patients may exhibit anergy to mycobacterial, mumps, candidal, trichophytin, and streptococcal antigens. Although potentially having increased susceptibility to infectious diseases, most patients do not have opportunistic infections concurrent with the initial diagnosis of HD. Natural killer cell–mediated cytotoxicity may be reduced in HD, but apparently B cell function is retained. Prior to splenectomy and systemic therapy, patients with HD develop humoral immune responses to a variety of antigens, including pneumococcal vaccine (Slivnick et al, 1990).

Hodgkin Disease in HIV-Infected Individuals

Many cases of HD have been described in patients with serologic evidence of HIV infection or in patients with AIDS (Gold et al, 1991; Levine, 1996; Levy et al, 1995; Monfardini et al, 1991; Tirelli et al, 1988). HD in HIV-infected patients has distinctive clinical and pathologic features. However, a direct link between HD and AIDS has not been definitively established. Epidemiologic studies have not proven an excess incidence of HD in HIV-infected individuals, and the current Centers for Disease Control and Prevention definition of AIDS is not met when an HIV-positive or immunosuppressed individual develops HD.

In the United States, most HIV-positive patients with HD are homosexuals. Fewer are intravenous drug users and even fewer are patients with other risk factors, such as hemophilia. The ratio of HD to other lymphomas in HIV-infected patients ranges from 1:5.2 to 1:6.8 in most studies from the United States. In Italy and Spain, this ratio is 1:2. In those countries, there is a much higher incidence of HIV acquisition by intravenous drug use, suggesting that the route of infection or other differences in the habits of homosexuals and intravenous drug abusers determines the risk for HD (Tirelli et al, 1988).

HD usually occurs in HIV-infected patients prior to the development of opportunistic infections or Kaposi sarcoma. However, at the time of diagnosis of HD, most HIV-infected individuals already have immunosuppression, as manifested by low peripheral blood CD4+ lymphocyte counts. Less than 65% of HIV-positive individuals who subsequently develop HD have progressive generalized lymphadenopathy with follicular hyperplasia.

HIV-infected patients with HD often present with B symptoms and high-stage disease (91% are in stage III or IV at diagnosis), owing to the frequency of marrow (50% of cases) and liver (11% of cases) involvement at diagnosis. In addition, HD in HIV-positive patients may not progress in the usual pattern from a lymph node group to the contiguous group. Mediastinal involvement is less frequent than in non–HIV-infected patients with HD. Involvement of anatomic sites unusual for HD (Waldeyer ring, colon, rectum, skin, pleura, central nervous system, and meninges) occurs with greater frequency in HIV-positive patients (Levine, 1996). The histologic features of the various types of HD is similar in HIV-positive and other individuals, but there is a much higher frequency of MCHD and LDHD in the former (Serraino et al, 1993).

PROGNOSIS

The progress in treatment of HD is an impressive accomplishment in oncology. A disease that once had a poor prognosis is now cured in 60–95% of patients with radiation therapy and/or chemotherapy (Kaufman & Longo, 1995; Rosenberg, 1996). Response to initial therapy and prognosis are both directly dependent on clinical stage and the presence or absence of constitutional symptoms. For example, low-bulk stage IA and IIA patients presenting with supradiaphragmatic disease have an initial response to radiation therapy that approaches 100% and a long-term (10 years or greater) survival between 80% and 95%. In contrast, 75–80% of patients with high-stage HD with constitutional symptoms have a complete response initially to chemotherapy, with a 60–65% anticipated cure rate.

Besides high stage, other risk factors for an adverse prognosis include extensive mediastinal disease, masses greater than 10 cm, low performance score, advanced age, and infection with HIV.

In contrast to these optimistic results, patients with HD and HIV have a 1-year survival rate of less than 30%, a median survival time of 8 months to 1 year, and frequent failure to achieve complete remission. There may be ambiguity from the epidemiologic studies regarding the prevalence of HD in HIV-infected patients, but it is clear that HD has very different clinical features and entails a very different prognosis in this population (Levine, 1996).

The enthusiasm over these therapeutic accomplishments has been tempered by the realization that there is an excess risk of therapy-induced second malignancies in patients with successfully treated HD (Bhatia et al, 1996; Sankila et al, 1996; Tucker, 1993). One of the first recognized was acute myelogenous leukemia, a complication with maximum risk 5 to 10 years following therapy. This leukemia occurs because of exposure to alkylating agents in MOPP (mechlorethamine, Oncovin [vincristine], procarbazine, and prednisone) and other chemotherapy regimens. The addition of radiation therapy probably increases the likelihood of leukemia. Patients receiving six to eight cycles of MOPP chemotherapy have an expected incidence of acute leukemia of 1.5–3%, an incidence that increases with dose and time of exposure to alkylating agents. Acute myelogenous leukemia in this setting is an aggressive disease and entails a very poor prognosis. Abnormalities involving chromosomes 5 and 7 are often present.

Compared to age-matched controls subjects, there is also an increase in the incidence B and T cell lymphomas in patients who have had HD, particularly LPHD (see "Lymphocyte-Predominant Hodgkin Disease"). In patients with HD of other types, the lymphomas are usually diffuse large-cell and immunoblastic B cell lymphomas that tend to involve extranodal sites, such as the gastrointestinal tract (Amini et al, 1997; Bennett et al, 1991; Casey et al, 1990; Hansmann et al, 1989; Zarate-Osorno et al, 1992). In this respect, they resemble the B and T cell lymphomas that occur in immunosuppressed individuals but differ in that the post-HD large-cell lymphomas have a lower frequency of EBV association. Probably the carcinogenic effects of therapy coupled with immunosuppression from HD have synergistic roles in the pathogenesis of these lymphomas that arise after treatment of HD.

Carcinomas of the lung, stomach, thyroid, and breast and malignant melanoma also occur at a younger age and higher frequency in successfully treated HD patients than to age-matched control subjects (Tucker, 1993). Smokers who have been treated for HD have a much higher incidence of lung cancer than do other smokers. Thyroid and breast cancers occur in patients treated with mantle irradiation, with the likelihood increasing over time to peak at 15 to 20 years. The risk increases if chemotherapy was given with radiation and when patients were children and young adults treated for HD. The risk for the development of posttherapy malignant melanomas is highest within the first 5 years following therapy but is not dependent on the specific therapy. The skin that develops melanomas is often outside radiation ports, suggesting that the immunosuppressive effects of HD and therapy predispose these patients to melanomas.

CLASSIFICATION AND HISTOPATHOLOGY OF HODGKIN DISEASE

The diagnostic criteria of HD in general include architectural effacement by a mixed cellular infiltrate that contains RS cells and large neoplastic cells with some features of RS cells, termed RS cell variants. A prominent inflammatory reaction, including varying numbers of small lymphocytes, macrophages, plasma cells, eosinophils, neutrophils, and fibroblasts is usually present (Lukes, 1971; Lukes & Butler, 1966). HD is an unusual neoplasm because the neoplastic RS cells and variants are outnumbered by the inflammatory host response. RS cells are large cells, 20–50μ in diameter, with bilobed or multilobed nuclei or multiple nuclei. Each nucleus or nuclear lobe has a thick nuclear membrane, with vesicular to partially clumped chromatin, and typically contains huge, inclusionlike nucleoli surrounded by a perinucleolar halo. The cytoplasm is abundant, eosinophilic to amphophilic, and homogeneous throughout, lacking the perinuclear clear zone or Golgi zone seen in immunoblasts (Fig. 13–1). The light microscopic features of RS cells mirror the ultrastructural characteristics of these cells, including the huge nucleoli, dispersed chromatin, polyribosome aggregates, and absence of haloed granules and filament bundles (Glick et al, 1976). In most cases of HD, a few RS cells appear to be partially degenerate or apoptotic and are termed mummified cells. They have indistinct nuclear membranes and smudged, homogeneous chromatin. The nucleolar borders merge with the nuclear chromatin, and the cytoplasm contracts and becomes intensely eosinophilic. Occasional cases of HD contain huge pleomorphic RS cells with multilobulated nuclei, very coarse heterochromatin, and multiple prominent nucleoli.

Although the presence of RS cells is a defining feature of HD, cells that are cytologically identical may be seen in reactive conditions, such as infectious mononucleosis (Reynolds et al, 1995; Tindle et al, 1972), and in other lymphomas. In addition, "diagnostic" RS cells are rare in LPHD and NSHD. Therefore, architectural effacement and associated inflammatory reaction are as important as RS cells in making the diagnosis of HD. Pathologists may distinguish cases of HD from other lymphomas containing RS-like cells by careful attention to the inflammatory cells, particularly the lymphocytes. In HD, there is a dimorphism between the Hodgkin cells and the small bland-appearing lymphocytes, whereas in other lymphomas there is often a population of lymphocytes with cytologic features intermediate between those of the RS-like cells and those of the smaller lymphocytes. The prominent host response in HD also complicates its separation from benign inflammatory processes. For example, granulomas containing multinucleated giant cells with or without central necrosis, abundant neutrophils, numerous eosinophils, granulation tissue, collagen deposition, and vascular proliferation are the hallmarks of the host immune response to a variety of infectious agents and may be seen as well in allergic reactions and autoimmune diseases. Since these features are present to varying degrees in HD, the differential diagnosis of HD is broad when assessing processes that initially appear inflammatory.

After the initial diagnostic features of HD are recognized, HD is subclassified based on the presence of particular types of RS cell variants and on the varying proportions of reacting inflammatory cells and fibrosis. With slight modification, the histologic system for diagnosis and classification of HD of Lukes, Butler, and Hicks (Lukes et al, 1966), still forms the basis of current practice (Fig. 13–2). The histologic types of HD, contracted into clinical groups at the Rye conference (Lukes et al, 1966), have been shown to predict the extent of disease. In general, LPHD and NSHD are correlated with low-stage disease, LDHD with advanced stages, and MCHD with intermediate-stage disease (Keller et al, 1968). The diagnostic importance of this classification is not diminished by the fact that clinical stage has as much prognostic significance as does the histologic type of HD. The biologic implications of the histologic diversity of HD will ultimately be determined,

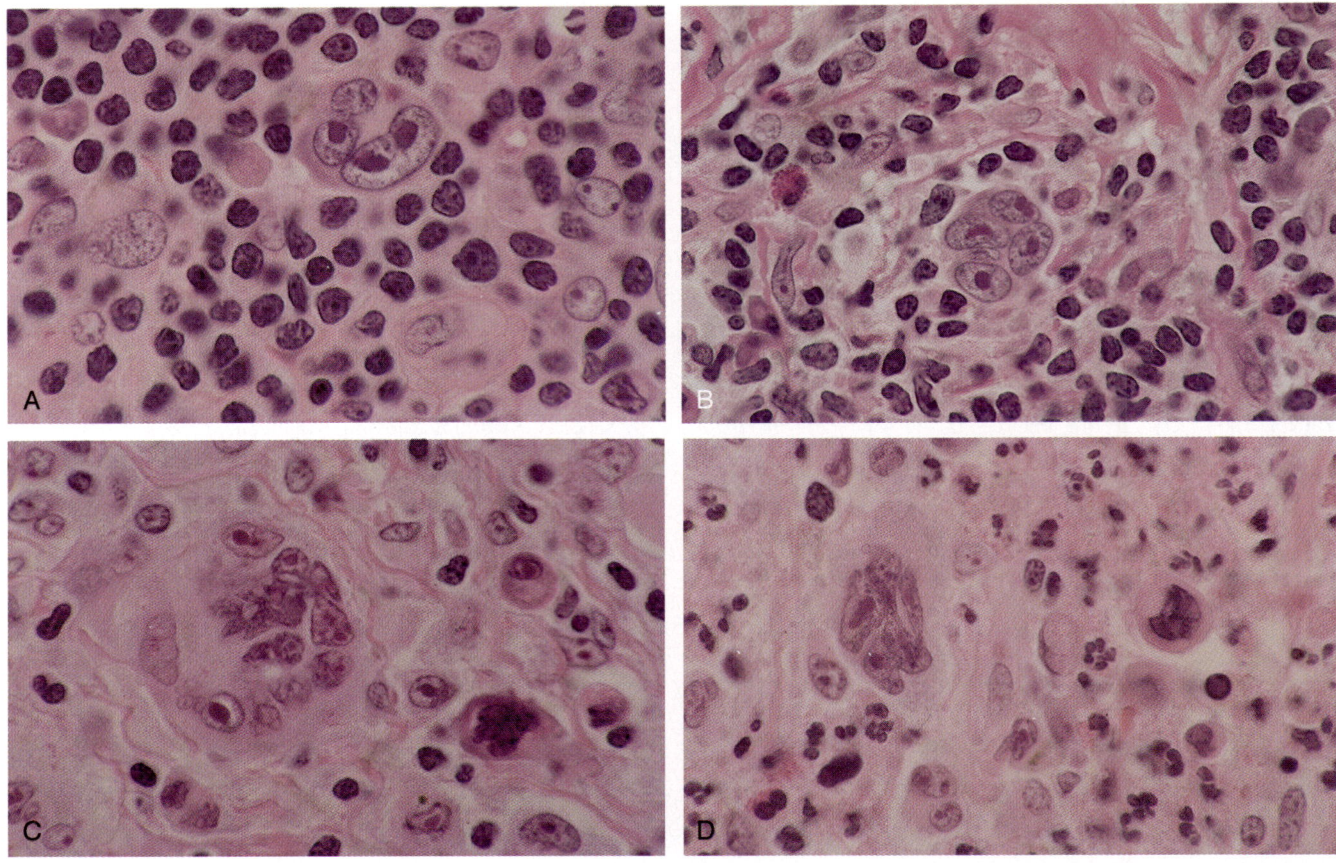

Figure 13–1

Hodgkin disease, various Reed-Sternberg cells. *A*, Diagnostic Reed-Sternberg cell with typical bilobed nucleus, large inclusion-like nucleoli, and ample eosinophilic cytoplasm. *B*, Diagnostic Reed-Sternberg cell with a multilobulated nucleus. *C*, A bizarre multinucleated Reed-Sternberg cell (*left*) and a mummified mononuclear variant (*right*). *D*, A pleomorphic diagnostic Reed-Sternberg cell and mononuclear variants, with a mummified cell on the right.

and clinicians may use the classification to predict the likelihood of advanced-stage disease. Since it has been established that the biologic features of LPHD are distinct from those of other histologic types, LPHD is considered later (see "Lymphocyte-Predominant Hodgkin Disease"). The histologic features of the various types of HD are compared in Table 13–1.

Mixed Cellularity Hodgkin Disease

MCHD is arguably the prototype of HD in exemplifying the essential diagnostic features found in these lymphomas, although cases not meeting accepted criteria for standard histologic subtypes are currently also placed in this category. The most characteristic cases show diffuse effacement of lymph node architecture by a reactive component of lymphocytes, plasma cells, eosinophils, and macrophages intermingled with RS cells and variants (Fig. 13–3). RS cells are easy to identify (Fig. 13–4). Collagen bands that thicken the lymph node capsule and define the borders of nodules are not present, although a delicate collagen fibrosis may be found. In addition, lacunar cells and L and H variants of RS cells are not identified. Within this basic morphologic framework, MCHD has a considerable histologic spectrum based on the relative numbers of RS cells and RS cell variants and the various types of reacting cells. This histologic spectrum also defines the differential diagnosis of MCHD.

Some cases of MCHD are characterized by areas with numerous RS cells and variants. The differential diagnosis of these cases includes the reticular variant of LDHD, CD30+ anaplastic large-cell lymphoma, and large-cell lymphomas of T and B cell types. The reticular variant of LDHD differs from MCHD in that all areas in the former contain numerous RS cells and variants. In MCHD a prominent reactive component is always present. MCHD with many RS cells may be distinguished from CD30+ anaplastic large-cell lymphoma (Frizzera, 1992) by involvement of lymph node sinuses in the latter by CD30+ neoplastic cells and other immunohistochemical findings (Table 13–2) (Fillipa et al, 1996). Large-cell lymphomas of B cell and T cell type are separated from MCHD with difficulty on morphologic grounds alone. Most B and T cell lymphomas with RS-like cells are accompanied by an atypical lymphocyte population that spans a cytologic continuum of small, regular lymphocytes, intermediate-sized cells with marked nuclear irregularity, and RS-like cells (Pinkus et al, 1990). This apparent spectrum of neoplastic cells stands in contrast to the dimorphism between the RS cells and the accompanying cytologically normal small lymphocytes. However, in most cases immunophenotypic studies are needed to separate these lymphomas definitely. In paraffin-section immunoperoxidase studies, the neoplastic small, medium, and

COMPARISONS OF CLASSIFICATIONS OF HODGKIN'S DISEASE

LUKES-BUTLER	RYE
Lymphocytic and/or histiocytic	
Nodular	Lymphocyte predominance
Diffuse	
Nodular sclerosis	Nodular sclerosis
Mixed	Mixed
Diffuse fibrosis	Lymphocyte depletion
Reticular	

Figure 13–2

Interrelationships between the Lukes, Butler, and Hicks classification of Hodgkin disease and the RYE Conference classification. (Lukes RJ, Craver LF, Hall TC: Report of the Nomenclature Committee. Cancer Res 26:1311, 1966.)

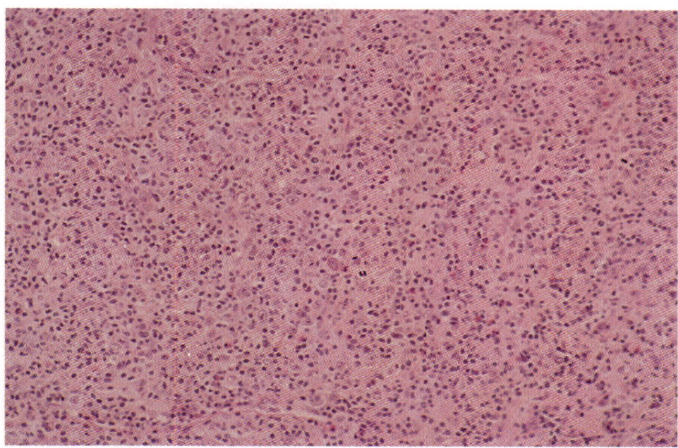

Figure 13–3

Mixed cellularity Hodgkin disease, lymph node. Note the diffuse architectural effacement without nodularity and without collagen band formation.

large cells in over 95% of cases of B and T cell lymphomas are positive for CD45 (leukocyte common antigen). Only in rare cases do the RS-like cells express CD15 and/or CD30. In contrast, RS cells characteristically lack CD45 expression and are positive for both CD15 and CD30 (Chittal et al, 1988). Demonstrating clonal immunoglobulin gene and T cell antigen receptor gene rearrangements by the Southern blot technique also supports diagnoses of B cell and T cell lineage lymphoma, respectively, and these rearrangements are usually not demonstrated in HD (Weiss & Chang, 1992).

Some cases of MCHD are rich in epithelioid macrophages (Fig. 13–5) (Patsouris et al, 1989b) and must be distinguished from various B and T cell lymphomas containing numerous macrophages, specifically certain large-cell lymphomas of B cell type (Delabie et al, 1992; Kojima et al, 1996), certain small-cell lymphocytic lymphomas with plasmacytic differentiation (Patsouris et al, 1990), and peripheral T cell lymphomas, particularly angioimmunoblastic T cell type and Lennert lymphoma (Patsouris et al, 1988; Patsouris et al, 1989a). These entities may be separated by careful attention to the cells between the histiocytes and by immunohistochemical studies. Histiocyte-rich lymphoplasmacytic lymphomas contain small lymphocytes, plasmacytoid lymphocytes (Dutcher bodies are usually present in periodic acid–Schiff–stained sections), and plasma cells that are readily shown to express monotypic surface and cytoplasmic immunoglobulin. Lymphocytes and plasma cells are, of course, polyclonal in HD. Occasional immunoblasts are noted, but they never develop the nucleolar features of RS cells. Peripheral T cell lymphomas contain a spectrum of small, medium, and large lymphocytes, usually with substantial nuclear irregularity, contrasting with the small lymphocyte–RS cell cytologic dichotomy. The neoplastic T cells in peripheral T cell lymphomas often have an aberrant phenotype (Picker et al, 1987), and T cell lymphomas have clonal T cell antigen receptor gene rearrangements (Greisser, 1995), as demonstrated by the Southern blot technique. In HD, the T cells are phenotypically normal, and clonal T cell antigen receptor gene rearrangements are rare.

Table 13–1
Classification of Hodgkin Disease in Relationship to Histologic Features

Type of Hodgkin Disease	Reed-Sternberg Cells and Mononuclear Variants	Host Response
Mixed cellularity	Frequent mononuclear variants and diagnostic RS cells	Lymphocytes, plasma cells, eosinophils, neutrophils, and macrophages
Nodular sclerosis	Lacunar cells and infrequent diagnostic RS cells	Lymphocytes, plasma cells, eosinophils, neutrophils, macrophages, and collagen bands that separate the cellular infiltrates into nodules
Lymphocyte depletion, diffuse fibrosis variant	Pleomorphic mononuclear variants and infrequent diagnostic RS cells	Disorderly collagen; depletion of all cellular elements
Lymphocyte depletion, reticular variant	Numerous pleomorphic mononuclear variants and frequent RS cells	Lymphocytes, plasma cells, neutrophils, macrophages, and disorderly granular-appearing collagen all less prominent than the RS cells
Lymphocyte predominant	L and H cells with very infrequent diagnostic RS cells	Small lymphocytes and macrophages; all other inflammatory cell types very infrequent

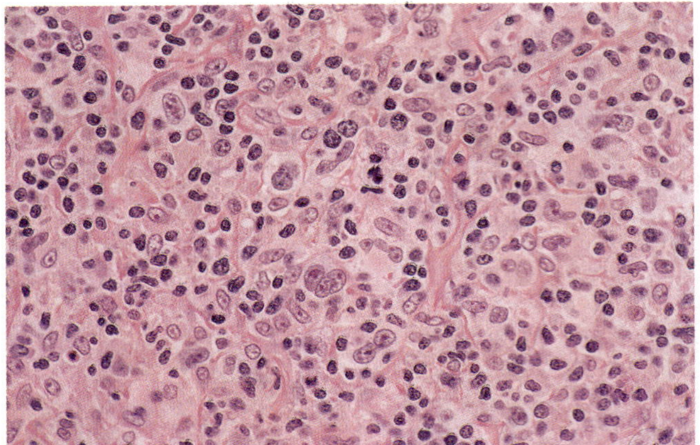

Figure 13–4

Mixed cellularity Hodgkin disease, lymph node. This appearance is typical, with numerous mononuclear variants and a polymorphous background cell population containing lymphocytes, histiocytes, plasma cells, and eosinophils.

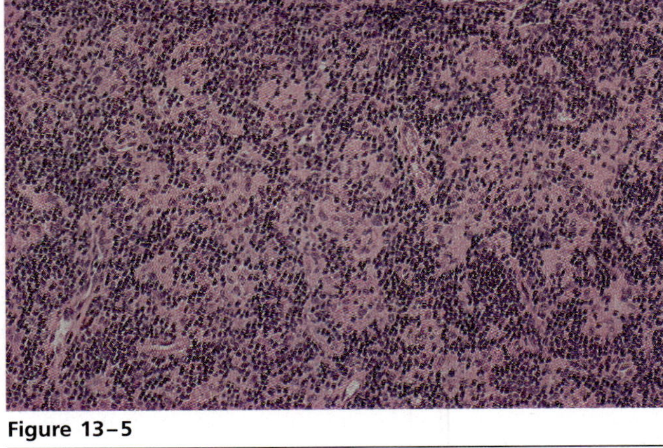

Figure 13–5

Mixed cellularity Hodgkin disease, lymph node. Numerous epithelioid histiocytes are seen. The small histiocyte clusters are distributed evenly throughout the lymph node, and mononuclear Reed-Sternberg cells are present between the benign histiocytes.

Rare cases of MCHD contain RS cells and variants that are positive for CD30 and CD15 and negative for CD45 but accompanied exclusively by small lymphocytes. These cases of MCHD are morphologically indistinguishable from the diffuse variant of LPHD and have been termed lymphocyte-rich classical HD in the Revised European-American Lymphoma (REAL) classification and the World Health Organization (WHO) lymphoma classification (Fig. 13–6) (Harris et al, 1994). They are defined by phenotype rather than by morphologic features and clinically are probably more akin to MCHD than to LPHD (von Wasielewski et al, 1997). These cases may also be distinguished by immunophenotype (Table 13–3) from large-cell lymphomas of B cell lineage with numerous intermixed nonneoplastic T cells ("T cell–rich B cell lymphoma") (Chittal et al, 1991; Macon et al, 1992; Ng et al, 1989; Ramsay et al, 1988; Rodriguez et al, 1993).

In some cases the infiltrates of HD are located between reactive germinal centers (Fig. 13–7), a pattern termed interfollicular HD (Doggett et al, 1983). In these cases, the reactive follicles usually predominate and are composed of the expected population of small and large cleaved and noncleaved lymphocytes, tingible-body macrophages, and frequent mitotic figures. Rarely, the follicles exhibit regressive transformation of germinal centers identical to the follicular changes in hyaline vascular Castleman disease (Fig. 13–8). The areas diagnostic of HD occur between the follicles and contain varying numbers of RS cells, small lymphocytes, macrophages, eosinophils, and plasma cells, and the diagnosis is suggested by finding, on low magnification, areas of interfollicular consolidation that result from the inflammatory reaction in which RS cells may be identified.

Interfollicular HD apparently is not a specific subtype, but probably represents partial lymph node involvement by one of the conventional types of HD. Supporting evidence for this hypothesis is that other lymph nodes removed concurrently or at staging laparotomy contain classical MCHD and NSHD. Furthermore, early nodal involvement by HD often occurs in the corticomedullary junction of lymph nodes unrelated to sinuses (Lukes, 1971; Strum & Rappaport, 1970).

Table 13–2

Distinction of Anaplastic Large-Cell Lymphoma (CD30+) from Hodgkin Disease by Immunophenotypic and Genetic Studies

Marker	Anaplastic Large-Cell Lymphoma (CD30+)	Hodgkin Disease
CD30	+ (strong, all cells)	+ (variable, cell subset)
CD45	+	–
CD15	–	+ (80%)
CD43	+(70%)	–
CD45RO	+ (50%)	–
CD3 (paraffin)	+ (50%)	–
EMA	+	–
CBF.78	+ (strong, all cells)	– (weak, cell subset)
BHN.9	+ (60%)	–
Clonal Ig or TCR gene rearrangements	+ (70%)	–
p80/ALK-1	+	–

Abbreviations: Ig, immunoglobulin; TCR, T cell receptor; EMA, epithelial membrane antigen; ALK, anaplastic lymphoma kinase.

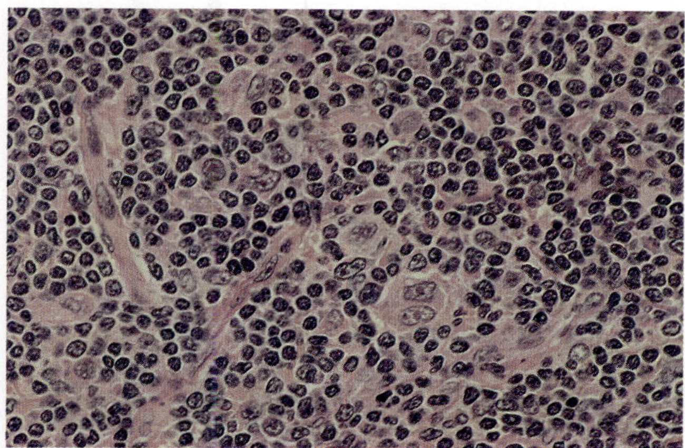

Figure 13–6

Mixed cellularity Hodgkin disease, lymph node. A background population is composed almost exclusively of lymphocytes.

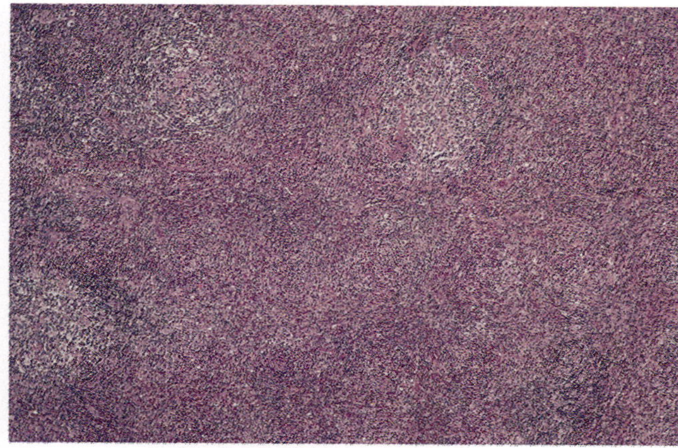

Figure 13–7

Mixed cellularity Hodgkin disease, interfollicular type, lymph node. The infiltrates are typically present between the reactive germinal centers and may be focal in distribution.

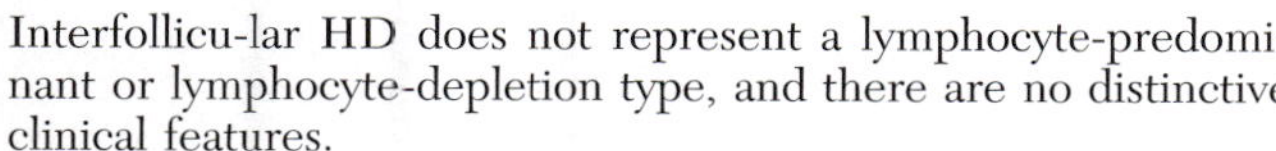

Interfollicu-lar HD does not represent a lymphocyte-predominant or lymphocyte-depletion type, and there are no distinctive clinical features.

Nodular Sclerosis Hodgkin Disease

NSHD is the most common histologic type of HD in the United States and the most reproducibly diagnosed. In addition to meeting the general criteria of HD—the presence of RS cells and the appropriate inflammatory reaction—two further criteria define this subtype: the presence of lacunar cells and collagen band formation. Lacunar cells have distinctive nuclear and cytoplasmic features (Lukes & Butler, 1966). The nuclei are hyperlobated, with delicate, lacy nuclear chromatin and small nucleoli, and the cytoplasm is abundant, pale staining to clear, with sharply demarcated peripheral margins. The distinctive cytologic features of lacunar cells are best appreciated in B5- or Zenker-fixed tissue sections (Fig. 13–9), but formalin-fixed sections demonstrate best the artifactual retraction of cytoplasm to form the lacunae for which these cells are named (Fig. 13–10). Lacunar cells may be very numerous in a single specimen, forming large aggregates or clusters, or they may be individually distributed. The earliest manifestation of NSHD in lymph nodes is the appearance of lacunar cells in the corticomedullary junction without collagen deposition. This is the cellular phase.

Collagen band formation begins in the lymph node capsule and extends into the cortex. At first a single collagen band accompanies the cellular reaction and lacunar cells (Fig. 13–11). Sclerosis then progresses to complete circumscription of the cellular nodules by collagen bands (Fig. 13–12) and obliterative sclerosis, in which the lymph node is virtually replaced by collagen (Fig. 13–13). There is dispute as to the minimal collagen sclerosis necessary to meet the diagnostic criteria for NSHD. It is clear from studies of interfollicular HD (Doggett et al, 1983) and the pathologic findings from staging laparotomy specimens (Strum, 1970) that NSHD is detectable as cellular infiltrate in nodes before collagen deposition occurs. However, in initial diagnostic biopsies, a minimum of focal lymph node capsular sclerosis and one cortical collagen band (see Fig. 13–11) are required to meet the sclerosis criteria in NSHD.

NSHD meeting these basic definitional criteria has a broad spectrum of histologic appearances, depending on the numbers of RS and lacunar cells, the amount of collagen sclerosis, the mix of inflammatory cells, and the extent of necrosis. Some cases with ill-defined nodules that are collagen poor are characterized by few RS and lacunar cells but abundant lymphocytes (Fig. 13–14). Such cases must be distinguished from

Table 13–3

Distinction by Immunophenotype between Lymphocyte-Predominant Hodgkin Disease (Diffuse), Mixed Cellularity Hodgkin Disease (with Many Lymphocytes), and T Cell–Rich B Cell Lymphoma

Feature	MCHD	LPHD, Diffuse	T Cell–Rich B Cell Lymphoma
CD45	−	+	+
CD30	+	±	−
CD15	+	−	−
κ and λ[a]	− or polyclonal	− or polyclonal	Clonal
Immunoglobulin genes[b]	Germ line	Germ line	Clonally rearranged

Abbreviations: LPHD, lymphocyte-predominant Hodgkin disease; MCHD, mixed cellularity Hodgkin disease.

[a]Paraffin-section immunohistochemical analysis.

[b]Southern blot technique.

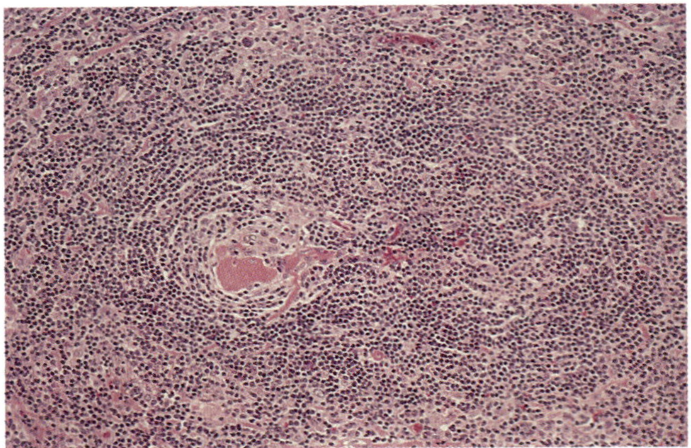

Figure 13–8

Mixed cellularity Hodgkin disease, interfollicular type, lymph node. The germinal centers show regressive transformation. An erroneous diagnosis of Castleman disease could be made in cases of this type unless Hodgkin disease is carefully searched for between these follicles.

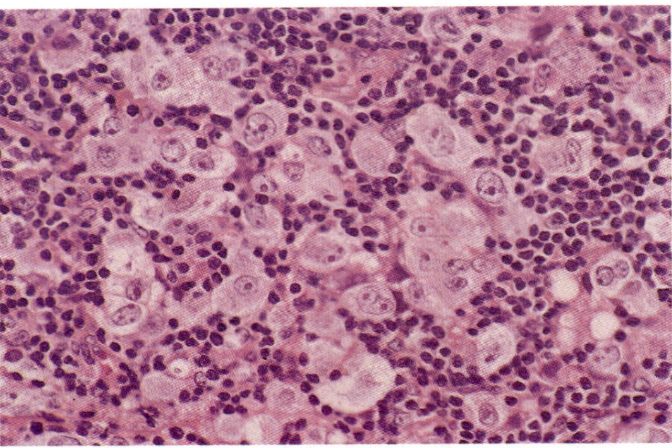

Figure 13–10

Nodular sclerosing Hodgkin disease, lymph node. In this formalin-fixed sample, the cytoplasm of the lacunar cells retracts artifactually, forming the lacunae for which these cells are named.

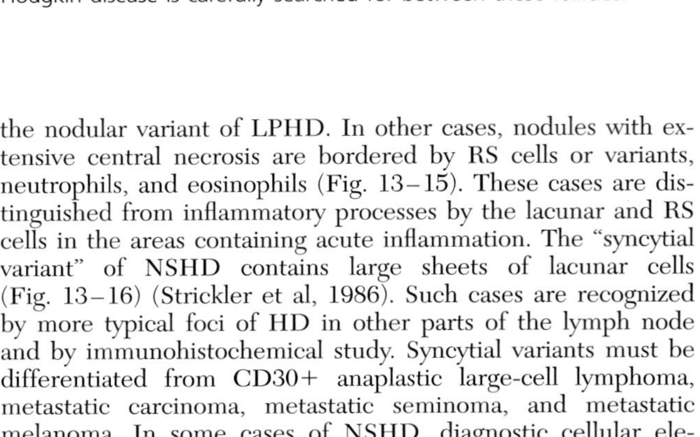

the nodular variant of LPHD. In other cases, nodules with extensive central necrosis are bordered by RS cells or variants, neutrophils, and eosinophils (Fig. 13–15). These cases are distinguished from inflammatory processes by the lacunar and RS cells in the areas containing acute inflammation. The "syncytial variant" of NSHD contains large sheets of lacunar cells (Fig. 13–16) (Strickler et al, 1986). Such cases are recognized by more typical foci of HD in other parts of the lymph node and by immunohistochemical study. Syncytial variants must be differentiated from CD30+ anaplastic large-cell lymphoma, metastatic carcinoma, metastatic seminoma, and metastatic melanoma. In some cases of NSHD, diagnostic cellular elements are embedded in such abundant hyalinized collagen that they are detected only by extensive sampling of the lymph node specimen. NSHD has diverse histopathologic features even when the basic elements of HD are combined with the presence of lacunar cells and collagen sclerosis.

Histologic grading schemes for NSHD have been devised in an attempt to define subgroups of patients with various prognoses. The British National Lymphoma Investigation (BNLI) (Bennett et al, 1981; MacLennan, 1989) grading criteria for NSHD have been adopted by the REAL classification authors. In the BNLI scheme, the cellular composition of the nodules determines the histologic grade. Features considered to indicate a higher grade include replacement of cellular nodules by bland-appearing fibroblasts and histiocytes with few RS cells and lacunar variants, uniform nodules of lacunar cells (the syncytial variant of NSHD), and nodules containing numerous lacunar cells as well as pleomorphic giant cells. NSHD cases that exhibit these features are designated grade II, while all others are designated grade I. Stage-matched, similarly treated patients with grade II NSHD have been reported as having a shorter survival times than those with grade I NSHD, but all study groups have not reproduced these data (Bennett et al,

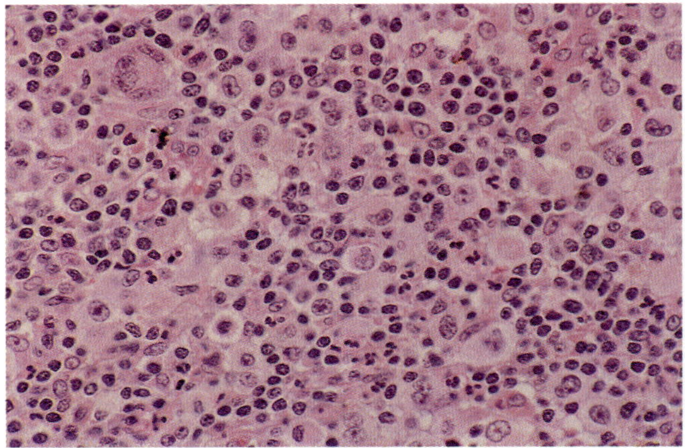

Figure 13–9

Nodular sclerosing Hodgkin disease, lymph node. The typical cytologic features of lacunar cells are seen in B5-fixed tissue sections.

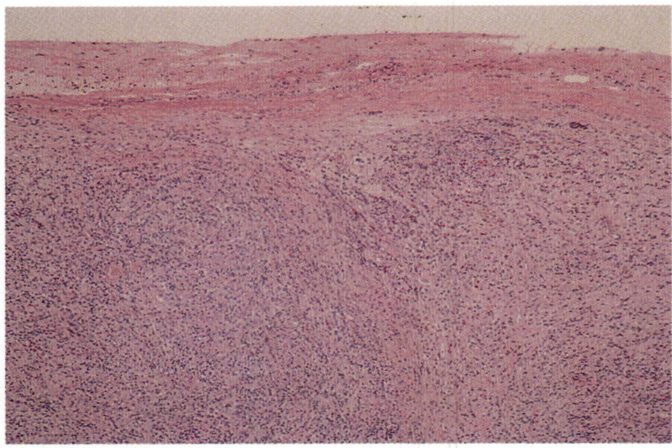

Figure 13–11

Nodular sclerosing Hodgkin disease, lymph node. The fibrosis apparently begins in the lymph node capsule and then extends into the nodal parenchyma along the lymph node sinuses. Note the collagen "spur" extending into the lymph node from the thickened capsule.

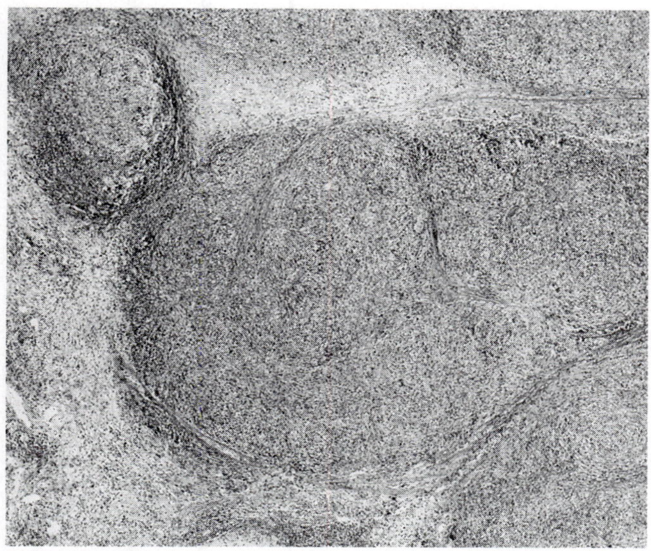

Figure 13–12

Nodular sclerosing Hodgkin disease, lymph node. The cellular nodules are separated by collagen bands in full-blown cases.

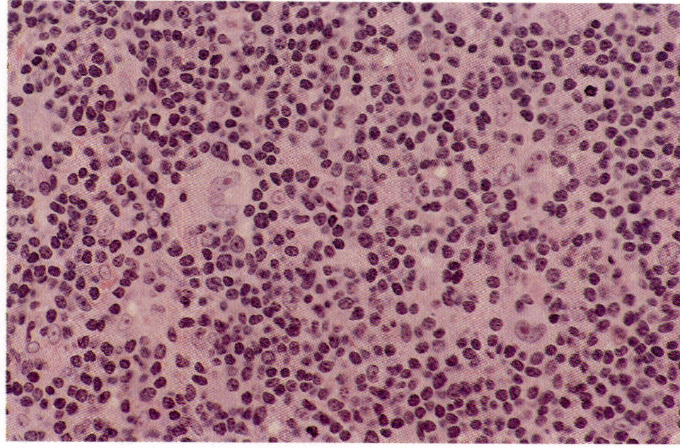

Figure 13–14

Nodular sclerosing Hodgkin disease, lymph node. The nodules in this case are composed of mononuclear variants and numerous lymphocytes. Lacunar cells, numerous Reed-Sternberg cells, and collagen bands separating the nodules *(not shown)* distinguish this example from lymphocyte-predominant Hodgkin disease.

1981; d'Amore et al, 1992; Ferry et al, 1993; Hess et al, 1994; MacLennan et al, 1989; Masih et al, 1992; van Spronsen et al, 1997; Wijlhuizen et al, 1989).

Lymphocyte-Depletion Hodgkin Disease

LDHD is the rarest type of HD. It is also the type most subject to definition by immunohistochemical study. The Rye conference on HD combined the original histologically defined categories of diffuse fibrosis type and reticular type (Lukes et al, 1966) into lymphocyte-depletion type, although retaining their separation has been useful to pathologists. The term *lymphocyte depletion* is perhaps more useful in concept than in reality, since it implies that this type of HD is defined by the scarcity of lymphocytes. In fact, the types are recognized by the numerous RS cells and variants or by the special type of collagen fibrosis with scattered RS cells. For these reasons, the distinction of reticular and diffuse fibrosis variants of LDHD will be maintained (Lukes, 1971; Lukes et al, 1966; Lukes & Butler, 1966; Neiman, 1978; Neiman et al, 1973).

The reticular variant of LDHD has two basic morphologic expressions. In each there are diffuse architectural effacement of the lymph node, absence of distinct nodularity, absence of birefringent collagen bands, absence of lacunar cells or L and H variants of RS cells, diminished numbers of lymphocytes, and a morphologic picture dominated by RS cells. In each, granular interstitial material may be found, and areas of

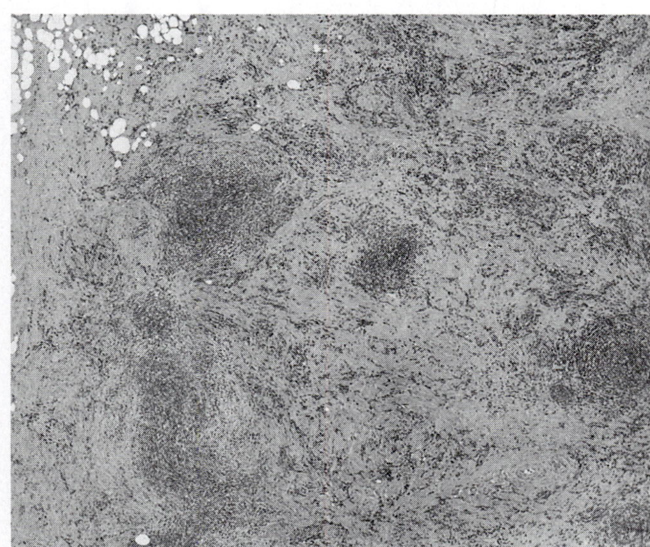

Figure 13–13

Nodular sclerosing Hodgkin disease, lymph node. Only a few cellular nodules of Hodgkin disease are present. Most of the node is obliterated by dense collagen.

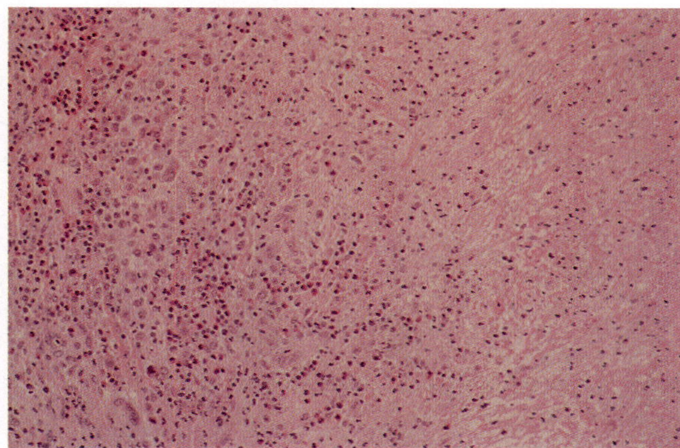

Figure 13–15

Nodular sclerosing Hodgkin disease, lymph node. The centers of the nodules are largely necrotic. Mononuclear variants are situated at the interface between the necrosis and the reactive cellular infiltrates, composed of lymphocytes, histiocytes, and eosinophils. Inflammatory processes with necrosis lack the mononuclear variants.

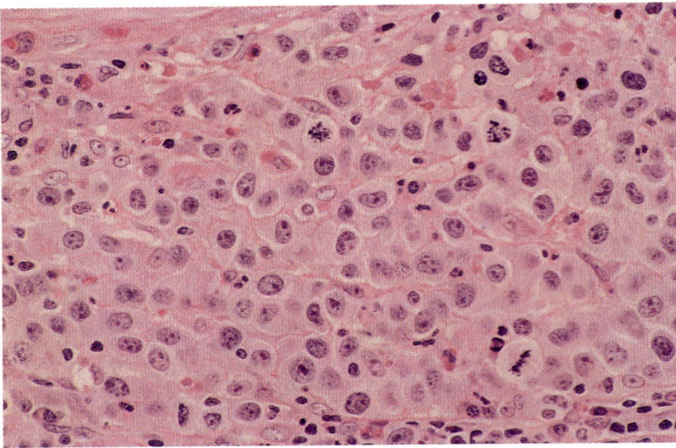

Figure 13–16

Nodular sclerosing Hodgkin disease, syncytial variant, lymph node. Nodules composed almost exclusively of lacunar cells and mononuclear variants are apparent.

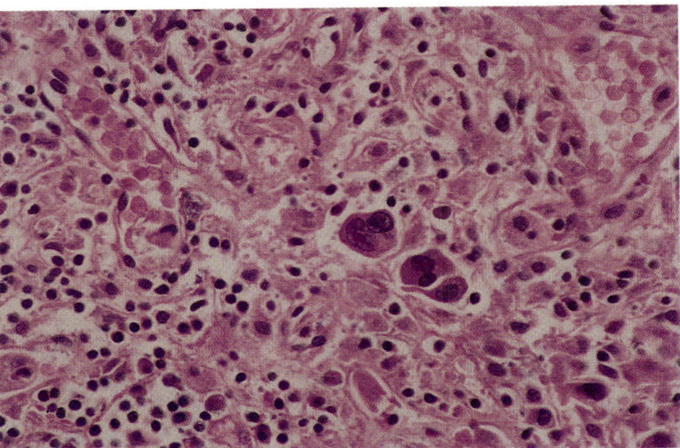

Figure 13–18

Lymphocyte-depletion Hodgkin disease, diffuse fibrosis variant, lymph node. Occasional diagnostic Reed-Sternberg cells and mononuclear variants are present, but there are very few intermixed inflammatory cells.

necrosis may be prominent. Numerous RS cells with large nucleoli predominate in one of these types, whereas, in the other, RS cells are extremely pleomorphic, even sarcomatoid. The reticular variant of LDHD has histologic features that overlap considerably with those of other lymphomas and pleomorphic malignancies. Thus, its diagnosis requires immunophenotypic confirmation. At a minimum, RS cells must be CD15+/CD30+ as well as CD45−, keratin negative, and S-100 negative. The reticular variant of LDHD is particularly difficult to distinguish from CD30+ anaplastic large-cell lymphoma, which usually requires immunohistochemical and/or molecular genetic studies. The nodules in NSHD may contain numerous RS cells and lacunar variants. Cases characterized by large numbers of RS cells should be classified as NSHD if collagen bands circumscribe these cells into distinct nodules and lacunar cells are present.

In the diffuse fibrosis variant, there is architectural effacement of the lymph nodes by abundant disorderly and nonbirefringent collagen admixed with relatively few RS cells and variants. There is diminished cellularity, and the process is particularly poor in lymphocytes (Figs. 13–17 and 13–18). In early stages, lymph nodes are usually small, with a depleted appearance. Fibrosis appears amorphous and occurs in the reticular framework of the node, sparing the lymph node sinuses and capsule. At the opposite end of the diffuse fibrosis spectrum, the entire lymph node is replaced by compact, hyalinized, disorderly collagen. In these late stages, RS cells and variants are actually quite infrequent. Cases with this appearance may be misinterpreted unless the infrequent, distorted RS cells lying in the abundant collagen are recognized. The differential diagnosis of the diffuse fibrosis type of LDHD includes "burned-out" inflammatory processes in lymph nodes, amyloidosis of lymph nodes, proteinaceous lymphadenopathy, and various sarcomas with hyalinization.

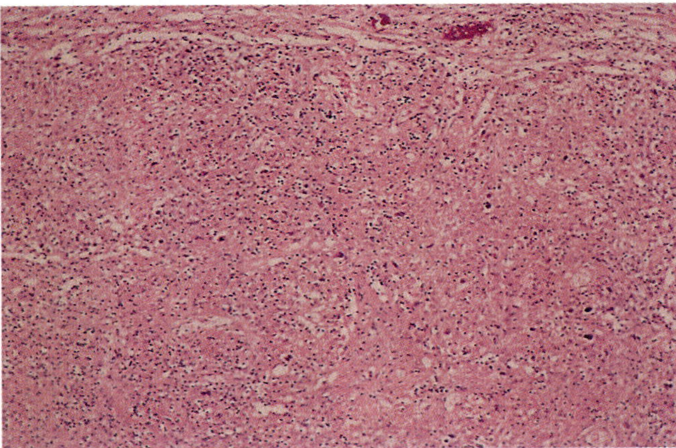

Figure 13–17

Lymphocyte-depletion Hodgkin disease, diffuse fibrosis variant, lymph node. The lymph node elements are completely replaced by disorderly nonbirefringent collagen and very sparse cellular elements.

PHENOTYPIC, CYTOGENETIC, AND MOLECULAR STUDIES IN HODGKIN DISEASE

Phenotypic Studies

Intensive study using phenotypic, cytogenetic, molecular genetic, and cell culture experiments have not precisely identified the cell or cells of origin of RS cells and their variants except in LPHD, which is discussed later. However, the cumulative evidence strongly suggests that RS cells are activated lymphocytes in a proliferative mode (Fig. 13–19). They test positively for CD30 (Fig. 13–20) (Hall et al, 1988; Hsu et al, 1985; Schwarting et al, 1989; Stein et al, 1982), CD70, CD25 (interleukin [IL]-2 receptors), CD71 (transferrin receptors) (Stein et al, 1982; Stein et al, 1985), CD40 (Carbone et al, 1995; Gruss et al, 1994; O'Grady et al, 1994), CD95 (APO-1/Fas) (Nguyen et al, 1996), CD80 (B7) (Munro et al, 1994), CD86 (B7-2) (Van Gool et al, 1997), and HLA-DR. CD15 is expressed in approximately 70–80% (Arber & Weiss, 1993) of cases, as assessed by paraffin-section immunohistochemical study (Fig. 13–21), but results are often negative for CD45 (leukocyte common antigen; (Fig. 13–22). This immunophenotype is quite distinctive and is reliably used (Table 13–4) to distinguish cases of HD from other lymphomas (Chittal et al, 1988).

RS cells in all types of HD also express a group of surface glycoproteins that are characteristically found on cells presenting antigen to T lymphocytes (Delabie et al, 1995; Gruss et al,

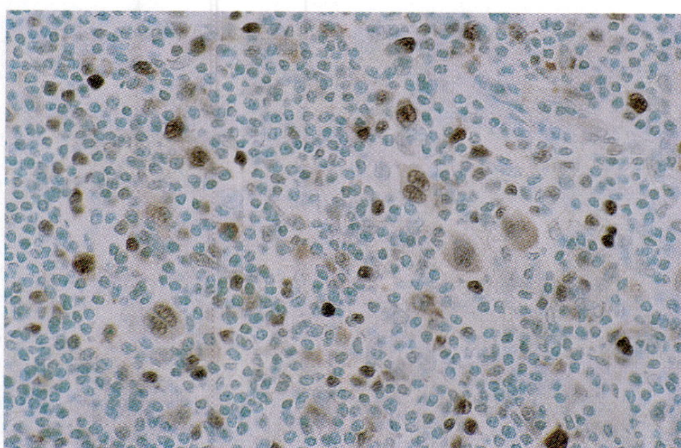

Figure 13–19

Mixed cellularity Hodgkin disease, lymph node, stained for proliferating cell nuclear antigen (PCNA). The nuclei of the mononuclear variants and Reed-Sternberg cells are strongly positive, demonstrating that they are in cell cycle.

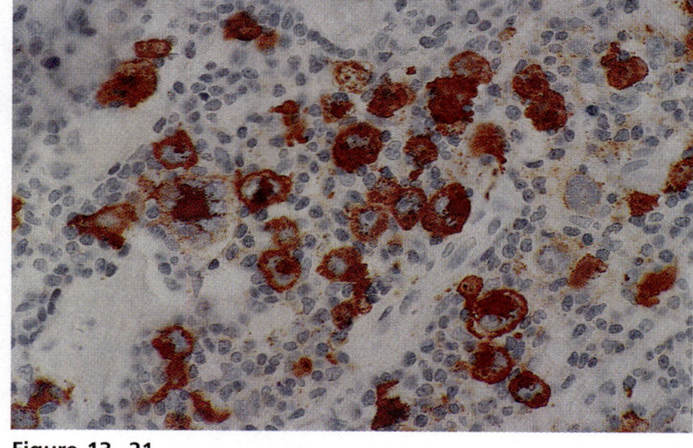

Figure 13–21

Nodular sclerosing Hodgkin disease, lymph node. Reed-Sternberg cells characteristically exhibit strong membrane and paranuclear globular staining for CD15, as illustrated here. CD15 by immunoperoxidase.

1997), including major histocompatibility complex class II molecules, fascin (Pinkus et al, 1997), the costimulatory cell surface glycoproteins CD80 (B7) and CD86 (B7-2), and the adhesion molecules CD58 (LFA-3) and CD54 (ICAM-1). Binding of these antigens with related antigens on T lymphocytes may facilitate adherence of T cells to RS cells and induce expression of T cell activation antigens. Resultant proliferation of T cells with elaboration of cytokines, including γ-interferon, and interleukin-4 may follow. This antigen-presenting cell phenotype in RS cells and variants found in all histologic types of HD may therefore explain the T cell immune response evoked in HD.

Expression of pan–B and pan–T cell markers by RS cells and variants differs from case to case. RS cells in individual cases have tested positively for the B cell–associated antigens CD19, CD20, CD22, and CD79a in 8–78% of cases (Fig. 13–23) (Casey et al, 1989; Falini et al, 1987; Kadin et al, 1988; Korkolopoulou et al, 1994; Kuzu et al, 1993; Schmid et al, 1991). In NSHD and MCHD, RS cells express CD2, CD3, CD4, and/or the T cell antigen receptor framework antigen, suggesting T cell lineage, in 45–55% of cases (Abdulaziz et al, 1984; Agnarsson & Kadin, 1989; Angel et al, 1987; Casey et al, 1989; Cibull et al, 1989; Falini et al, 1987). In a few cases, RS cells expressed granzyme B (Oudejans et al, 1996), suggesting an origin from activated cytotoxic T cells or natural killer cells. Except for CD15, RS cells have rarely contained antigens that are expressed on histiocytic or myelomonocytic cells. In summary, RS cells have been found to be variably marked in various series, some having features of T cells, some of B cells or natural killer cells. RS cells also have an activated phenotype and may function as antigen-presenting cells.

In addition to expressing receptors for IL-9 and IL-10, RS cells have expressed the genes for various cytokines, including IL-1, IL-3, IL-4, IL-5, IL-6, IL-7, IL-8, IL-9, IL-10, granulocyte-monocyte colony-stimulating factor, tumor necrosis factor α, tumor necrosis factor β, transforming growth factor β, and

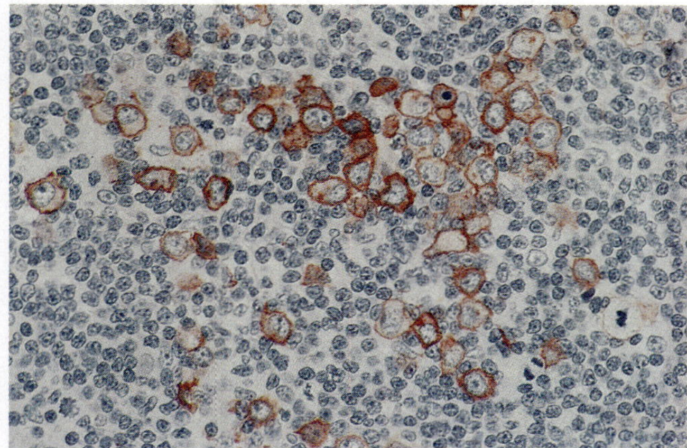

Figure 13–20

Mixed cellularity Hodgkin disease, lymph node. In this case, most of the mononuclear variants exhibit strong membrane staining, and some exhibit paranuclear globular staining for CD30. This is the typical pattern seen in cases of classic Hodgkin disease. CD30 by immunoperoxidase.

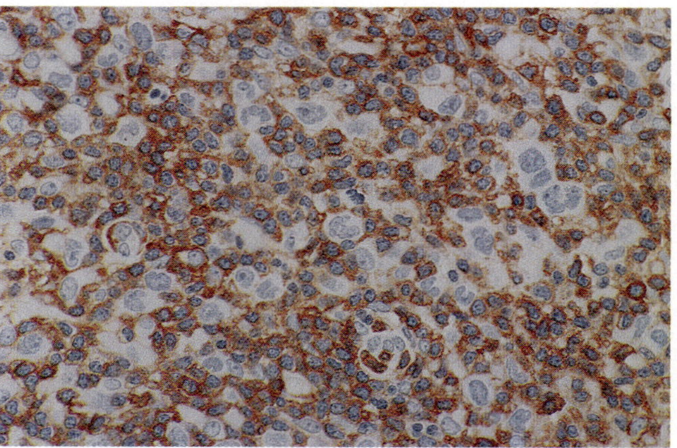

Figure 13–22

Mixed cellularity Hodgkin disease, lymph node. Staining reveals that the background small lymphocytes are strongly positive but the RS cells are consistently negative for CD45. CD45 by immunoperoxidase.

Table 13–4

Distinction of Hodgkin Disease from B and T Cell Lymphomas by Paraffin-Section Immunohistochemical Study

Antigen Expressed	Hodgkin Disease	B Cell Lymphoma	T Cell Lymphoma
CD45	−	+	+
CD30	+	±	±
CD15	+	−	±
CD20	±[a]	+[b]	−
CD3	−	−	+

[a]Often the positivity for CD20 is variable in intensity and present in only a subset of RS cells.

[b]CD20 positivity in B cell lymphomas is uniformly strongly positive in most neoplastic cells.

γ-interferon (Foss et al, 1996; Foss et al, 1995; Goss et al, 1993; Gruss et al, 1992a; Gruss et al, 1992b; Herbst et al, 1996; Merz et al, 1991; Newcom et al, 1992; Newcom & Gu, 1995; Ohshima et al, 1995; Ruco et al, 1990; Von Kalle & Diehl, 1992). Taken together, these findings suggest that RS cells have the potential to recruit cells in the host response, including T and B lymphocytes, plasma cells, macrophages, neutrophils, and eosinophils. Their cytokines may induce the fibrosis associated with NSHD as well as produce the systemic signs and symptoms seen in patients with HD (Gruss et al, 1997).

Molecular Genetic and Karyotypic Studies

Molecular genetic techniques of studying immunoglobulin and T cell antigen receptor gene configuration have not solved the questions relating to lineage and clonality of RS cells. Only a small number of cases of HD have been shown to exhibit clonal immunoglobulin or T cell antigen receptor gene rearrangements using the Southern blotting technique, even when cases containing numerous RS cells were selected (Angel et al, 1993; Brinker et al, 1987; Griesser et al, 1987; Roth et al, 1988; Sundeen et al, 1987; Weiss & Chang, 1992). Studies using polymerase chain reaction techniques performed on whole-tissue samples or on isolated RS cells have demonstrated clonal immunoglobulin gene rearrangements in approximately 25–50% of cases of MCHD (Delabie et al, 1996; Hummel et al, 1995; Küppers et al, 1994; Manzanal et al, 1995; Tamaru et al, 1994). Sequencing of the amplified immunoglobulin genes revealed abnormal rearrangements that would prevent translation into a functional immunoglobulin molecule, explaining the lack of immunoglobulin protein expression by these RS cells. An analysis of the gene sequences, from microdissected, single Hodgkin cells, demonstrated rearranged Ig genes that were clonal in all cases and that contained a high frequency of point mutations (Marafroti et al, 2000). Such studies have practical value when immunophenotyping is unable to distinguish HD from other lymphomas. Prominent clonal rearrangement bands revealed by Southern blot analysis of T cell antigen receptor or immunoglobulin genes virtually rule out HD, in which tissues usually produce germ line bands or very small clonal rearrangement bands accompanied by a polyclonal smear pattern.

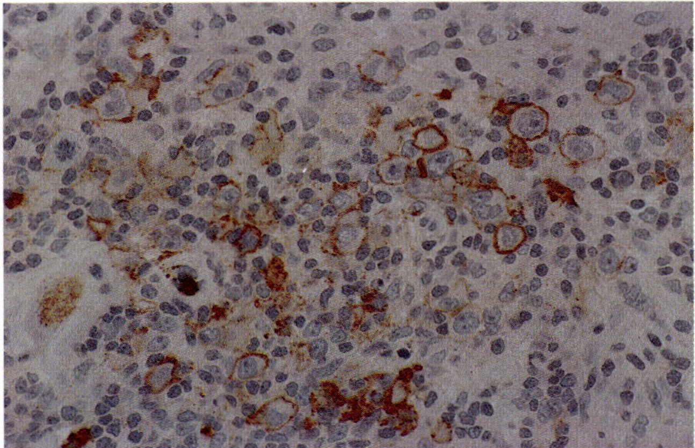

Figure 13–23

Nodular sclerosing Hodgkin disease, lymph node. Staining for CD20 reveals variable expression of intensity from cell to cell, a typical finding when RS cells are CD20+. CD20 by immunoperoxidase.

The most compelling evidence that RS cells are clonal comes from cytogenetic studies showing that karyotypes are abnormal and clonal in up to 82% of cases (Cabanillas et al, 1988; Koduru et al, 1993; Poppema et al, 1992; Schlegelberger et al, 1994). The most frequent abnormalities include hyperdiploidy, near triploidy, and near tetraploidy. When fluorescence immunophenotyping and in situ hybridization are combined with centromeric probes that recognize a number of different chromosomes, the CD30+ large cells in every studied case of HD contain clonal, numerical chromosomal abnormalities (Weber-Matthiesen et al, 1995a,b). Structural chromosomal abnormalities have also been identified, the most frequent being translocations, deletions, and inversions involving chromosomes 1p, 2p, 6q, 7q, 11q, 13q, 14q, and 19q. However, no consistent recurring karyotypic abnormality has been found, unlike the case in many other lymphomas. These results demonstrate that HD, like other malignant neoplasms, is composed of cells with clonal karyotypic abnormalities, but a common underlying molecular pathogenesis has not been found.

Epstein-Barr Virus and Hodgkin Disease

Several lines of evidence indicate a pathogenetic relationship between HD and EBV infection. Epidemiologic studies have shown that patients with HD are more likely to have had infectious mononucleosis than age-matched control subjects (Mueller, 1987; Rosdahl et al, 1974), and they also have higher antibody titers to EBV (Mueller et al, 1989). In addition, there are great morphologic and phenotypic similarities between RS-like cells in tissues from patients with mononucleosis and RS cells from patients with HD (Reynolds et al, 1995; Tindle et al, 1972).

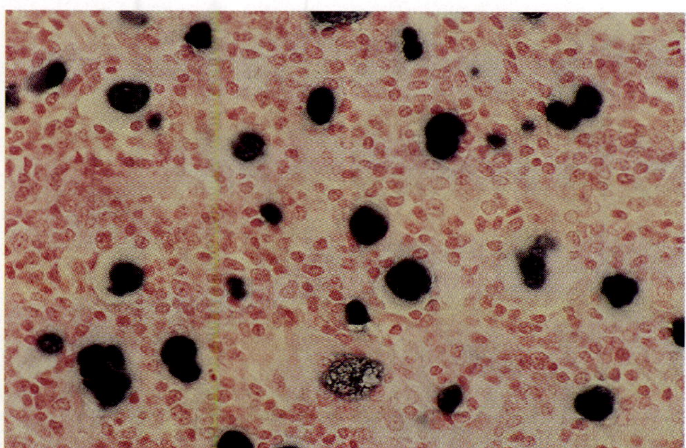

Figure 13–24

Mixed cellularity Hodgkin disease, lymph node. In situ hybridization for Epstein-Barr virus using Epstein-Barr virus–encoded RNA probes shows strong positivity in the Reed-Sternberg cells.

The presence of EBV in HD lesions has been effectively studied by in situ hybridization using probes that recognize EBV–encoded RNA, a transcript copied 10^6 to 10^7 times in cells latently infected with this virus. In these studies, EBV has been localized to the RS cells (Fig. 13–24). The frequency of cases of HD found to be EBV positive using this technique varies from <50% of cases in Western countries—with the highest frequency being detected in MCHD (Armstrong et al, 1992; Brousset et al, 1993; Herbst et al, 1990; Hummel et al, 1992; Khan et al, 1993; Khan et al, 1992; Weiss, 1992; Weiss et al, 1991)—to 100% in some underdeveloped countries (Ambinder et al, 1993; Chang et al, 1993; Huh et al, 1996; Khan et al, 1993; Leoncini et al, 1996; Weinreb et al, 1996; Zarate-Osorno et al, 1994). EBV has been found in RS cells in most cases of HD complicating HIV infections (Audouin et al, 1992; Herndier et al, 1993; Uccini et al, 1990). Immunohistochemical studies have shown that the RS cells in EBV-positive cases of HD express EBV latent membrane protein 1 and in many instances latent membrane protein 2A, but these cells lack the EBV proteins EBNA2, glycoprotein 350/250, viral capsid antigen, and early membrane antigen (Carbone et al, 1993; Deacon et al, 1993; Herbst et al, 1992; Isaacson et al, 1992; Joske et al, 1992; Khan & Naase, 1995; Niedobitek et al, 1997; Pallesen et al, 1991) These findings are consistent with a type II latent infectious state of EBV in the Hodgkin cells, but a pathogenetic relationship has not been established between EBV infection and development of Hodgkin disease.

Reed-Sternberg Cells and Other Lymphoproliferative Disorders

Clues about the origin of RS cells have come from studying immune reactions and lymphomas other than HD. For example, the lymph nodes and other tissues from patients with intense immune reactions were shown 25 years ago to contain cells cytologically identical to RS cells (Tindle et al, 1972). Later, these cells were shown to be CD30+ and may have either a T cell (e.g., infectious mononucleosis, Kikuchi histiocytic necrotizing lymphadenitis, adult Still disease, hypersensitivity reactions to drugs and vaccines, and lymphomatoid papulosis) or B cell phenotype (e.g., florid follicular hyperplasia and the immunoblastic reaction to EBV) (Lukes & Collins, 1992; Reynolds et al, 1995; Schwarting et al, 1989). Lymphomas of T and B cell lineage may contain activated neoplastic cells that cytologically resemble RS cells (Schwarting et al, 1989). CD30+ anaplastic large-cell lymphoma also provides an insight into the nature of RS cells. The neoplastic lymphocytes in CD30+ anaplastic large-cell lymphomas may be cytologically identical to RS cells as well as induce fibrosis and plasma cell infiltration (Agnarsson & Kadin, 1988; Chott et al, 1990), and macrophage infiltration (Pileri et al, 1990), similar to the immune response of HD. Cases of CD30+ anaplastic large-cell lymphoma may have a T cell, a B cell, or an undefined cell lineage, similar to RS cells. RS cells and cells of CD30+ anaplastic large-cell lymphoma express nearly identical activation antigens (O'Connor et al, 1987; Penny et al, 1991).

In summary, abundant cytologic and immunophenotypic evidence indicates that there is more than one HD and therefore that there are several types of RS cells in what are now called NSHD, MCHD, and LDHD. However, in all cases RS cells are clonal, activated, and proliferating and have the phenotypic characteristics predictive of antigen-presenting function. In addition, RS cells may express cytokines and cytokine receptors that can induce a host response to the oncogenic event.

LYMPHOCYTE-PREDOMINANT HODGKIN DISEASE

Lukes, Butler, and Hicks designated a category of HD termed lymphocytic and histiocytic type, which was characterized by an abundance of lymphocytes, varying numbers of macrophages, and a distinctive type of RS cell variant (Lukes et al, 1996). Lymphocytic and histiocytic–type HD was divided into two subcategories—nodular and diffuse—based on the architectural pattern in lymph node biopsy specimens. At the time of the Rye conference, these two subtypes of HD were combined in the lymphocyte predominance type (Lukes et al, 1966). Almost in parallel, Lennert and Mohri proposed that four subtypes of LPHD could be recognized (Lennert & Mohri, 1974). Their categories of nodular and diffuse paragranuloma corresponded to the nodular and diffuse forms of L and H types of HD described by Lukes and Butler. Most pathologists in the United States use the histologic criteria for L and H type HD of Lukes and Butler and apply the Rye conference terminology, *lymphocyte predominant type* modified by *nodular variant* or *diffuse variant*, based on the histologic pattern (Harris et al, 1994).

Clinical Features

LPHD is rare, making up an estimated 5% of all cases of HD in most large series (Colby et al, 1982; Poppema et al, 1979a). In contrast to other types of HD, there is a strong male predominance with a unimodal age peak in the fourth decade. LPHD usually involves peripheral lymph nodes, particularly in the axillary and cervical regions and much less commonly in the inguinal and femoral regions. Mediastinal lymphadenopathy is extremely unusual in LPHD, in contrast to its frequency in NSHD. Approximately 70% of LPHD cases are stage I or II at diagnosis. Very few patients are stage III or IV, and B symptoms occur in 10% of patients. The prognosis of patients with LPHD is good. There is a high complete remission rate following primary therapy and 80–90% 10-year survival in patients with stage I or II disease (Borg-Grech et al, 1989; Crennan et al, 1995; Hansmann et al, 1984; Pappa et al, 1995; Regula et al, 1988; Tefferi et al, 1990; Trudel et al, 1987). The nodular form of LPHD has been associated with late relapses, independent of stage or treatment, compared with few late relapses for the diffuse form (Regula et al, 1988), an outcome not confirmed in other studies (Borg-Grech et al, 1989; Tefferi et al, 1990).

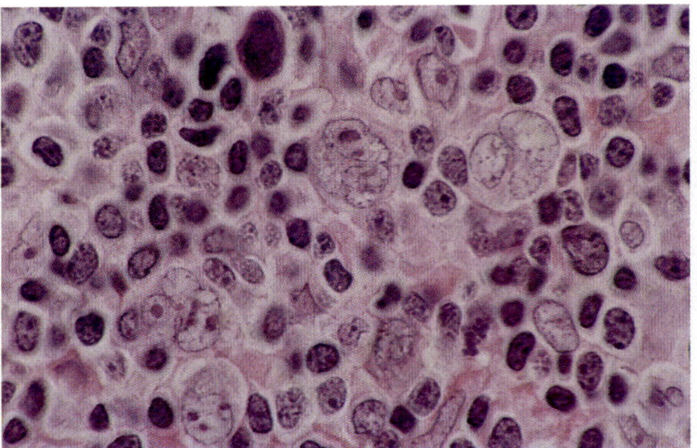

Figure 13–25

Lymphocyte-predominant Hodgkin disease, lymph node. The typical lobulated nuclei, delicate chromatin, small nucleoli, and delicate cytoplasm of L and H variants of Reed-Sternberg cells are illustrated.

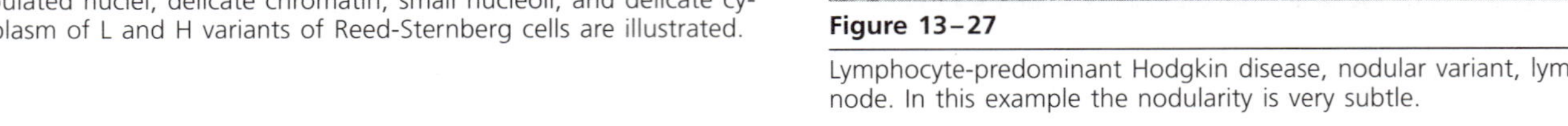

Figure 13–27

Lymphocyte-predominant Hodgkin disease, nodular variant, lymph node. In this example the nodularity is very subtle.

Histopathologic Features and Differential Diagnosis

LPHD is defined histologically by the presence of RS cell variants termed L and H cells and a host response rich in lymphocytes and macrophages (Lukes, 1971; Poppema, 1992). L and H cells are similar in size to other RS cell variants but have distinctly indented or lobulated nuclei (Fig. 13–25), a feature responsible for the appellation "popcorn cells." L and H cells are distinctive in having thin nuclear membranes, a very delicate chromatin, and small to intermediate-sized nucleoli that are sometimes multiple. Rarely are their nucleoli as prominent as in other types of RS cells. Most L and H cells have moderately abundant, pale, eosinophilic, feathery-appearing cytoplasm with indistinct borders that may rarely have an artifactual halo.

The nodular type of LPHD has a distinctive growth pattern owing to effaced architecture from macronodules most apparent on low magnification and in PAS-stained sections. Characteristically, these macronodules compress adjacent normal node in a portion of the section. These nodules are almost always larger than reactive follicles and may be missed when smaller. Early on, only a few nodules may be present, accompanied by follicular hyperplasia and progressively transformed germinal centers (Fig. 13–26). Later, the nodules may coalesce, so that the nodularity is almost imperceptible in advanced cases (Fig. 13–27). The macronodules in LPHD have a uniform appearance in most cases. Small lymphocytes predominate (Fig. 13–28). Epithelioid macrophages are distributed singly, in small clusters, or occasionally around the

Figure 13–26

Lymphocyte-predominant Hodgkin disease, nodular variant, lymph node. This example contains a hyperplastic follicle (*lower left*), a progressively transformed germinal center (*upper left*), and a well-defined nodule of Hodgkin disease.

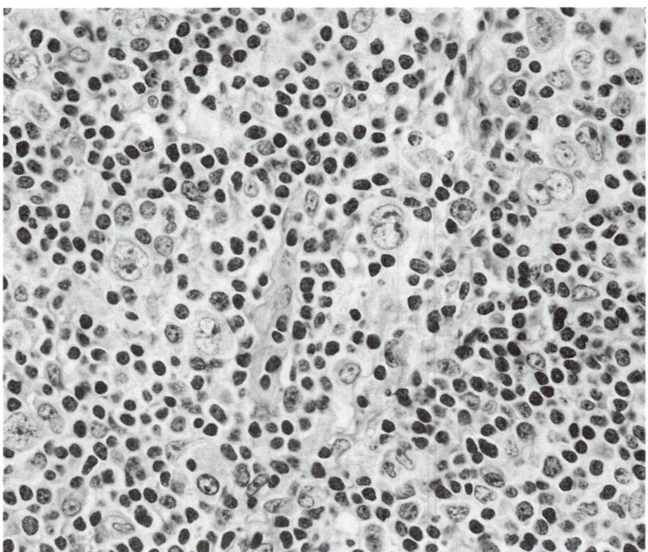

Figure 13–28

Lymphocyte-predominant Hodgkin disease, nodular variant, lymph node. The typical cellular composition of nodules is illustrated, including L and H variants of Reed-Sternberg cells, small lymphocytes, and occasional histiocytes. Note the absence of plasma cells and granulocytes.

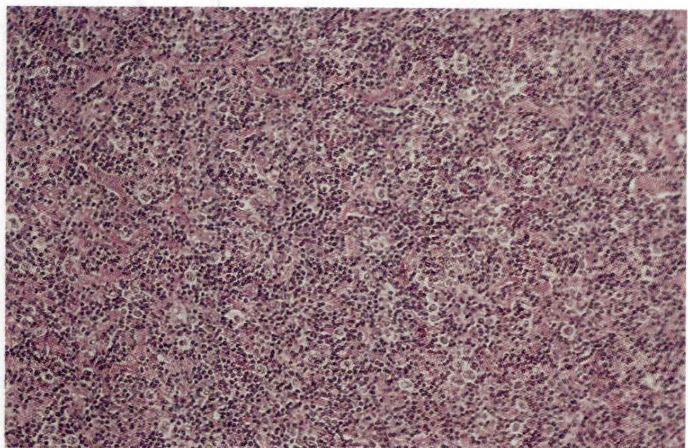

Figure 13–29

Lymphocyte-predominant Hodgkin disease, diffuse variant, lymph node. The architecture is completely effaced by a purely diffuse infiltrate of small lymphocytes, histiocytes, and L and H variants of Reed-Sternberg cells.

nodules in a wreathlike arrangement. Some macronodules may contain rare L and H variants, whereas in others these cells approach confluency. "Diagnostic" RS cells are extremely rare and are not required for diagnosis in cases with the typical growth pattern (described earlier) and immunophenotype (discussed in the next section). In contrast to other types of HD, plasma cells, eosinophils, and fibrosis are conspicuous by their absence.

Cases fitting the criteria of the diffuse type of LPHD are occasionally seen in large consultative practices (Fig. 13–29). This is not a popular diagnosis now, and cases in which diffuse LPHD was considered usually end up with other diagnoses owing to improved morphologic analysis and enhanced specificity of diagnosis resulting from experience and the benefits of immunoperoxidase panels.

The differential diagnosis of the nodular variant of LPHD includes toxoplasmic lymphadenitis, progressive transformation of germinal centers, follicular center cell lymphomas, and other types of HD. Toxoplasmic lymphadenitis is characterized by follicular hyperplasia, epithelioid macrophage clusters in interfollicular areas and follicular centers, and parafollicular (monocytoid) B cell hyperplasia (Dorfman & Remington, 1973; Dorfman & Warnke, 1974; Stansfeld, 1961). Follicular hyperplasia and epithelioid macrophage clusters are features shared with nodular LPHD, but in the latter the characteristic macronodules are seen, whereas the architecture of the lymph nodes is preserved in toxoplasmic lymphadenitis. Other differences are the prominent parafollicular B cells in toxoplasmosis and the progressive transformation of germinal centers in LPHD.

When fully developed, progressively transformed germinal centers (Burns et al, 1984; Poppema et al, 1979b) are easily recognized on low magnification by size (they are larger than normal follicular centers) and by their homogeneous population of small lymphocytes. In earlier stages, small lymphocytes may still predominate, but all progressively transformed germinal centers contain single and clustered follicular center cells of the various types and often contain scattered tingible-body macrophages as well as expanded dendritic reticulum meshworks. Progressively transformed germinal centers, in contrast to the nodules of LPHD, do not become confluent, do not efface lymph node architecture, and do not contain L- and H-type RS cells. Progressively transformed germinal centers may be seen in lymph nodes prior to, concurrent with, or following LPHD. Their coincidence clearly signifies a relationship between these two conditions (Hansmann et al, 1990; Osborne & Butler, 1984; Poppema et al, 1979b), but progressive transformation occurs most frequently as a reactive process accompanying follicular hyperplasia. Its presence does not de facto indicate a past or future risk for LPHD (Ferry et al, 1992).

Some follicular center cell lymphomas contain large neoplastic follicles with cloverleaf-shaped outlines that are architecturally similar to progressively transformed germinal centers and to the nodules of LPHD, a pattern that has been termed the floral variant of follicular lymphoma (Goates et al, 1994; Osborne & Butler, 1987). "Floral" follicular lymphomas may be distinguished from LPHD by the composition of the nodules. In follicular lymphomas, the neoplastic nodules generally contain cleaved follicular center cells but occasionally resemble HD if there are dysplastic large cells with polylobated nuclear outlines. In contrast, only small lymphoyctes and the occasional epithelioid macrophage accompany the L and H cells in the nodules of LPHD. Furthermore, follicular center cells in floral variants of follicular lymphomas express BCL2 in immunoperoxidase stains and may be clonal, while the small B cells in the nodules of LPHD are polyclonal.

Some cases of nodular LPHD contain large numbers of L and H variants, raising the possibility of a coexistent large-cell lymphoma (Sundeen, 1988) or progression to MCHD. The latter diagnosis should be made when RS cells with prominent nucleoli are found and when there are supporting immunophenotypic data (RS cells are CD45− CD15+/CD30+, and usually CD20−). A coexistent large-cell lymphoma is diagnosed when aggregates of transformed lymphocytes are found in cases with otherwise typical LPHD. These aggregates are almost uniformly B cell in phenotype and probably represent a tumorous mass of neoplastic L and H variants rather than as a composite lymphoma (Warnke et al, 1995).

The differential diagnosis of diffuse LPHD includes B cell lymphomas of large-cell type with abundant reactive T lymphocytes (T cell–rich B cell lymphomas) and/or macrophages (histiocyte-rich B cell lymphomas) and MCHD (see Table 13–3). T cell–and/or macrophage–rich lymphomas of B cell lineage may be extremely difficult to distinguish from diffuse LPHD (Chittal et al, 1991; Macon et al, 1992; Ng et al, 1989; Osborne et al, 1990; Ramsay et al, 1988; Rodriguez et al, 1993; Schmidt et al, 1995). In general, the L and H variants have more lobulated nuclear contours than do the large B cells (the neoplastic cell) in T cell–rich B cell lymphomas, and the latter cells often demonstrate light-chain restriction on paraffin-section immunoperoxidase staining. In contrast, the large cells of LPHD are polytypic or lack definite staining and often contain epithelial membrane antigen. T cell–rich B cell lymphomas usually exhibit clonal rearrangements of the immunoglobulin heavy- and light-chain genes, a finding that is unusual in LPHD. Some cases are phenotypically and morphologically almost indistinguishable. The clinical features, particularly widespread lymphadenopathy involving discontiguous sites; hepatic, splenic, and marrow involvement; and prominent B symptoms, are more likely to occur in T cell–rich B cell lymphomas than in diffuse LPHD.

MCHD may be distinguished from diffuse LPHD on histologic grounds, since the former contains numerous diagnostic RS cells, plasma cells, and eosinophils and lacks L and H variants. Immunophenotypic confirmation of MCHD is achieved when the RS cells are shown to CD15+/CD30+, and CD45−. They are negative for epithelial membrane antigen, and CD20 is usually absent. This phenotypic modification of the Lukes, Butler, and Hicks classification of HD has been accepted (Harris et al, 1994).

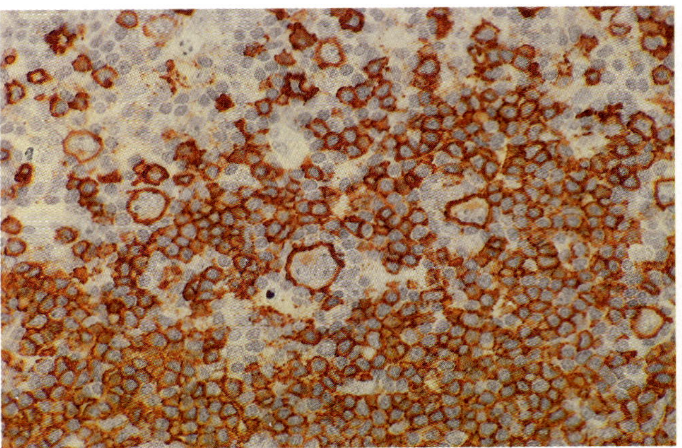

Figure 13–30

Lymphocyte-predominant Hodgkin disease, nodular variant, lymph node. The L and H cells, as well as numerous small B cells among the background lymphocyte population, exhibit strong staining for CD20. CD20 by immunoperoxidase.

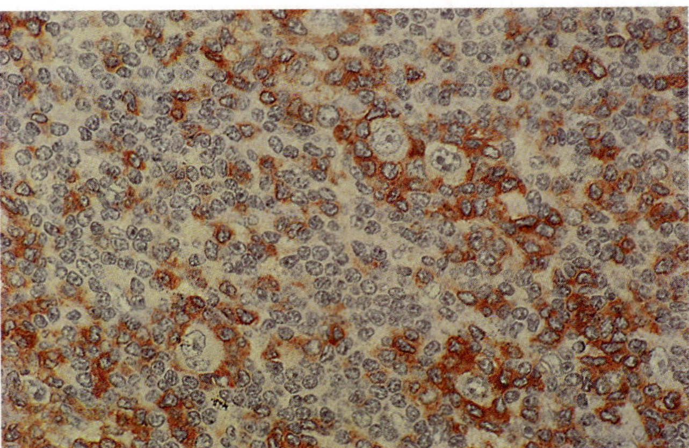

Figure 13–31

Lymphocyte-predominant Hodgkin disease, nodular variant, lymph node. CD3 positive T cells form rosettes around the L and H cells. CD3 by immunoperoxidase.

Phenotypic and Molecular Studies

Unlike other types of HD, L and H variants in nodular LPHD have a distinctive and consistent B cell phenotype, with positivity for CD19, CD20, CD22, and CD79a (Fig. 13–30) (Bishop et al, 1991; Coles et al, 1988; Hansmann et al, 1986; Korkolopoulou et al, 1994; Nicholas et al, 1990; Pinkus & Said, 1988; Pinkus & Said, 1985; Poppema, 1992; Poppema et al, 1985). L and H variants are also immunoreactive for the J chain, a polypeptide that joins monomeric into polymeric immunoglobulin and is synthesized exclusively by B lymphocytes (Poppema, 1980; Stein et al, 1986). Recently, BCL6, a zinc-finger protein normally expressed by follicular center cells, has been demonstrated in the nuclei of L and H variants (Falini et al, 1987; Flenghi et al, 1996). As in other types of HD, L and H variants are positive for the common framework antigen of the HLA-DR class II molecules (CD74). In contrast to other types of HD, L and H variants are frequently positive for CD45, lack staining for CD15, have variable staining for CD30, and in some cases express epithelial membrane antigen (Bishop et al, 1991; Nicholas et al, 1990).

The reactive lymphocytes in nodular LPHD are phenotypically different from those in other types of HD, since most are polyclonal B lymphocytes, express membrane IgM and IgD (similar to mantle zone lymphocytes), and are accompanied by numerous dendritic cells positive for CD21, CD23, and CD35 (Poppema, 1980; Poppema et al, 1985; Stein et al, 1986). The small lymphocytes forming "rosettes" around the L and H variants also have a distinctive phenotype (Falini et al, 1996; Hansmann et al, 1988; Poppema, 1989), since they are CD2+, CD3+, CD4+, and CD57+ and contain strong nuclear BCL6 positivity, features unique to LPHD (Fig. 13–31). Similar cells generally are not seen around the RS variants in other types of HD. Because of these findings, a follicular center cell origin of nodular LPHD seems likely.

Cases classified as diffuse LPHD by histologic criteria alone are phenotypically heterogeneous. In some cases, the phenotypes of the RS cell variants and the reacting lymphocyte population are very similar to those of the nodular variant of LPHD and therefore considered the diffuse counterpart of nodular LPHD (Bishop et al, 1991; Hansmann et al, 1991; Tefferi et al, 1990). Other cases of HD have reactive infiltrates very rich in T lymphocytes and RS cell variants that are CD15+/CD30+, CD45− and do not express B cell markers. These cases are phenotypically similar to MCHD and currently are classified as such. Therefore the diagnosis of the diffuse variant of LPHD requires phenotypic confirmation (Hansmann et al, 1991; von Wasielewski et al, 1997).

The molecular studies on tissue samples of LPHD have been difficult to interpret. In most studies, Southern blot techniques failed to reveal clonal rearrangements for immunoglobulin or T cell antigen receptor genes. However, using a sensitive in situ hybridization method, the L and H variants have been shown to be clonal, with light-chain restriction demonstrable in 80% of cases (Stoler et al, 1995). Polymerase chain reaction has been used to amplify the V-D-J joining regions of the IgH loci in single, isolated L and H cells from nodular and diffuse types of LPHD (Delabie et al, 1994). Different L and H cells from individual cases had V-D-J joining regions that lacked substantial sequence homology, strongly suggesting that the L and H variants in a given case are *not* clonal. Similar findings were described in 41 cases of nodular LPHD (Wickert et al, 1995; Pan et al, 1996). These results are in direct contrast with the demonstration of clonal IgH gene rearrangements in 14 of 21 cases of LPHD using a highly sensitive polymerase chain reaction–based assay on whole-tissue samples rather than on single cells (Tamaru et al, 1994). Clonality in this disorder has been established, using immunoglobulin gene sequencing from single L and H cells microdissected from lymphocyte predominant HD specimens (Ohno et al, 1997; Marafioti et al, 1997).

Large-Cell Lymphomas in Association with Lymphocyte-Predominant Hodgkin Disease

Several studies have addressed the issue of large–B cell lymphomas in patients with LPHD (Greiner et al, 1996; Hansmann et al, 1989; Miettinen et al, 1983; Sundeen et al, 1988). Monomorphous large-cell lymphomas complicating nodular LPHD may take three forms. In the first, there are sheets of cells cytologically identical to L and H variants; adjacent minor foci that resemble typical nodular LPHD are often present. The transformed cells in these sheets are CD19+, CD20+, and CD22+, but do not exhibit surface or cytoplasmic light-chain restriction. Clonal rearrangements of immunoglobulin or

T cell antigen receptor genes cannot be demonstrated, but this group presumably represents histologic progression of nodular LPHD, with sheetlike growth of L and H variants and a minimal lymphocyte and macrophage host response.

The second category of large-cell lymphomas complicating nodular LPHD includes B cell lymphomas of the large non-cleaved or immunoblastic type. In these cases, there is diffuse architectural effacement of the tissues by a monomorphous population. The neoplastic cells are CD19+, CD20+, and/or CD22+ and exhibit light-chain restriction and/or have clonal immunoglobulin gene rearrangements. In their appearance, these cases resemble conventional large-cell lymphomas more than HD, but in rare instances a clonal relationship to the RS cells of the antecedent HD biopsy specimen has been demonstrated.

Aggressive peripheral T cell lymphomas have been described in patients with well-documented nodular LPHD (Rysenga et al, 1995; Tefferi et al, 1992). In all cases, there was diffuse architectural effacement of nodes by small, medium, and large T cells that were cytologically atypical and phenotypically aberrant. In all cases, prominent clonal T cell antigen receptor rearrangement bands were identified by molecular studies. Despite aggressive therapy, this limited number of patients had a very poor survival time following the development of T cell lymphoma.

STAGING OF HODGKIN DISEASE AND PATHOLOGIC EVALUATION OF STAGING SPECIMENS

Staging of Hodgkin Disease

The distinct patterns of spread and relapse of HD fostered the development of our staging system (Rosenberg & Kaplan, 1966). Staging is the primary determinant of therapy type and prognosis in HD and should be initiated only after the histopathologic diagnosis of HD is rendered. Patients are staged by a detailed history, physical examination, chest radiograph, abdominal or pelvic computerized tomographic scans, and bilateral marrow trephine biopsies (Kaufman & Longo, 1995). Additional staging procedures may be performed as needed. For example, abnormal chest radiographs are usually followed by a computerized tomographic scan to delineate areas of intrathoracic lymph node or pulmonary involvement. Lymphangiography is rarely used now but has high diagnostic sensitivity and specificity in HD, exceeding that of computerized tomographic scans, in providing additional information about the spread of disease. Staging laparotomy, also used less regularly now than in the past, may be indicated in patients whose initial staging reveals supradiaphragmatic stage IA or IIA disease, since absence of intra-abdominal lymph node or splenic involvement may result in their receiving only radiation therapy.

The currently employed staging system for HD summarized in Table 13–5 (Lister et al, 1989) is based on proposals of the Ann Arbor conference (Carbone et al, 1971). Stage I disease is defined as involvement of a single lymph node group. Stage II disease involves two or more contiguous lymph node regions on the same side of the diaphragm. Stage III disease involves lymph nodes on both sides of the diaphragm or supradiaphragmatic lymph nodes and the spleen. The designation III_1 applies to patients whose intra-abdominal disease is confined to the spleen and/or splenic hilar, celiac, or portal lymph nodes and III_2 to patients whose intra-abdominal disease involves para-aortic, iliac, or mesenteric lymph nodes (lymph node involvement below the renal hila). Stage IV denotes hematogenous spread and is applied when patients have hepatic or marrow involvement. Involvement of more than one extranodal site also qualifies as stage IV.

Extranodal site involvement by HD, excluding liver and marrow, is indicated by adding E to the staging designation. The E designation is very rigidly defined in order to exclude extranodal site involvement owing to hematogenous dissemination. This designation is applied to a single extranodal mass that either is the only site of disease or results from direct extension from an involved lymph node group. Designation X is used for bulky disease, defined as a very large mediastinal mass (greater than one third of the transthoracic distance as measured on posteroanterior chest radiographs at the level of T5–T6) or as a nodal mass with a largest dimension ≧10 cm. The B designation in staging is applied when there are constitutional symptoms, including unexplained persistent fever in excess of 38°C, unintended loss of >10% of body weight, or recurrent drenching night sweats.

Evaluation of Staging Specimens in Hodgkin Disease

Pathologists play a critical role in the evaluation of tissue samples obtained to stage patients. After a staging laparotomy, these specimens include intra-abdominal lymph nodes, spleen, liver, and marrow samples. The diagnostic criteria for HD are

Table 13–5
Modified Ann Arbor Staging Classification for Hodgkin Disease

Ann Arbor Stage	Criteria
I	Involvement of a single lymph node group or localized involvement of a single extranodal site (IE)
II	Involvement of two or more lymph node groups on the same side of the diaphragm or localized involvement of an extranodal site and one or more lymph node groups on the same side of the diaphragm (IIE)
III	Involvement of lymph nodes on both sides of the diaphragm with splenic involvement (IIIS) or with localized involvement of an extranodal site (IIIE) or both (IIISE)
IV	Multiple extranodal organ involvement or disseminated involvement of an extranodal organ (usually bone marrow or liver) with or without lymph node involvement

Note: Each stage is further modified by designating the absence (A) or presence (B) of fever, night sweats, or unintended weight loss >10% of the body weight. Bulky disease is indicated by adding X to the staging designation.

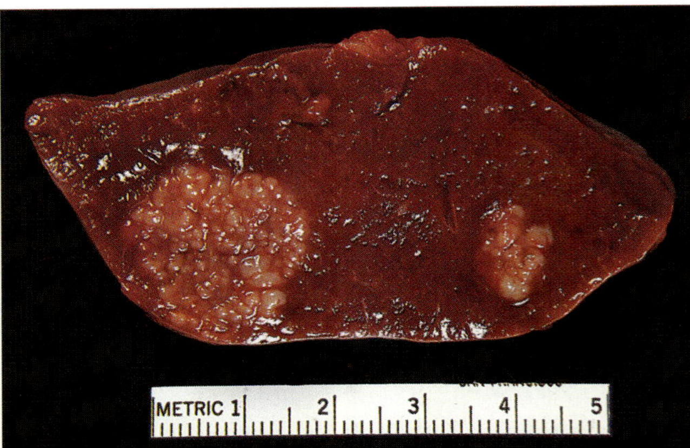

Figure 13–32

Hodgkin disease, spleen. A specimen removed at staging laparotomy reveals involvement by HD as discrete, yellow-tan nodules that bulge above the cut surface of the spleen.

modified when evaluating staging samples. The requisite criteria for diagnosing involvement in staging samples are the presence of the typical reactive inflammatory cellularity and the presence of RS cell variants (Lukes, 1971).

Accuracy of pathologic staging is operator dependent and greatly facilitated by proper handling of staging samples at the time of the gross examination. Frozen sections should not be prepared, and flow cytometric analysis is not indicated unless there is evidence of a composite lymphomatous process. Lymph nodes should be sectioned perpendicular to the long axis at 2-mm intervals, allowing optimal fixation and histologic evaluation. Accurate records of the anatomic location of each lymph node are necessary so that the final report documents the presence or absence of involvement in specific lymph node groups. Careful gross examination of the spleen is critical, requiring sectioning at 2-mm intervals. The small white nodules of potential HD (Fig. 13–32) may then be sampled for histologic examination. Fresh spleens may be briefly immersed in formalin if the fresh specimen cannot be sectioned readily into thin slabs. The number of nodules of HD in the spleen has prognostic significance, since the presence of six or more nodules confers a greater risk of recurrence following initial therapy (Hoppe et al, 1980). Physiologic or reactive aggregates of lymphocytes in the liver may be particularly difficult to evaluate in inadequately fixed wedge biopsy specimens or compressed needle biopsy specimens. Bilateral iliac crest marrow specimens ≧1.5 cm in length significantly increase the probability of detecting focal marrow involvement.

Assessing staging samples for HD presents problems that vary according to the anatomic site. In lymph nodes, the earliest foci of involvement by HD are at the junctions between follicles and the adjacent paracortex (Fig. 13–33) (Strum & Rappaport, 1970), where small, ill-defined nodules of inflammatory cells are mixed with minimal numbers of RS cell variants. Nodes from patients who have undergone lymphangiography exhibit histiocytic hyperplasia, with multinucleated histiocytes and lipogranulomas in the sinuses and paracortex that may obscure minimal foci. Eosinophilic response to the lymphangiogram dye may simulate the host response of HD. The latter circumstance has caused false-positive diagnoses of HD, whereas the lymphangiographic dye reaction has caused false-negative evaluations. In the spleen, the earliest foci of HD occur in the T cell zones of the white pulp (Fig. 13–34) (Burke, 1981; Kadin et al, 1971), a region that may undergo lymphocytic hyperplasia and immunoblastic proliferation as a part of the host response to HD (Burke & Osborne, 1983).

The importance of careful gross examination of the spleen cannot be overemphasized. All foci of HD should be recognized by this examination. Cluster or single immunoblasts have been incorrectly diagnosed as involvement, particularly when fixation is not ideal. In the liver, the host response to HD takes the form of periportal lymphocyte aggregates and Kupfer cell hyperplasia, the former being the regions most frequently involved by HD (Bagley et al, 1972; Dich et al, 1989). Mistakes may be avoided by having strict personal criteria for identifying RS cells. It helps to remember that hepatic involvement by HD is vanishingly rare in patients with uninvolved spleens. Sarcoid-type granulomas may be encountered in any tissue sample, but granulomas alone do not indicate the presence of HD and thus do not indicate a more advanced stage of the disease (Fig. 13–35) (Kadin et al, 1970; Sacks et al, 1978). However, sarcoid-type granulomas may reflect a local response to the immediate presence of HD and should always cause a careful search for RS cells and variants.

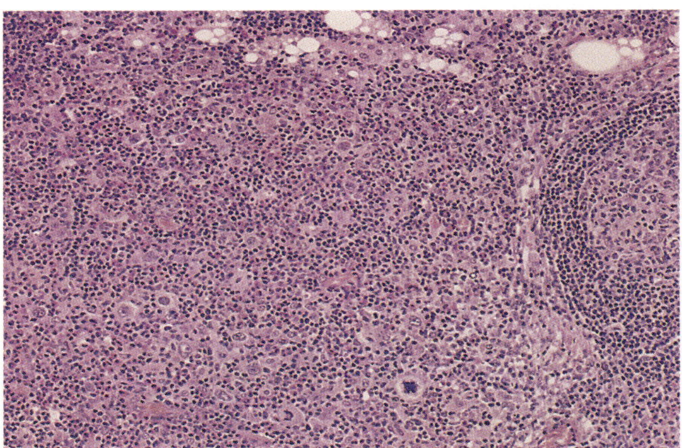

Figure 13–33

Hodgkin disease, celiac lymph node. This node exhibits involvement at the border of the germinal center, with lipogranulomas at the top of the photograph.

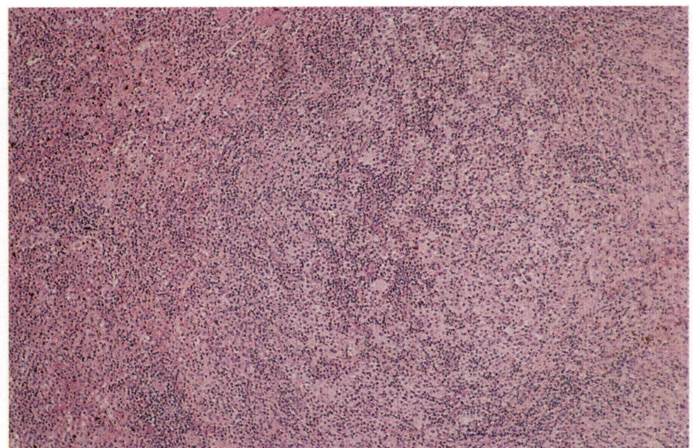

Figure 13–34

Hodgkin disease, spleen. Specimen removed at staging laparotomy exhibits involvement of the white pulp.

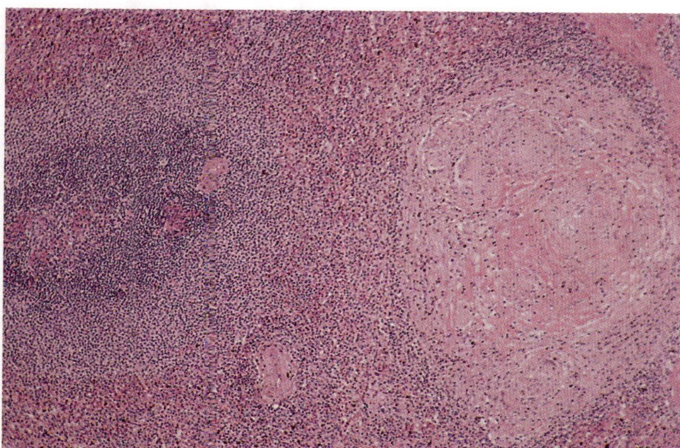

Figure 13–35

Spleen, staging laparotomy. Lymphocytic hyperplasia of the white pulp (*left*) and a noncaseating granuloma (*right*) are revealed. This spleen did not contain areas of involvement in the white pulp. Reed-Sternberg cells were not noted in association with the granulomas. Therefore, the spleen was determined not to be involved by Hodgkin disease.

Marrow involvement by HD in general is infrequent, occurring in 5–10% of cases at diagnosis. The frequency of marrow involvement varies with the histologic type of HD and is particularly low in LPHD (Chang et al, 1995; Siebert et al, 1995), in which there may be intertrabecular and paratrabecular aggregates of small lymphocytes admixed with macrophages and occasional L and H variants. The L and H cells may be found only in one or two levels of the biopsy specimen. Therefore, step sectioning of all lymphocyte aggregates in the marrow from patients with LPHD may be necessary to determine whether L and H cells are present.

The marrow is involved in 5%, 10%, and >50% of patients with NSHD, MCHD, and LDHD, respectively (Bartl et al, 1982; Foucar, 1995; Kinney et al, 1986; Macavei, 1990; Munker et al, 1995). The histologic pattern of marrow involvement in all types is so similar that the type of HD cannot be specified from marrow findings alone. Intertrabecular (Fig. 13–36) or paratrabecular (Fig. 13–37) aggregates of lymphocytes, macrophages, eosinophils, and plasma cells, together with a few RS cells, may be seen. Areas of involvement may be hypocellular but are usually cellular nodules associated with fibrosis and stellate borders. Histiocytes predominate in some cases, simulating granulomatous infiltrates (Fig. 13–38), whereas the fibrosis and eosinophilic infiltrates simulate systemic mastocytosis in others. In patients being staged for HD,

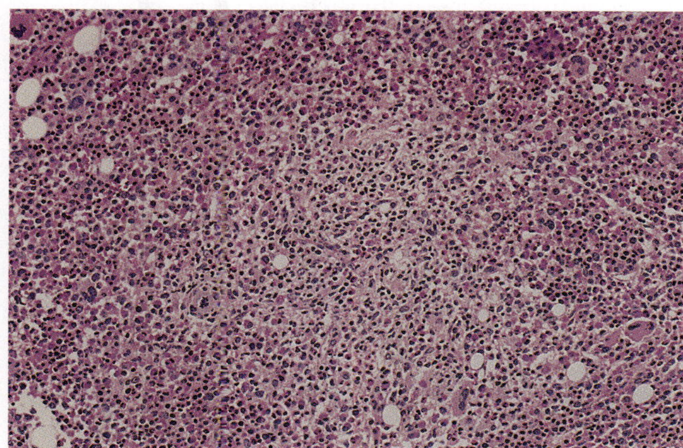

Figure 13–36

Hodgkin disease, marrow. Note the trilineage hyperplasia and the eosinophilia. The latter features represent the systemic host response to Hodgkin disease.

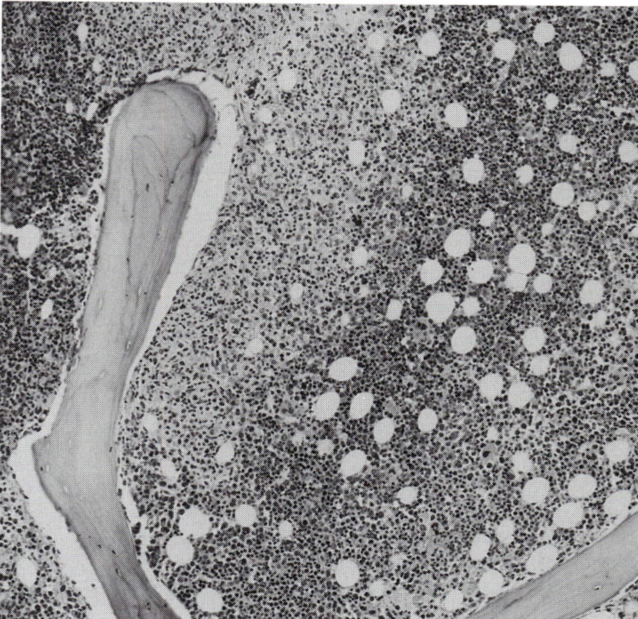

Figure 13–37

Hodgkin disease, marrow. Involvement by Hodgkin disease is paratrabecular.

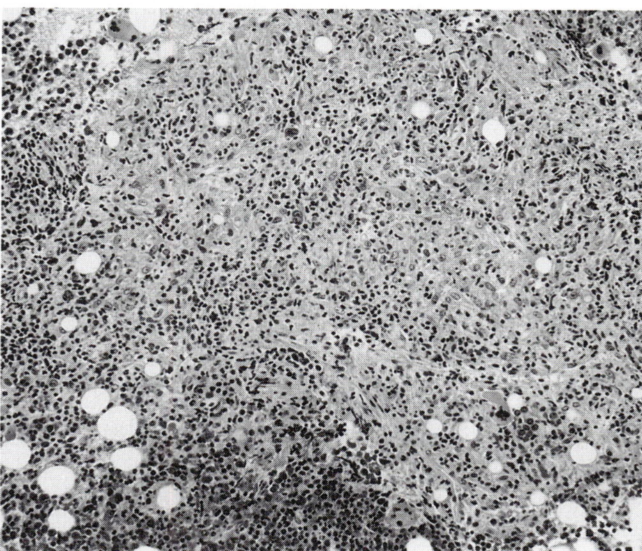

Figure 13–38

Hodgkin disease, marrow. Note the irregular borders of the areas of involvement and the numerous macrophages, simulating the appearance of a granuloma. Just above the center is a diagnostic Reed-Sternberg cell, establishing the nature of this infiltrate.

RS variants must be found in an inflammatory background in order to diagnose marrow involvement. Patients with HD and HIV infection or patients with LDHD (Kinney et al, 1986) may present with fever of undetermined origin and no peripheral adenopathy. The marrow is often the first site in which a diagnosis is established. In such cases, "diagnostic" RS cells must be found. Immunophenotypic confirmation of CD15/CD30 positivity and CD45 negativity should also be obtained, since marrow involvement by peripheral T cell lymphomas and T cell–rich B cell lymphomas closely simulates HD. The marrow in patients with HD may show trilineage hyperplasia, eosinophilic hyperplasia, benign lymphocytic aggregates, and noncaseating granulomas as a part of the host response or in some cases may reveal development of a second neoplasm, such as acute myelomonocytic leukemia or B or T cell lymphoma.

REFERENCES

Abdulaziz Z, Mason DY, Stein H, et al: An immunohistochemical study of the cellular constituents of Hodgkin's disease using an monoclonal antibody panel. Histopathology 8:1–25, 1984.

Agnarsson BA, Kadin ME: The immunophenotype of Reed-Sternberg cells: a study of 50 cases of Hodgkin's disease using fixed frozen tissues. Cancer 63:2083–2087, 1989.

Agnarsson BA, Kadin ME: Ki-1 positive large cell lymphoma: a morphologic and immunologic study of 19 cases. Am J Surg Pathol 12:264–274, 1988.

Ambinder RF, Browning PJ, Lorenzana I, et al: Epstein-Barr virus and childhood Hodgkin's disease in Honduras and the United States. Blood 81:462–467, 1993.

Amini R-M, Enblad G, Sunderstrom C, et al: Patients suffering from both Hodgkin's disease and non-Hodgkin's lymphoma: a clinicopathologic and immuno-histochemical population-based study of 32 patients. Int J Cancer 71:510–516, 1997.

Angel C, Pringle JH, Naylor J, et al: Analysis of antigen receptor genes in Hodgkin's disease. J Clin Pathol 46:337–340, 1993.

Angel CA, Warford A, Campbell AC, et al: The immunohistology of Hodgkin's disease: Reed-Sternberg cells and their variants. J Pathol 153:21–30, 1987.

Arber DA, Weiss LM: CD15: a review. Appl Immunohistochem 1:17–30, 1993.

Armstrong AA, Weiss LM, Gallagher A, et al: Criteria for the definition of Epstein-Barr virus association in Hodgkin's disease. Leukemia 6:869–874, 1992.

Audouin J, Diebold J, Pallesen G: Frequent expression of Epstein-Barr virus latent membrane protein-1 in tumor cells of Hodgkin's disease in HIV-positive patients. J Pathol 167:381–384, 1992.

Bagley C, Roth J, Thomas L, DeVita V: Liver biopsy in Hodgkin's disease: clinicopathologic correlations in 127 patients. Ann Intern Med 76:219–225, 1972.

Bartl R, Frisch B, Burkhardt R, et al: Assessment of bone marrow histology in Hodgkin's disease: correlation with clinical factors. Br J Haematol 51:345–360, 1982.

Bearman R, Pangalis G, Rappaport H: Hodgkin's disease, lymphocyte depletion type: a clinicopathologic study of 39 patients. Cancer 41:293–302, 1978.

Bennett MH, MacLennan KA, Vaughan-Hudson G, et al: Non-Hodgkin's lymphoma arising in patients treated for Hodgkin's disease in the BNLI: a 20-year experience. Ann Oncol 2:83–92, 1991.

Bennett M, Tu A, Hudson G: Analysis of grade I Hodgkin's disease. Clin Radiol 32:491–498, 1981.

Bhatia S, Robison LL, Oberlin O, et al: Breast cancer and other second neoplasms after childhood Hodgkin's disease. N Engl J Med 334:745–751, 1996.

Bishop PW, Harris M, Smith AP, et al: Immunophenotypic study of lymphocyte predominance Hodgkin's disease. Histopathology 18:19–24, 1991.

Borg-Grech A, Radford JA, Crowther D, et al: A comparative study of the nodular and diffuse variants of lymphocyte predominant Hodgkin's disease. J Clin Oncol 7:1303–1309, 1989.

Brinker MGL, Poppema S, Buys CHCM, et al: Clonal immunoglobulin gene rearrangements in tissues involved by Hodgkin's disease. Blood 70:186–191, 1987.

Brousset P, Rochaix P, Chittal S, et al: High incidence of Epstein-Barr virus detection in Hodgkin's disease and absence of detection in anaplastic large-cell lymphoma in children. Histopathology 23:189–191, 1993.

Burke J: Surgical pathology of the spleen: an approach to the differential diagnosis of splenic lymphomas and leukemias: I. Diseases of the white pulp. Am J Surg Pathol 5:551–563, 1981.

Burke J, Osborne B: Localized reactive lymphoid hyperplasia of the spleen simulating malignant lymphoma: a report of seven cases. Am J Surg Pathol 7:373–380, 1983.

Burns BF, Colby TV, Dorfman RF: Differential diagnostic features of nodular L and H Hodgkin's disease, including progressive transformation of germinal centers. 8:253–261, 1984.

Cabanillas F, Pathak S, Trujillo J, et al: Cytogenetic features of Hodgkin's disease suggest possible origin from a lymphocyte. Blood 71:1615–1617, 1988.

Carbone A, Gloghini A, Gattei V, et al: Expression of functional CD40 antigen on Reed-Sternberg cells and Hodgkin's disease cell lines. Blood 85:780–789, 1995.

Carbone A, Gloghini A, Zanette I, et al: Co-expression of Epstein-Barr virus latent membrane protein and vimentin in "aggressive" histological subtypes of Hodgkin's disease. Virchows Arch A Pathol Anat 422:39–45, 1993.

Carbone P, Kaplan H, Musshof K, et al: Report of the committee on the staging of Hodgkin's disease. Cancer Res 31:1860–1861, 1971.

Casey T, Cousar JB, Mangum M, et al: Monomorphic lymphomas arising in patients with Hodgkin's disease: correlation of morphologic, immunophenotypic, and molecular genetic findings in 12 cases. Am J Pathol 136:81–94, 1990.

Casey T, Olson SJ, Cousar JB, et al: Immunophenotypes of Reed-Sternberg cells: a study of 19 cases of Hodgkin's disease in plastic-embedded sections. Blood 74:2624–2628, 1989.

Chang KL, Albujar PF, Chen YY, et al: High prevalence of Epstein-Barr virus in the Reed-Sternberg cells of Hodgkin's disease occurring in Peru. Blood 81:496–501, 1993.

Chang K, Kamel O, Arber D, et al: Pathologic features of nodular lymphocyte predominance Hodgkin's disease in extranodal sites. Am J Surg Pathol 19:1313–1324, 1995.

Chittal SM, Brousset P, Voigt JJ, et al: Large B-cell lymphoma rich in T-cells and simulating Hodgkin's disease. Histopathology 19: 211–220, 1991.

Chittal SM, Caveriviere P, Schwarting R, et al: Monoclonal antibodies in the diagnosis of Hodgkin's disease: the search for a rational panel. Am J Surg Pathol 12:9–21, 1988.

Chott A, Kaserer K, Augustin I, et al: Ki-1 positive large cell lymphoma: a clinicopathologic study of 41 cases. Am J Surg Pathol 14:439–448, 1990.

Cibull ML, Stein H, Gatter KC, et al: The expression of the CD3 antigen in Hodgkin's disease. Histopathology 15:597–605, 1989.

Colby TV, Hoppe RT, Warnke RA: Hodgkin's disease: a clinicopathologic study of 659 cases. Cancer 49:1848, 1982.

Coles RB, Cartun RW, Pastuszak WT: Hodgkin's disease, lymphocyte-predominant type: immunoreactivity with B-cell antibodies. Mod Pathol 1:274–278, 1988.

Correa P, O'Connor G: Epidemiologic patterns of Hodgkin's disease. Int J Cancer 8:192–201, 1971.

Crennan E, D'Costa I, Liew KH, et al: Lymphocyte predominant Hodgkin's disease: a clinicopathologic comparative study of histologic and immunophenotypic subtypes. Int J Radiat Oncol Biol Phys 31:333–337, 1995.

d'Amore ESG, Lee CKK, Aeppli DM, et al: Lack of prognostic value of histopathologic parameters in Hodgkin's disease, nodular sclerosis type: a study of 123 patients with limited stage disease who had undergone laparotomy and were treated with radiation therapy. Arch Pathol Lab Med 116:856–861, 1992.

Deacon EM, Pallesen G, Niedobitek G, et al: Epstein-Barr virus and Hodgkin's disease: transcriptional analysis of virus latency in the malignant cells. J Exp Med 177:339–349, 1993.

Delabie J, Chan WC, Weisenburger DD, et al: The antigen-presenting cell function of Reed-Sternberg cells and the surrounding T-cell host response. Leuk Lymphoma 18:35–40, 1995.

Delabie J, Tiemens A, Wu G, et al: Lymphocyte predominance Hodgkin's disease: lineage and clonality determination using a single-cell assay. Blood 84:3291–3298, 1994.

Delabie J, Tierens A, Gavriil T, et al: Phenotype, genotype and clonality of Reed-Sternberg cells in nodular sclerosis Hodgkin's disease: results of a single-cell study. Br J Haematol 94:198–205, 1996.

Delabie J, Vanderberghe E, Kennes C, et al: Histiocyte-rich B-cell lymphoma: a distinct clinicopathologic entity possibly related to lymphocyte predominant Hodgkin's disease, paragranuloma subtype. Am J Surg Pathol 16:37–48, 1992.

Dich N, Goodman Z, Klein M: Hepatic involvement in Hodgkin's disease: clues to histologic diagnosis. Cancer 64:2121–2126, 1989.

Doggett RS, Colby TV, Dorfman RF: Interfollicular Hodgkin's disease. Am J Surg Pathol 7:145–149, 1983.

Dorfman R, Remington J: Value of lymph node biopsy in the diagnosis of acute acquired toxoplasmosis. N Engl J Med 289:878–881, 1973.

Dorfman R, Warnke R: Lymphadenopathy simulating the malignant lymphomas. Hum Pathol 5:519–550, 1974.

Falini B, Bigerna B, Pasqualucci L, et al: Distinctive expression pattern of the BCL-6 protein in nodular lymphocyte predominance Hodgkin's disease. Blood 87:465–471, 1996.

Falini B, Stein H, Pileri S, et al: Expression of lymphoid-associated antigens on Hodgkin's and Reed-Sternberg cells of Hodgkin's disease. Histopathology 11:1129–1242, 1987.

Ferry J, Linggood R, Convery K, et al: Hodgkin's disease, nodular sclerosis type: implications of histologic subclassification. Cancer 71: 457–463, 1993.

Ferry JA, Zukerberg LR, Harris WL: Florid progressive transformation of germinal centers: a syndrome affecting young men without early progression to nodular lymphocyte predominance Hodgkin's disease. Am J Surg Pathol 16:252–258, 1992.

Fillipa DA, Ladanyi M, Wollner N, et al: CD30 (Ki-1) positive malignant lymphomas: clinical, immunophenotypic, histologic, and genetic characteristics and differences with Hodgkin's disease. Blood 87:2905–2917, 1996.

Flenghi L, Bigerna B, Bizzotti M, et al: Monoclonal antibodies PG-B6a and PG-B6p recognize, respectively, a highly conserved and a formol-resistant epitope on the human BCL-6 protein amino-terminal region. Am J Pathol 148:1543–1555, 1996.

Foss HD, Herbst H, Gottstein S, et al: Interleukin-8 in Hodgkin's disease: preferential expression by reactive cells and association with neutrophil density. Am J Pathol 148:1229–1236, 1996.

Foss HD, Hummel M, Gottstein S, et al: Frequent expression of IL-7 gene transcripts in tumor cells of classical Hodgkin's disease. Am J Pathol 146:33–39, 1995.

Foucar K: Hodgkin's disease in bone marrow. In Foucar K (ed): Bone Marrow Pathology. ASCP Press, Chicago, pp 354–355, 1995.

Frizzera G: The distinction of Hodgkin's disease from anaplastic large cell lymphoma. Semin Diag Pathol 9:291–296, 1992.

Glaser S, Lin R, Stewart S, et al: Epstein-Barr virus–associated Hodgkin's disease: epidemiologic characteristics in international data. Int J Cancer 70:375–382, 1997.

Glick AD, Leech JH, Flexner JM, et al: Ultrastructural study of Reed-Sternberg cells: comparison with transformed lymphocytes and histiocytes. Am J Pathol 85:195–200, 1976.

Goates JJ, Kamel OW, LeBrun DP, et al: Floral variant of follicular lymphoma. Am J Surg Pathol 18:37–47, 1994.

Gold JE, Altarac D, Ree HJ, et al: HIV-associated Hodgkin disease: a clinical study of 18 cases and review of the literature. Am J Hematol 36:93–99, 1991.

Goss HD, Herbst H, Oelmann E, et al: Lymphotoxin, tumour necrosis factor and interleukin-6 gene transcripts are present in Hodgkin and Reed-Sternberg cells of most Hodgkin's disease cases. Br J Haematol 84:627–635, 1993.

Greer J, Kinney M, Cousar J, et al: Lymphocyte-depleted Hodgkin's disease: clinicopathologic review of 25 patients. Am J Med 81: 208–214, 1986.

Greiner TC, Gascoyner RD, Anderson ME, et al: Nodular lymphocyte-predominant Hodgkin's disease associated with large-cell lymphoma: analysis of Ig gene rearrangements by V-J polymerase chain reaction. Blood 88:657–666, 1996.

Greisser H: Gene rearrangements and chromosomal translocations in T-cell lymphoma: diagnostic applications and their limits. Virchows Archiv 426:323–338, 1995.

Griesser H, Feller AC, Mak TW, et al: Clonal rearrangements of T-cell receptor and immunoglobulin genes and immunophenotypic antigen expression in different subclasses of Hodgkin's disease. Int J Cancer 40:157–160, 1987.

Gruss HJ, Brach MA, Drexler HG, et al: Expression of cytokine genes, cytokine receptor genes, and transcription factors in cultured Hodgkin and Reed-Sternberg cells. Cancer Res 52:3353–3360, 1992a.

Gruss HJ, Brach MA, Drexler HG, et al: Interleukin 9 is expressed by primary and cultured Hodgkin and Reed-Sternberg cells. Cancer Res 52:1026–1031, 1992b.

Gruss HJ, Hirschstein D, Wright B, et al: Expression and function of CD40 on Hodgkin's and Reed-Sternberg cells and the possible relevance for Hodgkin's disease. Blood 84:2305–2314, 1994.

Gruss HJ, Pinto A, Duyster J, et al: Hodgkin's disease: a tumor with disturbed immunological pathways. Immunol Today 18:156–163, 1997.

Gulley ML, Eagen PA, Quintanilla-Martinez L: Epstein-Barr virus DNA is abundant and monoclonal in the Reed-Sternberg cells of Hodgkin's disease: association with mixed cellularity subtype and Hispanic American ethnicity. Blood 83:1595–1602, 1994.

Gutensohn N: Social class and age at diagnosis of Hodgkin's disease: new epidemiologic evidence for the "two disease hypothesis". Cancer Treat Rep 66:689–695, 1982.

Gutensohn N, Cole P: Childhood social environment and Hodgkin's disease. N Engl J Med 304:135–140, 1981.

Hall PA, D'Ardenne AJ, Stansfield AG: Paraffin section immunohistochemistry: II. Hodgkin's disease and large cell anaplastic (Ki-1) lymphoma. Histopathology 13:161–169, 1988.

Hansmann ML, Fellbaum C, Hui PK, et al: Correlation of content of B cells and Leu7-positive cells with subtype and stage in lymphocyte predominance type Hodgkin's disease. J Cancer Res Clin Oncol 114:405–410, 1988.

Hansmann ML, Fellbaum CH, Hui PK, et al: Morphological and immunohistochemical investigation of non-Hodgkin's lymphoma combined with Hodgkin's disease. Histopathology 15:35–48, 1989.

Hansmann ML, Fellbaum C, Hui PK, et al: Progressive transformation of germinal centers with and without association to Hodgkin's disease. Am J Clin Pathol 93:219–226, 1990.

Hansmann ML, Stein H, Dallenbach F, et al: Diffuse lymphocyte-predominant Hodgkin's disease (diffuse paraganglioma): a variant of the B-cell-derived nodular type. Am J Pathol 138:29–36, 1991.

Hansmann ML, Stein H, Fellbaum C, et al: Nodular paragranuloma can transform into high-grade malignant lymphoma of B type. Hum Pathol 20:1169–1175, 1989.

Hansmann ML, Wacker HH, Radzun HJ: Paragranuloma is a variant of Hodgkin's disease with predominance of B-cells. Virchows Arch A Pathol Anat 409:171–181, 1986.

Hansmann ML, Zwingers T, Böske A, et al: Clinical features of nodular paragranuloma (Hodgkin's disease, lymphocyte predominance type, nodular). J Cancer Res Clin Oncol 108:321–330, 1984.

Harris NL, Jaffe ES, Stein H, et al: A revised European-American classification of lymphoid neoplasms: a proposal from the International Lymphoma Study Group. Blood 84:1361–1392, 1994.

Herbst H, Foss HD, Samol J, et al: Frequent expression of interleukin-10 by Epstein-Barr virus–harboring tumor cells of Hodgkin's disease. Blood 87:2918–2929, 1996.

Herbst H, Niedobitek G, Kneba M, et al: High incidence of Epstein-Barr virus genomes in Hodgkin's disease. Am J Pathol 137:13–18, 1990.

Herbst H, Steinbrecher E, Niedobitek G, et al: Distribution and phenotype of Epstein-Barr virus–harboring cells in Hodgkin's disease. Blood 80:484–491, 1992.

Herndier BG, Sanchez HL, Chang KL, et al: High prevalence of Epstein-Barr virus in the Reed-Sternberg cells of HIV-associated Hodgkin's disease. Am J Pathol 142:1073–1079, 1993.

Hess JL, Bodis S, Pinkus G, et al: Histopathologic grading of nodular sclerosis Hodgkin's disease: lack of prognostic significance in 254 surgically staged patients. Cancer 74:708–714, 1994.

Hoppe R, Rosenberg S, Kaplan H, et al: Prognostic factors in pathological stage IIIA Hodgkin's disease. Cancer 46:1240–1246, 1980.

Hsu SM, Yang K, Jaffe ES: Phenotypic expression of Hodgkin's and Reed-Sternberg cells in Hodgkin's disease. Am J Pathol 118: 209–217, 1985.

Huh J, Park C, Juhng S, et al: A pathologic study of Hodgkin's disease in Korea and its association with the Epstein-Barr virus infection. Cancer 77:949–955, 1996.

Hummel M, Anagnostopoulos J, Dallenbach F, et al: EBV infection patterns in Hodgkin's disease and normal lymphoid tissue: expression and cellular localization of EBV gene products. Br J Haematol 82:689–694, 1992.

Hummel M, Ziemann K, Lammert H, et al: Hodgkin's disease with monoclonal and polyclonal populations of Reed-Sternberg cells. N Engl J Med 333:901–906, 1995.

Isaacson PG, Schmid C, Pan L, et al: Epstein-Barr virus latent membrane protein expression by Hodgkin and Reed-Sternberg-like cells in acute infectious mononucleosis. J Pathol 167:267–271, 1992.

Joske DJL, Emery-Goodman A, Bachmann E, et al: Epstein-Barr virus burden in Hodgkin's disease is related to latent membrane protein gene expression but not to active viral replication. Blood 80:2610–2613, 1992.

Kadin M, Donaldson S, Dorfman R: Isolated granulomas in Hodgkin's disease. N Engl J Med 283:859–861, 1970.

Kadin M, Glatstein E, Dorfman R: Clinicopathologic studies of 117 untreated patients subjected to laparotomy for the staging of Hodgkin's disease. Cancer 27:1277–1294, 1971.

Kadin ME, Muramoto L, Said J: Expression of T-cell antigens on Reed-Sternberg cells in a subset of patients with nodular sclerosing and mixed cellularity Hodgkin's disease. Am J Pathol 130: 345–353, 1988.

Kaplan HS: Patterns of anatomic distribution. In Hodgkin's Disease, 2nd ed. Harvard University Press, Cambridge, MA, pp 280–339, 1980.

Kaufman D, Longo D: Hodgkin's Disease. In Abeloff M, Armitage J, Lichter A, et al (eds): Clinical Oncology, Churchill Livingstone, New York, pp 2081–2107, 1995.

Keller AR, Kaplan HS, Lukes RJ, et al: Correlation of histopathology with other prognostic indicators in Hodgkin's disease. Cancer 22: 487–499, 1968.

Khan G, Coates PJ, Gupta RK, et al: Presence of Epstein-Barr virus in Hodgkin's disease is not exclusive to Reed-Sternberg cells. Am J Pathol 140:757–762, 1992.

Khan G, Naase MA: Down-regulation of Epstein-Barr virus nuclear antigen 1 in Reed-Sternberg cells of Hodgkin's disease. J Clin Pathol 48:845–848, 1995.

Khan G, Norton AJ, Slavin G: Epstein-Barr virus in Hodgkin disease: relation to age and subtype. Cancer 71:3124–3129, 1993.

Kinney M, Green J, Stein R, et al: Lymphocyte-depletion Hodgkin's disease: histopathologic diagnosis of marrow involvement. Am J Surg Pathol 10:219–226, 1986.

Koduru PRK, Susin M, Schulman P, et al: Phenotypic and genotypic characterization of Hodgkin's disease. Am J Hematol 44:117–124, 1993.

Kojima M, Nakamura S, Motoori T, et al: Centroblastic and centroblastic-centrocytic lymphomas associated with prominent epithelioid granulomatous response without plasma cell differentiation: a clinicopathologic study of 12 cases. Hum Pathol 27:660–667, 1996.

Korkolopoulou P, Cordell J, Jones M, et al: The expression of the B-cell marker Mb-1 (CD79a) in Hodgkin's disease. Histopathology 24:511–515, 1994.

Küppers R, Rajewsky K, Zhao M, et al: Hodgkin disease: Hodgkin and Reed-Sternberg cells picked from histological sections show clonal immunoglobulin gene rearrangements and appear to be derived from B cells at various stages of development. Proc Natl Acad Sci USA 91:10962–10966, 1994.

Kuzu I, Delsol G, Jones M, et al: Expression of the Ig associated heterodimer (Mb-1 and B29) in Hodgkin's disease. Histopathology 22:141–144, 1993.

Lennert K, Mohri N: Histological classification and occurrence of Hodgkin's disease. Internist 15:57–65, 1974.

Leoncini L, Spina D, Nyong'o A, et al: Neoplastic cells of Hodgkin's disease show differences in EBV expression between Kenya and Italy. Int J Cancer 65:781–784, 1996.

Levine AM: HIV-associated Hodgkin's disease: biologic and clinical aspects. Hemato Oncol Clin North Am 10:1135–1148, 1996.

Levy R, Colonna P, Tourani JM, et al: Human immunodeficiency virus associated Hodgkin's disease: report of 45 cases from the French Registry of HIV-Associated Tumors. Leuk Lymphoma 16:451–456, 1995.

Lister T, Crowther D, Sutcliffe S, et al: Report of a committee convened to discuss the evaluation and staging of patients with Hodgkin's disease: Cotswolds meeting. J Clin Oncol 7: 1630–1636, 1989.

Lukes R, Butler J: The pathology and nomenclature of Hodgkin's disease. Cancer Res 26:1063–1081, 1966.

Lukes RJ, Collins RD: Tumors of the hematopoietic system. In Hartman WH, Sobin LH (eds): Atlas of Tumor Pathology. Armed Forces Institute of Pathology, Washington, DC, p 225, 1992.

Lukes R, Craver L, Hall T, et al: Report of the nomenclature committee. Cancer Res. 26:1311–1326, 1966.

Lukes RJ: Criteria for involvement of lymph node, bone marrow, spleen, and liver in Hodgkin's disease. Cancer Res 31:1755–1767, 1971.

Lukes RJ, Butler JJ, Hicks EB: Natural history of Hodgkin's disease as related to its pathologic picture. Cancer 19:317–344, 1966.

Macavei M: Bone marrow biopsy (BMB): III. Bone marrow biopsy in Hodgkin's disease (HD). Morphol Embryol 36:25–32, 1990.

Macfarlane G, Evstifeeva T, Boyle P, et al: International patterns in the occurrence of Hodgkin's disease in children and young adult males. Int J Cancer 61:165–169, 1995.

Mack T, Cozen W, Shibata D, et al: Concordance for Hodgkin's disease in identical twins suggesting genetic susceptibility to the young-adult form of the disease. N Engl J Med 332:413–418, 1995.

MacLennan KA, Bennett MH, Tu A, et al: Relationship of histopathologic features to survival and relapse in nodular sclerosing Hodgkin's disease: a study of 1659 patients. Cancer 64: 1686–1693, 1989.

Macon WR, Williams ME, Greer JP, et al: T-cell–rich B-cell lymphomas: a clinicopathologic study of 19 cases. Am J Surg Pathol 16:351–363, 1992.

Manzanal A, Santon A, Oliva H, et al: Evaluation of clonal immunoglobulin heavy chain rearrangements in Hodgkin's disease using the polymerase chain reaction (PCR). Histopathology 27: 21–25, 1995.

Marafioti T, Hummel M, Anagnostopoulos I, et al: Origin of nodular lymphocyte-predominant Hodgkin's disease from a colnal expansion of highly mutated germinal-center B cells. N Engl J Med 14:453, 1997.

Marafioti T, Hummel M, Foss HD, et al: Hodgkin and Reed-Sternberg cells represent an expansion of a single clone originating from a germinal center B-cell with functional immunoglobulin gene rearrangements but defective immunoglobulin transcription. Blood 15:1443, 2000.

Masih A, Weisenburger D, Vose J, et al: Histologic grade does not predict prognosis in optimally treated, advanced-stage nodular sclerosing Hodgkin's disease. Cancer 69:228–232, 1992.

Medeiros L, Greiner T: Hodgkin's disease. Cancer 75(Suppl 1): 357–369, 1995.

Merz H, Houssiau FA, Orscheschek K, et al: Interleukin-9 expression in human malignant lymphomas: unique association with Hodgkin's disease and large cell anaplastic lymphoma. Blood 78:1311–1317, 1991.

Miettinen M, Franssila KO, Saxen E: Hodgkin's disease, lymphocytic predominance nodule: increased risk for subsequent non-Hodgkin's lymphomas. Cancer 51:2293–2300, 1983.

Momose H, Jaffe ES, Shin SS, et al: Chronic lymphocytic leukemia/small lymphocytic lymphoma with Reed-Sternberg-like cells and possible transformation to Hodgkin's disease: mediation by Epstein-Barr virus. Am J Surg Pathol 16:859–867, 1992.

Monfardini S, Tirelli U, Vaccher E: Hodgkin's disease in 63 intravenous drug users infected with HIV. Ann Oncol 2(Suppl 2):201, 1991.

Mueller N: Epidemiologic studies assessing the role of Epstein-Barr virus in Hodgkin's disease. Yale J Biol Med 60:321–332, 1987.

Mueller N, Evans A, Harris ML, et al: Hodgkin's disease and Epstein-Barr virus: altered antibody pattern before diagnosis. N Engl J Med 320:689–695, 1989.

Munker R, Hasenclever D, Brosteanu O, et al: Bone marrow involvement in Hodgkin's disease: an analysis of 135 consecutive cases. J Clin Oncol 13:403–409, 1995.

Munro JM, Freedman AS, Aster JC, et al: In vivo expression of the B7 costimulatory molecule by subsets of antigen-presenting cells and the malignant cells of Hodgkin's disease. Blood 83:793–798, 1994.

Neiman R: Current problems in the histopathologic diagnosis and classification of Hodgkin's disease. Pathol Ann 13:289–328, 1978.

Neiman R, Rosen P, Lukes R: Lymphocyte-depletion Hodgkin's disease: a clinicopathologic study. N Engl J Med 288:751–755, 1973.

Newcom SR, Ansari AA, Gu L: Interleukin-4 is an autocrine growth factor secreted by the L-428 Reed-Sternberg cell. Blood 79:191–197, 1992.

Newcom SR, Gu L: Transforming growth factor β1 messenger RNA in Reed-Sternberg cells in nodular sclerosing Hodgkin's disease. J Clin Pathol 48:160–163, 1995.

Ng CS, Chan JKC, Hui PK, et al: Large B-cell lymphomas with a high content of reactive T-cells. Hum Pathol 20:1145–1154, 1989.

Nguyen PL, Harris NL, Ritz J, et al: Expression of CD95 antigen and bcl-2 protein in non-Hodgkin's lymphomas and Hodgkin's disease. Am J Pathol 148:847–853, 1996.

Nicholas DS, Harris S, Wright DH: Lymphocyte predominance Hodgkin's disease: an immunohistochemical study. Histopathology 16:157–165, 1990.

Niedobitek G, Kremmer E, Herbst H, et al: Immunohistochemical detection of the Epstein-Barr virus–encoded latent membrane protein 2A in Hodgkin's disease and infectious mononucleosis. Blood 90:1664–1672, 1997.

O'Connor NTJ, Stein H, Gatter KC, et al: Genotypic analysis of large cell lymphomas which express the Ki-1 antigen. Histopathology 11:733–740, 1987.

O'Grady JT, Stewart S, Lowrey J, et al: CD40 expression in Hodgkin's disease. Am J Pathol 144:21–26, 1994.

Ohno T, Stribley JA, Wu G, Hinrichs SH, et al: Clonality in nodular lymphocyte-predominant Hodgkin's disease. N Engl J Med 14:459, 1997.

Ohshima K, Suzumiya J, Akamatu M, et al: Human and viral interleukin-10 in Hodgkin's disease, and its influence on CD4+ and CD8+ T lymphocytes. Int J Cancer 62:5–10, 1995.

Osborne BM, Butler JJ: Clinical implication of progressive transformation of germinal centers. Am J Surg Pathol 8:725, 1984.

Osborne BM, Butler JJ: Follicular lymphoma mimicking progressive transformation of germinal centers. Am J Clin Pathol 88: 264–269, 1987.

Osborne BM, Butler JJ, Pugh WC: The value of immunophenotyping on paraffin sections in the identification of T-cell rich B-cell large-cell lymphomas: lineage confirmed by J_H rearrangement. Am J Surg Pathol 14:933–938, 1990.

Oudejans JJ, Kummer JA, Jiwa M, et al: Granzyme B expression in Reed-Sternberg cells of Hodgkin's disease. Am J Pathol 148: 233–240, 1996.

Pallesen G, Sandvej K, Hamilton-Dutoit SJ, et al: Activation of Epstein-Barr virus replication in Hodgkin and Reed-Sternberg cells. Blood 78:1162–1165, 1991.

Pan LX, Diss TC, Peng HZ, et al: Nodular lymphocyte predominance Hodgkin's disease: a monoclonal or polyclonal B-cell disorder. Blood 87:2428–2434, 1996.

Pappa VI, Norton AJ, Gupta RK, et al: Nodular type of lymphocyte predominant Hodgkin's disease: a clinical study of 50 cases. Ann Oncol 6:559–565, 1995.

Parker S, Tong T, Bolden S, et al: Cancer statistics, 1996. CA Cancer J Clin 65:5–27, 1996.

Patsouris E, Nöel H, Lennert K: Angioimmunoblastic lymphadenopathy type of T-cell lymphoma with a high content of epithelioid cells: histopathology and comparison with lymphoepithelioid cell lymphoma. Am J Surg Pathol 13:262–275, 1989a.

Patsouris E, Nöel H, Lennert K: Cytohistologic and immunohistochemical findings in Hodgkin's disease, mixed cellularity type with a high content of epithelioid cells. Am J Surg Pathol 13: 1014–1022, 1989b.

Patsouris E, Nöel H, Lennert K: Histologic and immunohistologic findings in lymphoepithelioid cell lymphoma (Lennert's lymphoma). Am J Surg Pathol 12:341–350, 1988.

Patsouris E, Nöel H, Lennert K: Lymphoplasmacytic/lymphoplasmacytoid immunocytoma with a high content of epithelioid cells. Am J Surg Pathol 14:660–670, 1990.

Penny RJ, Blaustein JC, Longtine JA, et al: Ki-1 positive large cell lymphomas, a heterogeneous group of neoplasms: morphologic, immunophenotypic, genotypic, and clinical features of 24 cases. Cancer 68:362–373, 1991.

Picker L, Weiss L, Medeiros L, et al: Immunophenotypic criteria for the diagnosis of non-Hodgkin's lymphoma. Am J Pathol 128: 181–201, 1987.

Pileri S, Falini B, Delsol G, et al: Lymphohistiocytic T-cell lymphoma (anaplastic large cell lymphoma CD30+/Ki-1+ with a high content of reactive histiocytes). Histopathology 16:383–391, 1990.

Pinkus G, O'Hara C, Said J: Peripheral/post-thymic T-cell lymphomas: a spectrum of disease, clinical, pathologic, and immunologic features of 78 cases. Cancer 65:971–998, 1990.

Pinkus GS, Pinkus JL, Langhoff E, et al: Fascin, a sensitive new marker for Reed-Sternberg cells of Hodgkin's disease: evidence for a dendritic or B cell derivation? Am J Pathol 150:543–562, 1997.

Pinkus GS, Said JW: Hodgkin's disease, lymphocyte predominance type, nodular: a distinct entity? Unique staining profile for L and H variants of Reed-Sternberg cells defined by monoclonal antibodies to leukocyte common antigen, granulocyte-specific antigen, and B-cell-specific antigen. Am J Pathol 133:211–217, 1985.

Pinkus GS, Said JW: Hodgkin's disease, lymphocyte predominance type, nodular, further evidence for a B cell derivation: L and H variants of Reed-Sternberg cells express L26, a pan B cell marker. Am J Pathol 133:211–217, 1988.

Poppema S: The diversity of the immunohistological staining pattern of Sternberg-Reed cells. J Histochem Cytochem 28:788–791, 1980.

Poppema S: Lymphocyte-predominance Hodgkin's disease. Int Rev Exp Pathol 33:53–79, 1992.

Poppema S: The nature of the lymphocytes surrounding Reed-Sternberg cells in nodular lymphocyte predominance and in other types of Hodgkin's disease. Am J Pathol 135:351–357, 1989.

Poppema S, Kaiserling E, Lennert K: Epidemiology of nodular paragranuloma. J Cancer Res Clin Oncol 95:57, 1979a.

Poppema S, Kaiserling E, Lennert K: Hodgkin's disease with lymphocytic predominance, nodular type (nodular paragranuloma) and progressively transformed germinal centres: a cytohistological study. Histopathology 3:295–308, 1979b.

Poppema S, Kaleta J, Hepperle B: Chromosomal abnormalities in patients with Hodgkin's disease: evidence for frequent involvement of the 14q chromosomal region but infrequent bcl-2 gene rearrangement in Reed-Sternberg cells. J Natl Cancer Inst 84: 1789–1793, 1992.

Poppema S, Timens W, Visser L: Nodular lymphocyte predominance type of Hodgkin's disease is a B cell lymphoma. Adv Exp Med Biol 186:963–969, 1985.

Prazak J, Hermanska Z: Study of HLA antigens in patients with Hodgkin's disease. Eur J Haematol 43:50–53, 1989.

Ramsay AD, Smith WJ, Isaacson PG: T-cell–rich B-cell lymphoma. Am J Surg Pathol 12:433–443, 1988.

Regula DP, Hoppe RT, Weiss LM: Nodular and diffuse types of lymphocyte predominance Hodgkin's disease. N Engl J Med 318: 214–219, 1988.

Reynolds DJ, Banks PM, Gulley ML: New characterization of infectious mononucleosis and a phenotypic comparison with Hodgkin's disease. Am J Pathol 146:379–388, 1995.

Rodriguez J, Pugh WC, Cabanilla F: T-cell–rich B-cell lymphoma. Blood 82:1586–1589, 1993.

Rosdahl N, Larsen SO, Clemmesen J: Hodgkin's disease in patients with previous infectious mononucleosis: 30 years' experience. Br Med J 2:253–256, 1974.

Rosenberg S: The management of Hodgkin's disease: half a century of change. Ann Oncol 7:555–560, 1996.

Rosenberg S, Kaplan H: Evidence for an orderly progression in the spread of Hodgkin's disease. Cancer Res 26:1225–1231, 1966.

Roth MS, Schnitzer B, Bingham EL, et al: Rearrangement of immunoglobulin and T-cell receptor genes in Hodgkin's disease. Am J Pathol 131:331–338, 1988.

Ruco LP, Pomponi D, Pigott R, et al: Cytokine production (IL-1α, IL-1β, and TNFα) and endothelial cell activation (ELAM-1 and HLA-DR) in reactive lymphadenitis, Hodgkin's disease, and in non-Hodgkin's lymphomas: an immunocytochemical study. Am J Pathol 137:1163–1171, 1990.

Rysenga E, Linden MD, Carey JL, et al: Peripheral T-cell non-Hodgkin's lymphoma following treatment of nodular lymphocyte predominance Hodgkin's disease. Arch Pathol Lab Med 119: 88–91, 1995.

Sacks E, Donaldson S, Gordon J, et al: Epithelioid granulomas associated with Hodgkin's disease: clinical correlations in 55 previously untreated patients. Cancer, 1978.

Sankila R, Garwicz S, Olsen JH, et al: Risk of subsequent malignant neoplasms among 1,641 Hodgkin's disease patients diagnosed in childhood and adolescence: a population-based cohort study in the five Nordic countries. J Clin Oncol 14:1442–1446, 1996.

Schlegelberger B, Weber-Matthiesen K, Himmler A, et al: Cytogenetic findings and results of combined immunophenotyping and karyotyping in Hodgkin's disease. Leukemia 8:72–80, 1994.

Schmid C, Pan L, Diss T, et al: Expression of B-cell antigens by Hodgkin's and Reed-Sternberg cells. Am J Pathol 139:701–707, 1991.

Schmid U, Metz KA, Leder LD: T-cell–rich B-cell lymphoma and lymphocyte-predominant Hodgkin's disease: two closely related entities? Br J Haematol 90:398–403, 1995.

Schwarting R, Gerdes J, Dürkop H, et al: Ber-H2: A new anti-Ki-1 (CD30) monoclonal antibody directed at a formol-resistant epitope. Blood 74:1678–1689, 1989.

Serraino D, Carbone A, Franceschi S, et al: Increased frequency of lymphocyte depletion and mixed cellularity subtypes of Hodgkin's disease in HIV-infected patients. Eur J Cancer 29A:1948–1950, 1993.

Siebert J, Stuckey J, Kurtin P, et al: Extranodal lymphocyte predominance Hodgkin's disease: clinical and pathologic features. Am J Clin Pathol 103:485–491, 1995.

Slivnick J, Ellis T, Nawrocki J, et al: The impact of Hodgkin's disease on the immune system. Semin Oncol 17:673–682, 1990.

Stansfeld A: The histological diagnosis of toxoplasmic lymphadenitis. J Clin Pathol 14:565–573, 1961.

Stein H, Gerdes J, Schwab U, et al: Identification of Hodgkin and Sternberg-Reed cells as a unique cell type derived from a newly-detected small-cell population. Int J Cancer 30:445–459, 1982.

Stein H, Hansmann ML, Lennert K, et al: Reed-Sternberg and Hodgkin cells in lymphocyte-predominant Hodgkin's disease of nodular subtype contain J chain. Am J Clin Pathol 86:292–297, 1986.

Stein H, Mason DY, Gerdes J, et al: The expression of the Hodgkin's disease associated antigen Ki-1 in reactive and neoplastic lymphoid tissue: evidence that Reed-Sternberg cells and histiocytic malignancies are derived from activated lymphoid cells. Blood 66:848–858, 1985.

Stoler MH, Nichols GE, Symbula M, et al: Lymphocyte predominance Hodgkin's disease: evidence for a κ light chain–restricted monotypic B-cell neoplasm. Am J Pathol 146:812–818, 1995.

Strickler J, Miche S, Warnke R, et al: The "syncytial variant" of nodular sclerosing Hodgkin's disease. Am J Surg Pathol 10:470–477, 1986.

Strum S, Rappaport H: Significance of focal involvement of lymph nodes for the diagnosis and staging of Hodgkin's disease. Cancer 25:1314–1319, 1970.

Sundeen JT, Cossman J, Jaffe ES: Lymphocyte predominant Hodgkin's disease nodular subtype with coexistent "large cell lymphoma": histological progression or composite malignancy. Am J Surg Pathol 12:599–606, 1988.

Sundeen J, Lipford E, Uppenkamp M, et al: Rearranged antigen receptor genes in Hodgkin's disease. Blood 70:96–103, 1987.

Tamaru J, Hummel M, Zemlin M, et al: Hodgkin's disease with a B-cell phenotype often shows a VDJ rearrangement and somatic mutations in the V_H genes. Blood 84:708–715, 1994.

Tefferi A, Wiltsie JC, Kurtin PJ: Secondary T-cell lymphoma in the setting of nodular lymphocyte predominance Hodgkin's disease. Am J Hematol 40:232–233, 1992.

Tefferi A, Zellers RA, Banks PM, et al: Clinical correlates of distinct immunophenotypic and histologic subcategories of lymphocyte-predominance Hodgkin's disease. J Clin Oncol 8:1959–1965, 1990.

Tindle B, Parker J, Lukes R: "Reed-Sternberg cells" in infectious mononucleosis? Am J Clin Pathol 58:607–617, 1972.

Tirelli U, Vaccher E, Rezza G, et al: Hodgkin's disease and infection with the human immunodeficiency virus (HIV) in Italy. Ann Intern Med 108:309–310, 1988.

Trudel MA, Krikorian JG, Neiman RS: Lymphocyte predominance Hodgkin's disease: a clinicopathologic reassessment. Cancer 59:99–106, 1987.

Tsang WYW, Chan JKC, Ng CS: The nature of Reed-Sternberg-like cells in chronic lymphocytic leukemia. Am J Clin Pathol 99: 317–323, 1993.

Tucker M: Solid second cancers following Hodgkin's disease. Hematol Oncol Clin North Am 7:389–400, 1993.

Uccini S, Monardo F, Stoppacciaro A, et al: High frequency of Epstein-Barr virus genome detection in Hodgkin's disease of HIV-positive patients. Int J Cancer 46:581–585, 1990.

Van Gool S, Delabie J, Vandenberghe P, et al: Expression of B7-2 (CD86) molecules by Reed-Sternberg cells of Hodgkin's disease. Leukemia 11:846–851, 1997.

van Spronsen D, Vrints L, Hofstra G, et al: Disappearance of prognostic significance of histopathological grading of nodular sclerosing Hodgkin's disease for unselected patients, 1972–92. Br J Haematol 96:322–327, 1997.

Von Kalle C, Diehl V: Hodgkin's disease: analysis of cell line data. Int Rev Exp Pathol 33:185–203, 1992.

von Wasielewski R, Werner M, Fischer R, et al: Lymphocyte-predominant Hodgkin's disease: an immunohistochemical analysis of 208 reviewed Hodgkin's disease cases from the German Hodgkin Study Group. Am J Pathol 150:793–803, 1997.

Warnke RA, Weiss LM, Chan JKC, et al: Tumors of the lymph nodes and spleen. In Atlas of Tumor Pathology. Armed Forces Institute of Pathology, Washington, DC, p 277, 1995.

Weber-Matthiesen K, Deerberg J, Poetsch M, et al: Clarification of dubious karyotypes in Hodgkin's disease by simultaneous fluorescence immunophenotyping and interphase cytogenetics (FICTION). Cytogenet Cell Genet 70:243–245, 1995a.

Weber-Matthiesen K, Deerberg J, Poetsch M, et al: Numerical chromosome aberrations are present within the CD30+ Hodgkin and Reed-Sternberg cells in 100% of analyzed cases of Hodgkin's disease. Blood 86:1464–1468, 1995b.

Weinreb M, Day PJR, Niggli F, et al: The consistent association between Epstein-Barr virus and Hodgkin's disease in children in Kenya. Blood 87:3828–3836, 1996.

Weiss LM: Gene analysis and Epstein-Barr viral genome studies of Hodgkin's disease. Int Rev Exp Pathol 33:165–184, 1992.

Weiss LM, Chang KL: Molecular biologic studies of Hodgkin's disease. Semin Diag Pathol 9:272–278, 1992.

Weiss LM, Chen YY, Liu XF, et al: Epstein-Barr virus and Hodgkin's disease: a correlative *in situ* hybridization and polymerase chain reaction study. Am J Pathol 139:1259–1265, 1991.

Weiss LM, Strickler JG, Warnke RA, et al: Epstein-Barr viral DNA in tissues of Hodgkin's disease. Am J Pathol 129:86–91, 1987.

Wickert RS, Weisenburger DD, Tierens A, et al: Clonal relationship between lymphocytic predominance Hodgkin's disease and concurrent or subsequent large-cell lymphoma of B lineage. Blood 86:2312–2320, 1995.

Wijlhuizen T, Vrints L, Fairam R, et al: Grades of nodular sclerosis (NSI-NSII) in Hodgkin's disease: are they of independent prognostic value? Cancer 63:1150–1153, 1989.

Williams J, Schned A, Cotelingam JD, et al: Chronic lymphocytic leukemia with coexistant Hodgkin's disease: implications for the origin of the Reed-Sternberg cell. Am J Surg Pathol 15:33–42, 1991.

Zarate-Osorno A, Medeiros J, Longo DL, et al: Non-Hodgkin's lymphomas arising in patients successfully treated for Hodgkin's disease: a clinical, histologic, and immunophenotypic study of 14 cases. Am J Surg Pathol 16:885–895, 1992.

Zarate-Osorno A, Roman LN, Kingma DW, et al: Hodgkin's disease in Mexico: prevalence of Epstein-Barr virus sequences and correlations with histologic subtype. Cancer 75:1360–1366, 1994.

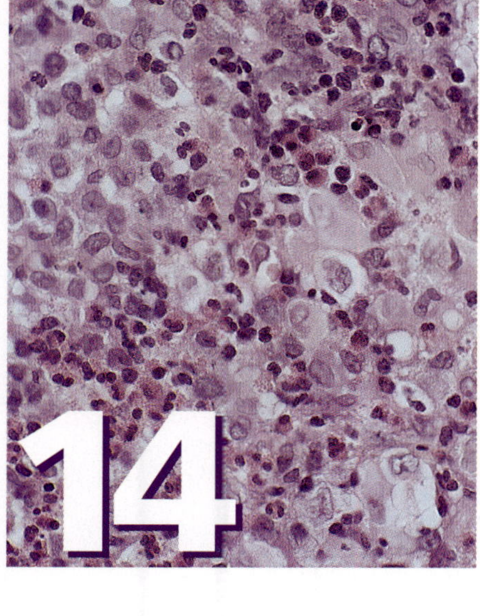

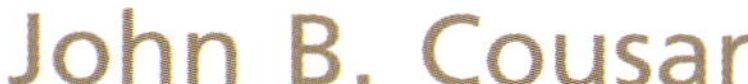
John B. Cousar

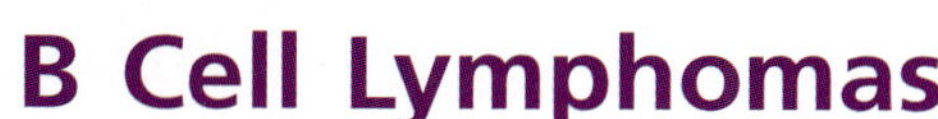

B Cell Lymphomas

Malignant lymphomas of B cell origin account for approximately 50–60% of lymphomas other than Hodgkin disease in children (Kjeldsberg et al, 1983; Murphy et al, 1989; Perkins et al, 1995; Sandlund et al, 1996; Wilson et al, 1984). In contrast to adults, childhood B cell lymphomas are almost exclusively aggressive, high-grade malignancies with a marked propensity for extranodal and advanced-stage presentation. Small transformed (noncleaved) cell lymphomas, including Burkitt and Burkitt-like lymphomas, are by far the most common types, followed by large B cell lymphomas. Children rarely develop follicular lymphomas, small lymphocytic lymphomas, or other types of low-grade B cell neoplasms.

The study of B cell lymphomas, particularly Burkitt lymphomas, in children has contributed greatly to our understanding of the biology and pathogenesis of all types of cancers. Technologic advances in flow cytometry, immunohistochemistry, cytogenetics, and molecular biology have improved diagnostic precision and led to the recognition of new clinicopathologic entities.

SMALL TRANSFORMED (NONCLEAVED) CELL LYMPHOMAS: BURKITT AND BURKITT-LIKE LYMPHOMAS

Equivalent Terms and Definitions

Small transformed cell lymphomas are B cell tumors, highly proliferative, and composed of monomorphic populations of blastic-appearing small noncleaved or transformed lymphocytes (Berard et al, 1969; Harris et al, 1994; Lennert & Feller, 1992; Lukes & Collins, 1992; Non-Hodgkin's Classification Project, 1982; Warnke et al, 1995). Small transformed cell lymphoma has two subtypes: Burkitt lymphoma (recognized by all classification systems) and similar lymphomas variously designated as Burkitt-like (Revised European-American Lymphoma (REAL) classification), non-Burkitt type (Lukes-Collins classification and Working Formulation), and undifferentiated non-Burkitt type (Rappaport classification).

Background

Burkitt tumor was first reported in 1958 as an unusual "sarcoma of the jaws" in children of equatorial Africa (Burkitt, 1958). Subsequently, this neoplasm was recognized as a malignant lymphoma (O'Conor & Davies, 1960). Later, childhood tumors histologically similar to Burkitt lymphoma were reported in the United States (O'Conor et al, 1965) and Europe. The morphologic features of Burkitt lymphoma were strictly defined by a World Health Organization (WHO)–sponsored group of experts in 1969 (Berard et al, 1969), and the neoplasm became a subtype of undifferentiated lymphomas in the Rappaport classification. The name *malignant lymphoma of small noncleaved follicular center cells* was proposed to emphasize the resemblance of the predominant cell in the tumor to a presumed counterpart in normal follicular centers (Lukes & Collins, 1974). Currently, most classification systems include two morphologic subtypes: Burkitt type, as defined by the WHO (Berard et al, 1969), and non-Burkitt type, which demonstrates more morphologic variability. The value of making the distinction between Burkitt and non-Burkitt small transformed cell lymphoma is controversial. In children, there is little to suggest that this histologic subdivision corresponds to significant clinical, phenotypic, karyotypic, or molecular differences (Magrath, 1997).

Investigations of Burkitt lymphoma have provided many seminal contributions to the pathogenesis and treatment of neoplasms (Magrath, 1991). Burkitt lymphoma was the first human cancer to be (1) associated with a virus (i.e., the Epstein-Barr virus [EBV]), (2) curable by chemotherapy alone, and (3) linked to a chromosomal translocation involved in its pathogenesis. Furthermore, it was the first lymphoma from which continuous cell culture lines were established and the first shown to express surface immunoglobulin.

Clinical Features

Burkitt lymphoma is endemic in equatorial Africa and New Guinea but is sporadic in its occurrence in North America and Western Europe. African (endemic) Burkitt lymphoma and Burkitt lymphoma occurring in the United States (sporadic) exhibit significant clinicopathologic differences (Table 14–1) (Arseneau et al, 1975; Burkitt & O'Conor, 1961; Levine et al, 1983, Levine et al, 1982; Levine et al., 1975; Magrath, 1997; Magrath, 1991; Shad & Magrath, 1997). The average annual incidence of Burkitt lymphoma in equatorial Africa is 10 in 100,000 children, and the tumor accounts for approximately 50% of childhood cancers (Shad & Magrath, 1997). In the United States, small transformed cell lymphoma is uncommon but represents 40–50% of childhood B and T cell lymphomas. The peak age for the occurrence of small transformed cell lymphoma in children is slightly older in the United States than in Africa, where very few cases occur after the age of 15 years. In both endemic and sporadic Burkitt lymphoma, the male-female incidence ratio is approximately 2:1.

Table 14–1
Comparison of Endemic and Sporadic Burkitt Lymphoma

Feature	Endemic	Sporadic
Annual incidence in children < 16 years	10 in 100,000	0.2 in 100,000
Peak age and sex	5–10 years More males than females	Slightly older More males than females
Geographic occurrence	Climatically determined (e.g., equatorial Africa, New Guinea); suggests malaria may play a role in pathogenesis	No relationship to climate
Common sites of tumor	Jaw, abdomen, central nervous system, cerebrospinal fluid	Abdomen, marrow, lymph nodes
Histopathologic features	Same	Same
Immunologic features	Usually IgM, κ or λ CD10+; no IgM paraprotein	Usually IgM, κ or λ CD10+; may secrete IgM
Presence of Epstein-Barr virus DNA in tumor cells	95%	15%[a]
Karyotype and molecular genetics		
Presence of t(8;14), t(2;8), or t(8,22)	Yes	Yes
Chromosome 8 break points	Upstream of MYC	Within MYC

[a]Recent evidence suggests that this estimate may be low (Razzouk et al, 1996).

Source: Modified from Shad A, Magrath I: Malignant non-Hodgkin's lymphomas in childhood. In Pizzo PA, Poplack DG (eds): Principles and Practice of Pediatric Oncology, 3rd ed. Lippincott-Raven, Philadelphia, pp 545–587, 1997.

The geographic distribution of Burkitt lymphoma in equatorial Africa suggested a climatically determined infectious cause (Burkitt, 1962). Investigation of this possibility led to the discovery of EBV (Epstein et al, 1964). EBV genome is found in virtually all cases of African Burkitt lymphoma but only in a minority of the tumors occurring in the United States. Since the distribution of Burkitt lymphoma in Africa corresponds to regions of holoendemic malaria (Shad & Magrath, 1997), it seems likely that African cases are related to coinfection with EBV and malaria. The contribution of EBV may be immortalization of B cells and polyclonal lymphoproliferation (Klein et al, 1976), whereas malaria likely causes immune suppression. EBV infection is ubiquitous, but its role in the pathogenesis of sporadic cases has not been established. African Burkitt lymphoma often involves the facial bones, particularly the mandible and maxilla. Abdominal involvement is also frequent. In the United States, children rarely have jaw involvement, but abdominal disease occurs in >90% of cases. Infiltration of the bowel, particularly the ileocecal region and abdominal lymph nodes, is frequent, and intussusception due to tumor is seen in as many as 30% of patients. Disease is detected in the cerebrospinal fluid in approximately 20% of patients with African Burkitt lymphoma and less often in sporadic cases. Marrow involvement appears commoner in sporadic Burkitt lymphoma.

Burkitt lymphoma is the most rapidly growing human neoplasm, with growth fractions approaching 100% in some cases (Magrath, 1997) and with doubling times of a few days. These cytokinetic features have important clinical consequences. As a result of the high tumor cell turnover, tumor lysis syndrome may develop, especially in patients with large tumor burden (Cohen et al, 1980). Hyperuricemia, with subsequent renal insufficiency, hyperkalemia, and hyperphosphatemia with hypocalcemia may occur shortly after the initiation of therapy (Magrath, 1997). The high growth fraction is also partly responsible for the excellent response of Burkitt lymphoma to chemotherapy (Magrath, 1997).

Histopathologic Features

Both Burkitt and non-Burkitt small transformed cell lymphomas characteristically demonstrate a diffuse infiltrative growth pattern (Fig. 14–1) (Berard et al, 1969; Lukes & Collins, 1992; Warnke et al, 1995). The infiltrate often extends into extranodal fat and soft tissues (Fig. 14–2) and frequently infiltrates the wall of the bowel (Fig. 14–3). Occasionally, the tumor may encase uninvolved nodes or other capsular organs (Berard et al, 1969; Banks et al, 1975) or focally involve nodes adjacent to a primary tumor mass (Pavlova et al, 1987).

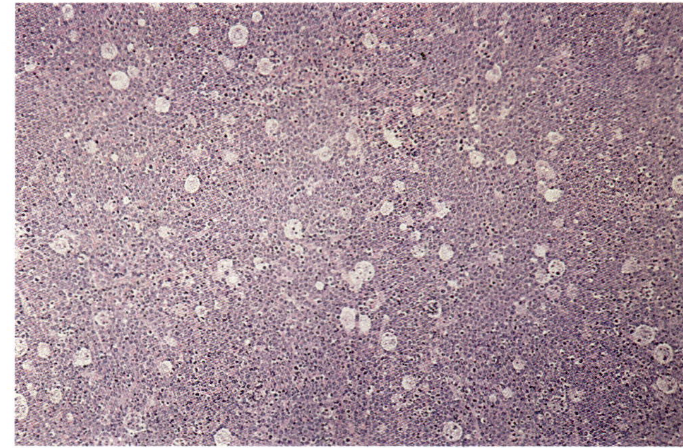

Figure 14–1

Small transformed cell lymphoma, Burkitt type, abdominal lymph node. At low magnification, the nodal architecture is effaced by a diffuse (nonfollicular) proliferation. Starry sky macrophages are prominent.

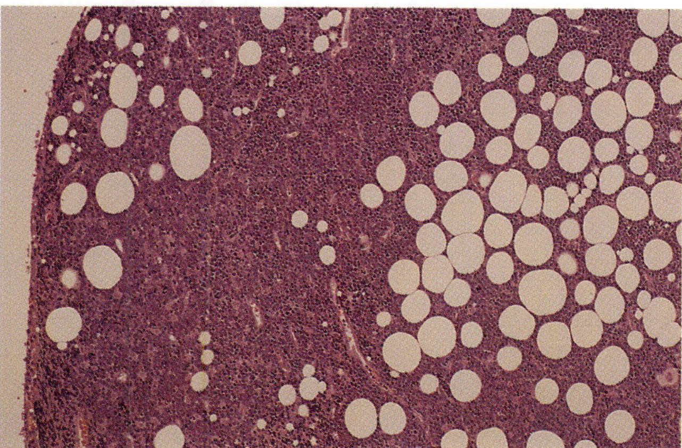

Figure 14–2

Small transformed cell lymphoma, Burkitt type, perinodal soft tissue and fat. This type of infiltrative pattern is often seen in Burkitt lymphoma.

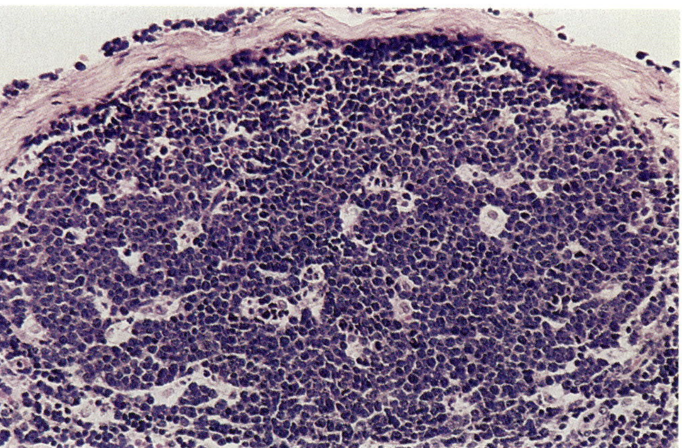

Figure 14–4

Small transformed cell lymphoma, Burkitt type, lymph node. There is selective involvement of follicles in an otherwise uninvolved node adjacent to a large tumor mass.

Infrequently, small transformed cell lymphoma may selectively involve follicular centers of nodes (Fig. 14–4) (Mann et al, 1976; Pavlova et al, 1987).

The distinction between the Burkitt and non-Burkitt types of small transformed cell lymphoma is based on the cytologic appearance of the tumor cells (Berard et al, 1969; Lukes & Collins, 1992; Pavlova et al, 1987; Warnke et al, 1995). In histologic sections, neoplastic cells of the Burkitt type are uniform in size, with nuclei no larger than those of reactive histiocytes (Fig. 14–5). The term *small transformed cell* refers to the overall size compared to that of large transformed cells. Nuclei are uniform and round, with distinct nuclear membranes. Two to five nucleoli are typical, and chromatin is finely granular, with areas of parachromatin clearing. Tumor cells have a thin rim of amphophilic cytoplasm around most of the nuclei. There is strong pyroninophilia owing to the abundance of polyribosomes (Fig. 14–6). Neoplastic cells may closely abut one another and have a cohesive or "jigsaw puzzle–like" appearance in formalin-fixed sections (Warnke et al, 1995). Mitotic figures are numerous, indicative of a highly proliferative tumor. Karyorrhexis is common, and macrophages containing cell debris or "tingible bodies" may impart a "starry sky" pattern (see Fig. 14–1).

In Wright-Giemsa smears or touch preparations, the neoplastic cells are 20–25 μ in diameter, with uniform nuclei containing stippled chromatin and prominent nucleoli (Fig. 14–7). Cytoplasm is intensely basophilic and often contains vacuoles, which are rich in lipid, as demonstrated with neutral fat stains.

Electron microscopic examination shows that the tumor cells of the Burkitt type are similar to small transformed cells of reactive follicular centers (Glick et al, 1974). Nuclei have round to irregular profiles and prominent nucleoli (Payne et al, 1987), and the cytoplasm contains abundant polyribosomes.

The neoplastic cells of the non-Burkitt type of small transformed cell lymphoma are more variable in size and are often admixed with multinucleated cells and large transformed cells

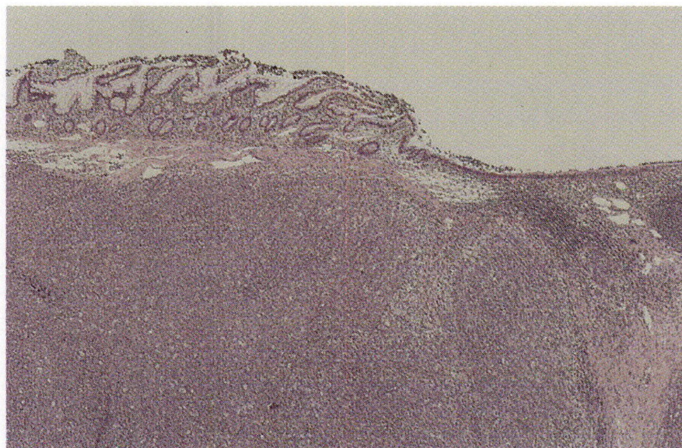

Figure 14–3

Small transformed cell lymphoma, bowel. At low magnification the tumor can be seen pushing up against the overlying uninvolved mucosa.

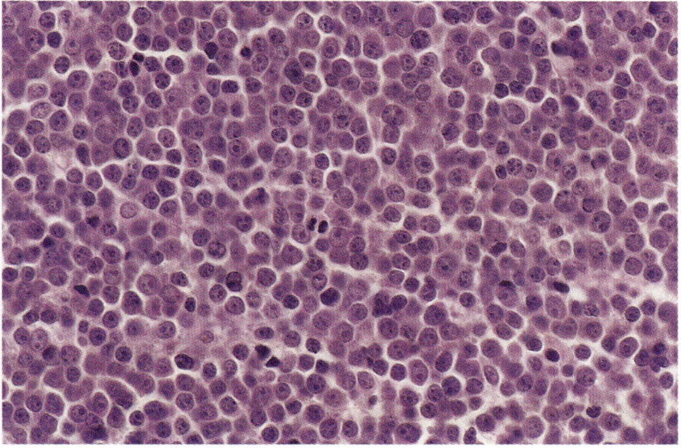

Figure 14–5

Small transformed cell lymphoma, Burkitt type, lymph node. At high magnification the neoplastic cells are uniform in size. Nuclear size is equivalent to or smaller than that of reactive histiocytes. Nucleoli are single or multiple and are often adjacent to the nuclear membrane. Mitoses are frequent.

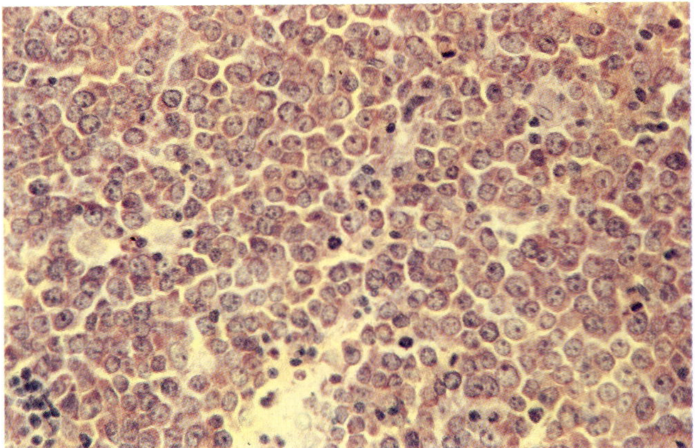

Figure 14–6

Small transformed cell lymphoma, Burkitt type. Strongly pyroninophilic cytoplasm rims most of the circumference of the nuclei. Methyl green pyronine.

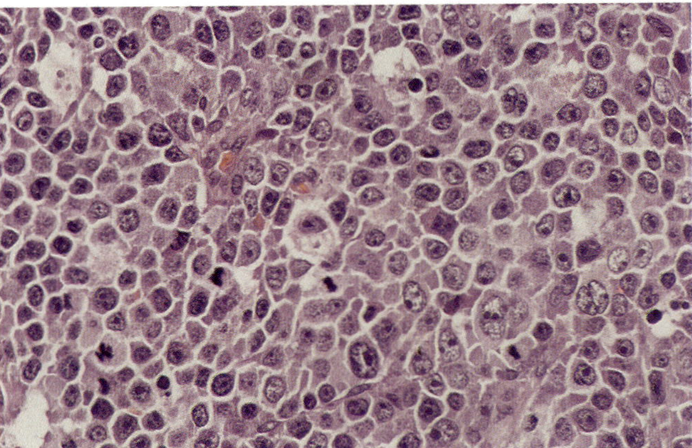

Figure 14–8

Small transformed cell lymphoma, non-Burkitt type. The neoplastic cells exhibit more variability in size and irregularity of nuclei. Nucleoli are more likely to be centrally placed than in Burkitt type. An admixture of larger tumor cells is also appreciated. Mitoses are frequent.

(Fig. 14–8) (Lukes & Collins, 1992; Pavlova et al, 1987; Warnke et al, 1995). Nuclear configurations are more irregular and nuclear membranes less prominent than in the Burkitt type. Nucleoli are usually fewer in number than in Burkitt type and often centrally placed. Cytoplasm is often more abundant in the non-Burkitt type of tumor.

By strict adherence to these guidelines, cases of small transformed cell lymphomas may be separated into Burkitt and non-Burkitt types (Pavlova et al, 1987), but diagnostic reproducibility is not high (Wilson et al, 1987). To date there are no clinical, phenotypic, or molecular genetic features in children that correspond to this subdivision (Shad & Magrath, 1997). In adults, the non-Burkitt variant is more clinically and cytogenetically heterogeneous and overlaps with large-cell lymphomas.

There is virtual morphologic and immunologic identity between small transformed cell lymphomas and the L3 type of acute lymphocytic leukemia (Brunning & McKenna, 1994; Flandrin et al, 1975) (see Chap. 4). L3 acute lymphocytic leukemia (Fig. 14–9) appears identical on Wright-Giemsa–stained smears to small transformed cell lymphoma and has a similar phenotype, with surface immunoglobulin and no terminal deoxyribonucleotidyl transferase. There is abundant evidence that L3 leukemia represents marrow and blood involvement by small transformed cell lymphoma in the absence of obvious extranodal disease (Warnke et al, 1995).

Immunophenotypic Features

Virtually all cases of childhood small transformed cell lymphoma demonstrate a B cell phenotype with surface immunoglobulin (Garcia et al, 1987; Grogan et al, 1982; Warnke et al, 1995; Yano et al, 1992). Most cases express IgM, with or without IgD, and only rarely IgG. Burkitt lymphoma characteristically expresses a number of B cell–specific antigens, including CD19, CD20 (Fig. 14–10), and CD22, as well

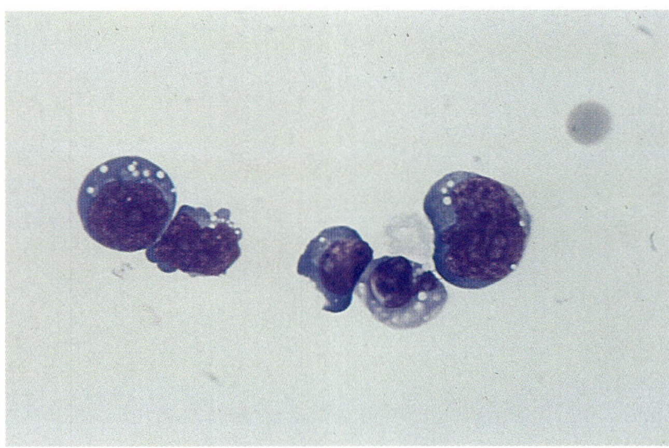

Figure 14–7

Small transformed cell lymphoma. A partially granular chromatin pattern, prominent nucleoli, and abundant, deeply basophilic cytoplasm containing vacuoles are apparent in this cytocentrifuged preparation. Wright stain.

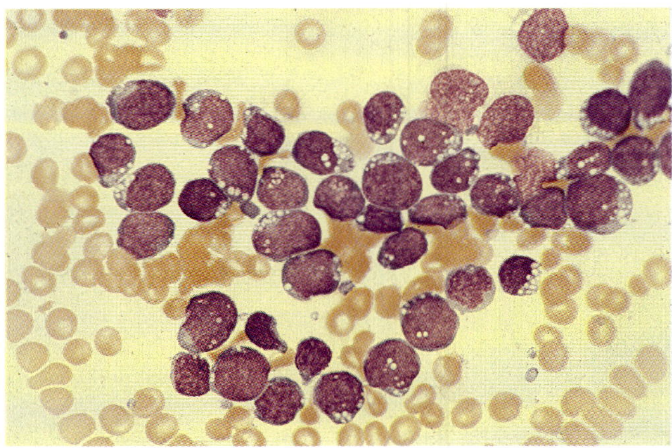

Figure 14–9

Small transformed cell lymphoma, marrow. This film shows cells that are cytologically identical to those in L3 acute lymphocytic leukemia. Wright stain.

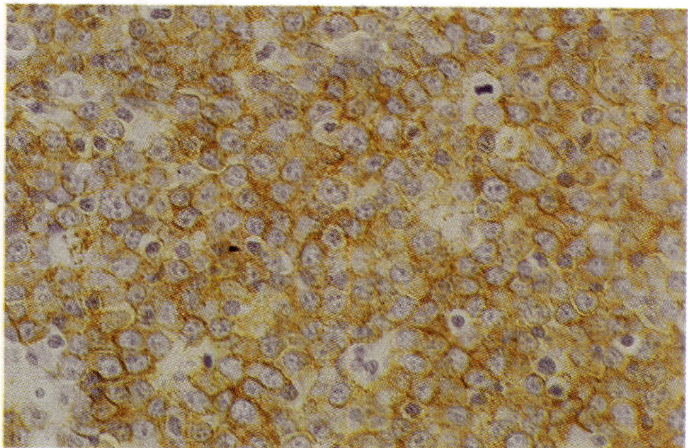

Figure 14–10

Small transformed cell lymphoma, Burkitt type. Strong membrane positivity for CD20 (L26) is revealed using a paraffin-embedded immunoperoxidase technique.

as nonlineage specific markers, such as HLA-DR. Most cases also demonstrate CD10, the common acute lymphocytic leukemia antigen). CD5 and CD23 expression are not seen. Activation markers, such as CD25 and CD30, generally are not present on small transformed cell lymphomas, although these lymphomas characteristically have a high Ki-67 index, indicative of a high proliferation ratio. Terminal deoxyribonucleotidyl transferase is not expressed. The absence of this marker helps differentiate small transformed cell lymphomas from neoplasms such as lymphoblastic lymphomas and leukemias, in which it is constantly expressed. The sporadic variant of Burkitt lymphoma is reported in some cases to secrete IgM in sufficient quantity to be detectable by protein electrophoresis (Shad & Magrath, 1997). African Burkitt lymphomas demonstrate no such paraproteinemia.

Cytogenetic and Molecular Genetic Features

Abundant information about the pathogenesis of small transformed cell lymphomas has been obtained from cytogenetic and molecular genetic studies. The great majority of small transformed cell lymphomas of childhood demonstrate a t(8;14)(q23;q21) translocation and, less frequently, variant translocations, t(8;22), and t(2;8) (Bernheim et al, 1981; Lenoir et al, 1982; Magrath & Bhatia, 1997; Manolov & Manolova, 1972). A unifying feature of these translocations is the involvement of chromosome 8 band q23, the site of the *MYC* oncogene. In Burkitt lymphoma, *MYC* on chromosome 8 is involved in a translocation with either the immunoglobulin heavy-chain locus at 14q32, the κ light-chain locus at 2p13, or the λ light-chain locus at 22q11. These translocations correlate with immunoglobulin light-chain expression by the tumor. Cases with t(8;14) express κ or λ light chains, and tumors containing t(2;8) or t(8;22) express κ or λ light chains (Lenoir et al, 1982).

The *MYC* oncogene (on chromosome 8) has a key role in cell proliferation and differentiation. Its translocation with chromosomes 2, 14, or 22 results in deregulation and overexpression of the *MYC* gene (Dalla-Favera et al, 1982) and probably maintains the affected cells in a proliferative state (Shad & Magrath, 1997).

The specific sites of break points on chromosome 8 involving the *MYC* locus appear to be correlated with the geographic origin of Burkitt lymphoma (Williams et al, 1995). In sporadic Burkitt lymphoma, the break points occur within or close to the *MYC* locus on chromosome 8, but in endemic cases the break points are mapped outside the *MYC* locus (Neri et al, 1988). It is unclear whether these differences reflect alterations occurring at different stages of B cell development.

Differential Diagnosis

Small transformed cell lymphomas resemble "small blue cell tumors" and must be distinguished from embryonal rhabdomyosarcoma, neuroblastoma, and Ewing sarcoma (see Chap. 16). Burkitt lymphoma can usually be easily differentiated from these neoplasms by morphologic features and immunohistochemical characteristics.

Differentiation of Burkitt lymphoma from lymphoblastic lymphoma is more difficult. However, the anatomic distribution of lymphoblastic lymphoma is nearly always supradiaphragmatic and mediastinal. Both sites are unusual at presentation in small transformed cell lymphoma. The neoplastic cells of lymphoblastic lymphoma have nuclei with more finely dispersed chromatin and less conspicuous nucleoli than do small transformed cells. The cytoplasm in lymphoblastic lymphoma is scant, not pyroninophilic, and is frequently evident only at one pole of the cell. Immunophenotypic studies are quite helpful in the distinction of lymphoblastic lymphoma from Burkitt lymphoma. Lymphoblastic lymphoma is usually of T lineage, with an immature phenotype, including terminal deoxyribonucleotidyl transferase positivity (see Chap. 15), in contrast to small transformed cell lymphoma, which has a B phenotype and is terminal deoxyribonucleotidyl transferase negative. Another hematopoietic tumor that must be distinguished from Burkitt lymphoma is granulocytic sarcoma. The distribution of disease can be quite similar, given the proclivity of granulocytic sarcoma for involving the orbital bones and the gonads. Leukemic infiltrates demonstrate more eosinophilic cytoplasm than seen in Burkitt lymphoma (Warnke et al, 1995) and are often observed around follicles. Cytochemical stains, including the Leder stain in tissue sections or immunohistochemical stains for myeloperoxidase, are helpful in identification of granulocytic sarcoma (see Chap. 16).

LARGE B CELL LYMPHOMAS

Equivalent Terms and Definitions

In children, large B cell lymphomas include lymphomas classified as large-cell and immunoblastic lymphomas (Working Formulation), large transformed (noncleaved) follicular center cell and immunoblastic lymphoma of B cells (Lukes and Collins classification), diffuse histiocytic lymphoma (Rappaport classification), centroblastic and immunoblastic lymphomas (Kiel classification), and diffuse large B cell lymphoma, including the primary mediastinal large B cell lymphoma subtype (REAL classification). Large B cell lymphomas are uncommon in children. They usually demonstrate a diffuse infiltrate composed of transformed B lymphocytes with nuclei larger than those of reactive histiocytes.

Background

Large-cell lymphomas in children and adults are clinically, morphologically, and immunophenotypically heterogeneous. In the past, these tumors were classified by morphologic features alone, as large cell, histiocytic, or immunoblastic (Kjeldsberg et al, 1983; Murphy et al, 1989; Wilson et al, 1984), and as a group represented 15–30% of childhood B and T cell lymphomas. The immunophenotype of childhood large-cell lymphomas has not been extensively studied (Hutchinson et al, 1995), but it is now recognized that anaplastic (Ki-1+) large-cell lymphoma (see Chap. 15) makes up approximately 30–40% of this group. The remainder are mostly of B cell type, and most large B cell lymphomas in children are classified as large transformed cell, centroblastic, and immunoblastic B (Nathwani et al, 1987; Reiter et al, 1995; Reiter & Riehm, 1997).

Clinical Features

Large B cell lymphomas occur most frequently in the 10- to 15-year-old age group and are rare under the age of 3 years (Reiter & Riehm, 1997). Males are affected slightly more frequently than are females. No genetic predispositions have been identified for large B cell lymphomas in children.

The clinical features of large B cell lymphomas in children are more diverse and less distinct than those of small transformed cell lymphoma (Link & Donaldson, 1998). Any node group, including mediastinal and retroperitoneal, may be involved. Extranodal disease may be seen in the intestine and in unusual sites, such as soft tissue and bone. The marrow and cerebrospinal fluid are rarely involved.

A distinct subtype of large B cell lymphoma often involves the mediastinum and is associated with sclerosis (Cazals-Hatem et al, 1996; Miller et al, 1981; Piiera et al, 1995). Commonly seen in young adults, it has been described in adolescents and children. Females are affected more frequently than are males. Patients with this lymphoma usually present with a mediastinal mass. This subtype has a proclivity for local invasion, and superior vena caval obstruction is common.

Histopathologic Features

There are few detailed morphologic studies of large B cell lymphomas in children. Most cases resemble the histopathologic variants described in adults. In a Pediatric Oncology Group study, large transformed and immunoblastic lymphoma B types represented the major categories (Nathwani et al, 1987).

Large transformed cell lymphomas resemble cells in follicular centers from which they presumably arise (Lukes & Collins, 1992). The growth pattern is usually diffuse, and the tumor is composed of neoplastic large lymphocytes with nuclei larger than those of reactive histiocytes (Figs. 14–11 and 14–12). Nucleoli are often multiple and characteristically located at the nuclear membrane. Cytoplasm is moderately abundant and pyroninophilic. Mitoses are easily found. In the background, small lymphocytes with irregular nuclei are often seen. Frequently, scattered binucleated or multinucleated tumor cells are found.

An unusual variant of large B cell lymphomas termed multilobated has been reported rarely in adolescents (O'Hara et al, 1986; van Baarlen et al, 1988; Weiss et al, 1985). The infiltrate is rich in neoplastic cells containing multilobated nuclei (Fig. 14–13). Immunohistochemical and ultrastructural evidence suggests that the neoplasm is of follicular center origin (O'Hara et al, 1986).

The growth pattern of immunoblastic lymphoma B is diffuse, and the neoplastic cells are large, with abundant amphophilic and pyroninophilic cytoplasm, often imparting a plasmacytic appearance (Fig. 14–14) (Lukes & Collins, 1992; Warnke et al, 1995). Nucleoli may be prominent and centrally placed or multiple and scattered. An admixture of immature

Figure 14–11

Large-cell lymphoma, lymph node. At low magnification the growth pattern is diffuse and completely effaces the node.

cells with plasmacytic features and plasma cells may be present. Mitotic figures are abundant.

Primary mediastinal (thymic) large B cell lymphomas usually demonstrate a diffuse large-cell proliferation (Cazals-Hatem et al, 1996; Warnke et al, 1995). Sclerosis is present in most cases but may be variable in degree (Fig. 14–15*A* and *B*). In some cases the sclerosis compartmentalizes groups of cells, whereas in others broad bands of fibrosis are seen. Necrosis may be present, and remnants of thymus may be recognized. The neoplastic cells in most cases have a large

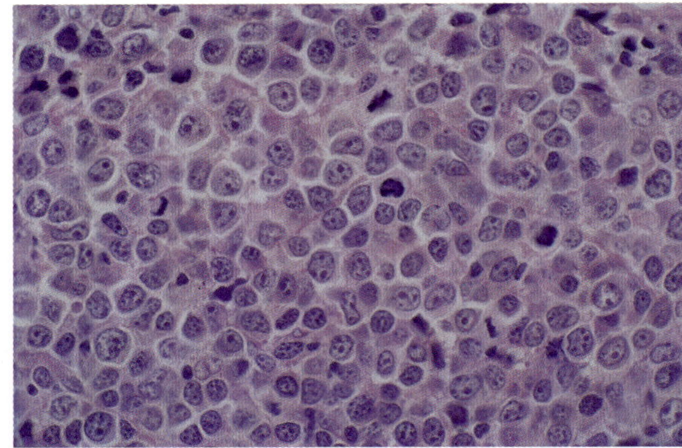

Figure 14–12

Large-cell lymphoma, lymph node. The neoplastic cells have abundant amphophilic cytoplasm and nuclei that are generally larger than those of reactive histiocytes. Chromatin is dispersed, and nucleoli are often adjacent to the nuclear membrane. Mitoses are frequent.

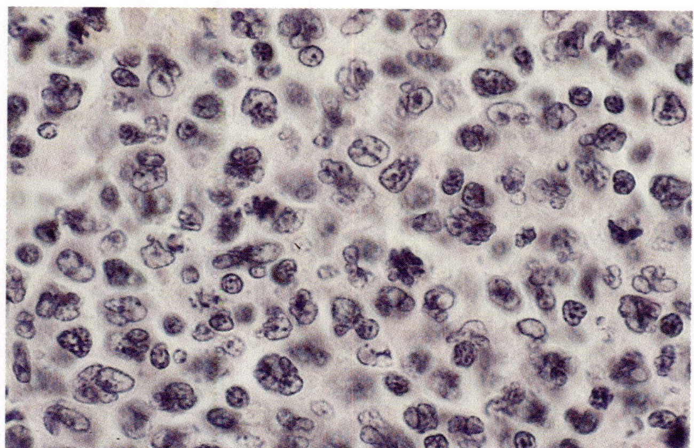

Figure 14–13

Multilobated large B cell lymphoma, lymph node. Note the characteristic nuclear lobation of the neoplastic cells.

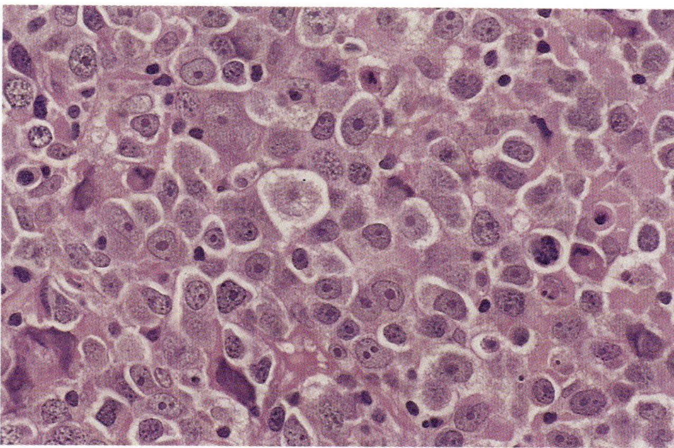

Figure 14–14

Immunoblastic lymphoma, B cell type. The neoplastic cells are large and have abundant cytoplasm, and nucleoli are centrally placed.

transformed cell appearance, whereas a smaller number of cases appear multilobated or contain clear cytoplasm.

IMMUNOLOGIC, CYTOGENETIC, AND MOLECULAR GENETIC FEATURES

Since childhood large B cell malignancies have not been investigated extensively by immunologic or molecular genetic techniques, information about these neoplasms is usually extrapolated from adult studies. Most cases express surface immunoglobulin and B lineage markers CD19, CD20, CD22, and CD79a (Warnke et al, 1995). Cytoplasmic immunoglobulin may be present in those cases with plasmacytic differentiation. Mediastinal large B cell tumors appear to arise from a B cell that normally resides in the medullary portion of the thymus. This cell type often fails to express surface immunoglobulin.

Some large B cell lymphomas have the same chromosomal features as small transformed cell lymphomas (Shad & Magrath, 1997), including a fraction with *MYC* or immunoglobulin rearrangement. The oncogenic t(14;18) chromosomal translocation at the locus associated with bcl-2 often seen in adult B cell lymphoma is rarely, if ever, seen in children.

Differential Diagnosis

The differential diagnosis of large B cell lymphoma of adults often includes carcinomas and melanomas, neoplasms that rarely occur in childhood and are easily recognized by immunohistochemical studies. Reactive conditions, especially nodal reactions secondary to EBV infection, drug reactions, and vaccinations, are more problematic. These conditions often produce a marked immunoblastic proliferation, often with bizarre large binucleated cells, and may mimic large-cell immunoblastic lymphomas and Hodgkin disease. The clinical history is often of paramount importance in arriving at the proper diagnosis. In reactive immunoblastic proliferations, the nodal architecture is usually partially preserved and demonstrates reactive follicles and patent sinuses. The immunoblastic

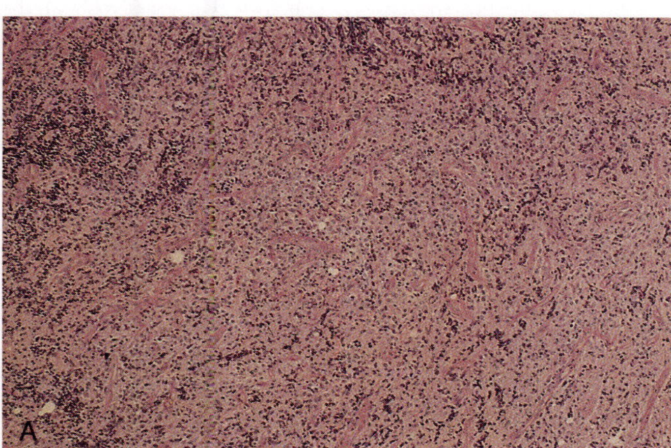

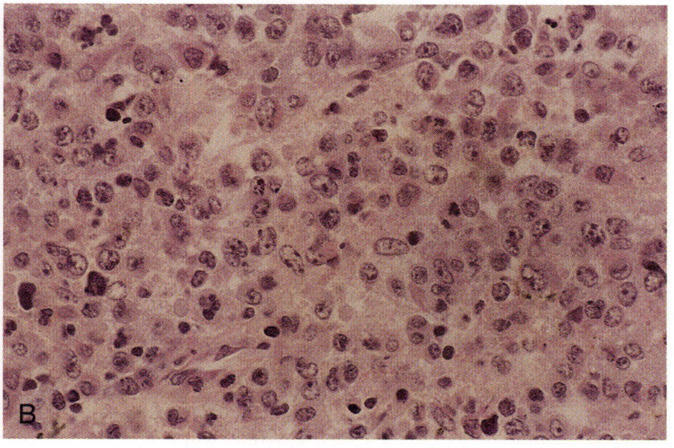

Figure 14–15

Primary large B cell lymphoma, mediastinum. *A,* The growth pattern is diffuse, and sclerosis is present. *B,* The neoplastic cells are large and occasionally have multilobated nuclei. The sclerosis that compartmentalizes groups of neoplastic cells is accentuated. PAS stain.

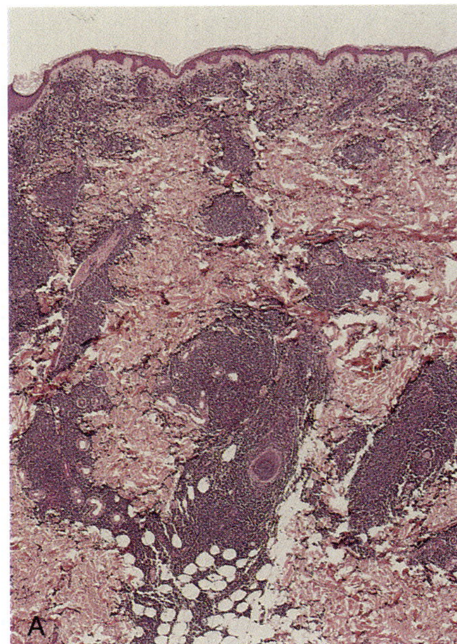

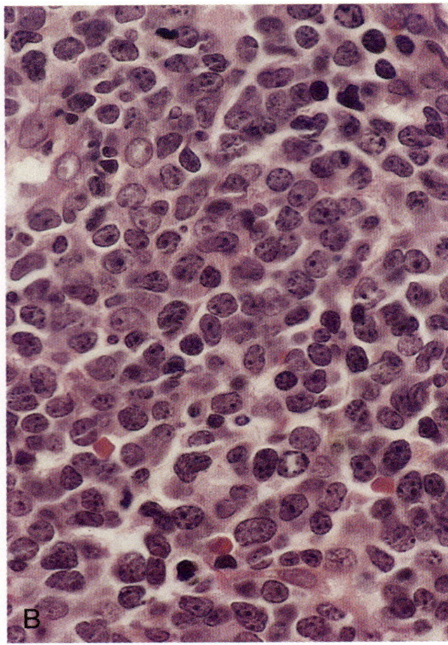

Figure 14–16

Lymphoblastic lymphoma, B cell type, skin. *A,* Note the deep dermal infiltrate. *B,* The neoplastic cells have cytologic features similar to those of T cell lymphoblastic lymphoma. Note the intermediate-sized cells with sparse cytoplasm. The nuclei are irregular, and the chromatin is finely dispersed. Nucleoli are not prominent.

proliferation appears more polymorphous than in most large-cell lymphomas. Immunologic and molecular genetic studies fail to reveal clonal B cell populations.

B Lymphoblastic Lymphoma

The large majority (90%) of lymphoblastic lymphomas of children and adults represent T cell neoplasms arising from immature thymic lymphocytes. Most children present with a mediastinal mass (see Chap. 15). However, a small number of cases have a pre–B cell phenotype identical to that of pre–B cell acute lymphocytic leukemia (see Chap. 4) (Bernard et al, 1982; Borowitz et al, 1983; Kamps & Poppema, 1985; Link et al, 1983; Sander et al, 1992). In contrast to T lymphoblastic lymphoma, B lymphoblastic lymphoma rarely involves the mediastinum, and females are more frequently affected. Skin lesions may be the presenting features or sites of involvement may be supra- or infradiaphragmatic (Fig. 14–16*A* and *B*).

Morphologically, these neoplasms are indistinguishable from T lymphoblastic lymphoma (see Fig. 14–16*A* and *B*) (see Chap. 15). Most B lymphoblastic lymphomas lack surface immunoglobulin but express the B lineage markers CD19, CD20, and CD10 as well as terminal deoxyribonucleotidyl transferase (Warnke et al, 1995).

Unusual or Rare Childhood B Cell Lymphomas

Adults have a diverse group of low-, intermediate-, and high-grade B lymphomas, but B cell lymphomas in children are almost exclusively small transformed cell and large-cell types. Low-grade B cell lymphomas are very rare in children and represent less than 2% of all childhood B and T cell lymphomas.

Follicular center cell lymphomas of low-grade types (follicular small cleaved and mixed cell types) rarely occur in children and adolescents (Frizzera & Murphy, 1979; Ribeiro et al, 1992; Winberg et al, 1981). The youngest patient in these series was 3 years old. In contrast to adults, children with low-grade follicular lymphomas are more likely to have localized nodal disease and longer disease-free survival.

Differentiation from follicular hyperplasia, a common cause of adenopathy in children, generally can be made by histopathologic examination. In contrast to hyperplasia, in which follicles are typically well separated and cortical in distribution, follicular lymphomas demonstrate crowded, back-to-back nodules that often extend to the capsule and pericapsular soft tissue (Warnke et al, 1995). Hyperplastic follicles typically exhibit cellular polarization, with dark and light zones. The cellular composition of follicular lymphoma is usually more homogeneous, and neoplastic cleaved cells often infiltrate the interfollicular region. In problematic cases, bcl-2 protein expression and immunologic or molecular genetic evidence of B cell clonality suggests a diagnosis of lymphoma.

Diffuse small lymphocytic lymphoma and B cell chronic lymphocytic leukemia are quite rare in children. Sonnier and colleagues (1983) reported a case of a chronic lymphocytic leukemia–like disease in a 10-year-old girl. The morphologic features were consistent with chronic lymphocytic leukemia–like disease, and the leukemic cells bore IgM-D, κ surface immunoglobulin, but the clinical course was aggressive, and the neoplasm exhibited an unusual chromosomal translocation, t(2;14). Two cases of parafollicular (monocytoid) B cell lymphoma in HIV-negative children 6 and 18 years of age (Elenitoba-Johnson et al, 1997) and one case of low-grade B cell lymphoma of mucosal-associated lymphocytic tissue in the lung of a 7-year-old HIV-positive girl (Teruya-Feldstein et al, 1995) have been reported.

REFERENCES

Arseneau JC, Canellos GP, Banks PM, et al: American Burkitt's lymphoma: a clinicopathologic study of 30 cases: I. Clinical factors relating to prolonged survival. Am J Med 58:314–321, 1975.

Banks PM, Arseneau JC, Gralnick HR, et al: American Burkitt's lymphoma: a clinico-pathologic study of 30 cases: II. Pathologic correlations. Am J Med 58:322–329, 1975.

Bennett JM, Catovsky D, Daniel MT, et al: The morphological classification of acute lymphoblastic leukemia: concordance among observers and clinical correlations. Br J Haematol 47:553–561, 1981.

Bennett JM, Catovsky D, Daniel MT, et al: Proposals for the classification of acute leukemias: French-American-British (FAB) Cooperative Group. Br J Haematol 33:451–458, 1976.

Berard CW: Reticuloendothelial system: an overview of neoplasia. In Rebuck JW, Berard CW, Abell MR (eds): The Reticuloendothelial System. Williams & Wilkins, Baltimore, pp 301–317, 1975.

Berard C, O'Conor GT, Thomas LB, et al: Histopathological definition of Burkitt's tumor. Bull World Health Organ 40:601–607, 1969.

Bernard A, Murphy SE, Melvin S, et al: Non-T, non-B lymphomas are rare in childhood and associated with cutaneous tumors. Blood 59:549–554, 1982.

Bernheim A, Berger R, Lenoir G: Cytogenetic studies on African Burkitt's lymphoma cell lines: t(8;14), t(2;8) and t(8;22) translocations. Cancer Genet Cytogenet 3:307–315, 1981.

Borowitz MJ, Croker BP, Metzgar RS: Lymphoblastic lymphoma with the phenotype of common acute lymphoblastic leukemia. Am J Clin Pathol 79:387–391, 1983.

Brunning RD, McKenna RW: Tumors of the bone marrow. In Atlas of Tumor Pathology, 3rd series, fascicle 9. Armed Forces Institute of Pathology, Washington, DC, pp 101–142, 1994.

Brunning RD, McKenna RW, Bloomfield CD, et al: Bone marrow involvement in Burkitt's lymphoma. Cancer 40:1771–1779, 1977.

Burkitt D: A children's cancer dependant on climatic factors. Nature 194:232–234, 1962.

Burkitt D: A sarcoma involving the jaws in African children. Br J Surg 46:218–223, 1958.

Burkitt D, O'Conor GT: Malignant lymphoma in African children: I. A clinical syndrome. Cancer 14:258–269, 1961.

Cazals-Hatem D, Lepage E, Brice P, et al: Primary mediastinal large B-cell lymphoma: a clinicopathologic study of 141 cases compared with 916 nonmediastinal large B-cell lymphomas, a GELA ("Group d'Etude des Lymphomes de l'Adulte") study. Am J Surg Pathol 20:877–888, 1996.

Cohen LF, Balow JE, Magrath IT, et al: Acute tumor lysis syndrome: a review of 37 patients with Burkitt's lymphoma. Am J Med 68:486–491, 1980.

Cotelingham JD, Witesby PF, Hsu SM, et al: Malignant lymphoma in patients with the Wiscott-Aldrich syndrome. Cancer Invest 3:515–523, 1985.

Crist WM, Kelly DR, Ragab AH, et al: Predictive ability of Lukes-Collins classification for immunologic phenotypes of childhood non-Hodgkin's lymphoma: an institutional series and literature review. Cancer 48:2070–2075, 1981.

Dalla-Favera R, Breyni M, Erikson J, et al: Human c-myc onc gene is located on the region of chromosome 8 that is translocated in Burkitt lymphoma cells. Proc Natl Acad Sci USA 79:7824–7827, 1982.

Elenitoba-Johnson KSJ, Kumar S, Lim MS, et al: Marginal zone B-cell lymphoma with monocytoid B-cell lymphocytes in pediatric patients without immunodeficiency: a report of two cases. Am J Clin Pathol 107:92–98, 1997.

Epstein MA, Achong BG, Barr YM: Virus particles in cultured lymphoblasts from Burkitt's lymphoma. Lancet 1:252–253, 1964.

Flandrin G, Brouet JC, Daniel MT, et al: Acute leukemia with Burkitt's tumor cells: a study of six cases with special reference to lymphocytic surface markers. Blood 45:183–188, 1975.

Frizzera G, Murphy SB: Follicular (nodular) lymphoma in childhood: a rare clinicopathological entity, report of eight cases from four cancer centers. Cancer 44:2718–2235, 1979.

Gaidano G, Ballerini P, Gong JZ, et al: p53 mutations in human lymphoid malignancies: association with Burkitt's lymphoma and chronic lymphocytic leukemia. Proc Natl Acad Sci USA 88:5413–5417, 1991.

Garcia CF, Weiss LM, Warnke RA: Small noncleaved cell lymphoma: an immunophenotypic study of 18 cases and comparison with large cell lymphoma. Hum Pathol 17:454–461, 1987.

Glick AD, Leech JH, Waldron JA, et al: Malignant lymphomas of follicular center cell origin in man: II. Ultrastructural and cytochemical studies. J Natl Cancer Inst 54:23–36, 1975.

Grogan TM, Warnke RA, Kaplan HS: A comparative study of Burkitt's and non-Burkitt's undifferentiated malignant lymphoma: immunologic, cytochemical, ultrastructural, cytologic, histopathologic, clinical and cell culture features. Cancer 49:1817–1828, 1982.

Harris NL, Jaffe ES, Stein H, et al: A revised European-American classification of lymphoid neoplasms: a proposal from the international lymphoma study group. Blood 84:1361–1392, 1994.

Hutchinson RE, Berard CW, Shusfer JJ, et al: B-cell lineage confers a favorable outcome among children and adolescents with large cell lymphoma: a Pediatric Oncology Group study. J Clin Oncol 13:2023–2032, 1995.

Hutchinson RE, Murphy SB, Fairclough DL, et al: Diffuse small noncleaved cell lymphoma in children, Burkitt's versus non-Burkitt's types: results from the Pediatric Oncology Group and St. Jude Children's Research Hospital. Cancer 64:23–28, 1989.

Iversen OH, Iverson U, Ziegler JL, et al: Cell kinetics in Burkitt's lymphoma. Eur J Cancer 10:155, 1974.

Kamps WA, Poppema S: Pre-B-cell non-Hodgkin's lymphoma in childhood: report of a case and review of the literature. Am J Clin Pathol 90:103–107, 1988.

Kelly DR, Nathawani BN, Griffith RC, et al: A morphologic study of childhood lymphoma of the undifferentiated type: the Pediatric Oncology Group experience. Cancer 59:1132–1137, 1987.

Kjeldsberg CR, Wilson JF, Berard CW: Non-Hodgkin's lymphoma in children. Hum Pathol 14:612–627, 1983.

Klein E, Klein G, Nad Karni JS, et al: Surface IgM-kappa specificity on a Burkitt lymphoma cell in vivo and in derived culture lines. Cancer Res 28:1300–1310, 1968.

Klein G, Svedmyr E, Jondal M, et al: EBV-determined nuclear antigen (EBNA) positive cells in the peripheral blood of infectious mononucleosis patients. Int J Cancer 17:21, 1976.

Lennert K, Feller AC: Histopathology of Non-Hodgkin's lymphomas (Based on the Updated Kiel Classification). 2nd ed. Springer-Verlag, New York, pp 43–45, 1992.

Lenoir GM, Preud'homme JL, Bernheim A, et al: Correlation between immunoglobulin light chain expression and variant translocation in Burkitt's lymphoma. Nature 298:474–476, 1982.

Levine AM: Acquired immunodeficiency syndrome-related lymphoma. Blood 80:8–20, 1992.

Levine AM, Pavlova Z, Pockros AW, et al: Small noncleaved follicular center cell (FCC) lymphoma: Burkitt and non-Burkitt variants in the United States: I. Clinical features. Cancer 52:1073–1079, 1983.

Levine PH, Connelly RR, Berard CW, et al: The American Burkitt lymphoma registry: a progress report. Ann Intern Med 83:31–36, 1975.

Levine PH, Kamaraju LS, Connelly RR, et al: The American Burkitt's lymphoma registry. Cancer 49:1016–1022, 1982.

Link MP, Donaldson SS: The lymphomas and lymphadenopathy. In Nathan DG, Orkin SH (eds): Hematology of Infancy and Childhood, 5th ed. W.B. Saunders Company, Philadelphia, pp 1373–1358, 1998.

Link MP, Roper M, Dorfman RF, et al: Cutaneous lymphoblastic lymphoma with pre-B markers. Blood 61:838–841, 1983.

Lukes RJ, Collins RD: Immunological characterization of human malignant lymphomas. Cancer 34:1488–1503, 1974.

Lukes RJ, Collins RD: Tumors of the hematopoietic system. In Atlas of Tumor Pathology, 2nd series, fascicle 28. Armed Forces Institute of Pathology, Washington, DC, pp 194–196, 1992.

Magrath IT: African Burkitt's lymphoma: history, biology, clinical features and treatment. Am J Pediatr Hematol Oncol 13:222–246, 1991.

Magrath IT: Small noncleaved cell lymphomas (Burkitt's and Burkitt-like lymphomas). In Magrath IT (ed): The Non-Hodgkin's Lymphomas, 2nd ed. Arnold, New York, pp 781–811, 1997.

Magrath IT, Bhatia K: Pathogenesis of small noncleaved cell lymphomas (Burkitt's lymphoma). In Magrath IT (ed): The Non-Hodgkin's Lymphomas, 2nd ed. Arnold, New York, pp 385–409, 1997.

Magrath IT, Lee YJ, Anderson T, et al: Prognostic features in Burkitt's lymphoma: importance of total tumor burden. Cancer 45:1507–1515, 1980.

Mann RB, Jaffe ES, Braylan RC, et al: Non-endemic Burkitt's lymphoma: a B-cell tumor related to germinal centers. N Engl J Med 295:685–691, 1976.

Manolov G, Manolova Y: Marker band in one chromosome 14 from Burkitt's lymphomas. Nature 237:33–34, 1972.

Miliauskas JR, Berard CW, Young RC, et al: Undifferentiated non-Hodgkin's lymphomas (Burkitt's and non-Burkitt's types): the relevance of making this histologic distinction. Cancer 50:2115–2121, 1982.

Miller JB, Variakojis D, Bitran JD, et al: Diffuse histiocytic lymphoma with sclerosis: a clinicopathologic entity frequently causing superior vena caval obstruction. Cancer 47:748–756, 1981.

Murphy SB, Fairclough DL, Hutchinson RE, et al: Non-Hodgkin's lymphomas of childhood: an analysis of the histology, staging and response to treatment of 338 cases at a single institution. J Clin Oncol 7:186–193, 1989.

Nathwani BN, Griffith RC, Kelly DR, et al: A morphologic study of childhood lymphoma of the diffuse "histiocytic" type: the Pediatric Oncology Group experience. Cancer 59:1138–1142, 1987.

Neri A, Barriga F, Knowles DM, et al: Different regions of the immunoglobulin heavy-chain focus are involved in chromosomal translocations in distinct pathogenetic forms of Burkitt lymphoma. Proc Natl Acad Sci USA 85:2748–2752, 1988.

Non-Hodgkin's Lymphoma Pathologic Classification Project: National Cancer Institute sponsored study of classifications of non-Hodgkin's lymphomas: summary and description of a working formulation for clinical usage. Cancer 49:2112–2135, 1982.

O'Conor GT, Davies JNP: Malignant tumors in African children with special reference to malignant lymphoma. J Pediatr 56:526–535, 1960.

O'Conor GT, Rappaport H, Smith EB: Childhood lymphoma resembling "Burkitt tumor" in the United States. Cancer 18:411–417, 1965.

O'Hara CJ, Said JW, Pinkus GS: Non-Hodgkin's lymphoma, multilobated B-cell type: report of nine cases with immunohistochemical and ultrastructural evidence for a follicular center cell derivation. Hum Pathol 17:593–599, 1986.

Pagano JS, Huang CH, Levine P: Absence of Epstein-Barr viral DNA in American Burkitt's lymphoma. N Engl J Med 289:1395–1399, 1973.

Pavlova A, Parker JW, Taylor CR, et al: Small noncleaved follicular center cell lymphoma: Burkitt's and non-Burkitt's variants in the US: II. Pathologic and immunologic features. Cancer 59:1892–1902, 1987.

Payne CM, Grogan TM, Cromey DW, et al: An ultrastructural morphometric and immunophenotypic evaluation of Burkitt's and Burkitt's-like lymphomas. Lab Invest 57:200–218, 1987.

Penn I: Cancer is a complication of severe immunosuppression. Surg Gynecol Obstet 162:603–610, 1986.

Perkins SL, Segal GS, Kjeldsberg CR: Classification of non-Hodgkin's lymphomas in children. Semin Diagn Pathol 12:303–313, 1985.

Piiera T, Perkins SL, Anderson JR, et al: Primary mediastinal large cell lymphoma in children: a report from the Children's Cancer Group. Pediatr Pathol Lab Med 15:561–570, 1995.

Pinto A, Hutchinson RE, Grant LH, et al: Follicular lymphoma in pediatric patients. Mod Pathol 3:308–313, 1990.

Purtilo DT, Stroback RS, Okano M, et al: Epstein-Barr virus–associated lymphoproliferative disorders. Lab Invest 67:5–23, 1992.

Razzouk BI, Srinivas S, Sample CE, et al: Epstein-Barr virus DNA recombination and loss in sporadic Burkitt's lymphoma. J Infect Dis 173:529–535, 1996.

Reiter A, Riehm H: Large cell lymphomas in children. In Magrath IT (ed): The Non-Hodgkin's Lymphomas, 2nd ed. Arnold, New York, pp 829–851, 1997.

Reiter A, Schrape M, Parwaresen T, et al: Non-Hodgkin's lymphomas of childhood and adolescence: results of a treatment stratified for biologic subtypes and stage—a report of the Berlin-Frankfurt-Munster Group. J Clin Oncol 13:359–372, 1995.

Ribeiro RC, Pin CH, Murphy SB, et al: Childhood malignant non-Hodgkin's lymphomas of uncommon histology. Leukemia 6:761–765, 1992.

Robinson JE, Brown N, Andiman W, et al: Diffuse polyclonal B-cell lymphoma during primary infection with Epstein-Barr virus. N Engl J Med 302:1293–1297, 1980.

Sander CA, Jaffe ES, Gebhardt FC, et al: Mediastinal lymphoblastic lymphoma with an immature B-cell immunophenotype. Am J Surg Pathol 16:300–305, 1992.

Sandlund JT, Downing JR, Crist WM: Non-Hodgkin's lymphomas in childhood. N Engl J Med 334:1238–1248, 1996.

Sandlund JT, Pui Ch, Santana VM, et al: Clinical features and treatment outcome for children with CD30+ large cell non-Hodgkin's lymphoma. J Clin Oncol 12:895–898, 1994.

Shad A, Magrath I: Malignant non-Hodgkin's lymphomas in childhood. In Pizzo PA, Poplack DG (eds): Principles and Practice of Pediatric Oncology, 3rd ed. Lippincott-Raven, Philadelphia, pp 545–587, 1997.

Smith SD, Rubin CM, Horvath A, et al: Non-Hodgkin's lymphoma in childhood. Semin Oncol 16:113–119, 1990.

Sonnier JA, Buchanan GR, Howard-Peebles P, et al: Chromosomal translocation involving the immunoglobulin kappa-chain and heavy-chain loci in a child with chronic lymphocytic leukemia. N Engl J Med 309:590–594, 1983.

Teruya-Feldstein J, Temeck BK, Sloas MM, et al: Pulmonary malignant lymphoma of mucosa-associated lymphoid tissue (MALT) arising in a pediatric HIV-positive patient. Am J Surg Pathol 19:357–363, 1995.

van Baarlen J, Schuurman H-J, van Unnik JAM: Multilobated non-Hodgkin's lymphoma: a clinicopathologic entity. Cancer 61:1371–1376, 1988.

Warnke RA, Weiss LM, Chan JKC, et al: Tumors of the lymph nodes and spleen. In Atlas of Tumor Pathology, 3rd series, fascicle 14. Armed Forces Institute of Pathology, Washington, DC, pp 221–232, 1995.

Weiss RL, Kjeldsberg CR, Colby TV, et al: Multilobated B-cell lymphomas: a study of seven cases. Hematol Oncol 3:79–86, 1985.

Williams SA, Suen Y, Cairo MS: Molecular biology and cytogenetics of non-Hodgkin's lymphoma in children. Semin Diagn Pathol 12:335–341, 1995.

Wilson JF, Jenkin RDT, Anderson JR, et al: Studies on the pathology of non-Hodgkin's lymphoma of childhood: I. The role of routine histopathology as a prognostic factor: a report from the Children's Cancer Study Group. Cancer 53:1695–1704, 1984.

Wilson JF, Kjeldsberg CR, Sposto R, et al: The pathology of non-Hodgkin's lymphoma of childhood: II. Reproducibility and relevance of the histologic classification of "undifferentiated" lymphomas (Burkitt's versus non-Burkitt's). Hum Pathol 18:1008–1014, 1987.

Winberg CD, Nathwani BN, Bearman RB, et al: Follicular (nodular) lymphomas during the first two decades of life: a clinicopathologic study of 12 patients. Cancer 48:2223–2235, 1981.

Yano T, vanKrieken J, Magrath I, et al: Histogenetic correlations between subcategories of small non-cleaved cell lymphomas. Blood 79:1282–1290, 1992.

Ziegler JL, Anderson M, Klein G, et al: Detection of Epstein-Barr virus DNA in American Burkitt's lymphoma. Int J Cancer 17:701–706, 1976.

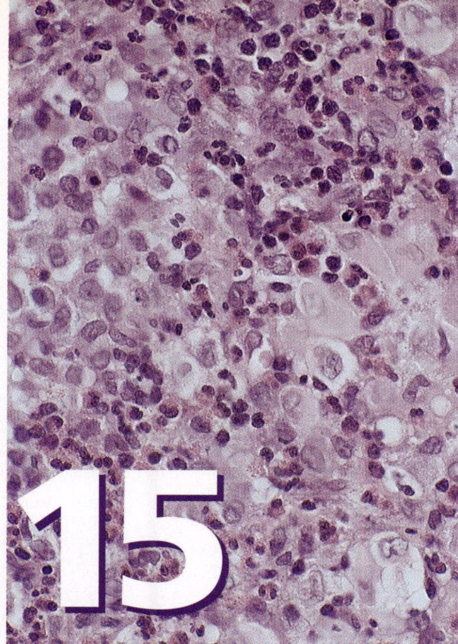

Marsha C. Kinney

T Cell Lymphomas and Natural Killer Cell Neoplasms

T cell lymphomas are biologically complex and clinically heterogeneous. They are also difficult to categorize precisely. Advances in immunology and molecular genetics over the last 10 to 15 years have led to better definition of these diverse processes and more precise correlation with clinical features. Natural killer (NK) cell neoplasms that have overlapping features with T cell lymphomas have been recognized. Understanding and recognizing T cell lymphomas are relevant to the care of pediatric patients, since these neoplasms are relatively common, are biologically aggressive, and are potentially curable. This chapter discusses T cell biology, the classification and diagnosis of T cell lymphomas, and their clinical features. Each T cell lymphoma is also discussed in detail.

T CELL BIOLOGY

T cells are identified by surface antigens, and some antigens are uniquely associated with specific lineages (Table 15–1). T cells (and B cells) express functional receptors that recognize antigen. Most peripheral T cells are T cell receptor (TCR)α/β+. Generally <5% of T cells express TCRγ/δ. The latter receptor has limited diversity, and is probably involved in the initial immune response at mucosal surfaces to nonpolymorphic "super antigens" such as those on bacteria.

T cell precursors, or prothymocytes, are CD7+, CD2−, CD3−, and TdT− and arise from multipotential cells in the marrow. Most of these cells migrate to the thymus where maturation occurs. The most immature cells (CD7+, CD2+, surface CD3−, cytoplasmic CD3+, CD4−, CD8−, CD1−, TCRα/β−, and TdT positive) are in the subcapsular sinus and upper part of the cortex. Common thymocytes (CD7+, CD2+, CD3+/−, CD4+, CD8+, CD1+, TdT+ cytoplasmic TCRα/β+ or TCRγ/δ+) are present in the cortex. Medullary thymocytes are either CD4+ or CD8+. They are TCRα/β+ and have lost CD1 and TdT. There also is a small population of mature CD4−, CD8−, TCRγ/δ+ cells in the medulla.

T cells have a distinct distribution or homing pattern in normal tissues, a feature that is useful in identifying and classifying T cell lymphomas. T cells are found in the paracortex (between follicles and in the deep cortex) of lymph nodes. In the spleen TCRα/β+ T cells are present in the periarteriolar lymphocyte sheaths, and TCRγ/δ+ T cells are preferentially located in the splenic sinuses. Minor populations of T cells are also present in the skin, gastrointestinal tract, and lung. Most of these cells are CD4+, but individual T cell populations (including CD4+ cells) may home to specific organs, where they have specific functions. TCRγ/δ+ T cell populations are relatively increased in the epithelium of the intestine.

T cells and NK cells arise from a common precursor but are distinct lineages (Lanier et al, 1992). Complex subsets of T cells that express NK cell antigens have been described in humans and mice (MacDonald, 1995). Malignancies, called NK-like T cell lymphomas, may arise in extramedullary sites from these subsets (see "Natural Killer and Natural Killer–Like T Cell Neoplasms").

CLASSIFICATION OF T CELL NEOPLASMS

T cell lymphomas as a group are difficult to classify. They are rare, averaging 1 for every 10 B cell lymphomas. Whereas most B cell lymphomas produce distinctive structures (neoplastic follicles) that greatly facilitate their recognition, the growth patterns and cytologic features of T cell lymphomas are much more difficult to recognize by microscopic examination. Diagnosis in all cases should be confirmed by flow cytometric analysis, immunophenotyping, or genetic studies. There are, however, two T cell lymphomas that general pathologists should diagnose with assurance: T lymphoblastic lymphoma and anaplastic large-cell (Ki-1+) lymphoma (ALCL).

Our classification systems of lymphomas are currently undergoing revision. The basic concept relating lymphomas to normal lymphocyte compartments, as in the Kiel and Lukes-Collins classifications, is now accepted by most hematopathologists, and is the case for the Revised European-American Lymphoma (REAL) classification (Harris et al, 1994). This classification included NK cell and NK-like T cell malignancies for the first time. T cell neoplasms are divided into precursor cell type (lymphoblastic) and peripheral or mature. The latter are divided into definite or provisional categories based on their identification as distinct clinicopathologic entities. The REAL system includes morphologic, immunophenotypic, and genotypic findings for each entity. The World Health Organization classification is being revised and has been presented in only a preliminary fashion (Jaffe et al, 1998).

DIAGNOSIS OF T CELL NEOPLASMS

Subclassification of T cell lymphomas is often a problem even for specialists. The distinction of T cell lymphoma from reactive processes and other neoplasms is often difficult in itself, owing to the rarity of T cell neoplasms and their

Table 15–1

Antigens Commonly Expressed on T cells That are Useful in Classifying T Cell Neoplasms

Antigen	Cellular Distribution
CD1	Immature T cells (common thymocyte stage); Langerhans granule histiocytes and other dendritic cells
CD2	Pan T cell; NK cells
CD3	Pan T cell; cytoplasmic expression may be seen in NK cells
CD4	Helper T cell subset; monocytes; histiocytes
CD5	Pan T cell; B cell subsets
CD7	Pan T cell; NK cells; subset granulocyte precursors
CD8	Suppressor T cells; NK cells
CD25	Activated T cells (IL-2 receptor); activated B cells and macrophages
CD30	Activated T cells; subset of activated B cells; Reed-Sternberg cells
CD43	T cells; granulocyte precursors; B cell subset
CD45RO	T cells; histiocytes
TCRα/β	T cells (framework antigen of TCRα/β protein)
TCRγ/δ	T cells (framework antigen of TCRγ/δ protein)

Abbreviations: IL-2, interleukin-2; NK, natural killer; TCR, T cell receptor.

morphologic diversity. The morphologic features of T cell lymphomas are usually not specific and may be mimicked by B cell neoplasms, malignant histiocytoses, carcinomas, or reactive processes. The infiltrate in T cell lymphomas is often heterogeneous, with tumor cells of various sizes and many admixed inflammatory cells, such as histiocytes, eosinophils, and sometimes plasma cells. Clonality is also more difficult to evaluate in T cell processes than in B cell proliferations. For these reasons, immunophenotyping, TCR gene rearrangement studies, and cytogenetic studies are often required to make a definitive diagnosis of T cell lymphoma. There is no surface marker of clonality, but in neoplastic processes there is often a marked predominance of one T cell subset (CD4 or CD8), and there may be loss of pan–T cell antigens, such as CD2, CD3, CD5, and CD7, indications that an abnormal T cell infiltrate is present. Caution must be exercised, since some T cell antigens, particularly CD7, may be lost in reactive processes (see "Mycosis Fungoides"). In addition, there is overlap between the immunophenotypes of T cells and NK cells, and expression of surface CD3 (not cytoplasmic) or the TCRα/β or TCRγ/δ framework antigen proteins is required to confirm a T cell origin (see "Natural Killer and Natural Killer–Like T Cell Lymphoma"). If tissue architecture is partially preserved and the infiltrate is heterogeneous without significant cellular dysplasia, tests of clonality, such as T cell gene rearrangement studies, may be required to make a diagnosis of lymphoma. Cytogenetics studies are also useful, particularly in NK cell proliferations where TCR rearrangements are not present.

Routine histologic examination remains the mainstay of diagnosis in hematopathology. The pattern of tissue architectural alteration often mirrors the normal distribution of T cells and provides a clue to the T cell nature of the neoplastic process. In the node, the distribution may be paracortical or sinus; in the spleen, periarteriolar or sinus; in the liver, peribiliary or sinusoid; and in the skin, epidermotropic or subcutaneous. In all tissue sites, vasocentricity with prominent vasodestruction and necrosis suggests a T or NK cell process. Other histologic features common to T cell neoplasms include vascular proliferation (particularly high endothelial venules), pleomorphic or clear cell morphologic features, giant cells with Reed-Sternberg–like morphologic features, and numerous admixed inflammatory cells. Immunophenotyping studies are required to confirm the T cell origin of the infiltrate.

CLINICAL FEATURES

The incidence of T cell lymphoma varies with age group and geographic location. In Western countries, approximately 50% of childhood lymphomas other than Hodgkin disease are T cell, compared with 10% in adults. In contrast, in Asia T cell lymphomas are more frequent in adults (30–70%) than in children (37%) (Shih & Liang, 1991). Sixty percent or more of childhood T cell lymphomas arise in the thymus and have a blastic appearance and immature phenotype. The mature or "peripheral" (to the thymus) lymphomas are largely represented by ALCL. Other peripheral T cell lymphomas are very rarely or never (Lennert lymphoma) seen in children.

Children and adolescents with T cell lymphomas most frequently present with a mediastinal mass (lymphoblastic lymphoma) or peripheral adenopathy (ALCL). Extranodal sites are common and include skin, bone, liver, spleen, lung, intestine, and testis. Central nervous system (CNS) and marrow involvement are uncommon except in lymphoblastic lymphoma, the small-cell variant of ALCL, and aggressive NK or NK-like T cell neoplasms. Constitutional symptoms are present in most patients. The presence of fever, lymphadenopathy, and hepatosplenomegaly in lymphoma suggests an infectious cause, and the diagnosis may be delayed (Lin et al, 1994). T cell lymphomas have been identified in adult patients with such underlying conditions as autoimmune disease, ataxia telangiectasia, such lymphoproliferative disorders as lymphomatoid papulosis, celiac disease, and immunodeficiency. After solid organ transplantation, children may develop T cell lymphomas, probably owing to Epstern-Barr virus (EBV) activation (Wiles et al, 1994). Other predisposing factors have not been identified.

T cell lymphomas are staged as follows. Stage I is a single extranodal or nodal site, with the exclusion of the mediastinum or abdomen. Stage II includes a single extranodal site with regional node involvement, two extranodal sites on the same side of the diaphragm, or a primary gastrointestinal tumor with or without mesenteric nodes (and completely resected). Intrathoracic, extensive unresectable abdominal, paraspinal, epidural, or extrathoracic disease on both sides of the diaphragm are stage III. Stage IV disease includes marrow or CNS involvement (Murphy, 1978; Murphy et al, 1989)

Patients with T lymphomas are usually given multiagent chemotherapy. Lymphoblastic lymphoma is treated with intensive sustained leukemia-type therapy, and large-cell lymphoma with short course regimens of varying intensity (Anderson et al, 1993). Survival is related to stage with over 85% 5 year event free survival in limited stage cases receiving short-course chemotherapy (Link et al, 1997). With more intensive regimens, advanced stage patients with lymphoblastic lymphoma are approaching a similar survival (Patte et al, 1992). In general, a patient with large B cell lymphoma has had a better prognosis than a patient with T cell large cell lymphoma except in systemic Ki-1+ anaplastic large cell lymphoma, which has an event free survival over 80% following short course chemotherapy (Hutchinson et al, 1995; Reiter et al, 1995). Radiation alone or in combination with chemotherapy does not appear to improve survival. Marrow transplantation is successful as salvage therapy.

T LINEAGE LYMPHOBLASTIC LYMPHOMA

Neoplasms of precursor T cells originate in the marrow as acute lymphoblastic leukemia or in the thymus as lymphoblastic lymphoma. These aggressive neoplasms disseminate rapidly, and it is often not possible to determine the site of origin—thymus or marrow—in individual cases (Nathwani et al, 1976). These two T neoplasms have nearly identical biologic features and therapeutic responses (Head & Behm, 1995). In the REAL classification T lymphoblastic lymphoma (T-LBL) and T acute lymphoblastic leukemia (T-ALL) are combined as precursor T cell neoplasms. They have been distinguished principally by clinical features and arbitrary criteria (e.g., >25% marrow blasts for the diagnosis of leukemia) (Kjeldsberg et al, 1983; Picozzi & Coleman, 1990). Most patients with T-LBL have a mediastinal mass or peripheral adenopathy without splenomegaly, whereas cytopenias and splenomegaly are more likely in T-ALL. Terminology for T-LBL in other classifications includes convoluted T lymphocytic (Lukes-Collins), T lymphoblastic (Kiel), lymphoblastic convoluted or nonconvoluted cell (Working Formulation).

Clinical Features

Lymphoblastic lymphoma (LBL) represents about 30% of B and T cell lymphomas in children and about 10% of those in adults. Most patients are children, adolescents, or young adults. Fifty to 70% of patients present with a mediastinal mass that may cause dyspnea, dysphagia, pain, and swelling of the neck, face, and upper extremities if superior vena caval obstruction is present. Pleural and pericardial effusions are common. Lymphadenopathy, usually in the neck, axilla, or supraclavicular area, is present in 50–80% of patients. Marrow involvement is common in disseminated disease, in which liver, spleen, kidney, and para-aortic nodes are often involved. CNS disease is uncommon at presentation but was a frequent site of relapse before the advent of CNS radiation for prophylaxis. There may be cranial nerve or meningeal infiltration. Other sites involved include the testes, particularly at relapse; bone (Niemann & Thomas, 1995); and skin, particularly in the head and neck region (Pesce et al, 1997; Sander et al, 1991; Zaatari et al, 1987).

The St. Jude's Children's Research Hospital system is used for staging (Murphy, 1980). Work-up after diagnosis includes chest and abdominal computed tomographic (CT) scan, magnetic resonance imaging (MRI) for examining the tumor relationship to the heart, bone scan, marrow biopsy, and cerebrospinal fluid (CSF) examination.

LBL is a high-grade neoplasm, and first-line treatment is multiagent chemotherapy (reviewed in Sandlund & Magrath, 1997). Radiation is not used in localized disease but may be indicated in special circumstances, such as life-threatening airway obstruction; CNS involvement, including spinal cord compression; and poor response to chemotherapy. Radiation has not been shown to improve survival, and it increases toxicity to chemotherapy, particularly to anthracyclines. Steroids have been given in emergencies and typically produce dramatic reduction in tumor bulk. Five-year event-free survival rate are in the 65–85% range (Sandlund & Magrath, 1997). The most reliable indicator of treatment outcome is tumor burden at di agnosis, as reflected in staging as well as in levels of biochemical tumor markers, such as lactic dehydrogenase and soluble interleukin-2 (IL-2) receptor levels. Conversion of the chest radiograph to normal within 60 days of treatment appears to identify good-risk patients in whom therapy may modified to a less intense regimen (Shepherd et al, 1995).

Malignant lymphomas arising in the mediastinum represent approximately 60% of all mediastinal tumors in children, two thirds of them B or T cell lymphomas and one third Hodgkin disease. The great majority of mediastinal B and T cell lymphomas are LBL in type, and large-cell lymphomas are rare (Piira et al, 1995).

Histopathologic Features

The growth pattern in nodes is paracortical or diffuse (Fig. 15–1*A* and *B*). Blasts are invasive and infiltrate the capsule and surrounding soft tissue in a single-file fashion. There is a high mitotic rate, and a "starry sky" pattern similar to that in Burkitt lymphoma, may be seen. Blasts are recognized by their high nuclear-cytoplasmic ratio and finely dispersed, homogeneous nuclear chromatin (see Figs. 15–1 and 15–2). LBL blasts have L1 or L2 morphologic features in the French-American-British (FAB) classification (Griffith et al, 1987) (see Fig. 15–2*A*). L1 blasts have relatively condensed, homogeneous chromatin and small or indistinct nucleoli. L2 blasts have more dispersed chromatin, prominent nucleoli, and moderate cytoplasm. Patients with the large-cell or L2 variant have a predisposition for abdominal disease (Kjeldsberg et al, 1983). T lymphoblasts often have prominent nuclear convolutions (Nathwani et al, 1976). Cytochemical studies demonstrate strong, focal cytoplasmic acid phosphatase reactivity (see Fig. 15–2*B*). The diagnosis may easily be made on effusions or fine-needle aspiration of lesions (Niemann & Thomas, 1995; Wakely & Kornstein, 1996) (see Chap. 2).

LBL may rarely be associated with eosinophilia, myeloid hyperplasia or myeloid malignancy, and a t(8;13) chromosomal translocation (Abruzzo et al, 1992; Inhorn et al, 1995). T-LBL has also been reported with histiocytic malignancies, interdigitating reticulum cell sarcoma (Horschowski et al, 1993) and malignant histiocytosis (Soslow et al, 1996).

Immunophenotype

Eighty to 90% of LBLs have a T cell phenotype and are TdT+, CD2+, CD7+, HLA-DR−. CD43, CD3, and TdT are detectable with paraffin immunoperoxidase staining (Orazi et al, 1994).

Most cases of T-LBL and T-ALL may be subclassified according to stage of thymic differentiation (Table 15–2) (Jennings & Foon, 1997). Compared with T-ALLs, T-LBLs are less likely to express an early thymocyte immunophenotype

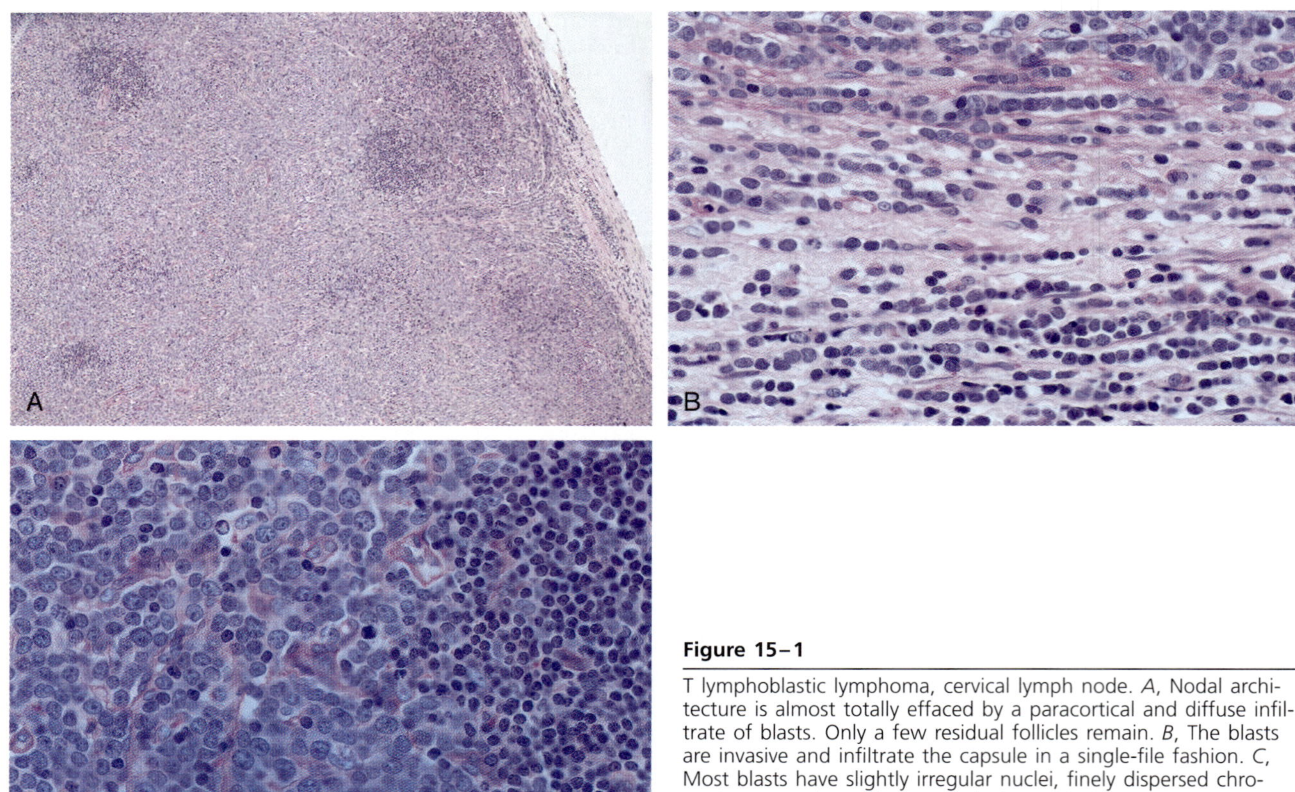

Figure 15–1

T lymphoblastic lymphoma, cervical lymph node. *A*, Nodal architecture is almost totally effaced by a paracortical and diffuse infiltrate of blasts. Only a few residual follicles remain. *B*, The blasts are invasive and infiltrate the capsule in a single-file fashion. *C*, Most blasts have slightly irregular nuclei, finely dispersed chromatin, somewhat indistinct nucleoli, and little cytoplasm. There is a high mitotic rate. Normal residual small lymphocytes are present at the right.

and are more often CD10 (CALLA)+ (Bernard et al, 1981; Crist et al, 1988; Weiss et al, 1986). Surface expression of TCRγ/δ appears to be more frequent in T-ALL and the TCRα/β in T-LBL (Gouttefangeas et al, 1990). T-ALL and T-LBL cells at the thymic or common stage (CD3+/−, CD4+, CD8+) express the CD21 antigen (a receptor for the C3d fragment of complement and EBV), in contrast to the pro-, or early, thymocyte stages, which are CD21− (Tatsumi et al, 1994). Rare cases express NK antigens (NK-like T cells and true NK cell neoplasms) (Ichinohasama et al, 1996; Koita et al, 1997; Nakamura et al, 1997; Sheibani et al, 1987b; Swerdlow et al, 1985).

Diagnostic Criteria

The diagnostic criteria for T-LBL are summarized in Table 15–3.

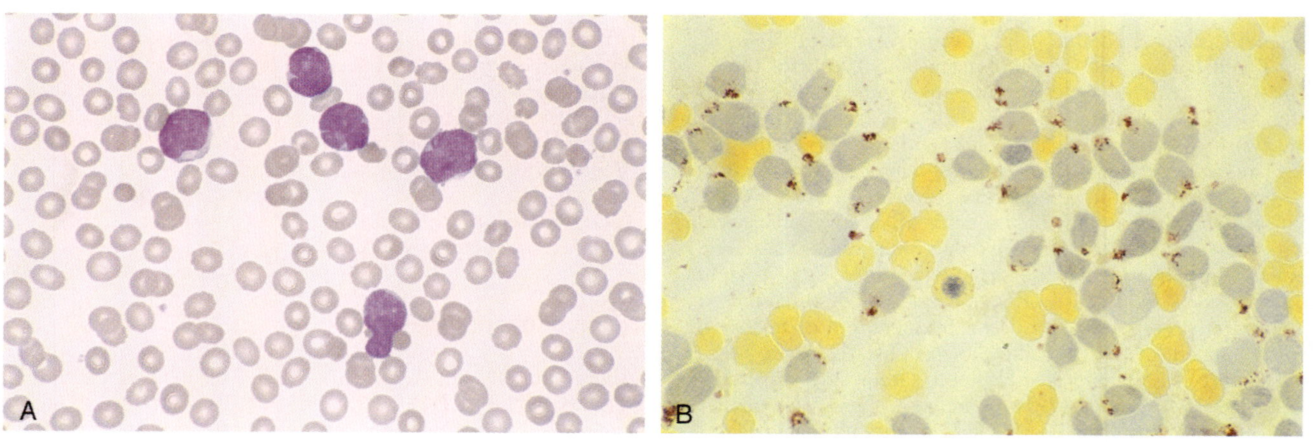

Figure 15–2

T acute lymphoblastic leukemia, blood and marrow aspirate. *A*, The lymphoblasts have a high nuclear-cytoplasmic ratio, folded nuclei with dense homogeneous chromatin, somewhat indistinct nucleoli, and relatively little cytoplasm. These morphologic features are typical of L1 blasts in French-American-British (FAB) classification. Wright stain. *B*, The lymphoblasts have strong focal cytoplasmic acid phosphatase reactivity.

Table 15–2

Stages of T Cell Differentiation in the Thymus in Relationship to Antigen Expression

Stage	Antigen Expression							
	CD1	CD2	CD5	CD7	CD3	CD4	CD8	TdT
I (immature, early cortical)	–	+	+/–	+	–	–	–	+
II (common, late cortical)	+	+	+	+	+/–	+	+	+
III (medullary)	–	+	+	+	+	+/–*	+/–*	+/–

*Mature phenotype, either CD4 or CD8 is expressed.

Differential Diagnosis

The differential diagnosis of T-LBL and T-ALL includes other "small blue cell tumors," such as B lineage ALL, acute nonlymphocytic leukemia, Burkitt lymphoma, rhabdomyosarcoma, neuroblastoma, and Ewing sarcoma. T-LBL and T-ALL have inconspicuous nucleoli and more indistinct cytoplasm. Burkitt lymphoma has prominent nucleoli and abundant pyroninophilic cytoplasm. Acute nonlymphocytic leukemia blasts have more open chromatin, prominent nucleoli, and abundant cytoplasm. Immature eosinophilic myelocytes may be present. Neuroblastoma has a more cohesive growth pattern and nuclear molding. Homer Wright rosettes are seen in about 25% of cases. Ewing sarcoma is periodic acid–schiff (PAS) positive. Embryonal rhabdomyosarcoma may have admixed larger cells with vesicular nuclei and eosinophilic cytoplasm in which cross-striations may be present. These neoplasms may also be readily distinguished by immunophenotypic and cytochemical studies (Table 15–4).

A B or pre–B cell phenotype is seen in approximately 1–10% of LBLs. The disease generally involves peripheral nodes, skin or subcutaneous tissue, and bone (Iravani et al, 1999; Link et al, 1983; Ozdemirli et al, 1998; Sander et al, 1991; Sheibani et al, 1987a; Stroup et al, 1990).

Pathogenesis and Biologic Characteristics

Specific epidemiologic factors have not been identified in the pathogenesis of LBL. It is not seen with increased frequency in immunocompromised patients or those exposed to irradiation. There is no evidence of viral induction.

The presumed mechanism of neoplastic transformation is the deregulated expression of oncogenes or tumor suppressor genes. There is overlap between the cytogenetic and molecular genetic lesions in T-ALL and T-LBL, but more information is available about the former. In T-ALL, chromosomal translocations are common and involve chromosome bands 14q11, 7q35, and 7p15 sites of the *TCRα/δ*, *TCRβ*, and *TCRδ* genes, respectively (Raimondi et al, 1988; Sandlund & Magrath, 1997). Errors in *TCR* gene rearrangements result in exchanges with other proto-oncogenes, including *LYL1* (19p13.1), *TAL1/SCL* (1p32–34), *TAL2* (9q32), *LMO1 (TTG1/RBTN1)* (11p15), *LMO2 (TTG2/RBTN2)* (11p13), *HOX11* (10q24), *TAN* (9q34.3), *LCK* (1p34), and *MYC* (8q24), leading to their aberrant expression (Schichman et al, 1997; Warnke et al, 1995). Structural alterations of the *TAL1/SCL* gene, resulting from translocations or more commonly deletions, are one of the most frequent. Defects in the DNA mismatch repair genes may also lead to abnormal expression of these proto-oncogenes (Lowsky et al, 1997). Most of these genes function as transcription factors (Cleary, 1991). The tumor suppressor gene *P16/MTSI/P*^{INK4A}, a cell cycle inhibitor, is altered by methylation or deletion and may be the most frequent genetic alteration in T-ALL (Batova et al, 1997; Kees et al, 1997)

Table 15–3

T Cell Lymphoblastic Lymphoma: Diagnostic Criteria

Homogeneous population of blasts with delicate nuclear chromatin, inconspicuous nucleoli, and scant cytoplasm; nuclear convolutions variable
High mitotic rate; tingible-body macrophages may give a "starry sky" appearance
Invasive growth pattern, with infiltration of thymic or nodal capsule
Immature T cell phenotype
<25% marrow blasts; mediastinal mass generally present

ANAPLASTIC LARGE-CELL LYMPHOMA

ALCL, the most common peripheral T cell lymphoma in children (Sandlund et al, 1994), was initially described in 45 patients, 8 (18%) of whom were children (Stein et al, 1985). The association of adenopathy and skin lesions in children has been emphasized (Kadin et al, 1986). ALCL is defined by morphologic, immunologic, and genetic features (Kinney & Kadin, 1999). In typical or classic ALCL, there is a pleomorphic large-cell lymphoma, with a characteristic paracortical or sinus growth pattern in nodes. Virtually all the tumor cells are CD30+ (as recognized by antibodies Ki-1 or Ber-H2). Prior to development of antibodies to CD30, these lymphomas were often misdiagnosed as malignant histiocytosis or metastatic carcinoma (Ornvold et al, 1992; Wilson et al, 1990). In classifications other than the REAL and updated Kiel, ALCL was classified as T immunoblastic sarcoma (Lukes-Collins) or diffuse large-cell, immunoblastic (Working Formulation). Other equivalent terms include sinusoidal large-cell lymphoma and regressing atypical histiocytosis.

Clinical Features and Prognosis

ALCL represents approximately 6–16% of all pediatric B and T cell lymphomas and 30–40% of large-cell lymphomas (Kadin et al, 1986; Murphy, 1994; Reiter et al, 1994; Sandlund et al,

Table 15–4

Differential Diagnosis of Lymphoblastic Lymphoma: Distinguishing Cytochemical and Immunologic Features

Neoplasm	Distinguishing Features
B lineage ALL	CD45 (LCA)+; B cell antigens (CD19)+
Acute nonlymphocytic leukemia	CD45 (LCA)+; Sudan black, myeloperoxidase+; CD13, CD33, CD14, CD68, CD15 (granulocyte markers)+
Burkitt lymphoma	CD45 (LCA)+; CD20 (B cell antigen)+; monoclonal surface immunoglobulin
Rhabdomyosarcoma	CD45 (LCA)−; desmin+
Neuroblastoma	CD45 (LCA)−; neuron specific enolase+; chromogranin+, synaptophysin+
Ewing sarcoma	PAS+; CD45 (LCA)−; glycoprotein p30/32^{MIC2}+*

*ALL and LBL may also express this antigen (Riopel et al, 1994; Weidner & Tjoe, 1994).

Abbreviations: ALL, acute lymphoblastic leukemia; LBL, lymphoblastic lymphoma; LCA, leukocyte common antigen; PAS, periodic acid–Schiff.

1994; Vecchi et al, 1993). Most series have a male predominance, and the median age ranges from 10 to 15 years (Brugières et al, 1998; Gordon et al, 1993; Heitger et al, 1989; Kadin et al, 1986; Reiter et al, 1994; Rubie et al, 1994; Sandlund et al, 1994; Vecchi et al, 1993). A few patients less than 1 year of age have been reported (Kinney et al, 1993; Reiter et al, 1994). B symptoms are present in 42–89% of patients (Heitger et al, 1989; Reiter et al, 1994; Vecchi et al, 1993). The most common presentation, peripheral adenopathy, is seen in 70–90% of patients, while mediastinal adenopathy is detected in only 5–39%. Involvement of extranodal sites, particularly the skin and soft tissue, is also common, occurring in one third to two thirds of cases at presentation. Skin lesions are usually solitary large tumor masses, but small papules and rashes may be present (Kinney et al, 1993; Meier et al, 1992). Erythema of the skin around affected lymph nodes (periadenitis) is occasionally seen (Massimino et al, 1995). Other sites of involvement, with percentages of affected patients, are marrow (5–15%), CNS (0–5%), bone (5–30%), lung (8–30%), peritoneal or pleural effusions (5–15%), gastrointestinal tract (5–10%), and kidney (0–5%). Very unusual presentations in childhood include a perirectal and buttock mass (Winter et al, 1991), a hard palate mass involving the nasal cartilage and floor of the orbit (Papadimitriou et al, 1996), bone pain with lytic bone lesions (Chan et al, 1991; Ishizawa et al, 1995), primary brain and spinal cord lymphoma (Havlioglu et al, 1995), and a polypoid gastric mass with ulceration and bleeding (Moubayed et al, 1987).

Roughly one third of patients present with stage I or II disease and two thirds with advanced stage (III or IV) disease. Treatment has been variable but generally involves combination chemotherapy. Most pediatric patients achieve complete remission, with survival in the range of 65–85% (Brugières et al, 1998; Greer et al, 1995; Murphy, 1994; Massimino et al, 1995; Reiter et al, 1995; Sandlund et al, 1994). Long-term (14–25 years) pediatric and adult survivors have been reported (Salhany et al, 1991). Approximately 10–35% of patients relapse, but salvage therapy is effective in most cases (Brugières et al, 1998; Greer et al, 1995; Heitger et al, 1989; Massimino et al, 1995; Murphy, 1994; Reiter et al, 1994; Sandlund et al, 1994). Marrow transplantation has been successful in attaining prolonged disease control in most patients (Chakravarti et al, 1990; Fanin et al, 1999; Gordon et al, 1994; Gordon et al, 1993; Takamura et al, 1995).

The treatment of limited-stage disease, particularly that confined to the skin, is controversial. Prognosis is excellent, and some patients are treated with simple excision and/or local radiotherapy if the lesions are solitary and localized (Beljaards et al, 1993; Beljaards et al, 1989; Bittencourt et al, 1992; De Bruin et al, 1993; Greer et al, 1995; Paulli et al, 1995; Tomaszewski et al, 1999). Spontaneous regression of skin lesions may occur (Bittencourt et al, 1992; Kadin et al, 1986). Factors associated with the risk of treatment failure in ALCL include liver and lung involvement (Massimino et al, 1995), the presence of B symptoms (Heitger et al, 1989), small-cell variant (SCV) histologic features (Whitlock et al, 1992), and visceral or mediastinal involvement and lactate dehydrogenase (LDH) level ≥ 800 IU/L (Brugières et al, 1998).

Histopathologic Features

Nodal architecture is effaced by a sinus, paracortical, or diffuse infiltrate of cohesive-appearing large tumor cells with a high mitotic rate (Fig. 15–3). Classic ALCL is broadly divided into two subtypes: pleomorphic and monomorphic. Pleomorphic ALCL is composed of large cells with irregular, indented, or embryoid nuclei. Nuclear chromatin is dispersed, and nucleoli are single or multiple and small to large. Multinucleated giant cells, which are often present, may have a wreathlike appearance. Cytoplasm is usually abundant and basophilic to clear. In the monomorphic variant, the cells are somewhat smaller and show minimal cytologic variation (Fig. 15–4) (Chott et al, 1990). Nuclei are round, oval, or slightly irregular. Their chromatin is dispersed, and nucleoli are prominent. Cytoplasm is moderately abundant, and multinucleated giant cells are absent or few in number. Admixed inflammatory cells are variably present in both subtypes of ALCL. Plasma cells frequently surround sheets of tumor cells and, rarely, eosinophils or neutrophils may be prominent (Mann et al, 1995).

A SCV of ALCL has a predominance of small, irregular lymphocytes and a minor population of large CD30+ cells (Kinney et al, 1993; Toren et al, 1996). A paracortical infiltrate partially effacing nodal architecture on low magnification is characteristic (Fig. 15–5). The SCV may be confused with a reactive process because the patients are often young and have symptoms suggesting infection, and involved sites may be extranodal. The large-cell component is difficult to identify until staining for CD30 (Ki-1) is performed. Transformation to ALCL histologic features, particularly of the monomorphic type, may occur in patients with the SCV (Hodges et al, 1999)

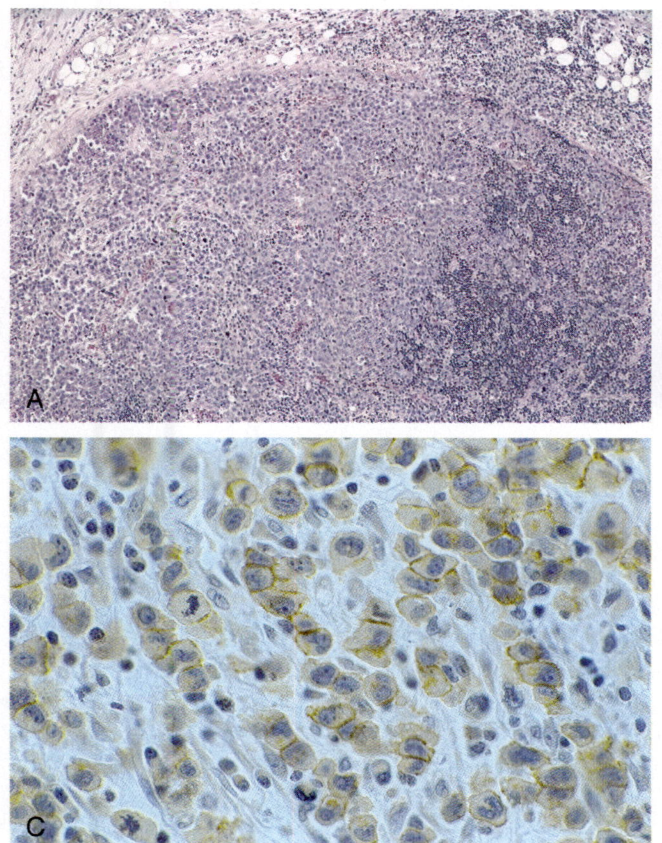

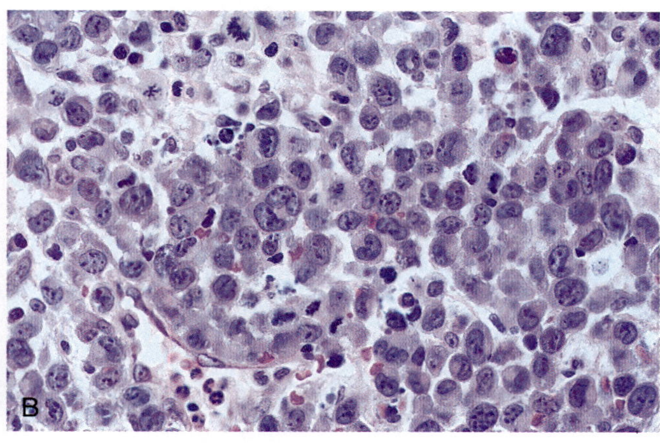

Figure 15–3

Anaplastic large-cell lymphoma, pleomorphic type, lymph node. *A*, Cohesive-appearing sheets of large tumor cells are present in the subcapsular sinus and the paracortical area. *B*, The cells are large and dysplastic with folded, indented nuclei, partially dispersed chromatin, prominent nucleoli, abundant cytoplasm, and a high mitotic rate. Occasional giant cells are present. There are few admixed inflammatory cells. *C*, Tumor cells uniformly exhibit strong membrane CD30 (Ber-H2) positivity. Some cells also stain in the paranuclear or Golgi region. CD30 by paraffin immunoperoxidase.

(Figs. 15–6, 15–7, and 15–8). The clinical course may be aggressive, regardless of whether transformation supervenes.

Rarely, ALCLs have spindle- and oval-shaped tumor cells with a storiform growth pattern that resembles a sarcoma, a form known as the sarcomatoid variant (Chan et al, 1990) (Fig. 15–9). There is also a lymphohistiocytic variant in which reactive histiocytes predominate; neoplastic cells are rare and somewhat smaller than in classic ALCL (Pileri et al, 1990).

ALCL may show overlap with Hodgkin disease (particularly reticular subtype of lymphocyte depleted or syncytial variant of nodular sclerosing) due to the presence of capsular thickening, fibrous tissue deposition, and Reed-Sternberg–like

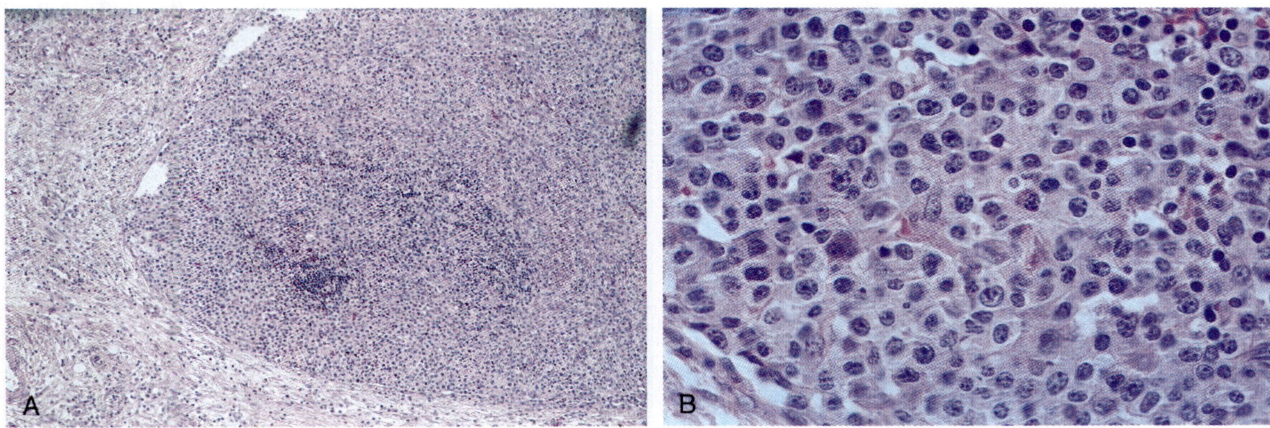

Figure 15–4

Anaplastic large-cell lymphoma (ALCL), monomorphic type, lymph node. *A*, Nodal architecture is effaced by a sinus and paracortical diffuse large-cell infiltrate. *B*, The tumor cells are large transformed lymphocytes with little variability from cell to cell. The nuclei are only slightly irregular. Tumor cells are smaller than in pleomorphic ALCL (see Fig. 15–3). This type of ALCL is distinguished from other large transformed cell lymphomas by its growth pattern (sinus or paracortical) and strong reactivity with antibodies against CD30 (not shown).

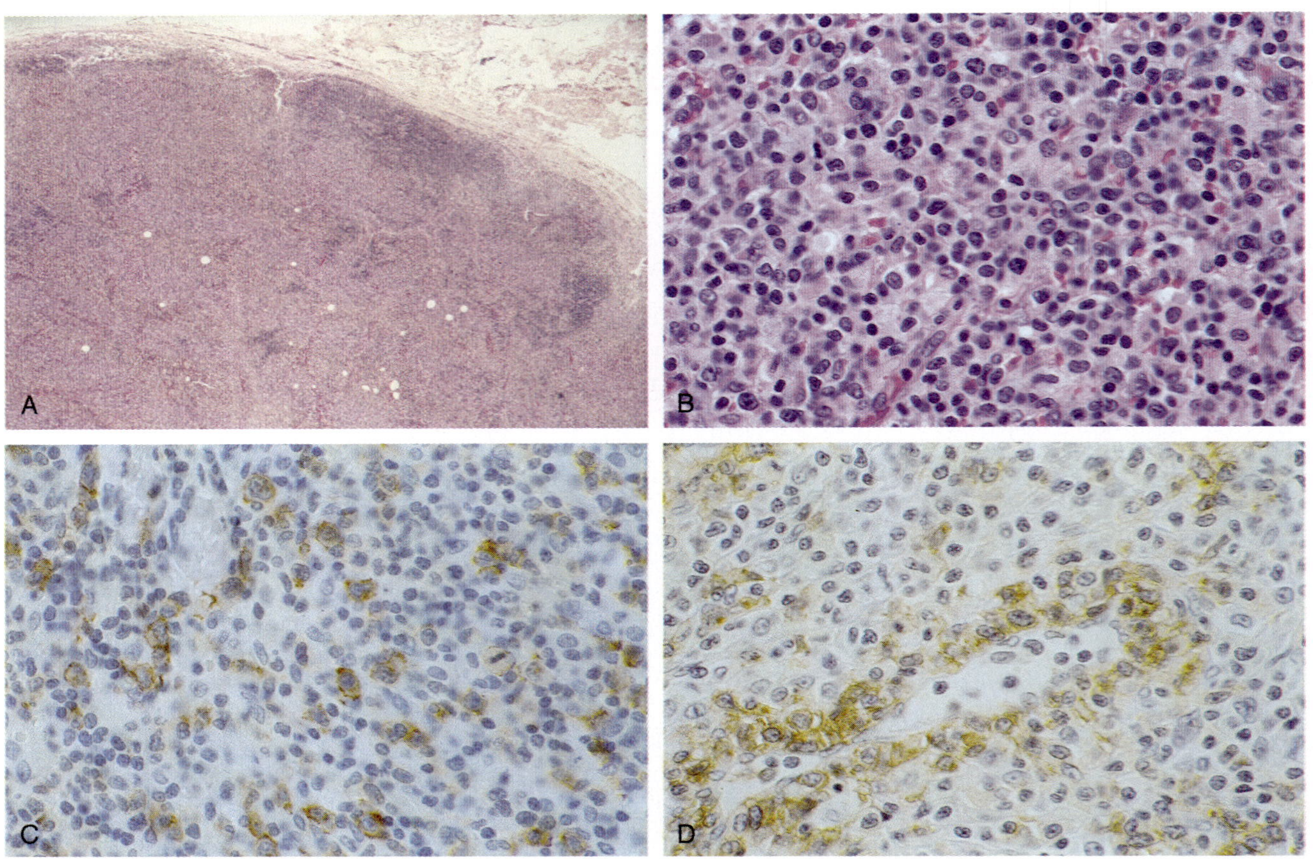

Figure 15–5

Anaplastic large-cell lymphoma, small-cell variant, lymph node. *A*, Nodal architecture is partially effaced by a paracortical and diffuse infiltrate. *B*, The infiltrate is composed predominantly of small, irregular lymphocytes with only a minor component of large transformed cells. *C*, The large transformed cells and a few smaller lymphocytes are CD30+ (Ber-H2+). Paraffin immunoperoxidase. *D*, The large tumor cells often show a predilection for blood vessels. CD30 by paraffin immunoperoxidase.

giant cells (Agnarsson & Kadin, 1988; Kinney & Kadin, 1999). The REAL classification has a provisional entity, ALCL Hodgkin's-Like (Hodgkin's-related) (Harris et al., 1994). Further study is required to define the relationship of these cases to ALCL and Hodgkin disease, but the WHO classification committee has suggested this tumor may be more closely related to the latter (Stein, 1997).

The appearance of the neoplastic infiltrate in skin lesions is variable, corresponding to the cytologic spectrum seen in nodes (Kadin, 1990; Kaudewitz et al, 1994; Krishnan et al, 1993; Macgrogan et al, 1996; Willemze & Beljaards, 1993). The pattern of tumor infiltration corresponds to the gross morphologic features. Mass lesions are often ulcerated and have a diffuse infiltrate of large cells that extends from the superficial to the deep dermis and into the subcutaneous fat (Fig. 15–10). With small nodules and rashes, the tumor infiltrate occurs around skin appendages and small vessels. With mass lesions or infiltrates, there may be focal epidermotropism and/or pseudoepitheliomatous hyperplasia so extensive as to be confused with squamous cell carcinoma (Krasne et al, 1988). Large numbers of histiocytes may be present. The term *regressing atypical histiocytosis* has been erroneously applied to such lesions (Flynn et al, 1982; Headington et al, 1987; Motley et al., 1992) (see Fig. 15–10).

ALCL may be very difficult to distinguish from lymphomatoid papulosis (Demierre et al, 1997; Kinney & Kadin, 1999; Tomaszewski et al, 1995). Patients with lymphomatoid papulosis typically have multiple disseminated small papules on the trunk and proximal extremities that regress with a hyperpigmented or hypopigmented scar, whereas a single, or, less commonly, multiple lesions localized to one anatomic site are seen in ALCL. Lesions in lymphomatoid papulosis are small (usually <1 cm) and produce a wedge-shaped infiltrate with a perivascular or periadnexal location that in most cases does not extend to the subcutaneous fat. ALCL produces a more diffuse infiltrate that does involve the subcutaneous tissue. Ulceration is seen in both lesions, but necrosis of the dermal infiltrate is much more common in ALCL. Both lesions have large dysplastic CD30+ cells. Epithelial membrane antigen is usually absent in lymphomatoid papulosis but is often not expressed in cutaneous ALCL of the primary type. Nodal involvement is not seen in lymphomatoid papulosis.

Marrow involvement is infrequent, except in the SCV (Fraga et al, 1995; Kinney et al, 1993). In ALCL, tumor cells are usually found singly or in very small clusters (Fig. 15–11). These cells are not readily apparent until immunoperoxidase staining with antibodies to CD30 is performed.

ALCL may be diagnosed in body fluids and fine-needle aspirates (Tani et al, 1989; Yazdi & Burns, 1991). The cytologic appearance is distinctive (see Fig. 15–8*C*). The tumor cells are noncohesive and may be very large, with round to irregular nuclei, dispersed chromatin, and prominent nucleoli. Multinucleated cells are often present. The cytoplasm is abundant

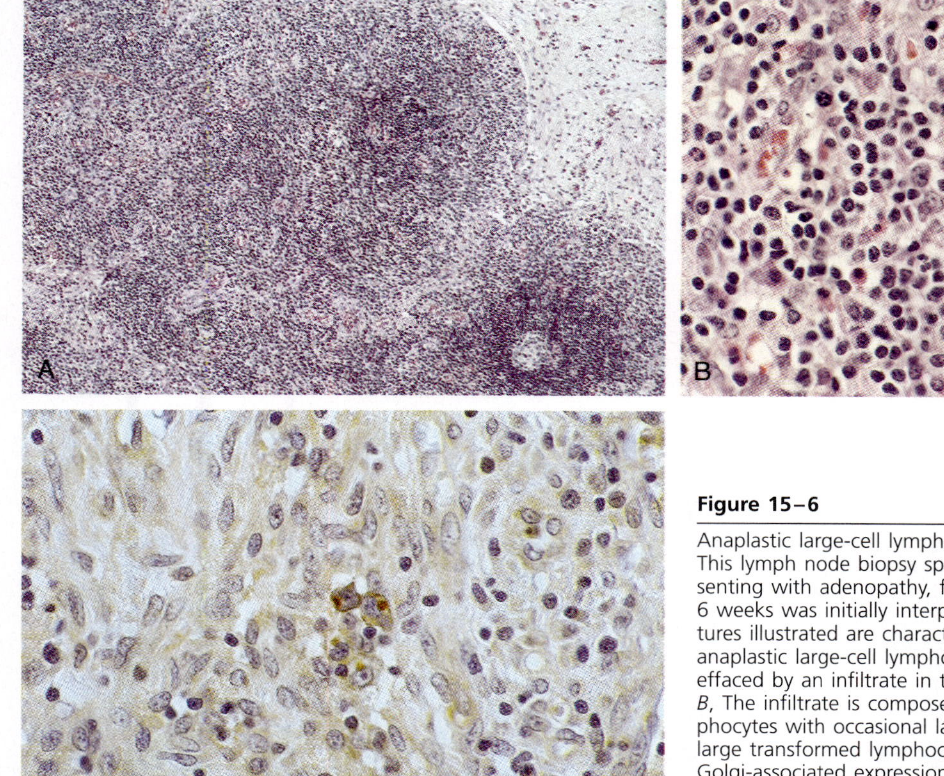

Figure 15–6

Anaplastic large-cell lymphoma, small-cell variant, lymph node. This lymph node biopsy specimen from a 14-year-old male presenting with adenopathy, fever, pharyngitis, and weight loss for 6 weeks was initially interpreted as a reactive process. The features illustrated are characteristic of the small-cell variant of anaplastic large-cell lymphoma. *A*, Nodal architecture is partially effaced by an infiltrate in the subcapsular sinus and paracortex. *B*, The infiltrate is composed principally of small, irregular lymphocytes with occasional large transformed cells. *C*, The marking large transformed lymphocytes have distinct membrane and Golgi-associated expression of CD30 in contrast to the weak background positivity. Ber-H2 staining, paraffin immunoperoxidase.

and very basophilic and has fine vacuoles, best appreciated with Wright stain.

Immunophenotype

Most ALCL cases have a T cell phenotype, 10–20% mark as B cells, and 15–25% have a null or unclassified phenotype. The B cell phenotype is seen in <5% of childhood ALCL (Reiter et al, 1994; Rubie et al, 1994; Sandlund et al, 1994; Vecchi et al, 1993) and should be grouped with other diffuse large B cell lymphomas. Virtually all tumor cells are CD30 (Ki-1)+. Epithelial membrane antigen (EMA) and cytolytic granule protein TIA-1 expression are particularly frequent in T cell and null ALCL (Delsol et al, 1988; Felgar et al, 1999). CD45 expression may be absent or weak and focal. Rare cases of ALCL exhibit weak cytokeratin expression (Gustmann et al, 1991). Approximately 15–20% of cases are CD15+. Immunologic study to detect CD45, EMA, cytokeratin, CD30, and B and T cell markers must be performed to avoid a misdiagnosis (Table 15–5). It should be emphasized that CD30 reactivity is not specific for neoplasms, since CD30 may be seen in reactive conditions such as infectious mononucleosis (Abbondanzo et al, 1990). Various neoplasms, including Hodgkin disease, B and T cell lymphomas (Stein et al, 1985), and carcinomas, particularly embryonal carcinomas (Pallesen & Hamilton-Dutoit, 1988; Schwarting et al, 1989), may be CD30+.

Diagnostic Criteria

The diagnostic criteria for ALCL are given in Table 15–6.

Differential Diagnosis

The differential diagnosis of ALCL includes Hodgkin disease with numerous Reed-Sternberg cells, microvillous B cell lymphoma (Kinney et al, 1990), metastatic carcinoma or melanoma, and malignant histiocytosis, all diseases that are distinguished from ALCL readily by immunohistochemical study (see Table 15–5). In distinguishing Hodgkin disease and ALCL, admixed inflammatory cells, inclusion-like nucleoli in the tumor cells, a lower mitotic rate, and little or no sinus involvement favor a diagnosis of Hodgkin disease. Conversely, a sheetlike growth pattern with few interspersed inflammatory cells (most surround the sheet of tumor), a high mitotic rate, nucleoli that are not inclusion like, and prominent sinus involvement favor ALCL. Microvillus lymphoma has a cohesive growth pattern with prominent sinus involvement. Compared to ALCL, the cells are round to oval with less nuclear folding and pleomorphism (Kinney et al, 1990). Metastatic carcinoma has a very cohesive growth pattern. Nasopharyngeal carcinoma has vesicular chromatin and a single prominent nucleolus. Melanoma cells have very prominent nucleoli, abundant eosinophilic cytoplasm, rarely cytoplasmic melanin, and stain with antibodies S-100 and HMB.45. Malignant histiocytosis is difficult to diagnose based on morphologic criteria. There are no distinguishing features, and immunologic or ultrastructural confirmation of a histiocytic neoplasm is required.

The SCV of ALCL may be confused with a reactive interfollicular infiltrate. Ki-1+, CD30+ large cells are present in reactive adenitis, but they are negative for EMA and ALK1 (antibody against anaplastic lymphoma kinase). In the SCV, the large CD30+ cells tend to surround blood vessels. Flow

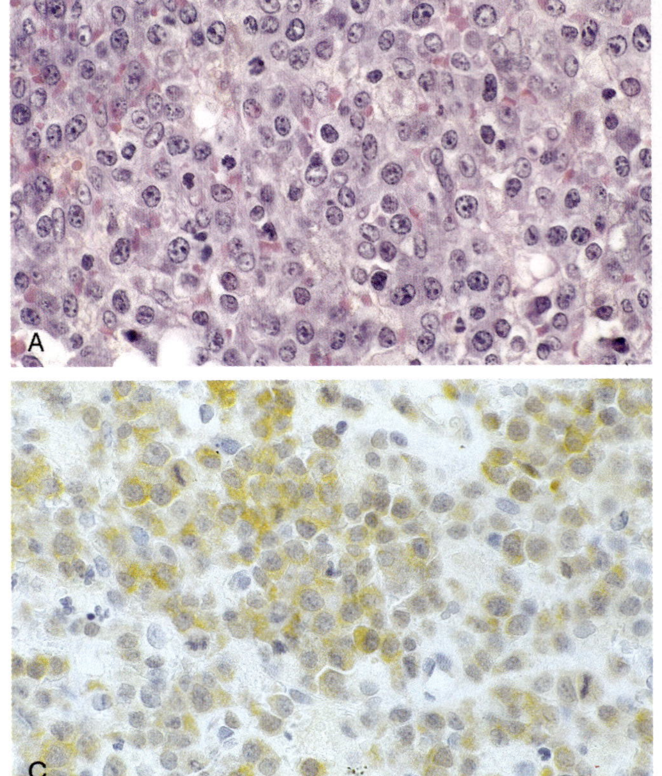

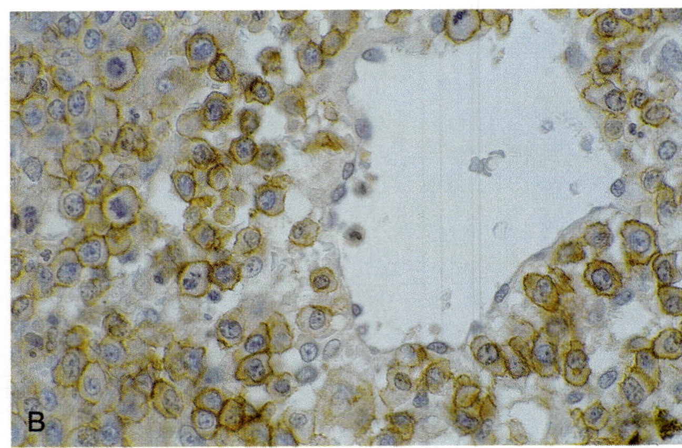

Figure 15–7

Anaplastic large-cell lymphoma, small-cell variant with transformation to large-cell lymphoma, axillary mass. A rapidly developing axillary mass was noted 4 weeks after obtaining the diagnostic lymph node biopsy specimen shown in Fig. 15–6. *A*, Subcutaneous tissue is diffusely involved by a homogenous infiltrate of large transformed lymphocytes with round to oval, slightly irregular nuclei and abundant cytoplasm. *B*, Virtually all tumor cells strongly express CD30. The features illustrated in *A* and here are diagnostic of monomorphic anaplastic large-cell lymphoma. Ber-H2 staining paraffin immunoperoxidase. *C*, The tumor cells are reactive with an antibody against the ALK kinase portion of the fusion protein p80$^{NPM/ALK}$, created by the t(2;5)(p23;q35). Paraffin immunoperoxidase.

cytometric studies in the SCV often reveal loss of pan–T cell antigens, particularly CD3.

Pathogenesis and Biologic Characteristics

ALCL is frequently associated with a nonrandom chromosomal translocation, t(2;5)(p23;q35). Cloning of the translocation has revealed involvement of the nucleophosmin *(NPM)* gene on chromosome 5 and the anaplastic lymphoma kinase *(ALK)* gene on chromosome 2 (Morris et al, 1994), with dysregulation of the latter presumably important in the pathogenesis of ALCL. The t(2;5) is detected by various molecular methods in 13–80% of ALCL (summarized in Elmberger et al, 1995). Antibodies (ALK1 and P80) to the anaplastic lymphoma kinase protein and the fusion protein p80 $^{NPM/ALK}$ have been developed. They provide an immunohistochemical method to detect the t(2;5), since ALK is not normally expressed in hematic or lymphocytic cells (Pulford et al, 1997; Shiota et al, 1994, 1995) (see Fig. 15-7*C*). ALK expression correlates most highly with T cell or null phenotype, young patient age, and monomorphic or SCV histologic features (Benharroch et al, 1998; Drexler et al, 2000; Falini et al, 1998; Kinney & Kadin, 1999; Kinney et al, 1996; Pittaluga et al, 1997; Shiota et al, 1995; Wellman et al, 1995). Most secondary Ki-1+ lymphomas, B cell ALCLs, Hodgkin-related ALCLs, and primary cutaneous ALCLs lack the t(2;5) (DeCoteau et al, 1996; Wellman et al, 1995). When these types of Ki-1+ lymphoma are excluded, the incidence of the t(2;5) increases to 65–80%. The overall incidence of the t(2;5) has been found to be approximately 30% using molecular genetic techniques and 40–60% using immunohistochemical studies.

Immunostaining for ALK-1 or p80 is nuclear and cytoplasmic in approximately 80% of positive cases. The nuclear staining results from the nuclear localization due to the NPM portion of the t(2;5) fusion protein. Cytoplasm only stains in the remaining 20% of cases, in which there are other genetic abnormalities: t(1;2)(q25;p23); t(2;3)(p23;q21); inv(2)(p23q35), which result in *ALK* gene dysregulation (Drexler et al, 2000; Ma et al, 2000; Touriol et al, 2000). The role of EBV in the pathogenesis of ALCL is controversial. Using immunohistochemical and molecular methods, the incidence of EBV infection in a series of adults and children has been shown to vary from 5 to 47% (Anagnostopoulos et al, 1989; Herbst et al, 1991; Herbst & Stein, 1993a; Lopategui et al, 1995; Nakagawa et al, 1997). Other studies suggest that EBV may be present in reactive cells in some of the polymerase chain reaction–positive cases (Kanavaros et al, 1992). In childhood ALCL, EBV is infrequent or absent (Brousset et al, 1993; Nakagawa et al, 1997). Human T cell lymphotropic virus-1 complete and incomplete proviruses have been detected in some cutaneous ALCLs (Herbst & Stein, 1993b).

ANGIOIMMUNOBLASTIC LYMPHADENOPATHY–LIKE T CELL LYMPHOMA

Immunoblastic lymphadenopathy (Lukes & Tindle, 1975), angioimmunoblastic lymphadenopathy with dysproteinemia (AILD) (Frizzera et al, 1974), and AILD-like T cell lymphoma (Nathwani et al, 1978; Shimoyama et al, 1979) are clinically and pathologically similar but are not identical. Patients have systemic disease with generalized adenopathy, fever, weight loss, rash, polyclonal hypergammaglobulinemia, and autoimmune

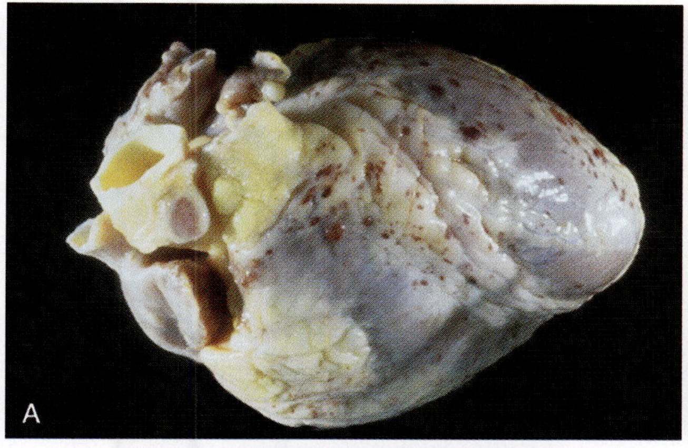

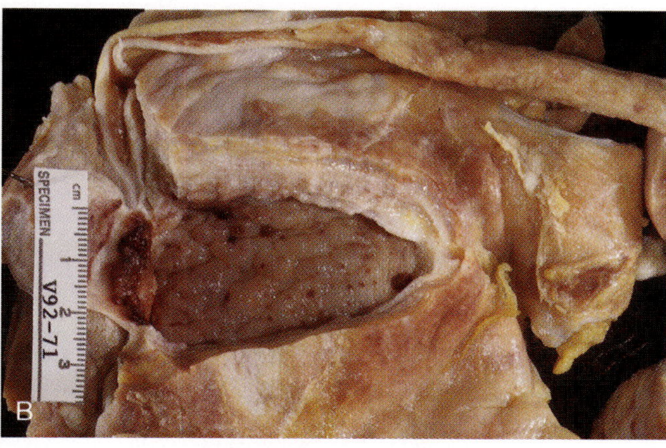

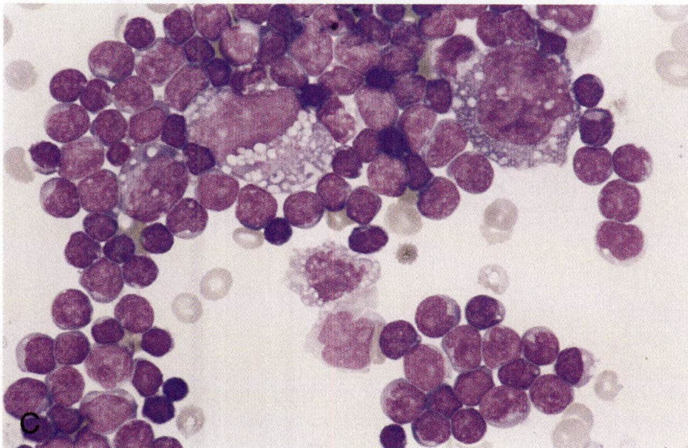

Figure 15–8

Anaplastic large-cell lymphoma, small-cell variant with transformation to large-cell lymphoma, autopsy. The patient died a few hours after the axillary biopsy (see Fig. 15–7) was performed. Autopsy revealed widespread, disseminated disease on the pleural, peritoneal, and pericardial surfaces and in most organs and nodes. *A*, The heart has hemorrhagic tumor nodules on the pericardial surface. *B*, The bladder exhibits tumor encasing the bladder wall and forming hemorrhagic nodules on the mucosal surface. *C*, The pleural fluid contains large tumor cells with abundant basophilic vacuolated cytoplasm. Numerous small dysplastic lymphocytes are also present. Wright stain. Figures 15–6 to 15–8 are from the same patient.

hemolytic anemia. Node biopsy reveals obliteration of nodal architecture owing to marked proliferation of branching vessels and a polymorphous infiltrate of small lymphocytes, plasma cells, and immunoblasts. Immunologic, cytogenetic, and genotypic data have been difficult to interpret in these cases because of varying diagnostic criteria. Most cases have exhibited clonality in TCR gene rearrangement studies (Weiss et al, 1986). Diseases carrying these diagnoses likely represent a spectrum of diseases from T cell dysplasia to peripheral T cell lymphoma (Frizzera et al, 1989; Smith et al, 2000; Watanabe et al, 1986). The majority are considered to be lymphomas and are classified as angioimmunoblastic T cell lymphomas in the REAL classification (Harris et al, 1994; Lennert & Feller, 1992; Nathwani & Jaffe, 1995). Equivalent terms include immunoblastic lymphadenopathy-like T cell lymphoma (Lukes-Collins); T cell angioimmunoblastic lymphoma (AILD; Kiel); and diffuse mixed small- and large-cell, diffuse large-cell, and large-cell immunoblastic lymphoma (Working Formulation).

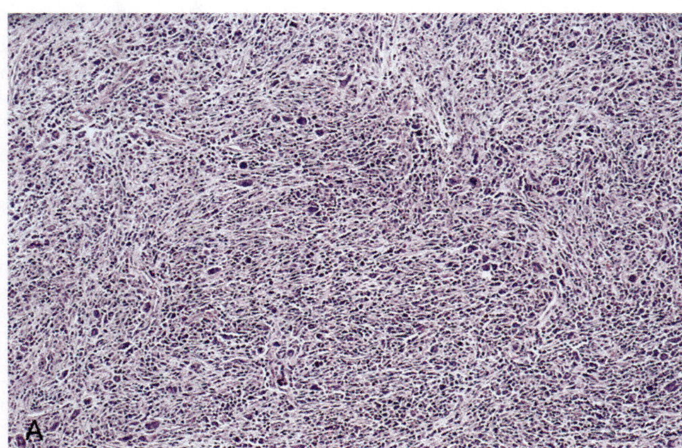

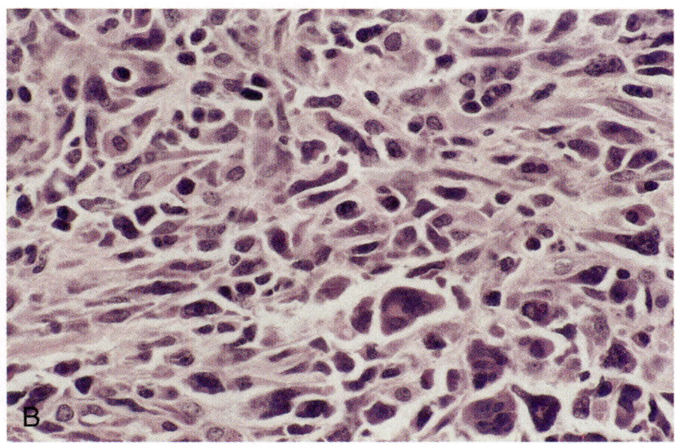

Figure 15–9

Anaplastic large-cell lymphoma, sarcomatoid variant, lymph node. This patient had skin and node involvement. *A*, The node is diffusely effaced by pleomorphic large cells with an interlacing or swirled growth pattern. *B*, The tumor cells are very anaplastic, and many are elongated or straplike, resembling a sarcoma.

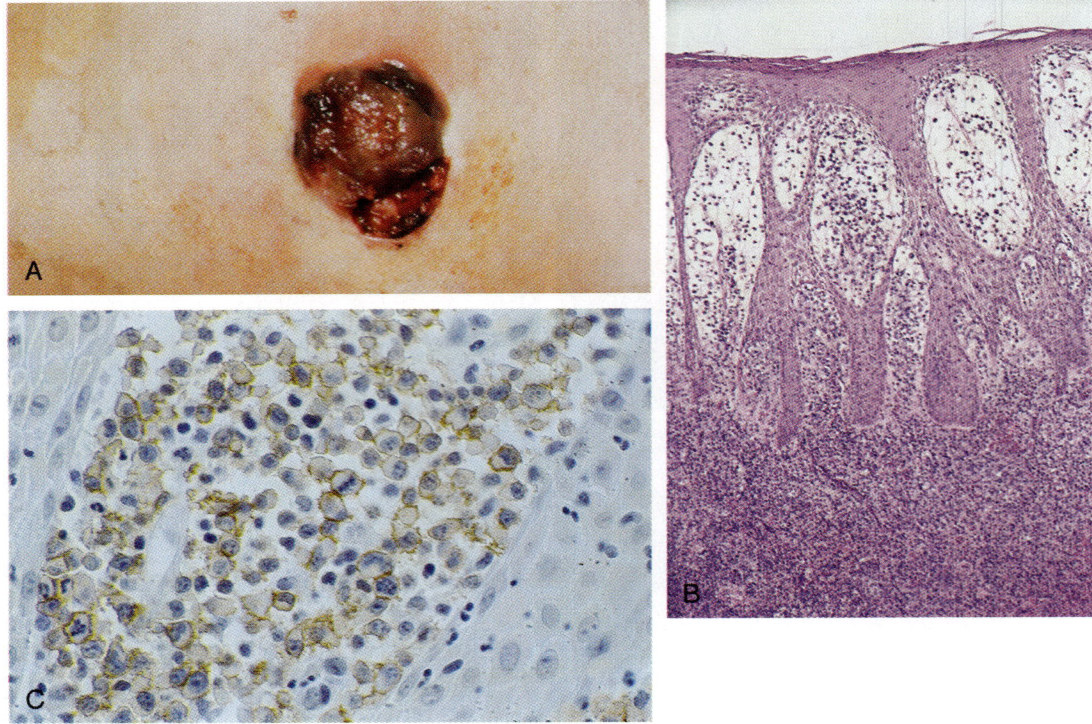

Figure 15–10

Anaplastic large-cell lymphoma, skin. *A*, Ulcerated tumor mass (5 × 4 cm) in a 16-year-old girl. This was the only site of disease. Several weeks after the biopsy, the lesion regressed, and the patient is disease free after 8 years. *B*, Histologic section reveals epidermal hyperplasia with a diffuse large-cell infiltrate that extends deep into the dermis and subcutaneous fat (not shown). *C*, The cells are anaplastic, resemble histiocytes, and strongly express CD30 (Ber-H2). This appearance was initially described as regressing atypical histiocytosis. Paraffin immunoperoxidase.

Clinical Features

AILD-like T cell lymphomas are rare in children. Fewer than 20 cases have been reported, with an age range from 5 months to 14 years (Geha et al, 1984; Howarth & Bird, 1976; Kissane, 1974; Nakazono et al, 1991; Nezelof & Virelizier, 1982; Stensvold et al, 1984). Fever, weight loss, generalized lymphadenopathy, hepatosplenomegaly, skin rash, and polyclonal hypergammaglobulinemia are described, as in adult patients.

Cases of AILD are also very rare in children and have a variable clinical course. Cases have shown spontaneous regression (Fiorillo et al, 1981), an indolent course with response to immunosuppression (Hirose et al, 1994), or a relapsing course (de Terlizzi et al, 1989). Progression from AILD to T cell lymphoma (immunoblastic and AILD-like) has been reported (Howarth & Bird, 1976; Nakazono et al, 1991). In both of these reports, the patients died in a year or less after the diagnosis of lymphoma, despite cytotoxic chemotherapy.

Histopathologic Features

In AILD-like T cell lymphoma, nodal architecture is effaced by a polymorphous infiltrate of small lymphocytes, immunoblasts and large transformed cells, plasma cells, and eosinophils with a diffuse or paracortical or interfollicular growth pattern, with loss of most sinuses and follicular structures (Fig. 15–12). There is marked proliferation of small vessels (high endothelial venules) that arborize and may extend into the capsule and surrounding tissue. Vessel lumina may be narrowed or obstructed by endothelial cell hyperplasia. Vessel walls in some cases may be hyalinized and periodic acid–Schiff (PAS) positive. Proliferation of follicular dendritic cells gives the appearance of burned-out follicles or a look of depletion. Burned-out or reactive follicles are more prominent in AILD. Hyperplastic follicles are rare; when they are prominent a drug reaction should be considered. A diagnosis of lymphoma is made when there are clusters or diffuse proliferations of immunoblasts, transformed cells, or pale cells with weakly staining or clear cytoplasm. Pale cells are generally medium to large but may be small (Nathwani & Jaffe, 1995; Tobinai et al, 1988). Clusters of epithelioid histiocytes may be seen and are rarely so prominent as to suggest lymphoepithelioid lymphoma (Lennert lymphoma) (Patsouris et al, 1989).

Extranodal involvement occurs in the skin, marrow, spleen, and liver (Nathwani et al, 1978). Infiltrates are similar to those in the nodes. Vessels are variably present. In the skin, infiltrates are around adnexal structures and blood vessels, in the marrow they are paratrabecular or interstitial, in the spleen they involve red and white pulp, and in the liver they surround portal tracts or are parenchymal.

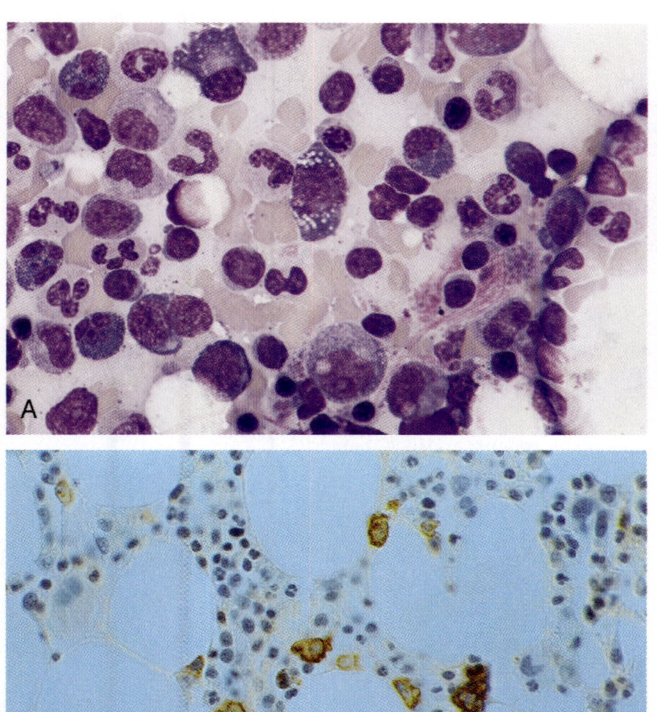

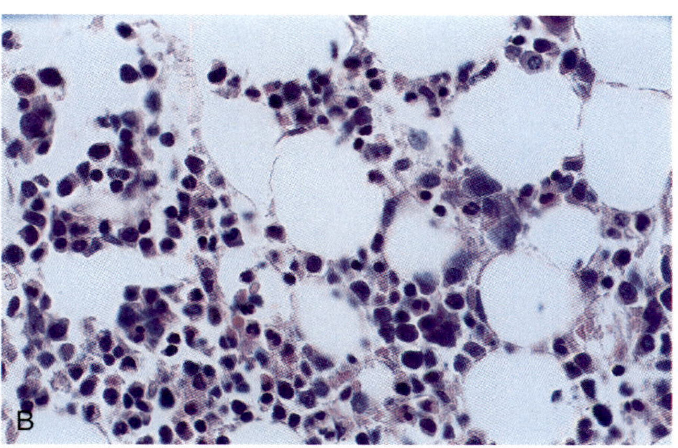

Figure 15–11

Anaplastic large-cell lymphoma, small-cell variant, marrow. *A*, Rare large, vacuolated basophilic tumor cells are identified on this marrow aspirate film. Wright stain. *B*, Tumor infiltration in tissue section is subtle, since there are no masses of tumor cells. *C*, CD30 (Ber-H2) staining shows scattered single tumor cells. Paraffin immunoperoxidase.

Immunophenotype

Tumors express T cell antigens, and approximately one half to two thirds are of the CD4+ subtype. The remainder are CD8+ or do not mark as to subtype. Anti-CD21 or -CD35 antibodies are useful in demonstrating the expanded clusters of follicular dendritic cells. A minor population of CD30+ large cells may be present (Stein et al, 1985).

Diagnostic Criteria

The diagnostic criteria for AILD-like T cell lymphoma are listed in Table 15–7.

Differential Diagnosis

The differential diagnosis of AILD-like T cell lymphoma includes reactive and neoplastic processes that expand the paracortex (interfollicular area) and result in varying degrees of destruction of the follicles and sinuses. As mentioned earlier, AILD-like T cell lymphoma and AILD are distinguished by the presence of clusters or sheets of atypical lymphocytes, with immunoblastic, transformed cell, or clear cell morphologic features in the former or more burned-out follicles or reactive follicles in the latter. Hodgkin disease may have an interfollicular growth pattern and may be difficult to distinguish morphologically from AILD-like T cell lymphoma (see Chap. 13). Immunoblasts or atypical small lymphocytes are absent in Hodgkin disease. Immunoperoxidase studies demonstrate that the large atypical cells are strongly CD15+, CD30+, and LCA− in Hodgkin disease. Scattered CD30+ cells may be present in AILD (Stein et al, 1985). Drug reactions and viral infections produce an immunoblastic proliferation in the paracortical area of nodes (see Chap. 16). Reactive hyperplastic follicular centers and eosinophils are usually prominent in drug reactions and are useful diagnostic features. Viral infections, particularly EBV infections, may cause profound immunoblastic proliferation with dysplastic cells resembling Reed-Sternberg cells. Clinical history is essential. Immunoperoxidase studies are useful and show a mixture of B and T cells and lack of CD15. Nodal sinuses are preserved; they contain immunoblasts and transformed and some small lymphocytes.

Pathogenesis and Biologic Characteristics

The presence of gene rearrangements (most often T cell and less frequently B cell) in most cases of AILD-like T cell lymphoma (Feller et al, 1988; Lipford et al, 1987; Weiss et al, 1986) implies that AILD is a neoplasm. However, it is probably simplistic to equate clonality with malignancy. Some investigators have failed to detect clonality and have suggested that AILD is a disorder of immunoregulation resulting in increased proliferation and increased susceptibility to genetic errors during cell division. EBV genomes are detected in many cases (Anagnostopoulos et al, 1992; Khan et al, 1993; Weiss et al, 1992), suggesting its involvement in the pathogenesis of this lymphoma. Karyotypic abnormalities include trisomy 3 and/or 5 and +X and a high frequency of cytogenetically unrelated clones (oligoclonal proliferations) (Schlegelberger et al, 1994; Schlegelberger et al, 1990). Some cases have been shown to have abnormal expression of *MYB* or *NRAS* (Knecht, 1989).

Table 15–5
Immunophenotypic Differentiation of ALCL from Other Large-Cell Neoplasms

	Antigen Expression*							
Tumor Type	CD30	CD15	CD45	EMA	Keratin	CD68	CD20	CD43
ALCL	+	−/+	+	+	−	−	−/+	+
Carcinoma	−/+	+/−	−	+	+	−	−	−
Malignant histiocytosis	−/+	−/+	+/−	−/+	−	+	−	−/+
Microvillus lymphoma	−	−	+	−	−	−	+	−
HD†	+	+	−/+	−/+	−	−	−/+	−/+

*+, >50% of cases; +/−, 25–50%; −/+, 5–24%; −, 0–4%.

†Other than lymphocyte predominant.

Abbreviations: ALCL, anaplastic large-cell lymphoma; EMA, epithelial membrane antigen; HD, Hodgkin disease.

MYCOSIS FUNGOIDES

Mycosis fungoides (MF) is a chronic lymphoproliferative disorder that arises in the skin and may involve the peripheral blood (Sézary syndrome). The tumor cell is presumably a skin-based T lymphocyte with cerebriform nuclei. The term *cutaneous T cell lymphoma* (CTCL) has been used synonymously with MF, but this broad and somewhat nonspecific term should be avoided, since it includes several T cell neoplasms with cutaneous involvement (ALCL, adult T cell leukemia or lymphoma, angiocentric T cell lymphoma, AILD-like T cell lymphoma, subcutaneous panniculitis-like T cell lymphoma). Equivalent terms include cerebriform T cell lymphoma (Lukes-Collins); small-cell, cerebriform T cell lymphoma (Kiel); and mycosis fungoides (Working Formulation).

Clinical Features and Prognosis

Skin lesions may be localized or generalized and produce patches, erythema, plaques, or tumors. Patches begin as red, circumscribed flat macules that generally coalesce to form patches. The plaque stage has palpable indurated, discrete lesions that may arise from preexisting patches, from confluence of papules, or *de novo*. Tumors are large nodules more than 1 cm in diameter that are frequently ulcerated or eroded.

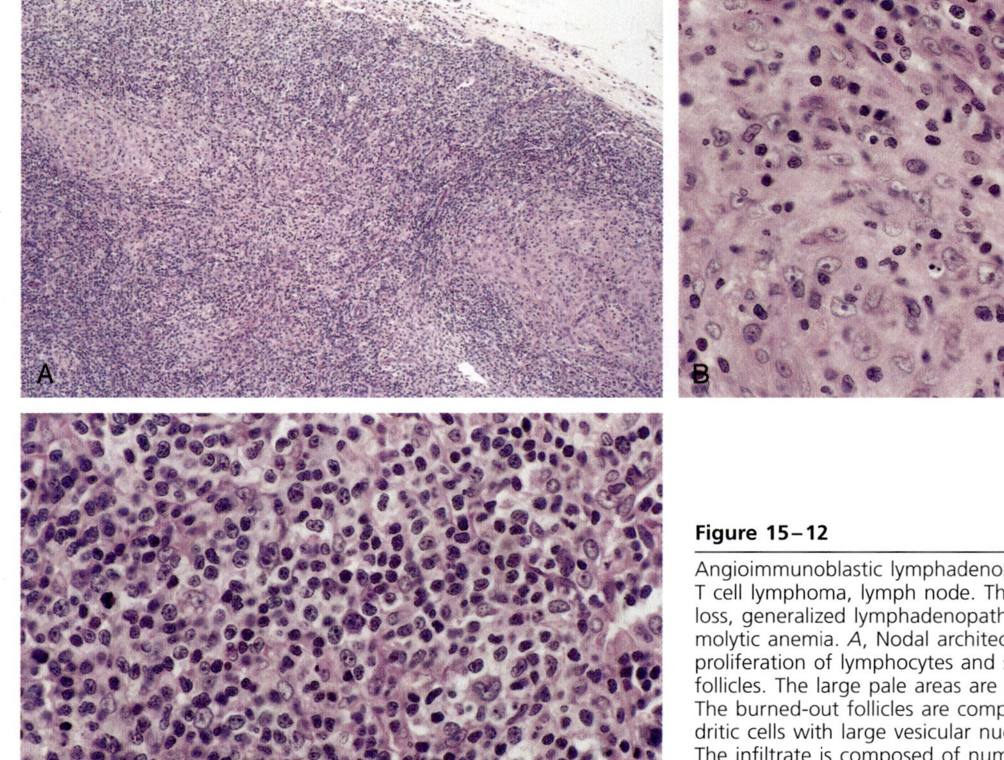

Figure 15–12

Angioimmunoblastic lymphadenopathy with dysproteinemia–like T cell lymphoma, lymph node. This patient had fever, weight loss, generalized lymphadenopathy, and a Coombs-positive hemolytic anemia. *A*, Nodal architecture is obliterated secondary to proliferation of lymphocytes and small vessels as well as loss of follicles. The large pale areas are burned-out follicular centers. *B*, The burned-out follicles are composed of sheets of follicular dendritic cells with large vesicular nuclei and prominent nucleoli. *C*, The infiltrate is composed of numerous small lymphocytes, transformed lymphocytes, and occasional large Reed-Sternberg–like cells. Some of the small and larger lymphocytes have clear cytoplasm.

Table 15–6
ALCL: Diagnostic Criteria

Cohesive large-cell infiltrate with pleomorphic or monomorphic cytologic features; a subset of patients with small-cell variant histologic features
Paracortical or sinus growth pattern
Strong expression of CD30 in virtually every tumor cell
T or null cell phenotype with frequent expression of EMA
t(2;5) or other evidence of *ALK* gene dysregulation in most pediatric cases

Abbreviations: ALCL, anaplastic large-cell lymphoma; EMA, epithelial membrane antigen.

Table 15–7
AILD-like T Cell Lymphoma: Diagnostic Criteria

Polymorphous infiltrate of lymphocytes, plasma cells, and eosinophils; clusters or diffuse proliferations of immunoblasts, transformed cells, or "pale cells" with clear or weakly staining cytoplasm
Total or near-total effacement of nodal architecture; absent or burned-out germinal centers; follicular dendritic cell proliferation present in most; increased numbers of branching venules often with PAS+ hyalinized walls
CD4+ >> CD8+; EBV+
T cell receptor rearrangements show clonality in most cases

Abbreviations: AILD, angioimmunoblastic lymphadenopathy with disproteinemia; EBV, Epstein-Barr virus; PAS, periodic acid–Schiff.

The erythrodermic form is characterized by generalized reddening of the skin. Some patients have superimposed plaques or tumors. The skin lesions of all types are often pruritic with scaling. The clinical course is usually indolent, with gradual progression of lesions.

Patients with MF have a median age of 55 to 65 years. The male-female ratio of MF is 2:1, and the incidence in blacks is twice as high as in whites. Children are rarely affected, representing 5% or less of MF cases (Koch et al, 1987; Peters et al, 1990). Their age range is 3 to 18 years. Most children have patch or plaque lesions, and the tumor stage is rare (Taniguchi et al, 1980; Tope et al, 1992). Sézary syndrome has been reported in an 11-year-old girl (Meister et al, 1993). Pagetoid reticulosis (Woringer-Kolopp disease), a clinical entity in which patients have single or multiple hyperkeratotic or verrucous plaques on hands or feet and a benign course (Burns et al, 1995; Deneau et al, 1984; Mielke et al, 1989), is considered a localized form of MF. This disease has been described in children and adolescents and is notable for prominent epidermotropism and little dermal involvement (Mandojana & Helwig, 1983). A more disseminated form (Ketron-Goodman disease) has a worse prognosis. A rare hypopigmented macular form of MF reported in black males aged 9 and 15 may be more common in young patients (Whitmore et al, 1994).

Most childhood MF arises *de novo*, but antecedent pityriasis lichenoides et varioliformis acuta and benign reactive lymphocytic hyperplasias have been reported (Fortson et al, 1990; Wilson et al, 1991). MF should be considered in the differential diagnosis of skin lesions in childhood, and skin biopsy should be performed in children and adolescents with chronic scaly eruptions and a lack of response to topical steroids (Koch et al, 1987).

MF and Sézary syndrome may be divided into three risk groups (Sausville et al, 1988). Patients with low-stage disease with plaques are a good risk group, with a median survival time of over 12 years. Patients in an intermediate risk group, with plaques and involvement of lymph nodes or blood or, alternatively, tumors or erythroderma without nodal involvement, have a median survival time of 5 years. Patients with visceral disease or node effacement by tumor have a median survival time of 2.5 years or less.

Treatment includes electron beam therapy, photochemotherapy with ingestion of the photosensitizing drug 8-methoxy-psoralen followed by exposure to ultraviolet A irradiation (Herrmann et al, 1995); extracorporeal photopheresis (Gollnick et al, 1995); topical chemotherapy, most commonly with nitrogen mustard (Kuzel et al, 1991); and systemic chemotherapy (Bunn et al, 1994).

Histopathologic Features

MF is diagnosed by finding dysplastic cerebriform cells invading the epidermis (Fig. 15–13). Ease of diagnosis varies with

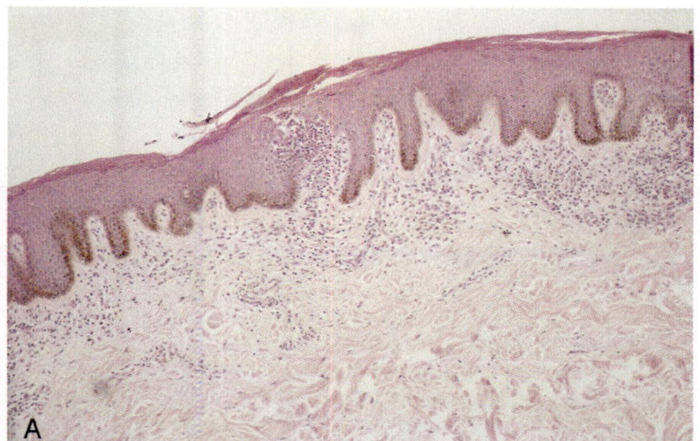

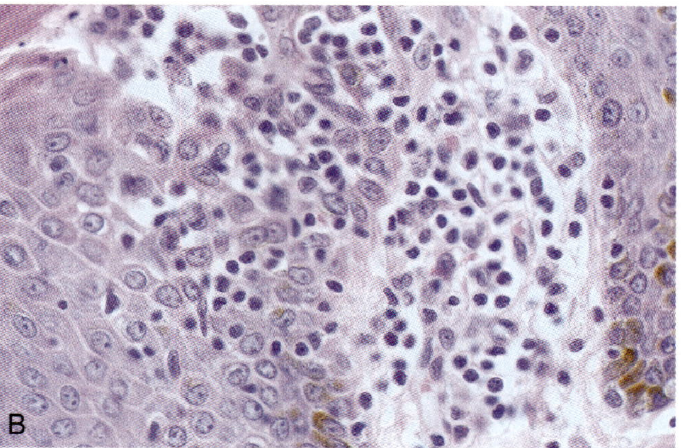

Figure 15–13

Mycosis fungoides, skin. *A*, A bandlike lymphocytic infiltrate is present in the superficial dermis. The epidermis is acanthotic with focal parakeratosis and little spongiosis. *B*, The lymphocytes are epidermotropic, and small intraepidermal collections of lymphocytes are present (Pautrier microabscesses). The lymphocytes have folded, cerebriform nuclei, and some are dysplastic, with enlarged, hyperchromatic nuclei.

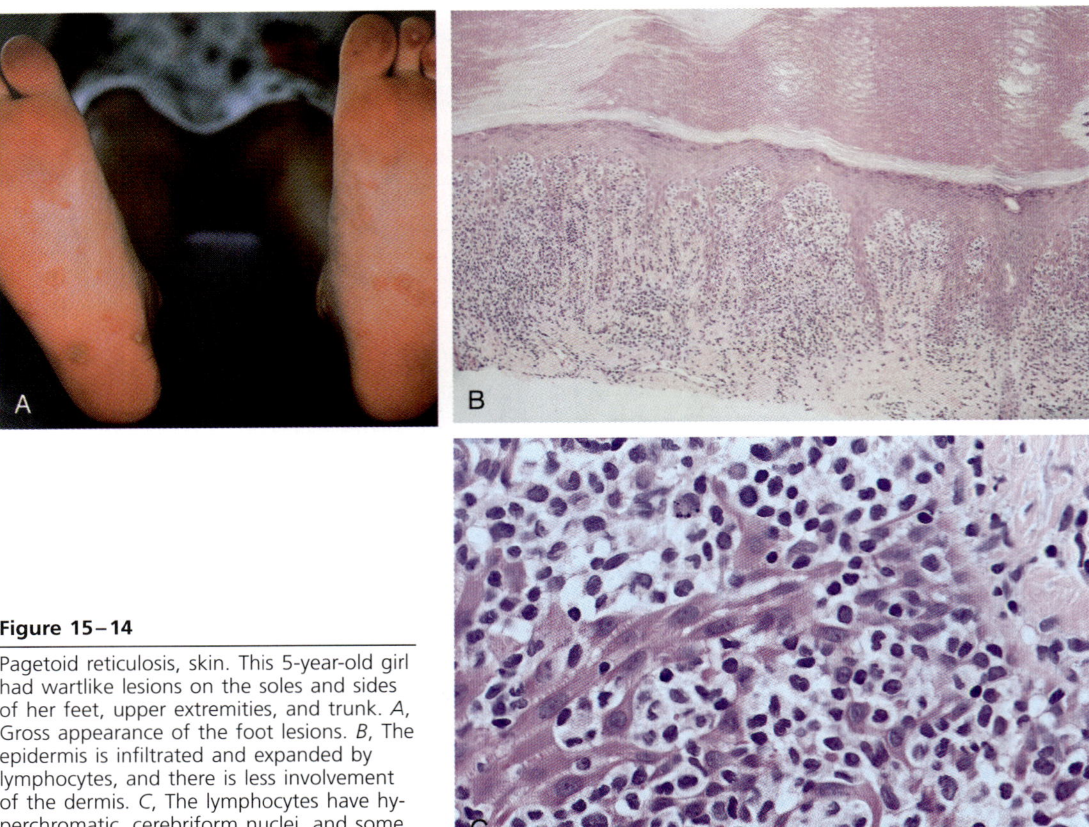

Figure 15–14

Pagetoid reticulosis, skin. This 5-year-old girl had wartlike lesions on the soles and sides of her feet, upper extremities, and trunk. *A*, Gross appearance of the foot lesions. *B*, The epidermis is infiltrated and expanded by lymphocytes, and there is less involvement of the dermis. *C*, The lymphocytes have hyperchromatic, cerebriform nuclei, and some are large with dysplastic features.

the stage of the disease. The earliest lesion, consisting of a sparse, superficial perivascular dermal lymphocytic infiltrate with little epidermal hyperplasia or epidermotropism, is difficult to distinguish from inflammatory dermatoses. Cerebriform lymphocytes along the basement membrane are a useful histologic feature in early patch MF. In the late patch and plaque stage, the epidermis is acanthotic, with ortho- or focal parakeratosis and little if any spongiosis. There is a moderate to marked inflammatory dermal infiltrate, often in a bandlike distribution. Dysplastic cerebriform lymphocytes with hyperchromatic nuclei are readily detected. Some are twice the size of a normal lymphocyte and are called mycosis cells. Cerebriform cells infiltrate the epidermis singly, in small groups, or in large clusters called Pautrier microabscesses. In pagetoid reticulosis (Woringer-Kolopp or Ketron-Goodman diseases) the epidermis is diffusely infiltrated with cerebriform cells, and there is scant dermal infiltrate (Fig. 15–14). Hair follicles in MF may be infiltrated, with subsequent disruption and mucinous degeneration of the outer hair shaft or sebaceous apparatus. This process is called follicular mucinosis (Mehregan et al, 1991). Admixed inflammatory cells include Langerhans granule histiocytes and variable numbers of plasma cells and eosinophils. In the tumor stage, cerebriform cells form nodules within the deeper dermis and subcutaneous tissue, and the epidermis may be eroded or ulcerated.

Transformation to a large-cell process with vesicular nuclei and prominent nucleoli may occur (Cerroni et al, 1992; Diamandidou et al, 1998; Dmitrovsky et al, 1987; Salhany et al, 1988). Transformed MF resembles large-cell lymphoma or Hodgkin disease. Residual cerebriform lymphocytes and Langerhans granule histiocytes are histologic clues that these lesions originated as MF.

Evaluation of nodes for MF is difficult because dermatopathic changes are present in about 70% of patients with MF, and scattered cerebriform cells are seen in various reactive dermatoses (see Chap. 21). Massive nodal involvement or the presence of clusters of cerebriform lymphocytes with >10 cells significantly worsens prognosis (Saussville et al, 1985). Marrow involvement is present in 2–10% of patients at diagnosis and in approximately 25% of cases at autopsy and may be difficult to recognize by light microscopic examination (Salhany et al, 1989).

Diagnostic Criteria

The diagnostic criteria for MF are listed in Table 15–8.

Table 15–8
Mycosis Fungoides: Diagnostic Criteria

Dense, often bandlike, superficial dermal cerebriform lymphocytic infiltrate with cytologic dysplasia (nuclear hyperchromatism, enlarged size) in some cells
Cerebriform lymphocytes (with halos) infiltrate the basal cell layer in early patch lesions
Epidermal hyperplasia with parakeratosis and little spongiosis
Epidermotropism with Pautrier microabscess formation in most cases
T cell phenotype; CD4 >>> CD8; CD7 expression often lost

Differential Diagnosis

Difficulties in establishing the diagnosis of MF are legendary among pathologists and clinicians. The reasons for these difficulties are complex but basically involve two issues. First, many inflammatory states mimic MF clinically and pathologically, and, second, MF may evolve out of previous inflammatory conditions. In borderline cases, it is generally helpful to have B5-fixed material to enhance cytologic detail. The diagnosis of MF should be made only when there are dense infiltrates of cerebriform cells, with both small and dysplastic forms readily demonstrated. Generally, diagnostic lesions have very few reacting cells of other types. Pathologists should err on the side of conservatism in diagnosis until dense infiltrates of cells, including dysplastic cells, are readily found. Virtually all of these cases also demonstrate epidermotropism.

Immunophenotype

MF cells are T cells (CD2+, CD3+, CD5+) that are predominantly helper cells (CD4+), although rare CD8+ MF cases have been reported (Agnarsson et al, 1990; Ralfkiaer et al, 1993). CD7 is often lost, but CD7 negativity cannot be used as a diagnostic criterion, since CD7−T cells may be identified in 10–20% of inflammatory skin lesions (Picker et al, 1987). In lymph nodes, CD7 negativity is very rare in benign T cell infiltrates. With advanced tumor-stage disease, other T cell antigens may be lost. After transformation of MF, the large cells may be Ki-1+ (45%) or LeuM1+ (25%) (Salhany et al, 1988).

Pathogenesis and Biologic Considerations

The pathogenesis of MF is unknown (Barcos, 1993). It is unlikely that skin exposure to chemicals or allergens is the cause (Teixeira et al, 1994). Some studies have suggested involvement of retroviruses HTLV-I or -II (Hall, 1994; Manca et al, 1994; Pancake et al, 1995).

Cytogenetic studies have shown extensive heteroploidy; break points in chromosomes 1, 9, 14, and 17; and abnormalities involving the gene for the TCRα (14q11) have been detected. No specific genetic lesion has been identified.

OTHER PERIPHERAL T CELL LYMPHOMAS

Pleomorphic T Cell Lymphomas

Pleomorphic T cell lymphomas are a heterogeneous group of lymphomas that includes adult T cell leukemia/lymphoma, NK and NK-like T cell proliferations, and the SCV of Ki-1+ ALCL. These lymphomas involve nodes and frequently skin. Histopathologic features vary from homogeneous populations of small cells with irregular, folded nuclei (pleomorphic, small-cell T cell lymphoma in the Kiel classification) to medium-sized or large cells with similar morphologic features (pleomorphic, medium-sized, and large-cell T cell lymphoma in the Kiel classification). The tumor cells most frequently have a CD4+ T cell phenotype and may or may not be associated with HTLV-1.

Subcutaneous Panniculitis-Like T Cell Lymphoma

A variant of peripheral T cell lymphoma, this subcutaneous T cell lymphoma appears to be a specific clinicopathologic entity (Gonzalez et al, 1991; Mehregan et al, 1994; Wang et al, 1996). Patients usually present with multiple subcutaneous nodules on the extremities and, less commonly, the trunk. Patients are predominantly middle-aged adults, but the age range is from 19 to 70 years. The clinical features suggest panniculitis or erythema nodosum. Systemic symptoms are present in patients with hemophagocytic syndrome. The course is aggressive with death from lymphoma or complications of hemophagocytosis. Responses to multiagent chemotherapy are usually seen, but the relapse and mortality rates are high.

Small to large lymphocytes with irregular, hyperchromatic nuclei infiltrate the subcutaneous fat in a lobular pattern (Fig. 15–15). The tumor cells may involve the lower to mid dermis, but the superficial dermis is spared. Vascular involvement is found in most cases but the infiltrate is not angiodestructive nor angiocentric. Karyorrhexis, necrosis, and benign histiocytes are present. Approximately 40% of patients have evidence of hemophagocytosis in the skin or marrow.

Cases mark as CD8+CD4−CD8−, or CD4+ T cell types. CD30 expression is reported in 43%. (Wang et al, 1996). Results of testing for EBV are negative. Gene rearrangements have shown TCR gene rearrangements of both a TCRα/β and a TCRγ/δ (approximately two thirds and one third, respectively) phenotype.

Diagnostic Criteria

The diagnostic criteria are summarized in Table 15–9.

Differential Diagnosis

The differential diagnosis includes ALCL, angiocentric lymphoma, and reactive panniculitis. ALCL generally exhibits greater involvement of the superficial dermis and a diffuse, rather than a lobular, pattern of infiltration and more strongly expresses CD30 (Monterroso et al, 1996). Systemic ALCL, unlike the type confined to the skin, exhibits EMA positivity and the presence of the t(2;5)(p23;q35). Angiocentric lymphoma is distinguished by vascular invasion and large areas of necrosis, EBV presence, and, frequently, expression of CD56. Benign panniculitis lacks cytologic atypia in the lymphocytes.

Adult T Cell Leukemia/Lymphoma

Patients with this HTLV-1–associated neoplasm may present with lymphomatous masses (50% of cases) and minimal or no involvement of the blood, with a leukemic phase (30% of cases), or as lymphoma or leukemia (20% of cases) (Franchini, 1995; Yamaguchi & Takatsuki, 1993). Adult T cell leukemia/lymphoma is most often diagnosed in patients from southwestern Japan and the Caribbean basin, where HTLV-1 is endemic. Sporadic cases have been identified in Africa and, rarely, in the southeastern United States (Catovsky et al, 1982; Swerdlow et al, 1984; Tajima et al, 1990).

Adult T leukemia/lymphoma is a disease of older adults in Japan (median age 55 to 60). Younger adults are affected in the Caribbean and southeastern United States (median age 34 to 39). Children are rarely affected (Foucar et al, 1985; Head et al, 1987; Kinoshita et al, 1982; Lin et al, 1997). Most childhood cases are from nonendemic areas and are HTLV-1+ or not tested. Children may have a mediastinal mass, an unusual feature in endemic cases but reported in 20% of sporadic cases.

In HTLV-1–endemic areas, adult T leukemia/lymphoma develops in 2–5% of patients with positive serologic results an estimated 20 to 30 years after infection. The clinical presentation is usually acute and aggressive, with systemic symptoms, disseminated disease (lymphadenopathy, hepatosplenomegaly, and lung

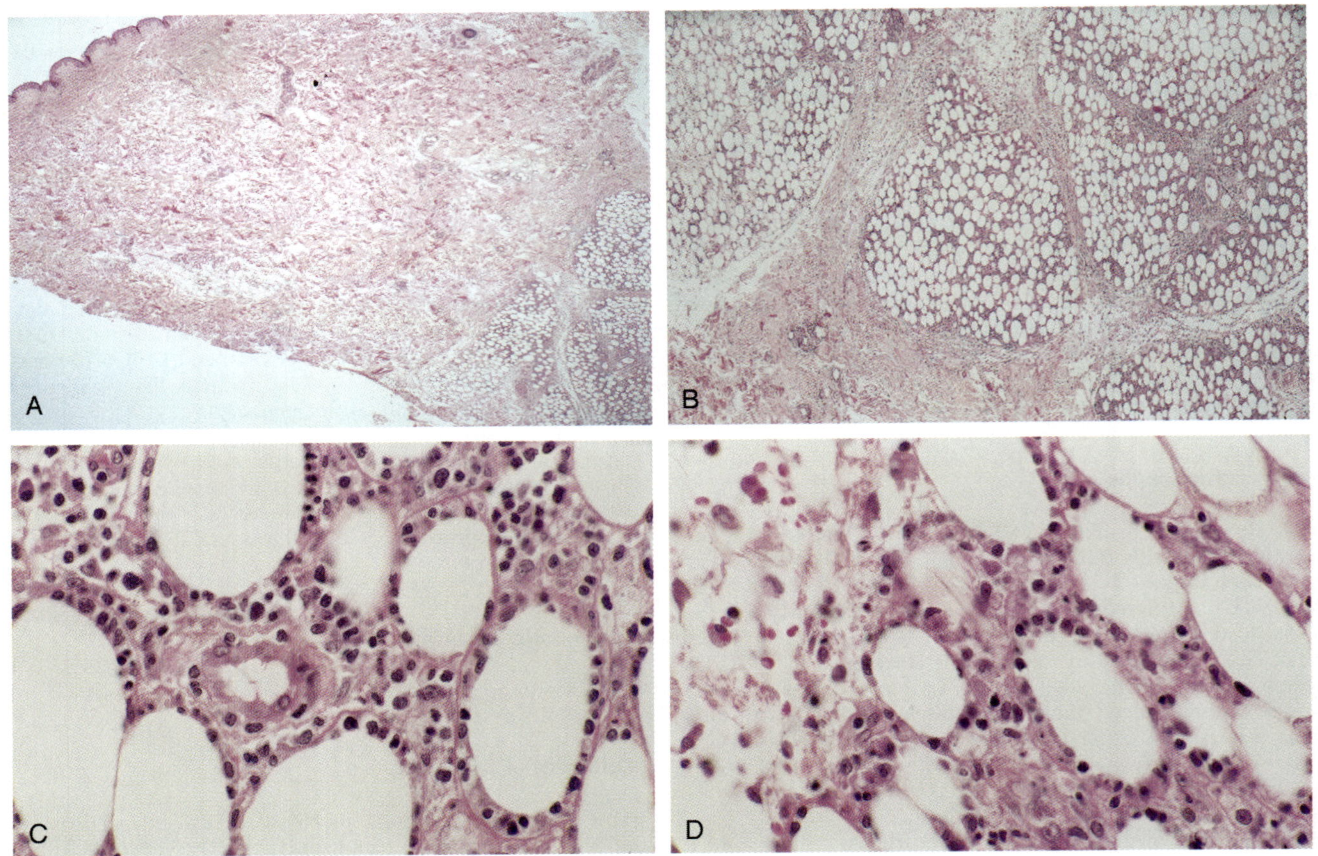

Figure 15–15

Panniculitis-like T cell lymphoma, skin. *A*, A lymphocyte infiltrate is present in the subcutaneous tissue and spares the epidermis and dermis. *B*, The lymphocytes are distributed in a lacelike lobular pattern, with little involvement of the septae. *C*, The lymphocytes are pleomorphic and medium to large in size. They infiltrate but do not destroy vessels. Note the characteristic rimming of fat spaces by tumor cells. *D*, Histiocytes have phagocytosed red blood cells, and there is focal necrosis.

and skin involvement), a leukemic phase, and hypercalcemia. Treatment response is poor, with a short median survival time. Chronic and smoldering forms also exist. They are distinguished by the absence of extranodal disease, except in skin and lung, and normal calcium levels. There is a defect in cell-mediated immunity that results in frequent opportunistic infections. Chronic and smoldering forms may transform to an acute phase.

Table 15–9

Subcutaneous Panniculitis-Like T Cell Lymphoma: Diagnostic Criteria

Pleomorphic small to large lymphocytic infiltrate with irregular, hyperchromatic nuclei infiltrating the subcutaneous fat in a lobular pattern
Vascular invasion without angiodestruction; focal necrosis and karyorrhexis
Hemophagocytosis present in the skin or marrow in 40% of patients
CD8+ > CD4−CD8− > CD4+; TCRα/β >> TCRγ/δ; CD30+ in approximately 40% of patients; EBV−
Multiple subcutaneous nodules

Abbreviations: EBV, Epstein-Barr virus; TCR, T cell receptor.

In the acute leukemic phase, Wright-stained blood films show lymphocytes with moderately condensed nuclear chromatin, inconspicuous nucleoli, and marked lobulation of the lymphocytic nuclei (Fig. 15–16*A*). Lymphocytes may be homogeneous or vary in size and degree of nuclear irregularity. Marrow infiltration is diffuse or focal and may be minimal when compared with the degree of peripheral blood involvement. Patients with hypercalcemia show bone resorption, with prominent osteoclastic activity, but tumor is usually absent from the marrow.

The pattern in nodes is diffuse, with variable cell types (Fig. 15–16*B* and *C*). The most frequent type is a mixture of small, medium, and large atypical lymphocytes, and other types have a predominance of one cell size (Jaffe, 1995; Jaffe et al, 1984). A more monomorphic large-cell form exists and may be confused with other transformed cell lymphomas. Reed-Sternberg–like cells may be seen. There are few background inflammatory cells, in contrast to other peripheral T cell lymphomas. Skin lesions are common (seen in two thirds of cases) and may show focal epidermal infiltration and/or Pautrier microabscesses, but acanthosis and hyperkeratosis, as seen in MF, are usually absent (Jaffe et al, 1984; Leong et al, 1980).

Tumor cells are CD2+, CD3+, CD5+ but usually CD7−. Most are CD4+, CD25+, but rare CD8+ cases have been reported. A subset of adult T lymphoma or leukemia may be CD30 (Ki-1)+ and have histologic features of ALCL or pleomorphic T cell lymphoma (Takeshita et al, 1995).

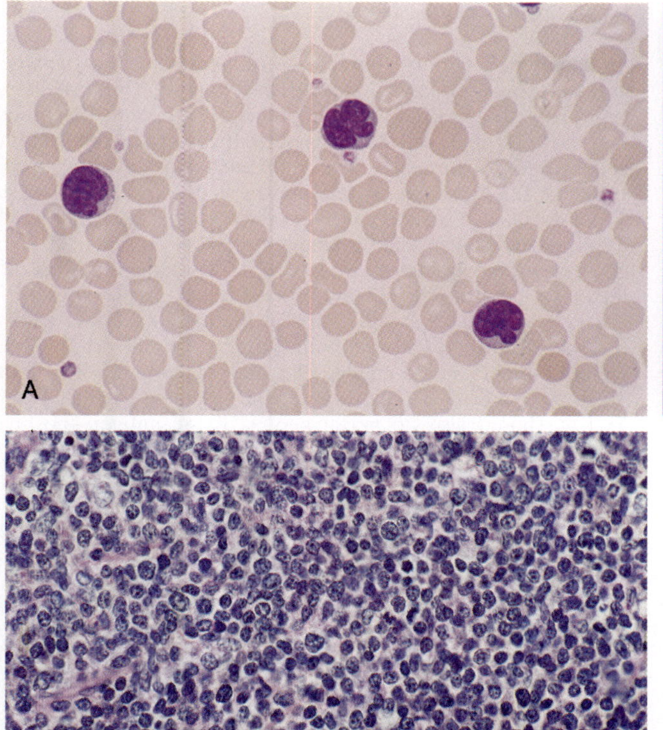

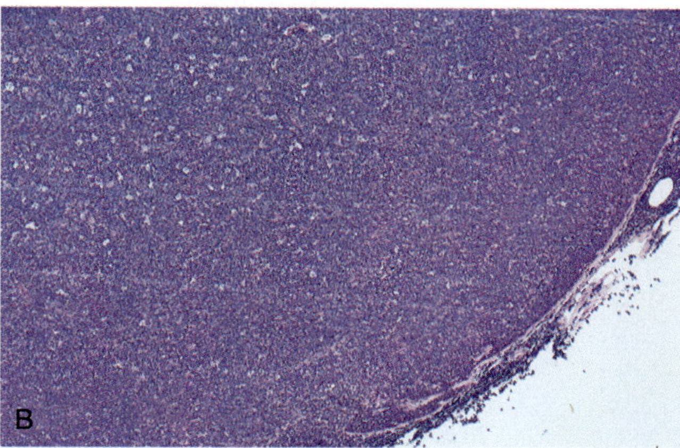

Figure 15–16

HTLV-1–associated T cell leukemia/lymphoma, blood and lymph node. *A*, The peripheral blood lymphocytes are predominantly small, with irregular nuclei. Occasional lymphocytes have very irregular, folded nuclei with a lobulated cloverleaf appearance. Wright stain. *B*, Nodal architecture is diffusely effaced by a neoplastic lymphocytic infiltrate. Wright stain. *C*, The infiltrate is composed of a relatively homogeneous population of small to medium-sized lymphocytes with irregular nuclei. Occasional lymphocytes have nucleoli. There are few admixed inflammatory cells compared with other T cell lymphomas. Wright stain.

Diagnostic Criteria

The diagnostic criteria are summarized in Table 15–10.

Differential Diagnosis

With blood, marrow, and mediastinal involvement, adult T leukemia/lymphoma may be distinguished from T-ALL and T-LBL by its coarser nuclear chromatin and marked nuclear lobulation, the frequent absence of CD7, and evidence of HTLV-1 infection.

If the skin is involved, the epidermotropism with Pautrier microabscesses seen in two thirds of cases may cause confusion with MF. In adult T leukemia/lymphoma, the acanthosis and hyperkeratosis often seen in MF are absent. Clinically, the course is acute, with absence of the chronic premycotic phase.

Table 15–10
Adult* T Cell Leukemia/Lymphoma: Diagnostic Criteria

Dysplastic lymphocytes with very irregular lobulated or cloverleaf nuclei and variable size
Few admixed inflammatory cells compared with other peripheral T cell lymphomas
May have focal epidermal infiltration and Pautrier microabscesses; acanthosis and hyperkeratosis absent
CD4+ >> CD8+; CD7−
HTLV-1+
Clinical features vary from acute aggressive leukemia and dissemination (liver, spleen, node, lung, skin) with hypercalcemia to chronic and smoldering forms with little extranodal disease other than skin

*This name is misleading in that several cases have been described in children.

Abbreviations: HTLV, human T cell lymphotropic virus.

NATURAL KILLER AND NATURAL KILLER–LIKE T CELL NEOPLASMS

NK and NK-like T cell neoplasms are a complex, heterogeneous group that are difficult to classify (Jaffe, 1996). These neoplasms vary in clinical spectrum from indolent to aggressive. Since NK markers have not been studied consistently in lymphomas, knowledge of neoplasms that express NK antigens is limited. Currently, this is an area of intense study. NK neoplasms are uncommon in the pediatric population. The pathogenetic mechanisms are not understood and are not discussed.

Natural Killer and Natural Killer–Like T Cell Biologic Characteristics

Many cytolytic or cytotoxic lymphocytes have the appearance of large granular lymphocytes (LGLs) with azurophilic granules. Cytolytic T cells may be divided into three groups: CD8+ T cells, NK-like T cells (T cells that express NK antigens), and true NK cells. The latter are ontogenetically related to T cells, sharing the same progenitor cell. However, NK cells are a separate lineage from T cells and therefore do not have rearranged TCR genes or express TCR proteins (Lanier et al,

Table 15–11
Immunophenotypic Comparison of T Cells and NK Cells

NK-like T Cell	NK Cell
CD2+	CD2+
Cytoplasmic CD3+	Cytoplasmic CD3+/−
Surface CD3+*	Surface CD3−
CD4−†	CD4−
CD8+	CD8+/−
CD5+/−	CD5−
CD7+	CD7+
CD16+/−	CD16+/−
CD57+/−	CD57+/−
CD56+/−	CD56+
TCR$\alpha\beta$+ or, less frequently, $\gamma\delta$+	TCR$\alpha\beta$− and $\gamma\delta$−

*May be absent in some T cell neoplasms.

†A small subset are CD4+, CD8−.

Abbreviations: NK, natural killer; TCR, T cell receptor.

1992; Spits et al, 1995). NK-like T cells are differentiated from NK cells by their surface immunophenotype and genotype (Table 15–11).

Most cytolytic T cells recognize antigens on target cells in the context of major histocompatibility complex (MHC), leading to specific killing. Most are CD8+ and recognize self class I MHC molecules. A minor population expresses CD4 and recognizes class II MHC. The majority of cytolytic T cells express TCRα/β, but a small population of γ/δ T cells has been identified in the mouse (Arase et al, 1995). NK-like T cells and NK cells do not require prior sensitization (previous exposure to the antigen) for reactivity, and the target cell does not have to express MHC antigen. This killing is "natural" in that it is broader, but it is not random.

There is immunologic overlap between NK-like T cells and NK cells (see Table 15–11). Both cell types express CD2 and CD7. Antigens CD16, CD56, and CD57 are expressed on NK cells. CD16 is usually expressed on both NK cells and NK-like T cells. Variable expression of CD56 and CD57 is seen in NK-like T cell and NK neoplasms.

NK-like T cells normally make up <5% of human peripheral blood lymphocytes and are present in the epithelium of the intestinal mucosa and in the hepatic sinuses. NK cells represent approximately 10–15% of peripheral blood lymphocytes and are principally found in the liver and spleen.

Histopathologic Features of Natural Killer and Natural Killer–Like T Cell Neoplasms

Touch imprints or Wright-stained blood or marrow films reveal small, medium, or large cells with fine to coarse azurophilic granules and condensed nuclear chromatin. The cytoplasm is abundant and pale or slightly basophilic. Occasional giant or large anaplastic cells may be present. Some large cells have dispersed chromatin and a blastic appearance, particularly in the more aggressive NK or NK-like T cell leukemia or lymphomas (DiGiuseppe et al, 1997). Tumor cells infiltrate tissue in a diffuse pattern. In some tissues, particularly those of the nose and skin, there is an angiocentric growth pattern. In the liver, the sinusoids and portal areas are infiltrated, and the infiltrate is mainly in the red pulp in the spleen. In the intestine, tumor cells are in the epithelium, and the adjacent mucosa may be atrophic.

Immunophenotypic Features

As mentioned earlier, there is considerable overlap between antigen expression in NK and NK-like T cells. Tumor cells recapitulate the normal immunophenotype, except that there may be loss of T cell antigens. For this reason, determining cell lineage in lymphoma may be difficult, particularly if loss of surface CD3 expression is revealed by flow cytometric analysis. Absolute lineage assignment in surface CD3− cases generally requires molecular genetic analysis for the presence of TCR gene rearrangements. Cytoplasmic CD3 expression, as detected by paraffin-reactive antibody studies, may be present in NK cells as well as T cells. Paraffin immunoperoxidase studies may be performed with antibodies against framework determinants of the β and δ chains βF1 and δ1 respectively, of the TCR to confirm T cell phenotype. Staining for βF1 and TCRδ1 should also be performed in T cell antigen–positive, CD56+, or CD57+ cases.

Large Granular Lymphocytic Leukemia Disease: T Cell and Natural Killer Types

The most frequent LGL disease is chronic lymphocytic leukemia (CLL), composed of lymphocytes with condensed chromatin, fine to coarse azurophilic granules, abundant pale or slightly basophilic cytoplasm, and little or no cytologic atypia (Loughran & Hammond, 1986) (Fig. 15–17). Chronic lymphoproliferative disorders of LGLs were recognized in the mid-1970s (Berliner, 1990; Brouet et al, 1975; McKenna et al, 1977) and have been variously called Tγ lymphocytosis, LGL leukemia, Tγ lymphoproliferative disease, T-CLL, and lymphoproliferative disorder of granular lymphocytes.

Patients with LGL are older (median age 57 years, range 4 to 88 years) (Loughran, 1993). The disease is rare in children, but it is apparent that the clonal abnormality may occur in childhood (Le Deist et al, 1991; Platanias et al, 1990). LGL leukemia has a chronic, indolent course often associated with neutropenia, recurrent infection, autoimmune disease (particularly rheumatoid arthritis), and splenomegaly in the absence of lymphadenopathy (Dhodapkar et al, 1994).

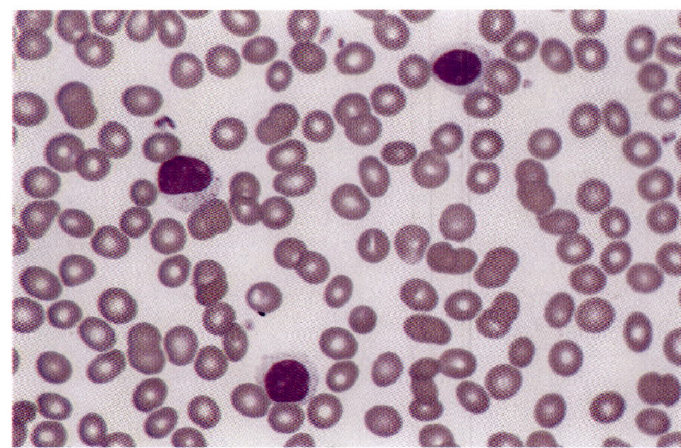

Figure 15–17

Large granular lymphocytes, blood. This patient had a history of rheumatoid arthritis. There is a slight peripheral blood lymphocytosis. The lymphocytes are medium to large, with clear or weakly basophilic cytoplasm containing multiple fine azurophilic granules. The nuclei are round to slightly irregular, and there is no cytologic atypia. Wright stain.

Table 15–12

Large Granular Lymphocytic Leukemia: Diagnostic Criteria

Increased large lymphocytes with azurophilic granules and little cytologic dysplasia in the blood film
Lymphocytic infiltrates, which may be subtle, are present in marrow, splenic red pulp, and liver sinusoids
80% mark as T cell (surface CD3+) and are usually CD16+, CD57+, CD8+; 20% mark as NK cell (surface CD3−) and are CD56+, CD16+, CD57+/−
Often associated with neutropenia, recurrent infection, autoimmune disease (particularly rheumatoid arthritis), splenomegaly, and an indolent course

Infiltrates of small lymphocytes are present in the marrow, liver sinusoids, and splenic red pulp. In the marrow the infiltrate may be diffuse and somewhat subtle or form small interstitial aggregates. In about 80% of cases, the cell of origin is a CD8+ T cell with expression of NK cell antigens, such as CD16 and CD57. Approximately 20% of cases are proliferations of true NK cells (Chan et al, 1992; Tefferi et al, 1994) that express CD16 and CD56 with or without CD57. Clonality studies, such as cytogenetic analysis, may be required to avoid confusion with reactive NK proliferations (Loughran, 1993; Taniwaki et al, 1990).

Diagnostic Criteria

The diagnostic criteria for LGL leukemia or lymphoma are summarized in Table 15–12.

Differential Diagnosis

In children the main differential diagnosis for LGL leukemia is a reactive lymphocytosis. CD8+ LGL cells proliferate in viral infections and may be accompanied by neutropenia. With viral infections, more "atypical" or activated lymphocytes with dispersed chromatin, prominent nucleoli, and abundant cytoplasm or with plasmacytoid differentiation are mixed in with the LGLs. The LGL proliferation with viral infections is usually self-limited and often associated with positive viral serologic test results. If the lymphocytosis persists after several months, cytogenetic and molecular genetic studies should be performed to rule out a clonal process.

Aggressive Large Granular Lymphocytic Leukemia/ Lymphoma: T Cell and Natural Killer Types

There are two rare aggressive LGL leukemias, one true NK (Imamura et al, 1990; Loughran, 1993; Sun et al, 1993) and the other NK-like T cell (Gentile et al., 1994; Macon et al, 1996; Sun et al, 1992). Patients have a leukemic phase, hepatosplenomegaly, and usually tumor in other tissue sites, resulting in the terms *NK* and *NK-like T cell leukemia/lymphoma* (Imamura et al, 1990). With NK cell neoplasms, in addition to hepatosplenomegaly there is a predilection for skin. Node involvement is seen in approximately 30–40% of cases (DiGiuseppe et al, 1997; Imamura et al, 1990; Nakamura et al, 1995; Sun et al, 1993). In NK-like T cell neoplasms, additional sites of involvement include the gastrointestinal tract, lung, and kidney (Emile et al, 1996; Gentile et al, 1994; Macon et al, 1996).

NK cell leukemia/lymphoma, reported in several adolescents (13 to 16 years old), may involve the liver, spleen, blood, marrow, and skin. Only one patient exhibited node involvement (Imamura et al, 1990; Sun et al, 1993). The tumor is very aggressive, with survival times ranging from 1 to 32 months. NK-like T cell neoplasms have been reported in four children and adolescents (range 9 to 18 years old) (Macon et al, 1996; Sun et al, 1992; Wong et al, 1992), who had liver, spleen, marrow, and blood involvement. Two of these children were immunosuppressed, one on prednisone for thrombocytopenia and the other for organ transplantation.

Some NK cell leukemias have an acute lymphoblastic leukemia–like or blastoid presentation (Chan et al, 1997; DiGiuseppe et al, 1997; Kaplan et al, 1986; Kawano et al, 1995; Pirruccello et al, 1989). LGL with NK features have also been reported (Ichinohasama et al, 1996; Koita et al, 1997; Swerdlow et al, 1985). Immature neoplasms with the CD7+CD5−, CD2+CD56+ phenotype may be of T or NK cell lineage, and gene rearrangement studies or TCR antigen analysis are required to differentiate between the two (Nakamura et al, 1997).

The tumor cells have cytologic dysplasia, with irregular, hyperchromatic nuclei or a blastic appearance, and a higher nuclear-cytoplasmic ratio, as opposed to the normal LGL cytologic features seen in chronic LGL proliferations (Figs. 15–18 and 15–19). Most NK tumors are CD3−, CD4−, CD8−. NK-like T cells are CD3+ and are most frequently CD4−/CD8+. Aggressive NK neoplasms are associated with EBV, whereas the aggressive NK-like T cell leukemia/lymphomas have not shown as high a degree of association with EBV (Chan et al, 1997). CD56 expression may be a marker for an aggressive course (Nichols et al, 1994).

Diagnostic Criteria

The diagnostic criteria for aggressive LGL leukemia/lymphoma are summarized in Table 15–13.

Differential Diagnosis

The differential diagnosis of aggressive LGL leukemia/lymphoma includes acute leukemia (primarily T-ALL), T-LBL, and other large T cell lymphomas with peripheral blood and organ involvement (e.g. the SCV of ALCL or transformed

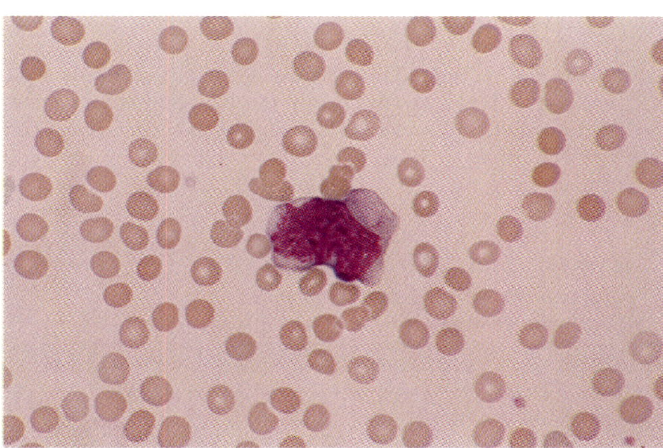

Figure 15–18

True natural killer cell leukemia/lymphoma, blood. The patient presented with splenomegaly, neutropenia, and lymphocytosis of true natural killer cell type. Wright-stained blood film showed large dysplastic lymphocytes with cytoplasmic granules. This is in contrast to the usual indolent T cell large granular lymphocytes where there is little or no cytologic atypia (see Fig. 15–17). Immunophenotypic and genotypic studies confirmed that these were true natural killer cells.

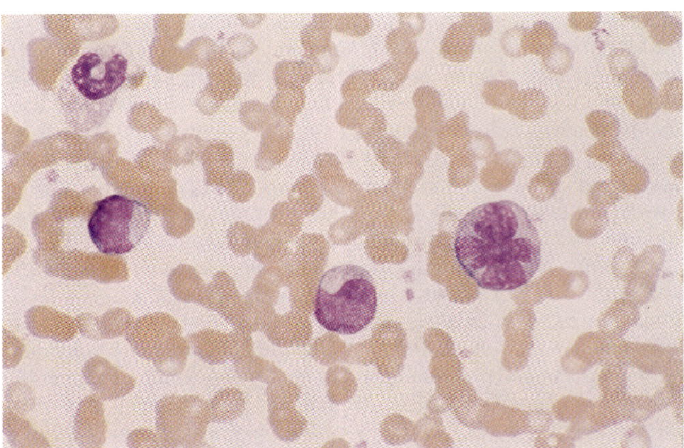

Figure 15–19

Natural killer-like T cell leukemia/lymphoma, blood. This 9-year-old had fever, lymphadenopathy, hepatosplenomegaly, and lymphocytosis. Peripheral blood contains irregular, dysplastic lymphocytes with scant fine granules.

MF–Sézary syndrome). LGL leukemia/lymphoma may be distinguished by the presence of azurophilic granules on Wright-stained smears or touch imprints and NK-associated antigen (CD16, CD56, and CD57) expression. In T-ALL and T-LBL, terminal deoxyribonucleotidyl transferase (TdT) is usually expressed, CD10 may be present, and azurophilic granules and CD56 expression are uncommon. In the disseminated, aggressive form of the SCV of ALCL, the tumor cells have basophilic cytoplasm with vacuoles and are CD30+ and EMA+ and have evidence of *ALK* gene dysregulation (P80+, *ALK*-1+). Transformed MF is very rare in chidren. The tumor cells have folded, cerebriform nuclear profiles and lack CD56 expression. *Ehrlichia* infections are associated with proliferation of atypical LGLs (Hamilton et al, 2000), but they may be distinguished from LGL neoplasms by a history of tick exposure and toxic changes in neutrophils.

Angiocentric (Nasal and Nasal-Type Natural Killer or T Cell) Lymphoma

Aside from the chronic leukemias of LGLs, the most common NK or NK-like T cell neoplasms are the lymphomas characterized by localized extranodal disease and angiocentric histologic features. There is a high incidence of nasal, lung, or skin involvement. Other extranodal sites include soft tissue, gastrointestinal tract, testis, CNS, and spleen (Chan et al, 1997). Angiocentric lymphomas were previously known by confusing terms, such as *lethal midline granuloma, polymorphic reticulosis, malignant midline granuloma* in the upper aerodigestive tract, and *lymphomatoid granulomatosis* in the lung. In 1985, the unifying term *angioimmunoproliferative lesion* or *angiocentric lymphoma* was proposed for these entities (Jaffe, 1985).

In angiocentric lymphomas, there is a wide range of patient age, with most patients in the fifth to seventh decades. Initially the disease is localized to the primary site, except with skin involvement, which is associated with extracutaneous disease (upper respiratory tract, nodes, liver, and spleen) in over half the cases (Chan et al, 1988). Clinical outcome correlates with histologic grade. High-grade tumors have a more aggressive course. Patients with low-grade tumors may not achieve a complete remission if they progress to a higher-grade lesion later (Lipford et al, 1988).

Childhood angiocentric lymphomas are rare (Agnarsson & Kadin, 1995). The pediatric age range for angiocentric lymphoma is from 13 months to 20 years. Tumors predominantly involve the lung and upper airway. Additional sites include the testis, submandibular gland, eyelid, and skin (Hsueh et al, 1993; Natkunam et al, 1999; Magaña et al, 1998; Millot et al, 1998). Immunophenotypic data are incomplete, since most cases were diagnosed in the late 1970s to early 1980s. Prognosis is poor, with survival time generally less than 1 year (Hsueh et al, 1993). In approximately half of the children, angiocentric lymphoma developed 1 month to 4.5 years after remission of acute lymphoblastic leukemia. One of these cases had a clearly documented immature T cell phenotype in the acute lymphoblastic leukemia and a mature T cell phenotype in the angiocentric lymphoma (Hsueh et al, 1993). Molecular studies to determine the relationship of these neoplasms (i.e., the same clone or different clones) have not been done.

Histologically, angiocentric lymphomas are characterized by a polymorphous lymphocytic infiltrate with varying degrees of cytologic atypia that surrounds, invades, and destroys blood vessels and causes necrosis (Fig. 15–20). The infiltrate is composed of a mixture of small lymphocytes and variable numbers of large atypical lymphocytes along with plasma cells, histiocytes, and often eosinophils. There is a histologic spectrum from benign lymphocytic vasculitis to frank lymphoma (Lipford et al, 1988). Grade I lesions are principally composed of small lymphocytes with minimal nuclear irregularity. Large lymphocytes are rare, and necrosis is usually absent. In grade II, cytologic atypia is present in the small lymphocytes, and there are infrequent large, atypical cells. Necrosis is more common than in grade I. In grade III, the infiltrate is obviously lymphomatous, an observation based on its monomorphism and the marked cytologic atypia in small and large cells. Necrosis is prominent. Wright-stained touch preparations reveal the presence of azurophilic granules (Aozasa et al, 1995).

Initially, immunologic typing studies in angiocentric lymphoma were interpreted as showing a T cell phenotype (Chan et al, 1987; Chott et al, 1988; Jaffe, 1985; Jaffe et al, 1989; Lipford et al, 1988). T cell antigens are present, but most cases lack TCR gene rearrangements and are more like NK cells (Kanavaros et al, 1993; Kaneko et al, 1995; Medeiros et al, 1991; Suzumiya et al, 1994; van Gorp et al, 1995). Consequently, the designation *nasal T/NK cell lymphoma* has been proposed for nasal lymphomas (polymorphic reticulosis midline malignant reticulosis and lethal midline granuloma) and *nasal-type T/NK cell lymphoma* for other sites (Jaffe et al, 1996). Angiocentric lesions in the lung (lymphomatoid granulomatosis) contain numerous T cells, but in >50% of cases the large dysplastic cells are B cells (Guinee et al, 1994; Myers

Table 15–13
Aggressive LGL Leukemia/Lymphoma: Diagnostic Criteria

Large granular lymphocytes with hyperchromatic, folded dysplastic nuclei or blastic appearance
Expression of NK antigens CD16, CD56; true NK (surface CD3−) or NK-like T cell (surface CD3+) phenotype; NK-like T cells most often CD4−, CD8+; NK cells CD4−, CD8−; EBV+ more often in NK phenotype
Disseminated disease with involvement of the liver, spleen, blood, and skin; nodal involvement more common in NK-like T cell; aggressive clinical course

Abbreviations: EBV, Epstein-Barr virus; NK, natural killer.

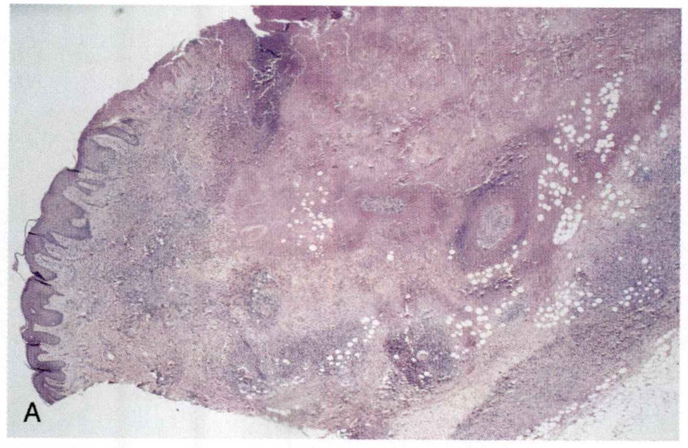

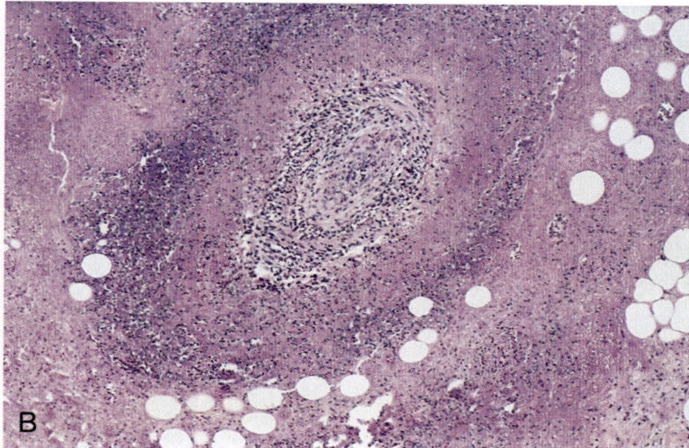

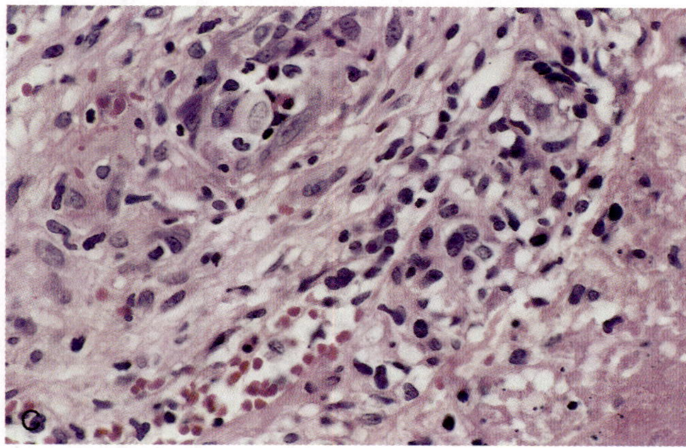

Figure 15–20

Angiocentric T cell lymphoma (T/NK cell lymphoma, nasal-type), skin. This patient presented with angiocentric lymphoma in the skin that later involved the nasopharynx. *A*, There is a lymphocytic infiltrate that extends deep into the subcutaneous tissue. Vascular invasion and destruction by the tumor cell infiltrate have produced large areas of dermal and epidermal necrosis and ulceration. *B*, Large vessel infiltrated by tumor cells. *C*, Higher magnification of vessel wall. The tumor cells are predominantly large, dysplastic lymphocytes with irregular, folded nuclei. There are few admixed inflammatory cells.

et al, 1995). Angiocentric lymphomas in extranodal sites other than the upper and lower respiratory tract also vary in immunophenotype (Nakamura et al, 1995).

There is frequent association with EBV (Emile et al, 1996; Harbuchi et al, 1990; Ho et al, 1990; Jaffe et al, 1996; Kanavaros et al, 1993; Medeiros et al, 1991; Nakamura et al, 1995; Strickler et al, 1994) and angiocentric lymphomas may be associated with hemophagocytosis (Chubachi et al, 1992; Jaffe et al, 1983; Ng et al, 1986).

CD56 (NCAM, neural cell adhesion molecule) is normally expressed on NK cells and is present in most angiocentric lymphomas with an NK phenotype and some with a T cell phenotype (Ho et al, 1990; Kanavaros et al, 1993; Nakamura et al, 1995; Ng et al, 1987; Suzumiya et al, 1994; van Gorp et al, 1995; Wong et al, 1994). CD56 positivity strongly correlates with immunoreactivity for granzyme B and the presence of cytoplasmic granules (van Gorp et al, 1995).

Diagnostic Criteria

The diagnostic criteria for angiocentric lymphoma are listed in Table 15–14.

Differential Diagnosis

The pathognomonic features of angiocentric lymphoma are angioinvasive and angiodestructive lesions. If the biopsy specimen is small and only necrosis, not angiocentric lesions, is present, the differential diagnosis includes any large-cell lymphoma. The extranodal anatomic site (nasal or paranasal, lung, skin, gastrointestinal tract, and testis), presence of azurophilic granules on Wright-stained touch imprints, CD56 expression, or association with EBV should be clues to the presence of an angiocentric (nasal or nasal-type T/NK cell lymphoma). The immunophenotype of the tumor cells varies with regard to the anatomic site. Lymphomas in the lung are predominantly B cell in type. T cell or NK cell phenotypes predominate in other sites. ALCL may have angioinvasion, particularly in cutaneous lesions. ALCL is distinguished by the presence of strong CD30 expression in virtually every tumor cell. EMA and ALK1 expression is often present unless the presentation is primarily cutaneous. Vascular infiltration is seen in subcutaneous panniculitis-like T cell lymphoma, but vasodestruction and evidence of EBV infection are absent.

Hepatosplenic $\gamma\delta$ T Cell Lymphoma

Hepatosplenic $\gamma\delta$ T cell lymphoma is a rare peripheral T cell lymphoma with features of NK-like $\gamma\delta$ T cells (frequent CD56+,

Table 15–14

Angiocentric (Nasal and Nasal-Type T/NK Cell) Lymphoma: Diagnostic Criteria

Angiocentric and angiodestructive pleomorphic, usually large-cell, lymphocytic infiltrate with necrosis; cytoplasmic azurophilic granules present
Involvement of extranodal sites predominantly nose or paranasal sinuses, lung, and skin; nodal involvement relatively rare
CD56 present in NK and T cell types; most NK cell types EBV+

Abbreviations: EBV, Epstein-Barr virus; NK, natural killer.

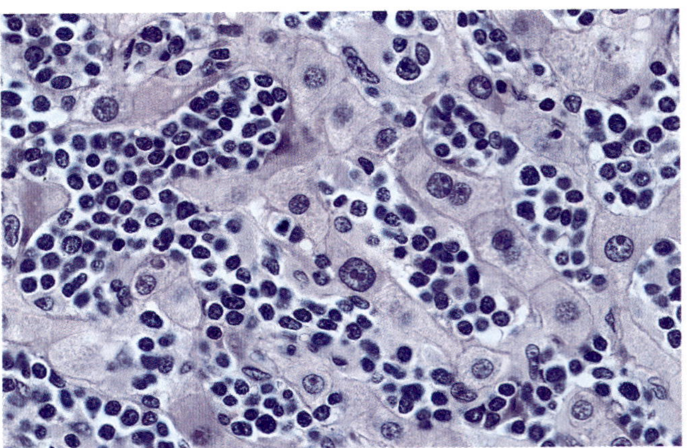

Figure 15–21

Hepatosplenic T cell lymphoma, liver. Liver sinusoids are expanded by a relatively monomorphic population of medium-sized lymphocytes with round to irregular nuclei and a small amount of cytoplasm. (Case provided by Terence T. Casey, MD.)

cytotoxic granule expression, and a tissue distribution similar to that of normal NK-like T cells) (Cooke et al, 1996; Farcet et al, 1990; Gaulard et al, 1990; Gaulard et al, 1986; Salhany et al, 1997; Wong et al, 1995). There is a marked predominance of young males, with a possible predilection for blacks (Cooke et al, 1996). Approximately 20–25% are pediatric cases (ages 8 to 19) (Cooke et al, 1996; Garcia-Sanchez et al, 1995; Macon et al, 1996). Patients have marked hepatosplenomegaly, marrow involvement with or without a peripheral blood lymphocytosis, and infrequent node involvement. Most patients die within 2 years despite aggressive chemotherapy.

The tumor cells are medium-sized lymphocytes with slightly irregular nuclei with partially dispersed chromatin, prominent nuclei, and eosinophilic cytoplasm. Tumor cells are present in the hepatic sinusoids, marrow sinuses, and splenic red pulp (Fig. 15–21). Azurophilic granules are usually absent, but most cases are CD56+. The tumor cells are usually CD4−/CD8− but also may be CD4−/CD8+. TCR$\gamma\delta$ is expressed in most cases and TCRα/β is in the minority. EBV results are negative. Isochromosome 7q has been reported in several cases, particularly in immunocompromised patients (François et al, 1997; Kraus et al, 1998; Macon et al, 1996; Wang et al, 1995).

Diagnostic Criteria

The diagnostic criteria for hepatosplenic $\gamma\delta$ T cell lymphoma are summarized in Table 15–15.

Table 15–15
Hepatosplenic $\gamma\delta$ T Cell Lymphoma: Diagnostic Criteria

- Infiltration of medium-sized lymphocytes with irregular nuclei, partially dispersed chromatin, and prominent nucleoli present in hepatic sinusoids, splenic red pulp, and marrow sinuses; azurophilic granules absent
- CD4−, CD8− or CD4−, CD8+ phenotype; TCR$\gamma\delta$+, CD56+, EBV−
- Marked hepatosplenomegaly and little adenopathy
- Isochromosome 7q reported in some cases

Abbreviations: EBV, Epstein-Barr virus; TCR, T cell receptor.

Differential Diagnosis

The differential diagnosis for hepatosplenic $\gamma\delta$ T cell lymphoma includes NK and NK-like T cell leukemia or lymphoma. Hepatosplenic $\gamma\delta$ T cell lymphoma has prominent hepatic sinusoid involvement, and most cases lack azurophilic granules, which are present in NK and NK-like T cell leukemia or lymphoma. Both tumors express CD56. There is overlap between some cases of NK-like T cell lymphoma and hepatosplenic $\gamma\delta$ T cell lymphoma (Jaffe, 1996). An NK cell origin is confirmed by the lack of surface CD3 and TCR rearrangement and TCR protein expression.

Intestinal T Cell Lymphoma With or Without Enteropathy

Intestinal T cell lymphomas are multifocal ulcerated tumors, usually in the jejenum and ileum, that are associated with celiac disease in approximately half of the cases (Chott et al, 1992). Patients are generally middle-aged adults who have abdominal pain and weight loss. Intestinal perforation and an acute abdomen occur in approximately one third of cases. Mesenteric nodes are frequently involved, but disseminated disease is unusual. The clinical course is aggressive. Celiac disease is relatively more frequent in children than in adults, but intestinal T cell lymphomas arising in this setting in children are rare. In a single case report, a child who responded to a gluten-free diet and had a normal small bowel mucosa developed an intestinal lymphoma and died despite chemotherapy (Arnaud-Battandier et al, 1983). In another case report, a child had no clinical pathologic features of enteropathy (Weiss et al, 1997).

Small, medium, or large pleomorphic lymphocytes diffusely infiltrate the gut mucosa and extend into or through the bowel wall (Chott et al, 1992; Chott et al, 1999) (Fig. 15–22). Tumor cells may invade the epithelium, forming Pautrier-like microabscesses. Most are classified as pleomorphic medium- and large-cell lymphoma. The mucosa may show villous atrophy and increased intraepithelial lymphocytes away from the tumor. The tumor cells are usually CD8+ or CD4−/CD8−, a phenotype similar to that of intraepithelial $\gamma\delta$ T cells. However, many are βF1 positive or have a TCRα/β rearrangement (Isaacson et al, 1985; Longacre et al, 1990; Murray et al, 1995). Azurophilic granules and CD56 and CD57 expression have been reported, suggesting an NK-like T cell phenotype (Kanavaros et al, 1988; Longacre et al, 1990; Weiss et al, 1997). CD30 expression is present in up to 80% of cases (Murray et al, 1995). The gut intraepithelial T cell–associated molecule HML-1 (CD103) is expressed in most cases. CD103 is not expressed in other peripheral T cell lymphomas (Falini et al, 1991). Test results for EBV are negative in most cases (Ilyas et al, 1995).

Diagnostic Criteria

The diagnostic criteria for intestinal T cell lymphoma are summarized in Table 15–16.

Differential Diagnosis

Primary small intestinal lymphomas may be of B or T cell type, the most common being mucosal-associated, follicular center low or high grade, Burkitt, pleomorphic medium- and large–T cell, and anaplastic large-cell (Domizio et al, 1993). Intestinal lymphoma accounts for approximately 44% of extranodal lymphoma in the pediatric population. The most common is Burkitt lymphoma, which is distinguished by a homogeneous population of small transformed cells, a "starry sky"

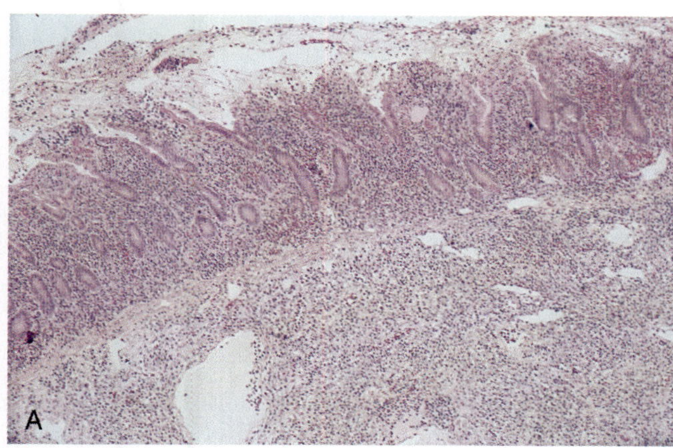

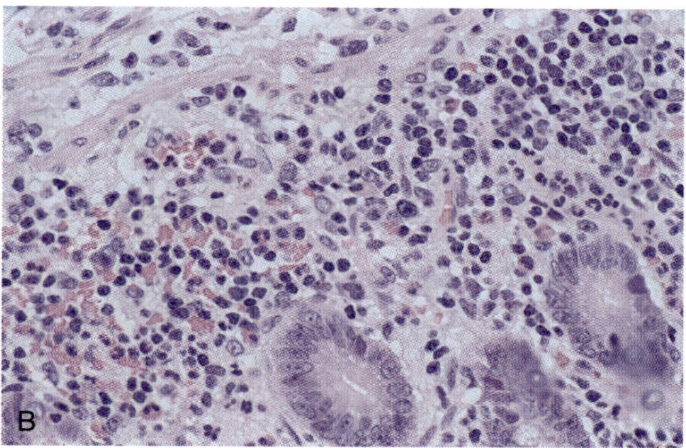

Figure 15–22

Intestinal T cell lymphoma, jejunum. A 6-year-old boy developed intestinal obstruction and a large retroperitoneal mass. There was no clinical or serologic evidence of gluten-sensitive enteropathy. *A*, The jejunal wall mucosa shows only slight villous blunting and a diffuse lymphocytic infiltrate. *B*, The lymphocytes are pleomorphic and are medium to large in size. (Case provided by Ronald L. Weiss, MD.)

pattern owing to tingible-body macrophages and mitoses, and a B cell phenotype. Small intestinal T cell lymphomas are most frequently pleomorphic medium- and large-cell type (including those with enteropathy), followed by ALCL (Domizio et al, 1993). CD30 may be present in both, making these lymphomas difficult to distinguish in some cases. *ALK* gene expression is useful in defining ALCL but has not been evaluated in a large number of intestinal lymphomas.

Precursor NK Cell Leukemia

CD56 has been detected in 13–41% of cases of acute myelogenous leukemia (Iizuka et al, 1992; Seymour et al, 1994; Vidriales et al, 1993). Two groups of myeloid or NK cell precursor acute leukemias have been described. CD56 expression has been identified in a subset (approximately 5%) of cases of acute myelogenous leukemia, with cytologic features of microgranular acute promyelocytic leukemia (FAB-M3v) (Scott et al, 1994). These myelocytic or NK cell leukemias are HLA-DR−, CD34−, CD33+, CD13+, CD56+, CD11a+, CD16−. Results of analysis for the t(15;17) and *PML/RAR*α have been negative in some cases (Scott et al, 1994) and positive in others (Paietta et al, 1994). These acute leukemias may arise from a precursor cell committed to myelocytic and NK cell differentiation (HLA-DR−, CD33+, CD56+, CD16−) and have been called precursor NK cell leukemia (Scott et al, 1994; Jaffe, 1996).

Table 15–16
Intestinal T Cell Lymphoma: Diagnostic Criteria

- Pleomorphic lymphocytic infiltrate diffusely involving the intestinal mucosa with extension to the bowel wall in some areas
- Multiple ulcers predominantly in the jejunum and ileum
- CD4−, CD8− or CD4−, CD8+ phenotype; most are EBV−, CD103
- Approximately one half the cases are associated with celiac disease

Abbreviations: EBV, Epstein-Barr virus.

Another group of CD56+ myeloid or NK cell precursor acute leukemias has been described with a more immature CD7+, CD33+, CD34+, CD56+, and HLA-DR+ phenotype (Suzuki et al, 1997). These patients ranged in age from 19 to 59 years and had extramedullary disease (adenopathy or mediastinal masses) with a lymphoblastic appearance, lack of cytoplasmic azurophilic granules, and a poor prognosis.

REFERENCES

Abbondanzo SL, Sato N, Straus SE, et al: Acute infectious mononucleosis: CD30 (Ki-1) antigen expression and histologic correlations. Am J Clin Pathol 93:698–702, 1990.

Abruzzo LV, Jaffe ES, Cotelingam JD, et al: T-cell lymphoblastic lymphoma with eosinophilia associated with subsequent myeloid malignancy. Am J Surg Pathol 16:236–245, 1992.

Agnarsson BA, Kadin ME: Ki-1 positive large cell lymphoma: a morphologic and immunologic study of 19 cases. Am J Surg Pathol 12:264–274, 1988.

Agnarsson BA, Kadin ME: Peripheral T-cell lymphomas in children. Semin Diagn Pathol 12:314–324, 1995.

Agnarsson BA, Vonderheid EC, Kadin ME: Cutaneous T cell lymphoma with suppressor/cytotoxic (CD8) phenotype: identification of rapidly progressive and chronic subtypes. J Am Acad Dermatol 22:569–577, 1990.

Anagnostopoulos I, Herbst H, Niedobitek G, et al: Demonstration of monoclonal EBV genomes in Hodgkin's disease and Ki-1-positive anaplastic large cell lymphoma by combined Southern blot and in situ hybridization. Blood 74:810–816, 1989.

Anagnostopoulos I, Hummel M, Finn T, et al: Heterogeneous Epstein-Barr virus infection patterns in peripheral T-cell lymphoma of angioimmunoblastic lymphadenopathy type. Blood 80:1804–1812, 1992.

Anderson JR, Jenkin RD, Wilson JF, et al: Long-term folow up of patients treated with COMP or LSA_2L_2 therapy for childhood non-Hodgkin's lymphoma: a report of CCG-551 from the Children's Cancer Group. J Clin Oncol 11:1024–1032, 1993.

Aozasa K, Oshawa M, Tomita Y, et al: Polymorphic reticulosis is a neoplasm of large granular lymphocytes with a CD3+ phenotype. Cancer 75:894–901, 1995.

Arase HS, Ono N, Arase SY, et al: Development arrest of NK1.1 T cell receptor (TCR)-α/β+ T-cells and expansion of NK1.1 TCR−γ/δ T-cell development of CD3ζ-deficient mice. J Exp Med 182:891–895, 1995.

Arnaud-Battandier F, Schmitz J, Ricour C, et al: Intestinal malignant lymphoma in a child with familial coeliac disease. J Paediatr Gastroenterol Nutr 2:320–323, 1983.

Barcos M. Mycosis fungoides: diagnosis and pathogenesis. Am J Clin Pathol 99:452–458, 1993.

Batova A, Diccianni MB, Yu JC, et al: Frequent and selective methylation of p15 and deletion of both p15 and p16 in T-cell acute lymphoblastic leukemia. Cancer Res 57:832–836, 1997.

Beljaards RC, Kaudewitz P, Berti E, et al: Primary cutaneous CD30-positive large cell lymphoma: definition of a new type of cutaneous lymphoma with a favorable prognosis. Cancer 71: 2097–2104, 1993.

Beljaards RC, Meijer CJLM, Scheffer E, et al: Prognostic significance of CD30 (Ki-1/Ber H2) expression in primary cutaneous large-cell lymphomas of T-cell origin: a clinicopathologic and immunohistochemical study in 20 patients. Am J Pathol 135:1169–1178, 1989.

Benharroch D, Meguerian-Bedoyan Z, Lamant L, et al: ALK-positive lymphoma: a single disease with a broad spectrum of morphology. Blood 91:2076–2084, 1998.

Berliner N: T gamma lymphocytosis and T cell chronic leukemias. Hematol Oncol Clin North Am 4:473–487, 1990.

Bernard A, Boumsell L, Reinherz EL, et al: Cell surface characterization of malignant T cells from lymphoblastic lymphoma using monoclonal antibodies: evidence for phenotypic differences between malignant T cells from patients with acute lymphoblastic leukemia and lymphoblastic lymphoma. Blood 57:1105–1110, 1981.

Bittencourt AL, Mendonça N, Rodrigues de Freitas LA: Ki-1 large cell lymphoma with regressing lesions in a child. Pediatr Dermatol 9:117–122, 1992.

Brouet JC, Sasportes M, Flandrin G, et al: Chronic lymphocytic leukaemia of T-cell origin: immunological and clinical evaluation in eleven patients. Lancet 2:890–893, 1975.

Brousset P, Rochaix P, Chittal S, et al: High incidence of Epstein-Barr virus detection in Hodgkin's disease and absence of detection in anaplastic large-cell lymphoma in children. Histopathology 23: 189–191, 1993.

Brugières L, LeDeley H, Pacquement H, et al: CD30+ anaplastic large-cell lymphoma in children: analysis of 82 patients enrolled in two consecutive studies of the French Society of Pediatric Oncology. Blood 92:3591–3598, 1998.

Bunn PA Jr, Hoffman SJ, Norris D, et al: Systemic therapy of cutaneous T-cell lymphomas (mycosis fungoides and the Sézary syndrome). Ann Intern Med 121:592–602, 1994.

Burns MK, Chan LS, Cooper KD: Woringer-Kolopp disease (localized pagetoid reticulosis) or unilesional mycosis fungoides? An analysis of eight cases with benign disease. Arch Dermatol 131:325–329, 1995.

Catovsky D, Greaves MF, Rose M, et al: Adult T-cell lymphoma-leukemia in blacks from the West Indies. Lancet 1:639–643, 1982.

Cerroni L, Rieger E, Hodl S, Kerl H: Clinicopathologic and immunologic features associated with transformation of mycosis fungoides to large-cell lymphoma. Am J Surg Pathol 16:543–552, 1992.

Chakravarti V, Kamani NR, Bayever E, et al: Bone marrow transplantation for childhood Ki-1 lymphoma. J Clin Oncol 8:657–690, 1990.

Chan JKC, Buchanan R, Fletcher CDM: Sarcomatoid variant of anaplastic large-cell Ki-1 lymphoma. Am J Surg Pathol 14: 983–988, 1990.

Chan JKC, Ng C-S, Hui P-K, et al: Anaplastic large cell Ki-1 lymphoma of bone. Cancer 68:2186–2191, 1991.

Chan JKC, Ng CS, Lau WH, et al: Most nasal/nasopharyngeal lymphomas are peripheral T-cell neoplasms. Am J Surg Pathol 11: 418–429, 1987.

Chan JKC, Ng CS, Ngan KC, et al: Angiocentric T-cell lymphoma of the skin: an aggressive lymphoma distinct from mycosis fungoides. Am J Surg Pathol 12:861–876, 1988.

Chan JKC, Sin VC, Wong KF, et al: Nonnasal lymphoma expressing the natural killer cell marker CD56: a clinicopathologic study of 49 cases of an uncommon aggressive neoplasm. Blood 89:4501–4513, 1997.

Chan WC, Gu LB, Masih A, et al: Large granular lymphocyte proliferation with the natural killer-cell phenotype. Am J Clin Pathol 97:353–358, 1992.

Chott A, Vesely M, Simonitsch I, et al: Classification of intestinal T-cell neoplasms and their differential diagnosis. Am J Clin Pathol 111:S68–S74, 1999.

Chott A, Dragosics B, Radaszkiewicz T: Peripheral T-cell lymphomas of the intestine. Am J Pathol 141:1361–1371, 1992.

Chott A, Kaserer K, Augustin I, et al: Ki-1 positive large cell lymphoma: a clinicopathologic study of 41 cases. Am J Surg Pathol 14:439–448, 1990.

Chott A, Rappersberger K, Schlossarek W, et al: Peripheral T cell lymphoma presenting primarily as lethal midline granuloma. Hum Pathol 19:1093–1101, 1988.

Chubachi A, Imai H, Nishimura S, et al: Nasal T-cell lymphoma associated with hemophagocytic syndrome: immunohistochemical and genotypic studies. Arch Pathol Lab Med 116:1209–1212, 1992.

Cleary ML: Oncogenic conversion of transcription factors by chromosomal translocations. Cell 66:619–622, 1991.

Cooke CB, Krenacs L, Stetler-Steveneson M, et al: Hepatosplenic T-cell lymphoma: a distinct clinicopathologic entity of cytotoxic $\gamma\delta$ T-cell origin. Blood 88:4265–4274, 1996.

Crist WM, Shuster JJ, Falletta J, et al: Clinical features and outcome in childhood T-cell leukemia-lymphoma according to stage of thymocyte differentiation: a Pediatric Oncology Group study. Blood 72:1891–1897, 1988.

De Bruin PC, Beljaards RC, Van Heerde P, et al: Differences in clinical behaviour and immunophenotype between primary cutaneous and primary nodal anaplastic large cell lymphoma of T-cell or null cell phenotype. Histopathology 23:127–135, 1993.

DeCoteau JF, Butmarc JR, Kinney MC, et al: The t(2;5) chromosomal translocation is not a common feature of primary cutaneous CD30+ lymphoproliferative disorders: comparison with anaplastic large-cell lymphoma of nodal origin. Blood 87:3437–3441, 1996.

Delsol G, Al Saati T, Gatter KC, et al: Coexpression of epithelial membrane antigen (EMA), Ki-1 and interleukin-2 receptor by anaplastic large cell lymphomas: diagnostic value is so-called malignant histiocytosis. Am J Pathol 130:59–70, 1988.

Demierre M-F, Goldberg LJ, Kadin ME, et al: Is it lymphoma or lymphomatoid papulosis? J Am Acad Dermatol 36:765–772, 1997.

Deneau DG, Wood GS, Beckstead J, et al: Woringer-Kolopp disease (pagetoid reticulosis): four cases with histopathologic, ultrastructural, and immunohistologic observations. Arch Dermatol 120: 1045–1051, 1984.

de Terlizzi M, Toma MG, Santostasi T, et al: Angioimmunoblastic lymphadenopathy with dysproteinemia: report of a case in infancy with review of literature. Pediatr Hematol Oncol 6:37–44, 1989.

Dhodapkar MV, Li C-Y, Lust JA, et al: Clinical spectrum of clonal proliferations of T-large granular lymphocytes: a T-cell clonopathy of undetermined significance? Blood 84:1620–1627, 1994.

Diamandidou E, Colome-Grimmer M, Fayad L, et al: Transformation of mycosis fungoides/Sezary syndrome: clinical characteristics and prognosis. Blood 92:1150–1159, 1998.

DiGiuseppe JA, Louie DC, Williams JE, et al: Blastic natural killer cell leukemia/lymphoma: a clinicopathologic study. Am J Surg Pathol 21:1223–1230, 1997.

Dmitrovsky E, Matthews MJ, Bunn PA, et al: Cytologic transformation in cutaneous T cell lymphoma: a clinicopathologic entity associated with poor prognosis. J Clin Oncol 5:208–215, 1987.

Domizio P, Owen RA, Shepherd NA, et al: Primary lymphoma of the small intestine: a clinicopathologic study of 119 cases. Am J Surg Pathol 17:429–442, 1993.

Drexler HG, Gignac SM, von Wasielewski R, et al: Pathobiology of *NPM-ALK* and variant fusion genes in anaplastic large cell lymphoma and other lymphomas. Leukemia 14:1533–1559, 2000.

Elmberger PG, Lozano MD, Weisenburger DD, et al: Transcripts of the *npm-alk* fusion gene in anaplastic large cell lymphoma, Hodgkin's disease, and reactive lymphoid lesions. Blood 86: 3517–3521, 1995.

Emile J-F, Boulland M-L, Haioun C, et al: CD5− CD56+ T-cell receptor silent peripheral T-cell lymphomas are natural killer cell lymphomas. Blood 87:1466–1473, 1996.

Falini B, Flenghi L, Fagioli M, et al: Expression of the intestinal T-lymphocyte associated molecule HML-1: analysis of 75 non-Hodgkin's lymphomas and desription of the first HML-1 positive T-lymphoblastic tumour. Histopathology 18:421–426, 1991.

Falini B, Bigerna B, Fizzotti M, et al: ALK expression defines a distinct group of T/null lymphomas ("ALK lymphomas") with a wide morphological spectrum. Am J Pathol 153:875–886, 1998.

Fanin R, Ruiz de Elvira MC, Sperotto A, et al: Autologous stem cell transplantation of T and null cell CD30-positive anaplastic large cell lymphoma: analysis of 64 adult and paediatric cases reported to the European Group for Blood and Marrow Transplantation (EBMT). Bone Marrow Transplant 23:437–442, 1999.

Farcet J-P, Gaulard P, Marolleau J-P, et al: Hepatosplenic T-cell lymphoma: sinusal/sinusoidal localization of malignant cells expressing the T-cell receptor $\gamma\delta$. Blood 75:2213–2219, 1990.

Felgar RE, Salhany KE, Macon WR, et al: The expression of TIA-1+ cytolytic-type granules and other cytolytic lymphocyte-associated markers in CD30+ anaplastic large cell lymphomas (ALCL): correlation with morphology, immunophenotype, ultrastructure, and clinical features. Hum Pathol 30:228–236, 1999.

Feller AC, Griesser H, Schilling CV, et al: Clonal gene rearrangement patterns correlate with immunophenotype and clinical parameters in patients with angioimmunoblastic lymphadenopathy. Am J Pathol 133:549–556, 1988.

Fiorillo A, Pettinato G, Raia V, et al: Angioimmunoblastic lymphadenopathy with dysproteinemia: report of the first case in childhood evolving toward spontaneous remission. Cancer 48: 1611–1114, 1981.

Flynn KJ, Dehner LP, Gajl-Pezalska KJ, et al: Regressing atypical histiocytosis: a cutaneous proliferation of atypical neoplastic histiocytes with unexpectedly indolent biologic behavior. Cancer 49: 959–970, 1982.

Fortson JS, Schroeter AL, Esterly NB: Cutaneous T-cell lymphoma (parapsoriasis en plaque): an association with pityriasis lichenoides et varioliformis acuta in young children. Arch Dermatol 126: 1449–1453, 1990.

Foucar K, Carroll TJ Jr, Tannous R, et al: Nonendemic adult T-cell leukemia/lymphoma in the United States: report of two cases and review of the literature. Am J Clin Pathol 83:18–26, 1985.

Fraga M, Brousset P, Schlaifer D, et al: Bone marrow involvement in anaplastic large cell lymphoma: immunohistochemical detection of minimal disease and its prognostic significance. Am J Clin Pathol 103:82–89, 1995.

Franchini G: Molecular mechanisms of human T-cell leukemia/lymphotropic virus type I infection. Blood 86:3619–3639, 1995.

François A, Lesesve J-F, Stamatoullas A, et al: Hepatosplenic gamma/delta T-cell lymphoma: a report of two cases in immunocompromised patients, associated with isochromsome 7q. Am J Surg Pathol 21:781–790, 1997.

Frizzera G, Kaneko Y, Sakurai M: Angioimmunoblastic lymphadenopathy and related disorders: a retrospective look in search of definitions. Leukemia 3:1–5, 1989.

Frizzera G, Moran EM, Rappaport H: Angio-immunoblastic lymphadenopathy with dysproteinaemia. Lancet 1:1070–1073, 1974.

Garcia-Sanchez F, Menárguez J, Cristobal E, et al: Hepatosplenic gamma-delta T-cell malignant lymphoma: report of the first case in childhood, including molecular minimal residual disease follow-up. Br J Haematol 90:943–946, 1995.

Gaulard P, Bourquelot P, Kanavaros P, et al: Expression of the alpha/beta and gamma/delta T-cell receptors in 57 cases of peripheral T-cell lymphomas: identification of a subset of γ/δ T-cell lymphomas. Am J Pathol 137:617–628, 1990.

Gaulard P, Zafrani ES, Mavier P, et al: Peripheral T-cell lymphoma presenting as predominant liver disease: a report of three cases. Hepatology 6:864–868, 1986.

Geha RS, Perez Atayde AR, Griscom T, et al: A 10-year-old boy with progressive lymphadenopathy, fever, and rash. Ann Allergy 53:381–389, 1984.

Gentile TC, Uner AH, Hutchison RE, et al: CD3+, CD56+ aggressive variant of large granular lymphocyte leukemia. Blood 84:2315–2321, 1994.

Gollnick HPM, Owsianowski M, Ramaker J, et al: Extracorporeal photophoresis: a new approach for the treatment of cutaneous T cell lymphomas. Recent Results Cancer Research 139:409–415, 1995.

Gonzalez CL, Medeiros LJ, Braziel RM, et al: T-cell lymphoma involving subcutaneous tissue: a clinicopathologic entity commonly associated with hemophagocytic syndrome. Am J Surg Pathol 15:17–27, 1991.

Gordon BG, Weisenberger DD, Sanger WG, et al: Peripheral T-cell lymphoma in children and adolescents: role of bone marrow transplantation. Leuk Lymphoma 14:1–10, 1994.

Gordon BG, Weisenburger DD, Warkentin PI, et al: Peripheral T-cell lymphoma in childhood and adolescence: a clinicopathologic study of 22 patients. Cancer 71:257–263, 1993.

Gouttefangeas C, Bensussan A, Boumsell L: Study of the CD3-associated T-cell receptors reveals further differences between T-cell acute lymphoblastic lymphoma and leukemia. Blood 75:931–934, 1990.

Greer JP, Whitlock JA, Kinney MC: Ki-1 positive anaplastic large cell lymphoma: a useful concept? In Armitage J, Newland A, Keating A, et al (eds): Cambridge Medical Reviews: Haematological Oncology, vol 4. Cambridge University Press, Cambridge, England, 89–117:1995.

Griffith RC, Kelly DR, Nathwani BN, et al: A morphologic study of childhood lymphoma of lymphoblastic type: the Pediatric Oncology Group experience. Cancer 59:1126–1131, 1987.

Guinee D, Jaffe E, Kingma D, et al: Pulmonary lymphomatoid granulomatosis: evidence for a proliferation of Epstein-Barr virus infected B-lymphocytes with a predominant T-cell component and vasculitis. Am J Surg Pathol 18:753–764, 1994.

Gustmann C, Altmannsberger M, Osborn M, et al: Cytokeratin expression and vimentin content in large cell anaplastic lymphomas and other non-Hodgkin's lymphomas. Am J Pathol 138:1413–1422, 1991.

Hall WW: Human T cell lymphotropic virus type I and cutaneous T cell leukemia//lymphoma. J Exp Med 180:1581–1585, 1994.

Hamilton KS, Standaert SM, Kinney MC: Characteristic peripheral blood findings in human ehrlichiosis. Mod Pathol 13:169A, 2000.

Harbuchi Y, Yamanaka N, Kataura A, et al: Epstein-Barr virus in nasal T-cell lymphomas in patients with lethal midline granuloma. Lancet 335:128–130, 1990.

Harris NL, Jaffe ES, Stein H, et al: A revised European-American classification of lymphoid neoplasms: a proposal from the International Lymphoma Study Group. Blood 84:1361–1392, 1994.

Havlioglu N, Manepalli A, Galindo L, et al: Primary Ki-1 (anaplastic large cell) lymphoma of the brain and spinal cord. Am J Clin Pathol 103:496–499, 1995.

Head DR, Behm FG: Acute lymphoblastic leukemia and the lymphoblastic lymphomas of childhood. Semin Diagn Pathol 12: 325–334, 1995.

Head DR, Kjeldsberg CR, Kadin ME, et al: Childhood T-cell malignancy resembling adult T-cell leukemia/lymphoma. Hematol Pathol 1:15–25, 1987.

Headington JT, Roth MS, Schnitzer B: Regressing atypical histiocytosis: a review and critical appraisal. Semin Diagn Pathol 4:28–37, 1987.

Heitger A, Gadner H, Bucsky P, et al: Das grosszellige anaplastische Lymphom im Kindesalter: klinische Erfahrungen bei einer histologisch neu definierten Entität. Klin Pädiatr 210:237–241, 1989.

Herbst H, Dallenbach F, Hummel M, et al: Epstein-Barr virus DNA and latent gene products in Ki-1 (CD30)-positive anaplastic large cell lymphomas. Blood 78:2666–2673, 1991.

Herbst H, Stein H: Epstein-Barr virus and CD30+ malignant lymphomas. Crit Rev Oncog 4:191–239, 1993a.

Herbst H, Stein H: Tumor viruses in CD30-positive anaplastic large cell lymphomas. Leuk Lymphoma 9:321–328, 1993b.

Herrmann JJ, Roenigk HH, Hurria A, et al: Treatment of mycosis fungoides with photochemotherapy (PUVA): long term follow-up. J Am Acad Dermatol 33:234–242, 1995.

Hirose M, Sano T, Takahashi Y, et al: Immunoblastic lymphadenopathy in a five-month-old girl: successful treatment with immunosuppressants. Jpn J Clin Oncol 24:228–232, 1994.

Ho FCS, Srivastava G, Loke SL, et al: Presence of Epstein-Barr virus DNA in nasal lymphomas of B and T cell type. Hematol Oncol 8:271–281, 1990.

Hodges KB, Collins RD, Greer JP, et al: Transformation of the small cell variant Ki-1+ lymphoma to anaplastic large cell lymphoma: pathologic and clinical features. Am J Surg Pathol 23:49–58, 1999.

Horschowski N, Guitard AM, Amoux I, et al: Interdigitating cell sarcoma: occurrence during incomplete remission of a lymphoblastic lymphoma. Pathol Biol 41:255–259, 1993.

Howarth CB, Bird CC: Immunoblastic sarcoma arising in child with immunoblastic lymphadenopathy. Lancet 2:747–748, 1976.

Hsueh C, Gonzalez-Crussi F, Murphy SB: Testicular angiocentric lymphoma of postthymic T-cell type in a child with T-cell acute lymphoblastic leukemia in remission. Cancer 72:1801–1805, 1993.

Hutchinson RE, Berard CW, Shuster JJ, et al: B-cell lineage confers a favorable outcome among children and adolescents with large-cell lymphoma: a pediatric oncology group study. J Clin Oncol 13:2023–2032, 1995.

Ichinohasama R, Endoh K, Ishizawa K, et al: Thymic lymphoblastic lymphoma of committed natural killer cell precursor origin: a case report. Cancer 77:2592–2603, 1996.

Iizuka Y, Aiso M, Oshimi K, et al: Myeloblastoma formation in acute myeloid leukemia. Leuk Res 16:665–671, 1992.

Ilyas M, Niedobitek G, Agathanggelou A, et al: Non-Hodgkin's lymphoma, coeliac disease, and Epstein-Barr virus: a study of 13 cases of enteropathy-associated T- and B-cell lymphoma. J Pathol 177:115–122, 1995.

Imamura N, Kusunoki Y, Kawa-Ha K, et al: Aggressive natural killer cell leukaemia/lymphoma: report of four cases and review of the literature: possible existence of a new clinical entity originating from the third lineage of lymphoid cells [see comments]. Br J Haematol 75:49–59, 1990.

Inhorn RC, Aster JC, Roach SA, et al: A syndrome of lymphoblastic lymphoma, eosinophilia, and myeloid hyperplasia/malignancy associated with t(8;13)(p11;q11): description of a distinctive clinicopathologic entity. Blood 85:1881–1887, 1995.

Iravani S, Singleton TP, Ross CW, et al: Precursor B lymphoblastic lymphoma presenting as lytic bone lesions. Am J Clin Pathol 112:836–843, 1999.

Isaacson PG, Spencer J, Connolly CE, et al: Malignant histiocytosis of the intestine: a T-cell lymphoma. Lancet 2:688–691, 1985.

Ishizawa M, Okabe H, Matsumoto K, et al: Anaplastic large cell Ki-1 lymphoma with bone involvement: report of two cases. Virchows Arch 427:105–110, 1995.

Jaffe ES: Classification of natural killer (NK) cell and NK-like T-cell malignancies. Blood 87:1207–1210, 1996.

Jaffe ES: Post-thymic lymphoid neoplasia. In Jaffe ES (ed): Surgical Pathology of the Lymph Node and Related Organs. WB Saunders Company, Philadelphia, pp 241–246, 1985.

Jaffe ES: Post-thymic T-cell lymphomas. In Jaffe ES (ed): Surgical Pathology of the Lymph Node and Related Organs, 2nd ed. WB Saunders Company, Philadelphia, pp 367–374, 1995.

Jaffe ES, Harris NL, Diebold J, Muller-Hermelink HK: World Health Organization Classification of lymphomas: work in progress. Ann Oncol 9:S25–S30, 1998.

Jaffe ES, Blattner WA, Blayney DW, et al: The pathologic spectrum of adult T-cell leukemia/lymphoma in the United States: human T-cell leukemia/lymphoma virus-associated lymphoid malignancies. Am J Surg Pathol 8:263–275, 1984.

Jaffe ES, Chan JKC, Su I-J, et al: Report of the workshop on nasal and related extranodal angiocentric T/natural killer cell lymphomas: definition, differential diagnosis, and epidemiology. Am J Surg Pathol 20:103–111, 1996.

Jaffe ES, Costa J, Fauci AS, et al: Malignant lymphoma and erythrophagocytosis simulating malignant histiocytosis. Am J Med 75:741–749, 1983.

Jaffe ES, Lipford EH, Margolick JB, et al: Lymphomatoid granulomatosis and angiocentric lymphoma: a spectrum of post-thymic T-cell proliferations. Semin Respir Med 10:167–172, 1989.

Jennings CD, Foon KA: Recent advances in flow cytometry: application to the diagnosis of hematologic malignancy. Blood 90: 2863–2892, 1997.

Kadin ME: The spectrum of Ki-1+ cutaneous lymphomas. Curr Probl Dermatol 19:132–143, 1990.

Kadin ME, Sako D, Berliner N, et al: Childhood Ki-1 lymphoma presenting with skin lesions and peripheral lymphadenopathy. Blood 68:1042–1049, 1986.

Kanavaros P, Jiwa NM, De Bruin PC, et al: High incidence of EBV genome in CD30-positive non-Hodgkin's lymphomas. J Pathol 168:307–315, 1992.

Kanavaros P, Lavergne A, Galian A, et al: A primary immunoblastic T-malignant lymphoma of the small bowel, with azurophilic intracytoplasmic granules: a histologic, immunologic, and electron microscopy study. Am J Surg Pathol 12:641–647, 1988.

Kanavaros P, Lescs M-C, Brière J, et al: Nasal T-cell lymphoma: a clinicopathologic entity associated with peculiar phenotype and with Epstein-Barr virus. Blood 81:2688–2695, 1993.

Kaneko T, Fukuda J, Yoshihara, T et al: Nasal natural killer (NK) cell lymphoma: report of a case with activated NK cells containing Epstein-Barr virus and expressing CD21 antigen, and comparative studies of their phenotype and cytotoxity with normal NK cells. Br J Haematol 91:355–361, 1995.

Kaplan J, Ravindranath Y, Inoue S: T-cell acute lymphoblastic leukemia with natural killer cell phenotype. Am J Hematol 22: 355–364, 1986.

Kaudewitz P, Kind P, Sander CA: CD30+ anaplastic large cell lymphomas. Semin Dermatol 13:180–186, 1994.

Kawano S, Tatsumi E, Yoneda N, et al: Novel leukemic lymphoma with probable derivation from immature stage of natural killer (NK) lineage. Hematol Oncol 13:1–11, 1995.

Kees UR, Burton PR, Lü C, et al: Homozygous deletion of the *p16/MTS1* gene in pediatric acute lymphoblastic leukemia is associated with unfavorable clinical outcome. Blood 89:4161–4166, 1997.

Khan G, Norton AJ, Slavin G: Epstein-Barr virus in angioimmunoblastic T-cell lymphomas. Histopathology 22:145–149, 1993.

Kinney MC, Collins RD, Greer JP, et al: A small-cell-predominant variant of primary Ki-1 (CD30+) T-cell lymphoma. Am J Surg Pathol 17:859–868, 1993.

Kinney MC, Glick AD, Stein H, et al: Comparison of anaplastic large cell (Ki-1) lymphomas and microvillous lymphomas in their immunologic and ultrastructural features. Am J Surg Pathol 14:1047–1060, 1990.

Kinney MC, Greer JP, Kadin ME, et al: $p80^{npm/alk}$ expression in Ki-1+ lymphomas: histologic and immunophenotypic correlation [abstract]. Lab Invest 74:114A, 1996.

Kinney MC, Kadin ME: The pathologic and clinical spectrum of anaplastic large cell lymphoma and correlation with *ALK* gene dysregulation, Am J Clin Pathol 111:S56–S67, 1999.

Kinoshita K, Kamihira S, Ikeda S, et al: Clinical, hematologic, and pathologic features of leukemic T-cell lymphoma. Cancer 50: 1554–1562, 1982.

Kissane JM: Lymphadenopathy in childhood: long-term follow-up in patients with nondiagnostic lymph node biopsies. Hum Pathol 5:431–439, 1974.

Kjeldsberg CR, Wilson JF, Berard CW: Non-Hodgkin's lymphoma in children. Hum Pathol 14:612–627, 1983.

Knecht H: Angioimmunoblastic lymphadenopathy: ten years' experience and state of current knowledge. Semin Hematol 26: 208–215, 1989.

Koch SE, Zackheim HS, Williams ML, et al: Mycosis fungoides beginning in childhood and adolescence. J Am Acad Dermatol 17: 563–570, 1987.

Koita H, Suzumiya J, Ohshima K, et al: Lymphoblastic lymphoma expressing natural killer cell phenotype with involvement of the mediastinum and nasal cavity. Am J Surg Pathol 21:242–248, 1997.

Krasne DL, Warnke RA, Weiss LM: Malignant lymphoma presenting as pseudoepitheliomatous hyperplasia: a report of two cases. Am J Surg Pathol 12:835–842, 1988.

Kraus MD, Crawford DF, Kaleem Z, et al: T γ/δ hepatosplenic lymphoma in a heart transplant patient after an Epstein-Barr virus positive lymphoproliferative disorder. Cancer 82:983–992, 1998.

Krishnan J, Tomaszewski M-M, Kao GF: Primary cutaneous CD30-positive anaplastic large cell lymphoma: report of 27 cases. J Cutan Pathol 20:193–202, 1993.

Kuzel TM, Roenigk HH, Rosen ST: Mycosis fungoides and the Sézary syndrome: a review of pathogenesis, diagnosis, and therapy. J Clin Oncol 9:1298–1313, 1991.

Lanier LL, Spits H, Phillips JH: The developmental relationship between NK cells and T cells. Immunol Today 13:392–395, 1992.

Le Deist F, de Saint Basile G, Coulombel L, et al: A familial occurrence of natural killer cell-T-lymphocyte proliferation disease in two children. Cancer 67:2610–2617, 1991.

Lennert K, Feller AC: Histopathology of Non-Hodgkin's Lymphomas (Based on the Updated Kiel Classification). Springer-Verlag, Berlin, 1992.

Leong AS-Y, Sage RF, Kinnear GC, et al: Preferential epidermotropism in adult T-cell leukemia-lymphoma. Am J Surg Pathol 4: 421–430, 1980.

Lin BT-Y, Musset M, Székaly A-M, et al: Human T-cell lymphotropic virus-1–positive T-cell leukemia/lymphoma in a child: report of a case and review of the literature. Arch Pathol Lab Med 121: 1282–1286, 1997.

Lin K-H, Su I-J, Chen R-L, et al: Peripheral T-cell lymphoma in childhood: a report of five cases in Taiwan. Med Pediatr Oncol 23: 26–35, 1994.

Link M, Schuster JJ, Donaldson SS, et al: Treatment of children and young adults with early-stage non-Hodgkin's lymphoma. N Engl J Med 337:1259–1266, 1997.

Link MP, Donaldson SS, Berard CW, et al: Results of treatment of childhood localized non-Hodgkin's lymphoma with combination chemotherapy with or without radiotherapy. N Engl J Med 322:1169–1174, 1990.

Link MP, Roper M, Dorfman RF, et al: Cutaneous lymphoblastic lymphoma with pre-B markers. Blood 61:838–841, 1983.

Lipford EH, Margolick JB, Longo DL, et al: Angiocentric immunoproliferative lesions: a clinicopathologic spectrum of post-thymic T-cell proliferations. Blood 72:1674–1681, 1988.

Lipford EH, Smith HR, Pittaluga S, et al: Clonality of angioimmunoblastic lymphadenopathy and implications for its evolution to malignant lymphoma. J Clin Invest 79:637–642, 1987.

Longacre TA, Listrom MB, Spigel JH, et al: Aggressive jejunal lymphoma of large granular lymphocytes: immunohistochemical, ultrastructural, molecular and DNA content analysis. Am J Clin Pathol 93:124–132, 1990.

Lopategui JR, Gaffey MJ, Chan JKC, et al: Infrequent association of Epstein-Barr virus with CD30-positive anaplastic large cell lymphomas from American and Asian patients. Am J Surg Pathol 19: 42–49, 1995.

Loughran TP: Clonal diseases of large granular lymphocytes. Blood 82:1–14, 1993.

Loughran TP, Hammond WP: Adult onset cyclic neutropenia is a benign neoplasm associated with clonal proliferation of large granular lymphocytes. J Exp Med 164:2089–2094, 1986.

Lowsky R, DeCoteau JF, Reitmair AH, et al: Defects of the mismatch repair gene MSH2 are implicated in the development of murine and human lymphoblastic lymphomas and are associated with the aberrant expression of rhombotin-2 (Lmo-2) and Tal-1 (SCL). Blood 89:2276–2282, 1997.

Lukes RJ, Tindle BH: Immunoblastic lymphadenopathy: a hyperimmune entity resembling Hodgkin's disease. N Engl Med 292:1–8, 1975.

Ma Z, Colls J, Marynen P, et al: Inv(2) (p23q35) in anaplastic large-cell lymphoma induces constitutive anaplastic lymphoma kinase (ALK) tyrosine activation by fusion to ATIC, an enzyme involved in purine nucleotide biosynthesis. Blood 95:2144–2149, 2000.

MacDonald HR: NK1.1+ T cell receptor-α/β+ cells: new clues to their origin, specificity, and function. J Exp Med 182:633–638, 1995.

Macgrogan G, Vergier B, Dubus P, et al: CD30-positive cutaneous large cell lymphomas: a comparative study of clinicopathologic and molecular features of 16 cases. Am J Clin Pathol 105: 440–450, 1996.

Macon WR, Williams ME, Greer JP, et al: Natural killer-like T-cell lymphomas: aggressive lymphomas of T-large granular lymphocytes. Blood 87:1474–1483, 1996.

Magaña M, Sangueza P, Gil-Beristain J, et al: Angiocentric cutaneous T-cell lymphoma of childhood (hydroa-like lymphoma): a distinctive type of cutaneous T-cell lymphoma. J Am Acad Dermatol 38:574–579, 1998.

Manca N, Piacentini E, Gelm M, et al: Persistence of human T cell lymphotropic virus type I (HTLV-1) sequences in peripheral blood mononuclear cells from patients with mycosis fungoides. J Exp Med 180:1973–1978, 1994.

Mandojana RM, Helwig EB: Localized epidermotropic reticulosis (Woringer-Kolopp disease). J Am Acad Dermatol 8:813–829, 1983.

Mann KP, Hall B, Kamino H, et al: Neutrophil-rich, Ki-1 positive anaplastic large-cell malignant lymphoma. Am J Surg Pathol 19:407–416, 1995.

Massimino M, Gasparini M, Giardini R: Ki-1 (CD30) anaplastic large-cell lymphoma in children. Ann Oncol 6:915–920, 1995.

McKenna RW, Parkin J, Kersey JH, et al: Chronic lymphoproliferative disorder with ususual clinical, morphologic, ultrastructural and membrane surface marker characteristics. Am J Med 62: 588–596, 1977.

Medeiros LJ, Peiper SC, Elwood L, et al: Angiocentric immunoproliferative lesions: a molecular analysis of eight cases. Hum Pathol 22:1150–1157, 1991.

Mehregan DA, Gibson LE, Muller SA: Follicular mucinosis: histopathologic review of 33 cases. Mayo Clin Proc 66:387–390, 1991.

Mehregan DA, Su WPD, Kurtin PJ: Subcutaneous T-cell lymphoma: a clinical, histopathologic, and immunohistochemical study of six cases. J Cutan Pathol 21:110–117, 1994.

Meier F, Schaumburg-Lever G, Kaiserling E, et al: Primary cutaneous large-cell anaplastic (Ki-1) lymphoma in a child. J Am Acad Dermatol 26:813–817, 1992.

Meister L, Duarte AM, Davis J, et al: Sézary syndrome in an 11-year-old girl. J Am Acad Dermatol 28:93–95, 1993.

Mielke V, Wolff HH, Winzer M, et al: Localized and disseminated pagetoid reticulosis: diagnostic and immunophenotypical findings. Arch Dermatol 125:402–406, 1989.

Millot F, Brizard F, Babin P, et al: t (3;17) (q21:q25) in Epstein-Barr virus associated peripheral T-cell lymphoma: a paediatric case. Br J Haematol 100:331–334, 1998.

Monterroso V, Bujan W, Jaramillo O, et al: Subcutaneous tissue involvement by T-cell lymphoma: a report of 2 cases. Arch Dermatol 132:1345–1350, 1996.

Morris SW, Kirstein MN, Valentine MB, et al: Fusion of a kinase gene, *ALK*, to a nucleolar protein gene, *NPM*, in non-Hodgkin's lymphoma. Science 263:1281–1284, 1994.

Motley RJ, Jasani B, Ford AM, et al: Regressing atypical histiocytosis, a regressing cutaneous phase of Ki-1-positive anaplastic large cell lymphoma: immunocytochemical, nucleic acid, and cytogenetic studies of a new case in view of current opinion. Cancer 70:476–483, 1992.

Moubayed P, Kaiserling E, Stein H: T-cell lymphomas of the stomach: morphological and immunologic studies characterizing two cases of T-cell lymphoma. Virchows Arch A 411:523–529, 1987.

Murphy SB: Childhood non-Hodgkin's lymphomas. N Engl J Med 299:1446–1448, 1978.

Murphy SB: Classification, staging and end results of treatment of childhood non-Hodgkin's lymphomas: dissimilarities from lymphomas in adults. Semin Oncol 7:332–339, 1980.

Murphy SB: Pediatric lymphomas: recent advances and commentary on Ki-1-positive anaplastic large-cell lymphomas of childhood. Ann Oncol 5:S31–S33, 1994.

Murphy SB, Fairclough DL, Hutchinson RE, et al: Non-Hodgkin's lymphomas of childhood: an analysis of the histology, staging, and response to treatment of 338 cases at a single institution. J Clin Oncol 7:186–193, 1989.

Murray A, Cuevas EC, Jones DB, et al: Study of the immunohistochemistry and T cell clonality of enteropathy-associated T cell lymphoma. Am J Pathol 146:509–519, 1995.

Myers JL, Kurtin PJ, Katzenstein A-LA, et al: Lymphomatoid granulomatosis: evidence of immunophenotypic diversity and relationship to Epstein-Barr virus infection. Am J Surg Pathol 19:1300–1312, 1995.

Nakagawa A, Nakamura S, Ito M, et al: CD30-positive anaplastic large cell lymphoma in childhood: expression of $p80^{npm/alk}$ and absence of Epstein-Barr virus. Mod Pathol 10:210–215, 1997.

Nakamura F, Tatsumi E, Kawano S, et al: Acute lymphoblastic leukemia/lymphoblastic lymphoma of natural killer (NK) lineage: quest for another NK-lineage neoplasm [letter]. Blood 89: 4665–4666, 1997.

Nakamura S, Suchi T, Koshikawa T, et al: Clinicopathologic study of CD56 (NCAM)-positive angiocentric lymphoma occurring in sites other than the upper and lower respratory tract. Am J Surg Pathol 19:284–296, 1995.

Nakazono S, Kitahara T, Takezaki T, et al: Immunoblastic lymphadenopathy (IBL)-like T-cell lymphoma in a child. Acta Paediatr Jpn 33:398–407, 1991.

Nathwani BN, Jaffe ES: Angioimmunoblastic lymphadenopathy (AILD) and AILD-like T-cell lymphomas. In Jaffe ES (ed): Surgical Pathology of the Lymph Nodes and Related Organs, vol 16 in Major Problems in Pathology, 2nd ed. WB Saunders Company, Philadelphia, pp 390–412, 1995.

Nathwani BN, Kim H, Rappaport H: Malignant lymphoma, lymphoblastic. Cancer 38:964–983, 1976.

Nathwani BN, Rappaport H, Moran EM, et al: Malignant lymphoma arising in angioimmunoblastic lymphadenopathy. Cancer 41:578–606, 1978.

Natkunam Y, Smoller R, Zehnder JL, et al: Aggressive cutaneous NK and NK-like T-cell lymphomas. Clinicopathologic, immunohistochemical, and molecular analyses of 12 cases. Am J Surg Pathol 23:571–581, 1999.

Nezelof C, Virelizier JL: Long lasting lymphadenopathy in childhood as an expression of a severe hyperimmune B lymphocyte disorder. Hematol Oncol 1:227–242, 1983.

Ng CS, Chan JKC, Cheng PNM, et al: Nasal T-cell lymphoma associated with hemophagocytic syndrome. Cancer 58:67–71, 1986.

Ng CS, Chan JKC, Lo STH: Expression of natural killer cell markers in non-Hodgkin's lymphomas. Hum Pathol 18:1257–1262, 1987.

Nichols GE, Normansell DE, Williams ME: Lymphoproliferative disorder of granular lymphocytes: nine cases including one with features of CD56(NKH1)-positive aggressive natural killer cell lymphoma. Mod Pathol 7:819–824, 1994.

Niemann TH, Thomas PA: Primary lymphoma of bone: diagnosis by fine-needle aspiration biopsy in a pediatric patient. Diagn Cytopathol 12:165–167, 1995.

Orazi A, Cattoretti G, John K, et al: Terminal deoxynucleotidyl transferase staining of malignant lymphoma in paraffin sections. Mod Pathol 5:582–585, 1994.

Ornvold K, Carstensen H, Junge J, et al: Tumours classified as "malignant histiocytosis" in children are T-cell neoplasms. APMIS 100: 558–566, 1992.

Ozdemirli M, Fanburg-Smith JC, Hartmann D-P, et al: Precursor B-lymphoblastic lymphoma presenting as a solitary bone tumor and mimicking Ewing's sarcoma. A report of four cases and review of the literature. Am J Surg Pathol 22:795–804, 1998.

Paietta, Gallagher RE, Wiernik PH: Myeloid/natural killer cell acute leukemia: a previously unrecognized from of acute leukemia potentially misdiagnosed as FAB M3. Blood 84:2824–2825, 1994.

Pallesen G, Hamilton-Dutoit SJ: Ki-1 (CD30) antigen is regularly expressed by tumor cells of embryonal carcinoma. Am J Pathol 133:509–519, 1988.

Pancake BA, Zucker-Franklin D, Coutavas EE: The cutaneous T cell lymphoma, mycosis fungoides, is a human T cell lymphotropic virus-associated disease: a study of 50 patients. J Clin Invest 95:547–554, 1995.

Papadimitriou JC, Abruzzo LV, Bourquin PM, et al: Correlation of light microscopic, immunocytochemical and ultrastructural cytomorphology of anaplastic large cell Ki-1 lymphoma, an activated lymphocyte phenotype: a case report. Acta Cytol 40:1283–1288, 1996.

Patsouris E, Noel H, Lennert K: Angioimmunoblastic lymphadenopathy-type T-cell lymphoma with a high content of epithelioid cells: histopathology and comparison with lymphoepithelioid cell lymphoma. Am J Surg Pathol 13:262–275, 1989.

Patte C, Kalifa C, Flamant F, et al: Results of the LMT81 protocol, a modified LSA_2L_2 protocol with high dose methotrexate, on 84 children with non-B-cell (lymphoblastic) lymphoma. Med Pediatr Oncol 20:105–113, 1992.

Paulli M, Berti E, Rosso R, et al: CD30/Ki-1-positive lymphoproliferative disorders of the skin—clinicopathologic correlation and statistical analysis of 86 cases: a multicentric study from the European Organization for Research and Treatment of Cancer Cutaneous Lymphoma Project Group. J Clin Oncol 13: 1343–1354, 1995.

Pesce K, Hoss DM, Berke A, et al: Metastatic lesions to the skin in children and adolescents. Adv Dermatol 12:237–274, 1997.

Peters MS, Thibodeau SN, White JW, et al: Mycosis fungoides in children and adolescents. J Am Acad Dermatol 22:1011–1018, 1990.

Picker LJ, Weiss LM, Medeiros LJ, et al: Immunophenotypic criteria for the diagnosis of non-Hodgkin's lymphoma. Am J Pathol 128: 181–201, 1987.

Picozzi VJ, Coleman CN: Lymphoblastic lymphoma. Semin Oncol 17:96–103, 1990.

Piira T, Perkins SL, Anderson JR, et al: Primary mediastinal large cell lymphoma in children: a report from the Children's Cancer Group. Pediatr Pathol Lab Med 15:561–570, 1995.

Pileri S, Falini B, Delsol G, et al: Lymphohistiocytic T-cell lymphoma (anaplastic large cell lymphoma CD30+/Ki-1+ with a high content of reactive histiocytes). Histopathology 16:383–391, 1990.

Pirruccello SJ, Bicak MS, Gordon BG, et al: Acute lymphoblastic leukemia of NK-cell lineage: responses to IL-2. Leuk Res 13: 735–743, 1989.

Pittaluga S, Wlodarska I, Pulford K, et al: The monoclonal antibody ALK1 identifies a distinct morphological subtype of anaplastic large cell lymphoma associated with *2p23/ALK* rearrangements. Am J Pathol 151:343–351, 1997.

Platanias LC, Larson RA, Vardiman JW, et al: Complex rearrangement of the T cell receptor in large granular lymphocytosis associated with myeloid suppression. Leukemia 4:863–865, 1990.

Pulford K, Lamant L, Morris SW, et al: Detection of anaplastic lymphoma kinase (ALK) and nucleolar protein nucleophosmin (NPM)-ALK proteins in normal and neoplastic cells with the monoclonal antibody ALK1. Blood 89:1394–1404, 1997.

Raimondi SC, Behm FG, Roberson PK, et al: Cytogenetics of childhood T-cell leukemia. Blood 72:1560–1566, 1988.

Ralfkiaer E, Wolff-Sneedorff A, Thomsen K, et al: Immunophenotypic studies in cutaneous T-cell lymphomas: clinical implications. Br J Dermatol 129:655–659, 1993.

Reiter A, Schrappe M, Tiemann M, et al: Successful treatment strategy for Ki-1 anaplastic large-cell lymphoma of childhood: a prospective analysis of 62 patients enrolled in three consecutive Berlin-Frankfurt-Munster group studies. J Clin Oncol 12:899–908, 1994.

Reiter A, Schrappe M, Parwaresch R, et al: Non-Hodgkin's lymphomas of childhood and adolescence: results of treatment stratified for biologic subtypes and stage—a report of the Berlin-Frankfurt-Munster Group. J Clin Oncol 13:359–372, 1995.

Riopel M, Dickman PS, Link MP, et al: MIC2 analysis in pediatric lymphomas and leukemias. Hum Pathol 25:396–399, 1994.

Rubie H, Gladieff L, Robert A, et al: Childhood anaplastic large cell lymphoma Ki-1/CD30: clinicopathologic features of 19 cases. Med Pediatr Oncol 22:155–161, 1994.

Salhany KE, Collins RD, Greer JP, et al: Long-term survival in Ki-1 lymphoma. Cancer 67:516–522, 1991.

Salhany KE, Cousar JB, Greer JP, et al: Transformation of cutaneous T-cell lymphoma to large cell lymphoma: a clinicopathologic and immunologic study. Am J Pathol 132:265–277, 1988.

Salhany KE, Feldman M, Kahn MJ, et al: Hepatosplenic $\gamma\delta$ T-cell lymphoma: ultrastructural, immunophenotypic, and functional evidence for cytotoxic T lymphocyte differentiation. Hum Pathol 28:674–685, 1997.

Salhany KE, Greer JP, Cousar JB, et al: Marrow involvement in cutaneous T-cell lymphoma: a clinicopathologic study of 60 cases. Am J Clin Pathol 92:747–754, 1989.

Sander CA, Medeiros LJ, Abruzzo LV, et al: Lymphoblastic lymphoma presenting in cutaneous sites: a clinicopathologic analysis of six cases. J Am Acad Dermatol 25:1023–1031, 1991.

Sandlund JT, Magrath IT: Lymphoblastic lymphoma. In Magrath IT (ed): The Non-Hodgkin's Lymphomas, 2nd ed. Arnold, London, pp 813–828, 1997.

Sandlund JT, Pui C-H, Santana VM, et al: Clinical features and treatment outcome for children with CD30+ large-cell non-Hodgkin's lymphoma. J Clin Oncol 12:895–898, 1994.

Sausville EA, Eddy JL, Makuch RW, et al: Histopathologic staging at initial diagnosis of mycosis fungoides and the Sézary syndrome: definition of three distinctive prognostic groups. Ann Intern Med 109:372–382, 1988.

Sausville EA, Worsham GF, Matthews MJ, et al: Histologic assessment of lymph nodes in mycosis fungoides/Sézary syndrome (cutaneous T-cell lymphoma): clinical correlations and prognostic import of a new classification system. Hum Pathol 16:1098–1109, 1985.

Schichman SA, Aplan PD, Neri A, et al: Pathogenesis of T-cell lymphomas. In Magrath IT (ed): The Non-Hodgkin's Lymphomas, 2nd ed. Arnold, London, pp 411–442, 1997.

Schlegelberger B, Feller A, Godde W, et al: Stepwise development of chromosomal abnormalities in angioimmunoblastic lymphadenopathy. Cancer Genet Cytogenet 50:15–29, 1990.

Schlegelberger B, Zhang Y, Weber-Matthiesen K, Grote W: Detection of aberrant clones in nearly all cases of angioimmunoblastic lymphadenopathy with dysproteinemia-type T-cell lymphoma by combined interphase and metaphase cytogenetics. Blood 84: 2640–2648, 1994.

Schwarting R, Gerdes J, Durkop H, et al: Ber-H2: a new monoclonal antibody directed at a formal-resistant epitope. Blood 74: 1678–1689, 1989.

Scott AA, Head DR, Kopecky KJ, et al: HLA-DR−, CD33+, CD56+, CD16− myeloid/natural killer cell acute leukemia: a previously unrecognized form of acute leukemia potentially misdiagnosed as French-American-British acute myeloid leukemia M3. Blood 84:244–255, 1994.

Seymour JF, Pierce SA, Kantarjian HM, et al: Investigation of karyotypic, morphologic and clinical features in patients with acute myeloid leukemia blast cells expressing the neural cell adhesion molecule (CD56). Leukemia 8:823–826, 1994.

Sheibani K, Nathwani BN, Winberg CD, et al: Antigentically defined subgroups of lymphoblastic lymphoma: relationship to clinical presentation and biologic behavior. Cancer 60:183–190, 1987a.

Sheibani K, Winberg CD, Burke JS, et al: Lymphoblastic lymphoma expressing natural killer–associated antigens: a clinicopathologic study of six cases. Leuk Res 11:371–377, 1987b.

Shepherd SF, A'Hern RP, Pinkerton CR: Childhood T-cell lymphoblastic lymphoma: Does early resolution of mediastinal mass predict for final outcome? The United Kingdom Children's Cancer Study Group (UKCCSG). Br J Cancer 72:752–756, 1995.

Shih L-Y, Liang D-C: Non-Hodgkin's lymphomas in Asia. Hematol Oncol Clin North Am 5:983–1001, 1991.

Shimoyama M, Minato K, Saito H, et al: Immunoblastic lymphadenopathy (IBL)–like T-cell lymphoma. Jpn J Clin Oncol 9(suppl 1):347–356, 1979.

Shiota M, Fujimoto J, Takenaga M, et al: Diagnosis of t(2;5)(p23;q35)-associated Ki-1 lymphoma with immunohistochemistry. Blood 84:3648–3652, 1994.

Shiota M, Nakamura S, Ichinohasama R, et al: Anaplastic large cell lymphomas expressing the novel chimeric protein $p80^{NPM/ALK}$: a distinct clinicopathologic entity. Blood 86:1954–1960, 1995.

Smith JL, Hodges E, Quin CT, et al: Frequent T and B cell oligoclones in histologically and immunophenotypically characterized angioimmunoblastic lymphadenopathy. Am J Pathol 156:661–669, 2000.

Soslow RA, Davis RE, Warnke RA, et al: True histiocytic lymphoma following therapy for lymphoblastic neoplasms. Blood 87:5207–5212, 1996.

Spits H, Lanier LL, Phillips JH: Development of human T and natural killer cells. Blood 85:2654–2670, 1995.

Stein, H: Society for Hematopathology Program. Am J Surg Pathol 21:114–121, 1997.

Stein H, Mason DY, Gerdes J, et al: The expression of the Hodgkin's disease associated antigen Ki-1 in reactive and neoplastic tissue: evidence that Reed-Sternberg cells and histiocytic malignancies are derived from activated lymphoid cells. Blood 66:848–858, 1985.

Stensvold K, Brandtzaeg P, Kvaloy S, et al: Immunoblastic lymphadenopathy with early onset in two boys: immunohistochemical study and indication of decreased proportion of circulating T-helper cells. Br J Haematol 56:417–430, 1984.

Strickler JG, Meneses MF, Habermann TM, et al: Polymorphic reticulosis: a reappraisal. Hum Pathol 25:659–665, 1994.

Stroup R, Sheibani K, Misset J-L, et al: Surface immunoglobulin-positive lymphoblastic lymphoma: a report of three cases. Cancer 65:2559–2563, 1990.

Sun T, Brody J, Susin M, et al: Aggressive natural killer cell lymphoma/leukemia: a recently recognized clinicopathologic entity. Am J Surg Pathol 17:1289–1299, 1993.

Sun T, Schulman P, Kolitz J, et al: A study of lymphoma of large granular lymphocytes with modern modalities: report of two cases and review of the literature. Am J Hematol 40:135–145, 1992.

Suzuki R, Yamamoto K, Seto M, et al: CD7+ and CD56+ myeloid/natural killer cell precursor acute leukemia: a distinct hematolymphoid disease entity. Blood 90:2417–2428, 1997.

Suzumiya J, Takeshita M, Kimura N, et al: Expression of adult and fetal natural killer cell markers in sinonasal lymphomas. Blood 83:2255–2260, 1994.

Swerdlow SH, Habeshaw JA, Richards MA, et al: T lymphoblastic lymphoma with Leu-7 positive phenotype and unusual clinical course: a multiparameter study. Leuk Res 9:167–173, 1985.

Swerdlow SH, Habeshaw JA, Rohatiner AZS, et al: Caribbean T-cell lymphoma/leukemia. Cancer 54:687–696, 1984.

Tajima K, The T- and B-cell Malignancy Study Group, et al: The 4th nation-wide study of adult T-cell leukemia/lymphoma (ATL) in Japan: estimates of risk of ATL and its geographical and clinical features. Int J Cancer 45:237–243, 1990.

Takamura M, Mugishima H, Nagata T, et al: Successful autologous bone marrow transplant for relapsed Ki-1 lymphoma. Acta Paediatr Jpn 37:541–544, 1995.

Takeshita M, Akamatsu M, Ohshima K, et al: CD30 (Ki-1) expression in adult T-cell leukaemia/lymphoma is associated with distinctive immunohistological and clinical characteristics. Histopatholgy 26:539–546, 1995.

Tani E, Löwhagen T, Nasiell K, et al: Fine needle aspiration cytology and immunocytochemistry of large cell lymphomas expressing the Ki-1 antigen. Acta Cytol 33:359–362. 1989.

Taniguchi S, Horio T, Komura J: Mycosis fungoides in the tumor stage treated by PUVA: a successful trial in a 12-year-old girl. Dermatologica 160:409–413, 1980.

Taniwaki M, Tagawa S, Nishigaki H, et al: Chromosomal abnormalities define clonal proliferation in CD3- large granular lymphocyte leukemia. Am J Hematol 33:32–38, 1990.

Tatsumi E, Yoneda N, Kawano S, et al: CD21 antigen in T-lineage neoplastic lymphoid cells: characteristic expression at thymic stage. Am J Hematol 45:150–155, 1994.

Tefferi A, Li C-Y, Witzig TE, et al: Chronic natural killer cell lymphocytosis: a descriptive clinical study. Blood 84:2721–2725, 1994.

Teixeira F, Ortiz-Plata A, Courtes-Franco R, et al: Do environmental factors play any role in the pathogenesis of mycosis fungoides and Sézary syndrome? Int J Dermatol 33:770–772, 1994.

Tobinai K, Minato K, Ohtsu T, et al: Clinicopathologic, immunophenotypic, and immunogenotypic analyses of immunoblastic lymphadenopathy-like T-cell lymphoma. Blood 72:1000–1006, 1988.

Tomaszewski M-M, Lupton GP, Krishnan J, et al: A comparison of clinical, morphological and immunohistochemical features of lymphomatoid papulosis and primary cutaneous CD30(Ki-1)-positive anaplastic large cell lymphoma. J Cutan Pathol 22:310–318, 1995.

Tomaszewski M-M, Moad JC, Lupton GP: Primary cutaneous Ki-1 (CD30) positive anaplastic large cell lymphoma in childhood. J Am Acad Dermatol 40:857–861, 1999.

Tope WD, White PF, Fransway AF, et al: Cutaneous tumor in a child: cutaneous T cell lymphoma (CTCL). Arch Dermatol 128: 681–682, 684–685, 1992.

Toren A, Neumann Y, Rosner E, et al: Pediatric small cell variant of Ki-1 (CD30)+ T-cell lymphoma with germ-line configuration of the T-cell receptor gene. Acta Oncol 35:243–245, 1996.

Touriol C, Greenland C, Lamant L, et al: Further demonstration of the diversity of chromosomal changes involving 2p23 in ALK-positive lymphoma: 2 cases expressing ALK kinase fused to CLTCL (clathrin chain polypeptide-like). Blood 95:3204–3207, 2000.

Van Gorp J, De Bruin PC, Sie-Go DMDS, et al: Nasal T-cell lymphoma: a clinicopathological and immunophenotypic analysis of 13 cases. Histopathology 27:139–148, 1995.

Vecchi V, Burnelli R, Pileri S, et al: Anaplastic large cell lymphoma (Ki-1+/CD30+) in childhood. Med Pediatr Oncol 21:402–410, 1993.

Vidriales MB, Orfao A, Gonzalez M, et al: Expression of NK and lymphoid-associated antigens in blast cells of acute myeloblastic leukemia. Leukemia 7:2026–2029, 1993.

Wakely PE Jr, Kornstein MJ: Aspiration cytopathology of lymphoblastic lymphoma and leukemia: the MCV experience. Pediatr Pathol Lab Med 16:243–252, 1996.

Wang C-YE, Daniel WP, Kurtin PJ: Subcutaneous panniculitic T-cell lymphoma. Int J Dermatol 35:1–8, 1996.

Wang CC, Tien HF, Lin M-T, et al: Consistent presence of isochromosome 7q in hepatosplenic T γ/δ lymphoma: a new cytogenetic-clinicopathologic entity. Genes Chromosomes Cancer 12: 161–164, 1995.

Warnke RA, Weiss LM, Chan JKC, et al: Tumors of the lymph nodes and spleen. In Rosai J (ed): Atlas of Tumor Pathology, 3rd series, fascicle 9. Armed Forces Institute of Pathology, Washington, DC, pp 239–240, 1995.

Watanabe S, Sato Y, Shimoyama M, et al: Immunoblastic lymphadenopathy, angioimmunoblastic lymphadenopathy, and IBL-like T-cell lymphoma: a spectrum of T-cell neoplasia. Cancer 58:2224–2232, 1986.

Weidner N, Tjoe J: Immunohistochemical profile of monoclonal antibody O13: antibody that recognizes glycoprotein p30/32MIC2 and is useful in diagnosing Ewing's sarcoma and peripheral neuroepithelioma. Am J Surg Pathol 18:486–494, 1994.

Weiss L, Jaffe E, Liu X, et al: Detection and localization of Epstein-Barr viral genomes in angioimmunoblastic lymphadenopathy and angioimmunoblastic lymphadenopathy-like lymphomas. Blood 79:1789–1795, 1992.

Weiss LM, Strickler JG, Dorfman RF, et al: Clonal T-cell populations in angioimmunoblastic lymphadenopathy and angioimmunoblastic lymphadenopathy-like lymphoma. Am J Pathol 122:392–397, 1986.

Weiss M, Bindl JM, Picozzi VJ, et al: Lymphoblastic lymphoma: an immunophenotypic study of 26 cases with comparison to T cell acute lymphoblastic leukemia. Blood 67:474–478, 1986.

Weiss RL, Lazarus KH, Macon WR, et al: Natural killer–like T-cell lymphoma in the small intestine of a child without evidence of enteropathy. Am J Surg Pathol 21:964–969, 1997.

Wellman A, Otsuki T, Vogelbruch M, et al: Analysis of the t(2;5)(p23;q35) translocation by reverse transcription-polymerase chain reaction in CD 30+ anaplastic large-cell lymphomas, in other non-Hodgkin's lymphomas of T-cell phenotype, and in Hodgkin's disease. Blood 86:2321–2328, 1995.

Whitlock JA, Kinney MC, Greer JP: Childhood Ki-1+ lymphoma: effect of small cell predominant histology on outcome. Blood 80(suppl 1): 43a, 1992.

Whitmore SE, Simmons-O'Brien E, Rotter FS: Hypopigmented mycosis fungoides. Arch Dermatol 130:476–480, 1994.

Wiles HB, Laver J, Baum D: T-cell lymphoma in a child after heart transplantation. J Heart Lung Transplant 13:1019–1023, 1994.

Willemze R, Beljaards RC: Spectrum of primary cutaneous CD30 (Ki-1)-positive lymphoproliferative disorders: a proposal for classification and guidelines for management and treatment. J Am Acad Dermatol 28:973–980, 1993.

Wilson AGM, Cotter FE, Lowe DG, et al: Mycosis fungoides in childhood: an unusual presentation. J Am Acad Dermatol 25:370–372, 1991.

Wilson MS, Weiss LM, Gatter KC, et al: Malignant histiocytosis: a reassessment of cases previously reported in 1975 based on paraffin section immunophenotyping studies. Cancer 66:530–536, 1990.

Winter SS, Duncan MH, Foucar E, et al: Childhood Ki-1 lymphoma: presentation as a buttock mass. Am J Pediatr Hematol Oncol 13:334–337, 1991.

Wong KF, Chan JKC, Matutes E, et al: Hepatosplenic $\gamma\delta$ T-cell lymphoma: a distinctive aggressive lymphoma type. Am J Surg Pathol 19:718–726, 1995.

Wong KF, Chan JKC, Ng CS: CD56 (NCAM)-positive malignant lymphoma. Leuk Lymphoma 14:29–36, 1994.

Wong KF, Chan JKC, Ng CS, et al: CD56 (NCAM)-positive hematolymphoid malignancies: an aggressive neoplasm featuring frequent cutaneous/mucosal involvement, cytoplasmic azurophilic granules, and angiocentricity. Hum Pathol 23:798–804, 1992.

Wood GS, Matthews MJ: Diagnosis of T-cell malignant lymphoproliferative disorders in the skin. In Jaffe ES (ed): Surgical Pathology of the Lymph Nodes and Related Organs, vol 16 in Major Problems in Pathology, 2nd ed. WB Saunders Company, Philadelphia, pp 413–447, 1995.

Yamaguchi K, Takatsuki K: Adult T-cell leukaemia/lymphoma. Baillieres Clin Haematol 6:899–915, 1993.

Yazdi HM, Burns BF: Fine needle aspiration biopsy of Ki-1 positive large cell "anaplastic" lymphoma. Acta Cytol 35:306–310, 1991.

Zaatari GS, Chan WC, Kim TH, et al: Malignant lymphoma of the skin in children. Cancer 59:1040–1045, 1987.

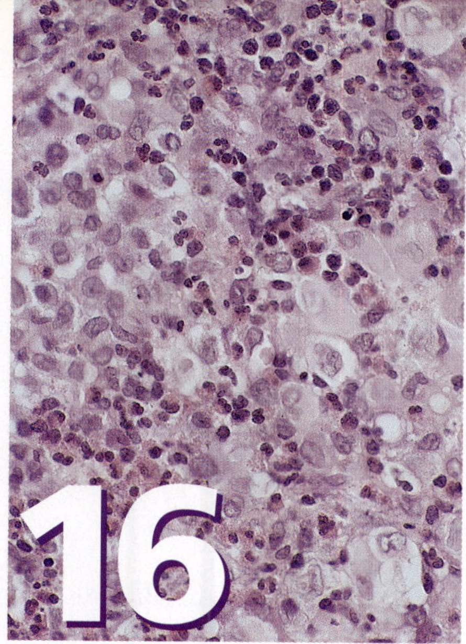

Steven H. Swerdlow

Lymph Nodes: Other Pathologic Conditions

SINUS HISTIOCYTOSIS WITH MASSIVE LYMPHADENOPATHY

Equivalent Terms

Rosai-Dorfman disease is another term for *sinus histiocytosis with massive lymphadenopathy* (SHML).

Definition

SHML is a benign nodal or extranodal proliferation of S-100+ histiocytes that demonstrate phagocytosis of lymphocytes and sometimes other inflammatory cells.

Clinical Features and Prognosis

SHML occurs in patients of all ages, ranging from neonates to older adults, although it is most frequent among children in their first decade (Rosai & Dorfman, 1972). The SHML registry reports a mean age of 20.6 ± 20.5 years (Foucar et al, 1990). There is a slight male predominance, with rare cases reported in identical twins or among family members. Patients present with massive lymphadenopathy often preceded by fever and pharyngitis. Cervical lymph nodes are most frequently affected, and a minority are painful or tender. The adenopathy is most frequently bilateral. Axillary, inguinal, or even mediastinal lymph node involvement is common. Extranodal involvement with or without nodal disease is reported in 43% of registry patients, but this extranodal frequency may be inflated artificially (Foucar et al, 1990). The most frequent extranodal sites include skin and soft tissue, nasal cavity and paranasal sinuses, eyelid and orbit, bone, salivary gland, and the central nervous system. Data from the SHML registry suggest that anemia is common at presentation (66% of cases), with granulocytosis in 34% and lymphopenia in 16%. Neutropenia and lymphocytosis are rare. Hypergammaglobulinemia is extremely common, but monoclonal paraproteins are rarely found. Hypoalbuminemia is seen in 60% of patients. A significant minority of patients have clinically evident immune disorders, with hematologic autoantibodies and joint disease the most common (Foucar et al, 1990).

SHML follows a benign course in the vast majority of patients, although many have stable but persistent disease. Follow-up for many reported cases has been incomplete. Complete remission of adenopathy may occur after a period of years. Some patients show remission and recurrence of adenopathy. These patients do not require specific therapy. A minority of patients show disease progression, and some die either with or of the disease. An "ideal" therapy is not reported for these patients, but they may require surgery, radiation, or chemotherapy (Komp, 1990). Adverse prognostic indicators include involvement of multiple lymph node groups and extranodal sites as well as the presence of immunologic abnormalities. Involvement of specific extranodal sites—the kidney, lower respiratory tract, and liver—is also associated with a markedly adverse prognosis (Foucar et al, 1990). Age does not appear to be an important prognostic variable, but the four patients who died of SHML had a mean age of onset of only 8.5 years.

SHML has occasionally been identified in lymph nodes with Hodgkin disease or B and T lymphomas (Maia & Dorfman, 1995). Rare patients are reported with subsequent lymphomas, but the occurrence of such lymphomas may be coincidental.

Pathologic Features

Lymph nodes demonstrate expansion of sinuses by large histiocytes, with frequent intracytoplasmic lymphocytes (lymphophagocytosis) (Fig. 16–1). Phagocytosed plasma cells, neutrophils, and red blood cells may also be identified. The histiocytes have round to oval vesicular nuclei and variably prominent nucleoli, and some appear atypical. Mitoses are usually infrequent but may be numerous. Indistinct cytoplasmic borders in hematoxylin-eosin–stained sections may complicate appreciation of the striking lymphophagocytosis in some cases. The sinuses also contain foamy or multinucleated histiocytes, neutrophils, lymphocytes, and plasma cells. Elsewhere, the lymph node exhibits a medullary plasmacytosis, but hyperplastic follicles and eosinophils are infrequent. Necrosis and microabscesses may be present. Sometimes the histiocytic proliferation extends beyond the sinuses and causes architectural effacement. Capsular and extracapsular fibrosis is also characteristic, but intranodal fibrosis is usually minimal. Extranodal cases often resemble nodes involved by SHML, even exhibiting sinuslike collections of histiocytes. However, there are usually more fibrosis, fewer typical SHML cells, and less lymphophagocytosis in extranodal cases.

Markers

The characteristic histiocytes in SHML have Langerhans cell features of S-100 positivity and also express many monocyte and

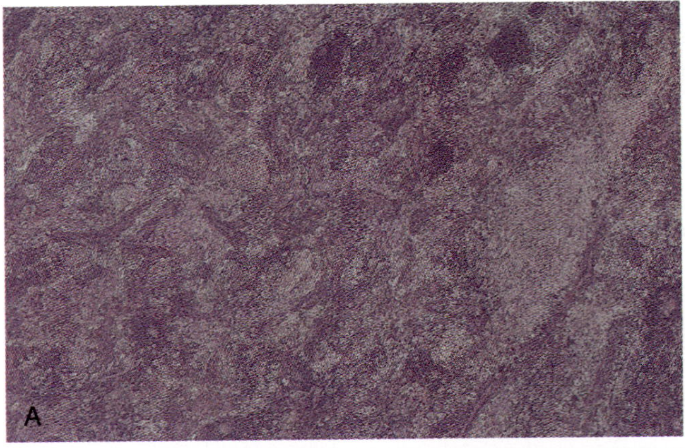

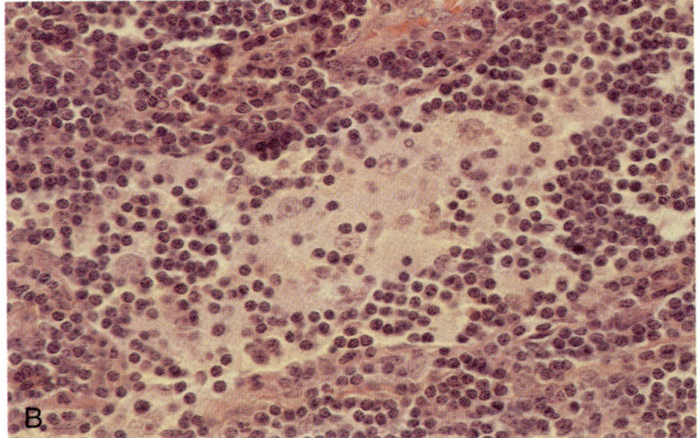

Figure 16–1

Sinus histiocytosis with massive lymphadenopathy, lymph node. *A*, Note the marked sinus expansion by histiocytes that on the right extend into the nodal parenchyma. The lymph node contains few follicles. *B*, Note several large histiocytes with prominent nucleoli and lymphophagocytosis. Their indistinct borders make definitive identification of the latter difficult.

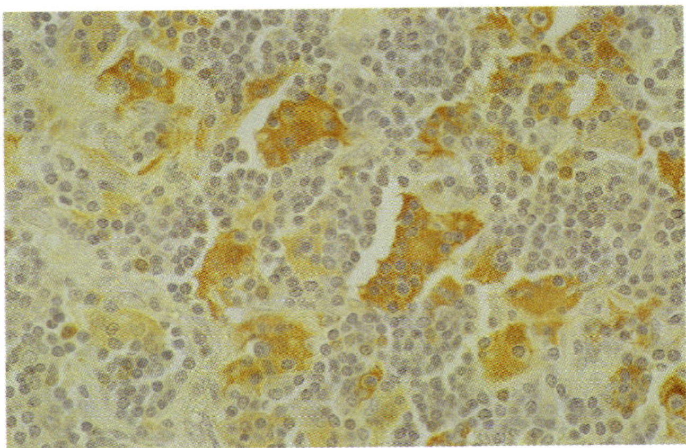

Figure 16–2

Sinus histiocytosis with massive lymphadenopathy, lymph node. The stain highlights the large histiocytes with lymphophagocytosis, confirming the diagnosis. S-100 immunostain.

macrophage antigens (e.g., CD11c, CD14, CD33, and CD68) (Eisen et al, 1990; Paulli et al, 1992) (Fig. 16–2). Langerhans cells and SHML histiocytes express cathepsin E (Paulli et al, 1994). The literature is inconsistent regarding their precise phenotype, with varying positivity using Mac-387, antilysozyme, CD11b, CD36, and α-1-antichymotrypsin antibodies. CD1a expression (a feature of Langerhans cells detected by the antibody O1O) also varies in positivity (Paulli et al, 1994). HLA-DR expression is variable, and half the cases exhibit CD30 positivity (Eisen et al, 1990). Sinuses and intersinusal areas also contain many intermediate-sized mononuclear cells with the phenotype of monocytes (S-100−, lysozyme positive, and HLA-DR+).

Genotypic Studies

Study of a very limited number of cases using the human androgen receptor gene assay (HUMARA) has shown that the

Table 16–1
Differential Diagnosis of SHML

Diagnosis	Comments
Nonspecific sinus histiocytosis and storage disorders	Sinus histiocytes have less prominent nucleoli, generally lack lymphophagocytosis, and lack strong S-100 positivity. Histiocytes in storage disorders should demonstrate a characteristic cytoplasm without lymphophagocytosis.
Langerhans cell histiocytosis	Also sinus based with S-100+ cells, but Langerhans cells have elongated and grooved nuclei (not round with nucleoli), definite CD1a positivity, and Birbeck granules (by electron microscopic examination). Lymphophagocytosis is absent.
Anaplastic large-cell lymphoma or metastatic carcinoma	Morphologic features of these neoplastic cells, together with immunophenotypic studies (not always necessary) will distinguish these malignant tumors from SHML. SHML may be CD30+.
Other hemophagocytic disorders	The clinicopathologic setting, predominance of phagocytized lymphocytes, and strong S-100 positivity help make the diagnosis of SHML.

Abbreviations: SHML, sinus histiocytosis with massive lymphadenopathy.

histiocytes in SHML are polyclonal (Paulli et al, 1995). Clonal populations of lymphocytes are also not detected.

Diagnostic Criteria

SHML is diagnosed by the presence of nodal or extranodal sinus or sinuslike expansion by large S-100–positive histiocytes exhibiting lymphophagocytosis.

Differential Diagnosis

The major differential diagnoses for SHML include "nonspecific" sinus histiocytosis and Langerhans cell histiocytosis (LCH; Table 16–1). One patient had both SHML and LCH (Foucar et al, 1990). Prominent lymphophagocytosis is one of the most helpful features in the diagnosis of SHML, but it is not a specific phenomenon. Other hemophagocytic and storage disorders that may be considered are discussed elsewhere (Chap. 8). Intrasinusal neoplastic proliferations, including anaplastic large-cell lymphomas and metastatic tumors, also may be considered in rare cases, especially since SHML histiocytes may be CD30+. Rare cases are described in which SHML coexist with a lymphoma.

Pathogenesis and Biologic Characteristics

The pathogenesis of SHML is unknown, although there are suggestions that it represents an exaggerated or abnormal immune response to an uncertain infection or immunodeficiency. Human herpesvirus 6 infection has been documented in most lymph nodes involved by SHML, but a causative role has not been established (Levine et al, 1992). Serologic study results are positive for Epstein-Barr virus (EBV) in a moderate number of patients, but infection in lymph nodes with SHML is uncommon (Levine et al, 1992; Tsang et al, 1994). Other infections, such as *Klebsiella rhinoscleroma* and subclinical *Brucella*, have been described in rare patients (Foucar et al, 1990).

PROGRESSIVE TRANSFORMATION OF GERMINAL CENTERS

Definition

Progressive transformation of germinal centers (PTGC) is diagnosed by a change in the appearance of one or more germinal centers due to replacement by small lymphocytes (see "Histopathologic Features"). Although benign, some cases are associated with Hodgkin disease (HD) usually nodular lymphocyte-predominant Hodgkin disease (LPHD). PTGC is found in about 3.6–10% of lymph nodes with chronic "nonspecific" lymphadenitis or follicular hyperplasia (Hansmann et al, 1990; Osborne et al, 1992).

Clinical Features and Prognosis

PTGC most commonly occurs in males in their second decade. About 20% of patients are 16 years or younger (Hansmann et al, 1990; Osborne et al, 1992). Affected children have a median age of 11 years, with a range of 4 to 16 years (Osborne et al, 1992). Most present with localized asymptomatic adenopathy. Cervical adenopathy is commonest, followed by inguinal and axillary adenopathy. Multifocal or generalized disease also occurs, particularly in children or young adults. Extranodal disease is rarely seen.

PTGC is a reactive disorder, but it does recur in 50% of children, compared to 23% of adults (Osborne et al, 1992). The median time to recurrence is 3 years. Nineteen percent of children had three or more biopsies revealing PTGC. Recurrences are usually in the same region as the original adenopathy. Some patients may have persistent disease for months to years. In a small series of "florid" PTGC in young men, persistent disease was described in patients with more than one site of involvement. There were no recurrences in those with localized disease (Ferry et al, 1992).

It is extremely important to recognize the association between PTGC and HD, although most do not consider PTGC prelymphomatous. Seventeen to 40% of PTGC cases in large series are associated with HD, including 30% of patients in a pediatric series (Hansmann et al, 1990, Osborne et al, 1992). The HD is usually nodular LPHD, which may precede, follow, or be concurrent with the PTGC. The former circumstance is most common in children with one or more biopsy specimens exhibiting PTGC weeks to several years following the HD. HD following PTGC occurs at <1 to 13 years (mean 4 years) (Ferry et al, 1992). PTGC is found in 18% of lymph nodes containing nodular LPHD (Burns et al, 1984).

Pathologic Features

Lymph nodes with PTGC are typically from >1 to 4 cm and demonstrate architectural preservation with follicular hyperplasia. One or more scattered transformed germinal centers stand out because they are about 3 to 4 times the size of the surrounding follicles (Fig. 16–3*A*). Half the cases have 3 or fewer transformed germinal centers per section, whereas 20% demonstrate 8 or more. "Florid" cases may have up to 29 per slide. Recurrent cases do not exhibit a consistent change in the number of transformed centers.

Progressively transformed germinal centers represent hyperplastic follicles with an ongoing infiltration of small mantle zone–type lymphocytes. They contain variably sized remnants of the frequently fragmented germinal centers, with their cleaved and noncleaved follicular center cells (Fig. 16–3*B*). In some transformed centers, germinal center remnants may be miniscule. Some cases may exhibit architectural distortion and occasional clusters of two or three transformed centers, but L– and H–type Reed-Sternberg cells are absent. Eosinophils are rare. Children, in particular, may have clusters of epithelioid or confluent histiocytes surrounding the transformed centers or other follicles (Fig. 16–3*C*). Results of staining for fungal and acid-fast organisms are negative. Transformed centers associated with HD cannot be distinguished from those that are not.

Markers

Transformed germinal centers are composed of polyclonal IgM+, IgD+ mantle cells with variably sized foci of IgD– follicular center cells. They typically also contain numerous T cells (mostly CD4+ type) as well as more CD57+ cells than seen in typical hyperplastic follicles. Immunostains for CD21 or CD23 also demonstrate the presence of a network of follicular dendritic cells that contains holes without dendritic processes similar to those in floridly hyperplastic follicles (Hansmann et al, 1990). In contrast to ordinary reactive follicles, the follicular dendritic cells are reportedly immunoglobulin negative

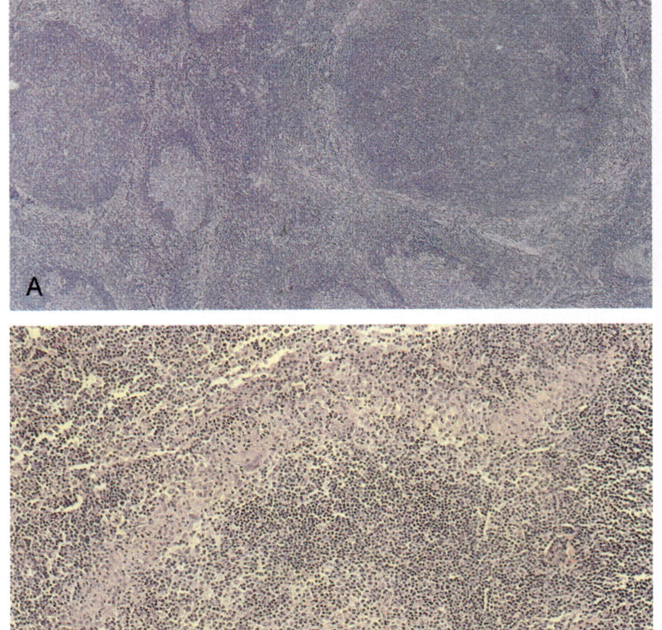

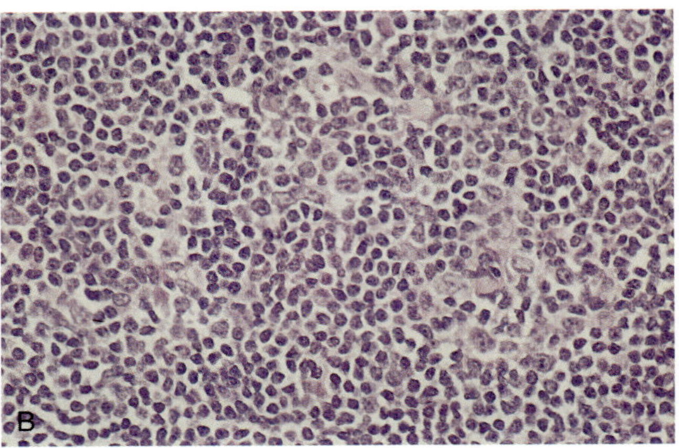

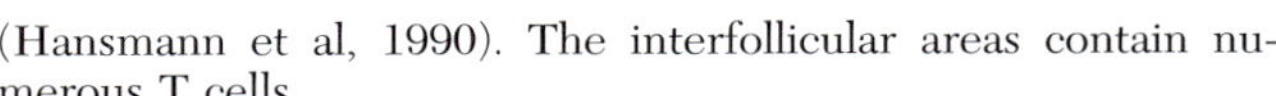

Figure 16–3

Progressive transformation of germinal centers, lymph node. *A*, Note the hyperplastic follicles and two much larger nodules composed predominantly of small mantle zone–like lymphocytes. *B*, Higher magnification of the largest progressively transformed germinal center reveals an ill-defined paler remnant of the hyperplastic follicle with large transformed follicular center cells. Most of the lymphocytes are small and relatively round. *C*, See the sinuous granuloma along the upper portion of one of the large follicles.

(Hansmann et al, 1990). The interfollicular areas contain numerous T cells.

Genotypic Studies

Genotypic studies are generally not used for diagnostic purposes in cases of suspected PTGC because they do not reveal the presence of clonal B or T cells.

Diagnostic Criteria

In PTGC, the nodal architecture is preserved, and there are follicular hyperplasia and large follicular nodules in which the germinal center has been partially or completely replaced by benign mantle zone lymphocytes. In a minority of cases the lymph node may also exhibit HD, usually of the nodular lymphocyte-predominant type.

Differential Diagnosis

In pediatric patients the major differential diagnosis is nodular LPHD (Table 16–2). Twenty-five percent of de novo childhood cases were originally diagnosed as HD (Osborne et al, 1992), and one of five cases was originally misdiagnosed as nodular LPHD (Ferry et al, 1992). Twenty-four percent of the PTGC cases in an early series had been misdiagnosed as either HD or a follicular lymphoma (Osborne & Butler, 1984). Experienced pathologists note that "detecting a sharp border between [nodular LPHD and PTGC] can be difficult" (Hansmann et al, 1990).

Pathogenesis and Biologic Characteristics

The pathogenesis of PTGC is unknown. Most interest has been focused on the association between PTGC and HD. As noted earlier, PTGC is generally not considered a preneoplastic disorder.

INFLAMMATORY PSEUDOTUMOR

Equivalent Terms

The term *plasma cell granuloma* is also used for inflammatory pseudotumor but is not usually used for nodal inflammatory pseudotumors.

Definition

Inflammatory pseudotumor of lymph nodes is a benign proliferation of spindle and inflammatory cells generally involving the connective tissue framework of the lymph node, often with extension into the nodal parenchyma and extranodal soft tissues.

Clinical Features and Prognosis

Inflammatory pseudotumors of lymph nodes occur mostly in adults, at a median age of 33 (Davis et al, 1991; Perrone et al, 1988). Affected children are in the second decade or latter part of the first decade. The onset may be acute or insidious, with several months' of adenopathy or other symptoms.

Table 16–2
Differential Diagnosis of PTGC

Diagnosis	Comments
NLPHD	Unlike PTGC, NLPHD should show some areas of nodal architectural effacement (sometimes with compressed adjacent normal lymph node) and must have "L and H" type RS cells.
NSHD	The nodules of NSHD usually do not demonstrate germinal center remnants and contain lacunar and other variant RS cells. In addition, partial or marked architectural effacement is present owing to the consolidative effects of Hodgkin disease.
Follicular lymphoma, especially with a "floral" growth pattern (Osborne & Butler, 1987)	Since follicular lymphomas are rare in childhood, this differential diagnosis is not usually a problem in pediatric pathology. Unlike PTGC and small cleaved FCC lymphomas, there is usually architectural effacement and a lack of hyperplastic follicles. The neoplastic follicular structures are composed of small cleaved and angulated lymphocytes, not round mantle cells. The "floral" type of FCC lymphomas have relatively homogeneous large noncleaved cell–predominant follicles divided into "petals" by small mantle lymphocytes. Reactive-appearing follicles are absent. Immunophenotypic or genotypic studies in follicular lymphomas demonstrate clonal B cells.
Angiofollicular hyperplasia	Aside from large nodules of small lymphocytes, angiofollicular hyperplasia should demonstrate either regressively transformed follicles or sheets of plasma cells. There is more architectural retention with PTGC than in localized angiofollicular hyperplasia.

Abbreviations: FCC, follicular center cell; NLPHD, nodular lymphocyte-predominant Hodgkin disease; NSHD, nodular sclerosis Hodgkin disease; PTGC, progressive transformation of germinal centers; RS, Reed-Sternberg.

Patients present with adenopathy that is often localized but that may be multifocal or even generalized. The adenopathy is often peripheral (frequently axillary, cervical, or supraclavicular), but mediastinal and abdominal disease also occurs. In some patients the adenopathy is tender. Hepatosplenomegaly is rare, and extranodal involvement usually does not occur.

About two thirds of patients with inflammatory pseudotumor have fever with or without sweats or weight loss. Other symptoms may include abdominal pain and vomiting. A minority of patients are completely asymptomatic except for adenopathy. The symptomatic patients are more likely to have more extensive adenopathy. Some also have nonspecific laboratory abnormalities, such as anemia, hypergammaglobulinemia, or an elevated sedimentation rate. Eosinophilia is rarely seen.

Patients with inflammatory pseudotumor do well, although some have persistent adenopathy or one or more relapses of the disease. In some, fever resolves with no therapy (other than the original biopsy). Antibiotics are of questionable value, but some patients apparently benefit from additional treatment, usually with steroids or nonsteroidal anti-inflammatory reagents (indomethacin). Rare patients have received chemotherapy. A study of cytokines suggests that all-*trans* retinoic acid might be of benefit (Menke et al, 1996).

Histopathologic Features

Lymph nodes are usually 3 cm or larger and may be grossly adherent to each other or adjacent structures. The histologic spectrum is more diversified than appreciated in its original descriptions (Davis et al, 1991; Perrone et al, 1988; Moran et al, 1997). The most distinguishing feature of inflammatory pseudotumor is the spindle and inflammatory cell proliferation that expands the connective tissue framework of the lymph node, including the hilum, trabeculae, and capsule. This proliferation extends into the nodal parenchyma, obliterating sinuses, and often into the perinodal soft tissues (Fig. 16–4). Only one portion of a lymph node may be involved, but ultimately the entire lymph node may be replaced, with only occasional follicles remaining. There are a small number of cases with just one or more small focal spindle and inflammatory cell masses (Moran et al, 1997). Inflammatory pseudotumor has been stratified as grade I, consisting of a very focal lesion; grade II, subtotal architectural effacement by a cellular proliferation; and grade III, total architectural effacement by a very sclerotic process (Moran et al, 1997).

The proliferation may be very cellular, edematous, or fibrotic, and in some cases the spindle cell component has a pronounced storiform growth pattern. The inflammatory cells include variable numbers of small lymphocytes, plasma cells, histiocytes, neutrophils, and large transformed cells or immunoblasts. The latter are typically not prominent, and there is no atypia among either the spindle or the inflammatory cells. Occasional cases have many eosinophils. Rarely, multinucleated giant cells are present, but granulomas are rare. Other very characteristic features include a prominent vascular proliferation and an infiltrative and/or obliterative vasculitis. The vasculitic process varies from lymphocyte infiltration of the intima and endothelium to a completely destructive proliferation of spindle and inflammatory cell elements causing luminal occlusion (Fig. 16–4*B*). Some cases exhibit vascular microthrombi, but fibrinoid necrosis and adjacent necrosis are infrequent. The remaining nodal parenchyma may demonstrate a number of hyperplastic patterns, including hypervascular paracortical expansion or follicular hyperplasia, even with progressively

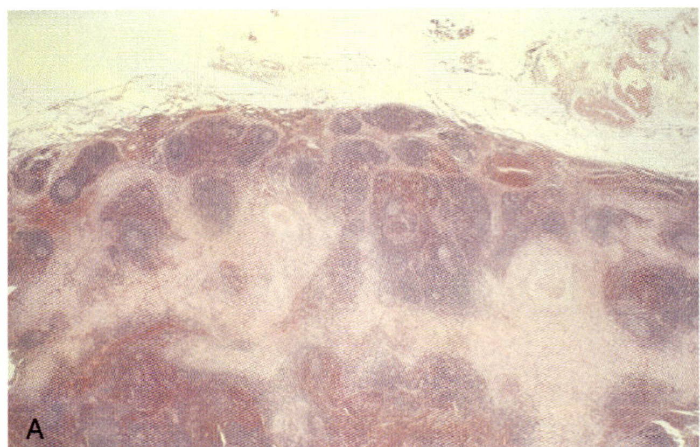

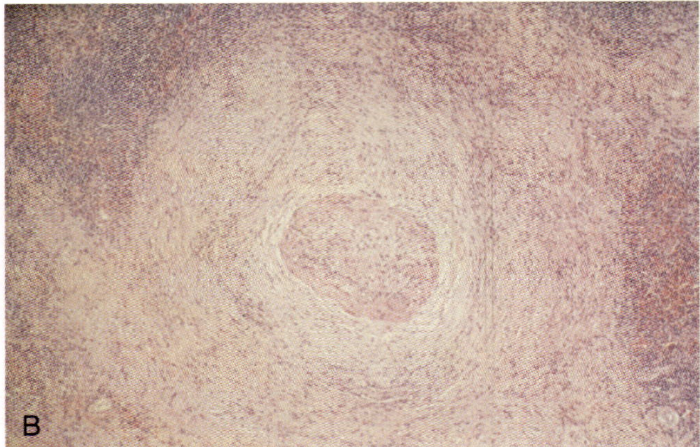

Figure 16–4

Inflammatory pseudotumor of lymph node. *A*, There is a marked fibrotic expansion of the lymph node connective tissue framework. *B*, At higher magnification the characteristic obliterative vascular lesion may be noted.

transformed germinal centers. Small amounts of hemosiderin are seen in a few cases.

Markers

The plasma cells and lymphocytes in inflammatory pseudotumor have been found to be polyclonal by immunostaining and limited genotypic studies (Facchetti et al, 1990; Menke et al, 1996; Moran et al, 1997; New et al, 1995; Perrone et al, 1988). Most of the lymphocytes are T cells. Approximately 20% of cases contain EBV-positive cells (Arber et al, 1995). CD68 (KP1) and Mac-387 highlight variable numbers of macrophages.

The spindle cells are vimentin positive, and variable proportions mark as myofibroblasts, as seen in granulation tissue (actin positive and desmin negative), and as histiocytes (actin negative, CD45+, and variable expression of macrophage-associated markers, e.g., CD68, Mac-387, and HAM-56) (Davis et al, 1991; Facchetti et al, 1990; Menke et al, 1996; Moran et al, 1997; New et al, 1995; Perrone et al, 1988). The histiocytes may also express HLA-DR. The spindle cells do not express antigens associated with either follicular dendritic or interdigitating reticulum cells (e.g., S-100). Desmin and actin stains also highlight the vasodestructive nature of inflammatory pseudotumor. CD34 highlights the vascular proliferation, but the frank spindle cell proliferation is CD34−.

Diagnostic Criteria

Inflammatory pseudotumor is diagnosed by the presence of expansion of the nodal connective tissue framework by a variably fibrotic spindle and mixed inflammatory cell proliferation that lacks atypia and that extends into both the lymph node parenchyma and the perinodal soft tissues. Hypervascularity and infiltrative and/or obliterative vasculitis are also characteristic.

Differential Diagnosis

The differential diagnosis of inflammatory pseudotumor is very lengthy, encompassing benign and malignant disorders in which a mixed inflammatory cell population, vascular proliferation, vasculitis, and/or fibrosis is prominent (Table 16–3) (Davis et al, 1991; Moran et al, 1997; New et al, 1995; Perrone et al, 1988). Almost one third of cases were originally diagnosed as or suspected to be HD or B and T cell lymphomas (New et al, 1995). Conversely, a case of nodular sclerosis HD, substantiated by a subsequent biopsy, was found among cases coded as inflammatory pseudotumor (Menke et al, 1996). Occasional cases have been diagnosed as other specific reactive disorders, including Kimura disease, with numerous eosinophils; possible angiofollicular lymph node hyperplasia, with vascular proliferation and sometimes numerous plasma cells; and Kikuchi lymphadenitis. Many other reactive adenopathies have also been included in the differential diagnosis, including viral infections, Kawasaki disease, autoimmune disorders, other vasculitides and panniculitides, sinus histiocytosis, SHML, and dermatopathic lymphadenopathy. Mycobacterial spindle cell pseudotumors should also be considered in the differential diagnosis. Neoplasms that should be considered in the differential diagnosis include mast cell disease, which can be associated with eosinophils and fibrosis, and other spindle cell proliferations (see Table 16–3).

The histologic features most useful in ruling out many of these disorders include the following:

- ☐ presence of the characteristic spindle and mixed inflammatory cell proliferation that extends from the connective tissue framework of the lymph node
- ☐ lack of atypia in the lymphocytes (unlike most B and T lymphomas) and in the spindle cells (unlike many spindle cell neoplasms)
- ☐ absence of Reed-Sternberg cells

Rarely, special stains or immunostains may be helpful in determining the nature of the spindle or other cells present.

Pathogenesis and Biologic Characteristics

The pathogenesis of inflammatory pseudotumor is unknown, but it is generally considered an abnormal inflammatory response to a number of various insults, with "mediators of inflammation" accounting for the pathologic changes and symptoms. Based on a study of procollagen-α_1 mRNA and IL-1β and IL-6, the spindle cells responsible for the fibrosis were thought to be consistent with monocyte-derived "neofibro-

Table 16–3
Differential Diagnosis of Inflammatory Pseudotumor of Lymph Node

Diagnosis	Comments
Hodgkin disease, especially nodular sclerosis	Architecture may be partially obliterated in inflammatory pseudotumor, but RS and lacunar variants are not detected by morphologic or immunophenotypic studies.
B and T cell lymphomas	The lymphocytes in inflammatory pseudotumor are not "atypical" and do not resemble any of the common pediatric lymphomas. Immunophenotypic studies may be helpful in problematic cases.
Other reactive disorders, including vasculidites	The characteristic inflammatory and spindle cell proliferation that extends from the nodal connective tissue framework is generally absent from other reactive disorders, even if they have fibrotic capsules and vasculitic features. Clinical features may have to be relied on in some cases of Kawasaki disease. Syphilitic nodes usually have more follicular hyperplasia. SHML may also have capsular fibrosis but has intrasinusal S-100+ histiocytes with lymphophagocytosis.
Spindle cell neoplasms, including dendritic (follicular and interdigitating) cell and fibrohistiocytic tumors, palisaded myofibroblastoma and Kaposi sarcoma	Inflammatory pseudotumors are expansions of the nodal connective tissue framework and lack the atypia seen in many spindle cell neoplasms.
Mastocytosis	A dense mast cell population is present in mastocytosis, although it is sometimes difficult to recognize because cells may be spindly and distorted by fibrosis. Toluidine blue and tryptase stains are helpful. Eosinophils are generally abundant in mastocytosis.
Mycobacterial pseudotumor	Usually not confused; results of AFB staining are negative in inflammatory pseudotumor.
Amyloid	The dense fibrosis in inflammatory pseudotumor is congo red negative.

Abbreviations: AFB, acid-fast bacillus; RS, Reed-Sternberg; SHML, sinus histiocytosis with massive lymphadenopathy.

blasts." Inflammatory pseudotumor may represent a sclerosing immune reaction, with IL-1β and IL-6 production by T lymphocytes possibly accounting for symptoms and the histopathologic features (Menke et al, 1996). Inflammatory pseudotumors involving nodes are distinct from pseudotumors in other locations and have a distinct pathogenesis (Arber et al, 1995; Davis et al, 1991).

ANGIOFOLLICULAR HYPERPLASIA

Equivalent Terms

Angiofollicular hyperplasia is also known as Castleman disease, angiofollicular lymph node hyperplasia, and giant lymph node hyperplasia.

Definition

Angiofollicular hyperplasia is an idiopathic nonneoplastic disorder with three variants. In the hyaline vascular type, regressively transformed follicles are surrounded by an interfollicular expansion with vascular proliferation and predominantly small lymphocytes. In the less common plasma cell type, hyperplastic follicles are surrounded, at least in part, by sheets of plasma cells, and the diagnosis is made after exclusion of other causes of follicular hyperplasia and plasmacytosis. In the multicentric or systemic type, patients have multicentric lymphadenopathy, and the lymph nodes demonstrate sinus retention and dilatation. Individual nodes are usually rich in plasma cells.

Clinical Features and Prognosis

Localized angiofollicular hyperplasia occurs in children and adults, with a median age of occurrence in the third or fourth decade and without a sex predilection (Frizzera, 1988), although a female predominance has been noted in the hyaline vascular form (Danon et al, 1993). Only 15 cases in children 13 years old or younger had been reported as of 1994 (Kinney et al, 1994). Occurrence in infants is very rare (Hunt & Anderson, 1989). Most patients present with large mediastinal nodal masses, and the abdomen is the second commonest site (Frizzera, 1988; Keller et al, 1972). Others describe cervical nodes as most commonly involved in the hyaline vascular form (Danon et al, 1993). Extranodal cases are uncommon.

Approximately 80–90% of cases are hyaline vascular type. Patients present with large (5–25 cm) solitary masses that are detected incidentally or because of compressive symptoms. Patients are usually otherwise asymptomatic, although rare cases have been associated with a variety of disorders, including growth retardation (Sethi & Kepes, 1971). Surgical excision is curative, and recurrences are rare.

Patients with plasma cell type usually have aggregates of enlarged lymph nodes measuring 3–15 cm in greatest dimension in the abdomen, particularly in the small bowel mesentery (Frizzera, 1988). Patients may present with constitutional symptoms, such as fever. Fifty to 90% have hematologic abnormalities, with anemia (mildly hypochromic and microcytic) and leukocytosis. Other laboratory abnormalities include an elevated sedimentation rate, hypergammaglobulinemia, and hypoalbuminemia. Many other disorders have been associated with plasma cell type angiofollicular hyperplasia, including growth retardation in pediatric cases (Buchanan et al, 1981; Frizzera, 1988; McCarty et al, 1995; Shahidi et al, 1995; Winter et al, 1996). Excisional surgery is curative and leads to normalization of laboratory parameters. Some patients have received steroid therapy.

An 8-year-old girl with localized hyaline vascular type in association with a vascular neoplasm has been described (Gerald et al, 1990). Follicular dendritic cell tumors may also rarely occur in adults (Chan et al, 1997).

The more recently described multicentric angiofollicular hyperplasia has a male predominance, is typically a disease of adults (median age in the sixth decade), and is associated with a much worse prognosis than the localized variants (Frizzera, 1988; Shahidi et al, 1995). Patients have constitutional symptoms and laboratory abnormalities similar to those seen with the plasma cell type. Hepatosplenomegaly is common. Kaposi sarcoma is reported in elderly patients (Chen, 1984). Multicentric angiofollicular hyperplasia in adults is also associated with HIV infection and disorders such as the POEMS (polyneuropathy, organomegaly, endocrinopathy, M protein, and skin changes) syndrome, a syndrome that perhaps is a separate entity (McCarty et al, 1995). Some HIV-negative patients may exhibit evidence of immunodeficiency (Ishiyama et al, 1994). Lymphomas develop in a significant minority of cases. The uncommon pediatric cases are like the adult cases except that most patients have done well following therapy, which usually included steroids (Smir et al, 1996). They have not demonstrated a male predominance. Some children have persistent or recurrent disease that may require further therapy, such as radiation or chemotherapy.

Histopathologic Features

Lymph nodes in localized angiofollicular hyperplasia exhibit architectural effacement, although in a few cases sinuses at the periphery of the lesions are retained. In the hyaline vascular form, mantle zones of differing thickness surround regressively transformed follicles (Fig. 16–5*A*) that are typically small, lymphocyte depleted, and penetrated by hyalinized vessels. These abnormal follicles may resemble Hassall corpuscles or a "lollipop" when the penetrating vessel is particularly prominent. The cells in the follicles are endothelial cells and follicular dendritic cells. Polypoid and dysplastic follicular dendritic cells may be seen in follicular centers or in the mantle zones in pediatric cases (Ruco et al, 1991) (Fig. 16–5*B*). The most characteristic mantle zones are widened and have onion skin–like concentric rings of small lymphocytes (Fig. 16–6). Sometimes large nodules of small lymphocytes include several of the regressively transformed follicles. Others are without any follicular center. The follicular structures make up half or more of the nodal area in pediatric cases. In some adult cases the interfollicular areas predominate (Danon et al, 1993). The interfollicular areas demonstrate a prominent capillary proliferation, with variable amounts of perivascular hyaline sclerosis (see Figs. 16–6 and 16–7). In two thirds of cases, numerous small lymphocytes are admixed with plasma cells and eosinophils. Plasma cells may be numerous but do not form sheets. Transformed lymphocytes and Reed-Sternberg–like cells may be present. The hyaline vascular form is one of the circumstances in which clusters of plasmacytoid monocytes (formerly plasmacytoid T cells) have been identified (Danon et al, 1993; Hsu et al, 1993; Menke et al, 1996) (Fig. 16–7). A small number of cases may have "nodular growths [that vary] from spindle cell foci to angio-histiocytic-[reticulum cell] proliferations" (Danon et al, 1993) and resemble follicular dendritic cell tumors. Bands of fibrosis may be present, and large areas of the lymph node may become sclerotic and even calcify. Adjacent lymph nodes may have similar changes or demonstrate partial involvement.

In the plasma cell type, the follicles are typically hyperplastic, and sheets of plasma cells are seen in some areas (Fig. 16–8). Regressively transformed follicles may also be present. Some classify occasional cases as "mixed" angiofollicular hyperplasia (hyaline vascular and plasma cell). Because of the nonspecific histopathologic appearance of these cases, it is important to rule out other autoimmune disorders or infections that can be associated with follicular hyperplasia and plasmacytosis.

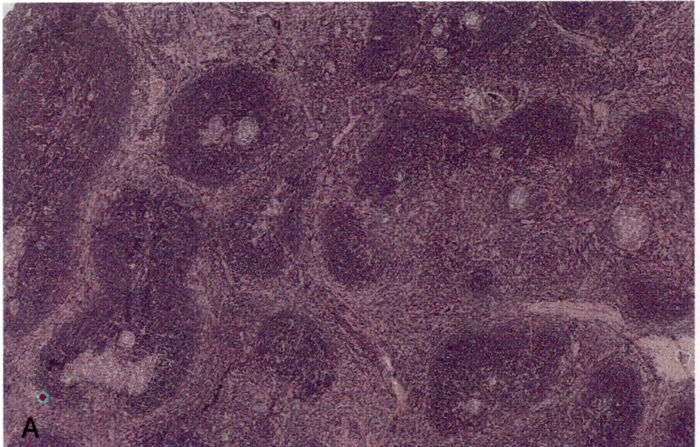

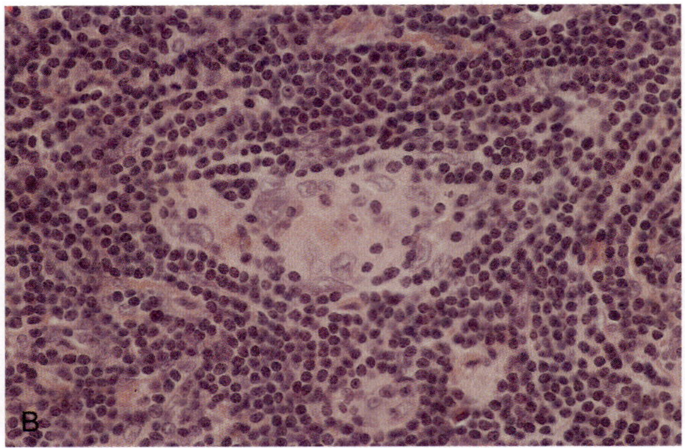

Figure 16–5

Angiofollicular hyperplasia, hyaline vascular type, lymph node. *A*, Note the large, primary-type follicles with scattered small, regressively transformed germinal centers. The interfollicular region demonstrates marked vascular proliferation. *B*, This unusual regressively transformed follicle contains abnormal-appearing follicular dendritic cells.

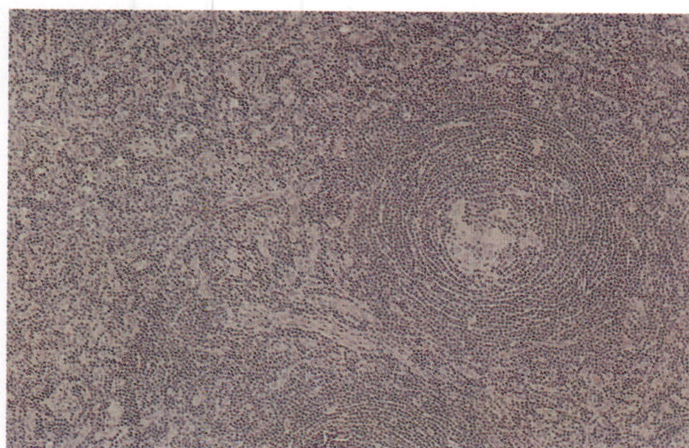

Figure 16–6

Angiofollicular hyperplasia, hyaline vascular type, lymph node. Note the striking onion skin–like mantle around a hyalinized remnant of a regressively transformed germinal center. There is also a marked interfollicular vascular proliferation.

In multicentric forms, lymph nodes resemble those described earlier, particularly in the plasma cell type, except that there is sinus retention and dilatation. In one series, three of eight of the pediatric cases were classified as hyaline vascular type (Smir et al, 1996). Other causes of follicular hyperplasia and plasmacytosis, such as HIV infection and autoimmune disorders, must be ruled out.

Markers

In the hyaline vascular form, the B lymphocytes surrounding the lymphocyte-depleted follicles are polyclonal. CD57+ cells are absent or present in small numbers, unlike the situation in normal follicles (Danon et al, 1993; Martin et al, 1985). The follicles contain cells that express endothelial cell antigens (e.g., factor VIII–related antigen) or follicular dendritic cell antigens (e.g., CD21). Atypical follicular dendritic cells in angiofollicular hyperplasia are also reported to be CD21+. Reed-Sternberg–like follicular dendritic cells as well as dendritic networks are reportedly CD15+ positive (Delsol et al, 1993). Mantle cells in angiofollicular hyperplasia are Ki-B3−, although normal mantle cells are Ki-B3+ (Menke et al, 1996). The interfollicular areas in hyaline vascular type contain many T cells and CD68+ plasmacytoid monocytes (Danon et al, 1993). The numerous plasma cells in most cases of the plasma cell type are polyclonal, but cases with monoclonal plasma cells are well described (Frizzera, 1988; Menke et al, 1996; York et al, 1981). Lambda monoclonal plasma cells have been noted in 7 of 21 cases of plasma cell type (all adults) (Radaszkiewicz et al, 1989), but a smaller proportion of monoclonal cases has also been reported (Menke et al, 1996). The monoclonal cases do not appear to be clinically distinct from the polyclonal cases. Clonal λ+ plasma cells are associated with POEMS-related multicentric angiofollicular hyperplasia. Genotypic studies in angiofollicular hyperplasia show clonal B cells in a minority of cases, in which the extent of the adenopathy was not specified (Menke et al, 1996). Pediatric multicentric cases have been shown to be polyclonal by immunohistologic staining.

EBV is identified in up to half of angiofollicular hyperplasia cases, including two of six pediatric cases. The pathogenetic significance of EBV is uncertain, however, owing to the small number of EBV-positive cells found in these studies (Luppi et al, 1996; Smir et al, 1996). Herpesvirus 8 has been found with multicentric angiofollicular hyperplasia, particularly in HIV-associated cases, but has not been found in pediatric cases (Luppi et al, 1996; Soulier et al, 1995a). Herpesvirus 8 has specifically been associated with a plasmablastic variant of angiofollicular hyperplasia and lymphoma in adults (Dupin et al, 2000).

Genotypic Studies

Localized angiofollicular hyperplasia lacks immunoglobulin or T cell receptor gene rearrangements, but the multicentric form may demonstrate immunoglobulin with or without associated T cell receptor gene rearrangements (Hanson et al, 1994; Soulier

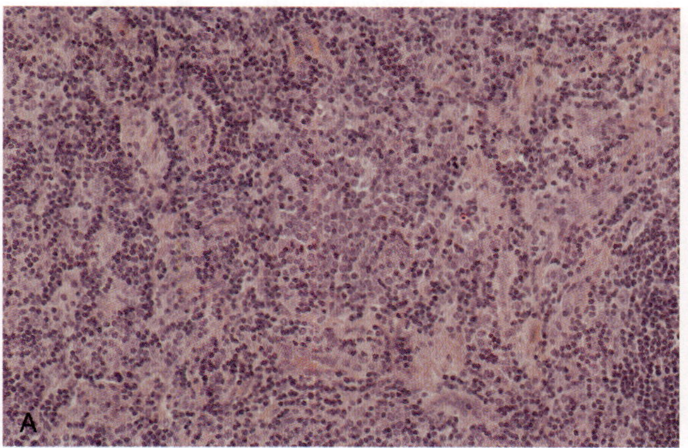

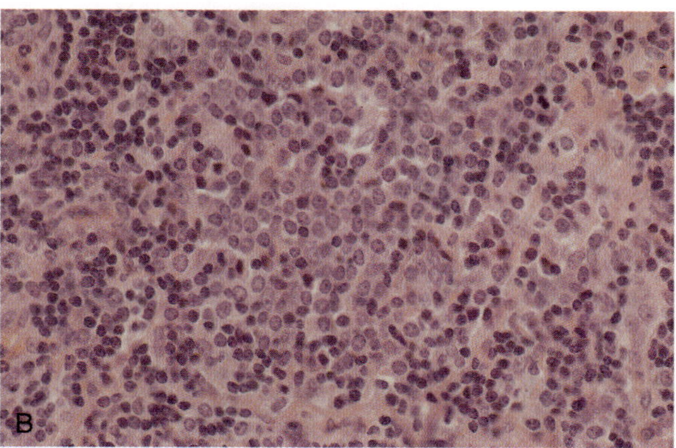

Figure 16–7

Angiofollicular hyperplasia, hyaline vascular type, lymph node. *A*, The interfollicular region demonstrates predominantly small lymphocytes. In the center is an ill-defined pale aggregate of plasmacytoid monocytes. *B*, The plasmacytoid monocytes have relatively dispersed chromatin and somewhat eccentric cytoplasm. They are associated with scattered pyknotic nuclei.

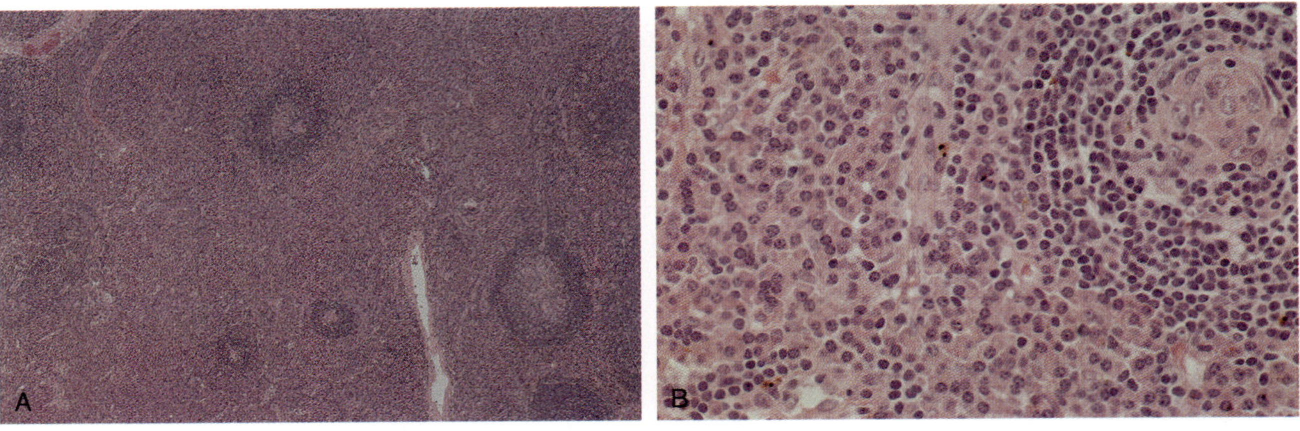

Figure 16–8

Angiofollicular hyperplasia, plasma cell type, mediastinal node. *A*, Scattered hyperplastic and regressively transformed follicles are surrounded by a sheet of plasma cells. *B*, At higher magnification numerous plasma cells surrounding the regressively transformed follicle are easily appreciated.

et al, 1995b). Presumably, those cases with monoclonal plasma cells would show immunoglobulin gene rearrangements. One of five pediatric multicentric cases with mild but persistent disease has been found to be clonal by polymerase chain reaction analysis (Smir et al, 1996).

Diagnostic Criteria

Localized angiofollicular hyperplasia demonstrates significant nodal architectural effacement with two major variants. In the hyaline vascular form, regressively transformed follicles are surrounded by wide mantle zones. There is interfollicular vascular proliferation, and small lymphocytes predominate. The plasma cell form exhibits hyperplastic follicles with aggregates or focal sheets of plasma cells. This diagnosis is made after excluding all other causes of follicular hyperplasia with plasmacytosis. Multicentric angiofollicular hyperplasia resembles the plasma cell form but usually demonstrates greater architectural preservation. This diagnosis is made only after excluding other possible causes of follicular hyperplasia and plasmacytosis.

Table 16–4

Differential Diagnosis of Angiofollicular Lymph Node Hyperplasia

Diagnosis	Comments
Nonspecific follicular hyperplasia with plasmacytosis, including infectious (e.g., HIV) and autoimmune disorders	Clinical data are required to diagnose the plasma cell variant of localized angiofollicular hyperplasia. The sheets of plasma cells and characteristic vascular proliferation are very helpful in recognizing angiofollicular hyperplasia, in which there is lessarchitectural preservation than in most reactive hyperplasias. Lymph nodes in patients with rheumatoid arthritis contain prominent reactive follicles and striking interfollicular plasmacytosis.
HD	HD with areas resembling angiofollicular hyperplasia has been reported. Interfollicular HD might resemble the plasma cell variant except that sheets of plasma cells are not present in the former. Regressively transformed follicles and marked vascular proliferation with hyalinization are not typical of HD. HD requires the presence of RS cells (not to be confused with dysplastic follicular dendritic cells).
Thymoma	Regressively transformed follicles must be distinguished from Hassall corpuscles. The other features characteristic of angiofollicular hyperplasia, e.g., vascular proliferation, are absent. Immunostains are useful in doubtful cases.

Abbreviations: HD, Hodgkin disease; RS, Reed-Sternberg.

Differential Diagnosis

The differential diagnosis of angiofollicular hyperplasia is summarized in Table 16–4. In general, the plasma cell and multicentric types are considered only after excluding the lengthy list of benign and neoplastic disorders associated with follicular hyperplasia and plasmacytosis, with or without clonal plasma cells. The classic regressively transformed follicles seen in the hyaline vascular type are nonspecific and may be seen in a variety of benign and neoplastic conditions. The most problematic cases with sinus preservation and clonal plasma cells are usually seen in adults.

Pathogenesis and Biologic Characteristics

Angiofollicular hyperplasia is a reactive, inflammatory, or dysregulated immunologic process that may be associated with some autoimmune phenomena. Its pathogenesis is uncertain, as are the relationships among the various types. Furthermore, explanations for the most characteristic feature—regressively transformed follicles—and abnormal follicular dendritic cells are not available. In the hyaline vascular form, antigenic stimuli may lead to a progressive accumulation of mantle zone–type lymphocytes (Danon et al, 1993) followed in some way by vascular and stromal proliferation. There are suggestions that the hyaline vascular form may be distinct from other types (Frizzera, 1988; Hsu et al, 1993).

Increased synthesis of interleukin-6 (IL-6) by lymph nodes may be important in causing angiofollicular hyperplasia of plasma cell or multicentric types, since IL-6 is a B cell stimulatory factor important in the differentiation of B cells into plasma cells (Kinney et al, 1994; Kishimoto, 1989; Shahidi et al, 1995; Yabuhara et al, 1989; Yoshizaki et al, 1989). Increased serum IL-6 levels have been detected in several patients following surgery for angiofollicular hyperplasia (Burger et al, 1994). Adult patients with plasma cell type or multicentric angiofollicular hyperplasia have responded to an anti-IL-6 antibody (Nishimoto et al, 2000; Beck et al, 1994).

Abnormal IL-6 production has been seen in follicular center B cells or dendritic cells (Hsu et al, 1993; Leger-Ravet et al, 1991; Yoshizaki et al, 1989), extrafollicular immunoblastic B cells (Hsu et al, 1993), marginal zone and other interfollicular cells (Kinney et al, 1994), and heterogeneous intersinusal cell types (Leger-Ravet et al, 1991). Interfollicular IL-6–positive cells in control lymph nodes were reportedly within sinuses. Dysregulated IL-6 production also causes a multicentric angiofollicular-like lesion in mice (Brandt et al, 1990), and increased expression of IL-6 receptor was documented in two of three patients with multicentric disease (Ishiyama et al, 1996).

IL-6 induces acute-phase proteins in hepatocytes and is capable of producing many of the systemic symptoms and laboratory abnormalities in the plasma cell and multicentric types, in addition to its effect on B cell development (Hsu et al, 1993; Yoshizaki et al, 1989). Furthermore, IL-6 may play a role in the vascular proliferation in some cases (Motro et al, 1990).

Other cytokines, including macrophage colony-stimulating factor, tumor necrosis factor α (TNFα), and IL-1, may also be important in multicentric angiofollicular hyperplasia (Lee et al, 1997; Leger-Ravet et al, 1991). Macrophage colony-stimulating factor has many activities, including increasing IL-6 and TNFα in monocytes in vitro (summarized in Lee et al, 1997). Activation of monocytes or macrophages may theoretically be an important factor in multicentric angiofollicular hyperplasia. Elevated levels of TNFβ and γ-interferon mRNA have also been reported in a pediatric case of the "mixed" angiofollicular hyperplasia type (Winter et al, 1996). Since multicentric angiofollicular hyperplasia has been associated with HIV infection, immunodeficiency may contribute to its development. The multicentric type (especially cases with HIV infection) is associated in some cases with EBV or human herpesvirus 8 (Kaposi sarcoma herpesvirus). Herpesvirus 8 encodes a homologue of IL-6, perhaps explaining its role in the pathogenesis of the multicentric type (Neipel et al, 1997; Nicholas et al, 1997).

SUGGESTED READINGS

Sinus Histiocytosis with Massive Lymphadenopathy

Foucar E, Rosai J, Dorfman R: Sinus histiocytosis with massive lymphadenopathy (Rosai-Dorfman disease): review of the entity. Semin Diagn Pathol 7:19, 1990. A review based on a registry established by Dr. Rosai, with an extensive description of extranodal disease.

Rosai J, Dorfman RF: Sinus histiocytosis with massive lymphadenopathy. Arch Pathol 87:63, 1969. The publication responsible for the eponym.

Rosai J, Dorfman RF: Sinus histiocytosis with massive lymphadenopathy: a pseudolymphomatous benign disorder, analysis of 34 cases. Cancer 30:1174, 1972. The original large series of cases.

Progressive Transformation of Germinal Centers

Hansmann M-L, Fellbaum C, Hui PK, et al: Progressive transformation of germinal centers with and without association to Hodgkin's disease. Am J Clin Pathol 93:219, 1990. A large clinicopathologic study with immunophenotypic data.

Osborne BM, Butler JJ, Gresik MV: Progressive transformation of germinal centers: comparison of 23 pediatric patients to the adult population. Mod Pathol 5:135, 1992. A pediatric study that includes an update on the extensive M.D. Anderson experience with progressive transformation of germinal centers.

Inflammatory Pseudotumor

Davis RE, Warnke RA, Dorfman RF: Inflammatory pseudotumor of lymph nodes: additional observations and evidence for an inflammatory etiology. Am J Surg Pathol 15:744, 1991. A large series with an expanded histologic description and immunophenotypic characterization.

Moran CA, Suster S, Abbondanzo SL: Inflammatory pseudotumor of lymph nodes: a study of 25 cases with emphasis on morphological heterogeneity. Hum Pathol 28:332, 1997. A large series and a histologic grading scheme.

Perrone T, de Wolf-Peeters C, Frizzera G: Inflammatory pseudotumor of lymph nodes: a distinctive pattern of nodal reaction. Am J Surg Pathol 12:351, 1988. The original series of cases of inflammatory pseudotumor of lymph nodes.

Angiofollicular Hyperplasia

Castleman B, Iverson L, Menendez VP: Localized mediastinal lymph-node hyperplasia resembling thymoma. Cancer 9:822, 1956. The explanation for the eponym.

Keller AR, Hochholzer L, Castleman B: Hyaline-vascular and plasma-cell types of giant lymph node hyperplasia of the mediastinum and other locations. Cancer 29:670, 1972. A large classic series with description of the plasma cell variant.

Frizzera G: Castleman's disease and related disorders. Semin Diagn Pathol 5:346, 1988. An important review.

Shahidi H, Myers JL, Kvale PA: Castleman's disease. Mayo Clin Proc 70:969, 1995. A review with a pictorial schema of the pathogenesis of angiofollicular hyperplasia.

Smir BN, Greiner TC, Weisenburger DD: Multicentric angiofollicular lymph node hyperplasia in children: a clinicopathologic study of eight patients. Mod Pathol 9:1135, 1996. A series dealing with pediatric cases of multicentric angiofollicular hyperplasia.

REFERENCES

Arber DA, Kamel OW, Van De Rijn M, et al: Frequent presence of the Epstein-Barr virus in inflammatory pseudotumor. Hum Pathol 26:1093, 1995.

Beck JT, Hsu S-M, Wijdenes J, et al: Brief report: alleviation of systemic manifestations of Castleman's disease by monoclonal anti-interleukin-6 antibody. N Engl J Med 330:602, 1994.

Brandt SJ, Bodine DM, Dunbar CE, et al: Dysregulated interleukin 6 expression produces a syndrome resembling Castleman's disease in mice. J Clin Invest 86:592, 1990.

Buchanan GR, Chipman JJ, Hamilton BL, et al: Angiomatous lymphoid hamartoma: inhibitory effects on erythropoiesis, growth, and primary hemostasis. J Pediatr 99:382, 1981.

Burger R, Wendler J, Antoni K, et al: Interleukin-6 production in B-cell neoplasias and Castleman's disease: evidence for an additional paracrine loop. Ann Hematol 69:25, 1994.

Burns BF, Colby TV, Dorfman RF: Differential diagnostic features of nodular L and H Hodgkin's disease, including progressive transformation of germinal centers. Am J Surg Pathol 8:253, 1984.

Chan JKC, Fletcher CDM, Nayler SJ, et al: Follicular dentritic cell sarcoma: clinicopathologic analysis of 17 cases suggesting a malignant potential higher than currently recognized. Cancer 79:294, 1997.

Chen KTK: Multicentric Castleman's disease and Kaposi's sarcoma. Am J Surg Pathol 8:287, 1984.

Danon AD, Kirshnan J, Frizzera G: Morpho-immunophenotypic diversity of Castleman's disease, hyaline-vascular type: with emphasis on a stroma-rich variant and a new pathogenetic hypothesis. Virchows Arch A Pathol Anat Histopathol 423:369, 1993.

Davis RE, Warnke RA, Dorfman RF: Inflammatory pseudotumor of lymph nodes: additional observations and evidence for an inflammatory etiology. Am J Surg Pathol 15:744, 1991.

Delsol G, Meggetto F, Brousset P, et al: Relation of follicular dendritic reticulum cells to Reed-Sternberg cells of Hodgkin's disease with emphasis on the expression of CD21 antigen. Am J Pathol 142:1729, 1993.

Dupin N, Diss TL, Kellam P, et al: HHV-8 is associated with a plasmablastic variant of Castleman disease that is linked to HHV-8-positive plasmablastic lymphoma. Blood 95:1406–1412, 2000.

Eisen RN, Buckley PJ, Rosai J: Immunophenotypic characterization of sinus histiocytosis with massive lymphadenopathy (Rosai-Dorfman disease). Semin Diagn Pathol 7:74, 1990.

Facchetti F, De Wolf Peeters C, De Wever I, et al: Inflammatory pseudotumor of lymph nodes: immunohistochemical evidence for its fibrohistiocytic nature. Am J Pathol 137:281, 1990.

Ferry JA, Zukerberg LR, Harris NL: Florid progressive transformation of germinal centers: a syndrome affecting young men, without early progression to nodular lymphocyte predominance Hodgkin's disease. Am J Surg Pathol 16:252, 1992.

Foucar E, Rosai J, Dorfman R: Sinus histiocytosis with massive lymphadenopathy (Rosai-Dorfman disease): review of the entity. Semin Diagn Pathol 7:19, 1990.

Frizzera G: Castleman's disease and related disorders. Semin Diagn Pathol 5:346, 1988.

Gerald W, Kostianovsky M, Rosai J: Development of vascular neoplasia in Castleman's disease: report of seven cases. Am J Surg Pathol 14:603, 1990.

Hansmann M-L, Fellbaum C, Hui PK, et al: Progressive transformation of germinal centers with and without association to Hodgkin's disease. Am J Clin Pathol 93:219, 1990.

Hsu S-M, Waldron JA, Xie S-S, et al: Expression of interleukin-6 in Castleman's disease. Hum Pathol 24:833, 1993.

Hunt SJ, Anderson WD: Giant lymph node hyperplasia of the hyaline vascular type with plasmacytoid T-cells and presentation in infancy. Am J Clin Pathol 91:344, 1989.

Ishiyama T, Koike M, Nakamura S, et al: Interleukin-6 receptor expression in the peripheral B cells of patients with multicentric Castleman's disease. Ann Hematol 73:179, 1996.

Ishiyama T, Nakamura S, Akimoto Y, et al: Immunodeficiency and IL-6 production by peripheral blood monocytes in multicentric Castleman's disease. Br J Haematol 86:483, 1994.

Keller AR, Hochholzer L, Castleman B: Hyaline-vascular and plasma-cell types of giant lymph node hyperplasia of the mediastinum and other locations. Cancer 29:670, 1972.

Kinney MC, Hummell DS, Villiger PM, et al: Increased interleukin-6 (IL-6) production in a young child with clinical and pathologic features of multicentric Castleman's disease. J Clin Immunol 14:382, 1994.

Kishimoto T: The biology of interleukin-6. Blood 74:1, 1989.

Komp DM: The treatment of sinus histiocytosis with massive lymphadenopathy (Rosai-Dorfman disease). Semin Diagn Pathol 7:83, 1990.

Lee M, Hirokawa M, Matuoka S, et al: Multicentric Castleman's disease with an increased serum level of macrophage colony-stimulating factor. Am J Hematol 54:321, 1997.

Leger-Ravet MB, Peuchmaur M, Devergne O, et al: Interleukin-6 gene expression in Castleman's disease. Blood 78:2923, 1991.

Levine PH, Jahan N, Murari P, et al: Detection of human herpesvirus 6 in tissues involved by sinus histiocytosis with massive lymphadenopathy (Rosai-Dorfman disease). J Infect Dis 166:291, 1992.

Luppi M, Barozzi P, Maiorana A, et al: Human herpesvirus-8 DNA sequences in human immunodeficiency virus-negative angioimmunoblastic lymphadenopathy and benign lymphadenopathy with giant germinal center hyperplasia and increased vascularity. Blood 87;3903-3909, 1996.

Maia DM, Dorfman RF: Focal changes of sinus histiocytosis with massive lymphadenopathy (Rosai-Dorfman disease) associated with nodular lymphocyte predominant Hodgkin's disease. Hum Pathol 26:1378, 1995.

Martin JME, Bell B, Ruether BA: Giant lymph node hyperplasia (Castleman's disease) of hyaline vascular type: clinical heterogeneity with immunohistologic uniformity. Am J Clin Pathol 84:439, 1985.

McCarty MJ, Vukelja SJ, Banks PM, et al: Angiofollicular lymph node hyperplasia (Castleman's disease). Cancer Treat Rev 21:291, 1995.

Menke DM, Tiemann M, Camoriano JK, et al: Diagnosis of Castleman's disease by identification of an immunophenotypically aberrant population of mantle zone B lymphocytes in paraffin-embedded lymph node biopsies. Am J Clin Pathol 105:268, 1996.

Moran CA, Suster S, Abbondanzo SL: Inflammatory pseudotumor of lymph nodes: a study of 25 cases with emphasis on morphological heterogeneity. Hum Pathol 28:332, 1997.

Motro B, Itin A, Sachs L, et al: Pattern of interleukin 6 gene expression in vivo suggests a role for this cytokine in angiogenesis. Proc Natl Acad Sci USA 87:3092, 1990.

Neipel F, Albrecht J-C, Ensser A, et al: Human herpesvirus 8 encodes a homolog of interleukin-6. J Virol 71:839, 1997.

New NE, Bishop PW, Stewart M, et al: Inflammatory pseudotumour of lymph nodes. J Clin Pathol 48:37, 1995.

Nicholas J, Ruvolo VR, Burns WH, et al: Kaposi's sarcoma-associated human herpesvirus-8 encodes homologues of macrophage inflammatory protein-1 and interleukin-6. Nature Med 3:287, 1997.

Nishimoto N, Sasai M, Shima Y, et al: Improvement in Castleman's disease by humanized anti-interleukin-6 receptor antibody therapy. Blood 95:56–61, 2000.

Osborne BM, Butler JJ: Clinical implications of progressive transformation of germinal centers. Am J Surg Pathol 8:725, 1984.

Osborne BM, Butler JJ, Gresik MV: Progressive transformation of germinal centers: comparison of 23 pediatric patients to the adult population. Mod Pathol 5:135, 1992.

Paulli M, Bergamaschi G, Tonon L, et al: Evidence for a polyclonal nature of the cell infiltrate in sinus histiocytosis with massive lymphadenopathy (Rosai-Dorfman disease). Br J Haematol 91:415, 1995.

Paulli M, Feller AC, Boveri E, et al: Cathepsin D and E co-expression in sinus histiocytosis with massive lymphadenopathy (Rosai-Dorfman disease) and Langerhans' cell histocytosis: further evidences of a phenotypic overlap between these histiocytic disorders. Virchows Arch A Pathol Anat Histopathol 424:601, 1994.

Paulli M, Rosso R, Kindl S, et al: Immunophenotypic characterization of the cell infiltrate in five cases of sinus histiocytosis with massive lymphadenopathy (Rosai-Dorfman Disease). Hum Pathol 23:647, 1992.

Perrone T, deWolf-Peeters C, Frizzera G: Inflammatory pseudotumor of lymph nodes: a distinctive pattern of nodal reaction. Am J Surg Pathol 12:351, 1988.

Radaszkiewicz T, Hansmann M-L, Lennert K: Monoclonality and polyclonality of plasma cells in Castleman's disease of the plasma cell variant. Histopathology 14:11, 1989.

Rosai J, Dorfman RF: Sinus histiocytosis with massive lymphadenopathy: a pseudolymphomatous benign disorder: analysis of 34 cases. Cancer 30:1174, 1972.

Ruco LP, Gearing AJH, Pigott R, et al: Expression of ICAM-1, VCAM-1 and ELAM-1 in angiofollicular lymph node hyperplasia

(Castleman's disease): evidence for dysplasia of follicular dendritic reticulum cells. Histopathology 19:523, 1991.

Sethi G, Kepes JJ: Intrathoracic angiomatous lymphoid hamartomas: a report of three cases, one of iron refractory anemia and retarded growth. J Thorac Cardiovasc Surg 61:657, 1971.

Shahidi H, Myers JL, Kvale PA: Castleman's disease. Mayo Clin Proc 70:969, 1995.

Smir BN, Greiner TC, Weisenburger DD: Multicentric angiofollicular lymph node hyperplasia in children: a clinicopathologic study of eight patients. Mod Pathol 9:1135, 1996.

Soulier J, Grollet L, Oksenhendler E, et al: Kaposi's sarcoma-associated herpesvirus-like DNA sequences in multicentric Castleman's disease. Blood 86:1276, 1995a.

Soulier J, Grollet L, Oksenhendler E, et al: Molecular analysis of clonality in Castleman's disease. Blood 86:1131, 1995b.

Tsang WYW, Yip TTC, Chan JKC: The Rosai-Dorfman disease histiocytes are not infected by Epstein-Barr virus. Histopathology 25:88, 1994.

Winter SS, Howard TA, Ritchey AK, et al: Elevated levels of tumor necrosis factor-beta, gamma-interferon, and IL-6 mRNA in Castleman's disease. Med Pediatr Oncol 26:48, 1996.

Yabuhara A, Yanagisawa M, Murata T, et al: Giant lymph node hyperplasia (Castleman's disease) with spontaneous production of high levels of B-cell differentiation factor activity. Cancer 63:260, 1989.

York JC, Taylor CR, Lukes RJ: Monoclonality in giant lymph node hyperplasia (abstract). Lab Invest 44:77A, 1981.

Yoshizaki K, Matsuda T, Nishimoto N, et al: Pathogenic significance of interleukin-6 (IL-6/BSF-2) in Castleman's disease. Blood 74:1360, 1989.

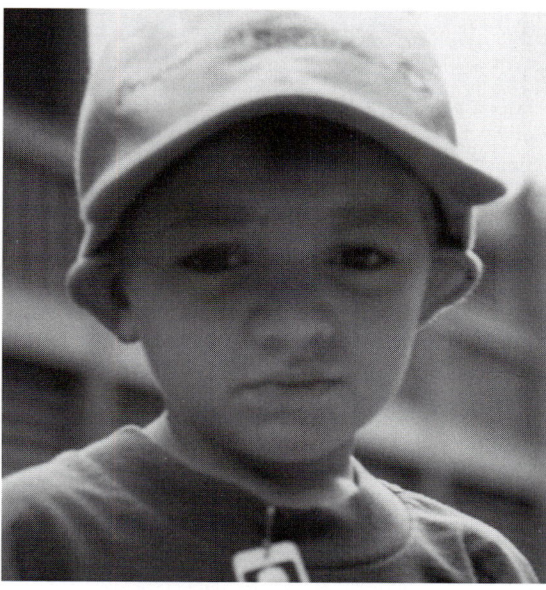

Camp Horizon, near Nashville. This child had stage III neuroblastoma with marrow involvement. He was treated with chemotherapy and total body irradiation as well as a marrow transplant. He was apparently cured, since this picture was taken more than 5 years later. His hair was dry and brittle; hence the cap. (Courtesy of Greg Kinney.)

Margie A. Scott

Infections Involving Lymph Nodes

DIAGNOSTIC APPROACH TO LYMPH NODE EVALUATION

Infectious disease of children, as well as adults, remains a leading cause of death worldwide as well as in developed countries. With little or no prodromal warning, systemic infections in children may rapidly progress to life-threatening illnesses. Lymph node biopsy may establish the diagnosis in some of these cases so that appropriate antimicrobial therapy may be given. A well-planned approach to lymph node handling and triage of tissue is required to facilitate appropriate diagnostic tests in cases of infectious lymphadenopathy (Collins, 1985; Perkins et al, 1995). Clinical information must be combined with a complete histologic or microbiologic investigation to yield maximum information and etiologic diagnoses. Tissue for cultures is best obtained by a surgeon under sterile operating conditions. If cultures have not been obtained, a 3- to 4-mm piece of tissue should be sliced from one pole of the lymph node with a sterile blade. Lymph node biopsy specimens in children should routinely be cultured for bacterial, fungal, and mycobacterial pathogens. Viral cultures should be obtained, particularly when there is extensive zonal necrosis or in the appropriate clinical setting (e.g., with a child who has a rash or is immunocompromised).

Serial sections 2 to 3 mm in thickness made across the long axis permit thorough gross examination for both diffuse and focal parenchymal changes. A hematoxylin-eosin–stained touch preparation is useful in determining the type of lymphadenopathy (Fig. 16–9). The common reaction patterns in infectious lymphadenopathy are readily recognized on touch preparations and include suppurative, granulomatous, histiocytic, and mixed lymphoplasmacytic patterns. Viral lymphadenitis specimens may demonstrate zonal necrosis accompanied by scattered, enlarged atypical cells with dense, smudged chromatin. After evaluation of the touch preparation, special stains and cultures may be ordered, and material may be set aside for such procedures as electron microscopic and molecular studies. Table 16–5 outlines a general approach to lymph node biopsy triage in infectious diseases based on evaluation of a hematoxylin-eosin–stained touch preparation.

If possible, one block of tissue should be fixed in 10% neutral buffered formalin and another in a mercuric-based fixative. Mercuric-based fixatives enhance cytologic morphologic features, allow maximum preservation of nuclear detail, and are optimal for study with hematoxylin-eosin, certain special stains, and immunoperoxidase. Mercuric-based fixatives are not suitable for silver stains, such as the Warthin-Starry and Steiner stains, which require 10% formalin–fixed tissue. Table 16–6 lists immunoperoxidase antibodies that are commercially available for identification and confirmation of infectious agents. Commercially available molecular tests for confirmation of infectious etiologic agents are outlined in Table 16–7.

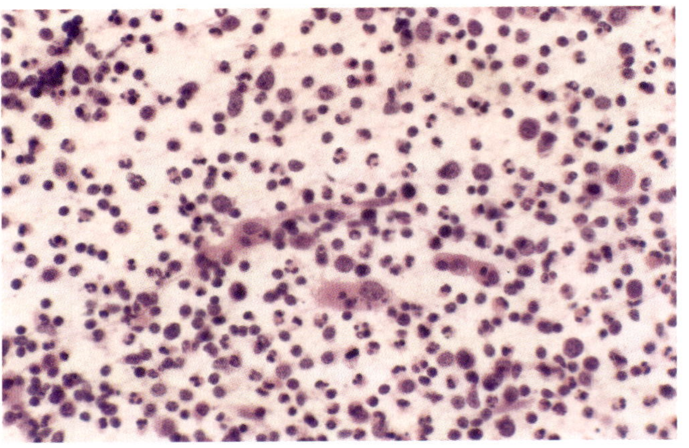

Figure 16–9

Subacute bacterial lymphadenitis, touch preparation. Note the abundance of neutrophils, tingible-body macrophages, and scattered lymphocytes.

Tissues fixed in 10% buffered formalin may be used for many molecular studies (Greer et al, 1991).

INFECTIONS IN IMMUNOCOMPETENT CHILDREN

Previously healthy children who present with infectious lymphadenopathy usually have unilateral regional lymphadenopathy or diffuse lymphadenopathy (Isaacs, 1996). Localized bacterial infections in immunocompetent children are usually subacute in presentation and related to a preceding event or injury, such as pharyngitis or a cat-scratch. With atypical mycobacterial infection of cervical nodes, a portal of entry is often not apparent. Diffuse or bilateral infectious lymphadenitis in previously healthy children most often represents viral infections, such as Epstein-Barr virus, cytomegalovirus, or acute HIV infection. These children are usually febrile and ill appearing and are likely to have hepatomegaly or splenomegaly.

INFECTIONS IN IMMUNOCOMPROMISED CHILDREN

Infectious lymphadenitis in immunocompromised children may represent a medical emergency. Initial symptoms may be blunted, and fever is not uniformly present. The expanded use of pediatric oncology protocols, marrow transplantation, and solid organ transplantation has increased the number of iatrogenically immunocompromised children. In addition, there is a distressing increase in childhood HIV infections. Congenital immunodeficiencies are also an important problem.

Children with multiple severe recurrent pyogenic bacterial infections occurring within a year should be evaluated for potential polymorphonuclear leukocyte defects or surface ligand deficiencies (Bowen et al, 1982). B or T cell functional deficiencies should be considered in children with multiple severe recurrent viral, fungal, or mycobacterial infections within a 1- to 3-year period (Rosen et al, 1995). A primary or acquired immunodeficiency may be responsible.

If lymph nodes are biopsied in immunocompromised children, material should routinely be processed for rapid special stains, cultures, and histologic sections, as well as possible electron microscopic or molecular studies. Duplicate air-dried touch preparations may be submitted for same-day special stains immediately after determining the tissue reaction pattern. Pathologists may thereby screen for etiologic agents prior to the bacterial culture reports and receipt of hematoxylin-eosin–stained tissue sections.

The distribution of the lymphadenopathy in immunocompromised children is often helpful in guiding the initial approach to pathogen identification. Mediastinal lymphadenopathy in the absence of superficial adenopathy most often results from infection by *Histoplasma capsulatum*, mycobacterial species, *Cryptococcus neoformans*, and occasionally *Pneumocystis carinii*. The last three types of infection are particularly frequent in children with AIDS. Mediastinal adenopathy may

Table 16–5
Guidelines for Pathologic Evaluation of Infectious Lymphadenopathy in Children

Tissue Reaction on Hematoxylin-Eosin–Stained Touch Preparation	Special Stains*	Cultures†	Tissue for Electron Microscopic Studies	Tissue for Molecular Studies
Neutrophilic	1. Gram 2. Fungal 3. Acid fast	1. Bacterial 2. Fungal 3. Mycobacterial	No	Yes
Granulomatous	1. Acid fast 2. Fungal 3. Gram	1. Mycobacterial 2. Fungal 3. Bacterial	No	Yes
Histiocytic	1. Gram 2. Acid fast 3. Fungal	1. Bacterial 2. Mycobacterial 3. Fungal	Yes	Yes
Mixed lymphocytic and/or plasmacytic	1. Silver precipitate 2. Fungal 3. Acid fast 4. Bacterial	1. Viral screen 2. Fungal 3. Mycobacterial 4. Bacterial	Yes	Yes

*Special stains and cultures are numbered in order of priority for the tissue reaction identified.

†Special stains may be used on air-dried touch preparation slides (use only smooth, not frosted, slides) or histologic sections.

Note: If there is extensive necrosis in association with any tissue reaction, tissues should be set aside for electron microscopic and molecular studies. The possibility of cat-scratch disease may be evaluated with Steiner silver stain, culture, and polymerase chain reaction techniques on paraffin blocks. The possibility of viral infections may be evaluated by herpes immunoperoxidase studies, viral cultures, and possibly by electron microscopic examination.

Table 16–6

Commercially Available Primary Antibodies Useful in Diagnosis of Various Infectious Agents in Paraffin-Embedded Tissues

Viral Agents		Bacterial Agents		Fungal and Protozoan Agents	
Organism	Antibody	Organism	Antibody	Organism	Antibody
Adenovirus	M	*Campylobacter jejuni*	M	*Aspergillus*	P
Cytomegalovirus	M	*Chlamydia*	M	*Blastomyces*	P
Epstein-Barr virus	M	*Mycobacterium bovis*	P	*Candida albicans*	P
Hepatitis B core, surface	P	*Helicobacter pylori*	P	*Coccidioides*	P
Hepatitis C virus	M	Mycobacteria	P	*Cryptococcus neoformans*	P
Herpes simplex 1 and 2	P	*Pseudomonas aeruginosa*	M	*Histoplasma capsulatum*	P
HIV, p24	M	*Salmonella*	P	*Pneumocystis carinii*	M
JC polyomavirus	M	*Shigella*	P	*Toxoplasma gondii*	P
Human papillomavirus	P,M	Staphylococci	P		
Parvovirus B19	M	Streptococci	P		
Respiratory syncytial virus	M				
Varicella zoster	M				

Abbreviations: M, monoclonal antibody P, polyclonal antibody.

occur with exudative pleural effusions. Positive pleural fluid culture results may help establish the infectious nature of mediastinal adenopathy. Of course, pleural fluid cultures may be falsely negative, particularly in children with fungal infections.

The commonest causes of cervical lymphadenitis in immunocompetent children are *Bartonella henselae*, in cat-scratch disease, and *Mycobacterium avium-intracellulare* complex, which has scrofula-like symptoms. Immunocompromised children may also have lymphadenitis caused by *Staphylococcus*, gram-negative bacilli, opportunistic fungi, protozoal agents, and viruses.

Table 16–7

Commercially Available Polymerase Chain Reaction and/or Southern Blot Testing to Detect Various Infectious Agents in Paraffin-Embedded Tissues

Viral Agents	Bacterial Agents
Cytomegalovirus	*Bartonella henselae*
Hepatitis C	*Bartonella quintana*
Hepatitis G	*Borrelia burgdorferi*
Herpes simplex	*Chlamydia pneumoniae*
HIV-1	*Legionella*
HIV-2	*Mycoplasma pneumoniae*
Human T cell lymphotrophic virus	*Mycobacterium* species
Parvovirus B19	*Mycobacterium tuberculosis*
Varicella zoster	*Mycobacterium avium-intracellulare* complex
Fungal and Protozoan Agents	*Mycobacterium kansasii*
	Mycobacterium gordonii
Histoplasma capsulatum	*Tropheryma whippleii*
Toxoplasma gondii	

Congenital Defects in Phagocytosis

Chronic granulomatous disease (CGD) of childhood is the prototypic example of congenital defects in phagocytic microbicidal activity (Harrison & Hanson, 1992). (For further discussion of this and other immunodeficiencies, see Chap. 3.) CGD represents a spectrum of X-linked recessive and autosomal recessive genetic defects that result in ineffective intracellular, oxygen-dependent microbial killing. The defective phagocytes are incapable of producing the hydrogen peroxide required for the microbicidal superoxide burst. Organisms that produce, but cannot inactivate, hydrogen peroxide are handled effectively by CGD phagocytes. Patients with CGD are plagued by organisms that produce catalase and thus can inactivate endogenous hydrogen peroxide. These catalase producers include *Staphylococcus aureus*, gram-negative enteric bacteria (Enterobacteriaceae), *Pseudomonas*, yeasts, most fungi (particularly *Aspergillus*), and *Nocardia*. The incidence of infections with catalase-negative organisms, such as *Streptococcus pneumoniae, Haemophilus influenzae,* and *Neisseria* is not increased in children with CGD. Chemotaxis, phagocytosis, and degranulation all occur normally in patients with CGD. Since cell-mediated immunity is also intact, viral infections are handled normally.

Cervical lymphadenitis is most often encountered in children with CGD, and the most frequently isolated organisms include *S. aureus* and *Aspergillus*, followed in frequency by *Pseudomonas, Klebsiella, Escherichia coli, Serratia*, and

Salmonella. Granuloma formation is a constant feature of CGD, even with gram-negative bacterial infections, and is usually mixed with areas of suppuration. Granulomas are probably induced by the persistent intracellular growth of pathogens, as in mycobacterial infections. Organisms may be sparsely and irregularly distributed, particularly in patients who are maintained on prophylactic antimicrobials. The search for pathogens may require cultures for bacterial, fungal, and mycobacterial agents as well as special stains on multiple tissue blocks or multiple levels. Degenerated, greatly distorted bacterial or fungal forms are frequently seen on tissue sections. Presumptive speciation in such a setting is inappropriate (Fig. 16–10).

Other congenital immunodeficiencies with leukocyte dysfunction may be associated with recurrent pyogenic infections, including myeloperoxidase deficiency, MAC-1 deficiency, Chédiak-Higashi syndrome, and hyper-IgE syndrome. Bacterial pathogens most often isolated include *Staphylococcus, Streptococcus, Haemophilus, Pseudomonas, Shigella, Salmonella*, and *Klebsiella. Candida* and *Aspergillus* are the commonest fungal isolates. The incidence of viral infections is not increased in patients with leukocyte dysfunction abnormalities.

Congenital Humoral Defects

Immunoglobulin deficiencies in children include X-linked agammaglobulinemia, common variable immunodeficiency, transient hypogammaglobulinemia of infancy, IgA deficiency, selective IgG deficiency, and hyper-IgM syndrome (Harrison & Hanson, 1992). Decreased levels of immunoglobulin result in inadequate mucosal barrier defenses, blunted complement activation, poor to absent opsonization, and ineffective phagocytosis. These children commonly present with progressive, refractory otitis media as well as acute, life-threatening pyogenic infections (e.g., sepsis or meningitis), and viral encephalitis. Arthritis may be the presenting illness in a small percentage of patients. Lymphadenitis is an atypical presentation in these patients but may be seen in association with widely disseminated infectious processes. The most common bacterial pathogens in these immunocompromised children include *Staphylococcus, Streptococcus, Haemophilus, Pseudomonas, Listeria*, gram-negative enteric bacteria, and *Mycoplasma*. Viruses cleared via antibody-dependent, cytotoxic killing pathways also cause problems for these patients. Particularly problematic are echovirus, coxsackie B, picornavirus, herpes simplex, measles, rotavirus, hepatitis B, and hepatitis C. Cultures are often necessary for diagnosis, since serologic responses in infections are blunted. Live viral vaccines should be avoided.

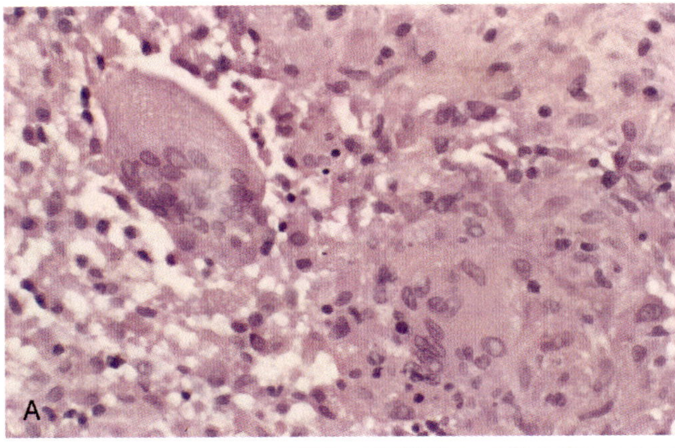

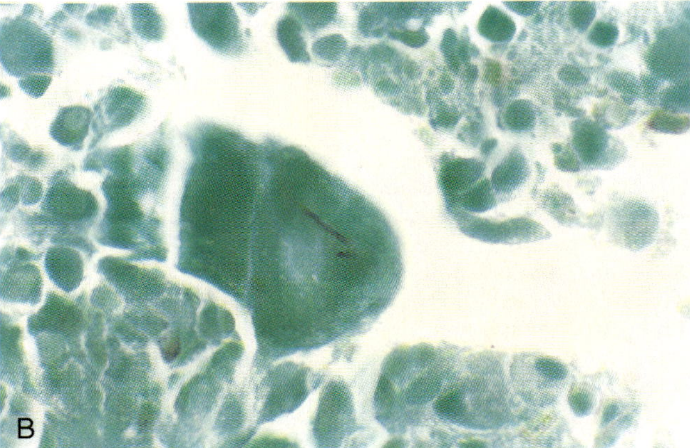

Figure 16–10

Chronic granulomatous disease, lymph node. *A*, Granulomatous reaction occuring in a child. *B*, Rare intracellular fragmented fungal hyphae were seen on staining. Culture subsequently grew *Pseudoallerichia boydii*. Methenamine silver.

Congenital Cell-Mediated Defects

Children with defects in cell-mediated immunity may have recurrent, severe, and sometimes fatal infections with fungal, viral, and bacterial pathogens (Harrison & Hanson, 1992). Cell-mediated defects include DiGeorge syndrome, severe combined immunodeficiency, Wiskott-Aldrich syndrome, and ataxia-telangiectasia. Lymphadenopathy often reflects a disseminated infectious process, but patients are also at increased risk for leukemia and lymphomas.

In the complete DiGeorge syndrome, infants are at significant risk for candidal infections, viral infections (adenovirus and rotavirus), and *Pneumocystis* infection. Bacterial pathogens are rarely a serious problem. Pathogens noted with increased frequency in patients with other cell-mediated immune defects include *Candida*, dermatophytes, and various protozoal agents. Since severe combined immunodeficiency and ataxia-telangiectasia are conditions with both cell-mediated and humoral defects, the spectrum of potential infectious agents includes pyogenic bacteria.

ACQUIRED IMMUNODEFICIENCY SYNDROME

AIDS is usually diagnosed in the pediatric population after failing T cell function leads to cellular immunodeficiency and secondary infections. In contrast to HIV in the adult population, HIV in children is often discovered during evaluation of recurrent bacterial infections (Fallon et al, 1989). Some of the opportunistic infectious organisms encountered are identical to those in the adult age group (*Pneumocystis carinii* pneumonia and disseminated *cytomegalovirus* disease), but children with AIDS also commonly present with recurrent *Streptococcus pneumoniae, Haemophilus influenzae* type b, and *Salmonella* infection (Krasinski et al, 1988). Children with HIV infection and AIDS rarely present with malignancies, but lymphocytic interstitial pneumonitis is reported as an unique presentation (Rubinstein et al, 1986).

BACTERIAL LYMPHADENITIS

Children with bacterial lymphadenitis may present with either a subacute febrile illness in which there is localized, tender lymphadenopathy associated with redness, edema, and surface warmth or a more acute sepsis-like syndrome with generalized lymphadenopathy. Recent or current antibiotic therapy may significantly alter detection of bacteria by culture or tissue staining. The great majority of cases of acute lymphadenitis in children are due to the pyogenic gram-positive cocci, group A beta-hemolytic *streptococci*, and *S. aureus*, followed by atypical mycobacteria. The two commonest causes of persistent regional lymphadenitis are *Mycobacterium avium* complex and *Bartonella henselae*, the agent of cat-scratch disease. Patients with these infections often fail multiple trials of antibiotics. Cat-scratch disease often suppurates, resulting in a fluctuant, pus-filled lymph node that may require therapeutic aspiration or excisional biopsy.

Gram-Positive Infections

Staphylococcus and *Streptococcus*

Lymphadenitis in children with tonsillitis, pharyngitis, or skin infections of the scalp or neck is usually due to gram-positive organisms. Cervical lymph nodes are most commonly involved. The characteristic etiologic agents include group A beta-hemolytic *Streptococcus* and *S. aureus* (Yamaucki et al, 1980). As organisms drain from the cutaneous or parapharyngeal soft tissues to the regional lymph node chain, swollen, tender lymphadenopathy develops. Most patients respond to initial antibiotic therapy, and biopsy is unnecessary. Some infections persist, and biopsies may be performed to exclude a neoplastic process. Incision and drainage of fluctuant lymph nodes in this setting should be avoided to minimize the potential complication of draining fistulas.

Touch preparations of lymphadenitis caused by pyogenic gram-positive cocci reveal numerous polymorphonuclear leukocytes and little else. Suppurative acute lymphadenitis usually begins as a focal lesion that is subcapsular or deep within the nodal parenchyma. *S. aureus* is the usual cause.

Tissue sections exhibit acute capsulitis and underlying abscesses in which gram-positive cocci are readily demonstrated. In general, clusters and chains of gram-positive organisms may be seen in tissue sections in both staphylococcal and streptococcal infections. Bacterial cultures are essential to confirm the genus and species of gram-positive organisms identified in lymph node biopsy specimens (Lane et al, 1980).

Actinomyces and *Nocardia*

The classic clinical course in actinomycosis is one of a slowly evolving chronic febrile illness with soft tissue mass formation, abscesses, pneumonia with or without cavitation, and smoldering lymphadenitis (Brown, 1973). Fistula formation and draining sinus tract occur in approximately one third of cases and should suggest the diagnosis. In the absence of draining sinuses, diagnoses have ranged from tuberculosis to systemic mycoses to disseminated bronchogenic carcinoma (Lane et al, 1980). Actinomycotic infection of the head and neck soft tissues may be associated with cervical lymphadenitis, and abdominal, appendiceal, and pelvic actinomycosis may be associated with mesenteric adenopathy. Actinomycotic infections above the diaphragm are more likely to form fistulae and sinus tracts.

Actinomyces in lymph nodes tend to grow in tight clusters and thus may be identified in a careful gross examination as pinpoint yellow "sulfur" granules. Microscopically, lymph nodes are seen to contain one or more abscesses with a characteristic central neutrophilic core surrounded by a scar or granulation tissue with a mixed inflammatory infiltrate. Sulfur granules are found in the center of abscesses. On hematoxylin-eosin–stained sections, they appear as an eosinophilic aggregate with "sun ray" or "starburst" edges (Fig. 16–11). Histiocytes and occasional giant cells may be seen, but the overall inflammatory reaction remains neutrophilic. Tissue Gram staining reveals tightly clustered, thin, filamentous, branching gram-positive bacilli that appear somewhat beaded. The filaments stain with Gomori methenamine silver and are not acid fast. When actinomycosis is suspected, multiple tissue levels should be examined for diagnostic organisms, since actively infected sites may be scattered among scar and chronically inflamed tissues. Since *Actinomyces* are extremely fastidious, cultures fail even when organisms have been seen in tissue sections. Strict anaerobic conditions are best for isolation of *Actinomyces*. Cultures may take 7–14 days to produce visible growth.

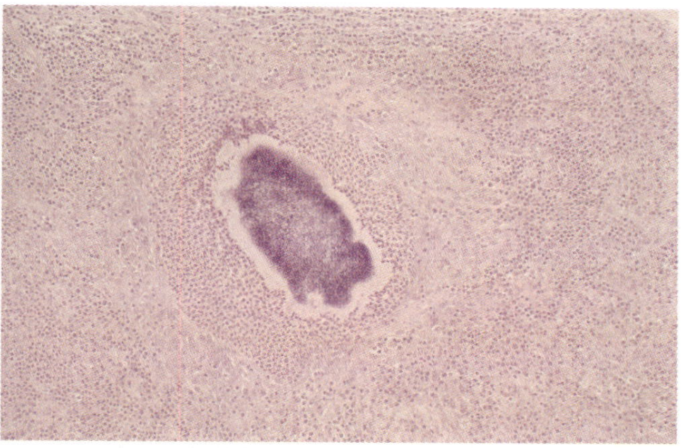

Figure 16–11

Actinomycosis, lymph node. A sulfur granule is surrounded by abundant neutrophils, fibrosis, and a few lymphocytes.

Systemic *Nocardia* infections very rarely cause suppurative lymphadenitis. Primary cutaneous infection may be accompanied by acute suppurative lymphadenitis that clinically simulates sporothricosis, with a subacute course of evolving cutaneolymphangitic nodules (von Lichtenberg, 1991). *Nocardia* elicits a tissue response similar to that of *Actinomyces*, with a few notable variations. *Nocardia* does not tend to cluster, and, thus, "sulfur" granules are not usually seen. In tissue sections dispersed, filamentous, beaded, gram-positive bacilli are noted on Gram staining. *Nocardia* stains moderately well with Gomori methenamine silver. In contrast to actinomycosis, *Nocardia* is partially acid fast when studied in modified acid-fast stains. Acid-fast methods modified with peanut oil immersion and shortened acid decolorization must be used to detect the partial acid-fast nature of *Nocardia*.

Rhodococcus equi

Rhodococcus equi is an opportunistic gram-positive coccobacillus that principally infects immunosuppressed patients (Scott et al, 1995). This agent is readily overlooked in cultures as a contaminating "diphtheroid," particularly if isolated from a nonsterile source, such as upper respiratory secretions. Isolation of "diphtheroids" from any sterile site, including lymph nodes, warrants work-up to rule out *Rhodococcus equi* infection. Pulmonary cavitary lesions are the commonest presentation, but lymphadenitis occurs in both immunocompetent and immunocompromised children (Thomsen et al, 1968; Van Etta et al, 1983). The clinical presentation often resembles that of mycobacterial infection or systemic mycosis. *Rhodococcus* produces an acute inflammatory infiltrate, as expected with gram-positive cocci. Rhodococcal lesions are distinctive in that they

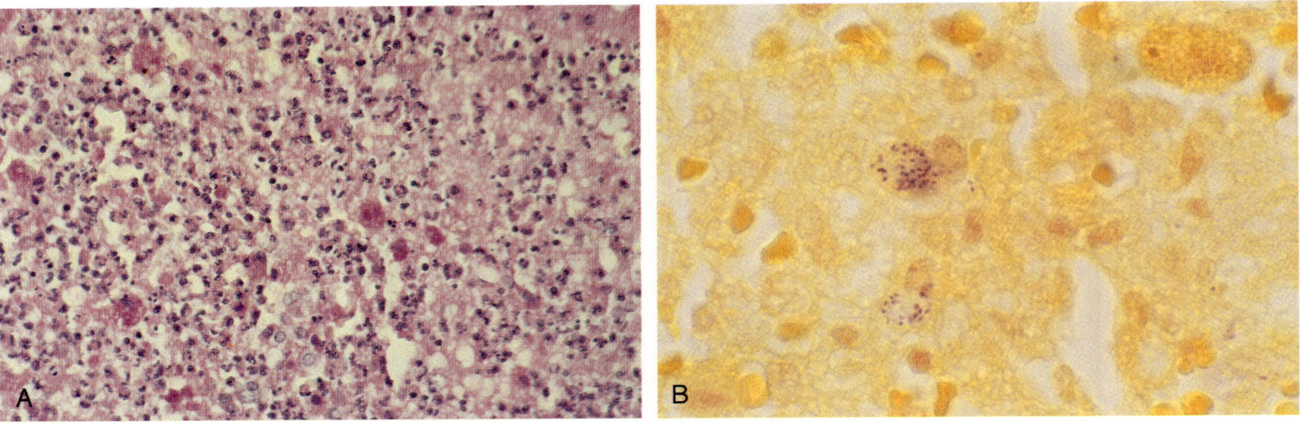

Figure 16–12

Rhodococcus equi infection, lymph node. *A*, Microabscesses are surrounded by positively staining histiocytes. Periodic acid–Schiff stain. *B*, Numerous pleomorphic gram-positive coccobacilli are demonstrated on a Gram-stained tissue sample.

contain histiocytes filled with organisms (Fig. 16–12). These histiocytes stain intensely with periodic acid–Schiff owing to the thick polysaccharide coat of the bacterial forms. *Rhodococcus* also stains easily with tissue Gram stains and Gomori methenamine silver stains and is acid fast. Its acid fastness is difficult to determine in tissue sections but is readily demonstrated on fresh touch preparations and fresh isolates grown on 5% sheep blood agar at 37°C for 48 h. *Rhodococcus equi* grows well on routine blood agar plates as salmon-pink colonies and on routine media used for mycobacteria.

Corynebacterium diphtheriae

Corynebacterium diphtheriae is a rare cause of lymphadenitis in children (Hodes, 1979), although the incidence of diphtheria has increased slightly since the 1970s. This virulent, phage-transfected, toxin-producing, gram-positive rod is highly contagious. In the United States, presentation as a localized cutaneous ulcer in children under 15 years of age is now commoner than the characteristic exudative pharyngitis. Either ulcer or pharygitis may be associated with regional lymphadenitis. In the malignant form of diphtheria, cervical lymphadenitis is so pronounced that the terms *bull neck* or *proconsular neck* are used. Soft tissue swelling extends from ear to ear, with the head somewhat thrown back to allow maximal laryngeal airflow. The local tissue response is an acute inflammatory exudate, with formation of a distinct green-yellow "membrane" of proteinaceous fibrin-rich debris, bacterial forms, and abundant neutrophils. Marked coagulative necrosis secondary to toxin production is the rule at local sites in diphtherial infection, while in myocardium and peripheral nerves the tissue response is that of toxin-induced coagulative necrosis with minimal inflammatory infiltrate. Myocardial conduction system and phrenic nerve involvement represent acute life-threatening complications. Lymph node biopsies are rarely performed and generally are not helpful. If performed, they reveal reactive follicular hyperplasia with areas of toxin-induced necrosis and minimal inflammatory infiltrates.

Culture and isolation of *C. diphtheriae* requires Löffler fibrin-enriched culture media (Krugman et al, 1977). Pathogenicity must be established in isolates by testing for toxin production. Treatment requires a dual approach of penicillin as an antibacterial agent and intravenous diphtherial antitoxin to neutralize the free circulating and unbound tissue toxin. Dosages of antitoxin vary with site of infection, size of membrane, and systemic symptoms.

Listeria monocytogenes

Listeria monocytogenes is ubiquitous in hoofed animals and has been documented in asymptomatic human carriers. Infection usually occurs after ingestion of contaminated milk, ice cream, or other food products. Outbreaks may often be traced to a single food source. Listeriosis in this setting is generally limited to mild gastroenteritis, but a hemolysin facilitates invasion through the gastrointestinal tract to cause a systemic febrile illness (Gellin & Broome, 1989; Gray & Killinger, 1966) that occasionally results in localized persistent lymphadenitis.

Listeria elicits a suppurative inflammatory reaction with abscess formation and central necrosis. Gram-positive or gram-variable bacterial rods may be identified in tissue sections. Organisms may not stain uniformly, with variations from red-purple to dark blue. Another helpful clue to the diagnosis is the aggregation of intracellular bacilli into "Chinese character" formations. Diagnosis of *Listeria* lymphadenitis depends on isolation in culture and biochemical classification.

Gram-Negative Infections

Lymphadenitis caused by gram-negative organisms may be associated with localized trauma or follow a sepsis episode in which organisms seed the lymphatic system. In the latter situation, patients are likely to be febrile and have generalized tender lymphadenopathy. The histologic tissue reaction pattern in gram-negative lymphadenitis is usually a dense neutrophilic infiltrate with microabscess formation. In general, lymphadenitis in gram-negative infections has more zonal necrosis than that in gram-positive infections because of the abundance of endotoxin in the gram-negative bacterial cell wall. All Enterobacteriaceae may cause acute suppurative lymphadenitis, but the most commonly encountered organisms in this setting are *E. coli* and *Serratia. Pseudomonas, Haemophilus, Neisseria,* and *Aeromonas* are other types of gram-negative bacteria that may cause acute suppurative lymphadentis in the setting of sepsis syndrome.

Pseudomonas

Pseudomonas is distinctive in eliciting two types of tissue response, depending largely on the immune status of the host. In immunocompetent children, *Pseudomonas* lymphadenitis has a neutrophil-rich microabscess pattern, with foci of coagulative

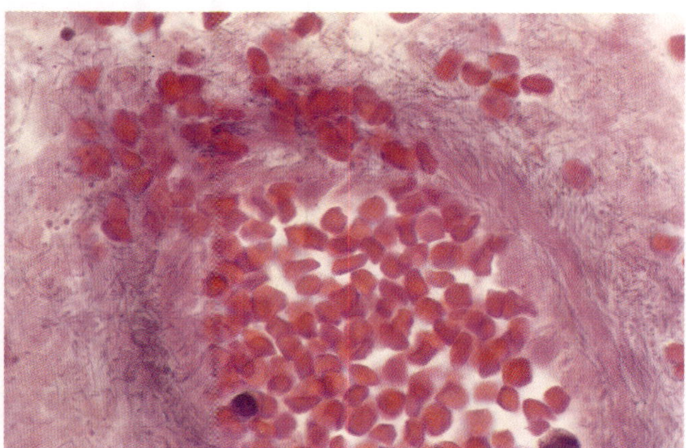

Figure 16–13

Pseudomonas aeruginosa vasculitis, lymph node. Note the innumerable bacterial rods surrounding and permeating a vessel in this neutropenic patient.

necrosis typical of most gram-negative bacilli. In contrast, in neutropenic children, *Pseudomonas* has a characteristic vasculitic presentation (Ziegler & Douglas, 1979). Innumerable gram-negative bacilli seen on routine hematoxylin-eosin stains swarm around and into the media of small veins and arteries (Fig. 16–13). This vascular lesion may clinically mimic pulmonary thromboembolism and produce wedge-shaped infarctions (Soave et al, 1978). Neutrophils in "*Pseudomonas* vasculitis" are sparse. This histologic pattern of infection in a neutropenic child is usually caused by *Pseudomonas*, although *Klebsiella pneumoniae* may produce similar-appearing lesions in the lung.

Salmonella typhi and *Salmonella enteritidis* (Typhoid Fever)

Both *Salmonella typhi* and *Salmonella enteritidis* cause typhoid fever, in which there is ulceration of the bowel wall, with periodic showering of gram-negative bacilli into the bloodstream accompanied by episodes of fever and bloody diarrhea. Blood cultures obtained during a febrile episode are diagnostic in 90% of cases. Typhoid fever lymphadenopathy is most pronounced in the mesenteric chain and is characterized by marked follicular hyperplasia and sinusal histiocytic aggregates displaying erythrophagocytosis. Necrosis may surround foci of fibrinous debris. On occasion suppurative necrosis may be the dominant histologic feature (Naqvi et al, 1988). Lymphohistiocytic "typhoid nodules" with central necrosis are rarely identified in nodes but are frequently seen in the liver and spleen. A granulomatous tissue reaction has also been described (Murray et al, 1994).

Yersinia pestis (Bubonic Plague)

Outbreaks and sporadic cases of plague in urban societies generally follow exposure to infected rodent excrement. *Yersinia pestis* lymphadenitis is, fortunately, a rare occurrence in the United States (Barnes et al, 1988). Most patients with plague present with regional lymphadenitis (hence, bubonic) with an identifiable site of entry, such as an ulcer of the foot or lower leg. Children may rarely contract *Yersinia* infection from their outdoor pets (Weniger et al, 1984). The pet is usually seriously ill or has died just prior to the appearance of illness in the child. *Yersinia pestis* lymphadenitis either accompanies or precedes a severe sepsis syndrome as the disease progresses. Peripheral blood leukocytosis with prominent left shift of neutrophils is noted. Organisms are usually abundant both in tissues and in peripheral blood films. Identification of organisms in the latter makes node biopsies superfluous. In addition, Gram- or Wright-stained preparations from cutaneous ulcers may reveal numerous short bacterial rods with the characteristic "safety pin" appearance. The suspicion of *Y. pestis* infection in a child is an indication for antimicrobial therapy of the child and the child's care giver. The clinical microbiology laboratory should also be immediately informed of the potential *Y. pestis* infection in order to ensure proper handling of blood and tissue cultures as well as to minimize exposure of laboratory workers.

The two forms of *Y. pestis* lymphadenitis are called plague major and minor. Plague major is the clinically virulent form of bubonic plague, in which there is complete obliteration of nodal parenchyma, marked histiocytosis in nodal sinuses, and numerous gram-negative "safety pin"–shaped organisms in the nodal sinuses and abscesses. Extensive hemorrhagic necrosis and abscess formation are noted. Organisms are so numerous that their presence may be predicted by an amphophilic to blue haze surrounding zones of suppurative necrosis seen with routine hematoxylin-eosin staining. Plague minor is clinically indolent, with subtle fever and mild localized lymphadenitis. The lymph nodes in plague minor exhibit only focal involvement. Scattered small abscesses and few organisms are seen with special stains.

Granulomatous Lymphadenitis with Stellate Microabscesses

A small group of non-Enterobacteriaceae gram-negative bacterial rods, including *Bartonella henselae, Yersinia enterocolitica, Yersinia pseudotuberculosis*, and *Francisella tularensis*, tend to elicit a necrotizing granulomatous lymphadenitis with stellate microabscesses surrounded by palisading histiocytes. The histologic lesions are so similar that a detailed history and notation of the distribution of disease are required to sort out the differential diagnosis. In children, most cases of subacute regional necrotizing lymphadentitis with stellate microabscess formation are due to cat-scratch disease.

Cat-Scratch Disease. Cat-scratch disease (CSD) is a common cause of subacute regional lymphadenitis in children. An estimated 120,000 to 150,000 cases are reported each year in the United States, with 2000 to 3000 hospitalizations annually for persistent or complicated infections in immunocompetent children. The diagnosis may usually be established by a history of cat exposure with a recent scratch or papule, tender regional lymphadenitis, CSD serologic positivity, and negative routine bacterial culture results (Carithers, 1970). The causative agent was first described in 1983 as small pleomorphic gram-negative bacilli proliferating within capillary walls and microabscesses of lymph nodes (Wear et al). Serologic data and molecular studies have subsequently shown that the great majority of CSD cases are caused by *Bartonella henselae* (Barka et al, 1993; Scott et al, 1996). The role of *Afipia felis*, another small pleomorphic gram-negative bacillus, remains unclear (Bergmans et al, 1995). *Bartonella henselae* DNA may be successfully detected in CSD in fresh tissue, freshly aspirated pus, or formalin-fixed lymph node biopsy tissues.

The site of the regional lymph node bed involved by CSD depends on whether the original bacterial inoculation occurred through a cat scratch or conjunctival mucosa exposure. Cervical lymph nodes are most often involved. Lymphadenitis usually lasts 3–8 weeks, but smoldering infections may persist up to 2 years. The tissue response in very early CSD is a

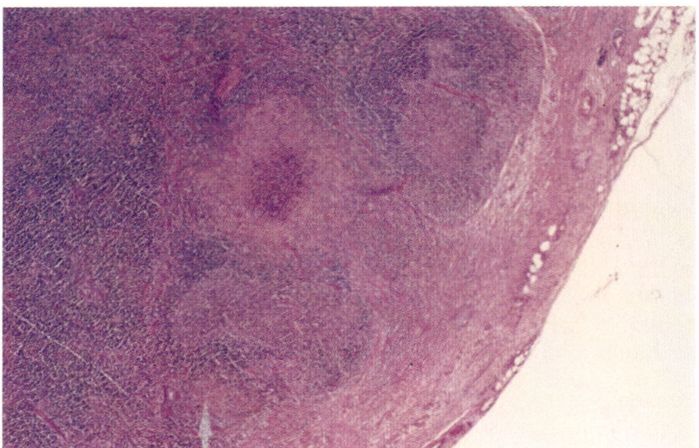

Figure 16–14

Cat-scratch disease, early, lymph node. Capsulitis and an underlying subcapsular abscess are surrounded by a few histiocytes. A brisk vascular proliferation surrounds the center of these early abscesses.

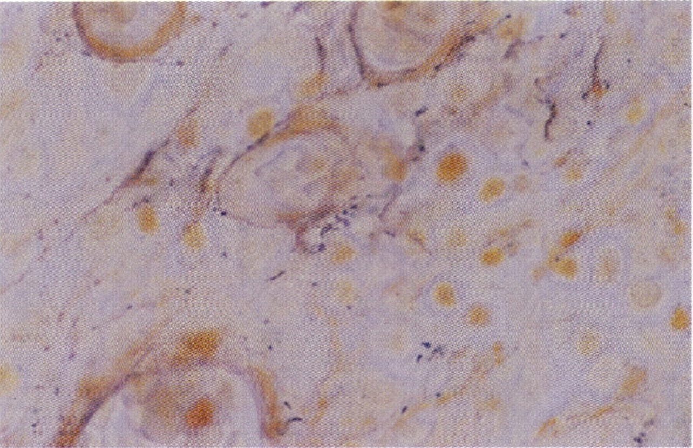

Figure 16–16

Cat-scratch disease, lymph node. This demonstrates the tiny pleomorphic bacterial rods characteristic of *Bartonella henselae*. Bacterial forms may be found in the center of microabscesses or surrounding the adventitia of the small vessels that proliferate around abscesses. Steiner stain.

localized, subcapsular microabscess (Fig. 16–14). The organism then spreads to adjacent nodal parenchyma, giving rise to the stellate lesions seen in later stages.

Biopsies are often performed 3–6 weeks after the onset of disease to rule out malignancy because one or more courses of antibiotics have had limited success. At gross examination, the lymph nodes of CSD are enlarged, with a somewhat thickened capsule. Serial sections through the nodes demonstrate multiple irregular microabscesses that may coalesce with time. Touch preparations reveal a mixture of neutrophils and histiocytes, whereas multinucleated giant cells are rarely seen. Sections exhibit stellate microabscesses with distinct zonation. A central aggregate of neutrophils is surrounded by palisading histiocytes and a lymphocyte-predominant inflammatory response (Fig. 16–15). Eosinophils and plasma cells may be seen in small numbers toward the periphery of these lesions. The overlying node capsule is fibrotic and contains a lymphocyte-predominant infiltrate with scattered plasma cells. The stellate microabscess surrounded by palisading histiocytes is a consistent unit lesion of *B. henselae* infection and has also been described in skin, liver, spleen, subcutaneous soft tissue, bone, and lung. The extranodal microabscesses of CSD, especially the hepatic lesions, are often surrounded by a dense zone of reactive fibrosis. It is occasionally possible to see the tiny pleomorphic cat-scratch bacilli by using specialized silver precipitate stains, such as the Warthin Starry or Steiner stains (Fig. 16–16). Organisms are most easily seen in the center of the microabscesses or in the adventitia of nearby proliferating vessels. These stains are optimal in formalin-fixed tissue and cannot be used on tissues fixed with mercuric- and zinc-based preparations because these heavy metals precipitate upon staining. In late stages of CSD, bacteria may be so scant that visualization of the organisms is even more problematic. Diagnosis may be confirmed if necessary by serologic studies for CSD or polymerase chain reaction or Southern blot confirmation of *B. henselae* DNA (Scott et al, 1996). It is equally important in suspected cases to document negative results with special stains for fungi, mycobacteria, and routine bacterial forms.

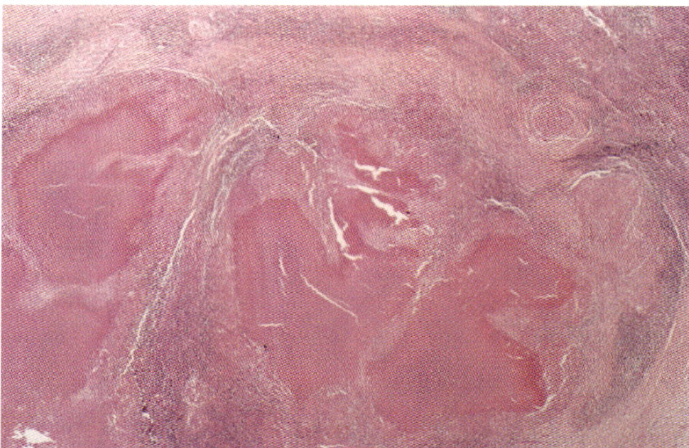

Figure 16–15

Cat-scratch disease, late, lymph node. Typical coalescent stellate microabscesses are surrounded by a zone of palisading histiocytes and lymphocytes.

Francisella tularensis

Clues to the diagnosis of *Francisella tularensis* lymphadenitis include a recent tick bite, hunting or hiking excursions, skinning of wild rabbits, or contact with a domestic animal that is an avid hunter (Evans et al, 1985). The ensuing febrile illness is often accompanied by regional lymphadenitis that is usually limited to the epitrochlear, axillary, and cervical nodes. Peripheral blood leukocytosis and left shift are typically absent.

If there are any suggestions that *F. tularensis* is the likely etiologic agent, the clinical microbiology laboratory should be immediately notified, since this infectious agent is highly contagious and virulent. The histopathologic features of lymphadenitis in tularemia is similar to that of CSD (Fig. 16–17), except that necrosis may be so extensive in tularemia as to mimic lesions of tuberculosis. The organisms are gram negative and stain well with Warthin Starry or Steiner silver precipitate stains. In addition, acridine orange fluorescent stains help detect these small bacilli in tissue sections. Diagnosis may depend on correlation of clinical history, lymph node histologic features, and the results of serologic studies for tularemia.

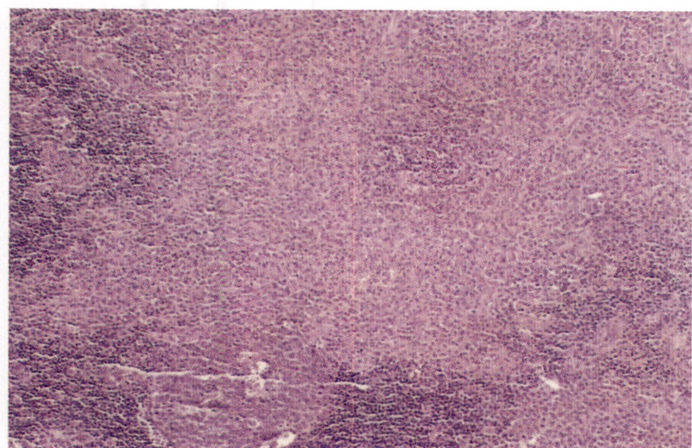

Figure 16–17

Francisella tularensis lymphadenitis. Note the similarity of the reaction pattern to that of early cat-scratch disease (compare with Fig. 16–14).

Yersinia enterocolitica and *Yersinia pseudotuberculosis*

Lymphadenitis due to *Yersinia enterocolitica* and *Yersinia pseudotuberculosis* has a characteristic presentation. Children have unexplained gastroenteritis that may mimic acute appendicitis or an acute abdomen. Intraoperatively, the small bowel, particularly the distal ileum, and appendix appear acutely inflamed. Associated mesenteric lymphadenitis is noted (Lee et al, 1990). Pathologists may receive appendices and mesenteric lymph nodes as well as portions of ileum (Saari & Triplett, 1974), in which necrotizing granulomas with stellate microabscess formation should suggest the possibility of *Y. enterocolitica* or *Y. pseudotuberculosis* infection. Follow-up serologic studies may be helpful, as may stool cultures incubated at room temperature to enhance recovery of these organisms.

The pathologic features of *Y. enterocolitica* and *Y. pseudotuberculosis* lymphadenitis are identical to the pattern described for *B. henselae* infection in CSD (Fig. 16–18). *Yersinia* is also gram-negative and stains well with Warthin Starry or Steiner silver precipitate stains. However, *Yersinia* may be as difficult to visualize as *Bartonella* by these methods, and an acridine orange fluorescent stain may be needed to detect organisms.

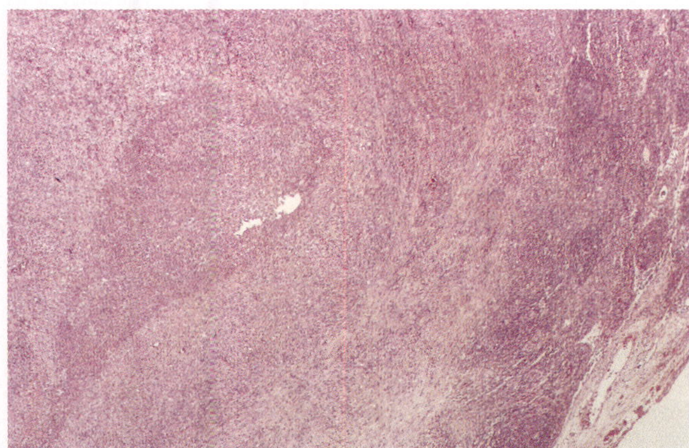

Figure 16–18

Yersinia enterocolitica mesenteric lymphadenitis. Compared with cat-scratch disease, there are fewer surrounding histiocytes. The capsulitis is generally not as developed.

Stenotrophomonas maltophilia

Stenotrophomonas (formerly *Xanthomonas*) *maltophilia* is a non-Enterobacteriaceae gram-negative rod that rarely causes disease in normal humans. However, immunocompromised patients being treated with broad-spectrum antibiotics are susceptible (Meier, 1997). Although rare, these infections are clinically significant because of their broad resistance to antimicrobial agents. Clinically and microbiologically, it is important to distinguish this organism from *Pseudomonas aeruginosa*. Clinical presentations are similar to those in other gram-negative infections. Patients with systemic disease often present with fever of unknown origin.

The pathologic features of systemic *Stenotrophomonas* infections is not well documented in the literature. This author has seen two previously healthy children with no evidence of immunocompromise that had nodular, ulcerative cutaneous lesions in which there was a giant cell–rich, granulomatous reaction with scant necrosis. Involved lymph nodes may demonstrate a pattern of granulomatous inflammation that may be confused with mycobacterial infection, fungal infection, or sarcoidosis. Progressive systemic disease may occur despite antimicrobial therapy owing to broad antimicrobial resistance of this organism. Cultural identification is necessary for diagnosis.

Brucella

Four species of *Brucella* cause human disease: *Brucella suis*, contracted from swine; *Brucella melitensis*, from goats; *Brucella abortus*, from cattle; and *Brucella canis*, from dogs. Exposure to these animals or improperly processed animal products is usually responsible for human brucellosis (Fox & Kaufmann, 1977). Patients with acute brucellosis present with acute onset of fever and chills that may be associated with pneumonia and systemic symptoms. Rapid antimicrobial therapy in most of these cases is usually curative, since *Brucella species* are susceptible to a wide spectrum of antimicrobial agents. Chronic forms of brucellosis are rare in industrialized countries, but in less severe or untreated cases progression to chronic brucellosis may occur. In this form, lesions within the lymph nodes, liver, spleen, and marrow become apparent as a chronic granulomatous infection with variable degrees of necrosis and limited abscess formation (Fig. 16–19). *Brucella abortus* is particularly known for eliciting nonnecrotizing

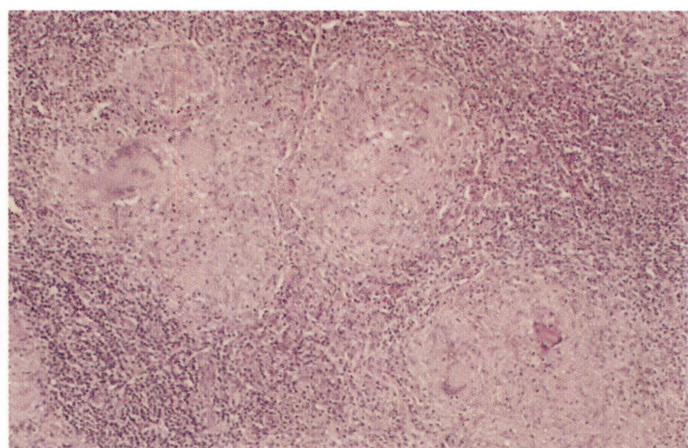

Figure 16–19

Brucella lymphadenitis. The most characteristic histopathologic features are nonnecrotizing granulomas with abundant giant cells, similar to the pattern seen in sarcoidosis. However, brucellosis is one of the few diseases causing intrafollicular aggregates of histiocytes and granulomas.

granulomas resembling sarcoidosis. Granulomas may become coalescent and form splenic or hepatic abnormalities detectable with imaging studies. Tests with special stains for mycobacteria and fungi are often performed because of the granulomas. Since *Brucella* is an intracellular gram-negative bacillus that is notoriously difficult to stain and visualize in tissue sections, culturing on specialized media is required for diagnosis. Brucellosis may be strongly considered in retrospect if the histopathologic changes described here are combined with negative special stain results, negative routine culture results, and positive *Brucella* serologic study results.

Spirochetes

Spirochetal lymphadenitis may be observed in *Treponema pallidum* and *Spirillum minus* infections. Both of these organisms are thin, coiled, gram-negative bacteria. The clinical presentation of patients with spirochetal lymphadenitis is preceded by a febrile illness that may be quite subtle in secondary stages of syphilis or quite abrupt in *S. minus* infection.

Syphilis is caused by direct transmission of *T. pallidum* from an infected person through compromised skin or mucous membranes (Sell & Norris, 1983). *T. pallidum* is a slender gram-negative bacillus with 4 to 14 loosely wound spirals. It is extremely virulent, and as few as three spirochetes may produce disease in an immunocompetent individual. Spirochetemia ensues and may persist for weeks, producing fever when the peripheral blood organism load approaches $1 \times 10^7/\text{ml}^3$. It is during this secondary or dissemination stage that clinical symptoms are most evident and palpable lymphadenopathy develops.

Lymph nodes in syphilis have a thickened, fibrotic capsule with a soft, congested parenchyma on sectioning. Touch preparations reveal a plasmacytic infiltrate without giant cells or significant numbers of neutrophils. A direct wet mount may demonstrate motile spirochetes under dark-field or phase microscopic examination. Sections exhibit chronic capsulitis with a dense plasmacytic infiltrate and obliteration of small vessels (Fig. 16–20). The underlying lymph node parenchyma demonstrates sinusal plasma cell infiltrates and scattered small vessels in which fibrointimal proliferation has obliterated the lumens. The combination of capsulitis and vascular lesions is indicative of syphilitic infection. Special stains, such as the Warthin Starry or Steiner silver precipitate stain, demonstrate organisms most readily in obliterated vessels or endothelium of newly infected vessels. Granulomas with focal central necrosis may be found later in the infection. Serologic confirmation may be helpful in cases in which the bacterial load is limited and organisms are not identified with special stains.

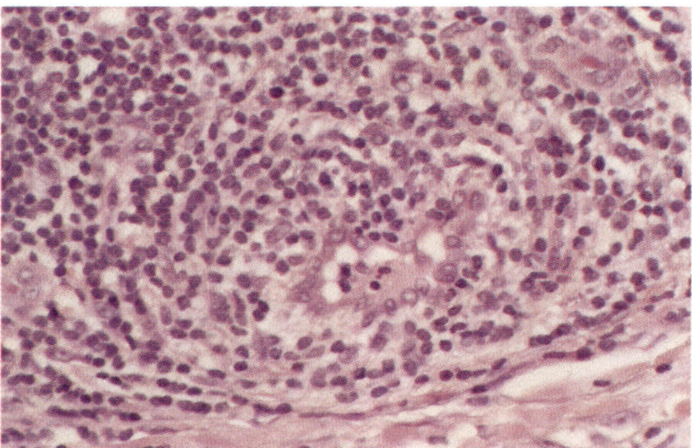

Figure 16–20

Syphilitic lymphadenitis. A prominent lymphoplasmacytic infiltrate is associated with obliteration of small vessels. Capsular scarring is typically seen in syphilitic lymphadenitis.

Patients coinfected with HIV and *T. pallidum* develop an accelerated course of syphilis with an increased risk of progression to neurosyphilis (Musher et al, 1990), perhaps because HIV cripples the very immune mechanism required to keep spirochetes in check. Penicillin treatment may fail in coinfected patients, with resultant meningeal and/or ocular disease.

Spirillum minus, formerly *Spirillum minor*, is a short, somewhat thick gram-negative bacillus with two to six tightly wound spirals that produces infection via a rat bite or scratch. The initial wound typically heals, but patients develop cyclic episodes of fever lasting 3 to 4 days followed by 3 to 9 days of quiescence (Dow et al, 1992). The recurrent febrile episodes are accompanied by acute regional suppurative lymphadenitis. Fine-needle aspirates of infected lymph nodes may be examined for spirochetes using wet preparations or Wright-stained smears. Exudates from the residual skin lesion may also be examined to confirm spirochete infection. *Spirillum minus* may be isolated by mice inoculation, but this test is not performed in clinical microbiology laboratories. No specific serologic test for *S. minus* is currently available. Penicillin is the antibiotic of choice. Without therapy the mortality rate may reach 10%.

FUNGAL LYMPHADENITIS

Only a few of the thousands of fungal species commonly infect humans. Granulomatous reactions are characteristic, but fungi may cause an acute inflammatory response (e.g., aspergillosis), chronic granulomatous reactions with microabscesses (e.g., blastomycosis), or prominent eosinophilic reactions (e.g., coccidioidomycosis).

Fungal infections activate cell-mediated responses that are central in controlling the spread of fungal organisms and resolution of infections. Therefore, children with defects in cell-mediated immunity, patients on corticosteroids or immunosuppressive agents, and AIDS patients are quite susceptible to fungal infections.

Culture isolation and definitive identification of fungal organisms may require 5–30 days using standard laboratory techniques. However, a presumptive diagnosis and initial therapeutic decisions may be made before cultural identification by correlating fungal morphologic features revealed by routine hematoxylin-eosin staining, periodic acid–Schiff staining, and methenamine silver staining.

The portal of entry of many fungal infections is the lungs. Fungi may cause local disease there or spread by lymphovascular dissemination. Four fungal pathogens that produce systemic infections in humans are *Histoplasma capsulatum, Blastomyces dermatitidis, Coccidioides immitis*, and *Cryptococcus neoformans*. The first three are dimorphic fungi existing both in a tissue-invasive budding yeast form at 37°C and an infectious but noninvasive mycelial form found in nature at 25°C. *Cryptococcus* exists only in a budding yeast phase.

Histoplasma capsulatum

Human infection by *Histoplasma capsulatum* is common in endemic areas such as the southeastern United States, where most adults have evidence of past infection (Goodwin et al, 1980). Infectious spores may be found in large numbers in blackbird roosts, chicken houses, chicken manure, and sites frequented by bats. Inhaled spores reach small bronchioles or alveoli and (at body temperature) produce the yeast form that is promptly phagocytized by macrophages (Goodwin & Des Prez, 1978). Dissemination to the spleen, liver, and mediastinal lymph nodes is common. With the acquisition of cell-mediated immunity, a granulomatous tissue reaction ensues, the organisms are walled off, and the lesions eventually calcify. The severity of infection depends on the size of the inoculum and the immune status of the patient. A heavy spore inoculum in a nonimmune child causes a flulike respiratory illness that resolves without treatment or may evolve to systemic disease with subsequent lymphadenopathy and hepatosplenomegaly. Common presenting symptoms include fever, gradual weight loss, weakness, and malaise. Oropharyngeal ulcers are common in disseminated histoplasmosis. Biopsies of such lesions are often diagnostic.

Lymphadenopathy involves only mediastinal lymph nodes in patients with histoplasmosis localized to the chest. Mediastinal lymphadenopathy may occasionally be so extreme as to push midline structures out of normal anatomic locations, mimicking a neoplastic process. Calcification is common in long-standing disease. All lymph node chains may be involved in disseminated disease, and many patients have generalized lymphadenopathy.

On gross examination, lymph nodes display firm, tan-white nodules and areas of necrosis. Touch preparations reveal a granulomatous tissue reaction with abundant giant cells and histocytes in which small intracellular yeast forms may be seen. The appearance of yeast forms may be mimicked on hematoxylin-eosin–stained touch preparations by intracytoplasmic vacuoles. Additional touch preparations may be used for Wright stain, periodic acid–Schiff stain, or methenamine silver stain to confirm the presence of fungi. *Histoplasma* is identified as an intracellular yeast with narrow buds measuring 2–8 μ in diameter that often cluster in giant cells and histiocytes. Wright stain or periodic acid–Schiff stain demonstrate a dotlike structure representing nuclear material in these yeast forms. Methenamine silver stain enhances the cell walls and facilitates their visualization.

Tissue sections exhibit granulomatous lymphadenitis and caseous necrosis. Multinucleated giant cells and yeast-filled histiocytes are abundant. Organisms are particularly abundant in children with chronic granulomatous disease or AIDS, to the extent that histiocytes filled with yeast forms may be readily identified on hematoxylin-eosin–stained tissue sections as "stippled" figures (Fig. 16–21). Periodic acid–Schiff and methenamine silver stains reveal cells filled with the 2- to 8-μ budding yeast forms (see Fig. 16–21).

The morphologic features of Histoplasma are sufficiently distinctive to allow presumptive diagnosis and initiation of therapy in most cases. The differential diagnosis includes mycobacterial infection (see "Mycobacterial Lymphadenitis") and other fungal infections (discussed in this section) as well as infections with *Torulopsis* and *Pneumocystis carinii*. *Torulopsis* is a small yeast measuring 4–10 μ in diameter that may be intra- and extracellular. Yeast forms of histoplasmosis, with central collapse of the cell wall due to immune killing or antimicrobial therapy, may rarely be difficult to distinguish morphologically from disseminated forms of *P. carinii*.

Blastomyces dermatitidis

Blastomycosis is a pyogranulomatous disease caused by the dimorphic fungus *Blastomyces dermatitidis*. The natural habitat of this fungus is soil enriched by organic material. A history of boating, camping, hunting, or contact with beaver dams is often elicited. As with other systemic fungi, initial infection is through inhalation of spores, followed by hematogenous dissemination. *Blastomyces* most often involves lungs, skin, bones, and genitourinary tract (Sarosi & Davies, 1979; Steele & Abernathy, 1983). Infectious lymphadenopathy may occur but is less common than in other systemic fungal infections. Disease may be limited to the lungs and mediastinal lymph nodes, or there may be dissemination to bone and/or skin. Skin lesions are verrucous, slowly enlarge, and then demonstrate central healing.

A presumptive diagnosis may be rendered and treatment initiated when the characteristic broad-based, budding yeast forms measuring 20–50 μ in diameter are seen. Yeast forms have a characteristic thick and refractile cell wall. Touch preparations of infected lymph nodes reveal a mixed neutrophilic and granulomatous tissue reaction. This pyogranulomatous reaction is characteristic of blastomycosis.

Tissue sections exhibit both microabscesses and granuloma formation. Budding yeast forms may be so scant that study of multiple levels, with careful examination of the microabscesses, may be required to demonstrate the organism. However, tissue examinations are rarely falsely negative in blastomycosis, in contrast to experience with other fungi and tuberculosis. Broad-based, budding yeast forms with a distinct double-wall contour and internal nuclear structure may be

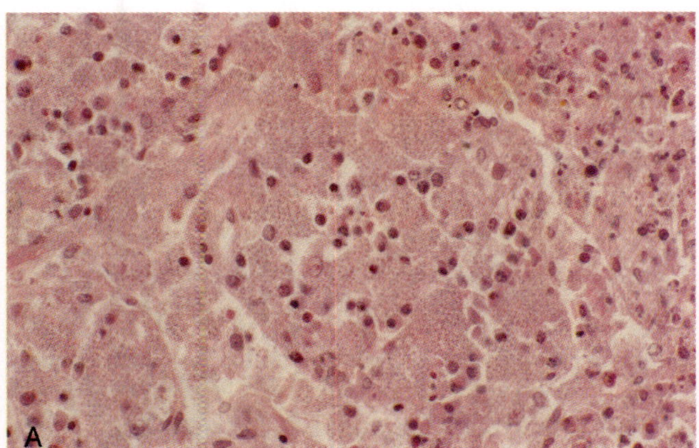

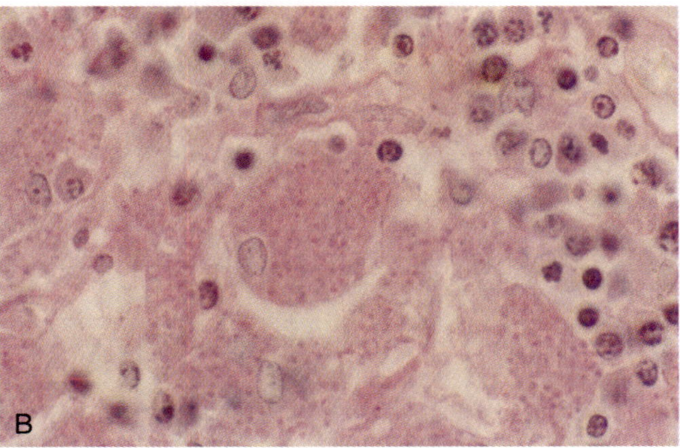

Figure 16–21

Histoplasmosis, disseminated, lymph node. *A*, Abundant yeast-filled histiocytes are noted on routine stains. *B*, Intracellular *Histoplasma* organisms show characteristic central dotlike positivity. Periodic acid–Schiff stain.

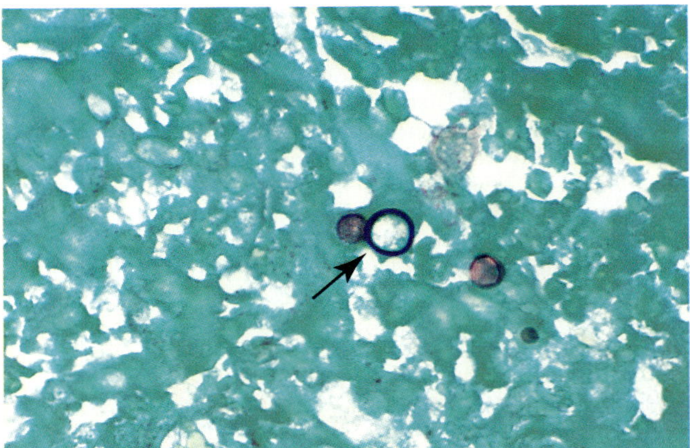

Figure 16–22

Blastomyces dermatitidis, lymph node. Characteristic broad-based budding is demonstrated (arrow). Methenamine silver.

confidently identified on routine hematoxylin-eosin–stained sections as *Blastomyces*, or special stains (methenamine silver or periodic acid–Schiff) may be used to facilitate their visualization (Fig. 16–22).

Coccidioides immitis

Coccidioidomycosis is caused by the dimorphic fungus *Coccidioides immitis*. This infection is endemic in the southwestern and western United States, particularly in the San Joaquin Valley (Ampel et al, 1989; Huntington, 1986). *Coccidioides* exists in the arid soil in its mycelial phase, which is characterized by highly infectious, alternate, barrel-shaped arthrospores along its hyphae.

After inhalation of arthrospores, spherulation and endosporulation occur in the pulmonary parenchyma. Most patients recall a flulike upper respiratory type of illness, which accounts for the name *valley fever*. Dissemination is more common among dark-skinned races and the immunocompromised. Dissemination often causes meningitis, although skin, muscles, bones, joints, and lymph nodes may also be involved.

The tissue response to coccidioidomycosis is largely granulomatous. The characteristic tissue form of the organism is the mature endosporulating spherule (Fig. 16–23), which, when seen in a biopsy specimen, is pathognomonic of coccidioidomycosis.

Diagnosis of disseminated disease may be extremely difficult. Detection of elevated levels of complement-fixing antibodies to *C. immitis* may be clinically helpful. In contrast, skin testing may not be useful because anergy is frequent in disseminated disease. Cultures should be handled with extreme caution because of the highly infectious nature of the arthrospores. Culture plates should be sealed and shipped to a reference facility if growth is noted.

Cryptococcus neoformans

Cryptococcus neoformans is a monomorphic fungus that exists only in the yeast phase (Lewis & Rabinovich, 1972). In nature, *Cryptococcus* is often found in soil or nests contaminated by pigeon excreta. This fungus is notorious for infecting both immunocompetent and immunocompromised humans (Kerkering et al, 1981). *Cryptococcus* is the most common cause of fungal meningitis and often complicates AIDS. The clinical manifestations of cryptococcosis are so ill-defined that diagnosis often relies on histopathologic findings, cytologic examination of cerebrospinal fluid, or serologic findings. The three clinical forms of cryptococcosis include meningoencephalitis, focal pneumonia, and acute disseminated infection. Lymphadenitis is seen with the latter. Focal pneumonia occurs in immunocompetent hosts and exhibits a mixed neutrophilic and granulomatous reaction, while acute disseminated cryptococcosis usually occurs in immunocompromised hosts and displays minimal or no tissue response to fungal growth. In such instances, myriad narrow-based, budding yeasts measuring 4–10 μ in diameter are identified and usually demonstrate a thick, mucicarmine-positive capsule (Fig. 16–24).

Lymph node biopsies demonstrate a soft, gelatinous cut surface. Cut surfaces may exhibit minute spaces, giving the tissue a spongelike appearance. Touch preparations exhibit numerous budding yeast forms surrounded by abundant clear spaces owing to exuberant capsule formation, a distinctive morphologic feature that is absent in capsule-deficient yeast forms found in patients treated for long-standing cryptococcosis. *Cryptococcus neoformans* is readily cultured and specifically identified in the clinical microbiology laboratory.

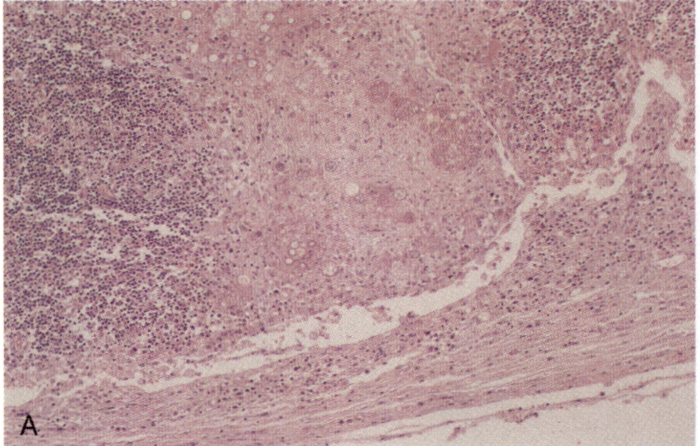

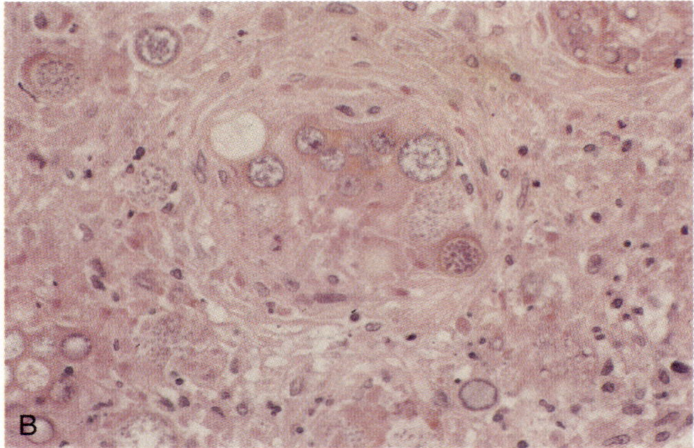

Figure 16–23

Coccidiodes immitis lymphadenitis. *A*, There is a neutrophilic and granulomatous tissue response. *B*, Higher magnification shows various stages of developing spherules, including the pathognomonic endospherules.

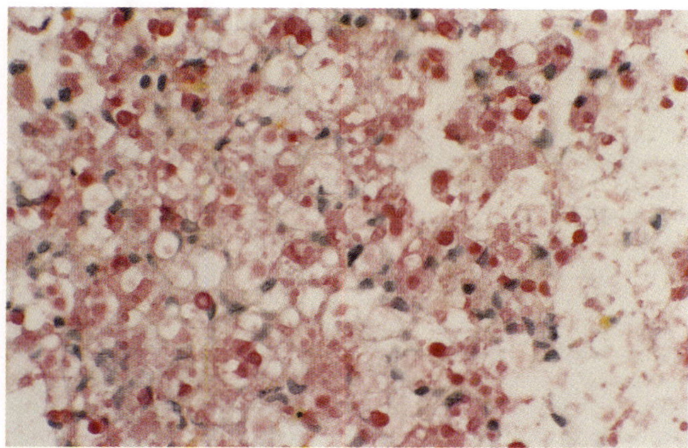

Figure 16–24

Cryptococcus neoformans. The demonstration of capsular material is helpful in recognizing this fungus. Capsule-negative forms may be seen in patients receiving therapy. Mucin stain.

OPPORTUNISTIC MYCOSES

Candida

Lymphadenitis only occurs in candidiasis when there is systemic infection in immunocompromised hosts (Myerowitz et al, 1977). Candida are unique in displaying reverse dimorphism. The hyphal phase represents the tissue invasive form, and budding yeasts represent the colonizing or noninvasive form. Systemic candidal infections are usually caused by *Candida albicans* or *Candida tropicalis*, with many other species accounting for 20–30% of cases. Speciation in the *Candida* group is possible only through culture and biochemical identification.

Systemic candidiasis is often preceded by superficial oropharyngeal or esophageal disease. Fungal plaques and ulcers may provide access to the lymphovascular system for this opportunistic fungus. Patients with systemic disease are seriously ill with fever, generalized lymphadenopathy, widespread skin lesions (maculopapular, erythemic, or ecthyma gangrenosum like), renal failure, and endocarditis. They may have abscesses in liver, spleen, and marrow. Retinal microabscesses have also been described in end-stage systemic candidiasis.

On gross examination, involved lymph nodes exhibit 1- to 3-mm miliary friable tan lesions surrounded by a hyperemic zone throughout the medulla and cortex. Each lesion represents a metastatic focus of *Candida*. Coalescent lesions are uncommon. Touch preparations demonstrate abundant neutrophils. Scattered hyphae and/or pseudohyphae may be identified on hematoxylin-eosin staining. If hyphal forms are not abundant, the touch preparation and clinical picture may suggest acute bacterial lymphadenitis.

On routine sections, lymph nodes may be seen to contain multiple microabscesses, with organisms easily identified in the center of the abscesses. Methenamine silver and periodic acid–Schiff stains highlight the morphologic features of these candidal organisms and allow distinction from those fungal infections in which organisms have septated hyphae. Tissue Gram staining is helpful because *Candida* hyphae and pseudohyphae stain intensely positive with a uniform uptake of stain, whereas true septated hyphae do not. Candidal organisms tend to indent at branch points, and small buds, rather than branches, may be seen in the pseudohyphal form. Walls of *Candida* hyphae are relatively uniform in thickness and contour. The presence of both hyphae or pseudohyphae and yeastlike blastospores is helpful in the identification of systemic candidiasis. Occasionally, yeastlike blastospore forms help distinguish this fungus from others, such as *Aspergillus*. Distinction between *Candida* and *Histoplasma* may be difficult if only blastospores are seen in tissue sections.

Candida grows rapidly and abundantly on routine microbiology media. Since even blood agar plates support its growth, appropriate subcultures and biochemical panels may be performed.

Torulopsis glabrata

Torulopsis glabrata (formerly *Candida glabrata*) is a rare opportunistic fungus closely related to *Candida* species that may be confused with *Histoplasma* and *Candida* in tissue sections. Toruloposis causes microabscesses resembling those of candidiasis. Sections show 3- to 10-μ blastospores without hyphae. *Torulopsis* blastospores, detected within histiocytes and extracellularly, resemble *Histoplasma capsulatum* in size and distribution. In difficult cases, it may be necessary to rely on culture isolation and identification.

Aspergillus

Aspergillus is one of a large family of fungi that has only a mycelial form. This fungus is ubiquitous in nature and is culturable from air samples, soil, dust particles, plants, and food materials. Construction or renovation projects in hospitals represent a particularly high risk for immunosuppressed patients because of exposure to contaminated dust. The species most commonly infecting humans are *Aspergillus fumigatus* and *Aspergillus flavus*. The four common forms of human infection include allergic aspergillosis, bronchopulmonary aspergillosis, aspergilloma, and disseminated aspergillosis. Fruiting bodies may form on bronchial lumina in the first three forms and are diagnostic of aspergillosis. However, disseminated disease is not associated with fruiting bodies and is often more difficult to diagnose (Rinaldi, 1983).

Disseminated aspergillosis, a life-threatening infection essentially limited to immunocompromised hosts, is the only form of aspergillosis associated with infectious lymphadenopathy. Disseminated aspergillosis begins with inhalation of hyphal forms by an immunosuppressed host, causing a suppurative necrotizing pneumonia. The severity of the pneumonic phase is highly dependent on the initial load of fungal forms inhaled. Hyphae quickly erode into adjacent blood vessels, causing thrombosis and initiating multiple emboli to virtually all organs or sites, including the central nervous system.

Touch preparations of infected lymph nodes demonstrate a neutrophilic inflammatory infiltrate, scattered eosinophils, and rare giant cells. On hematoxylin-eosin stains, scattered uniform septated hyphae may be identified, particularly if the microscope condenser is lowered to emphasize the refractile edges of the hyphae.

In tissue sections, the angioinvasive nature of disseminated aspergillosis is obvious, since fungal hyphae are readily identified in mural thrombi or penetrating the muscular media. Capillaries and small and medium-sized veins and arteries are often involved. The occluded degenerating vessels are surrounded by an intense neutrophilic inflammatory infiltrate. *Aspergillus* hyphae stain well with methenamine silver and periodic acid–Schiff. With these stains, the regularly spaced septations and 45°-angle dichotomous branching are easily appreciated. The branching pattern and distribution of *Aspergillus*, although not pathognomonic, are sufficiently characteristic to

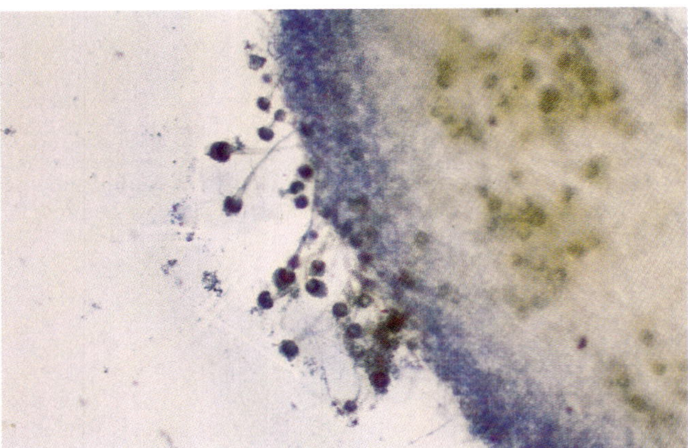

Figure 16–25

Aspergillus fumigatus. Typical morphologic features of cultured organisms are demonstrated. Lactophenol cotton blue.

allow a presumptive diagnosis from tissue sections. Diagnosis and species classification require culture, morphologic evaluation of fruiting bodies, heat stability testing, and limited biochemical testing (Fig. 16–25).

The major "look-alike" in the differential diagnosis of disseminated aspergillosis is the septate acute-angle–branching fungus *Pseudoallerichia*. *Pseudoallerichia* is distinctive in having swollen, round to club-shaped structures at the ends of its septate hyphae. These structures are not specific markers of *Pseudoallerichia*, as similar characteristics may be seen with other fungi after antifungal treatment or when hyphae degenerate. Therefore, this hyphal structure is best used for identification when abundant septate hyphae are present and the patient has not been recently treated with antifungal agents. An unusual feature of *Aspergillus* is its autofluorscence, which, in conjunction with immunoperoxidase antibodies, is helpful in identifying *Aspergillus* in difficult cases.

Pseudoallerichia and *Petriellidium*

Pseudoallerichia (Petriellidium and *Allescheria)* is commonly found in soil. Infection in humans is uncommon and essentially limited to immunocompromised hosts (Travis et al, 1985; Scherr et al, 1992). Disseminated disease has a pathogenesis similar to that of *Aspergillus*, with airway infection followed by vascular invasion and dissemination.

Touch preparations reveal a neutrophil-rich infiltrate without giant cells. Occasional septate hyphae may be identified on hematoxylin-eosin staining. Tissue sections demonstrate a pattern of tissue response identical to that of *Aspergillus*, and the septate hyphae have identical branching patterns. The distinguishing features of *Pseudoallerichia* are the bulbous, rounded hyphae and the lack of autofluorescence. An indirect immunofluorescent antibody test is available for identification of *Pseudoallerichia boydii* in tissue sections.

Sporotrichum

Sporotrichum schenckii, a dimorphic fungus normally found on plants, is a particular risk for immunocompromised patients who garden and might possibly handle rotting wood or sphagnum moss (Smith et al, 1981). *Sporotrichum* rarely causes systemic lesions but is well known for its involvement of skin and lymphatics. Penetrating skin injuries are the usual portal of entry, making thorned plants a particular risk. A localized mixed neutrophilic and granulomatous tissue reaction involves the soft tissues, followed by regional lymphatic spread of the organism. Characteristic "cord and nodule" lesions radiate from the original cutaneous injury, which persists as a nonhealing wound. The clinical picture and history are so characteristic that lymph node biopsy is rarely required for diagnosis.

Touch preparations and tissue sections demonstrate a mixed suppurative and granulomatous tissue reaction with scattered microabscesses. Organisms are usually scant in number and rarely identified on hematoxylin-eosin staining. Methenamine silver and periodic acid–Schiff stains reveal small budding yeast forms intra- and extracellularly. The yeast forms are unusual in that the daughter buds tend to be small and elongated in appearance. Hyphal forms are not seen in tissue section, and, if packed within macrophages or giant cells, *Sporotrichum* may be confused with *H. capsulatum*.

MYCOBACTERIAL LYMPHADENITIS

Mycobacterium tuberculosis

Mycobacterium tuberculosis is the most important bacterial pathogen worldwide owing to the high morbidity and mortality rates of tuberculosis. A menace to public health because of its communicability, tuberculosis is spread via inhalation. Fortunately, only a fraction of those infected with tuberculosis develop clinical disease, but, once infected, all remain at risk throughout life for reactivation of controlled foci of disease (Pitchenik et al, 1988). Virulence is related to a cell wall cord factor that inhibits phagosome-lysosome fusion and cell wall lipid components that initiate delayed cell-mediated hypersensitivity.

Almost all infections begin by inhalation of infective droplets, but tuberculosis may ultimately affect every organ system. Initially, mycobacteria multiply unimpeded for weeks in the initial pulmonary focus as well as in lymphohematogenous metastatic foci. Development of cell-mediated immunity controls the spread of individual lesions and initiates healing. Five to 15% of those infected develop active disease, and about half of these develop pulmonary cavitation and are thereby carriers. In the pediatric population, persistent cervical lymphadenopathy is a frequent manifestation of tuberculosis and one that often results in a diagnostic biopsy (Pinder & Colville, 1993). Patients with either *Mycobacterium tuberculosis* or *Mycobacterium avium-intracellular* complex may present with cervical adenopathy. Rare mixed tubercular infections have been reported (Piersimoni et al, 1991).

Lymph node biopsy specimens in tuberculosis are grossly abnormal. Granulomatous lesions appear as gray-white foci. Caseous necrosis or overt liquefaction with disruption may be noted. Recognition of tuberculosis by gross examination may avoid unnecessary contamination of a frozen-section apparatus and reduce risk of infection in laboratory personnel. Touch preparations are quite useful in revealing granulomas in these cases, since readily recognized giant cells are accompanied by scattered neutrophils and necrotic debris.

Tissue sections demonstrate well-formed granulomas with central caseation (Fig. 16–26), and acid-fast bacillus stains reveal the intracellular, slightly curved, beaded rods within giant cells and histiocytes. Occasional extracellular forms may be identified in areas of cell death and debris. Rapidly dividing mycobacterial organisms may also stain with methenamine silver. Demonstration of *rare* acid-fast bacilli in a caseating granulomatous reaction is virtually diagnostic of *M. tuberculosis*, but definitive speciation requires cultural isolation and identifi-

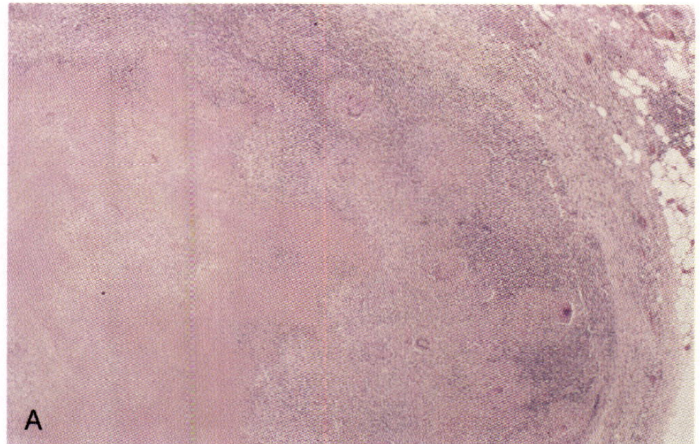
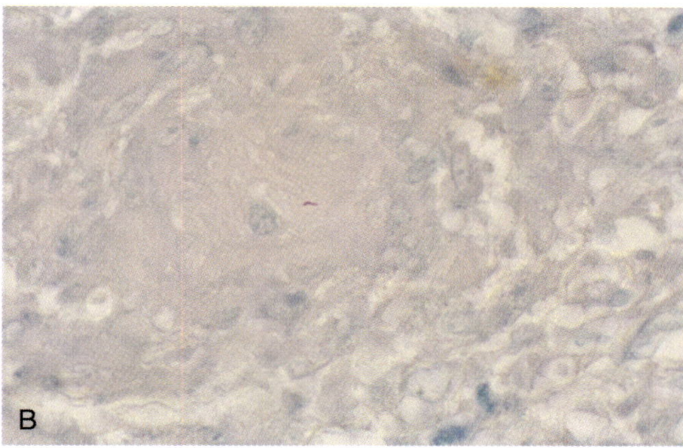

Figure 16–26

Mycobacterium tuberculosis lymphadenopathy. *A*, Prominent caseous necrosis and easily identified giant cells are noted. *B*, Organisms may be rare. Ziehl-Neelsen stain.

cation. The time for speciation of initial colony growths is significantly shortened by probe confirmation.

Mycobacterium avium-intracellulare

Mycobacterium avium-intracellulare (MAI) infection occurs in immunocompetent and immunocompromised children, with each having a distinct presentation. Special stains in both cases allow presumptive diagnosis and initiation of therapy. Confirmation by culture is readily accomplished.

MAI is the commonest cause of mycobacterial cervical lymphadenopathy, or scrofula, in immunocompetent children (Wolinsky, 1995). Scrofula is rarely caused by *Mycobacterium scrofulaceum*. Patients with scrofula present with unilateral, enlarged, somewhat tender cervical lymphadenopathy that may suppurate and drain. Touch preparations confirm the necrotic nature of these lesions and the presence of scattered giant cells. Tissue sections show caseating granulomatous lymphadenitis. Giant cells may be scant and necrosis prominent. Such cases may have scattered stellate microabscesses similar to those in cat-scratch disease. Organisms are typically scant in this form of mycobacterial infection. Search for acid-fast organisms is greatly facilitated by fluorescent microscopic studies. If mycobacteria are not identified, patients must wait up to 6 weeks for cultural confirmation. If cultures were not obtained on biopsy, the diagnosis may be confirmed using molecular methods on tissue blocks.

MAI infection in immunocompromised children usually occurs in AIDS. In these cases, since granulomas are often absent, touch preparations or tissue sections reveal abundant foamy macrophages, occasional neutrophils, eosinophils, and plasma cells. This pattern is most often identified in the gastrointestinal tract and lymph nodes. The histiocytes are packed with organisms that stain readily with acid-fast, periodic acid–Schiff, and methenamine silver stains (Fig. 16–27). Such histocytes are virtually diagnostic of MAI.

Mycobacterial infection may rarely cause a spindle cell reaction in immunocompromised patients (Fig. 16–28). The spindle cell pattern mimics a low-grade or benign spindle cell tumor, but the clinical history suggesting infection should alert pathologists to perform special stains. In this unusual tissue reaction, the spindle cells are histiocytes that contain numerous acid-fast bacilli, as revealed by special stains. Cultures confirm *MAI* infection in these cases.

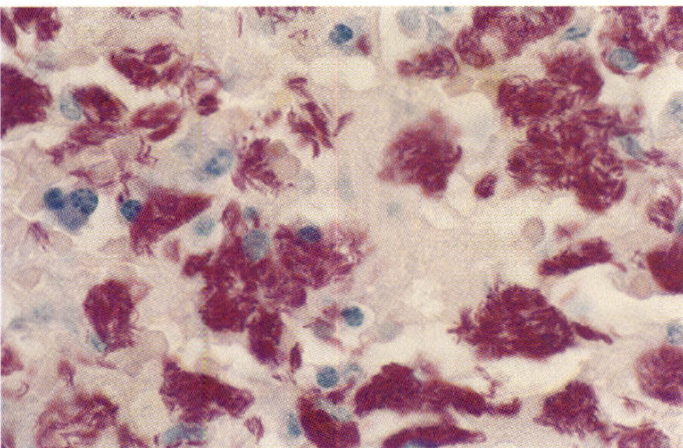

Figure 16–27

Mycobacterium avium complex lymphadenopathy. Numerous packeted intracellular acid-fast bacilli are identifiable on special stains in this immunocompromised patient. Bacterial forms may be difficult to identify in some cases of chronic cervical adenopathy (scrofula). Ziehl-Neelsen stain.

Other Atypical *Mycobacterium* Species

Other mycobacterial organisms causing infection in children and specifically infectious lymphadentitis include *Mycobacterium kansasii, M. gordonae*, and *M. scrofulaceum*. These mycobacteria generally elicit a granulomatous reaction with variable degrees of necrosis. Special stains reveal acid-fast bacilli, but confirmation of species requires culture and biochemical identification. Attribution of clinical disease to *M. gordonae* requires molecular confirmation of its presence in tissue, as this organism is a common contaminant in water.

VIRAL LYMPHADENITIS

Viral illnesses in children are frequent, may be serious, and are often difficult to treat. They are also difficult to diagnose etiologically. Viral lymphadenitis, either regional or diffuse, is seen

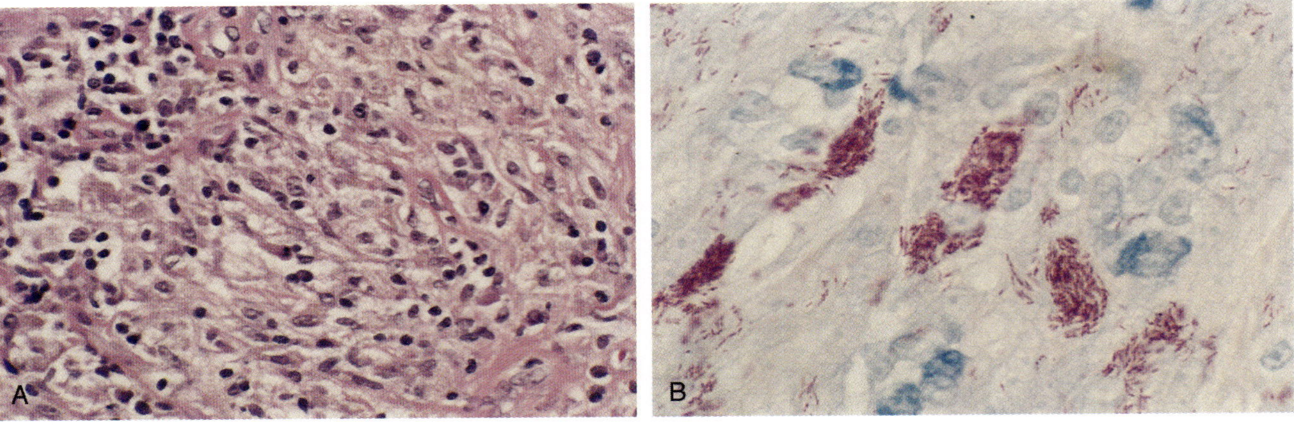

Figure 16–28

Mycobacterium avium complex lymphadenopathy. *A*, This spindle cell pattern may be encountered occasionally in immunocompromised patients. *B*, Numerous acid-fast forms are demonstrated. Ziehl-Neelsen stain.

in many viral syndromes. Histologic sections of nodes in viral lymphadenitis exhibit exuberant follicular hyperplasia, immunoblastic proliferation, and variable amounts of necrosis. Immunoblastic proliferation may be so extreme as to suggest malignancy. Although a few types of viral lymphadenitis may be specifically diagnosed by characteristic inclusions, most viral infections do not have cytopathic effects that are diagnostic of a particular agent. Additional diagnostic approaches include viral culture of lymph node biopsy specimens and/or serologic testing. Immunoperoxidase procedures and in situ hybridization studies directed toward specific viral antigens may also be quite helpful.

Epstein-Barr Virus

Epstein-Barr virus (EBV), a member of the Herpesviridae family of DNA viruses, was first seen by electron microsopic examination in Burkitt lymphoma tissue cultures (Epstein et al, 1964). This virus causes a wide assortment of human diseases (Fleisher, 1991), covered in several chapters in this book. This section focuses on EBV-caused infectious mononucleosis, a disease characterized by fatigue, fever, pharyngitis, lymphadenopathy, splenomegaly, and sometimes hepatomegaly. This infection is highly contagious and spreads readily from person to person through infected salivary droplets. Infectious mononucleosis may be asymptomatic, produce a very mild illness with pharyngitis and a low-grade fever, or produce the classic illness described here. Toddlers and children often have asymptomatic infections, whereas teenagers and young adults usually have more serious illnesses. The incubation period for EBV infection ranges from 40–60 days. Therefore, serologic markers are usually detectable at presentation. The clinical picture is often characteristic. Most diagnoses are confirmed by serologic tests showing active or recent EBV infection, thereby obviating the need for lymph node biopsies or other tissue studies (Table 16–8).

Heterophil antibodies may be detected quickly using one of the commercially available kits and are useful in evaluating a child or teenager with potential infectious mononucleosis. If EBV serologic studies fail to indicate active infection, cytomegalovirus (CMV) should be considered, since it occasionally causes an infectious mononucleosis–like syndrome (Oill et al, 1977; Rinaldo et al, 1980). Lymph node biopsies are usually performed when clinical features are atypical (e.g., minimal pharyngitis), enlarged nodes are in unusual locations (e.g., axilla or groin), or massive adenopathy or tonsillitis suggests a neoplastic process.

Lymph nodes in infectious mononucleosis are grossly enlarged, soft, and somewhat hyperemic with no focal lesions. Touch preparations or needle aspirates (see Chap. 3) demonstrate a mixed lymphocytic population that often includes a striking number of immunoblasts, plasma cells, and tingible-body macrophages. Cases characterized by large numbers of immunoblasts should undergo flow cytometric analysis even though clinical or cytologic features strongly indicate a reactive process. Polyclonal flow results may provide additional support for a reactive adenitis diagnosis if the immunoblastic reaction is particularly exuberant.

Tissue sections demonstrate marked follicular hyperplasia, with numerous immunoblasts within the nodal sinuses. Portions of nodal architecture are usually preserved, although large areas may be consolidated owing to immunoblastic proliferation. Large numbers of immunoblasts may be interspersed with small lymphocytes and plasma cells (Fig. 16–29). Reed-Sternberg–like cells, frequent mitoses, and foci of necrosis may be seen. Lymphadenopathy or enlarged tonsils in children have mistakenly been diagnosed as malignant lymphoma on the basis of an extensive immunoblastic infiltrate (see Fig. 16–29). EBV-driven reactive processes, however, are far more likely diagnoses, particularly if there is partial architectural preservation and immunoblasts are readily demonstrated in sinuses. Viral inclusions are not seen in EBV lymphadenitis. The diagnosis of EBV lymphadenitis is indicated by the constellation of partial architectural preservation, exuberant follicular hyperplasia, and paracortical immunoblastic proliferation that is shown to be polytypic on flow cytometric analysis. This histologic picture

Table 16–8

Serologic Testing for Epstein-Barr Virus Infection Status

Infection Type	Anti-VCA IgM	Anti-VCA IgG	Anti-EA	Anti-EBNA
Acute	+	+	+	−/+
Recent	+/−	+	+/−	−/+
Past	−	+	−	+

Abbreviations: anti-EA, antibodies to Epstein-Barr virus early antigens (cytoplasmic and/or nuclear nonstructural proteins); anti-EBNA, antibodies to Epstein-Barr virus nuclear antigens; anti-VCA, antibodies to Epstein-Barr virus capsular antigen.

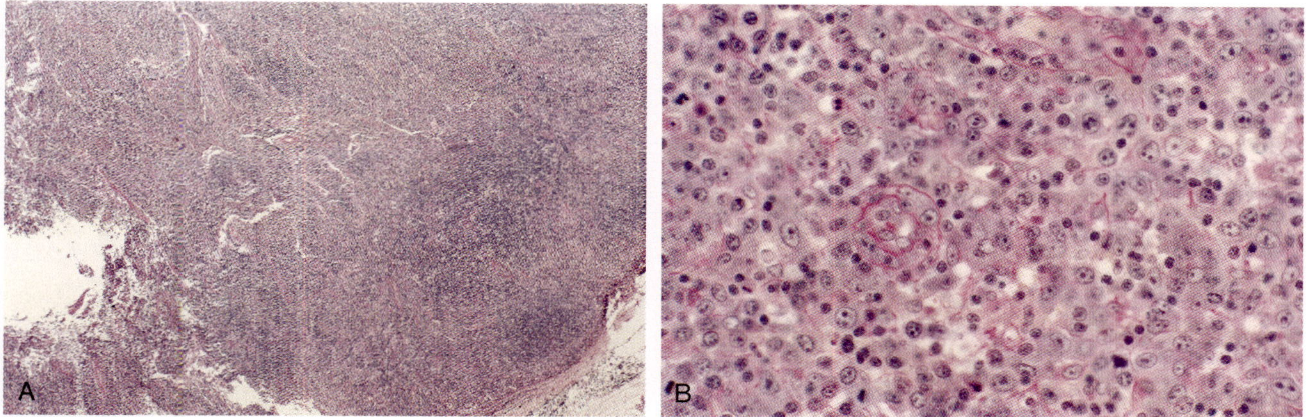

Figure 16–29

Infectious mononucleosis lymphadenopathy. *A,* Follicular hyperplasia, histiocytosis, and immunoblastic proliferation result in a ragged "moth-eaten" appearance. Periodic acid–Schiff stain. *B,* Prominent immunoblastic proliferation may mimic malignant lymphoma. Such mistaken diagnoses may be avoided by extreme caution when there is partial architectural preservation and by flow data showing a polyclonal process. Periodic acid–Schiff stain.

and serologic evidence of active EBV infection allow a diagnosis of infectious mononucleosis. Cultures for this viral pathogen are not currently available in routine laboratories, since EBV virus can only be cultivated in cord blood B lymphocytes.

Herpes Simplex

Herpes infections, described since antiquity, are caused by a DNA virus of the family Herpesviridae. After initial entry into the skin, herpes simplex virus (HSV) replicates locally in parabasal and intermediate epithelial cells, causes their lysis, and instigates a local inflammatory response. The characteristic creeping lesion of superficial cutaneous HSV infection results. Direct contact with infected material is apparently the principal mode of spread.

During primary infection, lymphatics and regional lymph nodes become involved, producing lymphadenopathy, pain, and fever. When associated with an erythematous blister, this clinical picture mimics a staphylococcal infection. The HSV finds its way to local nerves and ultimately the sensory nerve ganglia, where it may become latent and where it may reactivate to produce effects milder than those of primary infections if the host is immunocompetent. Complications of HSV infections include encephalitis, disseminated infection in immunocompromised hosts, and transmission to neonates. Herpetic lymphadenitis may occur as part of the primary or the reactivated infection (Corey & Spear, 1986; Gaffey et al, 1991; Tamaru et al, 1990).

Lymph nodes exhibit extensive zonal necrosis in well-developed HSV lymphadenitis. Touch preparations contain necrotic debris, scattered neutrophils, and a mixed lymphoplasmacytic infiltrate. Intranuclear inclusions may not be apparent on hematoxylin-eosin–stained touch preparations, and extensive necrosis is the cue that viral cultures are indicated.

Tissue sections in HSV lymphadenitis exhibit zones of coagulative necrosis with scattered nuclear inclusions (Fig. 16–30) that are often masked by extensive necrosis. Inclusions may be found most readily at the boundary between necrotic and reactive tissue. Immunoperoxidase studies for HSV may help establish the diagnosis in cases with unexplained zonal

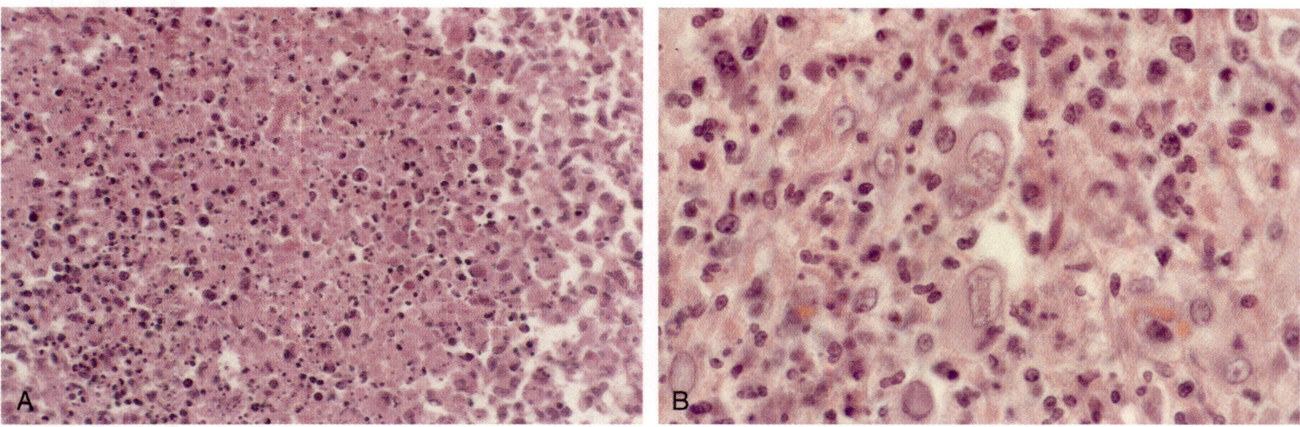

Figure 16–30

Herpes simplex lymphadenitis. *A,* Necrosis is the overriding feature. Nuclear inclusions may be sparse in some cases. *B,* Characteristic inclusions were seen in several areas.

lymph node necrosis. Antibodies are currently available for HSV-1 and HSV-2, both of which should be used as a "cocktail" in problem cases. Positive results should be reported only as "HSV positive," without mention of type, as extensive cross reactivity has been shown with these antibodies.

Infections from gram-negative bacilli also produce extensive necrosis of lymph nodes in children. Much less common causes of extensive necrosis are infarction from vascular compromise or vasculitis and Kickuchi-Fujimoto disease.

HSV infections may be diagnosed readily by viral cultures, which typically yield positive results in 1–3 days. In addition, herpetic infections may be confirmed by immunoperoxidase or molecular studies. Molecular methods are recommended to determine if HSV-1 or HSV-2 is the causative agent.

Cytomegalovirus

CMV is a DNA virus and member of the Herpesviridae family that was originally called the salivary gland virus. Long before identification of the causative virus, the presence of the disease was easily recognized by its prominent cytopathic effects and distinct nuclear or cytoplasmic viral inclusions.

CMV infections are particularly common in children in day care centers. As many as 21–59% become infected in this setting, as children acquire CMV at a younger age in crowded care arrangements (Murph et al, 1986; Pass et al, 1986; Pass & Hutto, 1986). Most initial infections are asymptomatic and are followed by viral latency. In summary, CMV infections are common, whereas symptomatic disease is rare. Reactivation of CMV may occur later, particularly when the host becomes immunocompromised. Clinical presentations of CMV disease include neonatal disease (Hanshaw, 1971), with a range of effects including encephalitis, pneumonia, hepatosplenomegaly, heterophil-negative infectious mononucleosis syndrome (Evans, 1978), postperfusion syndrome, hepatitis syndrome, chorioretinitis, and gastrointestinal syndromes.

CMV lymphadenopathy is seen in disseminated infections and may be the initial presentation of children with HIV infections. In the early stages of CMV lymphadenitis, the changes are nonspecific, with follicular hyperplasia, crowding of follicles, numerous tingible-body macrophages, immunoblastic proliferation, and apoptosis. Characteristic cytopathic changes of CMV are identified as the infection progresses. The initial change is nuclear enlargement in lymphocytes, macrophages, and endothelial cells as this DNA virus begins replication. As the nucleus fills with virions, the characteristic hyperchromatic "owl's eye" inclusion, measuring 8–10 μ, distends the nuclear space and is surrounded by a thin halo (Fig. 16–31). Basophilic cytoplasmic inclusions may appear as minute amphophilic granules. These inclusions reflect cytoplasmic viral replication. As viral inclusions develop, cells double or triple in size, justifying the term *cytomegalic*. After the cytoplasm fills with CMV virions, the cell dies and ruptures, freeing virions to infect other cells.

Immunoperoxidase studies with antibodies to CMV nuclear antigen may be helpful to confirm this diagnosis, particularly early in the infection when cytopathic effects are not as apparent. CMV immunopositivity is demonstrable as a signal from the entire nuclear surface area and cytoplasm in late infection, a signal from the entire nuclear surface area prior to the development of cytoplasmic inclusions, or focal nuclear block positivity in early infection.

Mumps Virus

Children and nonimmune adults with mumps virus, an RNA virus of the Paramyxoviridae family, usually present with painful parotitis. Infections are seasonal, with peak incidences occurring in the winter and spring months. On rare occasions, patients may present with orchitis, pancreatitis, or meningitis prior to classic parotitis. Cervical lymphadenopathy is seen in a small percentage of patients with mumps (<10%). The inflammatory infiltrate in the parotid is mononuclear, with a few lymphocytes and plasma cells around areas of necrosis. Cytoplasmic inclusions were demonstrated in acinar cells (Johnson & Goodpasture, 1936). Because mumps is clinically defined and treated without biopsy, detailed descriptions of mumps lesions in humans are not available.

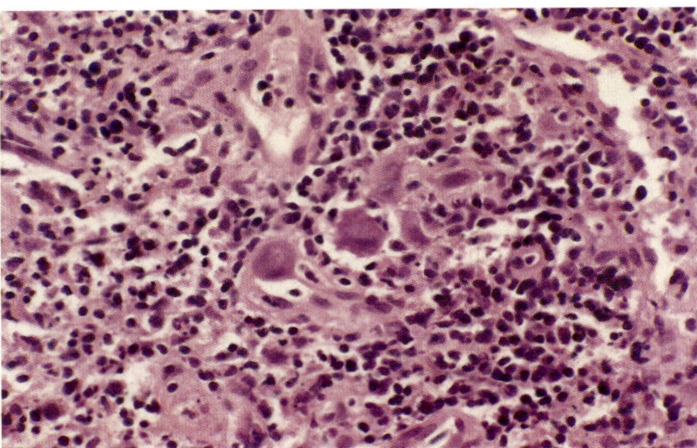

Figure 16–31

Cytomegalovirus lymphadenitis. Characteristic "owl's eye" nuclear inclusions are shown.

Human Immunodeficiency Virus and AIDS

AIDS is caused by infection with HIV-1, an enveloped RNA retrovirus. Over 21 million adults worldwide are infected with HIV, and approximately 8500 new HIV infections occur each day (Paul et al, 1996). It is estimated that 650,000 to 900,000 Americans are infected with HIV. Homosexual men represent two-thirds of these cases. The remaining one third occurs in intravenous drug users, female sexual partners of HIV-positive men, newborns of HIV-positive mothers, and hemophiliacs.

Cases of AIDS in children under 13 years of age are classified as pediatric AIDS by the Centers for Disease Control and Prevention. Infected expectant mothers who are untreated pass HIV to their children in 14–39% of cases (Blanche et al, 1989; Ryder et al, 1989). Intrauterine transmission is the most frequent route of infection in pediatric HIV infection, but viral infection also follows exposure to blood and body secretions during delivery and suckling of infected breast milk (Flynn & Shenep, 1992). The number of neonates, children, and teenagers with AIDS is increasing rapidly to near-epidemic levels. HIV infection in children follows a well-documented course of exposure, infection, and progression of disease. In this age group there is an unusually rapid progression into and through the "latent period." In addition, two distinct patterns of disease progression are described with HIV infection in children. Patients with HIV infections acquired perinatally have poor prognoses, with median survivals of only 38 months. An older age at diagnosis apparently favors a longer survival (Flynn & Shenep, 1992).

Acute HIV infections in the pediatric age group often go undetected unless there is high suspicion of HIV risk and ongoing surveillance. Acute HIV infection is characterized by a mononucleosis-like illness developing 2–3 weeks after pre-

Freeman TR, Stewart MA, Turner L: Illness after measles-mumps-rubella vaccination. Can Med Assoc J 149:1669, 1993.

Gaffey MJ, Ben-Ezra JM, Weiss LM: Herpes simplex lymphadenitis. Am J Clin Pathol 95:709, 1991.

Gellin BG, Broome CV: Listeriosis. JAMA 261:1313, 1989.

Goodwin RA, Des Prez RM: Histoplasmosis. Am Rev Respir Dis 117:929, 1978.

Goodwin RA, Shapiro JL, Thurman GH, et al: Disseminated histoplasmosis: clinical and pathologic correlations. Medicine 59:1, 1980.

Gray GF, Kimball AC, Kean BH: The posterior cervical lymph node in toxoplasmosis. Am J Pathol 69:349, 1972.

Gray ML, Killinger AH: *Listeria monocytogenes* and listeric infections. Bacteriol Rev 30:309, 1966.

Greer CE, Lund JK, Manos MM: PCR amplification from paraffin-embedded tissues: recommendations on fixatives for long-term storage and prospective studies. PCR Methods Appl 1:46, 1991.

Hanshaw JB: Congenital cytomegalovirus infection: a fifteen year perspective. J Infect Dis 123:555, 1971.

Harrison L F, Hanson I C: Congenital immunodeficiencies. In Patrick CC (ed): Infections in Immunocompromised Infants and Children. Churchill Livingstone, New York, p 179, 1992.

Hartsock JR: Postvaccinial lymphadenitis: hyperplasia of lymphoid tissue that simulates malignant lymphomas. Cancer 21:632, 1968.

Heyman MR, Rasmussen P: *Pneumocystis carinii* involvement of the bone marrow in acquired immunodeficiency syndrome. Am J Clin Pathol 87:780, 1987.

Hodes HL: Diphtheria. Pediatr Clin North Am 26:445, 1979.

Huntington RW: Coccidioidomycosis: a great imitator disease. Arch Pathol Lab Med 110:182, 1986.

Ioachim HL: Sinus histiocytosis with massive lymphadenopathy. In Lymph Node Pathology, Lippincott, Philadelphia, p 13, 1994.

Isaacs D: Cervical lymphadenopathy. In Isaacs D, Moxon ER (eds): A Practical Approach to Pediatric Infections. Churchill Livingstone, New York, p 87, 1996.

Johnson CD, Goodpasture EW: The histopathology of experimental mumps in the monkey, *Macacus rhesus*. Am J Pathol 12:495–510, 1936.

Kawasaki T: MCLS: clinical observations of 50 cases. Jpn J Allergy 16:178, 1967.

Kerkering TM, Duma RJ, Shadomy S: The evolution of pulmonary cryptococcosis: clincial implications from a study of 41 patients with and without compromising host factors. Ann Intern Med 94:611, 1981.

Kikuchi M: Histiocytic necrotizing lymphadenitis (Kikuchi-Fujimoto disease) in Japan. Am J Surg Pathol 15:197, 1991.

Krasinski K, Borkowsky W, Bonk S, et al: Bacterial infections in human immunodeficiency virus–infected children. Pediatr Infect Dis J 7:323, 1988.

Krugman S, Ward R, Katz SL: Diphtheria. In Infectious Diseases of Children, 6th ed. C.V. Mosby, Saint Louis, p 13, 1977.

Lane RJ, Keane WM, Potsic WP: Pediatric infectious lymphadenitis. Otolaryngol Head Neck Surg 88:332, 1980.

Layfield LJ, Glasgow BJ, DuPuis MH: Fine-needle aspiration of lymphadenopathy of suspected infectious etiology. Arch Pathol Lab Med 109:810, 1985.

Lee LA, Gerber AR, Lonsway DR, et al: *Yersinia enterocolitica* 0:3 infections in infants and children, associated with the household preparation of chitterlings. N Engl J Med 322:984, 1990.

Levin M, Tizard EJ, Killon MJ: Kawasaki disease: recent advances. Arch Dis Child 66:1369, 1991.

Lewis JL, Rabinovich S: The wide spectrum of cryptococcal infections. Am J Med 53:315, 1972.

Luft BJ, Naot Y, Araujo FG, et al: Primary and reactivated *Toxoplasma* infection in patients with cardiac transplants. Ann Intern Med 99:27, 1983.

Meier FA: *Pseudomonas aeruginosa*. In Connor DH, Chandler FW, Schwartz DA, et al (eds): Pathology of Infectious Diseases. Appleton & Lange, Stamford, CT, p 739, 1997.

Melish ME, Marchette NJ: Kawasaki syndrome. In Belsche RB (ed): Textbook of Human Virology. C.V. Mosby, St. Louis, p 1021, 1991.

Murph JR, Bale JF, Murray JC, et al: Cytomegalovirus transmission in a Midwest day care center: possible relationship to child care practices. J Pediatr 109:35, 1986.

Murray JC, Singh RR, Brandt ML, et al: Granulomatous submandibular lymphadenitis caused by *Salmonella* species in a healthy child. Clin Infect Dis 19:1175, 1994.

Musher DM, Hamill RJ, Baughn RE: Effect of human immunodeficiency virus (HIV) infection on the course of syphilis and on the response to treatment. Ann Intern Med 113:872, 1990.

Myerowitz RL, Pazin GJ, Allen CM: Disseminated candidiasis: changes in incidence, underlying disease, and pathology. Am J Clin Pathol 68:29, 1977.

Naqvi SH, Thobani S, Moazam F, et al: Generalized suppurative lymphadenitis with typhoidal salmonellosis. Pediatr Infect Dis J 7:882, 1988.

Nussinovitch M, Harel L, Varsano I: Arthritis after mumps and measles vaccination. Arch Dis Child 72:348, 1995.

Oill PA, Fiala M, Schofferman J, et al: Cytomegalovirus mononucleosis in a healthy adult: association with hepatitis, secondary Epstein-Barr virus antibody response and immunosuppression. Am J Med 62:413, 1977.

Owens DK, Holodniy M, McDonald TW, et al: A meta-analytic evaluation of the polymerase chain reaction for the diagnosis of HIV infection in infants. JAMA 275:1342, 1996.

Pass RF, Hutto C: Group day care and cytomegalovirus infections of mothers and children. Rev Infect Dis 8:599, 1986.

Pass RF, Hutto C, Ricks R, et al: Increased rate of cytomegalovirus among parents of children attending day care centers. N Engl J Med 314:1414, 1986.

Paul SM, Brown JW, Gorney M, et al: One world one hope AIDS 11th International Conference overview. Med Lab Observ 28:24, 1996.

Perkins SL, Segal GH, Kjeldsberg CR: Work-up of lymphadenopathy in children. Semin Diagn Pathol 12:284, 1995.

Piersimoni C, Felici L, Giorgi P, et al: Mixed mycobacterial infection of cervical lymph nodes. Pediatr Infect Dis J 10:544, 1991.

Pinder SE, Colville A: Mycobacterial cervical lymphadenitis in children: can histological assessment help differentiate infections caused by non-tuberulous mycobacteria from *Mycobacterium tuberculosis*? Histopathology 22:59, 1993.

Pitchenik AE, Fertel D, Bloch AB: Mycobacterial disease: epidemiology, diagnosis, treatment and prevention. Clin Chest Med 9:425, 1988.

Rinaldi MG: Invasive aspergillosis. Rev Infect Dis 5:1061, 1983.

Rinaldo CR, Carney WP, Richter BS, et al: Mechanisms of immunosuppression in cytomegaloviral mononucleosis. J Infect Dis 141:488, 1980.

Risdall RJ, McKenna RW, Nesbit ME, et al: Virus-associated hemophagocytic syndrome: a benign histiocytic proliferation distinct from malignant histiocytosis. Cancer 44:993, 1979.

Rosen FS, Cooper MD, Wedgwood RJP: The primary immunodeficiencies. N Engl J Med 333:431, 1995.

Rubinstein A, Morecki R, Silverman B, et al: Pulmonary disease in children with acquired immune deficiency syndrome and AIDS-related complex. J Pediatr 108:498, 1986.

Ryder RW, Nsa W, Hassig SE, et al: Perinatal transmission of the human immunodeficiency virus type 1 to infants of seropositive women in Zaire. N Engl J Med 320:1637, 1989.

Saari TN, Triplett DA: *Yersinia pseudotuberculosis* mesenteric adenitis. J Pediatr 85:656, 1974.

Said JW: Lymphoreticular system. In Nash G, Said JW (eds): Pathology of AIDS and HIV Infection, vol 26 in Major Problems in Pathology, W.B. Saunders Company, Philadelphia, p 35, 1992.

Sarosi GA, Davies SF: Blastomycosis. Am Rev Respir Dis 120:911, 1979.

Scherr GR, Evans SG, Kiyabu MT, et al: *Pseudoallescheria boydii* infection in the acquired immunodeficiency syndrome. Arch Pathol Lab Med 116:535, 1992.

Schultenover SJ, Ramzy I, Page CP, et al: Fine needle aspiration biopsy: role and limitations in surgical decision making. Am J Clin Pathol 82:405, 1984.

Scott MA, Graham BS, Verrall R, et al: *Rhodococcus equi*—an increasingly recognized opportunistic pathogen: report of 12 cases and review of 65 cases within the literature. Am J Clin Pathol 103:649, 1995.

Scott MA, McCurley TL, Vnencak-Jones CL, et al: Cat-scratch disease: detection of *Bartonella henselae* DNA in archival biopsies from patients with clinically, serologically, and histologically defined disease. Am J Pathol 149:2161, 1996.

Sell S, Norris SJ: The biology, pathology, and immunology of syphilis. Int Rev Exp Pathol 24:203, 1983.

Siegel RJ: Infection associated hemophagocytosis syndrome. In Connor DH, Chandler FW, et al (eds): Pathology of Infectious Diseases. Appleton & Lange, Stamford, CT, p 137, 1997.

Slavin MA, Meyers JD, Remington JS, et al: *Toxoplasma gondii* infection in marrow transplant recipients: a 20 year experience. Bone Marrow Transplant 13:549, 1994.

Smith PW, Loomis GW, Luckasen JL, et al: Disseminated cutaneous sporotrichosis: three illustrative cases. Arch Dermatol 117:143, 1981.

Soave R, Murrary HW, Litrenta MM: Bacterial invasion of pulmonary vessels: *Pseudomonas* bacteremia mimicking pulmonary thromboembolism with infarction. Am J Med 65:864, 1978.

Spector SA, Gleber RD, McGrath N, et al: A controlled trial of intravenous immune globulin for the prevention of serious bacterial infections in children receiving zidovudine for advanced human immunodeficiency virus infection. N Engl J Med 331:1181, 1994.

Steele RW, Abernathy RS: Systemic blastomycosis in children. Pediatr Infect Dis 2:304, 1983.

Tamaru J, Mikata A, Horie H, et al: Herpes simplex lymphadenitis: report of two cases with review of the literature. Am J Surg Pathol 14:571, 1990.

Thomsen F, Henriques U, Magnusson MM: *Corynebacterium equi manusson* isolated from a tuberculoid lesion in a child with adenitis colli. Dan Med Bull 15:135, 1968.

Tomita S, Kato H, Fujumoto T, et al: Cytopathogenic protein in filtrates from cultures of *Proprionobacterium acnes* isolated from patients with Kawasaki disease. Br Med J 295:1229, 1987.

Travis LB, Roberts GD, Wilson WR: Clinical significance of *pseudoallescheria boydii*: a review of 10 years experience. Mayo Clin Proc 60:531, 1985.

Tschirhart D, Klatt EC: Disseminated toxoplasmosis in the acquired immunodeficiency syndrome. Arch Pathol Lab Med 112:1237, 1988.

Turner RR, Martin J, Dorfman RF: Necrotizing lymphadenitis: a study of 30 cases. Am J Surg Pathol 7:115, 1983.

Van Etta LL, Filice GA, Ferguson M, et al: *Corynebacterium equi*: a review of 12 cases of human infection. Rev Infect Dis 5:1012, 1983.

von Lichtenberg F: Bacterial infections. In Pathology of Infectious Diseases. Raven Press, New York, p 96, 1991.

Wear DJ, Margileth AM, Hadfield TL, et al: Cat-scratch disease: a bacterial infection. Science 221:1403, 1983.

Weniger BG, Warren AJ, Forseth V, et al: Human bubonic plague transmitted by a domestic cat-scratch. JAMA 251:927, 1984.

Wolinsky E: Mycobacterial lymphadenitis in children: a prospective study of 105 nontuberculous cases with long-term follow-up. Clin Infect Dis 20:954, 1995.

Yamauchi T, Ferrieri P, Anthony BF: The aetiology of acute cervical adenitis in children: serological and bacteriological studies. J Med Microbiol 13:37, 1980.

Ziegler EJ, Douglas H: *Pseudomonas aeruginosa* vasculitis and bacteremia following conjuctivitis: a simple model of fatal *Pseudomonas* infection in neutropenia. J Infect Dis 139:288, 1979.

Sanya Sukpanichnant

Leishmaniasis, Melioidosis, Penicilliosis, and Typhoid Fever

LEISHMANIASIS

Equivalent Terms

Leishmaniasis is also known as uta, pian bois, chiclero ulcer (cutaneous leishmaniasis), and kala-azar (visceral leishmaniasis).

Definition

Leishmaniasis is an endemic infection caused by protozoan of the genus *Leishmania*, family Trypanosomatidae, and order Kinetoplastida that occurs predominantly in tropical and subtropical regions.

Clinical Features

Leishmaniasis has cutaneous, mucocutaneous, and visceral forms, the first two varying from a single, small, self-healing ulcer to disfigurement. Visceral leishmaniasis mainly affects children and young adults and has an incubation period of 2–4 months. Most infected individuals are asymptomatic (latent infection). However, some develop acute, subacute, or chronic disease. The risk factors for dissemination are usually young age and malnutrition. Children with classic visceral leishmaniasis are usually 3 to 4 years in age. Fever, weight loss, weakness, cough, diarrhea, and abdominal swelling are common. Skin pigmentation of the face, feet, and hands is noted, giving rise to the name kala-azar, or the "black sickness." The patients also have anemia, edema, bleeding disorders, and extreme hepatosplenomegaly. Generalized mild lymphadenopathy occurs in some cases. Multiple organ failure, superimposed infection, and hemorrhage are the common causes of death (Bittencourt & Barral-Netto, 1995).

Laboratory Features

Lymph nodes exhibit atrophy of follicles and hyperplasia of macrophages and plasma cells. Macrophages are loaded with leishmanial amastigotes, which in Giemsa- or Wright-stained preparations have pale-blue cytoplasm with a round nucleus and a rod-shaped kinetoplast (Fig. 16–38). In hematoxylin-eosin–stained sections, oil immersion is usually needed to see the characteristic kinetoplasts (Fig. 16–39).

The spleen is usually enlarged, weighing from 500 to 2000 g, mainly owing to enlargement of the red pulp by parasitized macrophages and plasma cells. Hemorrhagic infarcts and siderotic nodules are frequently seen (Veress et al, 1977). The white pulp is atrophic because of a loss of small lymphocytes. The marrow exhibits plasmacytosis and monocytic hyperplasia. Some patients are pancytopenic from decreased hematopoiesis and/or hemophagocytic syndrome. Granulomatous reactions, with caseous necrosis and fibrinoid deposits, are noted in the cutaneous and mucocutaneous forms (Bittencourt & Barral-Netto, 1995).

Cases with both negative results on direct examination and negative culture results may be diagnosed by serologic tests using enzyme-linked immunosorbent assay (ELISA) or indirect immunofluorescence assay. Cross-reactions with leprosy, Chagas disease, malaria, and schistosomiasis may be observed.

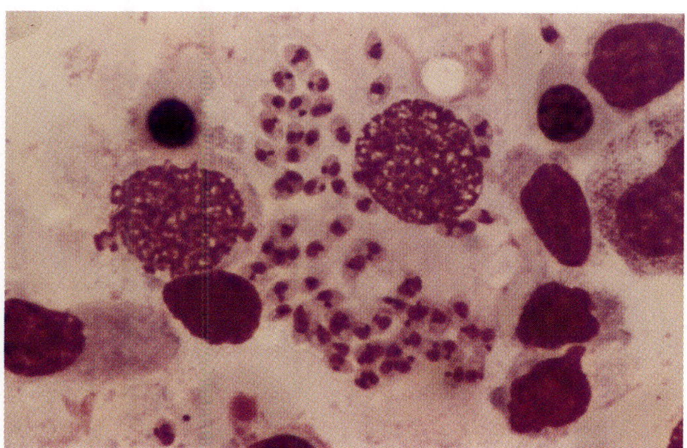

Figure 16–38

Leishmaniasis, marrow. Amastigotes of leishmaniasis are characterized by the presence of a nucleus and a rod-shaped kinetoplast. Wright stain.

The leishmaniasis skin test result is positive except in active visceral leishmaniasis, in which it becomes positive after treatment. Molecular techniques may also be used to identify the infectious agent (Howard et al, 1991).

Diagnostic Criteria

The diagnosis of leishmaniasis is made simply by the identification of the amastigote of leishmaniasis in Giemsa- or Wright-stained preparations from marrow, lymph node, or splenic biopsy (see Fig. 16–38). Confirmation in difficult cases is by using antiamastigote antibody or by culture. Serologic tests and skin tests are useful in detecting latent infections.

Differential Diagnosis

Many infections simulate leishmaniasis clinically, requiring tissue sections or a complete microbiologic investigation for exclusion.

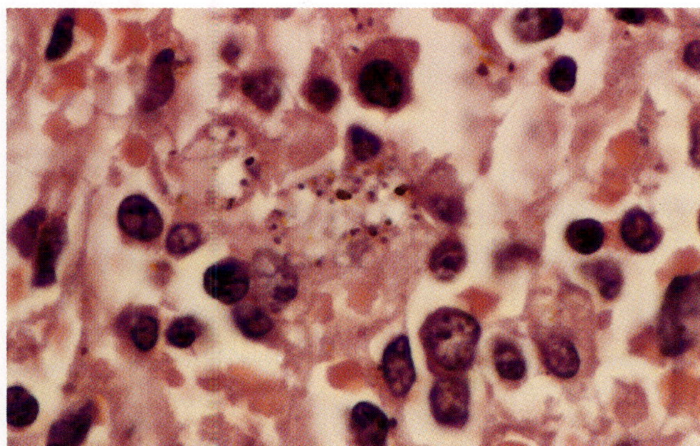

Figure 16–39

Leishmaniasis, lymph node. Amastigotes are noted in the cytoplasm of macrophages. The kinetoplast is less obvious than that in Wright- or Giemsa-stained smears.

Pathogenesis

Leishmaniasis is a zoonosis, in which the important vector is the sandfly. Promastigotes (flagellar forms) are inoculated into the skin and transform into amastigotes (aflagellar forms) inside macrophages. Depending on host immunity, the infection is controlled or disseminates to the hematopoietic organs. Suppression of cellular immunity during active disease may be due to a defect in accessory cell function, defective T cell function, or both (Bittencourt & Barral-Netto, 1995).

MELIOIDOSIS

Equivalent Terms

Melioidosis is also known as Whitmore disease.

Definition

Melioidosis is a tropical glanders-like disease caused by a gram-negative bacillus, *Burkholderia (Pseudomonas) pseudomallei*. The organisms are primarily found in water and soil. Melioidosis is most prevalent in Southeast Asia and northern Australia (Dance, 1991).

Clinical Features

Melioidosis has a broad spectrum of clinical manifestation, including inapparent infection, abscess formation, acute necrotizing pneumonia, and fulminant septicemia or chronic suppuration. The incubation period is not known. Primary infection often results in inapparent or mild illness with localized skin and lymph node lesions. At least half of the septicemic cases have chronic underlying diseases, such as liver or renal disease, malignancy, systemic lupus erythematosus, and immunodeficiency (Tanphaichitra, 1989).

The septicemic form has a very high mortality rate unless effective antibiotic therapy is administered. Relapse following appropriate antibiotic therapy occurs in 25% of patients with bacteremic disease (Chaowagul et al, 1993).

Laboratory Features

Suppurative lesions, sinus histiocytosis, and erythrophagocytosis may be seen in lymph nodes in acute melioidosis. Neutrophils accumulate in the center of the suppurative lesions (Fig. 16–40), and necrosis is constantly found at the advancing edge of the lesions. A hemorrhagic zone may be found in pulmonary lesions (Piggott & Hochholzer, 1970). Disseminated abscesses are noted in acute systemic disease. Gram-negative bipolar-staining bacilli may be demonstrated in this necrotic zone by the Brown and Hopps (tissue Gram) stain (Fig. 16–41). The organism also is visualized with Giemsa stains.

Chronic granulomatous inflammation is the hallmark of chronic melioidosis (Fig. 16–42). Central caseous necrosis may occur, mimicking tuberculosis. The causative organism is seldom identified in this form. Chronic melioidosis has been described in lungs, bone, soft tissue, liver, pancreas, urinary tract, testis, prostate, pleura, brain, and endocardium (Tanphaichitra, 1989).

Burkholderia pseudomallei may be cultivated from blood, pus, sputum, or affected organs. Direct immunofluorescent staining allows visualization of the organism in situ, and antibodies are detected by complement fixation, indirect hemagglutination,

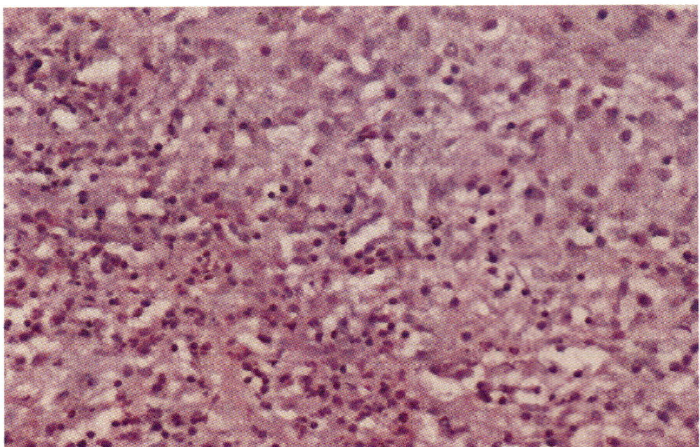

Figure 16–40

Acute melioidosis, lymph node. Accumulation of neutrophils is noted, as are macrophages. The necrotic area is not shown. (Courtesy Dr. Kanit Atisook.)

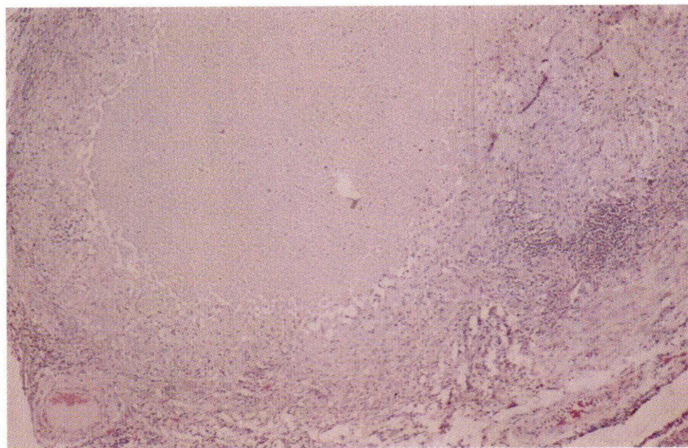

Figure 16–42

Chronic melioidosis, lymph node. This chronic granulomatous inflammation is not distinguishable from tuberculosis and other granulomatous infections. Central caseous necrosis is sometimes present in chronic melioidosis. (Courtesy Dr. Kanit Atisook.)

indirect immunofluorescence, and ELISA. A very sensitive avidin-biotin ELISA has been developed for antigens in serum (Isaäcson & Hale, 1995). Rapid detection by polymerase chain reaction is possible (Bauernfeind et al, 1998).

Diagnostic Criteria

The diagnosis of melioidosis is made by identification of the organism by Gram or Giemsa staining of infected material, with confirmation by culture and serologic tests.

Differential Diagnosis

Acute melioidosis is mimicked by acute suppurative inflammation from other infectious agents, whereas chronic melioidosis resembles tuberculosis, lymphogranuloma venereum, cat-scratch disease, and tularemia. Identification of the causative organism by Gram stain and culture is essential for diagnosis.

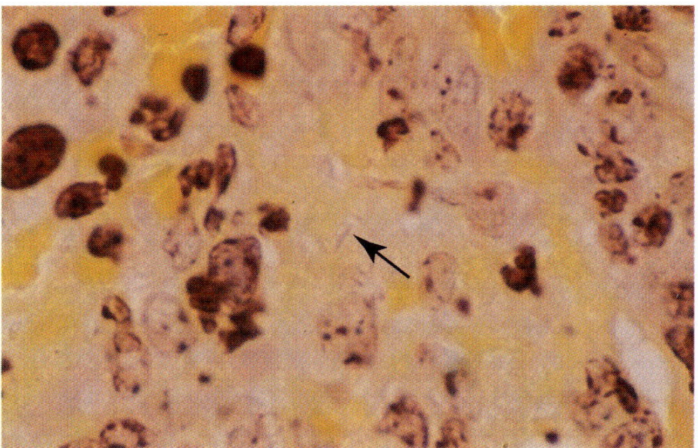

Figure 16–41

Burkholderia (Pseudomonas) pseudomallei, lymph node. A slender, slightly curved, gram-negative bacillus (*arrow*) is demonstrated in acute melioidosis. Brown and Hopps stain. (Courtesy Dr. Kanit Atisook.)

Pathogenesis

Burkholderia pseudomallei is an aerobic, non–spore-forming, small, motile, gram-negative rod that is straight or slightly curved. It is 1–5 μm long and 0.5–1 μm wide. The disease is acquired either by inhalation or by contact of cut or abraded skin with contaminated soil or water. *Burkholderia pseudomallei* (as well as *Mycobacterium tuberculosis*) survives and multiplies in macrophages (Pruksachartvuthi et al, 1990), accounting for the latency of infection in primary infection and recrudescence in other patients. Tissue necrosis consistently observed with large numbers of bacteria is probably due to production of heat-stable endotoxin, thermolabile exotoxin, and proteolytic enzymes. Effective cellular immunity is essential to control this intracellular organism.

PENICILLIOSIS

Equivalent Terms

Penicillium marneffei infection is also known as penicilliosis marneffei.

Definition

Penicillium marneffei infection is an opportunistic mycosis. Infection with this dimorphic fungus is endemic in Southeast Asia, where bamboo rats, the natural reservoir of this fungus, are found (Crissey et al, 1995).

Clinical Features

Penicillium marneffei infection is usually disseminated, because most patients are immunocompromised from HIV infection. Patients with other underlying diseases, such as tuberculosis, systemic lupus erythematosus, and lymphomas are also infected (Jayanetra et al, 1984). Subacute or chronic pyrexia is common. Other common clinical manifestations include anemia, weight loss, and skin and mucocutaneous lesions. The skin lesions vary from scattered erythematous papules, nodules, and pustules to deep-seated subcutaneous abscesses. Mucocu-

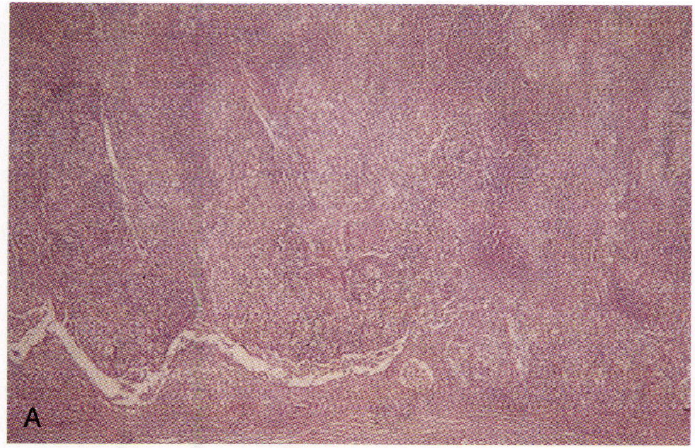

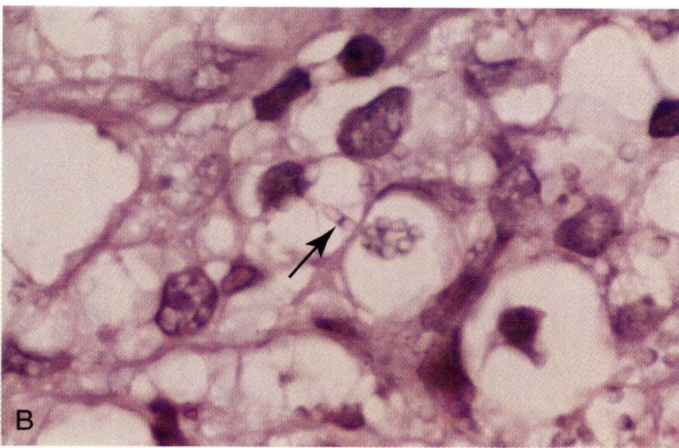

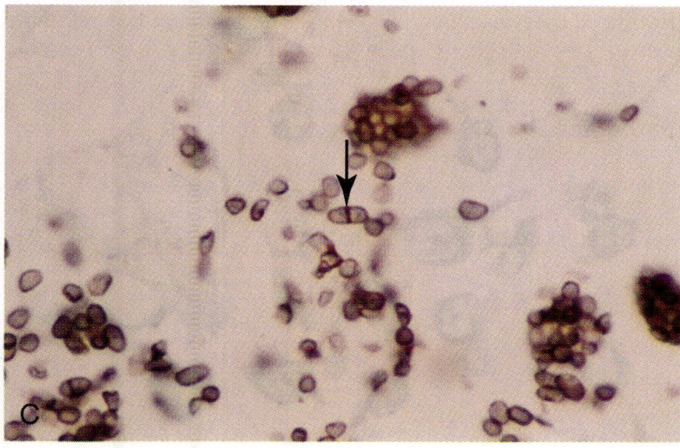

Figure 16–43

Penicillium marneffei, lymph node. *A*. Focal necrosis and accumulation of macrophages efface the lymph node architecture. The subcapsular sinus is partly preserved. *B*. Aggregates of yeast cells are noted in the cytoplasm of macrophages. In this case, a thick septation (binary fission) is demonstrated (*arrow*). *C*. Small yeast cells with some variation in size are noted. A typical thick septation is clearly demonstrated (*arrow*). Grocott methenamine silver.

taneous lesions may include oropharyngeal and genital ulcers. Infections may be widespread, involving lymph nodes, spleen, liver, intestine, lungs, pericardium, and marrow, with fatal outcomes in untreated patients.

Laboratory Features

Granulomatous inflammation and necrosis are the basic lesions (Fig. 16–43*A*). The infectious agents are yeastlike cells with thick septa universally found engulfed by macrophages (Fig. 16–43*B*) or lying free. They do not stain with hematoxylin-eosin but may be visualized by adjusting the contrast of the light microscope or staining with periodic acid–Schiff stain and Grocott methenamine silver (Fig. 16–43*C*). *Penicillium marneffei* measures 2×2 μm^2 to 3×6.5 μm^2 and does not exhibit budding. The somewhat elongated form with thick septation is unique to *P. marneffei*. Wright- or Giemsa-stained smears of peripheral blood, marrow aspirate, touch imprints of lymph node biopsy specimens, or aspirate of subcutaneous abscess may be used for identification (Fig. 16–44).

Cultures are needed for confirmation, or organisms may be identified by exoantigen assay (Sekhon et al, 1982). Serodiagnosis of *P. marneffei* infection is also possible (Crissey et al, 1995) as is identification of the organism by polymerase chain reaction (LoBuglio & Taylor, 1995).

Diagnostic Criteria

Penicillium marneffei infection should be suspected in immunocompromised residents or visitors in Southeast Asia if they develop fever, cough, weight loss, pulmonary infiltration, and skin and mucocutaneous lesions. Rapid diagnosis may be made by demonstrating *P. marneffei* yeastlike cells in the peripheral blood films or aspirates from abscesses. Cultural confirmation is useful unless the pathologists is familiar with the morphologic features of this organism.

Differential Diagnosis

The most important alternative diagnosis is histoplasmosis. *Histoplasma capsulatum* exhibits budding, rather than binary

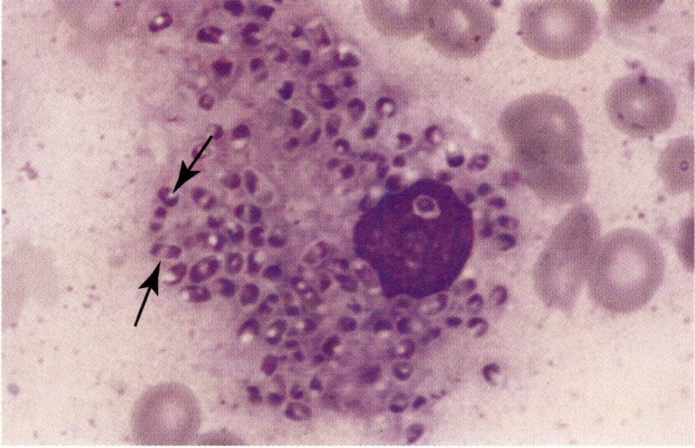

Figure 16–44

Penicillium marneffei, marrow. Many yeast cells are engulfed by a macrophage. Note that some forms are elongated and have thick, central, clear septations (*arrows*). Wright stain. (Courtesy Dr. Gavivann Veerakul.)

fission and does not septate. Less problematic differential diagnoses include *Pneumocystis carinii* and *Cryptococcus neoformans*. The former does not exhibit budding or septation, and the latter has a mucin-positive capsule.

Biologic Characteristics

Penicillium marneffei is closely related to species of the *Penicillium* subgenus *Biverticillium* and to sexual *Talaromyces* species with asexual biverticillate *Penicillium* states (LoBuglio & Taylor, 1995). It is the only true pathogen among members of the genus *Penicillium*. The portal of entry is probably pulmonary (Crissey et al, 1995).

TYPHOID FEVER

Equivalent Terms

Typhoid fever is also known as enteric fever.

Definition

Typhoid fever is a subacute systemic bacterial infection caused by *Salmonella typhi*, a gram-negative bacterium belonging to the Enterobacteriaceae (Isaäcson & Hale, 1995).

Clinical Features

The onset of illness is insidious. A prodrome for 1–3 weeks of malaise, fatigue, and headache is followed by fever with bradycardia, myalgia, anorexia, and lower abdominal pain. Rose spots, small pink maculopapular lesions, may appear transiently on the abdomen. Splenomegaly is observed in about half of the patients. Lymphadenopathy and hepatomegaly are less common. Fever remains for weeks. Complications include intestinal perforation, hemorrhage, disseminated intravascular coagulation, myocarditis, thrombophlebitis, peripheral vascular collapse, meningitis, pneumonia, and death. Common neuropsychiatric manifestations are confusion, delirium, coma, generalized myoclonus, parkinsonian rigidity, and psychosis.

Laboratory Features

The lymph node architecture may be partially effaced by typhoid nodules, which are most prominent in the paracortex (Fig. 16–45*A*). These nodules are characterized by numerous macrophages, known as Mallory cells (Fig. 16–45*B*), that exhibit abundant eosinophilic cytoplasm with distinct phagocytosis of lymphocytes, erythrocytes, and typhoid bacilli. Typhoid nodules tend to coalesce and exhibit central necrosis. Plasma cells and lymphocytes are prominent, whereas neutrophils are absent or rare. Typhoid nodules may be found in the red pulp of the spleen, liver parenchyma, marrow, testis, kidney, parotid gland, and brain. Ulceration in the ileum follows necrosis of Peyer patches and may lead to the dreaded complication of perforation or hemorrhage. Hemophagocytic syndrome may occur in typhoid fever (Smith, 1976).

Isolation of *S. typhi* from blood, stool, or urine is mandatory for diagnosis. Recent infections are confirmed by the Widal agglutination test on paired sera showing a fourfold rise in specific O (somatic) and H (flagellar) antibody titers. Carriers may have positive stool or urine cultures results but do not demonstrate such a change in serologic features.

Diagnostic Criteria

Most diagnoses of typhoid fever are made in patients of low socioeconomic status who have had a prolonged fever and other clinical features described earlier. Positive culture results and a fourfold rise in the Widal test confirm the diagnosis. Biopsies of node or marrow may provide helpful clues to the diagnosis.

Differential Diagnosis

Some patients with typhoid fever have the clinical features of fever of unknown origin, triggering consideration of autoimmune disease, hematologic malignancy, or other chronic infections.

Pathogenesis

Humans are the only reservoir, or carrier, of *S. typhi*. Carriers are commonly identified in developing areas with poor socioeconomic conditions. The portal of entry is the oral route. The

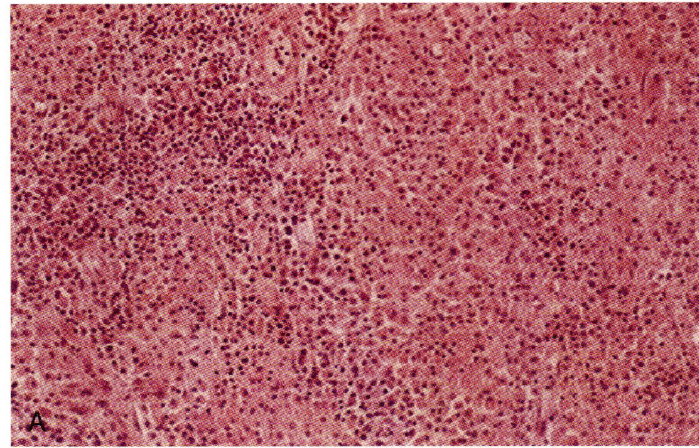

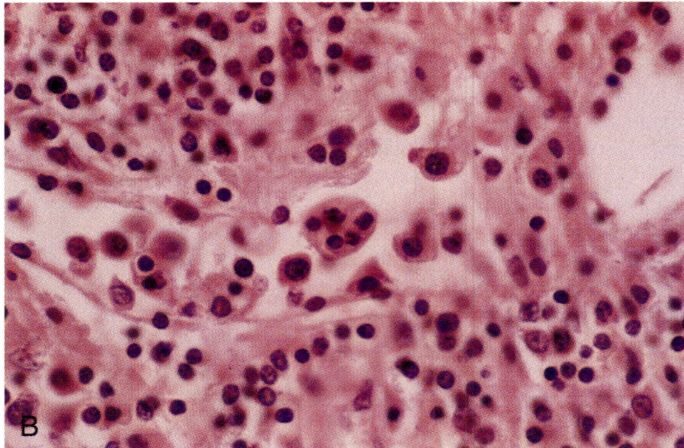

Figure 16–45

Typhoid fever, mesenteric lymph node. *A*, Many macrophages have accumulated, particularly in the paracortex. *B*, Macrophages with well-defined eosinophilic cytoplasm (Mallory cells) are noted. Some show phagocytic activity.

pathogenesis of typhoid fever is not fully elucidated. Apparently *S. typhi* enters the epithelial cells of the small intestine and initiates a mononuclear inflammatory infiltrate in the lamina propria. *Salmonella typhi* is an obligate intracellular parasite. Surviving within the cytoplasm of macrophages, organisms may disseminate to liver, spleen, and marrow. After proliferation in these cells during the incubation period, organisms are released into the circulation, resulting in septicemia (Hornick, 1985).

REFERENCES

Leishmaniasis

Bittencourt AL, Barral-Netto M: Leishmaniasis. In: Doerr W, Seifert G (eds): Tropical Pathology, 2nd ed. Springer-Verlag, Berlin, pp 597–651, 1995.

Howard MK, Kelly JM, Lane RP, et al: A sensitivity repetitive DNA probe that is specific to the *Leishmania donovani* complex and its use as an epidemic logical and diagnostic reagent. Mol Biochem Parasitol 44:63–72, 1991.

Veress B, Omer A, Satir AA, et al: Morphology of spleen and lymph nodes in fatal visceral leishmaniasis. Immunology 33:605–610, 1977.

Melioidosis

Bauernfeind A, Roller C, Meyer D, et al: Molecular procedure for rapid detection of *Burkholderia mallei* and *Burkholderia pseudomallei*. J Clin Microbiol 36:2737–2741, 1998.

Chaowagul W, Suputtamongkol Y, Dance DAB, et al: Relapse in melioidosis: incidence and risk factors. J Infect Dis 168:1181–1185, 1993.

Dance DAB: Melioidosis: the tip of the iceberg? Clin Microbiol Rev 4:52–60, 1991.

Isaäcson M, Hale MJ: Non-intestinal bacterial infections. In: Doerr W, Seifert G (eds): Tropical Pathology, 2nd ed. Springer-Verlag, Berlin, pp 179–222, 1995.

Piggot JA, Hochholzer L: Human melioidosis: a histopathologic study of acute and chronic melioidosis. Arch Pathol 90:101–111, 1970.

Pruksachartvuthi S, Aswapokee N, Thakerngpol K: Survival of *Pseudomonas pseudomallei* in human phagocytes. J Med Microbiol 31:109–114, 1990.

Tanphaichitra D: Tropical disease in the immunocompromised host: melioidosis and pythiosis. Rev Infect Dis 11(suppl 7):S1629–S1643, 1989.

Penicilliosis

Crissey JT, Lang H, Parish LC: Manual of Medical Mycology. Blackwell Scientific, MA, pp 232–234, 1995.

Jayanetra P, Nittiyanant P, Ajello A, et al: Penicilliosis marneffei in Thailand: report of five human cases. Am J Trop Med Hyg 33:637–644, 1984.

LoBuglio KF, Taylor JW: Phylogeny and PCR identification of the human pathogenic fungus *Penicillium marneffei*. J Clin Microbiol 33:85–89, 1995.

Sekhon AS, Li JSK, Garg AK: Penicillosis marneffei: serological and exoantigen studies. Mycopathologia 77:51–57, 1982.

Typhoid Fever

Hornick RB: Typhoid fever and other *Salmonella* infections. In: Warren KS, Mahamoud AFF (eds): Tropical and Geographical Medicine. McGraw-Hill, New York, pp 710–722, 1985.

Isaäcson M, Hale MJ: Intestinal bacterial infections. In: Doerr W, Seifert G (eds): Tropical Pathology, 2nd ed. Springer-Verlag, Berlin, pp 157–177, 1995.

Smith JH: Typhoid fever. In: Binford CH, Connor DH (eds): Pathology of Tropical and Extraordinary Diseases. Armed Forces Institute of Pathology, Washington, DC, pp 123–129, 1976.

John B. Cousar

Neoplasms Other Than Lymphomas in Lymph Nodes

Neoplasms other than lymphomas occur in lymph nodes in children. Metastatic sarcomas, carcinomas, and disseminated hematopoietic neoplasms, such as leukemia and Langerhans cell histiocytosis, may be seen. Surgical pathologists may be challenged to differentiate these processes from malignant lymphomas and then determine their origin (Blackshaw, 1992).

Histopathologic features suggesting metastatic carcinoma or sarcoma in nodes include partial nodal involvement, a sinusal distribution of the infiltrate, and a cohesive appearance of the neoplastic cells. These histiologic features are not specific, and ancillary studies, such as electron microscopic examination, flow cytometric analysis, immunohistochemical studies, and cytogenetic and molecular genetic analysis are usually necessary to establish the diagnosis.

NEUROBLASTOMA

Neuroblastoma, the fourth most common tumor of childhood, spreads to regional lymph nodes in as many as 35% of patients with localized disease. Multifocal adenopathy is seen in widely disseminated disease (Kelly & Joshi, 1996). Metastatic neuroblastoma may focally or totally replace nodal architecture (Fig. 16–46*A*). Neuroblasts are often aggregated in nests surrounded by characteristic fibrovascular septae. Neuroblasts may be surrounded by faintly eosinophilic, fibrillary neuropil. Homer-Wright rosettes are present in some cases (Fig. 16–46*B*). Individual tumor cells are intermediate-sized, with nuclei demonstrating a "salt and pepper" chromatin pattern (Kelly & Joshi, 1996; Triche & Askin, 1983). Neuroblasts are periodic acid–Schiff negative, a feature that is useful in distinguishing neuroblastoma from Ewing tumor and rhabdomyosarcoma. Immunohistochemical studies are often helpful in the recognition of neuroblastoma with neuron-specific enolase, the most commonly used marker (Kelly & Joshi, 1996). The typical staining pattern is one of moderately intense cytoplasmic and neuropil positivity regardless of the level of cytologic differentiation. Positivity may also be seen in primitive neuroectodermal tumors and rarely in rhabdomyosarcoma (Kelly & Joshi, 1996). S-100 marks Schwann cells in the fibrovascular stroma of neuroblastoma with ganglionic differentiation. Other markers useful in the recognition of neuroblastomas include chromogranin, synaptophysin, and neurofilament protein.

RHABDOMYOSARCOMA

Rhabdomyosarcoma accounts for approximately 5–8% of pediatric cancers (O'Shea, 1997). Most cases occur in children under 5 years of age. Since the head, neck, and orbital regions

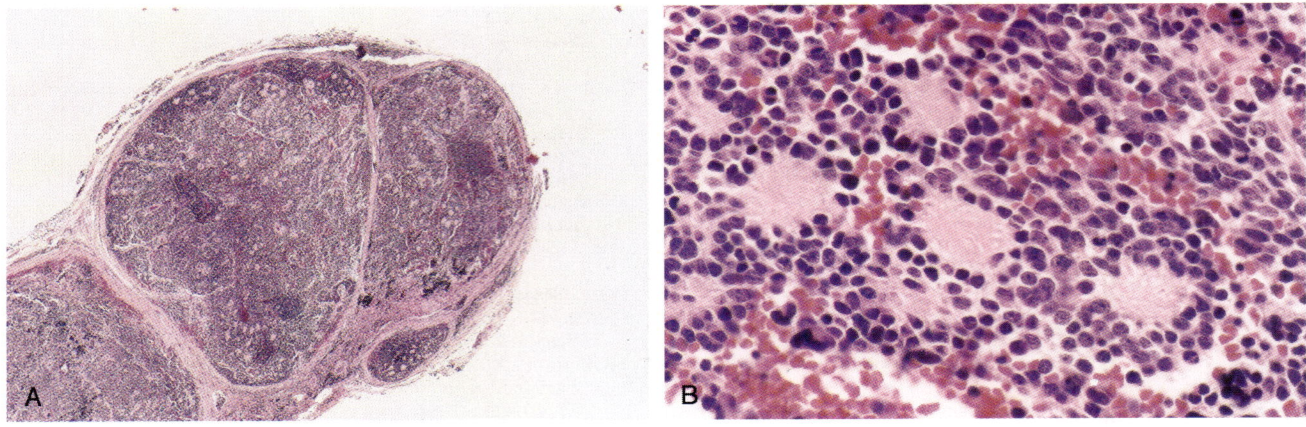

Figure 16–46

Metastatic neuroblastoma, abdominal lymph nodes. *A*, At low magnification the nodal architecture appears to be almost totally effaced, and the capsule is focally thickened. *B*, At high magnification the tumor cells form Homer-Wright rosettes. The neoplastic cells are intermediate in size and have dark nuclear chromatin.

are common locations for this neoplasm, children with rhabdomyosarcomas often present with cervical adenopathy. Rarely, patients with rhabdomyosarcoma present with a systemic illness with widespread dissemination mimicking lymphoma or leukemia (Almanaseer et al, 1984; Fitzmaurice et al, 1991; Nunez et al, 1983). Most rhabdomyosarcomas in children have either embryonal or alveolar features (O'Shea, 1997). Lymph node architecture may be partially (Fig. 16–47*A*) or completely effaced. The neoplastic cells may appear undifferentiated and closely resemble lymphocytes (Fig. 16–47*B*). Usually the tumor cells contain abundant cytoplasm that rarely contains striations. Occasionally, an alveolar pattern in the metastasis may be appreciated. Rhabdomyoblasts are typically periodic acid–Schiff positive. Immunohistochemical studies are particularly helpful in recognizing poorly differentiated rhabdomyosarcomas. In most cases, staining occurs with antibodies to muscle-specific actin, desmin, vimentin, and MyoD1, an antibody to myogenic regulatory protein. Staining with MyoD1 may be problematic in formalin-fixed material (O'Shea, 1997).

NASOPHARYNGEAL CARCINOMA

Nasopharyngeal carcinoma is common in adults and rare in children (Fernandez et al, 1976; Jaffe & Jaffe, 1973). Metastatic nasopharyngeal carcinoma in children is often misdiagnosed as lymphoma (Carbone & Michean, 1982; Giffler et al, 1977; Zarate-Osorno et al, 1992), since nasopharyngeal carcinomas are rare pediatric tumors and are inapparent as primary tumors owing in part to the inaccessibility of the nasopharnyx to direct examination. In addition, their growth pattern, their cytologic features, and the associated inflammatory response mimic those of large-cell lymphomas or Hodgkin disease. Lymph nodes involved by metastatic nasopharyngeal carcinoma demonstrate several histologic patterns (Fig. 16–48*A*). The neoplastic cells may form cohesive aggregates that are well demarcated within the lymphatic parenchyma and are readily recognized as carcinoma (so-called Regaude pattern). Other cases exhibit smaller nests of neoplastic cells intermixed with small lymphocytes, plasma cells, and eosinophils (Schmincke pattern). Sinusal growth of the tumor is seen in

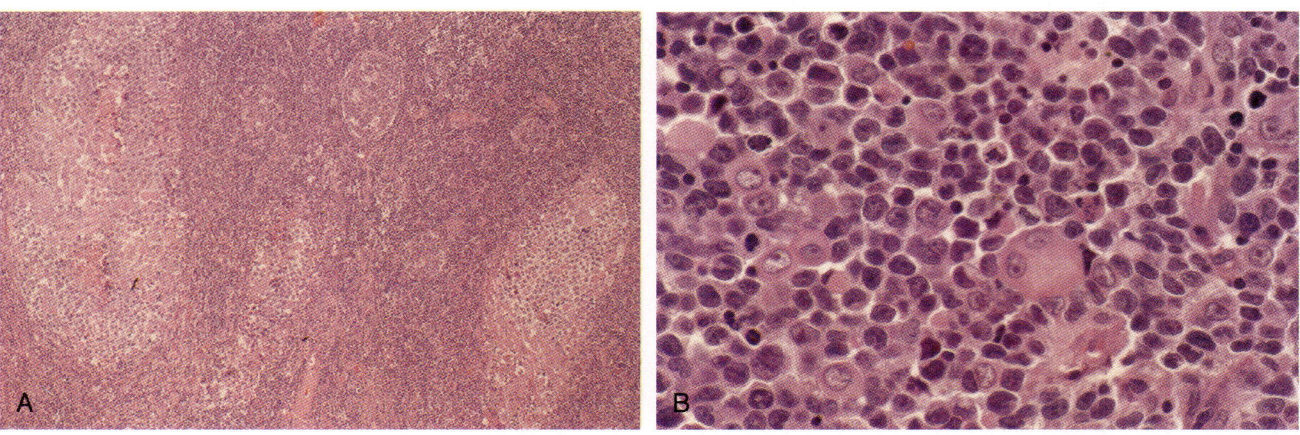

Figure 16–47

Metastatic rhabdomyosarcoma, cervical lymph node. *A*, At low magnification the node is partially involved, with nests of tumor expanding interfollicular sinuses. *B*, Many tumor cells are similar in appearance to lymphocytes. However, scattered large cells with abundant eosinophilic cytoplasm provide evidence of muscle differentiation.

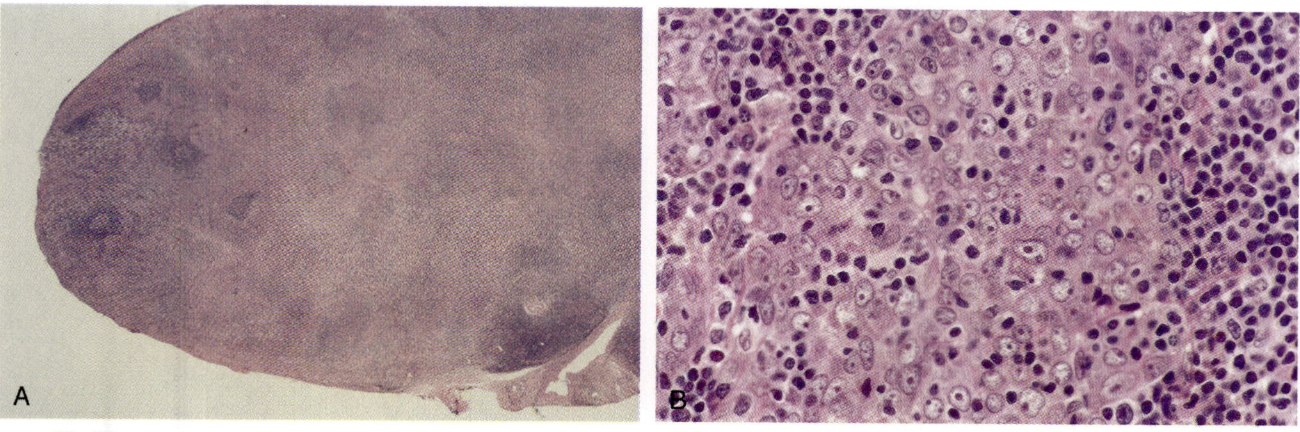

Figure 16–48

Metastatic nasopharyngeal carcinoma, cervical lymph node. *A*, Nodal architecture is extensively effaced by the tumor, with sparing of several reactive follicles. *B*, The neoplastic cells are arranged in loosely cohesive clusters, whereas small lymphocytes intermingle among the tumor cells. The malignant cells have large nuclei with prominent nucleoli, superficially resembling large transformed lymphocytes.

some cases. Neoplastic cells are usually uniform in shape, with large nuclei, dispersed chromatin, and prominent nucleoli (Fig. 16–48*B*), but occasional cells resemble mononuclear Reed-Sternberg cells or lacunar variants of Reed-Sternberg cells. Some cases also demonstrate parenchymal or capsular fibrosis and necrosis. These reactive patterns lead to the frequent misdiagnosis of undifferentiated nasopharyngeal carcinoma as nodular sclerosing Hodgkin disease. Immunohistochemical studies are diagnostic, since nasopharyngeal carcinoma cells react with anti-keratin antibodies and are CD45−.

EXTRAMEDULLARY LEUKEMIA (GRANULOCYTIC SARCOMA)

Localized extramedullary tumors of leukemic blasts may occur in virtually any site, including skin, bone, soft tissue, orbit, mediastinum, and nodes (Lukes & Collins 1992; Warnke et al, 1995). Extramedullary leukemia is rare in children, and lymph node involvement is infrequent. Patients with known acute leukemia or patients without evidence of marrow leukemia may be affected (Furebring-Freden et al, 1990; Meis et al, 1986; Neiman et al, 1981). Patients in the latter group usually develop marrow disease within a year.

Fresh nodes involved by acute myelogenous leukemia may exhibit a green sheen owing to the presence of myeloperoxidase, a feature that has given rise to the alternative name *chloroma*. Lymph nodes involved by leukemia typically demonstrate partial alteration of architecture, often with reactive-appearing follicles surrounded by infiltrates extending into the medulla (Fig. 16–49*A*). Invasion of blood vessels is common. Occasionally, the infiltrate is sinusal or perinodal in distribution. Tingible-body macrophages and mitoses are usually present. Leukemic blasts are small to intermediate in size and often have eosinophilic cytoplasm and finely dispersed chromatin (Fig. 16–49*B*). Nucleoli are usually inconspicuous. Eosinophilic myelocytes are present in some cases and provide a morphologic clue to the nature of the infiltrate. Touch imprints from fresh nodes may be helpful in recognizing leukemic blasts. Cytochemical stains, such as Sudan black B or myeloperoxidase, may be used on these preparations.

Histochemical and immunohistochemical staining is frequently necessary to confirm the leukemic nature of the infiltrate. Results of Leder staining (tissue chloroacetate esterase)

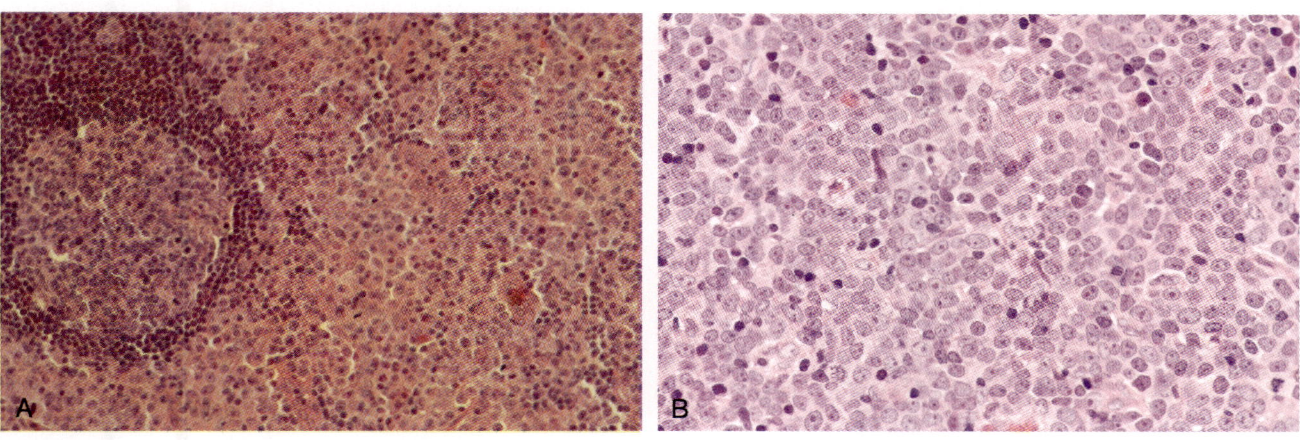

Figure 16–49

Acute myelogenous leukemia, lymph node. *A*, The infiltrate is characteristically interfollicular in distribution. *B*, At high magnification the blasts have finely dispersed chromatin, distinct nucleoli, and moderately abundant eosinophilic cytoplasm.

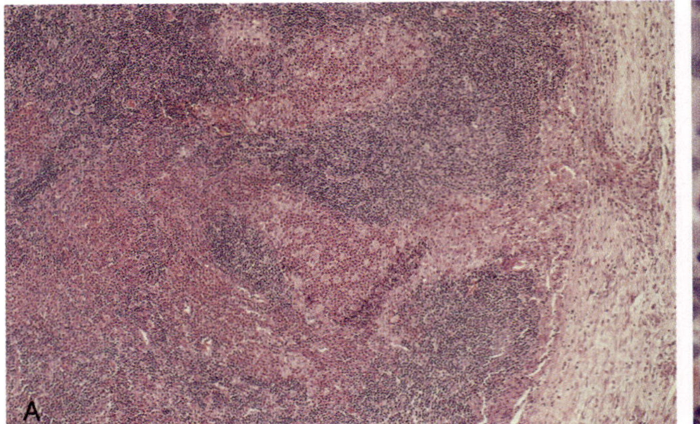

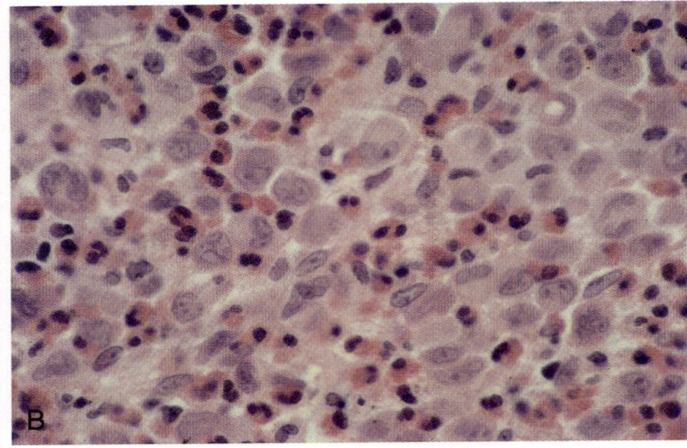

Figure 16–50

Langerhans cell histiocytosis, cervical lymph node. *A*, The histiocytic proliferation is typically sinusal in distribution, and numerous eosinophils are present. *B*, Note the characteristic cytologic feature of the Langerhans cell. The cytoplasm is abundant, and nuclei are often folded and typically demonstrate a deep linear groove. Nucleoli are generally small, and mitoses are infrequent.

are positive in most cases, but the stain does not work in Zenker-fixed or acid-decalcified tissues (Warnke et al, 1995).

Antimyeloperoxidase is the most sensitive and specific monoclonal antibody for recognition of immature myelocytes in paraffin-embedded material (Pinkus & Pinkus, 1990). Other monoclonal antibodies that may be useful are CD15 and CD68, but they lack the sensitivity and specificity of myeloperoxidase. CD43 is the only T and B cell antibody that may be present in extramedullary leukemia, and a "CD43-only" phenotype is reported as characteristic of leukemic infiltrates (Segal et al, 1992). Electron microscopic examination is now used infrequently but may detect dense primary and secondary granules that confirm the diagnosis of leukemic infiltrate.

The differential diagnosis of extramedullary leukemia principally includes B and T cell lymphomas. The interfollicular growth pattern is often a clue to the recognition of extramedullary leukemia. The eosinophilic cytoplasm and finely dispersed nuclear chromatin of leukemic blasts may suggest lymphoblastic lymphoma and the blastic variant of mantle cell lymphoma. Flow, electron microscopic, and immunohistochemical studies are often required for diagnosis.

LANGERHANS CELL HISTIOCYTOSIS

Langerhans cell histiocytosis (LCH) is a clonal proliferation (Willman et al, 1994) that occurs principally in children and may be focal or disseminated. In disseminated disease, sites of involvement include bone, skin, lungs, marrow, and lymph nodes (Favara et al, 1983). Lymphadenopathy is often the first sign of LCH and is usually associated with nearby skin or bone involvement. LCH rarely occurs as a solitary lesion of nodes without evidence of other organ involvement (Morganfeld & Schajowicz, 1971; Motoi et al, 1980; Reid et al, 1977; Williams & Dorfman, 1979). LCH of nodes may involve single or multiple node groups. Cervical and inguinal nodes are most often involved. Males are more often affected than females (Motoi et al, 1980).

In most cases, the node is partially involved, and reactive follicles are spared. The infiltrate is sinusal (Fig. 16–50*A*), may extend into the nodal parenchyma or perinodal soft tissue, and often is associated with capsular fibrosis. The proliferating cells of LCH are large, with abundant eosinophilic cytoplasm, and may be recognized by their nuclear features. The nuclei are folded and often demonstrate longitudinal grooves (Fig. 16–50*B*). The chromatin is fine, and nucleoli are generally not apparent. Eosinophils are always present and often form "eosinophilic abscesses" with necrotic centers in which Charcot-Leyden crystals are seen. Giant cells are often observed.

The proliferating cells in LCH are typically found to be S-100+, CD1a+, and vimentin positive on immunohistochemical study. Some cells express a granular CD68 positivity of variable intensity (Warnke et al, 1995). Langerhans cells are usually readily identified by electron microscopic study. Birbeck granules, racquet-shaped structures in the cytoplasm, are the most characteristic ultrastructural feature of Langerhans cells.

REFERENCES

Almanaseer IY, Trujllo YP, Taxy JB, et al: Systemic rhabdomyosarcoma with diffuse bone marrow involvement: case report of an unusual presentation. Am J Clin Pathol 82:349–353, 1984.

Ben-Ezra JM, Koo CH: Langerhans' cell histiocytosis and malignancies of the M-PIRE system. Am J Clin Pathol 99:464–471, 1992.

Blackshaw AJ: Metastatic tumours. In Stansfeld AG, d'Ardenne AJ (eds): Lymph Node Biopsy Interpretation, 2nd ed. Churchill Livingstone, New York, pp 421–439, 1992.

Carbone A, Michean C: Pitfalls in microscopic diagnosis of undifferentiated carcinoma of nasopharyngeal type (lymphoepithelioma). Cancer 50:1344–1351, 1982.

Davey FR, Olson S, Kurec AS, et al: The immunophenotyping of extramedullary myeloid cell tumors in paraffin-embedded tissue sections. Am J Surg Pathol 12:699–707, 1988.

Favara BE, Jaffe R: The histopathology of Langerhans' cell histiocytosis. Br J Cancer 70(suppl 23):S17–S23, 1994.

Favara BE, McCarthy RC, Mierau GW: Histiocytosis X. Hum Pathol 14:663–676, 1983.

Fellbaum C, Hansmann ML: Immunohistochemical differential diagnosis of granulocytic sarcoma and malignant lymphomas on formalin-fixed materials. Virchows Arch A 416:351–355, 1990.

Fernandez CH, Cangir A, Samaan NA, et al: Nasopharyngeal carcinoma in children. Cancer 37:2787–2791, 1976.

Fitzmaurice RJ, Johnson PRE, Liu Yin JA, et al: Rhabdomyosarcoma presenting as "acute leukemia." Histopathology 18:173–175, 1991.

Furebring-Freden M, Martinsson U, Sundstrom C: Myelosarcoma without acute leukemia: immunohistochemical and clinicopathologic characterization of 8 cases. Histopathology 16:243–250, 1990.

Giffler RF, Gillespie JJ, Ayala AG, et al: Lymphoepithelioma in cervical lymph nodes of children and young adults. Am J Surg Pathol 1:293–302, 1977.

Jaffe BF, Jaffe N: Head and neck tumors in children. Pediatrics 51:731–740, 1973.

Kelly DR, Joshi VV: Neuroblastoma and related tumors. In Parham DM (ed): Pediatric Neoplasia: Morphology and Biology. Lippincott-Raven, Philadelphia, pp 105–128, 1996.

Lukes RJ, Collins RD: Tumors of the hematopoietic system. In Atlas of Tumor Pathology, 2nd series, fascicle 28. Armed Forces Institute of Pathology, Washington, DC, pp 332–333, 1992.

Meis JM, Butler JJ, Osborne BM, et al: Granulocytic sarcoma in nonleukemic patients. Cancer 58:2697–2709, 1986.

Morganfeld MC, Schajowicz R: Solitary eosinophilic granuloma of lymph node: five-year follow-up. Pediatrics 48:301–305, 1971.

Motoi M, Itelbron D, Kaiserling E, et al: Eosinophilic granuloma of lymph nodes: a variant of histiocytosis X. Histopathology 4: 585–606, 1980.

Neiman RS, Barcos M, Berard C, et al: Granulocytic sarcoma: a clinicopathologic study of 61 biopsied cases. Cancer 48:1426–1437, 1981.

Nunez C, Abboud SL, Lemon NC, et al: Ovarian rhabdomyosarcoma presenting as leukemia: case report. Cancer 52:297–300, 1983.

O'Shea PA: Mycogenic tumors of soft tissue. In Coffin CM, Dehmer LP, O'Shea PA (eds): Pediatric Soft Tissue Tumors: A Clinical, Pathological, and Therapeutic Approach. Williams & Wilkins, Baltimore, pp 214–238, 1997.

Pinkus GS, Pinkus JL: Myeloperoxidase: a specific marker for myeloid cells in paraffin sections. Mod Pathol 6:733–741, 1991.

Reid H, Fox H, Whittaker JS: Eosinophilic granuloma of lymph nodes. Histopathology 1:31–37, 1977.

Segal GH, Stoler MH, Tubbs RR: The "CD43 only" phenotype: an aberrant, nonspecific immunophenotype requiring comprehensive analysis for lineage resolutions. Am J Clin Pathol 97:861–865, 1992.

Triche TJ, Askin FB: Neuroblastoma and the differential diagnosis of small-, round-, blue-cell tumors. Hum Pathol 14:569–595, 1983.

Warnke RA, Weiss LM, Chan JKC, et al: Tumors of the lymph nodes and spleen. In Hartmann WH, Sobin LH (eds): Atlas of Tumor Pathology, 3rd series, fascicle 14. Armed Forces Institute of Pathology, Washington, DC, pp 385–410, 1995.

Williams JW, Dorfman RF: Lymphadenopathy as the initial manifestation of histiocytosis X. Am J Surg Pathol 3:405, 1979.

Willman CL, Busque L, Griffith BB, et al: Langerhans'-cell histiocytosis (histiocytosis X) is a clonal proliferative disease. N Engl J Med 331:154–160, 1994.

Zarate-Osorno A, Jaffe ES, Medeiros JL: Metastatic nasopharyngeal carcinoma initially presenting as cervical lymphadenopathy: a report of two cases that resembled Hodgkin's disease. Arch Pathol Lab Med 116:862–865, 1992.

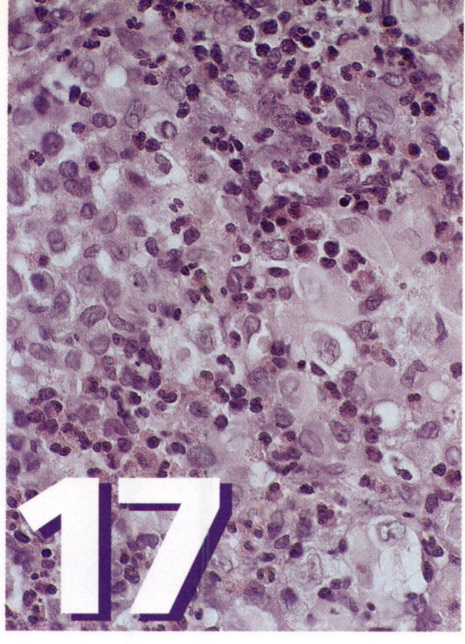

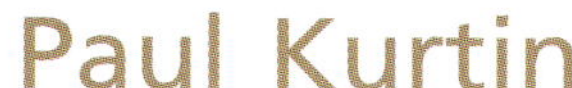

Paul Kurtin

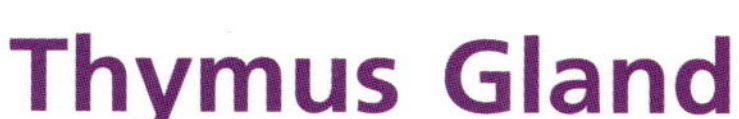

17 Thymus Gland

DEVELOPMENT, ANATOMY, HISTOLOGY, AND FUNCTION

The thymus is a derivative of the third and fourth pharyngeal pouches. During the sixth gestational week the endoderm of the third pharyngeal pouch forms a cystic protrusion that detaches from the pharyngeal pouch, forms the thymopharyngeal duct, and migrates in a caudal and medial direction. By the eighth gestational week, the left and right thymic primordia form bars of epithelium that fuse in the midline in the anterior mediastinum. The endodermally derived epithelium then breaks up into a stellate matrix that is encapsulated and separated into lobules by the ingrowth of mesenchymal elements. By the tenth gestational week, lymphocytes from the fetal liver and marrow begin to migrate into the thymus. The thymic cortex and medulla differentiate as successive waves of lymphocytes arrive in the thymus and as functional development of the thymic epithelium proceeds. The development of the thymic cortex and medulla is completed between the fourteenth and sixteenth gestational weeks. Tubular structures, termed medullary duct epithelia then appear and give rise to Hassall corpuscles. The thymus grows rapidly and before birth reaches a maximum weight (averaging 15 g) proportional to body weight (Shimosato & Kukai, 1997; Suster & Rosai, 1997; Suster & Rosai, 1990).

The mature thymus is an encapsulated organ consisting of two lateral lobes, often of varying size and configuration, connected by an isthmus of connective tissue and thymic parenchyma. Lying partly in the caudal neck and partly in the anterior superior mediastinum, the thymus extends superiorly from the caudal border of the thyroid gland to the level of the fourth costal cartilage inferiorly. It is immediately deep to the sternum and overlies the great vessels and the superior portion of the pericardium. The thymus receives its arterial blood supply from the internal thoracic artery as well as from the superior and inferior thyroid arteries, and the veins terminate in the left brachiocephalic and thyroid veins. The lymphatics drain into the anterior mediastinal, tracheobronchial, and sternal lymph nodes (Goss, 1973).

The thymus grows until puberty and then begins to involute, with progressive depletion of the lymphocytic and, to a lesser extent, the epithelial elements, followed by fatty replacement. Thymic weight varies considerably among individuals of similar ages (Table 17–1) (Suster & Rosai, 1997).

Histologically, the thymus has a lobulated architecture (Fig. 17–1), with the lobules separated by a delicate collagen and vascular framework. On low magnification the thymic lobules exhibit peripheral dark zones containing the thymic cortex. The paler central portions of the lobules, the thymic medulla, are contiguous with one another and contain whorls of nonkeratinized squamous epithelial cells, the Hassall corpuscles. Both thymic cortex and medulla contain a mixture of epithelial cells, lymphocytes, dendritic cells (including Langerhans cells), and macrophages. In addition, the thymus may contain hematopoietic precursors of all three cell lines. Hematopoietic cells are commoner in thymus glands from infants and children than in those from adults. Scattered mast cells are distributed in the capsule, septa, and the medulla and are associated with Hassall corpuscles (Suster & Rosai, 1990).

The thymic T lymphocytes vary in appearance among the microanatomic compartments of the thymus. In the outermost cortex, there is a population of lymphocytes with the cytologic characteristics of blasts: medium-sized to large cells with rounded nuclei; delicate, stippled chromatin; small nucleoli; and sparse cytoplasm (Fig. 17–2). They constitute about 15% of the cells of the thymus and represent the earliest T cell precursors. Cytologically, lymphocytes apparently form a gradient from the outermost cortex to the medulla. The larger blastlike cells become smaller, with more condensed chromatin and less prominent nucleoli. This cytologic change is accompanied by a progressive diminution of the numbers of mitotic figures and tingible-body macrophages from many in the cortex to few in the medulla. The medulla overall has fewer lymphocytes and more epithelial cells than the cortex (Fig. 17–3). These morphologic changes in lymphocytes parallel hierarchical expression of T lymphocyte–associated antigens that define the stages of intrathymic T cell maturation. The immunoarchitecture of the thymus is illustrated in Figs. 17–4*A* through *E*.

B lymphocytes are also normally found in the thymus distributed along the thymic septa and near blood vessels in the corticomedullary junction and the medulla. In addition, there is a population of phenotypically distinct B cells associated with Hassall corpuscles (Fig. 17–4*C*)(Isaacson et al, 1987). The normal thymus, particularly in children and young adults, may also contain germinal centers that are in perivascular spaces, separated by a basal lamina from the thymic parenchyma (Levine & Rosai, 1978; Suster & Rosai, 1990).

Three types of thymic epithelial cells may be recognized by light microscopic study. In the cortex, the epithelial cells have large, round to oval, vesicular nuclei with distinct nucleoli. In the medulla, the epithelial cells have a spindle shape and contain fusiform nuclei with more condensed chromatin,

Table 17–1
Normal Thymic Weights as a Function of Age

Age (years)	Mean Weight (g)	Standard Deviation (g)
0–1	27	16
1–4	28	19
5–9	22	22
10–14	21	21
15–19	20	19
20–24	22	23
25–29	23	24
30–34	26	28
35–44	22	22
45–54	25	26
55–64	21	24
65–84	24	26
85–90	18	20
91–107	12	13

Source: Modified from Suster S, Rosai J: Thymus. In Sternberg S (ed): Histology for Pathologists, 2nd ed. Lippincott-Raven, Philadelphia, 1997.

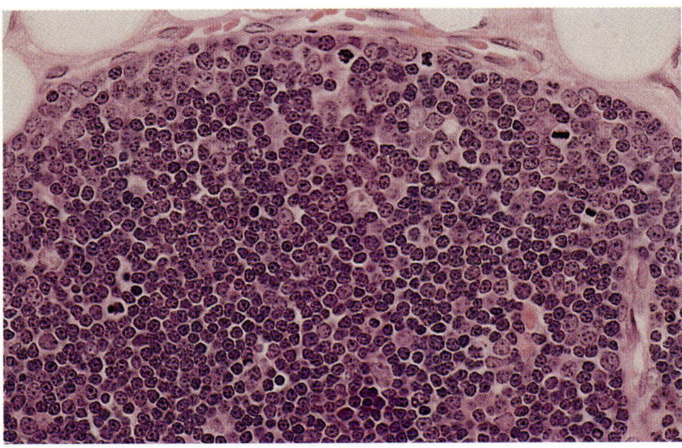

Figure 17–2

Normal thymus. The thymic cortex contains a population of larger blastlike thymocytes immediately adjacent to the capsule. The cytologic features of cortical thymocytes are illustrated.

inconspicuous nucleoli, and darkly staining interconnecting cell processes. Both cell types are present at the corticomedullary junction. The third general type of thymic epithelial cell is the nonkeratinized squamous cell of the Hassall corpuscle. Hassall corpuscles may show central keratinization, accumulation of central debris and microscopic cyst formation (Shimosato & Kukai, 1997; Suster & Rosai, 1990).

The apparent histologic simplicity of the thymic epithelium belies a phenotypic and ultrastructural complexity that is briefly described below. At the ultrastructural level, there are six types of thymic epithelial cells; the processes of one of these—the thymic nurse cell—encircle lymphocytes, presumably enabling the critical interaction between epithelial cells and lymphocytes required for T-lymphocyte maturation (van de Wijngaert, Kendall, Shuurman, Rademakers & Kater, 1984). Thymic epithelial cells may be separated into four or five different types by immunohistochemical expression of different constellations of surface antigens (Muller-Hermelink, Marino & Palestro, 1986). Four patterns of expression of different molecular weight keratin species are also demonstrated in murine thymic epithelial cells (Savino & Dardenne, 1988). The functional significance of the subtypes of thymic epithelial cells remains incompletely understood.

The thymus gland is critical to the normal functioning of the T cell arm of the immune system. In the thymus gland, T lymphocyte precursors develop the capacity to recognize antigen through the T cell antigen receptor. The thymus is critical to the development of T cells that recognize antigen in the context of self major histocompatibility complex (MHC) class I (usually CD4+) or MHC class II (usually CD8+) antigens. T cell tolerance to endogenous self MHC molecules and various exogenous antigens is induced in the thymus. These functions require interactions among the intrathymic lymphocytes, the thymic epithelial cells, and interdigitating cells that are mediated by adhesion molecules, functional cell surface receptor-ligand interactions, and various cytokines. Several models for these complex interactions have been proposed, and the coordination and precise role of each component remain incompletely understood (Anderson, 1997; Ardavin, 1997). T lymphocyte precursors apparently enter the thymus through high endothelial venules in the corticomedullary junction and migrate to the outermost cortex, where they proliferate and begin to coexpress CD4 and CD8 (double-positive cells). Cortical ep-

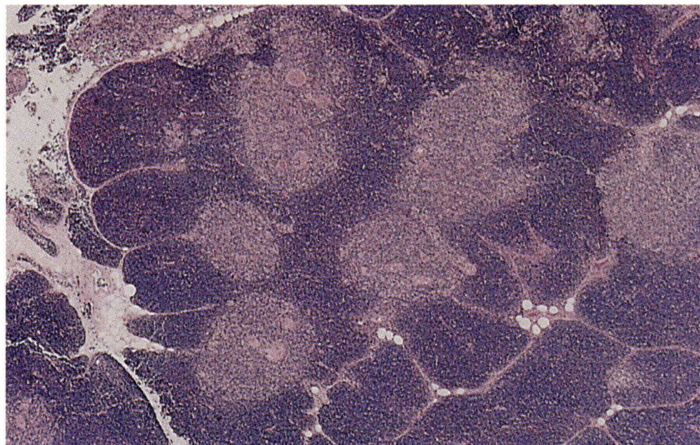

Figure 17–1

Normal thymus. The architecture is lobulated, with distinct cortical (dark) and medullary (pale) zones.

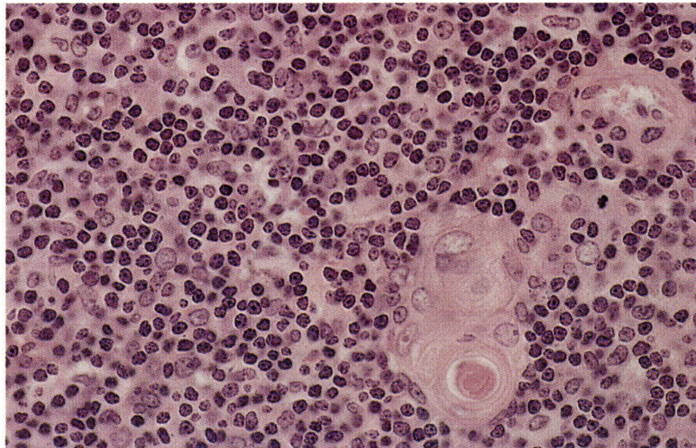

Figure 17–3

Normal thymus. The thymic medulla has a lower density of lymphocytes and greater numbers of thymic epithelial cells than the cortex. A Hassall corpuscle is illustrated at the lower right.

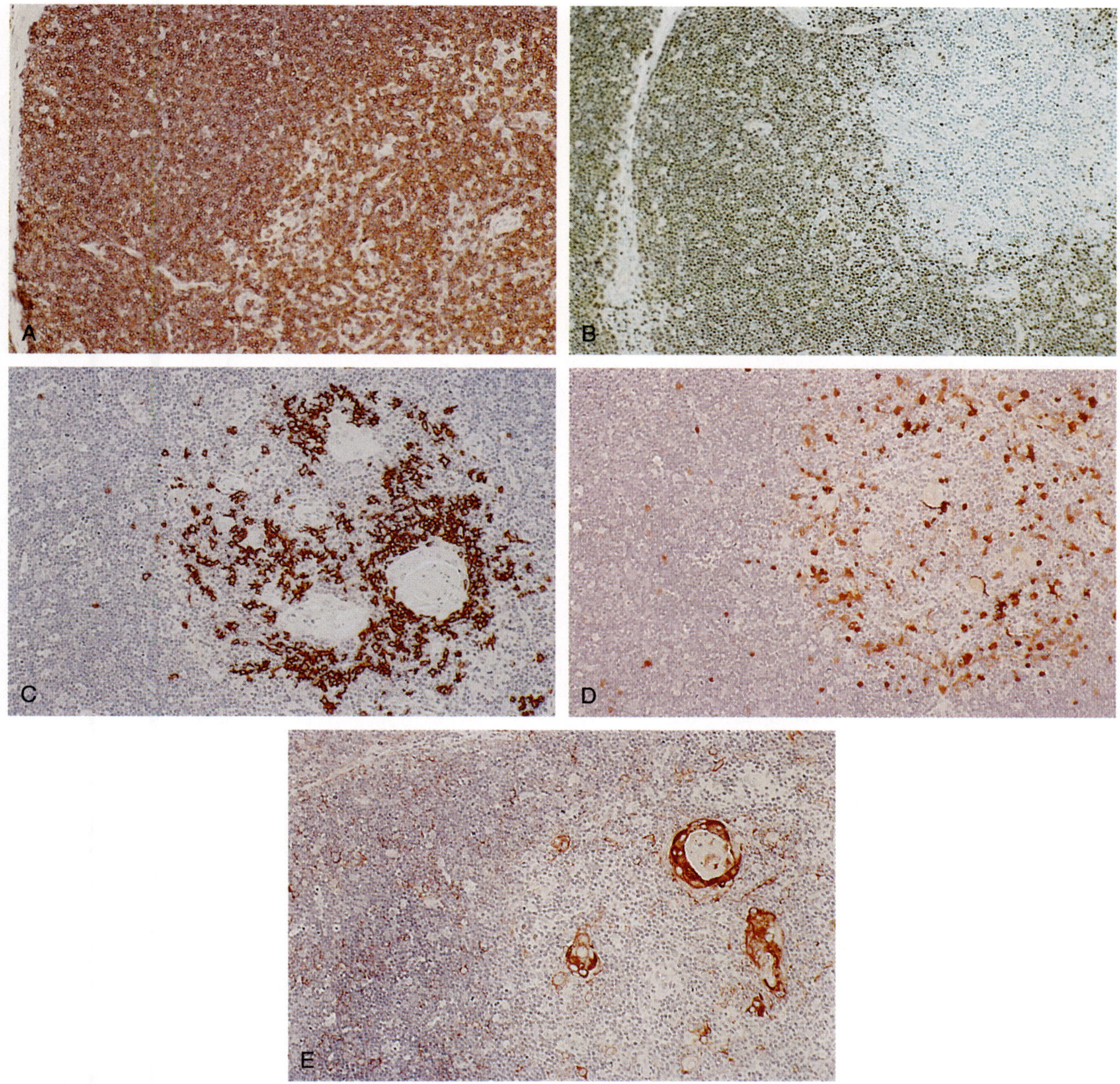

Figure 17–4

Immunoarchitecture of the normal thymus. In these photographs, the thymic cortex is to the left and the medulla to the right. *A*, Most of the lymphocytes in the thymic cortex and medulla are CD3 positive. Immunoperoxidase stain for CD3. *B*, Terminal deoxynucleotidyltransferase (TdT) is expressed in the immature T cells of the thymic cortex during the period when T cell antigen receptor gene rearrangments occur. Immunoperoxidase stain for TdT. *C*, Most thymic B cells are situated in the medulla around Hassall corpuscles and blood vessels near the corticomedullary junction. Immunoperoxidase stain for CD20. *D*, The thymus contains S-100 positive Langerhans cells and interdigitating reticulum cells, situated primarily in the medulla. Immunoperoxidase stain for S-100. *E*, The distribution and cytologic heterogeneity of keratin-positive thymic epithelial cells is highlighted. Immunoperoxidase stain for keratin (AE1/AE3).

ithelial cells interact with these double-positive T cells to select positively those with self MHC–restricted T cell receptors. These cells then migrate to the corticomedullary junction and the medulla. All other T cells undergo apoptosis, and their debris is phagocytosed by cortical macrophages. Some MHC class I–restricted thymocytes recognize endogenously synthesized peptides to which immunologic tolerance is desirable. These cells are clonally deleted by incompletely understood mechanisms that induce apoptosis. Thymic epithelial cells are also critical in the successful completion of this process. Past this checkpoint in T cell development, the remaining T cells encounter thymic dendritic cells (in corticomedullary and medullary areas) that allow the negative selection of T cell clones specific for antigens against which T cell tolerance cannot be induced by thymic epithelial cells. Usually, these are endogenous antigens synthesized by the dendritic cells or exogenous antigens phagocytosed and presented to the T cells by the thymic dendritic cells. The mature T cells that are positively and negatively selected, immunocompetent, CD4+, or CD8+ then leave the thymus through the high endothelial venules and migrate to the secondary lymphatic organs. The processes of selection and maturation of T cells in the thymus result in apoptosis of as many as 99% of the T lymphocytes that migrate to and proliferate in the thymus.

NONNEOPLASTIC CONDITIONS

Thymic Hyperplasia

The term *thymic hyperplasia* has been used for two forms of thymic enlargement that are clinically and pathologically distinct: follicular hyperplasia and thymic hyperplasia (hypertrophy). In some respects it is difficult to define precise morphologic criteria for follicular hyperplasia of the thymus, since apparently normal thymus glands may contain reactive germinal centers, as mentioned earlier. Follicular hyperplasia of the thymus occurs in autoimmune disorders, including systemic lupus erythematosus, rheumatoid arthritis, scleroderma, allergic vasculitis, and thyrotoxicosis (Table 17–2) (Suster & Rosai, 1990) as well as in the "thymitis" of HIV infection (Joshi et al, 1990; Joshi et al, 1986). Follicular hyperplasia is most frequent in patients with myasthenia gravis (Grody et al, 1986; Hankins et al, 1985). In myasthenia, the thymus gland is usually normal in size and configuration. The reactive germinal centers may be focally (Grody et al, 1986) or widely distributed in the gland. They are technically outside the thymic parenchyma, since they are centered at the thymic corticomedullary junction around blood vessel adventitia. They resemble reactive germinal centers of lymph nodes morphologically (Fig. 17–5) and phenotypically (Pizzighella et al, 1983). They are surrounded by T cells containing interdigitating reticulum cells that present antigen to T cells in lymph nodes. The thymus in myasthenia gravis may have normal (Gilcrease et al, 1997) or increased numbers of Langerhans cells in the corticomedullary vascular adventitia as well (Wekerle & Muller-Hermelink, 1986). Patients with myesthenia gravis and follicular hyperplasia have a more favorable clinical response to thymectomy, including a fall in antiacetylcholinesteresce antibody titers (Penn et al, 1981; Reinglass & Brickel, 1973).

In thymic hyperplasia, also referred to as thymic hypertrophy, there is a marked enlargement of morphologically normal thymic tissue (Fig. 17–6). In children this condition occurs most frequently between ages 7 and 14 years, and it is usually detected as an incidental finding on a chest radiograph (Lack, 1981). The resected thymus has an ovoid or lobulated gross appearance and histologically is normal, retaining a lobulated architecture, dark cortical zones, pale medullary zones, and Hassall corpuscles. The diagnosis is made only after demonstrating that the weight of the hyperplastic gland exceeds the maximum thymic weight in children and adolescents (see Table 17–1) (Lack, 1981). Hyperplasia produces thymic weights that are usually in the 200–500-g range. Thymic hyperplasia has also been described in patients after thermal burns (Gelfand et al, 1972), with hypothyroidism (Yulish & Owens, 1980), with hyperthyroidism (Rose & Lam, 1982), and after mediastinal radiation or systemic chemotherapy for various malignancies (Ford et al, 1987; Heron et al, 1988). Most cases are idiopathic, but the underlying pathphysiologic mechanism may be thymic hyperplasia following stress.

Table 17–2
Conditions Associated with Follicular Hyperplasia in the Thymus

Normal variant
Myasthenia gravis
Systemic lupus erythematosus
Rheumatoid arthritis
Scleroderma
Allergic vasculitis
Thyrotoxicosis
HIV-1 infection

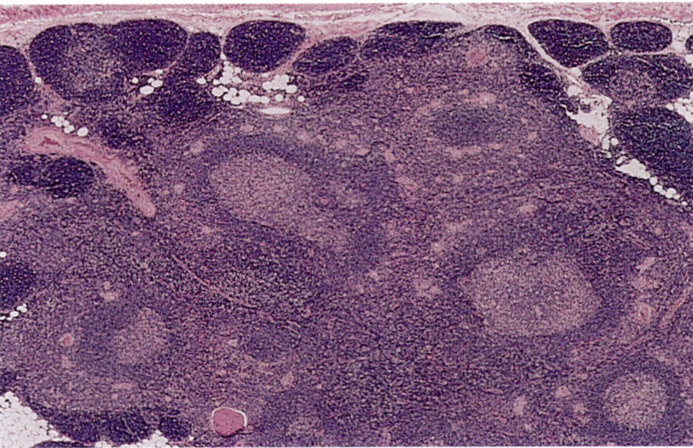

Figure 17–5

Follicular hyperplasia, thymus. This specimen was removed from a patient with myasthenia gravis.

The Thymus in Immunodeficiencies

Congenital immunodeficiencies are so rare that only a few investigators have had comprehensive experience with pathologic conditions of the thymus in these disorders. This section is based on the outstanding review by Nezelof (Nezelof, 1992). Since the thymus plays a key role in the development of immunocompetent T lymphocytes, it is not surprising that it has striking morphologic abnormalities in congenital and acquired immunodeficiencies, including thymic aplasia, thymic dysplasia, and thymic atrophy. Thymic aplasia is the complete absence of

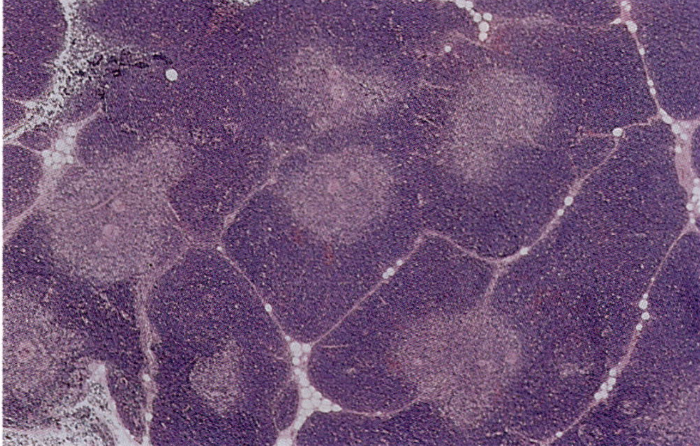

Figure 17–6

Hyperplasia, thymus. The architecture and cytologic composition of the thymus are normal, even though the gland weighed 435 g.

Table 17–3
Immunodeficiencies Associated with Thymic Dysplasia

Severe combined immunodeficiency
Reticular dysgenesis
Familial Omenn reticulosis with eosinophilia
Ataxia telangiectasia*
Adenosine deaminase deficiency*
Purine nucleosidase deficiency*

*Late stages of these disorders.

the thymus and is characteristically observed in Di George syndrome. Thymic dysplasia is present at birth, resulting from a prenatal failure or arrest in thymic development. It is characterized by a reduction in the size of the gland, a rudimentary histologic appearance, and a lack of maturation of thymic epithelial cells into Hassall corpuscles. Thymic dysplasia is always accompanied by a clinically apparent congenital immunodeficiency, but all congenital immunodeficiencies do not exhibit thymic dysplasia. Thymic atrophy refers to all regressive changes in the thymus. This depletion of lymphocytes and the secondary alteration of the thymic epithelial network occur after the initial development of a normal thymus. For additional discussion of immunodeficiencies, see Chap. 3.

Thymic Dysplasia

The thymus characteristically exhibits dysplasia in several genetic T cell immunodeficiencies, including severe combined immunodeficiency (Gitlin & Crain, 1963), reticular dysgenesis (Gitlin et al, 1964), familial Omenn reticulosis with eosinophilia (Jouan et al, 1987), and, in the late stages, ataxia telangiectasia, adenosine deaminase deficiency, and purine nucleosidase deficiency (Table 17–3) (Hirschhorn, 1983). Four types of thymic dysplasia have been recognized. In all the gland is smaller than normal. The commonest is simple thymic dysplasia, in which the gland has foliated lobules composed of polyhedral epithelial cells. There is no corticomedullary differentiation, no Hassall corpuscles are observed, and no CD1+, CD3+, CD4+, or CD8+ lymphocytes are present. In pseudoglandular thymic dysplasia, thymic lobules are present, but they have a primitive acinar appearance without lymphocytes and are lined by tall epithelial cells with basal nuclei. In thymic dysplasia with corticomedullary differentiation, thymic epithelial cells are condensed at the periphery of the thymic lobules, and there are no CD3+, CD4+, and CD8+ lymphocytes. Thymic pseudoatrophy has histologic features similar to those described for thymic atrophy in the next section. The most severe immunodeficiencies are associated with histologic patterns of pseudoglandular dysplasia and simple dysplasia (Nezelof, 1986; Nezelof, 1992).

Table 17–4
Conditions Associated with Thymic Atrophy

Bare lymphocyte syndrome
Wiskott-Aldrich disease
IL-2 deficiency
Acquired immunodeficiency (HIV-1)
Congenital rubella syndrome
Graft-versus-host disease
Prolonged administration of corticosteroids
Cytotoxic drugs
Cyclosporin A
Total-body irradiation
Severe protein calorie malnutrition
Langerhans cell histiocytosis

Thymic Atrophy

Atrophy is the characteristic thymic finding in some genetic immunodeficiencies, including bare lymphocyte syndrome (in which lymphocytes lack surface MHC class II molecules) (Touraine & Betuel, 1983), Wiskott-Aldrich disease (Cooper et al, 1968), and deficient production of interleukin-2 (Weinberg & Parkman, 1990). Thymic atrophy is also associated with acquired immunodeficiency syndromes (Table 17–4), including HIV infection (Grody et al, 1985; Joshi et al, 1990; Joshi et al, 1986; Schuurman et al, 1989; Seemayer et al, 1984); severe chronic viral infections, especially late-onset congenital rubella syndrome (Garcia et al, 1974; Rosenberg et al, 1986); graft-versus-host disease (Muller-Hermelink et al, 1987); prolonged administration of corticosteroids, cytotoxic drugs, and cyclosporin A; total-body irradiation; and severe, early protein calorie malnutrition (Durov, 1986; Mugerwa, 1971).

The severity of thymic atrophy is correlated more closely with the duration of the insult leading to the immunodeficiency than with the cause. It is not clear whether thymic atrophy contributes to the maintenance of an immunodeficient state. In thymic atrophy, thymic weight is decreased but usually not to the level of thymic dysplasia. Histologically, thymic lobules are present but appear collapsed (Fig. 17–7). Lobules are separated by connective tissue strands that often contain plasma cells. The perivascular spaces in atrophic thymus glands contain hyalinized collagen deposits. Hassall corpuscles may be absent, necrotic, or calcified. CD4+ and CD8+ T cells are present in reduced numbers in atrophic glands, whereas they are not present in dysplastic states (Nezelof, 1992). There is no fatty replacement of the thymic lobules in thymic atrophy, in contrast to the findings in physiologic involution.

Thymic Cysts

Cysts of the thymus gland are rare and may be congenital or acquired. They may be found in the anterior mediastinal location (Bieger & McAdams, 1966; McCafferty & Bahnson, 1982;

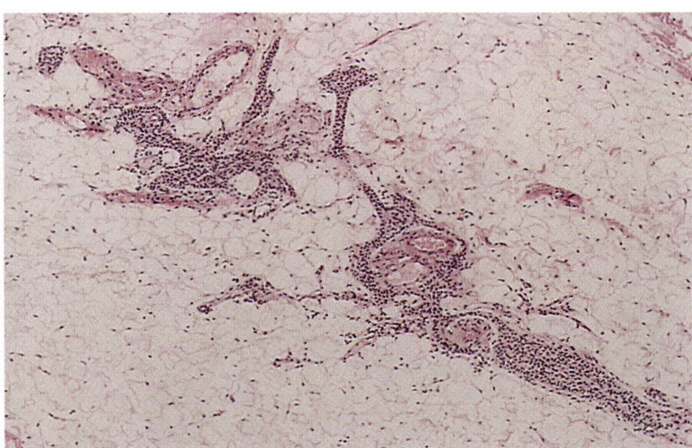

Figure 17–7

Atrophy, thymus. Note the absence of both lymphocytes and Hassall corpuscles in this example of severe atrophy.

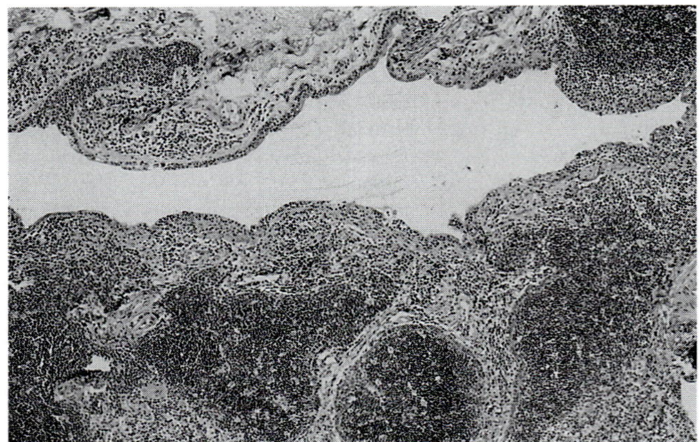

Figure 17–8

Cyst, ectopic cervical thymus. Note the stratified squamous epithelium–lined cyst in this ectopic thymus. The residual thymus gland is in the lower one-third of the photograph.

Rastegar et al, 1980; Zanca et al, 1965) or in ectopic tissue deposited anywhere along the path of migration of the thymic anlage (Lyons et al, 1989; Marra et al, 1995; Som et al, 1985; Stromme & Eraklis, 1977). Cysts may be found incidentally on chest radiographs, or they may produce symptoms by compressing adjacent structures. Thymic cysts have been associated with aplastic anemia (Moskowitz et al, 1980; Suster & Rosai, 1991). On radiographs they are well circumscribed, with sharp contours. Their cystic nature is demonstrable on computerized tomographic scans. Cysts vary in size, may contain serous fluid or keratinous material, and are surrounded by fubrous tissue. Linings are keratinizing or nonkeratinizing stratified squamous epithelium, ciliated columnar epithelium, or flattened cuboidal epithelium (Figs. 17–8 and 17–9). Remnants of normal or atrophic thymus occupy the cyst wall, which in some cases include parathyroid tissue, in keeping with the common developmental origin of the thymus and parathyroid glands (McCluggage et al, 1995). Cyst rupture and degenerative changes may be associated microscopically with cholesterol clefts and a granulomatous reaction.

Multilocular thymic cysts may be acquired, resulting from idiopathic inflammatory processes affecting the epithelium of Hassall corpuscles (Suster & Rosai, 1991), and probably differ thereby in pathogenesis from unilocular cysts. Multilocular cysts are often associated with inflammation or fibrosis extending outside the confines of the cyst, may recur after resection, and are seen in association with autoimmune disorders, HIV infections (discussed later), and neoplasms of the thymus. In contrast, congenital thymic cysts are derivatives of the thymopharyngeal duct, are usually unilocular, are not associated with inflammation, and are cured by resection.

Cyst formation is one of the ways in which the thymus gland responds to a variety of stimuli (Table 17–5) (Suster & Moran, 1995). Inflammatory processes and imunodeficiency disorders are accompanied by cystic thymic lesions, as discussed later. In addition, thymomas, B and T lymphomas, Hodgkin disease, and mediastinal germ cell tumors induce cystic changes in the thymus gland. Therefore, surgical pathologists should examine thymic cysts with multiple histologic sections to ensure that more serious lesions are not present.

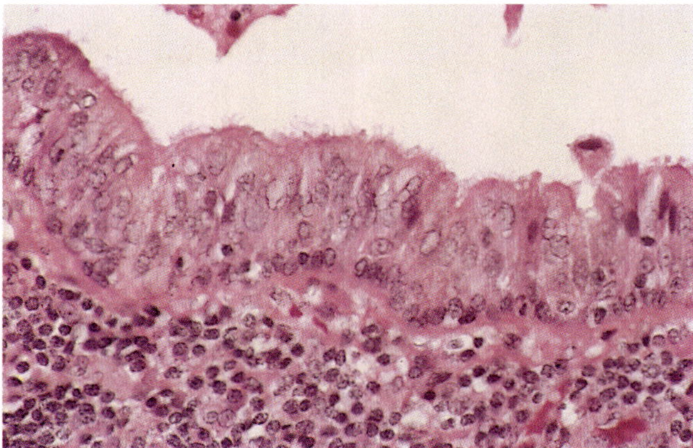

Figure 17–9

Cyst, thymus. A cyst may be lined by ciliated columnar epithelium, as in this case.

HIV-Associated Multilocular Thymic Cysts

A few children with HIV infections develop multilocular cysts of the thymus (Kontny et al, 1997; Leonidas et al, 1996; Mishalani et al, 1995). Symptoms related to a thymic mass are usually not present, and most cysts are detected incidentally by chest radiographs. These children have CD4+ cell counts that are low but never <100 cells/mm^3. Many also have generalized lymphadenopathy, lymphocytic interstitial pneumonitis, parotid gland cystic lymphocytic hyperplasia, hepatomegaly, or splenomegaly. With one exception, children with thymic cysts have not had opportunistic infections or other conditions satisfying the Centers for Disease Control and Prevention criteria for a diagnosis of AIDS. Histologically, resections or biopsies of thymus glands have revealed multiple cysts of varying sizes that are lined by nonkeratinizing squamous epithelium or ciliated columnar epithelium and are surrounded by reactive follicles with serpiginous borders and attenuated mantle zones. There is marked interfollicular plasmacytosis. Hassall corpuscles may be preserved or absent (Fig. 17–10). The B cells and plasma cells are polyclonal, whereas the interfollicular lymphocytes are mostly CD8+ T cells, with fewer CD4+ cells. HIV may be demonstrated by in situ hybridization in the follicular dendritic cells and a subset of the interfollicular T cells (Kontny et al, 1997). This morphologic and phenotypic pattern is similar to that observed in early-stage HIV-associated lymphadenopathy. In the patients in whom the cysts were biopsied, regression over several years occurred. Based on pathologic and clinical features, multilocular thymic cysts in HIV-positive individuals apparently have pathogenetic relationships to cystic lymphocytic hyperplasia of salivary glands (Labouyrie et al, 1993) and possibly to the diffuse infiltrative lymphocytosis syndrome as well (Itescu & Winchester, 1992).

Table 17–5
Conditions Associated with Thymic Cysts

Congenital eutopic or heterotopic thymic cysts
Multilocular cysts
Autoimmune disorders
HIV-1
Chemotherapy or radiation treatment
Thymoma
B and T cell lymphomas
Hodgkin disease
Germ cell tumors

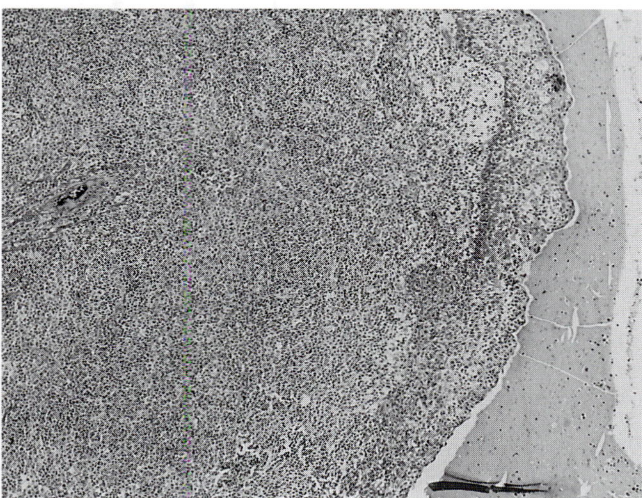

Figure 17–10

Cyst, thymus. This HIV-1–associated multilocular cyst demonstrates a stratified squamous epithelium lining and lymphocytic hyperplasia in the cyst wall.

Castleman Disease

Although the anterior mediastinum is the commonest location for Castleman disease (Keller et al, 1972), involvement of the thymus gland does occur rarely (Karcher et al, 1982; O'Reilly et al, 1993). In the thymus, Castleman disease has histologic features similar to those of the disease in lymph nodes and may be separated into hyaline vascular, plasma cell, and multicentric types by morphologic and clinical criteria. The clinical and pathologic features of Castleman disease are discussed in greater depth in Chap. 16.

The hallmark of all types of Castleman disease is the regressively transformed germinal center, a structure altered by decreased follicular center B lymphocytes, prominent follicular dendritic cells, and hypervascularity. Regressively transformed germinal centers are surrounded by aggregates of small lymphocytes that have many of the cytologic and phenotypic features of mantle zone lymphocytes. Often, a single "cloud" of mantle zone cells contains several regressively transformed germinal centers connected by a branched and hyalinized blood vessel (Fig. 17–11). In hyaline vascular Castleman disease, there is loss of normal thymic architecture. Regressively transformed germinal centers alternate with a vascularized stroma containing many small lymphocytes and few plasma cells, macrophages, and transformed lymphocytes (Fig. 17–12). In the plasma cell variant there is greater preservation of architecture, with large aggregates and sheets of plasma cells between the follicles (Fig. 17–13). Overlap between these two patterns sometimes occurs. Castleman disease–like changes may occur as part of the lymphocytic reaction in a number of processes, including HIV infections, various autoimmune diseases (especially rheumatoid arthritis) metastatic malignancies, and Hodgkin disease (Frizzera, 1988). Consequently, the diagnosis of Castleman disease should be made only on adequately sampled lesions, with an awareness of the clinical history.

MALIGNANT LYMPHOMAS INVOLVING THE THYMUS

In children, approximately 60% of mediastinal tumors are malignant lymphomas. Two thirds of these are B and T cell lymphomas (usually lymphoblastic type, with far fewer mediastinal

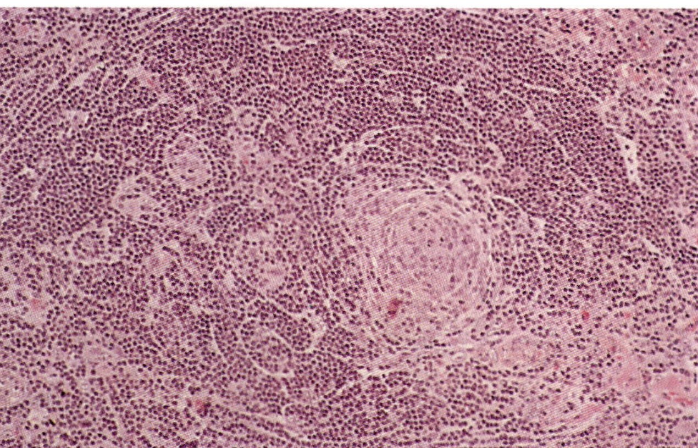

Figure 17–11

Castleman disease, hyaline vascular type, mediastinum. Note the regressively transformed germinal centers, several within one "cloud" of mantle zone cells, a feature that is characteristic of Castleman disease.

large–B cell type), and one third are Hodgkin disease. Most malignant lymphomas may potentially involve the mediastinum, but *primary* thymic involvement by lymphoma is uncommon, occurring only with lymphoblastic lymphoma of T cell lineage, large B cell lymphoma, and Hodgkin disease (Strickler & Kurtin, 1991). For more detailed coverage of these lymphomas, see Chap. 12.

T Lymphoblastic Lymphoma and Leukemia

Definition

T lymphoblastic lymphoma and leukemia is a neoplasm in which immature T progenitors predominate. When this neoplasm principally involves the marrow, it is conventionally referred to as acute lymphoblastic leukemia, T cell type. When it principally involves extramarrow sites, it is termed T lymphoblastic lymphoma or convoluted T cell lymphoma. Most T lymphoblastic lymphomas originate in the thymus, apparently because the thymus gland is normally the site of T cell maturation.

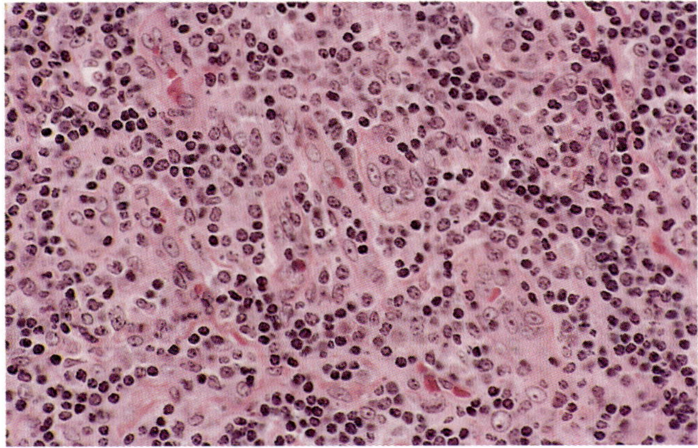

Figure 17–12

Castleman disease, hyaline vascular type. The interfollicular area contains prominent venules associated with mural collagen. Note also the relative absence of large cells and plasma cells.

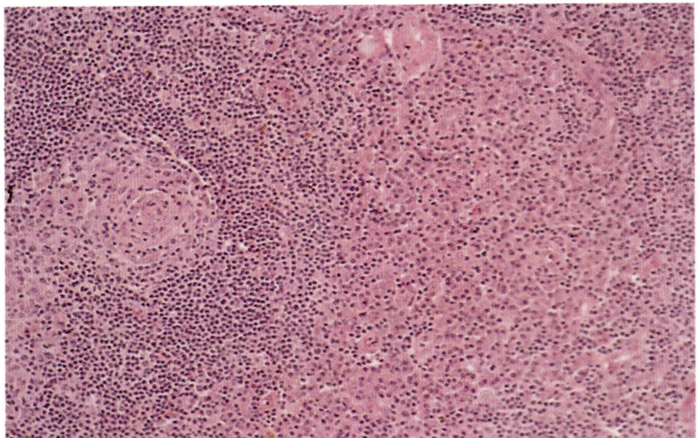

Figure 17–13

Castleman disease, plasma cell type, mediastinum. This patient was a 15-year-old girl. There is a regressively transformed germinal center on the left. The interfollicular areas, shown on the right, contain sheets of plasma cells.

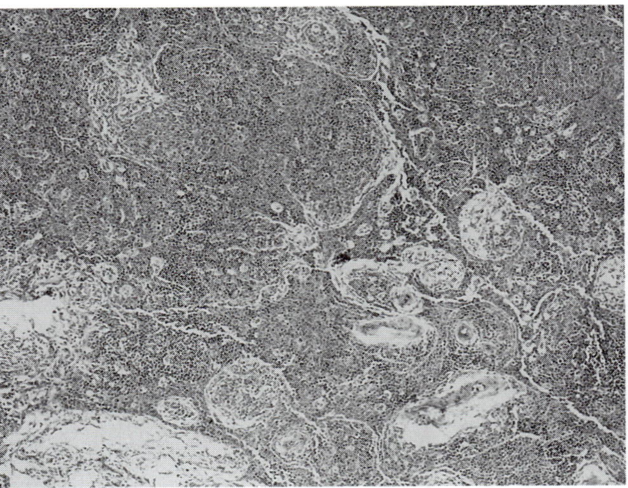

Figure 17–14

T lymphoblastic lymphoma, thymus. The unusual architectural pattern is due to infiltration of preexisting thymic lobules by neoplastic lymphoblasts.

Clinical Features

T lymphoblastic lymphoma has an age peak in the second and third decades, occurs more frequently in males, is the second commonest tumor of the mediastinum in children (Dehner, 1987), and is the commonest lymphoma involving the mediastinum in children. Sixty to 70% of T lymphoblastic lymphoma cases involve the mediastinum at the time of diagnosis (Griffith et al, 1987; Tubergen et al, 1995). Most patients have cough and chest pain. Many have as presenting symptoms shortness of breath or inspiratory pain related to pleural involvement by lymphoma. Likewise, infiltration into the pericardium may produce cardiac tamponade, or dysphagia may result from esophageal compression. Some patients present with superior vena cava syndrome or obstruction of large airways (Nathwani et al, 1976; Picozzi & Coleman, 1990). There are isolated reports of concurrent lymphoblastic lymphoma and myasthenia gravis (Liu et al, 1992). Patients treated with multiagent chemotherapy have a complete remission rate near 90%, with a 5-year median survival rate of about 70% (Eden et al, 1992; Picozzi, 1993; Picozzi & Coleman, 1990).

Histopathologic Features

T lymphoblastic lymphomas involving the thymus have a diffuse growth pattern with infiltrative borders, efface the thymic architecture, overrun thymic epithelium, and in many cases invade through the thymic capsule into adjacent soft tissues. In these instances, residual thymic epithelial cells may be found at the tumor periphery or in small clusters amid the tumor cells. They are often inapparent except in slides stained for keratin. In some cases thymic lobules are infiltrated and expanded (Fig. 17–14), with neoplastic lymphocytes interspersed among thymic epithelial cells and Hassall corpuscles. This pattern should not be mistaken for a thymoma, discussed later. In other cases collagen sclerosis (Fig. 17–15) or an unusual single-file arrangement of the neoplastic cells may be seen as the tumor involves the thymic capsule and interlobular septa. Cystic changes in the thymus are unusual in lymphoblastic lymphomas, although cysts occur as a reaction to other intrathymic neoplasms. These lymphomas are clinically aggressive and have high mitotic rates, frequent apoptotic cells, and a "starry sky" pattern produced by phagocytic histiocytes (Barcos & Lukes, 1975; Lukes & Collins, 1992; Nathwani et al, 1976; Stein et al, 1976; Warnke et al, 1995).

As described in Chap. 15, cells in lymphoblastic lymphomas are medium sized, with convoluted or ovoid nuclei, delicate chromatin, small nucleoli, and sparse cytoplasm (Fig. 17–16). They exhibit minimal pyroninophilia. Occasional cases are characterized by cells that do not have convoluted nuclei. A large-cell variety probably exists as well (Barcos & Lukes, 1975).

Phenotypic Features

As discussed in Chap. 15, lymphoblastic lymphomas are neoplasms of T cell precursors. Cells from an individual case often express a constellation of T cell antigens corresponding to the antigens on normal T cells at specific stages of maturation. However, "aberrant" phenotypes often occur, usually owing to loss of one or more expected antigens. For cases of lymphoblastic lymphoma involving the thymus, the phenotypes often closely match those found on cortical and medullary thymocytes. In addition, the cells in almost all cases of lymphoblastic

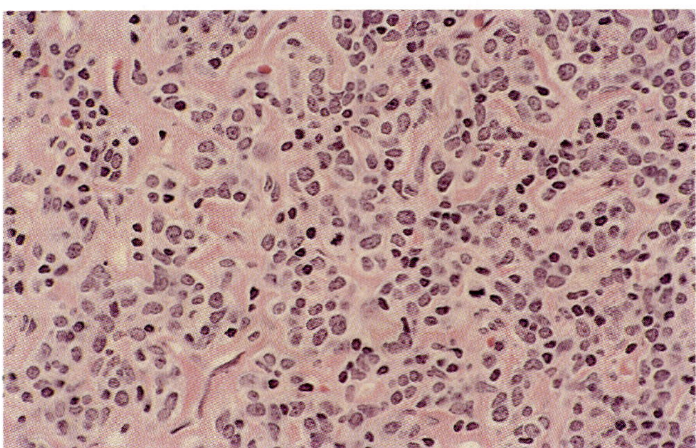

Figure 17–15

T lymphoblastic lymphoma, thymus. In this example there is the unusual finding of collagen sclerosis accompanying the neoplastic cells.

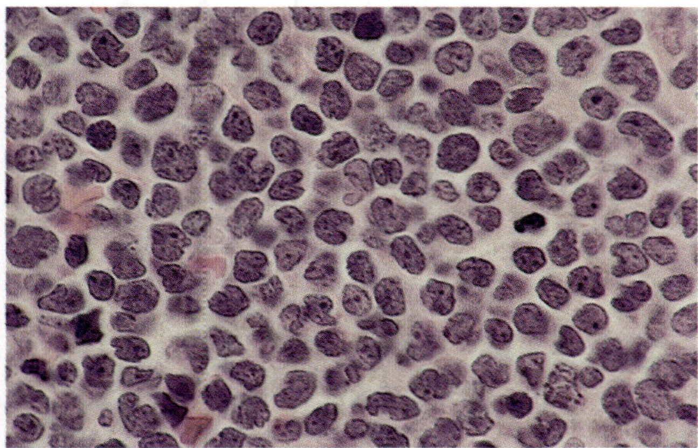

Figure 17–16

T lymphoblastic lymphoma, thymus. Typical cytologic features of the convoluted variant of this type of lymphoma are illustrated. Tumor cells are not cohesive and have dispersed chromatin and nuclear folds.

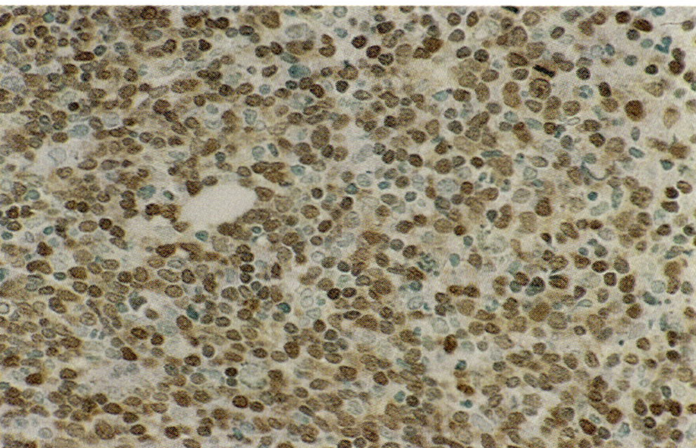

Figure 17–17

T lymphoblastic lymphoma, thymus. There is strong TdT positivity in almost all the neoplastic cells. Immunoperoxidase stain for TdT.

lymphoma express terminal deoxynucleotidyltransferase (Fig. 17–17) (Feller et al, 1986; Kaneko et al, 1989; Sheibani et al, 1987; Weiss et al, 1986).

Differential Diagnosis

The thymic tumor most closely resembling lymphoblastic lymphoma is lymphocyte-rich thymoma. Thymomas usually occur in adults, with a median age in the sixth decade, and are very uncommon in children (Lewis et al, 1987; Pescarmona et al, 1992; Ramon y Cajal & Suster, 1991). Since lymphoblastic lymphomas are uncommon in older adults, the age of the patient is a very important differential consideration. The features of these two tumors are compared and contrasted in Table 17–6. On low magnification thymomas have an organoid appearance, with lobulated borders, fibrous septa that circumscribe the lobules, and small blood vessels surrounded by perivascular spaces (Fig. 17–18). Lymphoblastic lymphomas have infiltrative borders, with single and clustered neoplastic lymphoblasts involving fat, collagen, and serous membranes. In lymphocyte-rich thymomas, the epithelial cells are large and have rounded nuclei, vesicular chromatin, small albeit distinct nucleoli, and inapparent cytoplasm (Fig. 17–19). These cells are usually single and rather uniformly distributed. Admixed lymphocytes have smaller nuclei, stippled chromatin, and small, inconspicuous nucleoli. The neoplastic epithelial cells in thymomas are highlighted by stains for keratin and characteristically form an interconnecting meshwork throughout the tumor (Fig. 17–20).

In lymphoblastic lymphoma, in contrast, keratin-positive residual epithelial cells are uncommon and are distributed singly and in small clusters. Lymphocyte-rich thymomas and lymphoblastic lymphomas may be associated with many mitotic figures, tingible-body macrophages, and a “starry sky” appearance. Lymphoblastic lymphoma cells have delicate chromatin and more pronounced nuclear convolutions in comparison to the lymphocytes in thymomas. The phenotype of lymphocytes in thymomas may be identical to that of the cells in lymphoblastic lymphoma, an obvious diagnostic pitfall, especially if the histologic features of the tumor are not carefully evaluated in well-fixed sections. Lymphoblastic lymphomas almost universally have clonal rearrangements of the T cell receptor genes, whereas lymphocyte-rich thymomas contain polyclonal T lymphocytes (Muller-Hermelink et al, 1986). In summary, distinction between thymoma and lymphoblastic lymphoma is not difficult unless the pathologist is unaware of the patient’s age or the tumor sample is small or distorted.

The differential diagnosis of lymphoblastic lymphoma also includes small transformed (noncleaved) cell processes of the Burkitt type. Patients with Burkitt-type lymphoma usually have an abdominal presentation (in Western countries), have a B cell phenotype, and are usually readily distinguished from lymphoblastic lymphoma. In tissue sections both are high grade and show diffusely infiltrative growth patterns, and neoplastic cells are similar in size. Burkitt-type cells are distinctly pyroninophilic and have readily recognized albeit small nucleoli. For further discussion of these two lymphomas, see Chaps. 14

Table 17–6

Distinction between Lymphoblastic Lymphoma and Lymphocyte-Rich Thymoma

Feature	Thymoma	Lymphoblastic Lymphoma
Architecture	Lobulated	Diffuse, infiltrative
Fibrous septa	Present	Absent
Perivascular spaces	Present	Absent
“Starry sky”	Present	Present
Epithelial cells	Latticework arrangement	Rare, scattered, clustered
Lymphocytes	Rounded nuclei	Convoluted nuclei
Lymphocyte phenotype	T precursor	T precursor
T cell receptor	Germ line or polyclonal	Clonal rearrangements

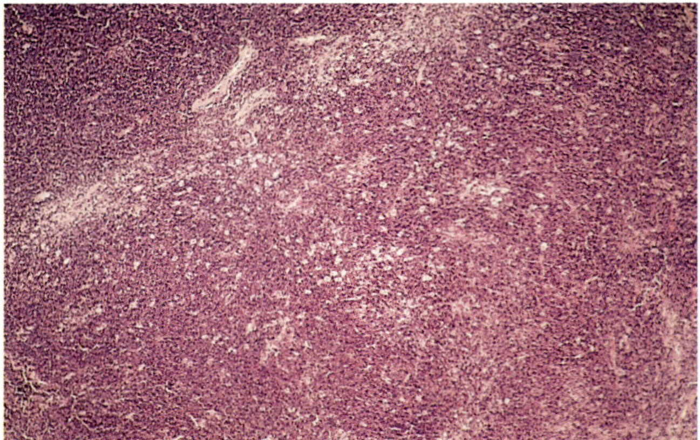

Figure 17–18

Thymoma, lymphocyte-rich type. The prominent "starry sky" appearance is similar to that seen with lymphoblastic lymphomas.

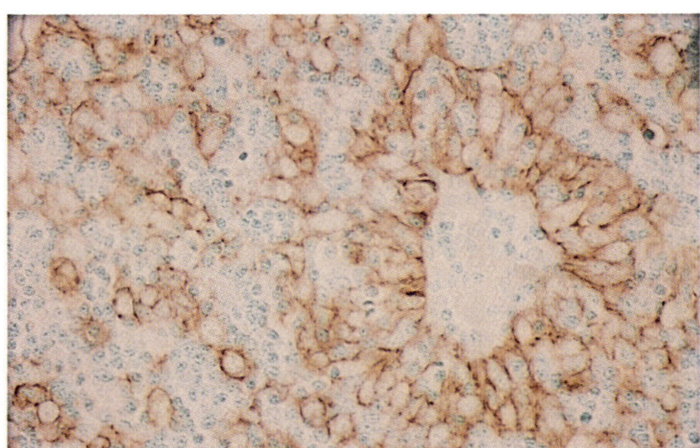

Figure 17–20

Thymoma, lymphocyte-rich type. The keratin-positive neoplastic thymic epithelial cells form an interconnecting meshwork throughout the tumor. Immunoperoxidase stain for keratin.

and 15. Specific diagnoses of these two processes may be made by examination of needle aspirates coupled with flow cytometric analysis (see Chap. 2).

Acute myelogenous leukemia rarely presents as an extramedullary tumor (granulocytic sarcoma) (Byrd et al, 1995; Meis et al, 1986; Neiman et al, 1981) and even more rarely involves the thymus gland at presentation (Liu et al, 1989; Mallick, 1987; Rege et al, 1993). Acute myelogenous leukemia and lymphoblastic lymphoma have morphologic similarities, including a high mitotic rate, intermixed tingible-body macrophages, and infiltrative growth patterns. Cytologically they are virtually indistinguishable (Fig. 17–21), since blasts in both are medium-sized cells with irregular nuclear contours, delicate chromatin, small nucleoli, and sparse cytoplasm. Extramedullary leukemias may contain eosinophilic myelocytes admixed with the myeloblasts, but lymphoblastic lymphomas may also be infiltrated by eosinophils. Flow studies readily differentiate between these two neoplasms. If fresh tissue is unavailable, paraffin-section immunohistochemical studies may be diagnostic. Cells of lymphoblastic lymphoma express TdT, CD43, and CD3, whereas myelogenous leukemia cells express CD34 (in a subset of cases), CD68, lysozyme, and myeloperoxidase (Fig. 17–22) (Chuang & Li, 1997; Davey et al, 1988; Pinkus & Pinkus, 1991; Roth et al, 1995). Electron miscroscopic study is also diagnostic in myelogenous leukemia.

Primary Mediastinal Large–B Cell Lymphoma

Equivalent Terms

Other terms for primary mediastinal B cell lymphoma are mediastinal large-cell lymphoma with sclerosis and clear cell lymphoma of the mediastinum.

Definition

Mediastinal large–B cell lymphoma is probably derived from intrathymic B cells and has distinct clinical, immunologic, and genetic features.

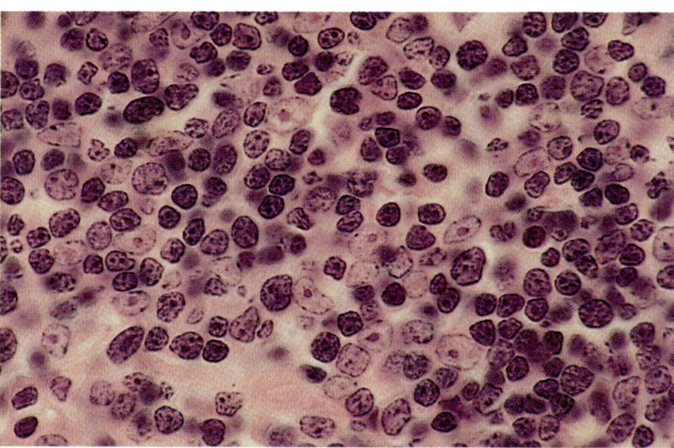

Figure 17–19

Thymoma, lymphocyte-rich type. Neoplastic thymic epithelial cells with large, round nuclei and vesicular chromatin are interspersed among the nonneoplastic lymphocytes. This appearance contrasts with that of T lymphoblastic lymphoma in Figs. 17–15 and 17–16.

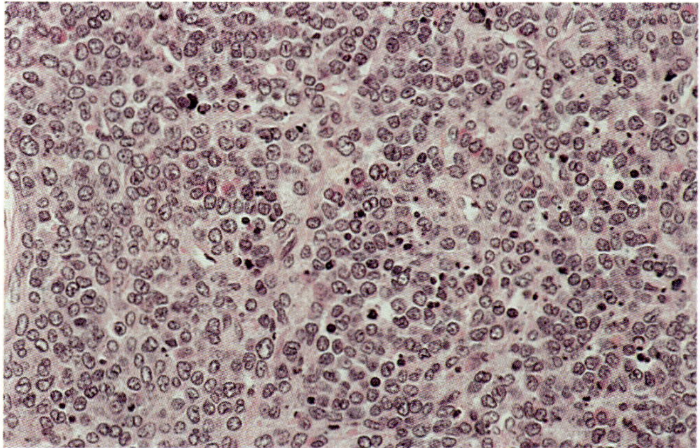

Figure 17–21

Acute myelogenous leukemia (extramedullary leukemia in mediastinum). The patient had superior vena cava syndrome secondary to massive anterior mediastinal involvement by acute leukemia. Most of the neoplastic cells have the characteristics of blasts, but occasional eosinophilic myelocytes are intermixed.

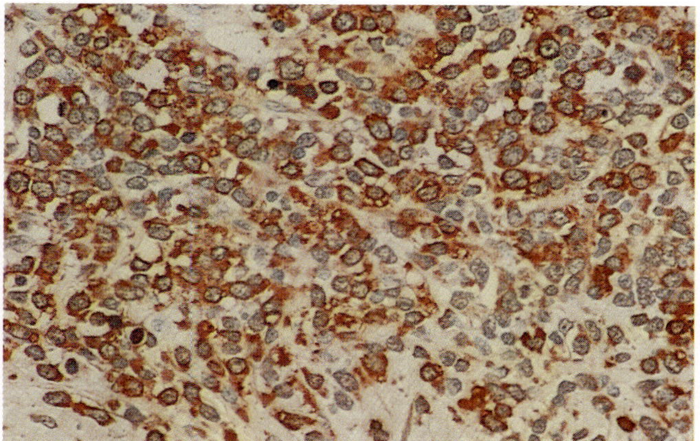

Figure 17–22

Acute myelogenous leukemia (extramedullary leukemia). The blasts are strongly myeloperoxidase positive. Immunoperoxidase stain for myeloperoxidase.

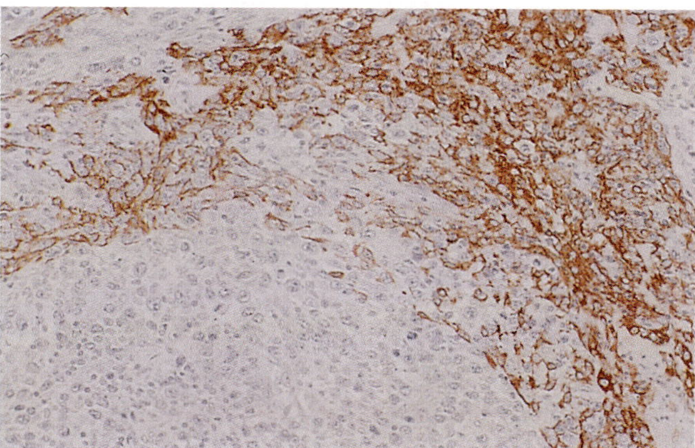

Figure 17–23

Large B cell lymphoma, mediastinum. The keratin stain highlights the proliferation of thymic epithelial cells as a reaction to thymic involvement by this lymphoma. A similar reaction occurs in Hodgkin disease. Immunoperoxidase stain for keratin (AE1/AE3).

Clinical Features and Prognosis

Besides Hodgkin disease, primary mediastinal B cell lymphoma is the commonest lymphoma arising in the mediastinum in adults in the United States. It also occurs in children (Bunin et al, 1986; Carr et al, 1993; Nathwani et al, 1987; Piira et al, 1995). The median age of occurrence is in the third and fourth decades. Some series have reported a bimodal age distribution, with one peak in young adult females and the second in older males. At presentation there is usually a large anterior mediastinal mass with cough, chest pain, and tightness. Structures adjacent to the thymus, including lung, pleura, pericardium, sternum, and chest wall, may be invaded. Resulting symptoms are hydrothorax, pericardial effusions, and superior vena cava syndrome. In most patients the lymphoma is confined to the chest at the time of presentation, but spread to kidney, adrenal, liver, pancreas, gastrointestinal tract, central nervous system, ovary, and retroperitoneal lymph nodes also occurs (Davis et al, 1990; Jacobson et al, 1988; Kirn et al, 1993; Perrone et al, 1986). This is an unusual lymphoma in that peripheral lymph node involvement is uncommon, either at presentation or at relapse.

Earlier series suggested that the prognosis of mediastinal large-cell lymphomas is poor (Haioun et al, 1989). However, adult patients treated with an anthracycline-based regimen equivalent to CHOP (cyclophosphamide, doxorubicin, vincristine, and prednisone) with or without radiation to the mediastinal mass may have rates of complete remission (80%) and disease-free survival at 5 years (59%) that are similar to those of patients with large–B cell lymphomas in other locations (Jacobson et al, 1988). Pediatric patients receiving multiagent chemotherapy and mediastinal radiation had rates of complete remission and disease-free survival at 4 years of 92% and 74%, respectively (Bunin et al, 1986). Relapses usually occur within 2 to 3 years of the initial diagnosis and often involve intraabdominal sites. In patients with disease confined to the chest, the major adverse prognostic factors are pleural effusions and a tumor diameter > 10 cm (Kirn et al, 1993).

Histopathologic Features

Most mediastinal large-cell lymphomas diffusely efface the thymic architecture and invade the adjacent fat, although rare cases involve only the thymic medulla. Histologic evidence of thymic involvement includes isolation of Hassall corpuscles or single thymic epithelial cells by neoplastic cells and thymic cysts lined with squamous epithelium amid a neoplastic infiltrate. Residual thymic epithelium may be recognizable only with keratin stains (Davis et al, 1990) (Fig. 17–23). Collagen deposition varies in mediastinal B cell lymphomas, although some collagen sclerosis is found in almost all adequately sampled cases. Collagen may form hyalinized strands that branch and taper, compartmentalizing the neoplastic cells into small groups (Fig. 17–24), or may form delicate interstitial fibers as well as broad sheets (Perrone et al, 1986). Necrosis may also be prominent and cause diagnostic difficulties with small biopsy specimens.

In many cases, the tumor cells have the appearance of large transformed (noncleaved) cells or centroblasts. They are medium to large cells with rounded nuclear contours; dispersed chromatin; variably prominent, multiple nucleoli; and abundant amphophilic cytoplasm (see Fig. 17–24). In other cases there is significant nuclear pleomorphism, with cells that resemble Reed-Sternberg cells, large cleaved lymphocytes, or B immunoblasts. Cytoplasmic clearing may be prominent (see Fig. 17–24), leading to the designation *clear cell lymphomas*. Clearing may be an artifact of formalin fixation because it is less frequent in B5- or Zenker-fixed tissue sections (Perrone et al, 1986; Strickler & Kurtin, 1991). A few cases have prominently lobated nuclei (see Fig. 17–24) (Lamarre et al, 1989; Perrone et al, 1986). Because of the cytologic variability (see Fig. 17–24), mediastinal large B cell lymphomas have been difficult to categorize in some lymphoma classifications (Lazzarino et al, 1993; Moller et al, 1986a).

Immunophenotype

The phenotypic profile of mediastinal large B cell lymphomas is similar to that of many other B cell lymphomas. They are positive for CD45, CD45RA, CD19, CD20 (Fig. 17–25), CD22 (Lamarre et al, 1989), CD37, CD40 (Moller et al, 1989), and CD79a (Kanavaros et al, 1995). They do not stain positively for CD30. Mediastinal large-cell lymphoma cells may not express surface immunoglobulin, in distinction to other types of B cell lymphomas. When they do, IgG and IgA are the most common isotypes. They are often positive for PC1 (plasma cell antigen) (Moller et al, 1987). In addition, they infrequently express CD21, are universally negative for CD10, and have a higher frequency of CD11c and CD23 positivity

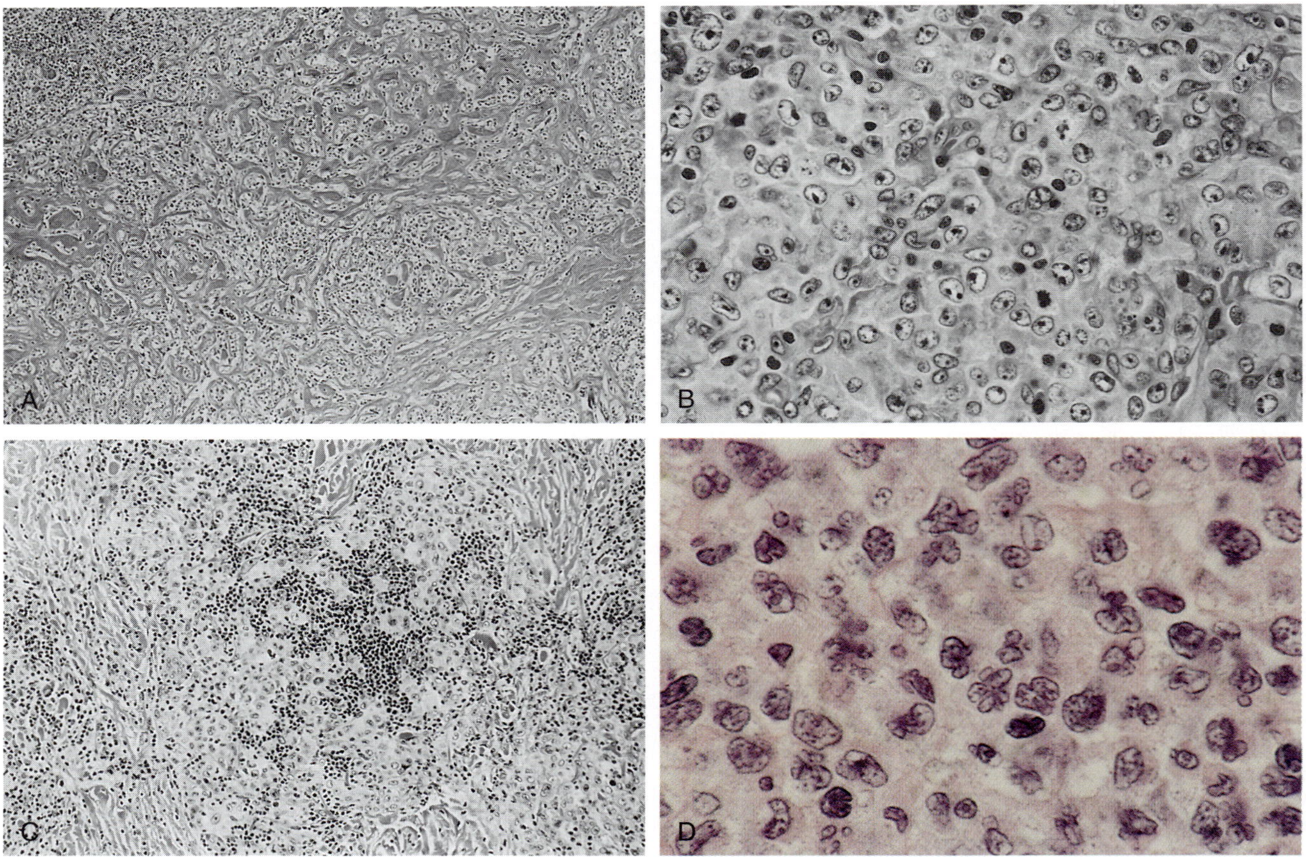

Figure 17–24

Mediastinal large B cell lymphoma. *A*, Collagen sclerosis is prominent. *B*, The characteristic cytologic features of this lymphoma are shown. There are back-to-back large cells, with abundant cytoplasm and prominent nucleoi. *C*, The neoplastic cells have abundant clear cytoplasm. *D*, Multilobated nuclei are a feature of this case.

than do follicular center cell lymphomas (Lamarre et al, 1989; Moller et al, 1989). Thus, the cells of mediastinal lymphomas antigenically resemble a population of normal thymic medullary B lymphocytes and monocytoid (parafollicular) B cells (Isaacson et al, 1987; Moller et al, 1989). Most cases of mediastinal large-cell lymphoma also have aberrant absence or diminished expression of HLA class I and II antigens compared with normal B cells and most B cell lymphomas (Moller et al, 1986b).

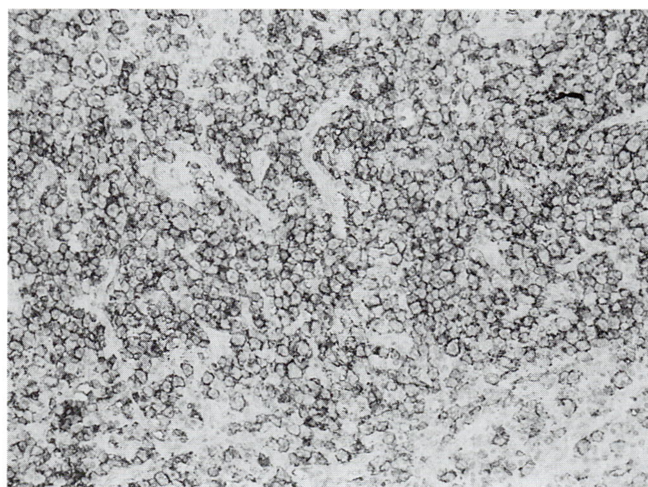

Figure 17–25

Mediastinal large B cell lymphoma. The lymphoma cells are strongly CD20 positive. Immunoperoxidase stain for CD20.

The adhesion molecule expression in mediastinal large-cell lymphomas has been comprehensively studied (Eichelmann et al, 1992). The pattern of β_1 integrin molecule expression is similar to that observed in intramedullary thymic B cells: negative for VLAα_1, -α_2, -α_3, -α_5, and -α_6; universally positive for ICAM-1; negative for CD11b; and exhibiting variable expression of VLAα_4, CD11a, CD11c, LFA-3, CD44, and LECAM. Local growth without dissemination of B cell lymphomas has been attributed to ICAM-1 expression and diminished CD44 and LECAM-1 expression (Eichelmann et al, 1992). In this regard, most cases of mediastinal B cell lymphomas are positive for ICAM-1 and lack expression of CD44 and LECAM-1, possibly providing an explanation for their localization to the thymus and mediastinum.

Genetic Features

Cytogenetic studies of mediastinal large-cell lymphomas are limited. Comparative genomic hybridization and fluorescence in situ hybridization showed gains of chromosomal material in 24 of 26 cases, with the most frequent abnormalities being additional material on chromosomes 9p, Xq, Xp, 12q, and 2p (Joos et al, 1996). These are novel findings compared with those in other types of lymphomas and further support the

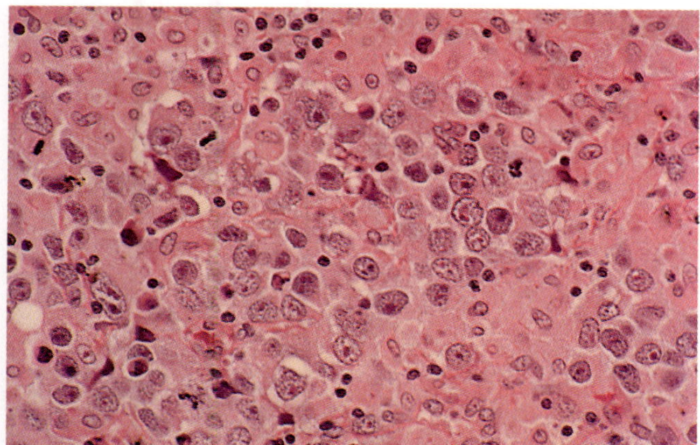

Figure 17–26

Seminoma, mediastinum. The cytologic features of seminomas overlap with those of large B cell lymphomas. Note the intermixed macrophage clusters, which may be seen in both neoplasms.

concept that primary mediastinal large–B cell lymphomas are a unique lymphoma subtype.

Clonal immunoglobulin gene rearrangements and lack of clonal T cell antigen receptor rearrangements may be demonstrated in almost all cases. Oncogene involvement in this tumor differs from that in most aggressive B cell lymphomas, since it lacks *MYC*, *BCL1*, and *BCL2* gene rearrangements. *BCL6* rearrangements were found in only 1 of 16 cases (Tsang et al, 1996). Occasional cases exhibit *MYC* or *P53* gene mutations, and no cases with N-*RAS* mutations have been described. Epstein-Barr virus is not considered to play a role in the pathogenesis of this type of lymphoma (Tsang et al, 1996).

Differential Diagnosis

Mediastinal large–B cell lymphomas exhibit abundant collagen sclerosis and clustering of cells with clear cytoplasm, features shared with mediastinal seminomas (Fig. 17–26). Seminomas are often accompanied by a distinct granulomatous host response or by yolk sac, embryonal, teratomatous, or choriocarcinomatous elements. Seminoma cells contain diastase-digestible periodic acid–Schiff–positive glycogen, whereas the clear cells of mediastinal lymphomas lack glycogen. In immunohistochemical studies of paraffin sections, B cell lymphomas have been found to express CD45 and B cell lineage antigens, such as CD20, whereas seminomas do not. Seminomas express placental alkaline phosphatase (Fig. 17–27) and in some cases low-molecular-weight keratin (Burke & Mostofi, 1988; Manivel et al, 1987; Wick et al, 1987).

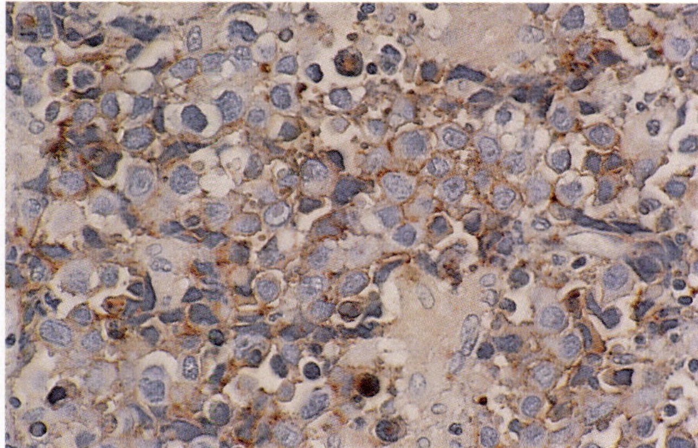

Figure 17–27

Seminoma, mediastinum. The tumor cells stain positively for placental alkaline phosphatase while large B cell lymphomas are negative. Immunoperoxidase stain for placental alkaline phosphatase.

Mediastinal large–B cell lymphomas may also be confused with Hodgkin disease, particularly the nodular sclerosis type. The reaction pattern in Hodgkin disease, including eosinophils, plasma cells, macrophages, and small lymphocytes, is characteristic and is not seen in large B cell lymphomas. Immunophenotypic studies are reliable in diagnosis, especially when biopsy specimens are small. In paraffin-section immunohistochemical studies, mediastinal large–B cell lymphomas are found to be CD45+, CD15−, and CD30−. Antibodies to CD20 strongly stain most cells in cases of mediastinal large–B cell lymphoma. In contrast, Reed-Sternberg cells and mononuclear variants are CD45−, CD15+, and/or CD30+. Reed-Sternberg cells and variants may be CD20+, especially in mediastinal cases, but the reactivity is variable from cell to cell and often weak and focal.

Hodgkin Disease

Clinical Features of Thymic Involvement

Mediastinal involvement by Hodgkin disease (HD) occurs in about 60% of cases at presentation (Colby et al, 1981; Lukes et al, 1966; Mauch et al, 1993; McClain et al, 1990; Patchefsky et al, 1973), but the frequency of thymic involvement is not known. In 60 pediatric patients, 58% had mediastinal involvement by HD at initial staging (Luker & Siegel, 1993). Seventeen (28%) of them had involvement of the thymus as well as mediastinal lymph node involvement in all but one case. In adults, the frequency of thymic HD is similar to that observed in children (Heron et al, 1988). In summary, mediastinal HD is very common, thymic HD is less common, and isolated primary thymic HD is rare. In terms of the realtionship of HD subtype to mediastinal involvement, nodular sclerosis type most frequently involves the mediastinum, followed by mixed cellularity type. Lymphocyte-predominant and lymphocyte-depletion types rarely involve the mediastinum and almost never involve the thymus. Thymic HD is invariably nodular sclerosis in type. The disease has a predilection for older adolescents and young adult females. A large mediastinal mass, occupying at least one third of the maximum intrathoracic diameter on conventional posteroanterior radiographs (Hoppe, 1989) (Fig. 17–28), is a significant adverse prognostic factor for stages I and II intrathoracic HD.

Some patients have a detectable thymic mass following therapy for mediastinal HD. Such masses are often not residual HD but probably are fibrous connective tissue, since serial computed tomographic scans of the chest in these cases are stable over time, and there is no mediastinal adenopathy (McClain et al, 1990; Murray & Parker, 1984). In other patients, particularly after chemotherapy or radiation therapy, the thymus undergoes rebound hyperplasia. Thymic hyperplasia usually occurs within several weeks following completion of therapy and most often regresses spontaneously or responds to a short course of corticosteroids (Ford et al, 1987; Heron et al, 1988). Residual thymic masses may also be due to thymic cysts that are presumably a reactive phenomenon in a previously diseased gland (Lindfors et al, 1985; Murray & Parker, 1984; Stolar et al, 1987).

Histopathologic Features

HD in the thymus gland has a cytologic appearance identical to that in other sites (see Chap. 13). Reed-Sternberg cells and

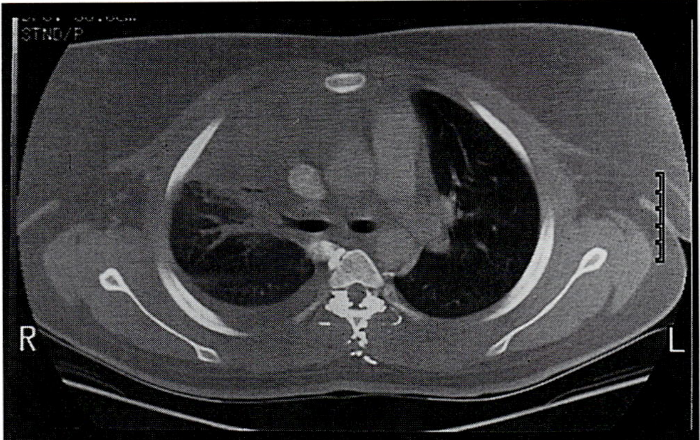

Figure 17–28

Hodgkin disease, mediastinum. A chest computed tomographic scan demonstrates a large anterior mediastinal mass.

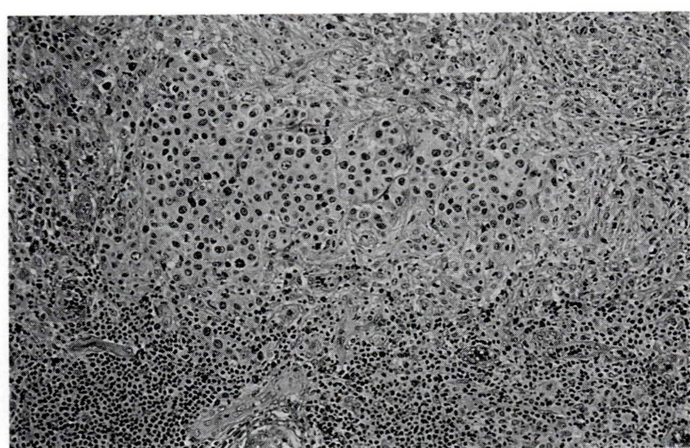

Figure 17–30

Hodgkin disease, nodular sclerosis type, syncytial variant, mediastinum. An area of necrosis (*top*) is surrounded by numerous lacunar cells.

mononuclear variants range from sparse (Fig. 17–29) to numerous (Fig. 17–30), and the host response includes varying proportions of lymphocytes, plasma cells, eosinophils, and macrophages. Fibrous bands usually circumscribe as well as transect the areas of HD in the thymus. Thymic remnants may usually be seen (Fechner, 1969; Katz & Lattes, 1969; Keller & Castleman, 1974). In some cases of HD there is a reactive epithelial proliferation that resembles the spindle cell component of thymomas (Suster & Moran, 1995). Thorough examination of the specimen may be required to detect the Reed-Sternberg cells and reactive components typical of HD. The thymus also reacts to HD by forming squamous epithelial cell–lined cysts that range in size from microscopic to very large (Fig. 17–31) (Federle & Callen, 1979; Lindfors et al, 1985; Nogues et al, 1987; Suster & Moran, 1995). Some cases are characterized by such large cysts that the lesion is indistinguishable from a benign thymic cyst on gross examination. Extensive sampling of thymic cysts is mandatory so that HD is not missed on microscopic examination. These thymic epithelial reactive processes originally led to the designation *granulomatous thymoma*, before the demonstration that HD was the underlying problem (Castleman, 1955).

Differential Diagnosis

The differential diagnosis of HD in the thymus includes Castleman disease, mediastinal large–B cell lymphoma, CD30+ anaplastic large-cell lymphoma, germ cell tumors (especially seminomas), thymic carcinomas, and thymoma. The distinction between HD and large B cell lymphomas was discussed earlier.

In some cases of HD, the diagnostic infiltrates occur between reactive germinal centers, a pattern termed interfollicular HD (Doggett et al, 1983), which may mimic Castleman disease. On low magnification of specimens containing interfollicular HD, the reactive follicles usually predominate, but in a small number of cases the follicles exhibit regressive transformation identical to the follicular changes in hyaline vascular–type Castleman disease (Zarate-Osorno et al, 1994). The diagnosis of interfollicular HD is confirmed by finding Reed-Sternberg cells and variants in ill-defined nodular lesions containing eosinophils, plasma cells, macrophages, and neutrophils located between the regressively transformed follicles. By contrast, the interfollicular areas of hyaline vascular

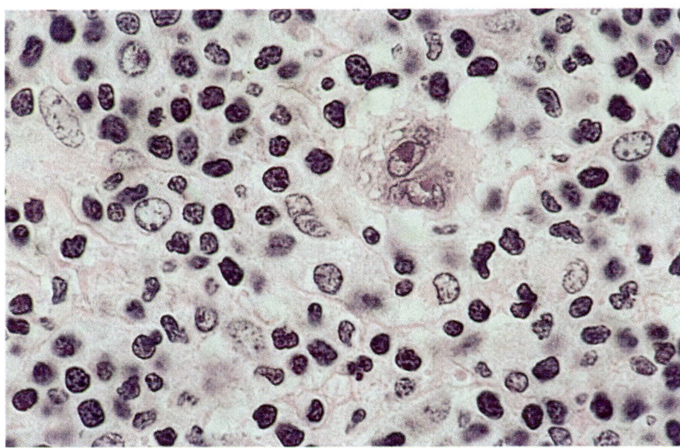

Figure 17–29

Hodgkin disease, nodular sclerosis type. A diagnostic Reed-Sternberg cell is intermixed with small lymphocytes and macrophages.

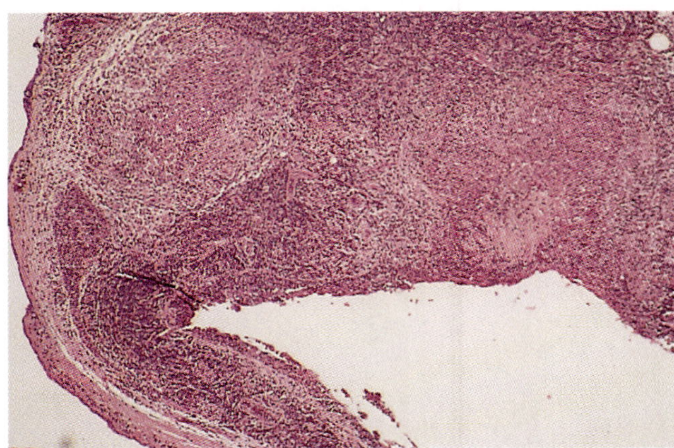

Figure 17–31

Hodgkin disease, mediastinum. Multiple intrathymic cysts are associated with septal infiltrates of the nodular sclerosis type of Hodgkin disease. The nodule (*upper left*) contains an area of Hodgkin disease. Lymphocystic hyperplasia is present in other areas of the cyst wall.

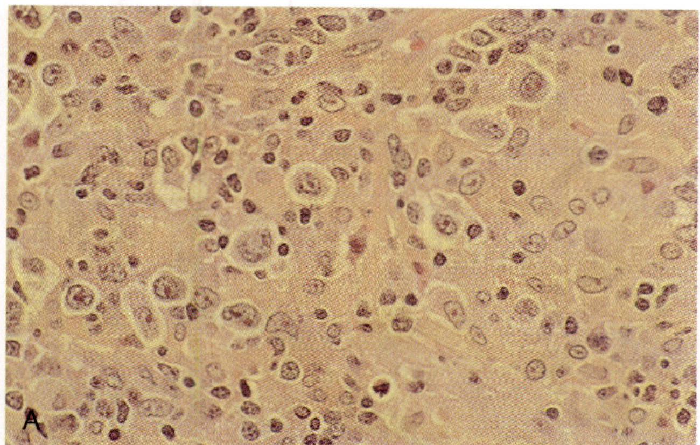

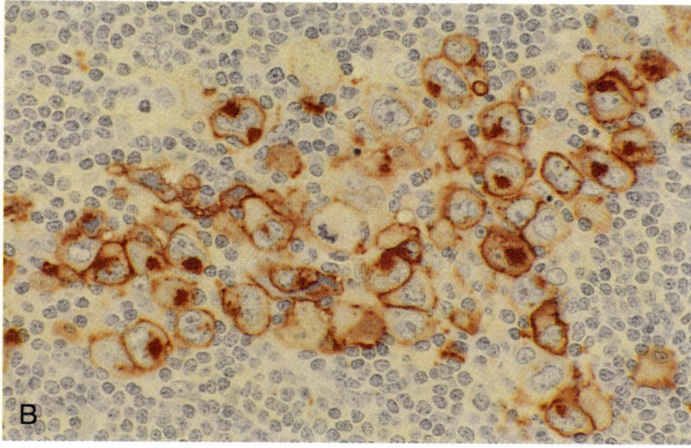

Figure 17–32

Hodgkin disease, mixed cellularity type, thymus. *A*, A granulomatous host response accompanies the Reed-Sternberg cells and variants, simulating a seminoma. *B*, The mononuclear variants stain strongly with antibodies to CD15. Immunoperoxidase stain for CD15.

type–Castleman disease contain sclerotic blood vessels, small lymphocytes, and few if any transformed lymphocytes, eosinophils, plasma cells, or macrophages. The interfollicular areas of the plasma cell variant of Castleman disease contain small lymphocytes and sheets of plasma cells but no Reed-Sternberg cells or mononuclear variants.

CD30+ anaplastic large-cell lymphoma closely resembles or is indistinguishable from cases of nodular sclerosing HD that contain many Reed-Sternberg cells and variants. Immunophenotypic studies are usually diagnostic, since tumor cells in the former are often positive for CD45, T cell lineage–associated antigens, epithelial membrane antigen, and p80/ALK-1. They are also strongly and uniformly CD30+, with a paranuclear globular and membrane staining pattern. In HD (excluding lymphocyte-predominant type) neoplastic cells are usually negative for CD45, T cell lineage antigens, epithelial membrane antigens, and p80/ALK-1, and they are typically positive for CD15 (Fig. 17–32). The pattern of CD30 expression (i.e., variable expression on a subset of the neoplastic cells) differs from that seen with CD30+ anaplastic large-cell lymphomas (Fillipa et al, 1996; Pileri et al, 1995; Zinzani et al, 1996). Lymphomas with numerous large cells resembling Reed-Sternberg cells have been classified as CD30+ anaplastic large-cell lymphoma, Hodgkin like, but critical review of follow-up and phenotypic data suggests that most of these cases are examples of nodular sclerosing HD.

Germ cell tumors, particularly seminomas, involving the mediastinum may mimic HD in their architectural and cytologic features as well as their granulomatous host response. Reed-Sternberg–like cells, eosinophils, and plasma cells are rare or not found in germ cell tumors (see Fig. 17–32). Seminoma cells contain glycogen, are positive for placental alkaline phosphatase and in some cases low-molecular-weight keratin proteins, and are negative for CD15 and CD30. However, the neoplastic cells in embryonal carcinomas may be positive for both CD30 and CD15, with a pattern similar to Reed-Sternberg cells. They may be identified by placental alkaline phosphatase and keratin positivity (Wick et al, 1987).

Cases of HD associated with thymic epithelial cell hyperplasia may be confused with thymomas (Suster & Moran, 1995). Clinically, thymomas are seen in older adults, whereas HD usually occurs in adolescents and young adults. Thymic epithelial neoplasms are usually not associated with eosinophils and plasma cells. In addition, thymic epithelial cells that are so cytologically atypical as to resemble mononuclear Reed-Sternberg cells retain their immunoreactivity for keratin. Rarely, HD forms a composite neoplasm with a thymoma (Ridell & Larsson, 1980).

MISCELLANEOUS CONDITIONS

Langerhans Cell Histiocytosis

Disseminated forms of Langerhans cell histiocytosis (LCH) may directly infiltrate the thymus gland or be associated with thymic atrophy or dysplasia. LCH may be found in thymus glands removed for myasthenia gravis. A few patients have had isolated involvement of the thymus (Bove et al, 1985; Segal et al, 1985). In most of these cases, thymic involvement was discovered incidentally, and the disease was limited to the thymus, to bone and thymus, or to thymus and adjacent intrathoracic structures. All of these patients had an indolent course. When the thymus is involved, Langerhans cells invade the thymic medulla, where they infiltrate and destroy the thymic epithelium and Hassall corpuscles. Microcystic changes and calcospherites may be found in association with LCH involvement (Bove et al, 1985). Cytologically, Langerhans cells are large, with folded nuclear contours, delicate chromatin, small but distinct nucleoli, and voluminous cytoplasm (Fig. 17–33). They are seen to contain Birbeck granules on electron microscopic examination and stain positively for S-100 protein and CD1a in immunoperoxidase preparations. Antibodies against CD1a (Fig. 17–34) have aided considerably in the recognition of Langerhans cells and their tumors in routinely processed paraffin-embedded tissue sections (Emile et al, 1995; Krenacs et al, 1993). Tissue infiltrates in LCH may be accompanied by multinucleated giant cells, foamy histiocytes, and numerous eosinophils. In one case there was depletion of thymic CD1+ and CD8+ lymphocytes (Bove et al, 1985). Patients with LCH frequently have decreased peripheral blood CD8+ T cells as well (Newton et al, 1987).

The thymus gland in patients with disseminated forms of LCH may exhibit thymic dysplasia or severe thymic atrophy similar to changes described in patients with immunodeficiencies (Hamoudi et al, 1982; Newton et al, 1987). These findings are apparently not related to the intensity of therapy, since the thymus gland in children treated for other malignancies does not exhibit the dysplastic changes seen in LCH patients.

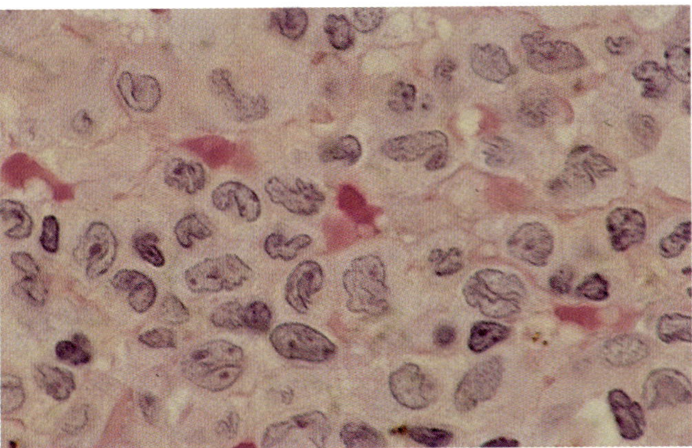

Figure 17–33

Langerhans cell histiocytosis. At high magnification, the characteristic folded and grooved nuclei, delicate chromatin, small nucleoli, and abundant pale cytoplasm are demonstrated.

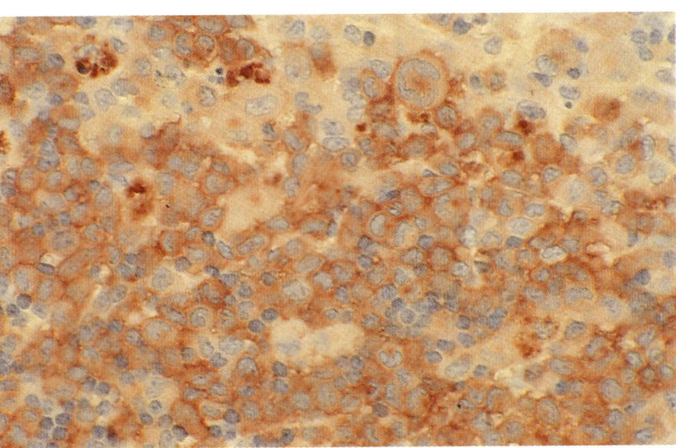

Figure 17–34

Langerhans cell histiocytosis. The tumor cells stain strongly with antibodies to CD1a. Immunoperoxidase stain for CD1a.

Rarely, patients with myasthenia gravis have follicular hyperplasia in the thymus and concurrent involvement by localized LCH (Bramwell & Burns, 1986; Gilcrease et al, 1997; Pescarmona et al, 1989). The autoimmune phenomena that characterize myasthenia gravis may be initiated by the presentation of acetylcholine receptor protein from the thymic myoid cells to the adjacent T cells by interdigitating cells and Langerhans cells. Loss of immunoregulation in the thymus might allow for the proliferation of Langerhans cells (Newton et al, 1987) and follicular hyperplasia in the myasthenic thymus.

Mediastinal Germ Cell Tumors Associated with Acute Myelogenous Leukemia

The thymus may contain aberrantly localized primordial germ cell elements that persist postnatally. These derivatives of the yolk sac normally give rise to both the testicular or ovarian germ cells and the marrow elements and are also thought to be the progenitors of mediastinal germ cell tumors. Mediastinal germ cell tumors other than seminomas, particularly those with yolk sac elements, are associated with the development of acute myelogenous leukemia and malignant histiocytosis (Chiganti et al, 1989; DeMent et al, 1985; Orazi et al, 1993) (Fig. 17–35). Hematopoietic precursors may be demonstrated in the yolk sac components of certain mediastinal germ cell tumors by microscopic and immunohistochemical studies. Acute leukemias may occur in untreated patients with germ cell tumors or may follow therapy for the germ cell tumor. The French-American-British classification types of acute leukemia associated with this phenomenon include M2, M4, M5, M6, M7, and mixed lineage. Some of the cases may represent therapy-related acute leukemias, and they have abnormalities of chromosomes 5 and 7. Others are clearly related to the germ cell tumor, since either the leukemic cells or the germ cell tumor and the leukemic blasts have a chromosomal abnormality, i(12p), almost exclusively encountered in germ cell tumors (Heim & Mietlman, 1987).

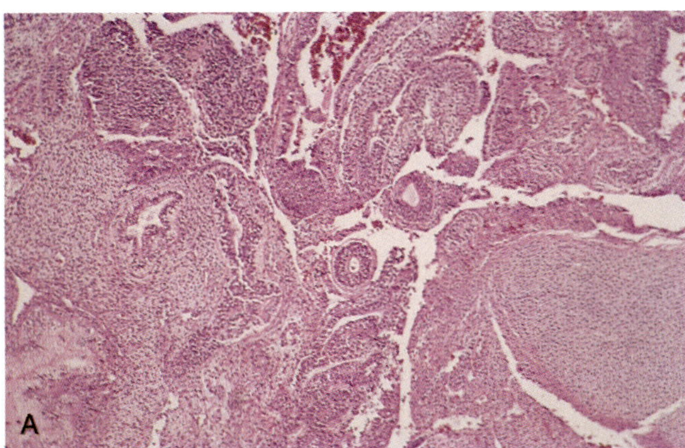

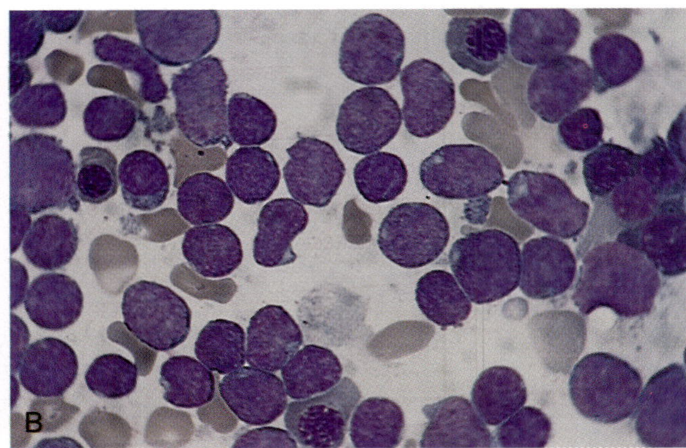

Figure 17–35

Germ cell tumor, mediastinum, associated with acute leukemia. *A*, This patient with a mixed germ cell tumor comprised of teratomatous, yolk sac, and embryonal carcinomatous elements developed acute monoblastic leukemia. The blasts exhibited the chromosome abnormality i(12p). In cases such as this, the acute leukemia is thought to arise from yolk sac elements in the germ cell tumor. *B*, The marrow from this patient exhibits acute monoblastic leukemia.

REFERENCES

Anderson G: Piecing together the thymic puzzle. Immunol Today 18:363–364, 1977.

Ardavin C: Thymic dendritic cells. Immunol Today 18:350–361, 1997.

Barcos M, Lukes R: Malignant lymphoma of convoluted lymphocytes: a new entity of possible T-cell type. In Sinks L, Gooden J (eds): Conflicts in Childhood Cancer: An Evaluation of Current Management. Liss, New York, pp 147–178, 1975.

Berrih S, Morel E, Gaud C, et al: Anti-AChR antibodies, thymic histology and T cell subsets in myasthenia gravis. Neurology 34:66–71, 1984.

Bieger R, Mc Adams A: (1966). Thymic cysts. Arch Pathol 82: 535–541, 1966.

Bove K, Hubertise P, Wong K: Thymus in untreated systemic histiocytosis X. Pediatr Pathol 4:99–115, 1985.

Bramwell N, Burns B: Histiocytosis X of the thymus in association with myasthenia gravis. Am J Clin Pathol 86:224–227, 1986.

Bunin N, Hvizdala E, Link M, et al: Mediastinal nonlymphoblastic lymphomas in children: a clinicopathologic study. J Clin Oncol 4:154–159, 1986.

Burke A, Mostofi K: Placental alkaline phosphatase immunohistochemistry of intratubular malignant germ cells and associated testicular germ cell tumors. Hum Pathol 19:663–670, 1988.

Byrd J, Edenfield J, Sheilds D, et al: Extramedullary myeloid cell tumors in acute nonlymphocytic leukemia: a clinical review. J Clin Oncol 13:1800–1816, 1995.

Carr T, Lockwood L, Stevens R, et al: Childood B cell lymphomas arising in the mediastinum. J Clin Pathol 46:513–516, 1993.

Castleman B: Tumors of the thymus gland. Fascicle 19, Atlas of Tumor Pathology. Armed Forces Institute of Pathology, Washington, DC, 1955.

Chiganti R, Ladanyi M, Samaniego F, et al: Leukemic differentiation of a mediastinal germ cell tumor. Genes Chromosomes Cancer 1:83–87, 1989.

Chuang S-S, Li C-Y: Useful panel of antibodies for the classification of acute leukemia by immunohistochemical methods in bone marrow trephine biopsy specimens. Am J Clin Pathol 107:410–418, 1997.

Colby T, Hoppe R, Warnke R: Hodgkin's disease: a clinicopathologic study of 659 cases. Cancer 49:1848–1858, 1981.

Cooper M, Chase H, Lowman J, et al: Immunologic defects in patients with Wiskott-Aldrich syndrome. Birth Defects 4:378–387, 1968.

Davey F, Olson S, Kurec A, et al: The immunophenotyping of extramedullary myeloid cell tumors in paraffin-embedded tissue sections. Am J Surg Pathol 12:699–707, 1988.

Davis R, Dorfman R, Warnke R: Primary large-cell lymphoma of the thymus: a diffuse B-cell neoplasm presenting as primary mediastinal lymphoma. Hum Pathol 21:1262–1268, 1990.

Dehner L: Mediastinum, lungs and cardiovascular system. In Pediatric Surgical Pathology. Williams & Wilkins, Baltimore, pp 229–231, 1987.

DeMent S, Eggleston J, Spivak J: Association between mediastinal germ cell tumors and hematologic malignancies: report of two cases and review of the literature. Am J Surg Pathol 9:23–30, 1985.

DiLoreto C, Mariuzzi L, DeGrassi A, et al: B-cell lymphoma of the thymus and salivary gland. J Clin Pathol 49:595–597, 1996.

Doggett R, Colby T, Dorfman R: Interfollicular Hodgkin's disease. Am J Surg Pathol 7:145–149, 1983.

Durov N: Thymic atrophy and immune deficiency in malnutrition. In Muller-Hermelink H (ed): The human thymus. Curr Top Pathol 75:127–146, 1986.

Eden O, Hann I, Imeson J, et al: Treatment of advanced stage T cell lymphoblastic lymphoma: results of the United Kingdom Children's Cancer Study Group (UKCCSG) protocol 8503. Br J Haematol 82:310–316, 1992.

Eichelmann A, Koretz K, Mechtersheimer G, et al: Adhesion receptor profile of thymic B-cell lymphoma. Am J Pathol 141:729–741, 1992.

Emile J-F, Wechsler J, Brousse N, et al: Langerhans' cell histiocytosis: definitive diagnosis with the use of monoclonal antibody O10 on routinely paraffin-embedded samples. Am J Surg Pathol 19: 636–641.

Fechner R: Hodgkin's disease of the thymus. Cancer 23:16–23, 1969.

Federle M, Callen P: Cystic Hodgkin's lymphoma of the thymus: computed tomography appearence. J Comput Asst Tomogr 3: 542–544, 1979.

Feller A, Parwaresch M, Stein H, et al: Immunophenotyping of T-lymphoblastic lymphoma/leukemia: correlation with normal T-cell maturation. Leuk Res, 10, 1025–1031, 1986.

Fillipa D, Ladanyi M, Wollner N, et al: CD30 (Ki-1) positive malignant lymphomas: clinical, immunophenotypic, histologic, and genetic characteristics and differences with Hodgkin's disease. Blood 87:2905–2917, 1996.

Ford E, Lockhart S, Sullivan M, et al: Mediastinal mass following chemotherapeutic treatment of Hodgkin's disease: recurrent tumor or thymic hyperplasia. J Pediatr Surg 22:1155–1159, 1987.

Frizzera G: Castleman's disease and related disorders. Semin Diagn Pathol 5:346–364, 1988.

Garcia A, Olinto F, Fortes T: Thymic hypoplasia due to congenital rubella. Arch Dis Child 49:181–185, 1974.

Gelfand D, Goldman A, Law E, et al: Thymic hyperplasia in children recovering from thermal burns. J Trauma 12:813–817, 1972.

Gilcrease M, Rajan B, Ostrowski M, et al: Localized thymic Langerhans' cell histiocytosis and its relationship with myasthenia gravis: immunohistochemical, ultrastructural and cytometric studies. Arch Pathol Lab Med 121:134–138, 1997.

Gitlin D, Crain J: The thymus and other lymphoid tissues in congential agammaglobulinemia: thymic alymphoplasia and lymphocytic hypoplasia and their relation to infection. Pediatrics 32:517–530, 1963.

Gitlin D, Vawter G, Craig J: Thymic alymphoplasia and congenital aleukocytosis. Pediatrics 33:184–192, 1964.

Goss C: Gray's Anatomy of the Human Body, 29th ed. Lea & Febiger, Philadelphia, 1973.

Griffith R, Kelly D, Nathwani B, et al: A morphologic study of childhood lymphoma of the lymphoblastic type: the Pediatric Oncology Group experience. Cancer 59:1126–1131, 1987.

Grody W, Fligiel S, Naeim F: Thymus involution in the acquired immunodeficiency syndrome. Am J Clin Pathol 84:85–95, 1985.

Grody W, Jobst S, Keesey J, et al: Pathologic evaluation of thymic hyperplasia in myasthenia gravis and Lambert-Eaton myasthenic syndrome. Arch Pathol Lab Med 110:843–846, 1986.

Haioun C, Gaulard P, Roudot-Thoraval F, et al: Mediastinal diffuse large-cell lymphoma with sclerosis: a condition with a poor prognosis. Am J Clin Oncol 12:425–429, 1989.

Hamoudi A, Newton W, Mancer K, et al: Thymic changes in histiocytosis. Am J Clin Pathol 77:169–173, 1982.

Hankins J, Mayer R, Satterfield J, et al: Thymectomy for myasthenia gravis: a 14 year experience. Ann Surg 201:618–625, 1985.

Heim S, Mietlman F: Cancer Cytogenetics. Alan R Liss, New York, 1987.

Heron C, Husband J, Williams M: Hodgkin's disease: CT of the thymus. Radiology 167:647–651, 1988.

Hirschhorn R: Genetic deficiencies of adenosine deaminase and purine nucleoside phosphorylase: overview, genetic heterogeneity and therapy. Birth Defects 19:74–81, 1983.

Hoppe R: The management of bulky mediastinal Hodgkin's disease. Hematol Oncol Clin North Am 3:265–276, 1989.

Isaacson P, Chan JK, Tang C, Addis BJ: Low grade B-cell lymphoma of mucosa-associated lymphoid tissue arising in the thymus: a thymic lymphoma mimicking myoepithelial sialadenitis. Am J Surg Pathol 14:342–351, 1990.

Isaacson P, Norton A, Addis B: The human thymus contains a novel population of B-lymphocytes. Lancet 2:1488–1491, 1987.

Itescu S, Winchester R: Diffuse infiltrative lymphocytosis syndrome: a disorder occurring in human immunodeficiency virus-1 infection that may present as a sicca syndrome. Rheum Clin North Am 18:683–697, 1992.

Jacobson J, Aisenberg A, Lamarre L, et al: Mediastinal large cell lymphoma: an uncommon subset of adult lymphoma curable with combined modality therapy. Cancer 62:1893–1898, 1988.

Joos S, Otano-Joos M, Ziegler S, et al: Primary mediastinal (thymic) B-cell lymphoma is characterized by gains of chromosomal material including 9p and amplification of the REL gene. Blood 87:1571–1578, 1996.

Joshi V, Oleske J, Connor E: Morphologic findings in children with acquired immunodeficiency syndrome: pathogenesis and clinical implications. Pediatr Pathol 10:155–165, 1990.

Joshi V, Oleske J, Saad S, et al: Thymus biopsy in children with acquired immunodeficiency syndrome. Arch Pathol Lab Med 110:837–842, 1986.

Jouan H, LeDeist F, Nezelof C: Omenn's syndrome: pathologic arguments in favor of a graft versus host pathogenesis: a report of nine cases. Hum Pathol 18:1101–1108, 1987.

Kanavaros P, Gaulard P, Charlotte F, et al: Discordant expression of immunoglobulin and its associated molecule mb-1/CD79a is frequently found in mediastinal large B-cell lymphomas. Am J Pathol 146:735–741, 1995.

Kaneko Y, Frizzera G, Shikano T, et al: Chromosomal and immunophenotypic patterns in T-cell acute lymphoblastic leukemia (T-ALL) and lymphoblastic lymphoma. Leukemia 3:886–892, 1989.

Karcher D, Pearson C, Butler W, et al: Giant lymph node hyperplasia involving the thymus with associated nephrotic syndrome and myelofibrosis. Am J Clin Pathol 77:100–104, 1982.

Katz A, Lattes R: Granulomatous thymoma or Hodgkin's disease of the thymus? A clinical and histologic study and a reevaluation. Cancer 23:1–15, 1969.

Keller A, Castleman B: Hodgkin's disease of the thymus gland. Cancer 33:1615–1623, 1974.

Keller A, Hochholzer L, Castleman B: Hyaline-vascular and plasma-cell types of giant lymph node hyperplasia of the mediastinum and other locations. Cancer 29:670–683, 1972.

Kirn D, Mauch P, Shaffer K, et al: Large-cell and immunoblastic lymphoma of the mediastinum: prognostic features and treatment outcome in 57 patients. J Clin Oncol 11:1336–1343, 1993.

Kontny H, Sleasman J, Kingma D, et al: Multilocular thymic cysts in children with human immunodeficiency virus infection: clinical and pathologic aspects. J Pediatr 131:264–270, 1997.

Krenacs L, Tiszalvicz L, Krenacs T, et al: Immunohistochemical detection of CD1a antigen in formalin-fixed and paraffin-embedded tissue sections with monoclonal antibody O10. J Pathol 171: 99–104, 1993.

Labouyrie E, Merlio J, Beylot-Barry M, et al: Human immunodeficiency virus type 1 replication within cystic lymphoepithelial lesion of the salivary gland. Am J Clin Pathol 100:41–46, 1993.

Lack E: Thymic hyperplasia with massive enlargement: report of two cases with review of diagnostic criteria. J Thorac Cardiovasc Surg 81:741–746, 1981.

Lamarre L, Jacobson J, Aisenberg A, et al: Primary large cell lymphoma of the mediastinum: a histologic and immunophenotypic study of 29 cases. Am J Surg Pathol 13:730–739, 1989.

Lazzarino M, Orlandi E, Paulli M, et al: Primary mediastinal B-cell lymphoma with sclerosis: an aggressive tumor with distinctive clinical and pathologic features. J Clin Oncol 11:2306–2313, 1993.

Leonidas J, Berdon W, Valderrama E, et al: Human immunodeficiency virus infection and multilocular thymic cysts. Radiology 198: 337–339, 1996.

Levine G, Rosai J: Thymic hyperplasia and neoplasia: a review of current concepts. Hum Pathol 9:495–515, 1978.

Lewis J, Wick M, Scheithauer B, et al: Thymoma: a clinicopathologic review of 283 cases. Cancer 60:2727–2743, 1987.

Lindfors K, Meyer J, Dedrick C, et al: Thymic cysts in mediastinal Hodgkin disease. Radiology 156:37–41, 1985.

Liu H, Wong K, Chan T, et al: Superior vena cava syndrome: a rare presenting feature of acute myeloid leukemia. Acta Haematol 79:213–216, 1989.

Liu K, Herbrecht R, Tranchant C, et al: Malignant thymic lymphoblastic lymphoma and myasthenia gravis: an exceptional association. Nouv Rev Fr Hematol 34:221–223, 1992.

Luker G, Siegel M: Mediastinal Hodgkin disease in children: response to therapy. Radiology 189:737–740, 1993.

Lukes R, Butler J, Hicks E: Natural history of Hodgkin's disease as related to its pathologic picture. Cancer 19:317–344, 1966.

Lukes R, Collins R: Convoluted (lymphoblastic) T-cell lymphoma. In Hartmann WH, Sobin LH (eds): Atlas of Tumor Pathology, 2nd series, fascicle 28. Armed Forces Institute of Pathology, Washington, DC, pp 147–178, 1992.

Lyons T, Disckson J, Variend S: (1989). Cervical thymic cysts. J Pediatr Surg, 24, 241–243, 1989.

Mallick B: An unusual presentation of acute myeloid leukemia. J Indian Med Assoc 85:244–245, 1987.

Manivel J, Jessurun J, Wick M, et al: Placental alkaline phosphatase immunoreactivity in testicular germ-cell neoplasms. Am J Surg Pathol 11:21–29, 1987.

Marra S, Hotaling A, Raslan W: Cervical thymic cyst. Otolaryngol Head Neck Surg 112:338–340, 1995.

Mauch P, Kalish L, Kadin M, et al: Patterns of presentation of Hodgkin disease: implications for etiology and pathogenesis. Cancer, 71, 2062–2071, 1993.

McCafferty M, Bahnson H: Thymic cyst extending into the pericardium: a case report. Ann Thorac Surg 33:503–506, 1982.

McClain K, Heise R, Day D, et al: Hodgkin's disease in children: correlation of clinical characteristics, staging procedures and treatment at the University of Minnesota. Am J Pediatr Hematol Oncol, 12:147–154, 1990.

McCluggage W, Russell C, Tlner P: Parathyroid cyst of the thymus. Thorax 50:913–914, 1995.

Meis J, Butler J, Osborne B, et al: Granulocytic sarcoma in non-leukemic patients. Cancer 58:2697–2709, 1986.

Mishalani S, Lones M, Said J: Multilocular thymic cyst: a novel thymic lesion associated with human immunodeficiency virus infection. Arch Pathol Lab Med 119:467–470, 1995.

Moller P, Lammler B, Eberlein-Gonska M, et al: Primary mediastinal clear cell lymphoma of B-cell type. Virchows Archiv A Pathol Anat 409:79–92, 1986a.

Moller P, Lammler B, Herrmann B, et al: The primary mediastinal clear cell lymphoma of B-cell type has variable defects in MHC antigen expression. Immunology 59:411–417, 1986b.

Moller P, Matthaei-Maurer D, Hofmann et al: Immunophenotypic similarities of mediastinal clear-cell lymphoma and sinusoidal (monocytoid) B-cells. Int J Cancer 43:10–16, 1989.

Moller P, Moldenhauer G, Momburg F, et al: Mediastinal lymphoma of clear cell type is a tumor corresponding to terminal steps of B-cell differentiation. Blood 69:1087–1095, 1987.

Moskowitz P, Noon M, McAlister W, et al: Thymic cyst hemorrhage: a cause of acute, symptomatic mediastinal widening in children with aplastic anemia. AJR 134:832–836, 1980.

Mugerwa J: The lympohreticular system in kwashiorkor. J Pathol 195:105–108, 1971.

Muller-Hermelink H, Marino M, Palestro G: Pathology of thymic epithelial tumors. In Muller-Hermelink H (ed): The human thymus. Curr Top Pathol 75:207–268, 1986.

Muller-Hermelink H, Sale G, Borisch B, et al: Pathology of the thymus after allogeneic bone marrow transplantation in man. Am J Pathol 129:119–134, 1987.

Murray J, Parker A: Mediastinal Hodgkin's disease and thymic cysts. Acta Haematol 71:282–284, 1984.

Nathwani B, Griffith R, Kelly D, et al: A morphologic study of childhood lymphoma of the diffuse "histiocytic" type: the Pediatric Oncology Group experience. Cancer 59:1138–1142, 1987.

Nathwani B, Kim H, Rappaport H: Malignant lymphoma, lympoblastic. Cancer 38:964–983, 1976.

Neiman R, Barcos M, Berard C, et al: Granulocytic sarcoma: a clinicopathologic study of 61 biopsied cases. Cancer 48:1426–1437, 1981.

Newton W, Hamoudi A, Shannon B: Role of the thymus in histiocytosis X. Hematol Oncol Clin North Am 1:63–74, 1987.

Nezelof C: Pathology of the thymus in immunodeficiency states. In Muller-Hermelink H (ed): The human thymus. Curr Top Pathol 75:151–177, 1986.

Nezelof C: Thymic pathology in primary and secondary immunodeficiencies. Histopathology 21:499–511, 1992.

Nogues A, Tovar J, Sunol M, et al: Hodgkin's disease of the thymus: a rare mediastinal cystic mass. J Pediatr Surg 22:996–997, 1987.

Orazi A, Neiman R, Ulbright T, et al: Hematopoietic precursor cells within the yolk sac tumor component are the source of secondary hematopoietic malignancies in patients with mediastinal germ cell tumors. Cancer 71:3873–3881, 1993.

O'Reilly P, Joshi V, Holbrook C, et al: Multicentric Castleman's disease in a child with prominent thymic involvement: a case report and brief review of the literature. Mod Pathol 6:776–780, 1993.

Patchefsky A, Brodovsky H, Soughard M, et al: Hodgkin's disease: a clinical and pathologic study of 235 cases. Cancer 32:150–161, 1973.

Penn A, Jaretzki A, Wolff M, et al: Thymic abnormalities: antigen or antibody? Response to thymectomy in myasthenia gravis. Ann NY Acad Sci 377:786–804, 1981.

Perrone T, Frizzera G, Rosai J: Mediastinal diffuse large-cell lymphoma with sclerosis: a clinicopathologic study of 60 cases. Am J Surg Pathol 10:176–191, 1986.

Pescarmona E, Giardini R, Brisgotti M, et al: Thymoma in childhood: a clinicopathological study of five cases. Histopathology 21:65–68, 1992.

Pescarmona E, Rendina E, Ricci C, et al: Histiocytosis X and lymphoid follicular hyperplasia of the thymus in myasthenia gravis. Histopathology 14:565–570, 1989.

Picozzi V: Lymphoblastic lymphoma. Cancer Treat Res 66:81–94, 1993.

Picozzi V, Coleman C: Lymphoblastic lymphoma. Semin Oncol 17:96–103, 1990.

Piira T, Perkins S, Anderson J, et al: Primary mediastinal large cell lymphoma in children: a report from the Childrens Cancer Group. Pediatr Pathol Lab Med 15:561–570, 1995.

Pileri S, Piccaluga A, Poggi S, et al: Anaplastic large cell lymphoma, update of findings. Leukemia and Lymphoma, 18:17–25, 1995.

Pinkus G, Pinkus J: Myeloperoxidase: a specific marker for myeloid cells in paraffin sections. Mod Pathol 4:733–741, 1991.

Pizzighella S, Riviera A, Tridente G: Thymic involvement in myasthenia gravis: study by immunofluorescent and immunoperoxidase staining. J Neuroimmunol 4:117–127, 1983.

Ramon y Cajal S, Suster S: Primary thymic epithelial neoplasms in children. Am J Surg Pathol 15:466–474, 1991.

Rastegar H, Arger P, Harken A: Evaluation and therapy of mediastinal thymic cyst. Am Surg 46:236–238, 1980.

Rege K, Powles R, Norton J, et al: An unusual presentation of acute myeloid leukaemia with pericardial and pleural effusions due to granulocyteic sarcoma. Leuk Lymphoma, 11, 305–307, 1993.

Reinglass J, Brickel C: The prognostic significance of thymic germinal center proliferation in myasthenia gravis. Neurology 23:69–72, 1973.

Ridell B, Larsson S: Coexistence of a thymoma and Hodgkin's disease of the thymus: a case report. Acta Pathol Microbiol Scand A Pathol 88:1–4, 1980.

Rose J, Lam C: Thymic enlargement in association with hyperthyroidism. Pediatr Radiol 12:37–38, 1982.

Rosenberg H, Oppenheimer E, Esterly J: Congenital rubella syndrome: the late effects and their relation to early lesions. Persp Pediatr Pathol 6:183–202, 1986.

Roth M, Medeiros J, Elenitoba-Johnson K, et al: Extramedullary myeloid cell tumors: an immunohistochemical study of 29 cases using routinely fixed and processed paraffin-embedded tissue sections. Arch Pathol Lab Med 119:790–798, 1995.

Savino W, Dardenne M: Developmental studies on expression of monoclonal antibody-defined cytokeratins by thymic epithelial cells from normal and autoimmune mice. J Histochem Cytochem 36:1123–1129, 1988.

Schuurman H, Krone W, Broekhuizen R, et al: The thymus in acquired immune deficiency syndrome: comparison with other types of immunodeficiency diseases, and presence of components of human immunodeficiency virus type 1. Am J Pathol 134: 1329–1338, 1989.

Seemayer T, Laroche A, Russo P, et al: Precocious thymic involution manifested by epithelial injury in the acquired immune deficiency syndrome. Hum Pathol 15:469–474, 1984.

Segal G, Dehner L, Rosai J: Histiocytosis X (Langerhans' cell histiocytosis) of the thymus: a clinicopathologic study of four childhood cases. Am J Surg Pathol 9:117–124, 1985.

Sheibani K, Nathwani B, Winberg CO, et al: Antigenically defined subgroups of lymphoblastic lymphoma: relationship to clinical presentation and biologic behavior. Cancer, 60, 183–190, 1987.

Shimosato Y, Kukai K: Tumors of the mediastinum. In Rosai J, Sobin LH (eds): Atlas of Tumor Pathology, 3rd Series, fascicle 21. Armed Forces Institute of Pathology, Washington, DC, pp 1–22, 1997.

Som P, Sacher M, Lanzieri C, et al: Parenchymal cysts of the lower neck. Radiology, 157:399–406, 1985.

Stein H, Petersen N, Gaedicke G, et al: Lymphoblastic lymphoma of convoluted or acid phosphatase type: a tumor of T-precursor cells. Int J Cancer 17:292–295, 1976.

Stolar C, Garvin J, Rustad D, et al: Residual or recurent chest mass in pediatric Hodgkin's disease: a surgical problem? Am J Pediatr Hematol Oncol 9:289–294, 1987.

Strickler J, Kurtin P: Mediastinal lymphoma. Semin Diagn Pathol 8:2–13, 1991.

Stromme M, Eraklis A: Thymic cysts in the neck. Laryngoscope 87:1645–1649, 1977.

Suster S, Moran C: Malignant thymic neoplasms that may mimic benign conditions. Semin Diagn Pathol 12:98–104, 1995.

Suster S, Rosai J: Histology of the normal thymus. Am J Surg Pathol 14:284–303, 1990.

Suster S, Rosai J: Multilocular thymic cyst: an acquired reactive process: study of 18 cases. Am J Surg Pathol 15:388–398, 1991.

Suster S, Rosai J: Thymus. In Sternberg S (ed): Histology for Pathologists, 2nd ed. Lippincott-Raven, Philadelphia, pp 687–706, 1997.

Takagi N, Nakamura S, Yamamoto K, et al: Malignant lymphoma of mucosa-associated lymphoid tissue arising in the thymus of a patient with Sjögren's syndrome. Cancer 69:1347–1355, 1992.

Touraine J, Betuel H: The bare lymphocyte syndrome: immunodeficiency resulting from the lack of HLA expression antigens. Birth Defects 19:1101–1108, 1983.

Tsang P, Cesarman E, Chadburn A, et al: Molecular characterization of primary mediastinal B-cell lymphoma. Am J Pathol 148: 2017–2025, 1996.

Tubergen D, Krailo M, Meadows A, et al: Comparison of treatment regimens for pediatric lymphoblastic non-Hodgkin's lymphoma: a Childrens Cancer Group study. J Clin Oncol 13:1368–1376, 1995.

van de Wijngaert F, Kendall M, Shuurman H, et al: Heterogeneity of epithelial cells in the human thymus: an ultrastructural study. Cell Tissue Res 237:227–237, 1984.

Warnke R, Weiss L, Chan J, et al: Malignant lymphoma, lymphoblastic. In Rosai J, Sobin LH (eds): Atlas of Tumor Pathology, 3rd series, fascicle 14. Armed Forces Institute of Pathology, Washington, DC, pp 223–244, 1995.

Weinberg K, Parkman R: Severe combined immunodeficiency due to a specific defect in the production of interleukin-2. N Engl J Med 322:1718–1723, 1990.

Weiss L, Bindl J, Pixozzi V, et al: Lymphoblastic lymphoma: an immunophenotype study of 26 cases with comparison to T-cell acute lymphoblastic leukemia. Blood 67:474–478, 1986.

Wekerle H, Muller-Hermelink H: The thymus in myasthenia gravis. In Muller-Hermelink H (ed): The human thymus. Curr Top Pathol 75:179–206, 1986.

Wick J, Swanson P, Manivel J: (1987). Placental-like alkaline phosphatase reactivity in human tumors: an immunohistochemical study of 520 cases. Hum Pathol 18:946–954, 1987.

Yulish B, Owens R: Thymic enlargement in a child during therapy for primary hypothyroidism. AJR 135:157–158, 1980.

Zanca P, Chuang T, DeAvila R, et al: True congenital mediastinal thymic cyst. Pediatrics 36:615–619, 1965.

Zarate-Osorno A, Medeiros L, Danon A, et al: Hodgkin's disease with coexistent Castleman-like histologic features: a report of three cases. Arch Pathol Lab Med 118:270–274, 1994.

Zinzani P, Bandandi M, Maretlli M, et al: Anaplastic large-cell lymphoma: clinical and prognostic evaluation of 90 adult patients. J Clin Oncol 14:955–962, 1996.

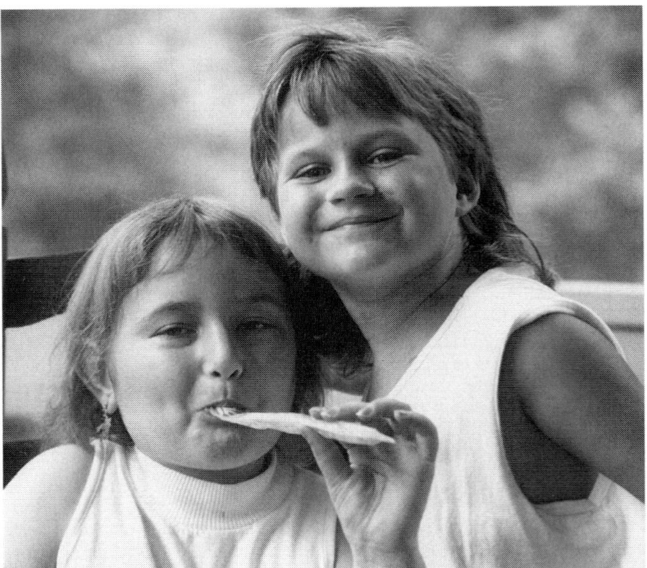

Camp Horizon, near Nashville. Both of these girls had acute lymphocytic leukemia and were in remission at the time of this writing. (Courtesy Greg Kinney.)

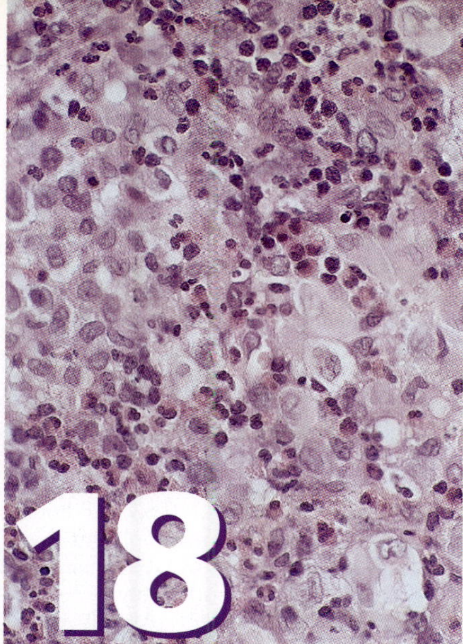

Robert D. Collins

Spleen

Most discussions of the spleen begin with an acknowledgment of its mysteriousness. It is an organ that was deemed unessential well into the 1950s, since it was usually removed with impunity. However, we now know that in a few patients its absence causes an illness of astonishing brevity from well-being to death and that this outcome may follow years of apparent health. One wonders how often these patients have been at risk for similar episodes and about the conditions enabling them to escape previously. If not mysterious, it is at least wondrous that a few encapsulated bacteria may wreak such havoc after splenectomy.

The spleen is also an organ that receives short shrift in most surgical and autopsy pathology laboratory reports. The term *congested* is often applied in the absence of a specific diagnosis (Butler, 1983). Few pathologists specialize in splenic diseases, and perhaps the spleen has not received the detailed study of its counterparts receiving lymph rather than blood. A number of important diseases arise in or affect the spleen, however, and they may be diagnosed with assurance with modest investments in fixation, staining, and background reading.

NORMAL STRUCTURE AND FUNCTION

The lymphatic tissue of the spleen is stationed along small vessels and usually consists of follicular centers that are distinctive owing to a clear marginal zone of small lymphocytes adjacent to the red pulp (Fig. 18–1). In humans, marginal zones are seen readily only around follicular centers in the spleen. Marginal zone cells are B cells with key roles in initial trapping and processing of antigen, particularly carbohydrate antigens. Follicular centers in the spleen and elsewhere produce plasma cell precursors. In the case of the spleen these precursors are responding to antigen delivered by the bloodstream. Another component of the lymphocyte system is the population of small T lymphocytes gathered along the penicilliary arteries, presumably as modulators of the B compartment immune response. The spleen also contains both $\alpha\beta$ and $\gamma\delta$ T cells, the latter preferentially located in splenic sinuses (Falini et al, 1989). Natural killer–like T cells have been identified in the spleen in murine models and are probably present in humans as well. Traffic of all lymphocyte populations is apparently brisk.

Blood passes through the spleen in adults at a rate of approximately 2 l/min. Normally, most of that amount goes directly into splenic sinuses. A small fraction is discharged into Billroth cords, a low-flow area in which cells are submitted to macrophage surveillance while transiting the fenestra of splenic sinuses and endothelial gaps before flowing freely again in the venous system (van Krieken et al, 1985). The fenestra are formed by connective tissue fibers that ring splenic sinuses and thereby create a sievelike apparatus, readily visible with a periodic acid–Schiff stain (Fig. 18–2). Since the sieve gaps are 3μ or less, only pliant red cells free of nuclear inclusions pass readily. Others are detained, pitted of inclusions, or phagocytosed by macrophages.

In addition to its immunologic and filtration functions, the human spleen stores platelets and granulocytes. Up to one third of the platelet mass, as well as large numbers of granulocytes, may be found in the red pulp. Less than 50 ml of blood is stored in the spleen. These storage functions apparently account for the commonly observed and usually transient post-splenectomy thrombocytosis and granulocytosis.

Extramedullary hematopoiesis (EMH) occurs in the spleen and is generally attributed to reactivation of hematopoiesis observed in fetuses. Hematopoietic stem cells have been demonstrated in the spleen of a child with prominent EMH associated with osteopetrosis, whereas various enlarged spleens without EMH did not contain such stem cells (Freedman & Sanders, 1981).

Under physiologic circumstances, the spleen produces a phagocytosis-stimulating peptide named tuftsin, an oligopeptide that stimulates phagocytosis, mobility, and bactericidal activity in phagocytic cells. Tuftsin levels are reduced after splenic removal or in conditions associated with splenic hypofunction, probably accounting for increased susceptibility to infections under such circumstances (Zoli et al, 1994). The spleen reaches adult size in individuals in their mid-teens. It may weigh 25 g or less until 1 year of age. Newborns and young infants have splenic weights of 6–15 g.

HYPOSPLENISM

Hyposplenism is the commonest abnormality in function. Hyposplenism is usually due to splenectomy after trauma, although some patients retain function via splenosis (discussed later). It may also be anticipated in children with sickle cell diseases or sickle–hemoglobin C disease. Less frequent causes of hyposplenism are congenital absence, hypoplasia (Kevy et al, 1968), irradiation (Dailey et al, 1981), systemic lupus erythematosus (Malleson et al, 1988), malabsorption, nephrotic syndrome (McVicar et al, 1986), neoplasms (Budke et al, 1995), and chemotherapy. It has been postulated that the increased susceptibility to infection of children with nephrotic syndrome might be related to splenic hypofunction (McVicar et al, 1986). Some support for this possibility was found using uptake of

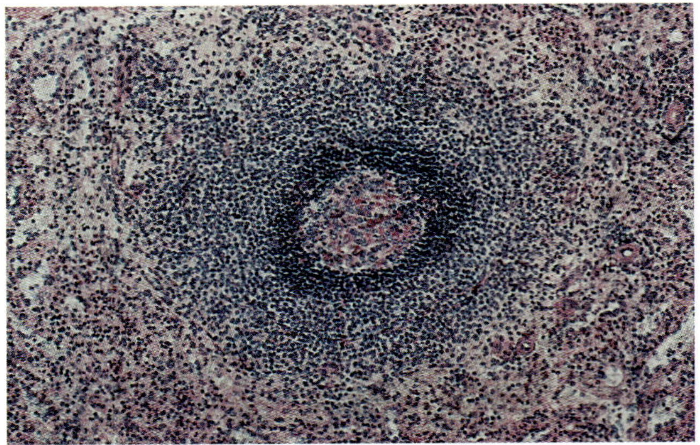

Figure 18–1

White pulp, spleen. This photomicrograph shows a normal follicular center surrounded by a mantle zone, with the paler-staining marginal zone at the interface between white and red pulp.

labeled, heat-treated autologous red cells as an indicator of splenic function, but subsequent studies using pocked red cells as a marker did not reveal significant hypofunction of the spleen. The possibility of hyposplenism may be evaluated in the laboratory most readily by evidence of inadequate red cell surveillance, including Howell-Jolly bodies, pocks or pits in red cells, and other nuclear inclusions. After splenectomy, phase contrast studies reveal that up to 50% of red cells have pocks, structures thought to represent excess red cell membrane. An alternative method for evaluating splenic function is to place a silver stain on air-dried blood films or Wright-stained films and count the number of red cells with one or more silver-staining inclusions. Results with this method (Fig. 18–3) correlate well with pocked erythrocyte counts in evaluating splenic function (Tham et al, 1996).

A dissociation between filtration and immunologic function is possible. The latter may be selectively depressed in general immunodeficient states or after irradiation or chemotherapy.

Infections in patients with hyposplenism are remarkable for their fulminance. Septicemia, shock, massive disseminated intravascular coagulation, and death may all occur in a few hours (Fig. 18–4). Most of these patients have no premonitory symptoms indicating infection at the usual portals of entry. At least two thirds of these infections are caused by uncommon serotypes of *Streptococcus pneumoniae*, to which the host was presumably not exposed while the spleen was functional. There is no apparent predisposition to viral and fungal infections after splenectomy.

HYPERSPLENISM

Four criteria were proposed in 1955 for hypersplenism: splenomegaly, cytopenia in one or more peripheral blood elements, hyperplasia of the corresponding precursors in the marrow, and correction by splenectomy. In 1962, another approach was somewhat more direct: hypersplenism encompasses all disorders in which the spleen causes destruction of circulating cells, with the resultant cytopenias ameliorated or corrected by splenectomy. The latter definition includes many cases of idiopathic thrombocytopenia in the category of hypersplenism, even though the spleen is carrying out its expected function of removing abnormal elements from the blood. Some agree with Crosby's definition. By this definition, there may be sequestration of abnormal cells in a normal spleen, as in spherocytosis and elliptocytosis; hemoglobinopathies; autoimmune disorders affecting red cells, granulocytes, or platelets; and parasitosis of red cells (e.g., malaria and babesiosis). Alternatively, the spleen may be abnormal, with sequestration of normal marrow elements, as in storage diseases or neoplasms, portal hypertension, and miscellaneous causes of splenomegaly, such as infections or cysts.

Pathologic examination in hypersplenism usually does not reveal dramatic diagnostic or prognostic information, with a few exceptions, such as in storage diseases or neoplasms. In idiopathic thrombocytopenic purpura, the spleen weight and follicle size were in the normal range in methylmethacrylate-embedded specimens (van Krieken et al, 1983), although prominent secondary follicles and foamy macrophages have been described in some patients (Chang et al, 1993), and patients with splenic follicles $>500\ \mu$ were more likely to relapse or develop additional autoimmune disorders (Arendt et al, 1988).

SPLENIC FUNCTION AFTER VARIOUS TREATMENTS AND PROCEDURES

Splenectomies are performed in children for treatment of various disorders, including congenital hemolytic anemias, chronic autoimmune disorders, immune thrombocytopenic purpura, autoimmune hemolytic anemia (Fig. 18–5), hypersplenism from portal vein thrombosis or liver disease, storage diseases, splenic tumors, and cysts (Lane, 1995). Splenic trauma is the most common indication for splenectomy. Splenectomy is occasionally performed in sequestration crises in the hemoglobinopathies. Splenectomies were commonly performed in the past as staging procedures in lymphoma, such as Hodgkin disease.

Complete splenectomy after trauma, for staging purposes, or as treatment, ablates splenic filtration activities as well as some immune function. The former may be partially assumed by the mononuclear phagocyte system of the liver. Chemotherapy, with its general suppression of the immune system, also affects the spleen. Irradiation in patients with lymphoma produced atrophy of the spleen and fibrosis with a wrinkled, thick capsule; rare patients after splenic irradiation have developed pneumococcal sepsis (Dailey et al, 1981).

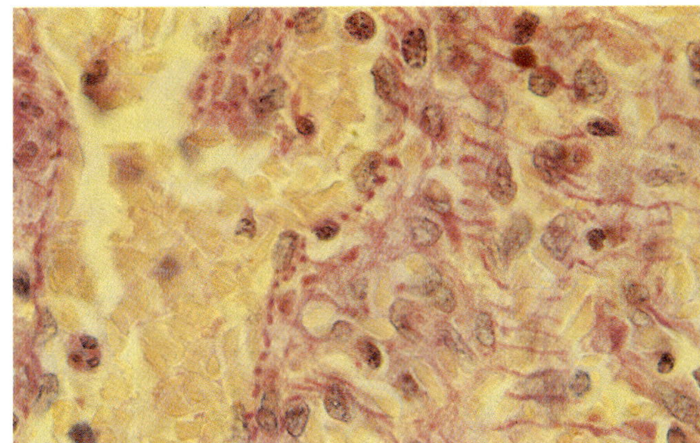

Figure 18–2

Sieve apparatus, spleen. High magnification reveals the sieve cut in cross section as well as tangentially. The gaps are 3–5 μ. Blood entering Billroth cords must return to the splenic sinuses and thence the general circulation by percolating through this sieve. Periodic acid–Schiff stain.

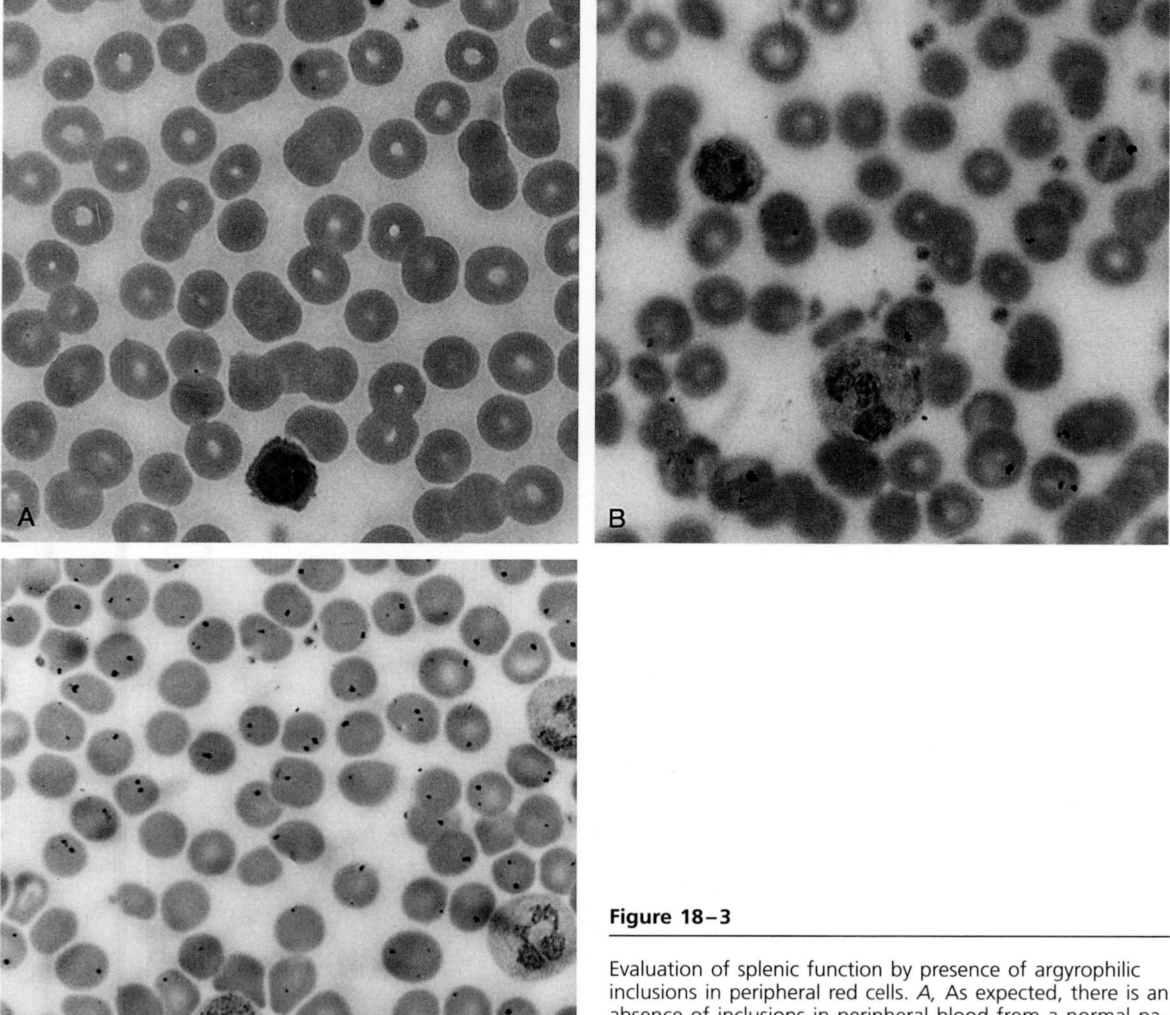

Figure 18–3

Evaluation of splenic function by presence of argyrophilic inclusions in peripheral red cells. *A,* As expected, there is an absence of inclusions in peripheral blood from a normal patient. Numerous inclusions are present in the blood from a child (*B*) with sickle cell disease, and (*C*) after splenectomy. (Courtesy Dr. K.T. Tham, Department of Pathology, Vanderbilt University Medical Center, Nashville, TN.)

Graft-versus-host (GVH) disease is seen clinically when immunodeficient hosts receive immunocompetent grafts or cells that are incompatible with the host. GVH disease thus occurs in immunodeficiency syndromes, immunodeficiency of prematurity, and immunodeficiencies secondary to chemotherapy or irradiation, malignancies, or viral infections. Immunocompetent cells may be derived from the maternal circulation, blood transfusions, or organ transplantation.

Animal models have greatly facilitated our understanding of GVH disease. Splenomegaly is pronounced and used as a marker indicating its presence. Animals also have weight loss, hepatomegaly, transient lymphadenopathy, and skin lesions varying from unkempt fur to epidermal necrosis. The severity of manifestations varies with the extent of histoincompatibility between host and graft.

Target organs of GVH reactions include skin (alopecia, desquamation, or epidermolysis), liver (hepatitis or bile retention), bowel (epithelial injury), and lung (pneumonitis). Lymphadenopathy and splenomegaly are typical owing to immune activation, underlying disease, or secondary infection.

Parenteral nutrition via intravenous administration of sterile fat emulsions is a valuable component of various treatment programs. These emulsions contain particles approximately 0.5 μ in size that are cleared by the mononuclear phagocyte system. Rare patients develop fever, hepatosplenomegaly, coagulopathy, and organ dysfunction owing to sudden elevation of serum triglyceride levels, a disorder called fat overload syndrome (Haber et al, 1988). In a single autopsied case the spleen was enlarged and pale, and the cords were distended by fat. Other autopsied cases have revealed necrotizing changes in the spleen, probably related to intravascular coagulation as well as widespread fat emboli.

CONGENITAL ABNORMALITIES

Congenital abnormalities of the spleen range from the rare asplenia to the common presence of single or multiple accessory spleens, found in splenic hilum, tail of pancreas, and, less frequently, omentum or intestinal mesentery (Wolf & Neiman,

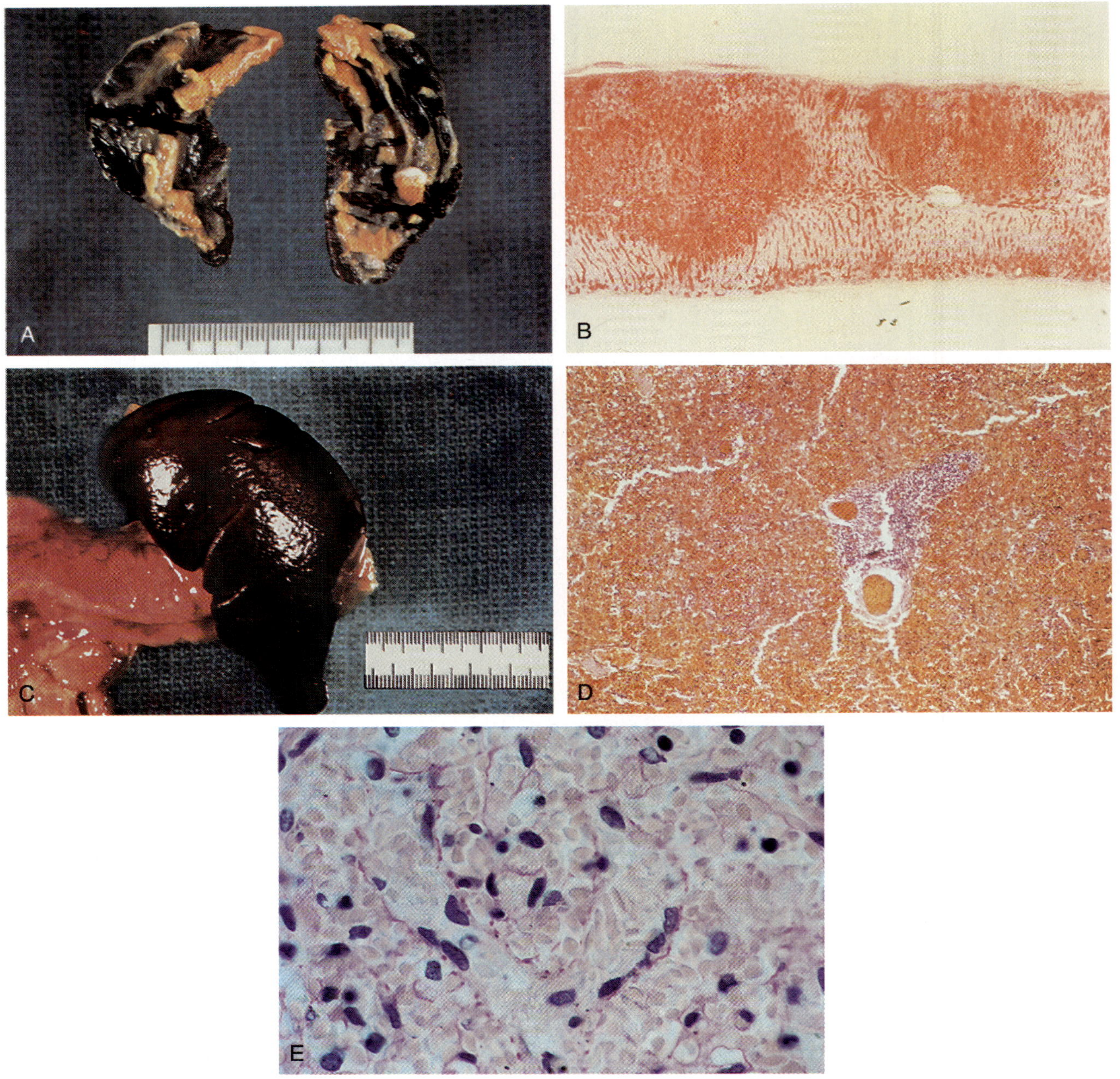

Figure 18–4

Sickle cell crisis and pneumococcal sepsis. The patient was a 3-year-old girl with sickle cell disease manifested only as dactylitis. She had polyvalent pneumococcal vaccine administered at age 2. In March of her third year, she suddenly developed a fever of 104°F, obtundation, and episodes of apnea with shock and irreversible ventricular fibrillation after an illness of 12 h. Type 6 pneumococcus was cultured from the blood premortem, and Howell-Jolly bodies were easily demonstrated in peripheral films. Autopsy showed evidence of Waterhouse-Friderichsen syndrome with hemorrhagic adrenals as well as an enlarged spleen engorged with numerous sickled cells. Sickling was also apparent in splenic sinuses. *A,* Massive hemorrhage is demonstrated in both adrenals. *B,* Microscopic examination reveals the typical multifocal hemorrhage often seen in early Waterhouse-Friderichsen syndrome. *C,* The spleen is dark and engorged, weighing 80 g, approximately twice normal weight. *D,* Low magnification reveals marked engorgement of the spleen and no white pulp. *E,* High magnification reveals numerous sickled cells in the spleen.

1989). In addition to the usual single reniform mass, spleens may be lobated, divided into discrete masses (polysplenia), wander from position, misplaced altogether, or fused with pancreatic tissue in trisomy 13 (Hashida et al, 1983) or with gonadal tissue (Wolf & Neiman, 1989). These congenital abnormalities, albeit rare, have clinical significance (Table 18–1), although biologic mechanisms responsible for the abnormalities are not known. Splenic malformations are often associated with complex congenital malformations of the heart but are not universally present and may not be used as a guide

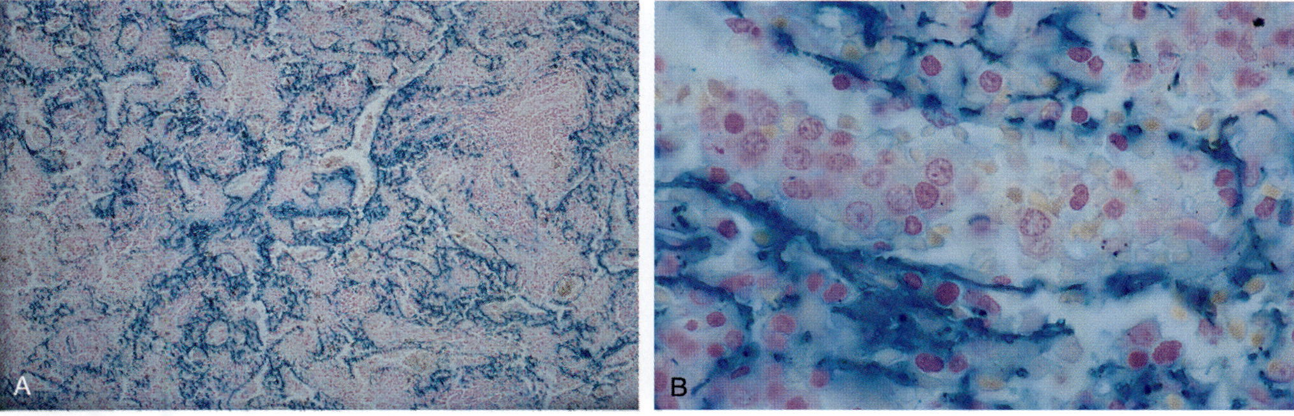

Figure 18–5

Siderosis of the spleen associated with autoimmune hemolytic anemia. This child had splenomegaly and persistent anemia, occasioning a splenectomy. The spleen weighed 500 g. *A,* Massive iron deposition is seen, with localization in the splenic sinuses. *B,* At high magnification the sieve apparatus is outlined by iron. This pattern of iron deposition is common in chronic hemolytic anemias.

as to the type of cardiac abnormality (Anderson et al, 1990). Splenic abnormalities seen in patients with heart disease include accessory spleens, multiple spleens, and absent spleens.

HAMARTOMAS

Hamartomas are infrequent, essentially asymptomatic, and therefore diagnosed incidentally. Falk and Stutte (1989) described a series of 20 cases in which 5 were in children. Spleen weight varied from 120 to 400 g, and hamartomas measured 3–7 cm in diameter. The lesions in children were all single. Hamartomas were well circumscribed, bulged from the cut surface, were dark in color in the smaller lesions, and had areas of remote hemorrhage in the larger. Microscopic sections consistently demonstrated tortuous vascular channels and scar, and lymphocytic tissue was absent. Some hamartomas exhibited plasmacytosis, foam cells, evidence of hemorrhage and extramedullary hemopoiesis.

SPLENIC CYSTS

Cysts without epithelial lining may occur in children and in some cases are associated with trauma. Some are sufficiently large to be symptomatic or may rupture and produce hemoperitoneum. Walls are often fibrotic, may calcify, and contain evidence of previous hemorrhage in the form of hemosiderin and cholesterol clefts. Cysts with epithelial lining are usually unilocular and may measure up to 10 cm in diameter, with nonkeratinizing squamous epithelium as the usual lining (Warnke et al, 1995). These cysts are most often found in children or young adults, in whom they may produce pressure symptoms or, less likely, rupture or become secondarily infected.

VASCULAR TUMORS

Lymphangiomas

Lymphangiomas are reportedly more common in the subcapsular region or around large trabeculae (Garvin & King, 1981). They contain proteinaceous fluid and are lined by flattened cells. Single or multiple lesions may be present in the spleen. Lymphangiomatosis has been reported (Ramani et al, 1993) as a rare condition affecting male infants and boys 9 months to 11 years of age. All four patients presented with respiratory symptoms, owing in part to chylothorax or chylopericardium. Widespread lesions were seen on imaging studies or at autopsy (three cases) in lung, spleen, bone, and mediastinum.

Table 18–1
Various Congenital Abnormalities of the Spleen and Their Clinical Significance

Abnormality	Comment
Asplenia	Predisposition to sepsis with encapsulated bacteria; associated with cardiovascular abnormalities
Accessory spleen	Should be removed with the spleen in patients undergoing splenectomy for hypersplenism; rarely subject to torsion
Polysplenia	Associated with cardiac abnormalities; no increase in infections (Peoples et al, 1983)
Wandering spleen	Subject to torsion; prolonged venous occlusion may cause perisplenitis and venous thrombosis; in 21 children with splenic weight stated, mean weight of spleen subject to venous occlusion was 566 g (Buehner et al, 1992)
Malposition	Clinical confusion in interpreting imaging studies
Splenic-gonadal fusion	May produce a painful scrotal or inguinal mass

Hemangiomas, Hemangioendotheliomas, Littoral Cell Angiomas, and Angiosarcoma

Vasoformative neoplasms in the spleen in children are extremely rare, ranging from processes designated as hemangiomas, hemangioendotheliomas (these cases may have areas justifying the terms *epithelioid* or *spindly*) (Suster, 1992), or littoral cell angiomas from the tall lining cells (Falk et al, 1991) to angiosarcomas. Hyposplenism has been described as a complication of epithelioid hemangioendothelioma (Budke et al, 1995), and spindle cell hemangioendotheliomas or hemangiomas may occur in association with multiple enchondromas (Mafucci syndrome) (Fanberg et al, 1995). One of the cases of littoral cell angioma reviewed by Falk et al (1991) was in a 3-year-old male who presented with splenomegaly. These cases had solid and papillary areas suggestive of angiosarcoma.

Peliosis

A review of the literature in 1983 dealing with peliosis of the spleen revealed one case in a child. This 9-year-old had aplastic anemia, with no history of drug treatment (Diebold & Aundouin, 1983).

TRAUMATIC EFFECTS

Blunt abdominal trauma after automobile accidents, falls, or blows may cause splenic injury or rupture. In a study of 413 children undergoing laparotomy for suspected splenic rupture between 1968 an 1977, the spleen was ruptured and not bleeding in 193, bleeding in 87, crushed in 99, normal in 1, and had a subcapsular hematoma in 5 (Wahlby et al, 1981). Ten of these children (2.4%) subsequently developed sepsis over the following 8 years, with 5 dying. The splenic weight and the amount of lymphocyte tissue in spleens removed for trauma are slightly greater than normal (van Krieken et al, 1983), suggesting that spleens with lymphocytic stimulation were more prone to injury after trauma.

Splenic tissue dispersed by injury may regrow on peritoneal surfaces and, less frequently, on pericardial surfaces or in the skin scar. These nodules of splenic tissue (splenosis) are usually small and encapsulated by fibrous tissue and may be sessile. Microscopic examination shows both red pulp and lymphocytic tissue. Pearson and associates (1978) showed that, in 13 of 22 children with emergency splenectomy for trauma, there was a low percentage of pocked red cells. In 5 of these children, a colloid scan demonstrated multiple nodules of splenic tissue. The relatively low incidence of sepsis after splenectomy following trauma was attributed to the frequent development of splenosis. After splenectomy, tuftsin activity is correlated with evidence of residual splenic function (Zoli et al, 1994). As a phagocyte-promoting peptide, tuftsin may be responsible, at least in part, for protection against infection in these circumstances. Tesluk and colleagues (1984) described an interesting patient who had autologous splenic transplantation (anterior rectus compartment). Eight years later he died from an overwhelming pneumococcal infection. The splenic transplants were fibrotic and congested. Howell-Jolly bodies were not seen in peripheral blood films just before death.

EFFECTS OF LIVER DISEASE

Splenomegaly owing to splenic engorgement is described in children with various causes of portal hypertension, including α_1-antitrypsin deficiency (Alagille, 1984), sclerosing cholangitis (Debray et al, 1994; Wilschanski et al, 1995), and hepatoportal sclerosis (Maksoud et al, 1986). Sclerosing cholangitis may be seen in children with inflammatory bowel disease and also with Langerhans cell histiocytosis. Splenomegaly ultimately occurs in most of these children, and death from portal hypertension is common. Some of the children with hepatoportal sclerosis have had omphalitis or umbilical catheterization.

HEMOGLOBINOPATHIES

Splenic function is a determinant of morbidity and mortality rates in the hemoglobinopathies. Abnormally shaped red cells develop "logjams" in the splenic microcirculation, particularly since the slow flow and hypoxic conditions apparently exaggerate sickling of red cells. Resultant engorgement, scarring, and infarctions produce hemolysis, splenomegaly (when dramatic, patients may develop one or more episodes of splenic sequestration with massive red cell trapping and potentially fatal outcome), and inevitably functional asplenia. Splenic injury may begin as early as 3 months of age as hemoglobin F levels diminish. However, Hegyi et al (1977) described evidence of a sickle cell crisis in a child dying at 5 days of age. Hemosiderosis was demonstrated in the liver, spleen, kidney, and pancreas, but the cause of death was probably related to a necrotizing enterocolitis, from which an etiologic agent was not isolated.

The proportion of children with hemoglobinopathies who have hyposplenia, as estimated by evaluation of red cell pocking, is 14% at 6 months, 28% at 1 year, 58% at 2 years, 78% at 3 years, and 94% at 5 years (Brown et al, 1994; Lane, 1995). Using pocked red cells as an indicator of splenic function, Pearson and colleages (1985) in a cooperative study of 2086 patients showed that development of splenic hypofunction was fastest and most severe in hemoglobin SS disease, considerably slower in hemoglobin SC disease, and intermediate in hemoglobin S β-thalassemia. Patients with hemoglobin S β-thalassemia had no detectable dysfunction. The level of pocked red cells was inversely associated with fetal hemoglobin levels and directly associated with age.

It is not surprising that bacterial infection is the leading cause of death in children when they have sickling disorders (Leikin et al, 1989).

Splenic injury may occur in any of the hemoglobinopathies, even in patients with sickle trait. Children with sickle trait rarely have any manifestations of disease, although adults hypoxic from altitude or exertion may develop typical sickling complications. Fatal bacterial infections in hemoglobin SC disease usually occur in older children or adolescents. Lane and colleagues described seven children with pneumococcal sepsis and hemoglobin SC disease ranging from a 1-year-old with congenital heart disease to patients 15 years of age. In four cases the spleens were considerably enlarged, with a maximum of 1500 g. Microscopic sections revealed congestion. Patients with hemoglobin S β-thalassemia may develop hyposplenia, but fatal bacterial infection is apparently exceedingly rare (Fig. 18–6). Parvovirus B19 infections may occur in various hemoglobinopathies and trigger fat embolism syndromes with massive marrow necrosis (Kolquist et al, 1996) or aplastic crises (Serjeant et al, 1993) as well as splenic sequestration syndromes (Mallouh & Qudah, 1993).

The natural history of sickle cell anemia has been altered dramatically by advances in management. In the past, as many as 20% of children died within the first 3 years, but 85–90% now survive to 20 years, and median ages at death are 42 and 48 years for males and females, respectively.

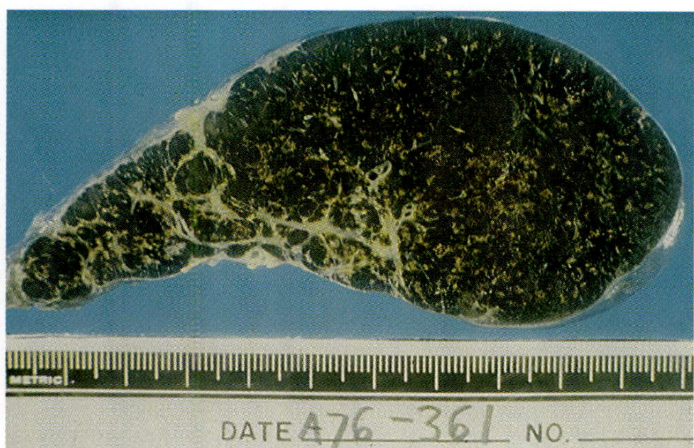

Figure 18–6

Siderofibrotic changes in the spleen associated with hemoglobin S thalassemia. This 18-year-old black female had a 200-g spleen at autopsy. The siderofibrotic changes shown here may be seen in various hemoglobinopathies. The spleens of patients with hemoglobin S thalassemia are typically larger than those of comparably aged patients with hemoglobin SS disease. (Courtesy Dr. L. W. Diggs, Division of Hematology/Oncology, University of Tennessee Medical Center, Memphis, TN.)

PATHOLOGY OF THE SPLEEN IN SICKLE CELL DISEASE

Descriptions of splenic pathology in sickle cell disease are largely based on the work of Diggs (1934, 1935, and 1965), who made original and useful observations about sickle cell disease and sickle trait for over 50 years. He recognized that the spleen may undergo dramatic changes leading to its destruction as a functional organ and provided detailed descriptions of the intermediary events (Fig. 18–7).

Late Phase

The spleen is reduced to a wrinkled mass and buried in adhesions, with a greatly thickened and hyalinized capsule. The splenic mass in the late stages has been recorded at 2.4 g in a 49-year-old woman, and Diggs described a 51-year-old man in whom no remnant of spleen was found at autopsy, a finding frequently recorded in single cases reported in the early literature.

Microscopically, in this stage, red and white pulp are replaced by scar, thick-walled calcified vessels abound, and numerous siderofibrotic nodules are present. A colorful array of pigmented structures are noted, owing in part to encrustations of iron, calcium, and perhaps bilirubin derivatives on trabeculae, vessels, and scar, resulting in refractile masses colored brown, yellow, green, and black. Attempts at phagocytosis of various encrusted forms led at an earlier time to speculation about fungal superinfections. Spleens weighing <10 g have been found in young children, but the extreme destructive late changes are usually found in adolescents or adults.

Intermediary Phase

Spleens are often enlarged, dark red, and diffusely engorged, or may contain hemorrhages, infarcts of varying size and age, and fibrosiderotic nodules and have a nodular surface owing to scar. Diggs (1935) noted average spleen weight in eight autopsied children under 5 years of age to be 240 g, including a 621-g spleen in a 4-year-old boy.

Microscopic sections reveal engorged sinuses, hemorrhages, infarcts, scarring, and granulation tissue. These lesions may be present individually or in various combinations and are interspersed with remnants of red and white pulp. Various pigmentary deposits are prominent, usually enhanced by a background of fresh hemorrhage or intense engorgement. Hemosiderin-rich scars or Gamna-Gandy bodies are similar to structures found in patients with other types of hemolytic disease or portal hypertension. Refractile encrustations of yellow, brown, and green pigment may be interspersed with numerous giant cells in the process of attempted phagocytosis. "Logjams" of sickled erythrocytes are demonstrable, particularly in formaldehyde-fixed spleens.

Early Phase

Spleens may be normal in size to moderately enlarged by engorgement of the red pulp. Sickled red cells may be demonstrated singly or as "logjams" in formaldehyde-fixed specimens. White pulp may be normal or atrophic. The capsule and trabeculae are thin and inconspicuous. Fresh hemorrhages or infarctions may be present, even in infants. Lane (1996) notes that splenic injury in hemoglobin SS disease begins as early as 3 to 6 months of life, although these children may be asymptomatic.

Splenic Sequestration

Splenic sequestration is a well-named complication, and its association with sicklemia is apparently unique. Over a few hours, a large amount of blood is trapped in the spleen, causing acute anemia and circulatory failure (Emond et al, 1985; Gill et al, 1995; Leikin et al, 1989). The conditions precipitating the sequestration crisis and the reasons for preferential susceptibility of some patients are not clearly established. However, in many cases parvovirus B19 is the triggering agent

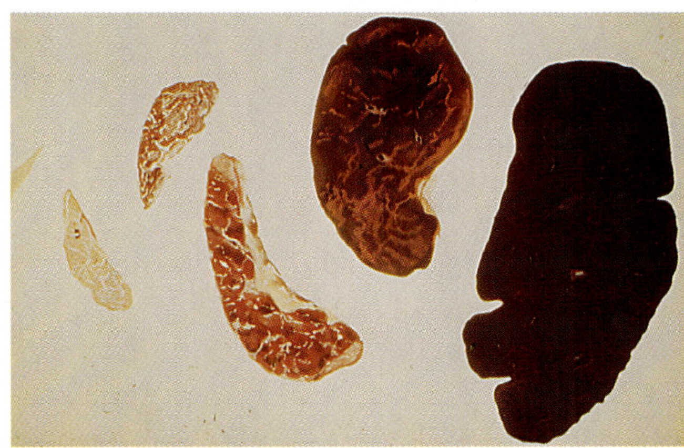

Figure 18–7

Changes in appearance over time of spleens obtained at autopsy from patients with sickle cell disease. The largest spleens are from infants and young children. There is a progressive loss of parenchyma, with replacement by fibrous tissue. In rare cases, only minute splenic remnants are found. (Illustration by Alice Diggs Sullivan, Courtesy Dr. L. W. Diggs, Division of Hematology/Oncology, University of Tennessee Medical Center, Memphis, TN.)

for splenic sequestration (Mallouh & Qudah, 1993). In a comprehensive analysis of this complication, Emond and colleagues found that 89 of 308 children with homozygous disease experienced 132 clinically significant attacks of acute splenic sequestration over a 10-year period. There were 13 fatalities, 11 during the first attack. Most episodes were associated with a febrile illness, but bacterial agents were infrequently isolated, and neither penicillin prophylaxis nor pneumococcal vaccination were preventive.

In a multicenter longitudinal study, Gill and associates (1995) studied clinical events in the first decade of life in 694 children with sickle cell anemia, hemoglobin SC disease, and hemoglobin S β-thalassemia. Twenty children, all of whom had hemoglobin SS disease, died, usually from infection. Forty-three patients had a total of 61 acute splenic sequestration crises, requiring splenectomy in 16. Two of the children with sequestration died. Pathologically, the spleen undergoes acute, marked enlargement, trapping a significant portion of the red cell mass (Fig. 18–8) (Serjeant, 1992). Splenic sequestration has also been described in patients with sickle cell trait and hereditary spherocytosis (Yang et al, 1992). Rarely, acute splenic sequestration may occur in the absence of palpable splenomegaly (Casey et al, 1994).

DISORDERS IN IMMUNE FUNCTION

Immunodeficiency Syndromes

Allegedly rare diseases, immunodeficiency syndromes are surely underreported. It is likely that only the most overt abnormalities are recognized and that myriad subtle and perhaps transient deficiencies exist. In patients with immunodeficiency, the relative frequency has been estimated at 50% for B cell deficiencies, 40% for T cell deficiencies (30% for B and T combined and 10% for pure T), 6% for deficiencies in phagocytosis, and 4% for complement deficiencies. Since abnormalities in the spleen are rarely of specific clinical or diagnostic importance in immunodeficiencies, few morphologic studies have been reported. Spleens usually become available for study after splenectomy for thrombocytopenia or at autopsy. For the principal discussion of immunodeficiency syndromes, see Chap. 3.

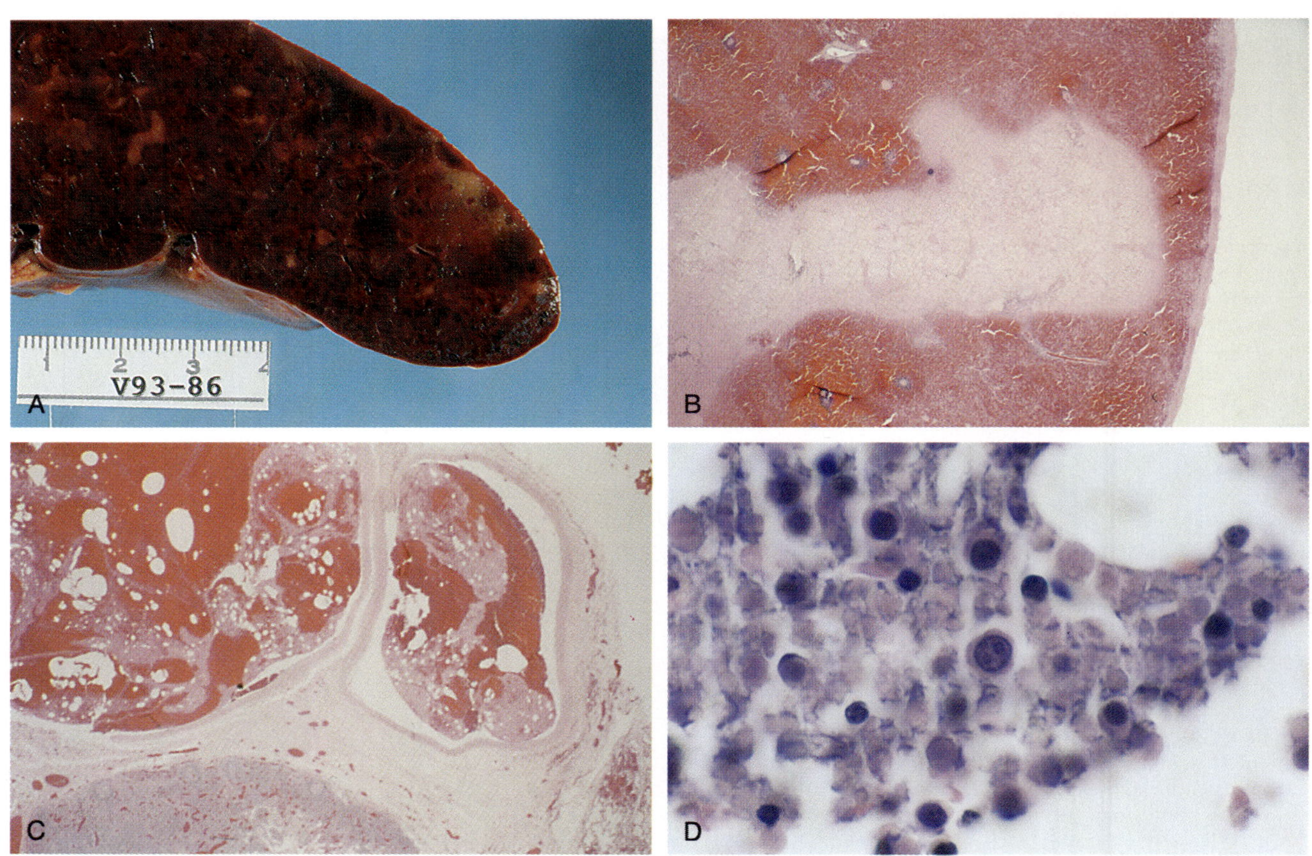

Figure 18–8

Parvovirus B19 infection in a patient with hemoglobin S β-thalassemia. A 14-year-old black girl developed headache, backache, abdominal discomfort, and respiratory distress over a 2-day period. She rapidly progressed to shock, with severe anemia and a reticulocyte count of 0.2%, dying on day 4 of hospitalization. Her 10-year-old brother died with a similar illness 1 week before but was not autopsied. Autopsy on this patient showed massive marrow necrosis and multiple pulmonary thromboemboli containing fat, necrotic marrow, and clot. Parvovirus B19 was identified by polymerase chain reaction in serum and multiple organs, including marrow and spleen. This case is an example of the splenic sequestration syndrome and massive marrow necrosis with fat or marrow emboli due to parvovirus B19 infection. The patient's brother presumably died from a similar infection (Kolquist et al, 1996). *A,* The spleen weighed 500 and was a dark purple-red color. *B,* A microscopic section of the spleen reveals marked engorgement and a central area of necrosis. *C,* Many small pulmonary arteries contained clots composed of fibrin, blood, and fat (clear spaces in this section). Fragments of necrotic marrow were also present. *D,* Marrow sections at autopsy showed extensive necrosis and enlargement of pronormoblasts of the type seen in parvovirus B19 infection.

B Cell Deficiencies

Boys with X-linked infantile agammaglobulinemia have low or absent immunoglobulins, absent plasma cells, and normal T cells. Lymph nodes, and presumably spleen, exhibit no germinal centers, primary follicles, or plasma cells. A kindred group has been described in which 10 of 22 members in three generations had massive splenomegaly in infancy and hypergammaglobulinemia, some with hemolytic anemia or thrombocytopenia. The pattern of inheritance was autosomal dominant. Immunodeficiency was evidenced as recurrent bacterial infection (Weisdorf & Krivit, 1982). Spleen weights varied from 480 g in a 16-month-old child to 605 g in a 10-year-old child. Spleen sections uniformly exhibited absent germinal centers, dilated sinuses, and hyperplastic red pulp. Splenic hilar lymph nodes were normal. The anatomic findings, coupled with immune deficits, suggested similarities to abnormalities in bursectomized chickens. The massive splenomegaly was attributed to compensation for splenic hypofunction. This condition has been referred to as empty spleen syndrome.

X-linked immunodeficiency with hyper decreased IgM affects young boys. Patients have absent or low levels of IgG, IgA, and IgE; elevated or normal levels of IgM; lymphadenopathy; hepatosplenomegaly; and enlarged tonsils. Recurrent bacterial infections are typical, and gingivitis is seen in patients with neutropenia. Lymphatic tissue may contain plasma cells, although they are often reduced in numbers, whereas germinal centers and primary follicles are absent.

Common variable immunodeficiency usually affects patients in the second or third decade. This somewhat heterogeneous group of patients has recurrent bacterial infections, markedly decreased serum immunoglobulin levels, and impaired antibody responses. Some patients have hepatosplenomegaly and lymphadenopathy. Others have hypoplastic lymphatic tissue. Plasma cells and germinal centers are decreased to absent, whereas T cells are normal or decreased (Snover et al, 1981).

Selective immunoglobulin deficiencies have been associated with IgM, IgA, IgE, IgG subclass, or light-chain deficiencies (Stiehm et al, 1980). In IgM deficiency, there are hypoplastic follicles without germinal centers. Plasma cells were present. A 3-month-old infant with low IgG3 had increased susceptibility to infection but had germinal centers in nodes with normal plasma cell numbers after antigenic stimulation. IgA deficiency is often associated with abnormal T cell function. Patients may appear normal but may have associated autoimmune diseases or T cell immunodeficiencies. One patient had hypersplenism and thrombocytopenia. No specific abnormalities are described in IgE deficiency. Elevated IgE levels may be associated with striking eosinophilia, as in one boy with traumatic rupture of the spleen. In addition to having eczema, he had recurrent staphylococcal infections (Stiehm et al, 1980).

Patients with the X-linked lymphoproliferative disorder are particularly susceptible to Epstein-Barr virus (EBV) infections. The mortality rate is high, reaching 85% by 10 years of age. EBV infections may be directly fatal or may trigger significant immune deficits, marrow failure, and development of lymphoma. Significant laboratory abnormalities include hypogammaglobulinemia and lack of antibody to EBV nuclear antigen. Sections exhibit immunoblastic proliferation in fatal cases in liver, spleen, and nodes. Lymphomas developing in these cases are usually high grade and may be widespread.

Transient hypogammaglobulinemia of infancy particularly affects premature infants and is associated with recurrent otitis media, bronchitis, and pneumonia. Node biopsy specimens exhibit small or absent germinal centers, with only a few plasma cells. Recovery is expected between 18 and 36 months of age.

T Cell Deficiencies

Immunodeficiency with generalized hematopoietic hypoplasia presents in the first few days of life and is rapidly fatal, with few patients surviving beyond 3 months. Lymphocytic depletion has been noted in spleen and other tissues at autopsy.

Thymic hypoplasia is characterized by hypocalcemia, congenital heart disease, increased susceptibility to infections, partial or complete T cell deficiencies, and normal B cell function. The thymus and parathyroids are absent in these patients, and T cells are absent in nodes and spleen. Germinal centers and plasma cells are normal.

Some patients with combined immunodeficiency syndrome have deficiencies of both T and B cell systems. These patients may have recurrent bacterial infections, oral candidiasis, skin infections, seborrheic dermatitis, chronic diarrhea, or chronic hepatitis. Node or spleen examination reveals areas of absence of T and B cells, with no plasma cells.

Patients with familial reticuloendotheliosis and eosinophilia (Omenn syndrome) have a rapidly fatal illness that may present in the first week of life with diarrhea, extensive skin lesions, hepatosplenomegaly, and eosinophilia. There is evidence of immune deficits involving both B and T systems, and pathologic arguments favor GVH pathogenesis (Jouan et al, 1987). Pathologic examination in nine cases revealed nodes enlarged by histiocyte proliferation, decreased follicles, no germinal centers, and lesions reminiscent of those seen in GVH disease. Spleen sections were similar to those in GVH, with depletion of lymphocytic tissue around arterioles and absent germinal centers. Despite this lymphocytic depletion, spleens were enlarged by hyperplasia of the red pulp.

Immunodeficiency with enzyme (adenosine deaminase) deficiency produces partial or complete B and T cell deficiencies, and most patients have manifestations of combined immunodeficiencies. Infections with all classes of organisms are life threatening for the first few weeks of life. Hepatosplenomegaly has been noted clinically, and one would expect these patients to have absent T cells and germinal centers.

Immunodeficiency with eczema and thrombocytopenias is also known as the Wiskott-Aldrich syndrome. This X-linked recessive process is characterized by thrombocytopenia, eczema, recurrent infections, defective T cell function, defective antibody response, markedly elevated IgA and IgE levels, and low IgM levels. Hepatosplenomegaly and lymphadenopathy are often present. Snover and associates (1981) reviewed the pathologic features of 17 lymph nodes and 13 spleens from 15 patients ranging in age from 4 to 96 months. Spleens weighed 20–102 g in the 13 cases and uniformly exhibited depleted T cell areas, normal or decreased germinal centers, and plasma cells. Patients were susceptible to development of lymphoma. A recent report of 12 cases (Vermi et al, 1999) described a significant depletion of the white pulp in all areas, but the marginal zone cells seemed particularly affected.

Immunodeficiency with ataxia telangiectasia is a combination of the conditions in its name and is autosomal recessive in transmission. The combined immunodeficiency, often with selective IgA deficiency, results in sinopulmonary infections and bronchiectasis. Spleen and node sections demonstrate decreased or absent T cells, normal or decreased germinal centers, and plasma cells.

Deficiencies of Neutrophils and Monocytes

Chronic granulomatous disease of childhood is a disorder of leukocyte dysfunction with an X-linked recessive inheritance pattern. Most patients are males and have widespread infections, particularly in skin, lung, and nodes. Secondary effects

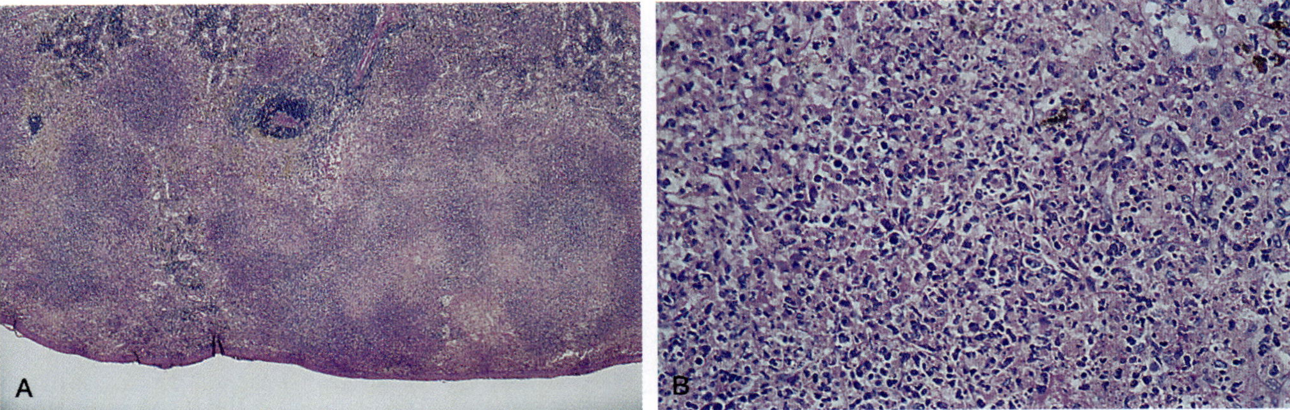

Figure 18–9

Chronic granulomatous disease, splenic abscess. This 6-year-old patient with recurrent fevers had a rectal fissure at 1 year of age and failure to thrive because of recurrent infections. Chronic granulomatous disease was suspected. Confirmation of the diagnosis was delayed because of a falsely negative nitroblue tetrazolium test result. A splenectomy was performed when the patient developed splenomegaly and sepsis. *A,* Low magnification reveals partial destruction of splenic architecture by multiple abscesses. *B,* High magnification reveals extensive acute inflammation. *Streptococcus constellatus* was cultured in this case.

are hypergammaglobulinemia, leukocytosis, and anemia. Unit lesions vary somewhat, depending on the infectious agent involved, but most show a combination of necrosis, suppuration, and granuloma formation (Fig. 18–9). Infectious agents may be of low virulence and initially discounted as contaminants. Often, lesions contain very few bacteria or fungi. Hepatosplenomegaly is a constant finding. Spread of infections to the spleen often occurs.

Autoimmune Diseases

A fatal pneumococcal infection in a 10-year-old was attributed to functional asplenia associated with systemic lupus erythematosus (Malleson et al, 1988). There was evidence of hyposplenism in the form of premortem Howell-Jolly bodies in peripheral blood. The spleen at autopsy was small (one half normal weight) and fibrotic, with decreased white pulp. Hemoglobinopathy and prior infection were not excluded in this girl of East Indian origin who had received chronic corticosteroid therapy. Another patient with active lupus had a transient reduction in colloid uptake by the spleen as well as transient Howell-Jolly bodies in peripheral films during a lupus flare. Eleven other children with lupus had no evidence of splenic dysfunction.

Infections

Specific infections are only occasionally diagnosed by splenic histopathologic examination after splenectomy or at autopsy. Recognizing splenic infectious lesions therefore is rarely of clinical significance, except when the spleen is the only or major site of involvement. Involvement of the spleen in infections is expected in generalized processes, and splenic lesions may be useful indicators of the presence of certain infections. Since functional or structural absence of the spleen may lead to the most devastating and clinically significant infections, splenic evaluation also is occasionally useful in understanding the pathogenesis of certain infections. In all cases, fixation of some blocks in B5 and periodic acid–Schiff stain facilitate visualization of key structural changes, such as distribution of lesions, presence of viral inclusions, and evidence of underlying disease.

Infections Involving the Spleen in Children with Intact Host Defenses

The likelihood that the spleen or any other organ will be involved by a particular infection is dependent on the geographic location or travel history of the patient, his or her age and immune status, and any medical treatments, procedures, and medications. This information is often not available to pathologists, despite its obvious predictive value in terms of diagnosis. Many of the infections affecting the spleen are described in a more general fashion in discussions of infection in lymph nodes (see Chap. 16) and infections in the Far East (see Chap. 16).

Infections Involving the Spleen in Children with Defective Host Defenses

Involvement of the spleen by infection is evidence of a widespread, blood-borne process. Such infections usually produce splenomegaly. Defective host defenses may be the underlying problem when infections produce splenomegaly under the following circumstances (Table 18–2): rapidly progressive, life-threatening illnesses of viral, bacterial, fungal, or protozoal cause; repeated or prolonged infection; and infections with agents that are usually not pathogenic. Specific defects in host defense are shown in Table 18–2 in relationship to expected infectious agents. The table does not list one of the commonest defects in host defense associated with overwhelming infection: the postsplenectomy or autosplenectomy syndrome, in which pneumococcal sepsis is often fatal.

Histopathologic Effects of Infection

Abscess. Abscesses are rare in the spleen in normal children. Bloodstream seeding of bacteria or fungi, as occurs in endocarditis or central line infections, as well as immunocompromise from chemotherapy or HIV infection (Smith et al, 1993) usually are the background condition for abcesses. Infectious agents found in abscesses are typically bacteria, although *Candida* species are also capable of inducing abscess formation. Stellate microabscesses typical of cat-scratch disease (see Chap. 16) presumably occur in the spleen (Larsen and Patrick, 1992) in disseminated disease, since these patients with hepatosplenomegaly have typical lesions on liver biopsy (Lamps et al, 1996). Abscesses are more frequent in patients with

Table 18–2

Defective Host Defenses Associated with Specific Widespread Infections Involving the Spleen

Defective Host Defense	Infection	Reference
X-linked lymphoproliferative disease	EBV	Iijima et al, 1992 Mroczek et al, 1987
Hypogammaglobulinemia, small thymus	*Pneumocystis carinii*	LeGolvan et al, 1973
Absent germinal centers	Echovirus 7	Ho-Yen et al, 1989
AIDS	Adenovirus Cat-scratch disease Splenic abscess Tuberculosis, including *Mycobacterium avium-intracellulare* *Candida* CMV, herpes Toxoplasmosis	Janner et al, 1990 Schwartzman et al, 1990 Smith et al, 1993
Chemotherapy	Varicella Splenic abscess *Pneumocystis carinii*	Miliauskas et al, 1984 Smith et al, 1993
Glucose-6-phosphate dehydrogenase deficiency	Rocky Mountain spotted fever	Walker et al, 1983
Chronic granulomatous disease	*Staphylococcus aureus* *Aspergillus* species *Pseudomonas aeruginosa* *Serratia marcescens*	
Hemoglobinopathies	Parvovirus B19	Mallouh & Qudah, 1993
Newborn*	Tuberculosis Congenital rubella Herpes, CMV	Schaaf et al, 1993 Singer et al, 1967
Malnutrition*	Miliary tuberculosis	Hussey et al, 1991

*Newborn and malnourished patients have variable degrees of immaturity of the immune system.

Abbreviations: CMV, cytomegalovirus; EBV, Epstein-Barr virus.

hemoglobinopathies, perhaps due to their frequent infections or superinfection of splenic hematomas (Nelken et al, 1987).

Granulomas. Histoplasmosis and tuberculosis often disseminate in their initial stages to the spleen. The resultant lesions are focal and clinically insignificant and gradually heal to produce calcified spherules. Active granulomas occur in miliary tuberculosis (Hussey and Chisholm, 1991; Schaaf et al, 1993), disseminated histoplasmosis, blastomycosis (Palmer et al, 1968), brucellosis (Hunt and Bothwell, 1967), Q fever (Laufer et al, 1986), and disseminated *Pneumocystis* infection (Le Golvan and Heidelberger, 1973). Splenomegaly occurs in approximately 50% of disseminated tuberculosis in children under 3 months (Schaff et al, 1993) and in malnourished children (Hussey and Chisholm, 1991). Necrotizing granulomas are rarely found in the spleen in patients with febrile illnesses in whom an infectious agent is not found (Collins and Neiman, 1983).

Histiocytic or Spindle Cell Proliferation. Histiocytic proliferation occurs in the spleen in several disorders not clearly associated with an infectious agent (Collins and Neiman, 1983). Infection-caused histiocytosis, particularly with spindle cell features, is frequently due to overwhelming infection with *Mycobacterium avium-intracellulare* or other "atypical" mycobacteria. These infections are readily detectible by periodic acid–Schiff staining, which is convenient for pathologists using this stain routinely to facilitate examination of splenic structures.

Necrosis or Infarctions. Focal necrosis may be found in disseminated viral infections, such as herpes or cytomegalovirus, and in bacterial infections, such as plague (Finegold, 1968). Intravascular coagulation in splenic sinuses induced by various infections may produce parenchymal necrosis. Multifocal splenic necrosis has also been described in fulminant Rocky Mountain spotted fever (Walker et al, 1983) as well as disseminated varicella in children with cancer (Miliauskas and Webber, 1984).

Immunoblastic Proliferation. The term *acute splenic tumor* was once used to describe rapid enlargement of the spleen in various infections. The word *tumor* now has a different connotation, and serious bacterial infections are not as prevalent. However, the spleen still responds to blood-borne antigenic stimuli by immunoblastic proliferation, plasmacytic differentiation, and varying degrees of histiocytic proliferation. Immunoblastic proliferation is now usually apparent in viral infections, with EBV leading the list. Rarer causes of immunoblastic proliferation are hantavirus (Nolte et al, 1995) and chronic EBV infection (Ishihara et al, 1995). The latter report is of interest, since these children did not have X-linked lymphoproliferative disease. Splenomegaly was present in 87%.

Calcification. Pathologists are familiar with the small spherular calcifications signaling remote histoplasmosis or tuberculosis. Calcifications probably occur to some extent after all chronic inflammatory processes, but calcifications recognizable by radiographic or ultrasound techniques are reported in patients with brucellosis (McGarity and Serafin, 1968) and cat-scratch disease (Larsen et al, 1992).

"Spontaneous" Rupture. *Atraumatic rupture* is a more precise term than *spontaneous rupture*. This condition is very rare and yet constitutes the commonest cause of death in patients with acute infectious mononucleosis. There were 9 (5 documented and 4 suspected) cases among 8116 patients with infectious mononucleosis seen at the Mayo Clinic over a 40-year period (Farley et al, 1992). Patient's ages in the documented cases were 16, 17, 18, 28, and 33 years. All had single capsular tears, from which they were actively bleeding at exploratory celiotomy. The four other cases in this series that were possibly attributable to infectious mononucleosis were interesting in that rupture occurred 2 weeks to 2 months after the acute illness. Patients with infectious mononucleosis–associated rupture often have splenomegaly in the 700-g range and exhibit hyperplasia of the white pulp, immunoblastic proliferation, and a diffuse mononuclear infiltrate that may involve the trabeculae and capsule. Rupture is presumably related to the rapid expansion of the spleen, its softness, and perhaps loss of capsular or trabecular integrity from cellular infiltrate.

Extramedullary Hematopoiesis. Extramedullary hematopoiesis may be seen in the spleen in stressed infants from a variety of causes, and its presence in infection probably has no diagnostic value. Nevertheless, extramedullary hematopoiesis has been described in the spleen in disseminated cytomegalovirus infection (Naeye et al, 1967) and congenital rubella syndrome (Singer et al, 1967).

LYMPHOPROLIFERATIVE DISORDERS

Multifocal Angiofollicular Hyperplasia

Angiofollicular hyperplasia usually occurs as a solitary mediastinal or mesenteric mass that is not associated with constitutional symptoms. The multicentric form, in contrast, is manifested by B symptoms, lymphadenopathy, hepatosplenomegaly, cytopenias, hyperglobulinemias, and renal and hepatic dysfunction. This disease is uncommon in children, but Smir et al (1996) have described eight children from the Angiofollicular Lymph Node Hyperplasia Registry at the University of Nebraska Medical Center. The ages were 2 to 17 years, and the male-female ratio was 1:3. All patients had constitutional symptoms, such as fever, weight loss, arthralgia, and pruritus. Lymphadenopathy, skin rash, hepatomegaly, and splenomegaly were noted in most. The spleen in one case showed marked hyperplasia of follicular centers and marginal zones, with occasional vascularized follicles similar to those in nodes. In contrast to adults, treatment (usually with prednisone) was effective in stabilizing the disease.

Autoimmune Lymphoproliferative Disease from Mutation of *FAS* Gene

Nine patients with autoimmune lymphoproliferative disease from mutation of the *FAS* gene and their families were extensively studied by Sneller and colleagues (1997). Patients ranged in age from 2 months to 5 years at presentation, with an equal sex distribution. Lymphadenopathy often involved multiple chains of nodes and was described as massive in five patients. Splenomegaly was equally marked. Many patients had hemolytic anemia, urticarial rash, thrombocytopenia, or glomerulonephritis.

Laboratory studies showed hypergammoglobulinemia, autoimmunity, B cell lymphocytosis, and expansion of a CD4−, CD8− T cell population expressing the α/β T cell receptor. Defective lymphocyte apoptosis was demonstrated in vitro in all cases. Heterozygous mutations of the *FAS* gene were found in eight of nine patients. Healthy relatives often had similar mutations but no clinical expression of disease, indicating that other factors are required before the mutation produces disease. Two members of one family had developed lymphoma. This lymphoproliferative disease in humans is very similar to a disease of mice homozygous for *LPR* or *GLD* mutations. These mutations render T cells resistant to activation-induced apoptosis (Cohen & Eisenberg, 1991).

Microscopic sections of the nodes and spleen in one case revealed a florid reactive follicular hyperplasia and immunoblastic proliferation. Numerous plasma cells were seen in the paracortex of the nodes. Noticeably absent in this hyperplasia were histiocytes containing apoptotic bodies.

Chronic Lymphadeno-Hepatosplenomegaly Syndrome in Children

Nezelof and associates (1989) reported three cases beginning early in life and having a chronic course of up to 25 years. Patients had hypergammaglobulinemia, massive splenomegaly, and lymphadenopathy, with spleen weights from 800 to 2400 g. The histologic features were distinctive, consisting of gradual depletion of follicular centers and marked infiltration of immunoblasts and plasma cells. A family history was obtained in one case. Generalized immunodeficiency, local depletion of T cells, or dendritic cells were not observed.

MALIGNANT LYMPHOMA

The lymphomas involving the spleen in children all apparently arise in other sites, with the possible exception of natural killer–like T cell lymphomas. Splenic involvement in lymphomas is rarely significant clinically, although patients with lymphoma occasionally present with hypersplenism. Now that staging laparotomy is infrequently performed, many fewer cases are likely to appear in the surgical pathology laboratory. However, Mendenhall and colleagues (1993) found in a group of pediatric cases of Hodgkin disease that the use of modern imaging techniques resulted in unacceptably high false-negative and false-positive rates for the presence of lymphoma. In this study, the actual frequency of splenic involvement by lymphocyte-predominant Hodgkin disease was 7%, by nodular sclerosing Hodgkin disease 30%, and by mixed cellularity Hodgkin disease 34%, with false-negative imaging study results in 20% and false-positive imaging study results in 32%. Splenic weight was not a sensitive predictor of involvement by Hodgkin disease in a series of 825 children and adults from Stanford (Hancock et al, 1993). The average weight of uninvolved spleens in that series was 169 g, with a range of 41–1400 g.

Hodgkin Disease

See Chap. 13 for a detailed discussion of Hodgkin disease.

Nodular Sclerosing Type

Thirty-five to 40% of cases have splenic involvement (Warnke et al, 1995). Involved spleens are often normal in size or slightly enlarged. Macroscopic lesions 1–3 mm in diameter are readily detected on thinly sectioned spleens as white, firm nodules bulging from the cut surface. Since single lesions may be present (Wolf & Neiman, 1989), careful gross examination is essential for declaration of a negative status. Microscopic involvement by nodular sclerosing Hodgkin disease is not found in the absence of gross involvement. White pulp exhibits multinodular foci easily detected at low magnification and having the usual morphologic features seen in nodes. However, classification of Hodgkin disease by splenic pathologic features is usually not warranted, since the appearance of the nodal lesion takes precedence.

Lymphocyte-Predominant Type

Ten to 25% of cases of lymphocyte-predominant Hodgkin disease have splenic involvement. Wolf and Neiman (1989) noted that in some cases small clusters of histiocytes may be found at the edge of follicles with L and H variants therein. Their illustration shows a focus of splenic consolidation that probably facilitated recognition of involvement.

Mixed-Cellularity Type

As noted in Chap. 13, mixed-cellularity Hodgkin disease is particularly common in developing countries and rare elsewhere. Splenic involvement is frequent, particularly at autopsy.

B Cell Lymphomas

For a detailed discussion of B cell lymphomas in children, see Chap. 14. Splenic involvement is very rare in children with any of the B cell lymphomas.

T Cell Lymphomas

For a detailed discussion of T cell lymphomas in children, see Chap. 15.

Natural Killer–Like T Cell Lymphoma

Children with fever, lymphadenopathy, marked hepatosplenomegaly, and normal or elevated white cell counts have been shown in a few cases to have a natural killer–like T cell lymphoma. The tumor cells are CD3+, CD8+, and CD56+ and are speculated to arise in the liver or intestine (Macon et al, 1995). Splenomegaly in these cases is presumably related to tumor, but histologic examinations have not been performed.

MYELOPROLIFERATIVE DISORDERS

Extramedullary Hemopoiesis

Extramedullary hemopoiesis in the spleen is most readily demonstrated in periodic acid–Schiff–stained sections, in which megakaryocytes are highlighted by their intrasinus location and periodic acid–Schiff cytoplasmic positivity. Clusters of nucleated red cells are also readily detected. Mature myelocytes may be part of the resident population, but immature cells, as detected by mononucleation, likely represent extramedullary hemopoiesis.

Extramedullary hemopoiesis may produce slight to massive splenomegaly in children, particularly in rare cases of widespread marrow involvement by neuroblastoma or the uncommon pediatric diseases agnogenic myeloid metaplasia and osteopetrosis (Tesluk et al, 1984). Splenectomy apparently does not affect survival in patients with agnogenic myeloid metaplasia, unless performed in those with thrombocytosis, and may provide symptomatic relief (Weinstein, 1991).

MARROW NEOPLASMS

For a major discussion of acute leukemias, see Chap. 4. For a discussion of chronic leukemias, see Chap. 5.

Chronic Leukemias

Chronic myelogenous leukemia is unusual in children but is apparently associated with prominent splenomegaly (Savage et al, 1997). In a review of 430 patients seen at a referral center at diagnosis, 8.8% were <20 years of age. Overall, the spleen was palpable in 75.8% of patients.

Juvenile chronic myelomonocytic leukemia is apparently associated with monosomy 7 karyotypic abnormality. This disorder is well recognized in children and may even occur in infants. Leukocytosis and thrombocytopenia are found in children with skin lesions and hepatosplenomegaly. In many children this condition evolves into overt acute myelogenous leukemia. Sections of marrow and spleen demonstrate increased immature myelocytes and monocytes, with rare blasts. Megakaryocytes and immature red cells may be present in the spleen. See Chap. 5 for more details.

Acute Leukemias

Splenomegaly is common in all types of acute leukemia (Fig. 18–10). The presence of splenomegaly apparently does not have diagnostic significance in the classification of leukemia, but it does signify adverse prognosis in acute lymphoblastic leukemia (Shuster et al, 1990). Massive splenomegaly is often reported, but rupture of the spleen as a complication of acute leukemia is very rare. A review of the English literature in 1996 (Giagounidis et al) identified only 45 cases of pathologic rupture owing to acute leukemia since 1861. Virtually all cases were in adults. One case is of particular interest because it was managed successfully without splenectomy. A 13-year-old with acute lymphoblastic leukemia and splenomegaly developed

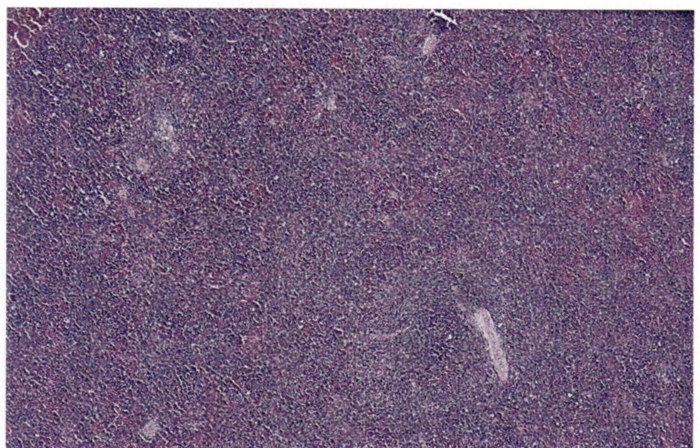

Figure 18–10

Spleen, acute lymphocytic leukemia. This adolescent had a short illness manifested by headache and dizziness before a peripheral white blood count of 800,000 cells/mm^3 was discovered. Ninety-three percent of the cells were blasts, and acute lymphocytic leukemia was diagnosed. During work-up the patient developed intracranial hemorrhage owing to leukostasis and died without treatment. At autopsy the spleen weighed 700 g. This section exhibits diffuse infiltration of blasts, with blurring of the distinction between red and white pulp.

abdominal pain with clinical evidence of hemoperitoneum attributed to splenic rupture (Soorya et al, 1980).

HISTIOCYTIC DISORDERS

The spleen is often involved in histiocytic disorders, with splenomegaly a dominant clinical feature. Consequently, splenectomies may provide initial diagnostic tissue. The understanding of histiocytic diseases has been hampered by the complexities of histiocyte biology, the rarity of many diseases, and terminologic confusion. Histiocyte accumulation is the central feature by which many histiocytic diseases are recognized. Functional deficiencies must occur but are incompletely defined. Histiocytes accumulate because of inborn errors of metabolism that cause storage of membrane breakdown products (e.g., in Gaucher and Niemann-Pick diseases), because unknown stimuli cause proliferation and phagocytosis of cellular elements (e.g., in infection-associated hemophagocytosis), or because of clonal growths (e.g., in Langerhans cell histiocytosis and malignant histiocytosis). There are many benign, localized clonal histiocytic proliferations and many circumstances in which histiocytes proliferate in response to stimulation. Nevertheless, there are few malignant neoplasms of these cells. For a major discussion of histiocyte disorders, see Chap. 10.

Storage Diseases: Glucocerebroside (Gaucher), Sphingomyelin or Cholesterol (Niemann-Pick), Cholesterol Ester (Wolman), and Ethanolaminosis

Storage diseases are rare, generally autosomal recessive, and have variable clinical severity that reflects in large part the aggregation of breakdown products in organs housing the histiocytic system. Animal models in some cases precisely mimic the human disorders. Patients with glucocerebroside accumulation, or Gaucher disease, have hepatosplenomegaly, marrow insufficiency, and in some cases a progressive neurologic disorder (Peters et al, 1977). A group of neonates with a rapid clinical course was recognized as having Gaucher disease by the resemblance to a mouse model in which the glucocerebrosidase gene was disrupted (Sidransky et al, 1992). These infants had ichthyosis, hydrops, and hepatosplenomegaly and died in hours to days. Glucocerebrosides in individual patients probably come from local breakdown of neural tissue and erythrocyte membranes, but leukocytes are the most important source. Thus, Gaucher-like cells may be found in chronic myelogenous leukemia. The diagnostic hallmark of this disease is the Gaucher cell, a macrophage distended with linear inclusions. Gaucher cells are periodic acid–Schiff–positive, contain iron, and are autofluorescent. Results of fat staining are essentially negative, but acid phosphatase is increased. The appearance in films and sections is distinctive (Fig. 18–11), as are the ultrastructural features.

Niemann-Pick disease has proven to be several disorders that differ in biochemical abnormalities (Vanier, 1983; Vanier et al, 1991) and to a certain extent in clinical expression and therapeutic implications. Sphingomyelin is a major lipid in cell membranes. Sphingomyelinase deficiency results in accumulation of sphingomyelin in neurons and visceral histiocytes (Niemann-Pick type A), principally in viscera (Niemann-Pick type B). A mouse model of type A has been described (Otterbach et al, 1995). Its potential value in understanding this and similar diseases is illustrated by the dramatic changes in Purkinje cells in this model. Within 60–90 days, homozygous mice exhibit packing of Purkinje cells with lipid-laden lysosomes followed by progressive destruction. The reason for the particular predilection of Purkinje cells to massive sphingomyelin accumulation is probably related to cell turnover rates. Niemann-Pick type C has been extensively studied by Vanier and colleagues (1991), who characterize this disorder as a complex lipidosis with a moderate increase of sphingomyelin and unesterified cholesterol. Niemann-Pick type C varies dramatically in age of onset and extent of neurologic disease. It is noteworthy that biochemical lipid analysis of formalin-fixed tissue may be used to establish the diagnosis (Vanier et al, 1991). The accumulation of histiocytes in all forms is remarkable for distention of the cytoplasm by uniform small vacuoles. These cells stain with oil red O or Sudan black B. Sea-blue histiocytes may also be found.

Cholesterol ester storage disease is inherited in an autosomal recessive pattern. Acid lipase deficiency causes failure to thrive and hepatomegaly. Liver biopsies show distention of hepatocytes by small vacuoles and cholesterol crystals. Splenomegaly is apparently due to portal hypertension. Wolman disease is an aggressive form that is usually fatal in

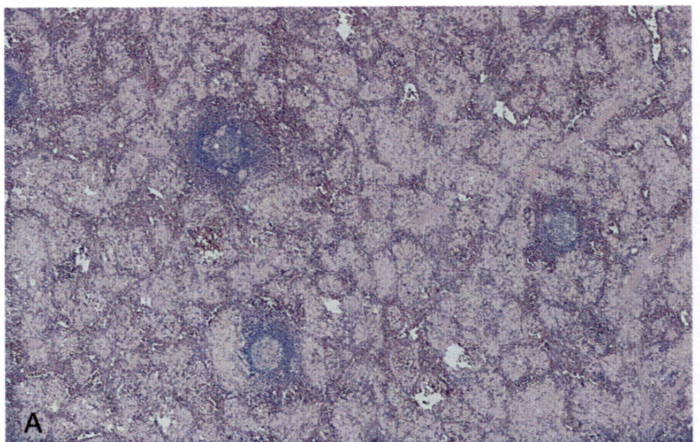

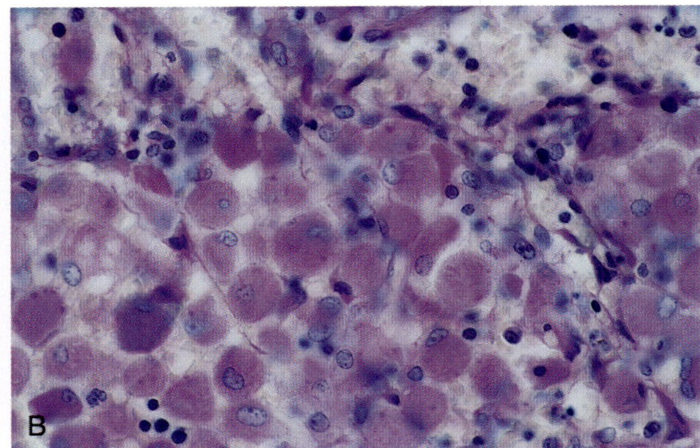

Figure 18–11

Gaucher disease, spleen. *A*, This section exhibits the typical distortion of architecture seen in spleens involved by Gaucher disease. There is reduced white pulp, and three follicular centers are surrounded by aggregates of histiocytes. Periodic acid–Schiff stain. *B*, High magnification reveals the typical morphologic features of Gaucher cells. Histiocytes have a finely striated and fibrillary cytoplasm with a moderately positive-staining background. There are few, if any, inflammatory cells of other types. Periodic acid–Schiff stain.

the first year (D'Agostino et al, 1988). Recognition of these rare diseases may be facilitated by the accelerated atherosclerosis and associated adrenal calcification.

Ethanolaminosis is a storage disease with cardiomegaly, hypotonia, cerebral dysfunction, failure to thrive and early death (Vietor et al, 1977). A periodic acid–Schiff–positive, diastase-resistant material is deposited in muscle, hepatocytes, Kupffer cells, and splenic macrophages. A predilection for periarteriolar macrophage distribution and atrophic follicles have been described.

Ceroid Storage (Sea-Blue Histiocytosis)

Clusters of macrophages with many of the cytochemical features of ceroids have been described in various hematologic conditions, including chronic myelogenous leukemia, thalassemia, hyperlipemia, idiopathic thrombocytopenic purpura, and congenital dyserythropoietic anemia. It is interesting to note that foam cells are not conspicuous in hereditary spherocytosis or sickle cell anemia. Ceroid-containing cells are usually brown tinged on hematoxylin-eosin–stained sections, sea blue in Giemsa-stained preparations, periodic acid–Schiff–positive after diastase, and iron containing. They probably have no significance other than indicating excess cell breakdown.

Tuberous Sclerosis

Three neonates with tuberous sclerosis were found to have collections of large cells in the spleen resembling brain lesions (Bender and Yunis, 1981). Cytoplasm was abundant, eosinophilic, and periodic acid–Schiff–positive and did not autofluoresce. Ultrastructurally, the splenic cells differed in several ways from those in the central nervous system.

Infection-Associated Hemophagocytosis

Infection-associated hemophagocytosis (IAHS) is a group of diseases that represent, in most cases, a dramatic complication of an underlying inherited or acquired immunodeficiency. The clinical and pathologic features are indistinguishable from familial erythrophagocytic lymphohistiocytosis, as described later. IAHS often occurs in patients with complex life-threatening illnesses, but even in this setting physicians may notice a dramatic worsening in clinical course, with fever, severe constitutional symptoms, lymphadenopathy, hepatosplenomegaly, pancytopenia, coagulopathy, and evidence of hepatic injury. In some patients there is evidence of a recent viral infection, concurrent bacterial or fungal infection, or administration of immunosuppressive medication. Approximately 85% of patients with Chédiak-Higashi syndrome enter an accelerated phase with clinical and morphologic similarities to IAHS (Rubin et al, 1985).

The diagnosis of IAHS is based on demonstrating a widespread hyperplasia of histiocytes, particularly in marrow, nodes, spleen, and liver. Rather bland-appearing histiocytes are actively phagocytosing red cells, nuclei, platelets, debris, and vacuoles. Examination of marrow films may be particularly useful in recognizing this histiocytic proliferation and phagocytosis as well as differentiating this process from the far rarer malignant histiocytosis, in which dysplastic nuclear features are required for diagnosis.

Familial Hemophagocytic Lymphohistiocytosis

Familial hemophagocytic lymphohistiocytosis is a rare, fatal autosomal recessive disease of early infancy characterized by fever, hepatosplenomegaly, lymphadenopathy, cytopenia, hypertriglyceridemia, hypofibrinogenemia, central nervous system involvement, and absence of bone or soft tissue lesions. The diagnosis should be considered only if proliferating histiocytes have a bland appearance (Arico et al, 1996; Goldberg and Nezelof, 1989; Henter et al, 1991). The diagnosis is often not made until autopsy, and there is considerable clinical and pathologic overlap with infection-associated hemophagocytosis, as discussed in the previous section. In this regard, there is no family history in one half of the cases, and hemophagocytosis may be detected at diagnosis in only 75%. Evidence of infection by various viral agents is documented in around 40% of cases (Henter et al, 1991). Entrance criteria for this series excluded children with fevers due to bacterial, rickettsial, protozoal, or spirochetal infection. Chromosomal abnormalities have not been found. The outcome is usually rapidly fatal from bleeding, infection, or progressive central nervous system disease despite treatment with steroids and cytotoxic drugs.

Pathologic findings have been summarized by Goldberg and Nezelof (1989). Most tissues were infiltrated by lymphocytes and immunoblasts, accompanied by bland histiocytes that demonstrated erythrophagocytosis. The latter phenomenon was particularly common in autopsy material. Lymph nodes and spleen showed depletion of follicular centers, with histiocytes involved in erythrophagocytosis. The role of lymphocytes in this disease as targets or effectors is difficult to evaluate. Natural killer cell activity has been described as impaired (Arico et al, 1996), but it is not clear whether lymphocytes directly cause any of the clinical or pathologic findings. The histiocytes are phagocytic and not Langerhans in type.

Histiocytoses

Langerhans Cell Type

Splenic involvement in Langerhans cell histiocytosis (LCH) is rarely significant clinically, even in cases in which there is extensive histiocytosis (Egeler & D'Angio, 1995). Hepatosplenomegaly occurs in those few patients with multiple site involvement. There is some evidence that splenic enlargement is secondary to portal hypertension. Of 64 patients from Children's Hospital of Philadelphia, nine had widespread disease and four splenomegaly. Three of the latter died with cytopenia, presumably from hypersplenism (Raney & D'Angio; 1989).

Favara and Jaffe (1994) have emphasized the potential variability of the LCH lesion owing to varying numbers of macrophages, eosinophils, and giant cells. They point out that LCH cells may be abundant or scarce. Further, Birbeck granules may be found in the minority or majority of lesional cells. In well-fixed tissues, however, LCH cells are readily identified in sections by their nuclear grooves. See Chap. 10 for a more detailed discussion of Langerhans histiocytosis.

Other Histiocytoses

A probable histiocytic proliferation with an unusual growth pattern has been described in a single case report (Russo & Seidman, 1990). This $2^1/_2$-month-old female was discovered to have asymptomatic splenomegaly at 3 weeks of age. Splenomegaly progressed, hepatomegaly followed, and a liver biopsy was performed. Sections exhibited large cells with widespread permeation of hepatic sinusoids and cellular thrombi in portal veins. Proliferating cells did not mark as B or T cells and demonstrated reactivity for leukocyte common antigen and S-100 protein. Ultrastructural studies demonstrated lysosomal granules, no cytoplasmic filaments, and no Birbeck granules. Chemotherapy was followed by gradual resolution of hepatosplenomegaly that was sustained for 27 months at the time of the report. The authors speculated that the case represented an unusual proliferation of histiocytic cells and that clinical improvement may have been due to self-healing as well as chemotherapy.

Systemic Juvenile Xanthogranuloma

Juvenile xanthogranuloma is usually limited to the skin, but 36 cases with systemic disease have been reviewed (Freyer et al, 1996). The median age of the 36 patients was 0.3 years, with a range from birth to 12 years. Skin or subcutaneous lesions were present in most patients, although two had abdominal disease without skin lesions. Eight of 36 had hepatic and/or splenic involvement.

The skin lesions in juvenile xanthogranuloma contain a monomorphous infiltrate of histiocytes that may extend into subcutaneous tissue. Areas with spindled and elongated forms may be present, as may single or numerous Touton giant cells. Eosinophils may be present, but these lesions may be distinguished from Langerhans histiocytosis by cytologic features (Langerhans cells have a distinctive nuclear groove), their nonreactivity with S-100 and CD1A protein, and absent Birbeck granules. Most children with system juvenile xanthogranulomatosis have a good prognosis, and disease regression in treated patients apparently parallels that in untreated patients.

REFERENCES

Alagille D: α-1-Antitrypsin deficiency. Hepatology 4:11S–14S, 1984.

Alt B, Hafez GR, Trigg M, et al: Angiosarcoma of the liver and spleen in an infant. Pediatr Pathol 4:331–339, 1985.

Anderson C, Devine WA, Anderson RH, et al: Abnormalities of the spleen in relation to congenital malformations of the heart: a survey of necropsy findings in children. Br Heart J 63:122–128, 1990.

Arendt T, Nizze H, Konrad H: Prognostic significance of splenic follicle size in splenectomized idiopathic thrombocytopenic purpura patients. Blut 57:347–349, 1988.

Arico M, Janka G, Fischer A, et al: Hemophagocytic lymphohistiocytosis: report of 122 children from the international registry. Leukemia 10:197–203, 1996.

Bender BL, Yunis EJ: Splenic involvement in tuberous sclerosis. Virchows Arch A Pathol Anat 391:363–369, 1981.

Brown AK, Sleeper LA, Miller ST, et al: Reference values and hematologic changes from birth to 5 years in patients with sickle cell disease. Arch Pediatr Adolesc Med 148:796–804, 1994.

Brunning RD, McKenna RW: Tumors of the bone marrow. In Rosai J (ed): Atlas of Tumor Pathology, 3rd series, fascicle 9. Armed Forces Institute of Pathology, Washington, DC, 1994.

Budke HL, Breitfeld PP, Neiman RS: Functional hyposplenism due to a primary epithelioid hemangioendothelioma of the spleen. Arch Pathol Lab Med 119:755–757, 1995.

Buehner M, Baker MS: The wandering spleen. Surg Gynecol Obstet 175:373–387, 1992.

Burke JS: Surgical pathology of the spleen: an approach to the differential diagnosis of splenic lymphomas and leukemias. Am J Surg Pathol 5:551–563, 1981.

Butler JJ: Pathology of the spleen in benign and malignant conditions. Histopathology 7:453–474, 1983.

Casey JR, Kinney TR, Ware RE: Acute splenic sequestration in the absence of palpable splenomegaly. Am J Pediatr Hematol Oncol 16:181–182, 1994.

Chang C-S, Li C-Y Cha SS: Chronic idiopathic thrombocytopenic purpura. Arch Pathol Lab Med 117:981–985, 1993.

Chang C-S, Li C-Y, Liang Y-H, et al: Clinical features and splenic pathologic changes in patients with autoimmune hemolytic anemia and congenital hemolytic anemia. Mayo Clinic Proc 68:757–762, 1993.

Chang KL, Kamel OW, Arber DA, et al: Pathologic features of nodular lymphocyte predominance Hodgkin disease in extranodal sites. Am J Surg Pathol 19:1313–1324, 1995.

Chilcote RR, Brown E, Rowley JD: Lymphoblastic leukemia with lymphomatous features associated with abnormalities of the short arm of chromosome 9. N Eng J Med 5:286–291, 1985.

Coetzee T: Clinical anatomy and physiology of the spleen. S. Afr Med J 15:737–746, 1982.

Cohen PL, Eisenberg RA: *Lpr* and *gld*: single gene models of systemic autoimmunity and lymphoproliferative disease. Ann Rev Immunol 9:243–269, 1991.

Collins RD, Neiman RS: Granulomatous diseases of the spleen. In Ioachim HL (ed): Pathology of Granulomas. Raven Press, New York, pp 188–190, 1983.

D'Agostino D, Bay L, Gallo G, et al: Cholesterol ester storage disease: clinical, biochemical and pathological studies of four new cases. J Pediatr Gastroenterol Nutr 7:446–450, 1988.

Dailey MO, Coleman CN, Fajardo LF: Splenic injury caused by therapeutic irradiation. Am J Surg Pathol 5:325–331, 1981.

Dawson JH, Roberts NG: Management of the wandering spleen. Aust NZ J Surg 64:441–444, 1994.

Debray D, Pariente D, Urvoas E, et al: Sclerosing cholangitis in children. J Pediatr 124:49–56, 1994.

Diebold J, Audouin J: Peliosis of the spleen: report of a case associated with chronic myelomonocytic leukemia, presenting with spontaneous splenic rupture. Am J Surg Pathol 7:197–204, 1983.

Diggs LW: Sickle cell crises: Ward Burdick Award contribution. Am J Clin Pathol 44:1–19, 1965.

Diggs LW: Siderofibrosis of the spleen in sickle cell anemia. JAMA 104:538–541, 1935.

Diggs LW, Ching RE: Pathology of sickle cell anemia. South Med J 27:839–845, 1934.

Egeler RM, D'Angio GJ: Langerhans cell histiocytosis. J Pediatr 127:1–11, 1995.

Emond AM, Collis R, Darvill D, et al: Acute splenic sequestration in homozygous sickle cell disease: natural history and management. J Pediatr 107:201–206, 1985.

Eyster ME, Saletan SL, Rabellino EM, et al: Familial essential thrombocythemia. Am J Surg 80:497–502, 1986.

Falini B, Flenghi L, Piteri S, et al: Distribution of T cells bearing different forms of the T-cell receptor γ/δ in normal and pathological human tissues. J Immunol 143:2480–2488, 1989.

Falk S, Stutte HJ: Hamartomas of the spleen: a study of 20 biopsy cases. Histopathology 14:603–612, 1989.

Falk S, Stutte HJ, Frizzera G: Littoral cell angioma: a novel splenic vascular lesion demonstrating histiocytic differentiation. Am J Surg Pathol 15:1023–1033, 1991.

Fanburg JC, Meis-Kindblom JM, Rosenberg AE: Multiple enchondromas associated with spindle-cell hemangioendotheliomas: an overlooked variant of Maffucci's syndrome. Am J Surg Pathol 19:1029–1038, 1995.

Farley DR, Zietlow SP, Bannon MP, et al: Spentaneous rupture of the spleen due to infectious mononucleosis. Mayo Clin Proc 67:846–853, 1992.

Favara BE, Jaffe R: The histopathology of Langerhans cell histiocytosis. Cancer 70:S17–S24, 1994.

Finegold M: Pathogenesis of plague: a review of plague deaths in the United States during the last decade. Am J Med 45:549–554, 1968.

Freedman MH, Saunders EF: Hematopoiesis in the human spleen. Am J Hematol 11:271–275, 1981.

Freyer DR, Kennedy R, Bostrom BC, et al: Juvenile xanthogranuloma: forms of systemic disease and their clinical implications. J Pediatr 129:227–237, 1996.

Frizzera G, Rosai J, Dehner LP, et al: Lymphoreticular disorders in primary immunodeficiencies: new findings based on an up-to-date histologic classification of 35 cases. Cancer 46:692–699, 1980.

Garvin DF, King FM: Cysts and nonlymphomatous tumors of the spleen. Pathol Annu 1:61–80, 1981.

Giagounidis AA, Burk M, Meckenstock G, et al: Pathologic rupture of the spleen in hematologic malignancies: two additional cases. Ann Hematol 73:297–302, 1996.

Gill FM, Sleeper LA, Weiner SJ, et al: Clinical events in the first decade in a cohort of infants with sickle cell disease. Blood 86:776–783, 1995.

Glueck CJ, Lichtenstein P, Trent T, et al: Safety and efficacy of treatment of pediatric cholesteryl ester storage disease with lovastatin. Pediatr Res 32:559–565, 1992.

Goldberg JC, Nezelof C: Familial lymphohistiocytosis: the pathologist's view. Pediatr Hematol Oncol 6:199–205, 1989.
Gottesman G, Vanunu D, Maayan M, et al: Childhood brucellosis in Israel. Pediatr Infect Dis J 15:610–615, 1996.
Haber LM, Hawkins EP, Seilheimer DK, et al: Fat overload syndrome: an autopsy study with evaluation of the coagulation. Single Case Rep 90:223–227, 1988.
Hancock SL, Scidmore NS, Hopkins KL, et al: Computed tomography assessment of splenic size as a predictor of splenic weight and disease involvement in laparotomy staged Hodgkin disease. Int J Radiat Oncol Biol Phys 28:93–99, 1993.
Hashida Y, Jaffe R, Yunis EJ: Pancreatic pathology in trisomy 13: specificity of the morphologic lesion. Pediatr Pathol 1:169–178, 1983.
Hegyi T, Delphin ES, Bank A, et al: Sickle cell anemia in the newborn. Pediatrics 60:213–216, 1977.
Henter JI, Elinder G, Soder O, et al: Incidence in Sweden and clinical features of familial hemophagocytic lymphohistiocytosis. Acta Paediatr Scand 80:428–435, 1991.
Ho-Yen DO, Hardie R, McClure J, et al: Fatal outcome of echovirus 7 infection. Scand J Infect Dis 21:459–461, 1989.
Hunt AC, Bothwell PW: Histological findings in human brucellosis. J Clin Pathol 20:267–272, 1967.
Hussey G, Chisholm T: Miliary tuberculosis in children: a review of 94 cases. Pediatr Infect Dis J 10:832–836, 1991.
Iijima T, Sumazaki R, Mori N, et al: A pathological and immunohistological case report of fatal infectious mononucleosis, Epstein-Barr virus infection, demonstrated by in situ and Southern blot hybridization. Virchows Arch A Pathol Anat 421:73–78, 1992.
Ishihara S, Okada S, Wakiguchi H, et al: Chronic active Epstein-Barr virus infection in children in Japan. Acta Paediatr 84:1271–1275, 1995.
Janner D, Petru AM, Belchis D, et al: Fatal adenovirus infection in a child with acquired immunodeficiency syndrome. Pediatr Infect Dis 9:434–436, 1990.
Jouan H, Le Deist F, Nezelof C: Omenn's syndrome—pathologic arguments in favor of a graft versus host pathogenesis: a report of nine cases. Hum Pathol 18:1101–1108, 1987.
Kelly DA, Portmann B, Mowat AP, et al: Niemann-Pick disease type C: diagnosis and outcome in children, with particular reference to liver disease. J Pediatr 123:245–247, 1993.
Kevy Sherwin V, Tefft M, Vawter GF, et al: Hereditary splenic hypoplasia. Pediatrics 42:752–757, 1968.
Klatt EC, Meyer PR: Pathology of the spleen in the acquired immunodeficiency syndrome. Arch Pathol Lab Med 3:1050–1053, 1987.
Kolquist KA, Vnencak-Jones CL, Swift L, et al: Fatal fat embolism syndrome in a child with undiagnosed hemoglobulin S/β^+ thalassemia: a complication of acute parvovirus B19 infection. Pediatr Pathol Lab Med 16:71–82, 1996.
Lamps LW, Gray GF, Scott MA: The histologic spectrum of hepatic cat-scratch disease: a series of six cases with confirmed *Bartonella henselae* infection. Am J Surg Pathol 20:1253–1259, 1996.
Lane PA: Sickle cell disease. Pediatr Hematolo 43:639–664, 1996.
Lane PA: The spleen in children. Curr Opin Pediatr 7:36–41, 1995.
Lane PA, Rogers ZR, Woods GM, et al: Fatal pneumococcal septicemia in hemoglobin SC disease. J Pediatr 124:859–862, 1994.
Larsen C, Patrick LE: Abdominal (liver, spleen) and bone manifestations of cat scratch disease. Pediatr Radiol 22:353–355, 1992.
Laufer D, Lew PD, Oberhansli I, et al: Chronic Q fever endocarditis with massive splenomegaly in childhood. J Pediatr 108:535–539, 1986.
LeGolvan DP, Heidelberger KP: Disseminated, granulomatous *Pneumocystis carinii* pneumonia. Arch Pathol 95:344–348, 1973.
Leikin S, Gallagher D, Kinney TR, et al: Mortality in children and adolescents with sickle cell disease. Pediatrics 84:500–508, 1989.
Macon WR, Williams ME, Greer JP, et al: Natural killer–like T-cell lymphomas: aggressive lymphomas of T–large granular lymphocytes. Blood 87:1474–1483, 1995.
Maksoud JG, Mies S, da Costa Gayotto LC: Hepatoportal sclerosis in childhood. Am J Surg 151:484–488, 1986.
Malleson P, Petty RE, Nadel H, et al: Functional asplenia in childhood onset systemic lupus erythematosus. Rheumatol 15:1648–1652, 1988.
Mallouh AA, Qudah A: Acute splenic sequestration together with aplastic crises caused by human parvovirus B19 in patients with sickle cell disease. J Pediatr 122:593–595, 1993.
McGarity WC, Serafin D: Brucellosis: indications for splenectomy. Am J Surg 115:355–363, 1968.
McVicar MI, Chandra M, Margouleff D, et al: Splenic hypofunction in the nephrotic syndrome of childhood. Am J Kid Dis 7:395–401, 1986.
Mendenhall NP, Cantor AB, Williams JL, et al: With modern imaging techniques, is staging laparotomy necessary in pediatric Hodgkin's disease? A Pediatric Oncology Group study. J Clin Oncol 11:2218–2225, 1993.
Miliauskas JR, Webber BL: Disseminated varicella at autopsy in children with cancer. Cancer 53:1518–1525, 1984.
Mroczek EC, Weisenburger DD, Grierson H Lipscomb, et al: Fatal infectious mononucleosis and virus-associated hemophagocytic syndrome. Arch Pathol Lab Med 111:530–535, 1987.
Naeye RL: Cytomegalic inclusion disease: the fetal disease. Am J Clin Pathol 47:738–744, 1967.
Nelken N, Ignatius J, Skinner M, et al: Changing clinical spectrum of splenic abscess: a multicenter study and review of the literature. Am J Surg 154:27–34, 1987.
Nezelof C, Maupas C, Griscelli C: The disappearance of germinal centers in chronic lymphadeno-hepato-splenomegaly syndrome in childhood: report of three cases. Pediatr Pathol 9:57–71, 1989.
Nolte KB, Feddersen RM, Foucar K, et al: Hantavirus pulmonary syndrome in the United States: a pathological description of a disease caused by a new agent. Hum Pathol 26:110–120, 1995.
Ohshio G, Furukawa F, Fujiwara H, et al: Hepatomegaly and splenomegaly in Kawasaki disease. Pediatr Pathol 4:257–264, 1985.
Otterbach B, Stoffel W: Acid sphingomyelinase-deficient mice mimic the neurovisceral form of human lysomal storage disease (Niemann-Pick disease). Cell 81:1053–1051, 1995.
Palmer PE, McFadden SW: Blastomycosis: report of an unusual case. N Engl J Med 279:979–983, 1968.
Pearson HA, Gallagher D, Chilcote R, et al: The cooperative study of sickle cell disease. Pediatrics 76:392–397, 1985.
Pearson HA, Johnston D, Smith KA, et al: The born-again spleen: return of splenic function after splenectomy for trauma. N Eng J Med 298:1389–1392, 1978.
Peoples WM, Moller JH, Edwards JE: Polysplenia: a review of 146 cases. Pediatr Cardiol 4:129–137, 1983.
Peters SP, Lee RE, Glew RH: Gaucher's disease, a review. Medicine 56:425–442, 1977.
Ramani P, Path MRC, Shah A: Lymphangiomatosis: histologic and immunohistochemical analysis of four cases. Am J Surg Pathol 17:329–335, 1993.
Raney RB Jr, D'Angio, GJ: Langerhans cell histiocytosis (histiocytosis X): experience at the Children's Hospital of Philadelphia, 1970–1984. Med Pediatr Oncol 17:20–28, 1989.
Rubin CM, Burke BA, McKenna RW, et al: The accelerated phase of Chédiak-Higashi syndrome: an expression of the virus-associated hemophagocytic syndrome? Cancer 56:524–530, 1985.
Russo PA, Seidman E: An unusual histiocytoid proliferation in infancy. Hum Pathol 21:564, 1990.
Satti MB, Melha AA, Al-Sohaibani MO, et al: Splenic foam cells: a clinic-pathology analysis of 92 splenectomized patients. Acta Haematol 83:9–15, 1990.
Savage DG, Szydlo RM, Goldman JM: Clinical features at diagnosis in 430 patients with chronic myeloid leukaemia seen at a referral centre over a 16-year period. Br J Haematol 96:111–116, 1997.
Schaaf HS, Gie RP, Beyers N, et al: Tuberculosis in infants less than 3 months of age. Arch Dis Child 69:371–374, 1993.
Shuster JJ, Falletta JM, Pullen DJ, et al: Prognostic factors in childhood T-cell acute lymphoblastic leukemia: a Pediatric Oncology Group study. Blood 75:166–173, 1990.
Schwartzman WA, Marchevsky A, Meyer RD: Epithelioid angiomatosis or cat-scratch disease with splenic and hepatic abnormalities in AIDS: case report and review of the literature. Scand J Infect Dis 22:121–133, 1990.
Serjeant GR: Sickle Cell Disease, 2nd ed. Oxford University Press, New York, pp 134–152, 1992.
Serjeant GR, Serjeant BE, Thomas PW, et al: Human parvovirus infection in homozygous sickle cell disease. Lancet 341:1237–1240, 1993.
Sidransky E, Sherer DM, Ginns EI: Gaucher disease in the neonate: a distinct Gaucher phenotype is analogous to a mouse model

created by targeted disruption of the glucocerebrosidase gene. Pediatr Res 32:494–498, 1992.

Singer DB, Rudolph AJ, Rosenberg HS, et al: Pathology of the congenital rubella syndrome. J Pediatr 71:665–675, 1967.

Smir BN, Greiner TC, Weisenburger DD: Multicentric angiofollicular lymph node hyperplasia in children: a clinicopathologic study of eight patients. Mod Pathol 9:1135, 1996.

Smith MD Jr, Nio M, Camel JE, et al: Management of splenic abscess in immunocomprised children. J Pediatr Surg 28:823–826, 1993.

Sneller MC, Wang J, Dale JK, et al: Clinical, immunologic, and genetic features of an autoimmune lymphoproliferative syndrome associated with abnormal lymphocyte apoptosis. Blood 89:1341–1348, 1997.

Snover DC, Frizzera G, Spector BD, et al: Wiskott-Aldrich syndrome: histopathologic findings in the lymph nodes and spleens of 15 patients. Hum Pathol 12:821–831, 1981.

Soorya DT, Ravindranath Y, Philippart A: Spontaneous splenic rupture in acute lymphoblastic leukemia: successful nonoperative management. Am J Dis Child 134:201–202, 1980.

Stiehm ER, Fulginiti VA: Immunologic Disorders in Infants and Children, 2nd ed. W.B. Saunders Company, Philadelphia, pp 183–327, 1980.

Suster S: Epithelioid and spindle-cell hemangioendothelioma of the spleen: report of a distinctive splenic vascular neoplasm of childhood. Am J Surg Pathol 16:785–792, 1992.

Tesluk G, Thomas CG Jr, Benjamin JT, et al: Fatal overwhelming postsplenectomy sepsis following autologous splenic transplantation in severe congenital osteopetrosis. J Pediatr Surg 19:269–272, 1984.

Tham KT, Teague MW, Howard CA, A simple splenic reticuloendothelial function test: counting erythrocytes with argyrophilic inclusions. Hematopathology 105:548–552, 1996.

van Krieken JHJM, Te Velden J, Hermans J, et al: The amount of red pulp: a histomorphometrical study in splenectomy specimens embedded in methylmethacrylate. Histopathology 9:401–416, 1985.

van Krieken JHJM, Te Velden J, Hermans J, et al: The amount of white pulp in the spleen: a morphometrical study done in methacrylate-embedded splenectomy specimens. Histopathology 7:767–782, 1983.

Vanier MT: Biochemical studies in Niemann-Pick disease. Biochim Biophys Acta 750:178–194, 1983.

Vanier MT, Rodriguez-Lafrasse C, Rousson R, et al: Type C Niemann-Pick disease: biochemical aspects and phenotypic heterogeneity. Dev Neurosci 13:307–314, 1991.

Vermi W, Blanzuoli L, Kraus MD, et al: The spleen in the Wiskott-Aldrich syndrome: histopathologic abnormalities of the white pulp correlate with the clinical phenotype of the disease. Am J Surg Pathol 23:182–191, 1999.

Vietor KW, Havsteen B, Harms D, et al: Ethanolaminosis: a newly recognized, generalized storage disease with cardiomegaly cerebral dysfunction and early death. Eur J Pediatr 126:61–75, 1977.

Wahlby L, Domellof L: Splenectomy after blunt abdominal trauma: a retrospective study of 413 children. Acta Chir Scand 147:131–135, 1981.

Walker DH, Hawkins HK, Hudson P: Fulminant Rocky Mountain spotted fever. Arch Pathol Lab Med 107:121–125, 1983.

Warnke RA, Weiss LM, Chan JKC, et al: Tumors of the lymph nodes and spleen. In Rosai J (ed): In Atlas of Tumor Pathology, 3rd series, fascicle 14. Armed Forces Institute of Pathology, Washington, DC, 1995.

Weinstein IM: Idiopathic myelofibrosis: historical review, diagnosis and management. Blood Rev 98–104, 1991.

Weisdorf SA, Krivit W: Paucity of splenic germinal centers: a new and unique splenomegaly syndrome including dysfunctional immune system. Clin Immunol Immunopathol 23:492–500, 1982.

Willman CL, Busque L, Griffith BB, et al: Langerhans'-cell histiocytosis (histiocytosis X): a clonal proliferative disease. N Eng J Med 21:154, 1994.

Wilschanski M, Chait P, Wade JA, et al: Primary sclerosing cholangitis in 32 children: clinical, laboratory, and radiographic features, with survival analysis. Hepatology 22:1415–1422, 1995.

Winberg CD, Nathwani BN, Bearman RM, et al: Follicular (nodular) lymphoma during the first two decades of life: a clinicopathologic study of 12 patients. Cancer 48:2223–2235, 1981.

Wolf BC, Neiman R: Disorders of the Spleen: vol 20 in Major Problems in Pathology. W.B. Saunders Company, Philadelphia, 1989.

Yam LT, Li C-Y: The spleen. In Emburg SH, et al (eds): Sickle Cell Disease: Basic Principles and Clinical Practice. Raven Press, New York, pp 555–566, 1994.

Yang Y-M, Donnell C, Wilborn W, et al: Splenic sequestration associated with sickle cell trait and hereditary spherocytosis. Am J Hemato 40:110–116, 1992.

Zoli G, Corazza GR, D'Amato G, et al: Splenic autotransplantation after splenectomy: tuftsin activity correlates with residual splenic function. Br J Surg 81:716–718, 1994.

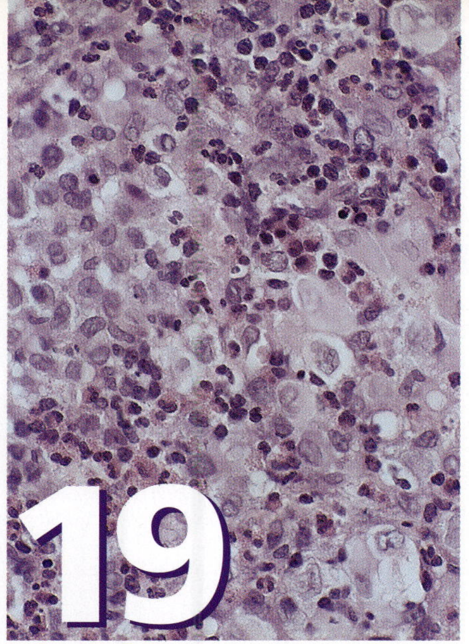

Laura W. Lamps
Kay Washington

Gastrointestinal Tract and Liver

NORMAL STRUCTURE AND FUNCTION OF THE GASTROINTESTINAL TRACT

The components of the digestive tract—the esophagus, stomach, small intestine, and large intestine—have a common structural organization consisting of a hollow tube with a wall of four principal layers: the mucosa, submucosa, muscularis propria, and serosal or adventitial tissue. The mucosa of each component is distinctive and varies according to the primary function of the site. For instance, the esophagus is lined by nonabsorptive squamous epithelium, since it functions principally as a conduit from mouth to stomach. Gastric epithelial cells are more varied, reflecting their multiple functions, such as secretion of gastric acid and pepsinogen. Small intestinal enterocytes are specialized for absorptive functions. The principal functions of the colon are absorption of water from the fecal stream and evacuation of waste, and thus the epithelial lining contains absorptive cells and mucin-secreting goblet cells.

The inflammatory and immune cells normally present in gastrointestinal (GI) mucosa are of major interest to hematopathologists. With the exception of the esophagus, the contents of the digestive tract are separated from the intestinal wall by only a single layer of epithelium. Accordingly, various specialized defenses have been developed to prevent infectious agents and harmful substances from gaining entrance through the GI mucosa. One component of these defenses is the intraepithelial lymphocyte, present in varying numbers at all levels of the digestive tract. These lymphocytes differ in phenotype from peripheral and lamina propria lymphocytes. Almost all intraepithelial lymphocytes are T cells, and most are CD8+ (Shanahan, 1997). Secretory IgA, so important for mucosal defense, is produced by plasma cells in the lamina propria, an area that also contains T and B lymphocytes, eosinophils, and mast cells. Lesser numbers of plasma cells secreting IgM are present, and there are few IgG-producing cells (Dhesi et al, 1984).

Normal esophageal mucosa contains scattered intraepithelial lymphocytes, often called squiggle cells because of their distorted nuclei. Langherans cells are also present, but neutrophils and eosinophils are not found in normal esophageal mucosa. Normal gastric mucosa contains a more varied inflammatory and immune population that is relatively rare in the lamina propria in children but increases in number with age. Occasional lamina propria lymphocytes and plasma cells should not prompt a diagnosis of chronic gastritis, although minimal criteria for diagnosis of chronic gastritis remain a matter of individual judgment. The presence of germinal centers in gastric mucosa is suggestive of chronic gastritis and should prompt a search for *Helicobacter pylori*. Scattered eosinophils and mast cells are also present in the lamina propria in the normal stomach. Intraepithelial lymphocytes are rare in gastric mucosa.

The normal small intestinal mucosa contains plasma cells, lymphocytes, eosinophils, macrophages, and mast cells in the lamina propria. Both B and T cells are in the lymphocytic infiltrate, with CD4+ T cells the most common subset of lamina propria T cells. Aggregates and nodules of lymphocytes are common, particularly in the distal small intestine. The overlying surface epithelium has fewer goblet cells and contains scattered specialized columnar epithelial cells, known as M cells, that deliver antigens across the epithelium to the underlying lymphocytic tissue. Intraepithelial lymphocytes are more prominent than in the gastric or colonic mucosa and are present in a ratio of up to one lymphocyte per five epithelial cells (Dobbins, 1986). A similar prominent infiltrate is present in the lamina propria of the colon, but fewer intraepithelial lymphocytes are normally present in the colon. Neutrophils are not a normal constituent of the inflammatory infiltrate in the small intestine and colon.

NONNEOPLASTIC DISORDERS OF THE GASTROINTESTINAL TRACT

Gastrointestinal Manifestations of Primary Immunodeficiencies

The primary immunodeficiencies are often associated with GI lesions (Table 19–1) that are infectious in etiology, but chronic conditions resembling inflammatory bowel disease are seen in many patients with antibody deficiencies. All patients with primary immunodeficiencies are at increased risk for neoplasia, most commonly B and T cell lymphomas. The GI tract is often the primary site. Few lymphomas in patients with primary immunodeficiencies are associated with Epstein-Barr virus (EBV) infection, in contrast to the almost universal association of EBV with posttransplant lymphoproliferative disorders (Fili-povich et al, 1994). In addition to a lymphoma risk, patients with IgA deficiency, common variable immunodeficiency (CVID), and ataxia-telangiectasia are at increased risk for gastric adenocarcinoma (Filipovich et al, 1994), and patients with X-linked agammaglobulinemia may be at increased risk for co-lorectal carcinoma (van der Meer et al, 1993). See Chap. 3 for general descriptions of immunodeficiencies.

Table 19–1
Gastrointestinal Findings in Primary Immunodeficiency

Site	CGD	SCID	XLAG	CVID
Esophagus	Obstruction	Reflux		
Stomach	Gastric outlet obstruction			Pernicious anemia, atrophic gastritis adenocarcinoma
Small bowel	Crohn-like pigmented macrophages	Viral infections	*Giardia*, Crohn like	Villous atrophy, *Giardia*
Lymphocytic system				Nodular hyperplasia, lymphoma
Large bowel	Colitis (UC like and Crohn like), pigmented macrophages		Adenocarcinoma	Colitis (UC like, GVHD like, or lymphocytic colitis like)
Anus	Perianal fistula		Perianal abscess	

Abbreviations: CGD, chronic granulomatous disease; CVID, common variable immunodeficiency; GVHD, graft-versus-host disease; SCID, severe combined immunodeficiency disease; UC, ulcerative colitis; XLAG, X-linked agammaglobulinemia.

Common Variable Immunodeficiency

Patients with CVID frequently develop chronic GI inflammatory disorders and malignancies. The former are in some cases a result of acute or chronic infections, but in others the GI lesions are probably a manifestation of autoimmunity (Washington et al, 1996). In one large clinical study, 20% of patients with CVID had one or more autoimmune diseases, most commonly idiopathic thrombocytopenic purpura and autoimmune hemolytic anemia (Cunningham-Rundles, 1989). Thirteen percent of these CVID patients developed cancer, with 9% (of the 103 patients) developing lymphoma. Most of the cancers occurred in older patients, but one child was diagnosed with lymphoma at age 12.

The stomach exhibits increased lymphocytes in the lamina propria in some patients with CVID, as well as increased apoptosis of gastric epithelial cells. Older children and adults with CVID may develop atrophic gastritis and pernicious anemia. Adults with CVID are at increased risk for gastric adenocarcinoma, whereas children with CVID are rarely affected (Conley et al, 1988).

In the small bowel, some patients with CVID develop a spruelike lesion with villous blunting (Fig. 19–1) that is associated with severe malabsorption. This lesion may be indistinguishable on biopsy from celiac disease, although it differs from celiac disease in its relative lack of crypt hyperplasia. Some CVID patients with this small bowel lesion respond to a gluten-free diet. Chronic giardiasis is a common problem in CVID and may cause clinical symptoms. Small bowel mucosal abnormalities seen in *Giardia* infection in this population include villous blunting, increased numbers of intraepithelial lymphocytes, and nodular lymphocytic hyperplasia. The latter is characterized by multiple discrete aggregates of lymphocytes in the lamina propria and submucosa of the small and/or large intestine (Fig. 19–2). Nodular hyperplasia of lymphocytes is often associated with CVID but may also be seen in giardiasis without antibody deficiency (Ward et al, 1983). Nodular hyperplasia of lymphocytes is not a malignant disorder, although a clonal immunoglobulin gene rearrangement has been demonstrated in such lesions in the GI tract in a child with CVID (Laszewski et al, 1990). Therefore, it is to be expected that malignant lymphomas of the GI tract in patients with immunodeficiencies often arise in a background of nodular hyperplasia of lymphocytes. The most common malignancies arising in the GI tract in CVID patients are B and T cell lymphomas of the small bowel. Most of them are of B cell origin and are diffuse large-cell or mixed small- and large-cell lymphomas.

Patients with CVID may develop chronic inflammatory processes of the small or large bowel that are clinically similar to chronic inflammatory bowel disease. In some cases, the small bowel is the main site of involvement and the lesions resemble Crohn disease, with transmural inflammation and small bowel obstruction. Rarely, granulomatous inflammation may involve the GI tract and other organs in CVID (Hermaszewski & Webster, 1993; Mike et al, 1991).

The morphologic features of colitis in CVID patients are variable and in some patients clinically mimic ulcerative colitis. Mucosal architectural distortion with crypt destruction is present but is generally milder than in most cases of ulcerative colitis. Neutrophils may be present in the lamina propria and crypt epithelium. In some cases, the crypt destruction and mucosal distortion are accompanied by increased apoptosis, lesions similar to those of colonic graft-versus-host disease (GVHD) (Washington et al, 1996). Milder cases of colitis in

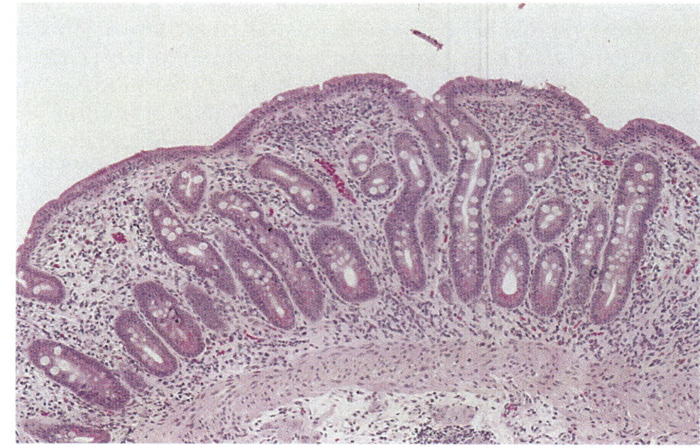

Figure 19–1

Common variable immunodeficiency, small intestine. Villous atrophy reminiscent of celiac disease is present.

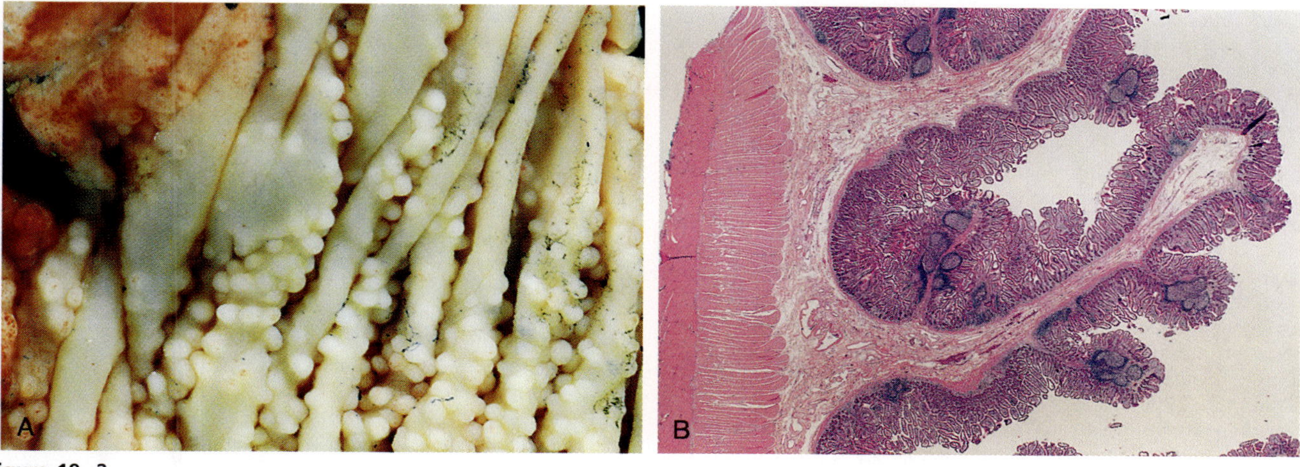

Figure 19–2

Common variable immunodeficiency, nodular lymphoid hyperplasia, small intestine. *A,* Low magnification shows numerous submucosal nodules. *B,* The lymphocytic nodules are present in the lamina propria and may involve the submucosa.

these patients resemble lymphocytic colitis, in which there are increased numbers of intraepithelial lymphocytes and minimal mucosal distortion (Teahon et al, 1994). The cause and pathogenesis of colitis in these patients remain largely unknown, but the association of chronic GI inflammatory disorders and autoimmune disorders in these patients, producing lesions that resemble those in other disorders of immune dysregulation, suggests that the colitis of CVID may be autoimmune in origin.

X-Linked Agammaglobulinemia

Patients with X-linked agammaglobulinemia (XLA) have fewer chronic GI problems than do patients with CVID. The onset of GI symptoms is earlier than in CVID patients, but autoimmune diseases are less common. Small intestinal and colonic mucosal biopsies in the XLA patient without GI symptoms reveal normal architecture and no villous blunting. However, there are no plasma cells. Approximately one third of patients present with GI symptoms, usually diarrhea or perirectal abscess (Lederman & Winkelstein, 1985). Up to 10% may have chronic GI symptoms secondary to bacterial overgrowth or infection with *Giardia lamblia*, *Salmonella*, and enteropathic *Escherichia coli*. Chronic diarrhea is unexplained in half the patients (Lederman & Winkelstein, 1985). In addition to GI infections, patients with XLA may develop a chronic, ulcerating, inflammatory condition clinically similar to Crohn disease that is manifested by recurrent diarrhea, malabsorption, ulcers, and small bowel strictures. A prominent lymphocytic infiltrate without plasma cells or granulomas is seen in affected mucosa (Abramowsky & Sorensen, 1988; Washington et al, 1996). Patients with XLA are at increased risk for malignancy, even in childhood. The most common malignancies are B and T cell lymphomas, often involving the GI tract. Many of these cases occur in children under the age of 10 years (Lavillia et al, 1993). There are rare cases of gastric adenocarcinoma (Lavillia et al, 1993) and colorectal adenocarcinoma (van der Meer et al, 1993) in young adults with XLA.

IgA Deficiency

Patients with IgA deficiency may have celiac disease, and their condition may improve on a gluten-free diet. Chronic giardiasis may occur. IgA deficiency is also associated with increased risk of gastric adenocarcinoma and intestinal lymphoma (Filipovich et al, 1994).

Severe Combined Immunodeficiency

Children with deficiencies of both T and B cell function may develop profound diarrhea early in life. GI biopsies reveal a hypocellular lamina propria without plasma cells. Since these patients are susceptible to viral infections, examination of stool for viral particles may be indicated. Rotavirus, normally a self-limited infection, in particular causes chronic diarrhea in children with severe combined immunodeficiency (SCID). Villous blunting occurs in acute rotavirus infection in normal children (Davidson & Barnes, 1979) and in animal models (Salim et al, 1995), but the GI pathologic features of chronic rotavirus infection in SCID patients have not been described. Other viral infectious agents identifiable on GI biopsy are cytomegalovirus (CMV) and adenovirus. *Salmonella* may also cause chronic GI infection in SCID patients. SCID patients receiving nonirradiated blood products or allogeneic marrow transplants are susceptible to GVHD, but patients who have not received these treatments may also develop a similar-appearing process in the colon and small intestine (Snover et al, 1985; Lee et al, 1991). Children with SCID apparently have a higher incidence of reflux esophagitis, for reasons unknown. (Boeck, Buckley, & Schiff, 1997).

Chronic Granulomatous Disease

GI manifestations are rare in chronic granulomatous disease (CGD) but may be broadly grouped into obstructive and inflammatory categories. Obstruction may occur from esophageal or small bowel lesions in CGD. In some cases obstruction is due to aggregates of pigment-laden macrophages, the histologic hallmark of CGD, or to granulomatous inflammation. In others, obstruction is attributed to a functional disturbance in GI motility, although deep infiltrates by macrophages often cannot be excluded. A few CGD patients have esophageal obstruction. Biopsies of the esophageal mucosa generally reveal only reflux esophagitis or scattered pigmented macrophages. Pyloric obstruction is more common and may be the first manifestation of CGD. Granulomas, giant cells, and pigment-laden macrophages are frequently present in gastric biopsy specimens, but only "nonspecific" inflammation is seen in some cases. Small bowel obstruction is rare in CGD but occasionally results from an inflammatory process.

Inflammatory lesions affecting the small and large bowel in CGD patients may mimic inflammatory bowel disease (Sloan et al, 1996). The small bowel in CGD may be involved by fistulas, stenosis, and nonnecrotizing granulomatous inflammation that is mistaken for Crohn disease. However, granulomas are not present in all cases. One CGD patient had an acute and chronic inflammatory infiltrate confined to the colonic mucosa. Crypt abscesses and lack of granulomas were more suggestive of ulcerative colitis than Crohn disease. However, mucosal architectural distortion and ulceration were not as prominent as usually seen in ulcerative colitis, and pigmented macrophages were present in the lamina propria (Sloan et al, 1996).

Even asymptomatic CGD patients have infiltration of the intestinal mucosa by pigmented macrophages. In a group of CGD patients with GI dysfunction, small bowel biopsy specimens from seven of eight patients revealed macrophages with yellow-brown pigment in the lamina propria. Eight patients had a similar infiltrate in rectal mucosa (Ament & Ochs, 1973). The pigmented macrophages were generally found in the lamina propria adjacent to crypts but were occasionally present high in the villus. The results of small bowel biopsies were negative, but rectal biopsy specimens revealed granulomas with giant cells in five of eight patients.

Autoimmune and Allergic Disorders

Allergic processes, particularly cow's milk–sensitive enteropathy and allergic proctocolitis, cause distinctive clinical syndromes likely to occasion GI biopsies in infants and children.

Cow's Milk–Sensitive Enteropathy

Occurring in early infancy, cow's milk–sensitive enteropathy is characterized by diarrhea leading to malabsorption and failure to thrive. Small intestinal biopsy shows villous atrophy with a mild degree of crypt hyperplasia, increased lamina propria chronic inflammation, and increased numbers of intraepithelial lymphocytes. Increased numbers of eosinophils are found in the crypts and surface epithelium but not in the lamina propria. Mucosal lesions are patchy and milder than in celiac disease. The mucosa is also thinner, since there is less crypt hyperplasia (Maluenda et al, 1984). The diagnosis may be made if mucosal abnormalities resolve with withdrawal of cow's milk and recur with rechallenge (Salazar de Sousa et al, 1986).

Allergic Proctocolitis

A disease of infants, allergic proctocolitis is clinically characterized by rectal bleeding that usually begins in the first 2 months of life (Machida et al, 1994). Prevalence is estimated at up to 7.5% of otherwise normal infants (Odze et al, 1995). Immune-mediated reactions to foreign proteins, most commonly cow's milk, are presumably causal, although the condition may also occur in breast-fed infants, probably due to maternal ingestion of milk or other allergens.

The lesions in allergic colitis are more common in the rectosigmoid but may involve any part of the colon. The mucosa appears friable and erythematous on endoscopic examination. Erosions may be seen, although ulcers are rare. Microscopically, the mucosal architecture is normal, with no features of chronicity, such as crypt loss or branching crypts. The most characteristic feature of allergic proctocolitis is the presence of large numbers of eosinophils (>60/10 high power fields) in the lamina propria. Eosinophils may also infiltrate crypt or surface epithelium or the muscularis mucosae. Eosinophilic infiltrate may be so patchy that examination of multiple sections is necessary for detection (Odze et al, 1995). Crypt abscesses occur in severe cases and typically contain eosinophils intermixed with neutrophils.

Celiac Disease

Celiac disease, also known as gluten-sensitive enteropathy and nontropical sprue, is an immune-mediated injury of the small bowel mucosa due to gliadin, the alcohol-soluble fraction of wheat gluten. Celiac disease is diagnosed by demonstrating the characteristic atrophy of the villi of the upper small intestine and restoration of normal mucosal architecture by a gluten-free diet. Mucosal abnormalities recur upon dietary challenge with gluten.

Clinical features vary but commonly include symptoms of malabsorption, such as diarrhea, weight loss, and flatulence. Impaired iron absorption from the proximal small intestine or occult GI bleeding (Fine, 1996) may lead to iron deficiency anemia. Growth retardation is commonly seen in children with untreated celiac disease and may be the only symptom. The incidence of autoimmune disorders, such as diabetes mellitus, thyroid disease, and inflammatory bowel disease, is increased in patients with celiac disease. Children with celiac disease in the past had high mortality rates, but with gluten-free diets their survival approaches that of the general pediatric population. Adults with celiac disease have an approximately two-fold increase in mortality rate, related to increased incidence of malignancy, infection, and problems associated with malabsorption (Holmes, 1996). Adult patients are at increased risk for malignancy, most commonly enteropathy-associated T cell lymphomas in the small bowel (Ferguson & Kingstone, 1996). A T cell–rich B cell lymphoma has been reported in a child (Stenhammar & Masreliez, 1993). Adults also have an increased risk of esophageal carcinoma, pharyngeal carcinoma, and adenocarcinoma of the small intestine (Ferguson & Kingstone, 1996).

Histopathologic Features. The proximal jejunum is affected more than other portions of the small intestine. Most descriptions of the histologic features of celiac disease are based on jejunal biopsy specimens, but the diagnosis is now usually made on the basis of duodenal biopsies. Accurate interpretation of villous changes in small endoscopic biopsies requires optimal sample orientation.

In general, the finding of four adjacent normal small intestinal villi rules out villous atrophy. In celiac disease villi are atrophic to a variable extent from enterocyte damage. However, increased proliferation within the crypts keeps overall mucosal thickness normal. The net result is the characteristic but not specific "crypt hyperplasia, villous atrophy pattern" seen in celiac disease (Fig. 19–3). Increased mitotic activity is present in the crypt zone. Enterocytes on the luminal surface are damaged, and villous tips are shorter than normal. Goblet cells are decreased in number. One of the key histopathologic features of celiac disease is a lymphocytosis in the surface epithelium. In the normal small intestine, approximately 20 intraepithelial lymphocytes are found per 100 enterocytes (Dobbins, 1986). In celiac disease as many as 50 to 60 lymphocytes per 100 enterocytes have been reported (Leonard et al, 1997). They are mostly CD8+ cells. The lamina propria contains increased numbers of plasma cells and lymphocytes. Rarely, a small number of neutrophils is present (Leonard et al, 1997). Ulcers and superficial erosions are not typically a feature of celiac disease but have been reported in children (Eltumi et al, 1996). Gastric metaplasia in the duodenum occasionally is present focally in cases of celiac dis-

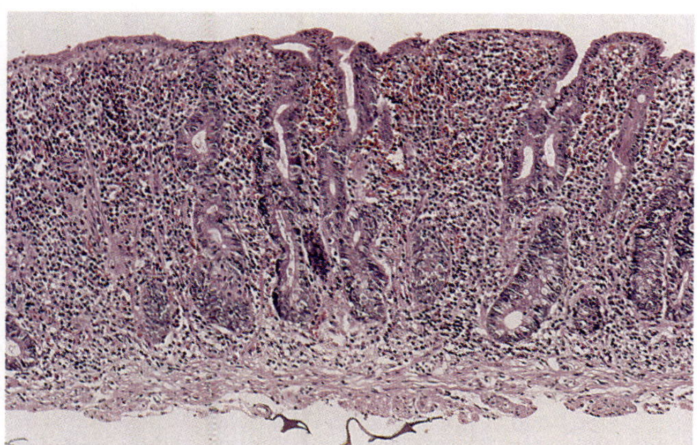

Figure 19–3

Celiac disease, small intestine. Marked villous atrophy with crypt hyperplasia is seen. The lamina propria contains a dense lymphocytic infiltrate. The superficial epithelium is flattened and contains numerous intraepithelial lymphocytes.

ease, although it is more often seen in peptic duodenitis (Leonard et al, 1997).

Serologic Studies. In establishing the diagnosis of celiac disease, serologic studies may be helpful. Antigliadin antibodies, both IgA and IgG, are present in most patients with celiac disease. IgA antibodies are more specific than are IgG antibodies but are relatively insensitive. Antiendomysial antibodies, especially IgA, are the most reliable for diagnostic purposes and are generally highly specific (98%) as well as sensitive (97%). IgA endomysial antibody titers correlate well with histologic abnormalities in the small bowel (Lerner et al, 1994). Serologic studies are useful for screening. However, patients with positive serologic test results should have confirmatory small bowel biopsies prior to institution of life-long dietary restrictions.

Diagnostic Criteria for Celiac Disease. Correlation of histologic features, clinical features, serologic study results, and response to a gluten-free diet is required to diagnose celiac disease. Morphologic changes in the small bowel that support the diagnosis of celiac disease are villous atrophy with crypt hyperplasia, numerous intraepithelial lymphocytes, and increased numbers of plasma cells or lymphocytes in the lamina propria.

Differential Diagnosis. Other causes of villous atrophy to be considered include patchy villous blunting from cow's milk intolerance, protein-calorie malnutrition, bacterial overgrowth, and various primary immunodeficiencies, such as common variable immunodeficiency and IgA deficiency. The mucosal changes associated with intolerance to cow's milk protein are less severe than those in celiac disease. The mucosa is relatively thin because the crypt hyperplasia is less extensive, villous atrophy is patchy and less pronounced, and intraepithelial lymphocytes, albeit increased in number, are not as numerous as in celiac disease (Stern et al, 1982). An increase in the numbers of intraepithelial eosinophils but not lamina propria eosinophils is noted upon challenge with cow's milk protein (Maluenda et al, 1984). Bacterial overgrowth rarely causes the degree of villous atrophy seen in celiac disease, and numbers of intraepithelial lymphocytes are increased only slightly. Malnutrition is associated with villous atrophy but does not cause crypt hyperplasia or increased intraepithelial lymphocytes. GI pathologic features of common variable immunodeficiency and IgA deficiency were discussed earlier.

Pathogenesis and Biologic Characteristics. The pathogenesis of celiac disease is complex. Genetic, environmental, and immunologic factors all play a role. Since 90% of patients with celiac disease have a specific HLA-DQ a/b heterodimer, there is compelling evidence for a genetic basis (Scott et al, 1997). The initiating event has not been identified, and the mechanisms for immune-mediated injury triggered by gluten exposure have not been fully elucidated. However, in a genetically predisposed individual, exposure to gluten may activate CD4+ T cells in the lamina propria of the small intestine. Cytokines released by these activated CD4+ cells damage small intestinal epithelial cells, activate macrophages, and promote antibody production by activated B cells.

Autoimmune Enteropathy

The term *autoimmune enteropathy* has been applied to cases of intractable diarrhea in which there are circulating autoantibodies directed against small intestinal epithelial cells. The disorder is relatively rare and is reported almost exclusively in children under 2 years of age (Hill et al, 1991). Diarrhea is so severe that most patients are dependent on total parenteral nutrition. Many patients with autoimmune enteropathy have other autoimmune diseases, such as diabetes mellitus, juvenile rheumatoid arthritis, and hypothyroidism (Mirakian et al, 1986). Subtotal or partial villous atrophy is seen in small bowel biopsy specimens, with lymphocytosis in the lamina propria in most cases. The histologic features in some cases of autoimmune enteropathy are indistinguishable from those in celiac disease, but in other cases the villous atrophy is less severe, and there are fewer intraepithelial lymphocytes than typically seen in celiac disease. Mild to severe colitis has also been reported in children with autoimmune enteropathy (Hill et al, 1991).

Gastrointestinal Infections

This discussion focuses on infectious agents likely in children with primary immunodeficiencies and on bacterial infections involving lymphatic tissue of the GI tract. GI changes in HIV infections are discussed with infections disorders of the liver later in this chapter.

Giardiasis

Infection by *Giardia intestinalis*, often called *Giardia lamblia* when isolated from humans, is the most common GI protozoal disease, with a prevalence of 2–7% in industrialized countries and up to 40% in tropical countries (Oberhuber et al, 1997). Infection is particularly common in children, with infection rates up to 90% in children in day care centers (Craft, 1982). Giardiasis is self-limiting in most patients, but chronic infection may occur in patients with immunodeficiencies, primarily agammaglobulinemia or CVID. Chronic infection with *Giardia* is not a major clinical problem in AIDS patients (Farthing, 1996).

Giardia exists as a motile trophozoite (the form identified in GI biopsy specimens) and in a nonmotile cyst form responsible for the transmission of infection (Farthing, 1996). Trophozoites are pear-shaped and have two central nuclei and a longitudinal cytoplasmic structure called the median body. They attach to GI mucosa by their ventral disc and possibly by a lectin-mediated mechanism. *Giardia* is not tissue invasive. Organisms are typically found near the apical

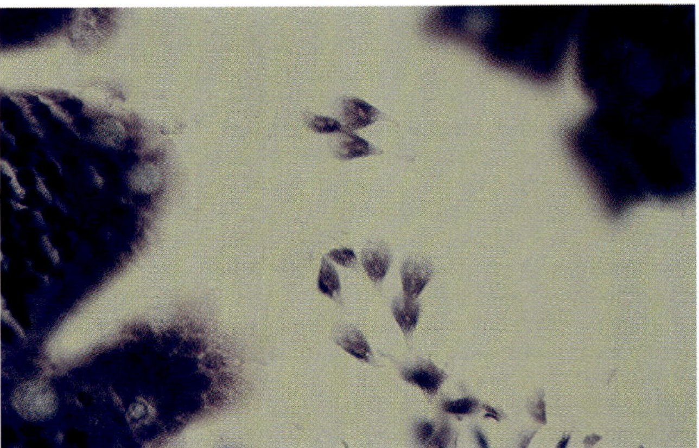

Figure 19–4

Giardiasis, small intestine. Organisms are usually found near the surface epithelium and may be numerous in patients with common variable immunodeficiency. This oil immersion photomicrograph shows the typical morphologic features of *Giardia*.

surface of enterocytes (Fig. 19–4), although they are occasionally found in lumens of the small intestinal crypts. The organism is most often identified in duodenal or jejunal biopsy specimens and occasionally in gastric antral and ileal mucosal biopsies but is not found in the gastric body. Duodenal mucosal architecture is generally normal in *Giardia* infection. Less than 5% of cases have mild villous shortening with crypt hyperplasia, moderate intraepithelial lymphocytosis, and increased mixed inflammatory infiltrate in the lamina propria (Oberhuber et al, 1997). Ultrastructural changes include shortening and disruption of intestinal microvilli, perhaps accounting for the diarrhea and malabsorption. Nodular lymphocytic hyperplasia of the small bowel may be associated with chronic giardiasis and with immunodeficiency (Farthing, 1996).

Typhoid Fever

Salmonella infections of the GI tract may produce mild ileitis with enlarged Peyer patches and acute self-limited colitis. Typhoid fever is due to infection with *Salmonella typhi* or, less commonly, *Salmonella paratyphi*. The former produces more severe symptoms and morphologic changes in the GI tract. *Salmonella* enters the small bowel through Peyer patches and disseminates systemically. After approximately 2 weeks, the organisms are released from mononuclear phagocyte cells (Kupffer cells) and are excreted via bile into the small intestine, where they recolonize Peyer patches. At this point Peyer patches become hyperplastic. The mucosa sloughs, producing the characteristic oval ulcers of typhoid. These ulcers may extend deep into the submucosa or muscularis propria and commonly perforate. Rarely, GI hemorrhage occurs (Reyes et al, 1986). Microscopically, neutrophils are rare, but numerous macrophages ("typhoid cells") containing red cells, cellular debris, and bacteria are present (Rowland, 1974).

Yersinia Infections

Yersinia infections of the GI tract produce acute enteritis and ileitis with diarrhea as well as mesenteric adenitis and appendiceal involvement mimicking acute appendicitis (Fig. 19–5). *Yersinia enterocolitica* produces multiple effects on GI mucosa. *Yersinia* gains entry by invasion of Peyer patches via M cells, with subsequent recruitment of neutrophils and destruction of follicle-associated epithelium. After day 5 in experimental models, abscesses are found in mesenteric lymph nodes (Autenrieth & Firsching, 1996). Goblet cell hyperplasia is most pronounced in the ileocecal region, where mucosal injury is most severe (Mantle et al, 1991), and brush border injury also occurs (Buret et al, 1990). Elongated ulcers overlying Peyer patches, with smaller punctate apthous ulcers and thickening of the distal ileal wall, are reported in resection specimens mistaken at surgery for Crohn disease (Gleason & Patterson, 1982). Enteric infection with *Yersinia pseudotuberculosis* mimics acute appendicitis. Mesenteric lymphadenitis, usually without appendiceal involvement, is found at surgery. Granulomas with microabscesses and central necrosis in a pattern similar to

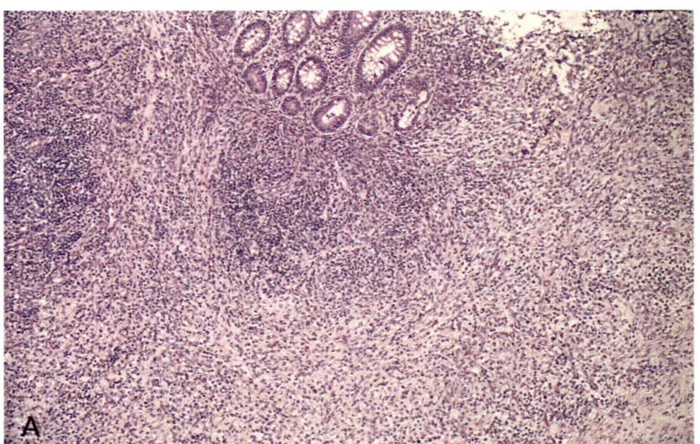

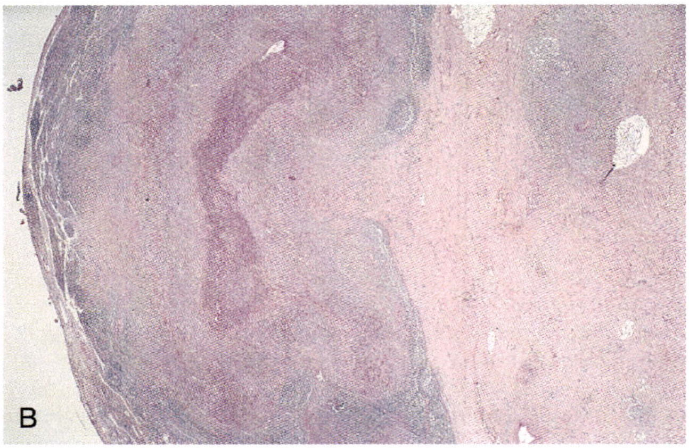

Figure 19–5

Yersinia infection. *A,* The appendix contains a dense inflammatory infiltrate with a focal mucosal erosion. *B,* A periappendiceal lymph node shows central necrosis similar to that seen in cat-scratch disease.

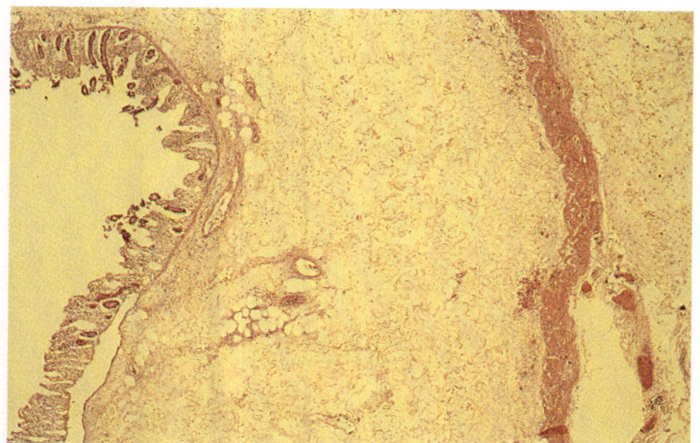

Figure 19–6

Neutropenic enterocolitis, cecum. No significant inflammatory infiltrate is present. Submucosal edema is prominent.

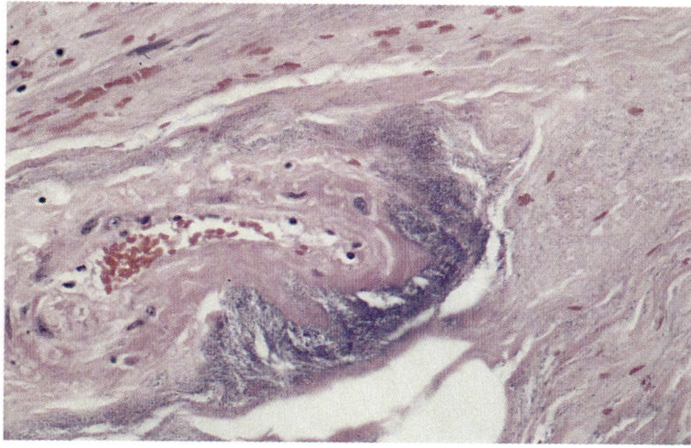

Figure 19–7

Neutropenic enterocolitis. Vessels are often surrounded by swarms of bacteria, which are *Pseudomonas* species.

cat-scratch disease are found in lymph nodes (Fig. 19–6) (El-Maraghi & Mair, 1979).

IATROGENIC DISORDERS

Neutropenic Enterocolitis (Typhlitis)

Hemorrhagic necrosis of the cecum has been termed typhlitis. Neutropenic enterocolitis applies when other areas of the GI tract such, as appendix, terminal ileum, or ascending colon, are involved. This disorder is usually seen in patients with absolute neutrophil counts $<1500/mm^3$. Most patients have acute leukemia and have received chemotherapy in the previous 30 days (Katz et al, 1990). However, typhlitis is seen in patients with other hematologic malignancies, patients with aplastic anemia, and renal transplant patients. Patients may present clinically with acute appendicitis, fever, and right lower quadrant pain. One third have GI hemorrhage (Katz et al, 1990), and, rarely, a right lower quadrant mass is palpated. The cecum and other affected portions of the GI tract are dilated, edematous, and congested or hemorrhagic. Pneumatosis intestinalis is rare. The mucosa is hemorrhagic and covered with granular necrotic material. There is no significant inflammation, but swarms of bacteria are present (Fig. 19–7).

The initiating factor in the pathogenesis of typhlitis is mucosal injury, chiefly related to recent administration of chemotherapeutic agents. The complicating neutropenia facilitates bacterial invasion of the injured mucosa, with *Clostridium* and *Pseudomonas* species the major offenders. Fungi, such as *Candida* species, may also cause or contribute to typhlitis. Microbial toxin–induced edema necrosis and distention of the bowel wall lead to decreased blood flow, adding an element of ischemic injury. Most patients become septicemic. The prognosis is grave in untreated typhlitis. Patients may survive with optimal medical and surgical management if adequate neutrophil counts return.

Graft-versus-Host Disease

Skin, liver, and GI tract are commonly involved in acute GVHD after allogeneic marrow transplantation. Symptoms indicative of GI involvement include profuse diarrhea, crampy abdominal pain, GI hemorrhage, anorexia, nausea, and vomiting. Involvement of the upper GI tract is slightly commoner than involvement of the large bowel, although simultaneous involvement is common (Roy et al, 1991). The major features of GVHD in the GI tract are epithelial apoptosis and a sparse mononuclear inflammatory infiltrate (Fig. 19–8). Apoptotic epithelial cells are found principally in the actively regenerating compartments, such as the crypts in the colon and small intestine and the neck area of gastric glands. The apoptotic cells in the colon are particularly conspicuous. They are termed exploding crypt cells (Fig. 19–9) and contain cytoplasmic vacuoles filled with karyorrhectic nuclear debris (Sale et al, 1979). Apoptotic cells are smaller and less conspicuous in the gastric mucosa. In severe cases of acute GVHD, crypt abscesses, with destruction and loss of crypts, are seen. In the most severe cases, mucosal sloughing and extensive ulceration occur. In the stomach, granular, eosinophilic, necrotic cellular debris without neutrophils may be present in the lumens of injured glands (Washington et al, 1997). Villous blunting is commonly seen in small bowel GVHD. A grading system for acute GVHD affecting the colon has been proposed (Table 19–2) (Sale et al, 1979), but such grading has poor correlation with clinical symptoms and patient outcome.

The GI tract is less often involved in chronic GVHD, which occurs >100 days after transplantation. The esophagus is more commonly affected than other portions of the GI tract. Findings include submucosal and lamina propria fibrosis, with minimal mucosal changes (Shulman et al, 1980).

Acute GVHD in the liver is diagnosed by demonstrating interlobular bile duct injury (Fig. 19–10). Changes may be patchy in mild hepatic GVHD, but affected bile ducts have reactive changes in bile duct epithelial cells, such as nuclear enlargement, pleomorphism, cytoplasmic vacuolization, and irregular distribution of epithelial cell nuclei. These changes are presumably secondary to biliary epithelial necrosis. Segmental necrosis of bile ducts may be seen in severe cases of acute hepatic GVHD, such as those associated with transfusion in immunodeficiency children (Washington et al, 1993). The portal lymphocytic infiltrate is usually sparse. Intraepithelial lymphocytes may be present. Spotty hepatocyte necrosis may be seen early in the course of GVHD. In prolonged cases, cholestasis and ballooning degeneration of hepatocytes may be prominent.

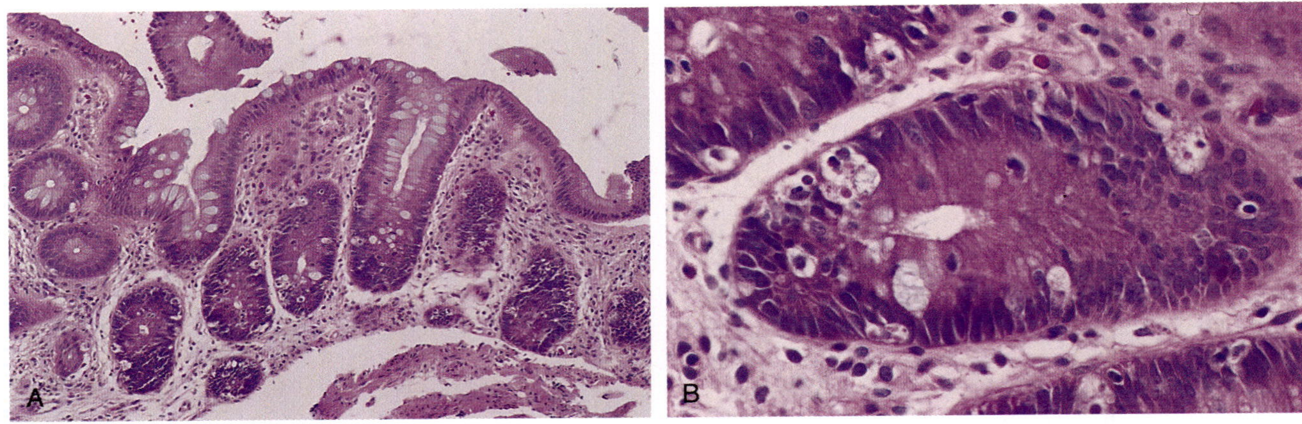

Figure 19–8

Acute graft-versus-host disease, colon. *A,* A sparse inflammatory infiltrate is present. No crypt destruction is seen in this field. *B,* Numerous apoptotic bodies are present in crypt epithelial cells ("exploding crypt cells").

Chronic hepatic GVHD develops after day 100, as mentioned earlier. Bile duct changes are similar to those seen in acute GVHD except that loss of bile ducts is more common, and the interlobular bile ducts often appear angular and distorted. Portal tracts usually show increased fibrosis, and bile ductular proliferation may be seen. The portal lymphocytic infiltrate is variable, and lobular changes are generally mild.

Differential Diagnosis of Graft-versus-Host Disease

The changes occurring in the GI tract in acute GVHD are not specific. Similar changes are reported in colonic biopsies from patients with severe T cell deficiencies (Snover et al, 1985) and CVID (Washington et al, 1996). The effects of cytoreductive therapy after marrow transplantation resemble the changes of GVHD of the GI tract in the early posttransplant period. Thus, a diagnosis of GVHD must be made with caution prior to 21 days after transplantation. CMV infection may produce mucosal damage with apoptotic epithelial cells, mimicking GVHD (Snover, 1985). Since GVHD and CMV infection may occur concurrently, it may be difficult to distinguish the effects of each process on the GI tract. The differential diagnosis of acute hepatic GVHD includes nonspecific hepatitis if the biopsy is performed early in GVHD, before the bile duct injury is well developed (Shulman et al, 1988). The bile duct lesions are not specific for GVHD. Bile duct injury may be seen in many conditions, including chronic hepatitis C infection, primary biliary cirrhosis, and drug reactions. Knowledge of the clinical setting is helpful in eliminating many of these possibilities, and the finding of bile duct injury out of proportion to the degree of portal inflammation is considered diagnostic of GVHD (Snover et al, 1984).

The distinction of chronic hepatic GVHD from chronic hepatitis may be difficult; however, distortion and loss of bile ducts with relatively sparse inflammatory infiltrate favors the former. The relatively stringent criterion of loss of bile ducts in over half of portal triads has been required for diagnosis of chronic GVHD in problematic cases (Shulman et al., 1988).

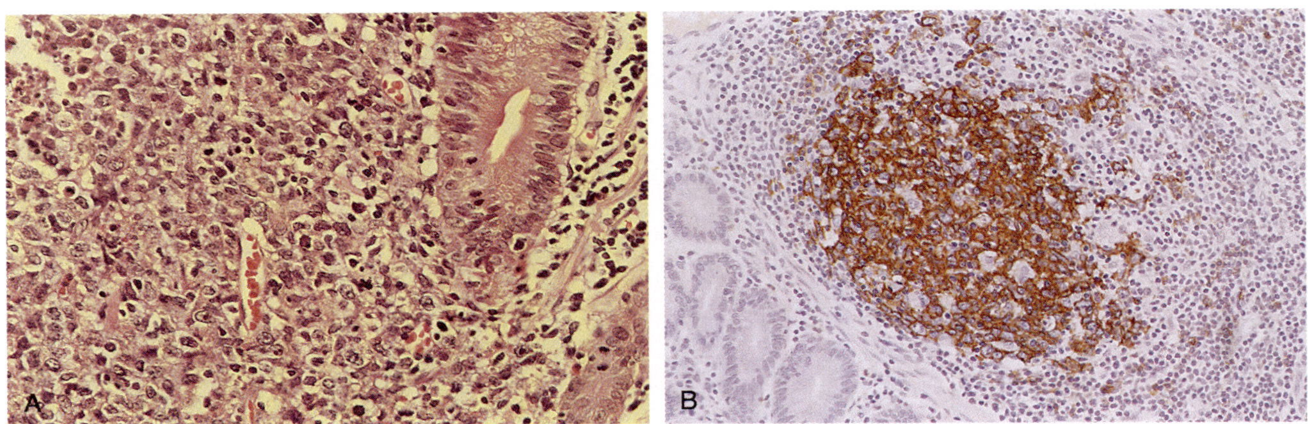

Figure 19–9

Diffuse large-cell lymphoma, small intestine. *A,* This patient had common variable immunodeficiency. A diffuse growth of large cells is apparent. *B,* Many of these lymphomas are B cell in type, as shown by this immunoperoxidase preparation using antibodies to CD20.

Table 19–2
Grading of Acute Graft-versus-Host Disease of the Colon

Grade	Histologic Features
I	Rare apoptotic cells, without crypt loss
II	Loss of individual crypts
III	Loss of two or more contiguous crypts
IV	No identifiable crypts (mucosal ulceration)

Source: Sale GE, McDonald GB, Shulman HM, et al: Gastrointestinal graft-versus-host disease in man. Am J Surg Pathol 3:219–229, 1979.

Short Bowel Syndrome

Partial small bowel resection is followed by mucosal changes in the remaining small bowel. The villi become elongated and increased microvillous height is seen on ultrastructural examination; these hyperplastic responses serve to increase the absorptive surface area in the remaining bowel (Whang et al., 1996). Anemia is one of the many complications of short bowel syndrome; if the entire duodenum is resected or bypassed, anemia may occur due to decreased absorption of iron or folate. Macrocytic anemia secondary to inadequate absorption of vitamin B12 often follows total total ileal resection. B12 deficiency may also complicate use of the lower GI tract as a urinary tract substitute, but anemia appears to be rare in this setting (Steiner and Morton, 1991).

NEOPLASTIC DISORDERS OF THE GASTROINTESTINAL TRACT

Leukemia

Leukemic infiltration of the GI tract was formerly a common finding at autopsy but has become less prevalent, probably as a result of more effective treatment. Early studies reported GI involvement in over 50% of autopsy cases, with 25% having grossly evident lesions (Prolla & Kirsner, 1964), but later studies report an incidence of only 4–12% (Barcos et al, 1987). Leukemic infiltration is rarely observed in surgical pathology specimens. GI involvement is usually seen in the setting of widespread involvement of other organ systems, but isolated gastroduodenal recurrence has been reported with acute lymphoblastic leukemia (Weisdorf et al, 1989), which is slightly more likely to involve the GI tract than is acute or chronic myelogenous leukemia. The lesions in leukemia include flat hemorrhagic areas, diffuse polypoid lesions, mucosal plaques, and ulcers. The esophagus is involved in roughly 27% of autopsied cases of leukemia and lymphoma (Givler, 1970), but clinically apparent involvement of this organ is rare (Agha & Schnitzer, 1985). Leukemic infiltrates in the stomach may cause diffuse thickening of the rugal folds or multiple white plaques (Kothur et al, 1990). Extramedullary myelogenous leukemia has been described in the stomach, where lesions may ulcerate and bleed. Leukemic infiltration is commoner in the distal small intestine, whereas colonic involvement may result in flat hemorrhagic lesions or multiple polypoid excrescences (Kothur et al, 1990). Microscopic examination reveals erosion and destruction of crypt epithelium by the leukemic infiltrate. The most common serious complication of GI involvement is hemorrhage. Rarely, patients present with typhlitis as an initial manifestation of acute leukemia (Kaste et al, 1997). See "Neutropenic Enterocolitis," earlier in this chapter, for a discussion of typhlitis following neutropenia.

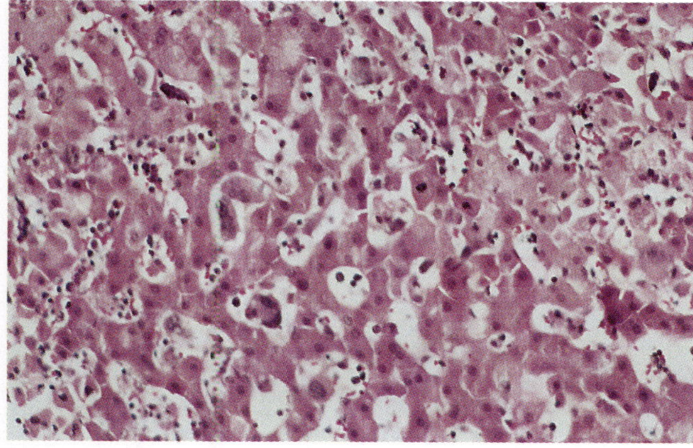

Figure 19–10

Extramedullary hematopoiesis, liver. Megakaryocytes and rare erythrocyte precursors are seen.

Malignant Lymphoma

The commonest site of extranodal lymphomas is the GI tract. Lymphoma is the most common GI malignancy in children. GI lymphomas are more common in boys than in girls (Berry & Keeling, 1970), with a mean age of approximately 9 years (Takahashi & Hansmann, 1990). In children without known immunodeficiencies, the commonest site of involvement is the region of the ileocecal valve (Berry & Keeling, 1970; Takahashi & Hansmann, 1990), where the lymphomas arise in Peyer patches. Other sites of origin are, in order of decreasing frequency, the small intestine, large intestine, and stomach (Takahashi & Hansmann, 1990). Most GI lymphomas in children, as in adults, are B cell malignancies that are usually classified as small transformed (noncleaved) cell lymphomas of the Burkitt (the commoner) or non-Burkitt type. Other, rarely reported histologic types include centroblastic lymphoma and immunoblastic lymphoma (Takahashi & Hansmann, 1990). Natural killer–like T cell lymphoma in the small intestine has been reported in a 6-year-old child without clinical or histologic evidence of enteropathy (Weiss et al, 1997). Peripheral T cell lymphomas arising in the intestine are generally associated with celiac disease and are extremely rare in children. Prognosis for GI lymphomas in children is related to stage at diagnosis and may be related to primary site, with lymphomas arising in the large intestine and ileocecal region having a better prognosis than those arising in the small intestine (Takahashi & Hansmann, 1990). Most patients have regional lymph node involvement at the time of diagnosis and many have widespread disease.

Malignant lymphomas may arise throughout the small or large intestine in immunodeficient patients, with no apparent preference for the ileocecal region. EBV is a major cofactor in most B cell lymphoproliferative disorders in children with immunodeficiency (Filipovich et al, 1994). B and T cell lymphomas arise at very young ages in children with SCID (median age 1.6 years) but are seen in older patients (median age 23 years) with CVID (Filipovich et al, 1994). The median age for 240 patients with lymphoma in all categories of immunodeficiency was approximately 7 years (Filipovich et al, 1994). The GI tract was the primary site in 8.8% of the 240 patients

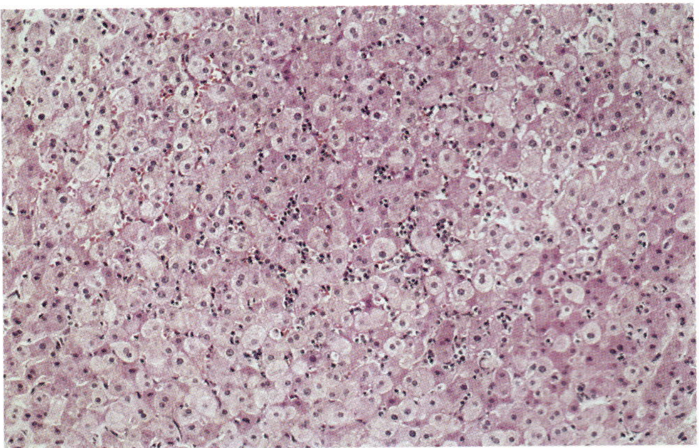

Figure 19–11

Epstein-Barr virus hepatitis. A diffuse lymphocytic sinusoidal infiltrate is characteristically seen.

(Filipovich et al, 1994). Most of the extranodal lymphomas arising in immunodeficient patients, including those arising in children, are classified as diffuse large-cell or diffuse mixed small- and large-cell lymphomas (Fig. 19–11) (Cunningham-Rundles et al, 1991). Posttransplant lymphoproliferative disorder, malignant histiocytosis, and mastocytosis may involve either the GI tract or the liver and are discussed later in this chapter.

NORMAL STRUCTURE AND FUNCTION OF THE LIVER

The liver as the single largest organ constitutes one fiftieth of adult body weight and one twentieth of newborn body weight. The larger relative size in neonates is due to the fetal blood-forming activity of the liver. Hepatocytes are arranged in plates two cells thick until 5 to 6 years of age and one cell thick thereafter. Hepatocytes contain abundant glycogen, and numerous glycogenated nuclei are normally present in children as well. The hepatic parenchymal cords are separated by the sinusoids, lined by Kupffer cells and endothelial cells. Kupffer cells, members of the monocyte-macrophage family, are most prominent near the portal tracts. They contain numerous lysosomes and phagosomes and respond to various insults by enlargement and proliferation. Perisinusoidal cells, such as hepatic stellate cells (also termed Ito or interstitial fat storage cells) and pit cells, lie in the space of Disse, between the endothelium and hepatocytes. The hepatic stellate cells store fat and vitamin A and produce collagen. Pit cells, which have been characterized only ultrastructurally, may correspond to large granular lymphocytes in other areas of the body.

In addition to bile ducts, hepatic artery branches, and portal vein branches, portal triads normally contain scattered lymphocytes, mast cells, and histiocytes. The number of these cells considered normal increases with age. Portal fibrous tissue is also more prominent in adults than in children (Gerber & Thung, 1987).

Extramedullary Hematopoiesis

Hematopoiesis is a normal feature of human embryonic and fetal liver beginning at about 6 weeks of gestational age. The liver is the major site of hematopoiesis from the twelfth week until the fifth month of gestation, when the marrow becomes active. Hematopoiesis normally ceases by 5–6 weeks postpartum and is considered abnormal thereafter. Hepatic hematopoiesis is largely erythropoietic, although granulocytes, monocytes, and megakaryocytes may also be seen (see Fig. 19–10). Erythrocyte precursors are usually located within the hepatic lobule, while leukocyte precursors are often at the edges of the portal triads. Extramedullary hematopoiesis is found in numerous illnesses, most commonly neonatal hepatitis and anemia of any cause (McSween, 1994), and is seen infrequently in neonatal lupus erythematosus (Laxer, 1990). Extramedullary hepatic hematopoiesis is usually a diffuse, interstitial process but rarely may form tumorlike nodules mimicking neoplasms (Lemos et al, 1997).

NONNEOPLASTIC DISORDERS OF THE LIVER

Infectious Disorders

This discussion focuses on infections characteristically associated with underlying hematopoietic diseases, infections complicating inherited or acquired immunodeficiencies, or infections mimicking hematopoietic neoplasms.

Epstein-Barr Viral Hepatitis

The liver is affected in >90% of cases of EBV infectious mononucleosis. Hepatitis may be diagnosed by elevated aminotransferase levels (Kilpatrick, 1966), although jaundice is detected in a minority of patients. The typical histologic picture in the liver features a diffuse lymphocytic sinusoidal infiltrate (see Fig. 19–11) that occasionally contains transformed lymphocytes, suggesting a lymphoproliferative disorder (Lucas, 1994). Focal apoptotic hepatocytes and steatosis may be seen, but cholestasis is not characteristic (Kilpatrick, 1966; Lucas, 1994). Rarely, scattered noncaseating granulomas are found (Ishak, 1983). Progression to chronic hepatitis or cirrhosis rarely, if ever, occurs.

The spectrum of hepatic involvement by EBV in children ranges from inapparent to fulminant liver failure with disseminated intravascular coagulation and aplastic anemia (Lau et al, 1994; Lloyd-Still et al, 1986). Patients with X-linked lymphoproliferative syndrome are particularly susceptible to fulminant hepatic failure complicating EBV infection (Purtilo et al, 1977) and may have florid portal infiltrates of small lymphocytes, transformed lymphocytes, and plasma cells. (For additional details, see Chap. 3.) Failure has also been reported in patients with immunodeficiency diseases and in previously healthy children (Deutsch et al, 1986; Shaw & Evans, 1988). In these patients, hepatic failure due to EBV infection may not be accompanied by the typical features of infectious mononucleosis, such as pharyngitis and "atypical" lymphocytosis (Shaw & Evans, 1988).

EBV infection is a major determinant of course and outcome in solid organ transplant recipients. Children have more complications related to EBV infection because they are more likely to be EBV seronegative at the time of transplant. In one large pediatric series, 77% of children who were seronegative before liver transplant demonstrated serologic evidence of EBV infection after transplantion, whereas 48% of children who were seropositive had evidence of EBV reactivation later (Ho et al, 1988).

Infection-Associated Hemophagocytic Syndrome

The syndrome of benign histiocytic hyperplasia with marked hemophagocytosis is well documented in children and is usually accompanied by fever, hepatomegaly, splenomegaly, pe-

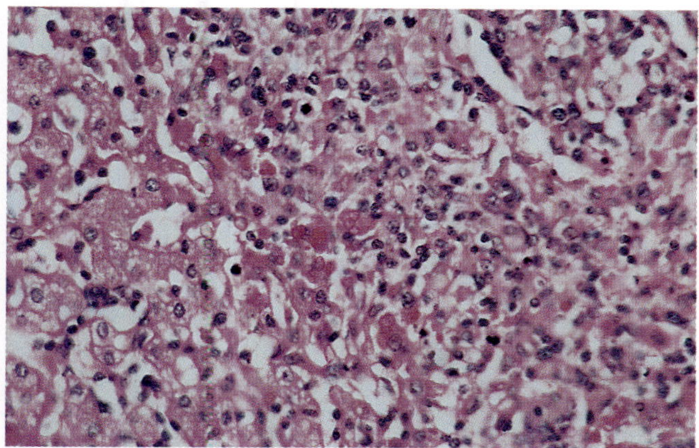

Figure 19–12

Infection-associated hemophagocytosis, liver. Cytologically benign histiocytes in the sinusoid contain numerous red blood cells.

ripheral blood cytopenias, and lymphadenopathy. Rash and pulmonary infiltrates may also be present. This clinical syndrome is strongly associated with infection, especially viral infection. EBV infection is most often implicated, although other viruses, including herpes, hepatitis B, hepatitis C, adenovirus, HIV, and CMV, have been described (Faurschou et al, 1999; Okano & Gross, 1996; Risdall et al, 1979). Infection-associated hemophagocytic syndrome is often seen in patients who have undergone organ transplants, have underlying lymphomas, or have other immunodeficiencies (Stephan & Galambrun, 2000). Most patients recover, but there are rare reports of fatal hemophagocytic syndrome associated with EBV infection in children with underlying immunodeficiencies (Okano & Gross 1996).

The histologic features within the liver typically include cytologically benign histiocytes displaying hemophagocytosis within the portal tracts and sinusoids of the liver (Fig. 19–12). Kupffer cells may be hypertrophic and also demonstrate hemophagocytosis and/or siderosis. Patchy hepatocyte necrosis may also be seen, as may perivenular hemorrhage and venous endothelial cell enlargment. Viral inclusions are seldom identified in tissue sections. There is no correlation between the degree of hepatic hemophagocytosis and the severity of peripheral cytopenia (Favara, 1996; Risdall et al, 1979; Tsui et al, 1992). The histologic features of infection-associated hemophagocytic syndrome and malignant histiocytosis may overlap, as discussed later. In general, the histiocytes in the former are bland in appearance, hemophagocytosis is much more prominent, and fibrosis is rare (Favara, 1996; Risdall et al, 1979).

Familial hemophagocytic syndrome has a clinical presentation and histopathologic features so similar to infection-associated hemophagocytic syndrome that the two syndromes may be very difficult to differentiate, although the familial disorder is almost uniformly fatal (Buckley et al, 1992). A family history and lack of an associated infection make the familial disorder more likely. Further, the histiocytes in the familial type have a characteristic immunophenotype of CD35, CD21, CD11b, CD36, CD25, and CD30 positivity.

Bacterial and Fungal Infections

Bacterial and fungal infections may cause abscesses and/or granulomas in the liver. Patients present with fever, malaise, and weight loss. In some cases, neoplasms are mimicked by the multiple liver lesions and associated abdominal lymphadenopathy. *Bartonella henselae*, the etiologic agent of cat-scratch disease, causes this clinical scenario in a minority of patients. Visceral cat-scratch disease usually affects children. Patients rarely have typical skin papules or superficial lymphadenopathy. They are generally immunocompetent, and the pathogeneis of visceral distribution has not been accounted for by host or microbial factors. The typical lesion consists of multiple granulomas with central stellate abscesses surrounded by three distinct zones: an inner layer of palisading histiocytes, an intermediate zone of lymphocytes, and an outer zone of fibrosis (Fig. 19–13) (Lamps et al, 1996). Both *B. henselae* and *B. quintana* may also be associated with hepatic epithelioid angiomatosis and bacillary peliosis hepatis, usually in immunocompromised hosts (Adal et al, 1996; Kemper et al, 1990). These lesions rarely occur in children.

Hepatic abscesses may be caused by numerous organisms including *Klebsiella, E. coli, Enterococcus* species, *Yersinia enterocolitica, Francisella tularensis, Actinomycetes*, mycobacterial species, and other agents (Greenstein et al, 1984; Lamps et al, 1996; Lucas, 1994). *Candida albicans* may cause large

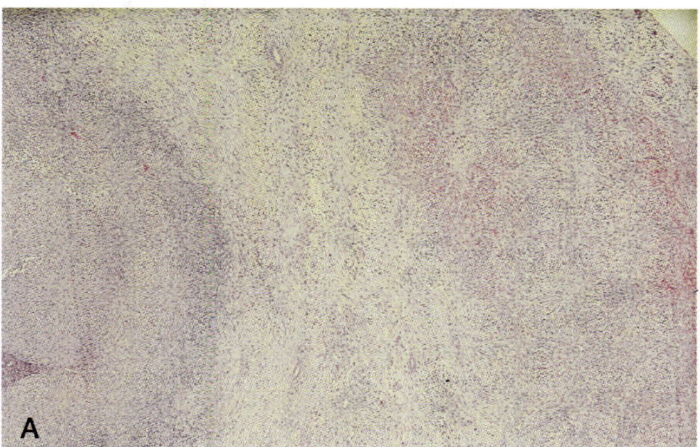

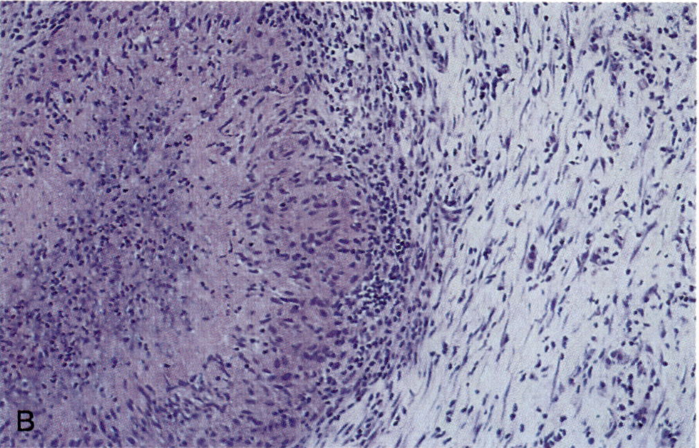

Figure 19–13

Hepatic cat-scratch disease. *A*, The edge of a granuloma with central stellate abscess is shown. *B*, Abscess is surrounded by an inner layer of palisading histiocytes, an intermediate zone of lymphocytes, and an outer zone of fibrosis.

abscesses with granulomas in immunocompromised hosts (Johnson et al, 1988), and hepatosplenic candidiasis has been well documented in neutropenic children following chemotherapy for acute leukemia (Carstensen et al, 1990). Factors influencing mortality rates for liver abscesses include presence of jaundice, positive results on blood culture, biliary origin of infection, and polymicrobial infection (Greenstein et al, 1984).

Acquired Immunodeficiency Syndrome

Children at special risk for AIDS include hemophiliacs, children of high-risk parents, and recipients of blood transfusions. Pediatric AIDS patients often have GI complaints, including diarrhea, malnutrition, abdominal distention, weight loss, and GI hemorrhage. This discussion focuses on hepatic and GI manifestations of AIDS that are common or particularly problematic in the pediatric population.

The opportunistic infectious agents involving the GI tract of AIDS patients include *Candida* species, herpes simplex viruses, *Histoplasma*, CMV, *Mycobacterium avium-intracellulare* (MAI), *Cryptosporidium, Microsporidium*, and numerous bacteria. The spectrum of infectious organisms affecting children with AIDS is similar to that in adults (Clayton & Clayton, 1997; Kahn, 1997). Cryptosporidiosis is very common in the pediatric AIDS population and is typically present in the small bowel and colon, although it may also involve the stomach, biliary tree, and esophagus (Clayton & Clayton, 1997). MAI infection of the GI tract has been described in children, as has severe involvement by CMV infection. Other GI diseases described in children with AIDS include a severe villous atrophy similar to celiac sprue, pseudomembranous necrotizing enterocolitis associated with *Klebsiella* infection, and *Serratia marcescens* cholecystitis with perforation of the gallbladder (McLoughlin et al, 1987).

The spectrum of hepatic lesions in children with HIV mirrors that in adults. Common viral pathogens found in the livers of AIDS patients include CMV, adenovirus, herpes simplex viruses, and EBV. Two viral infections deserve special mention, since they may cause unusual patterns of disease in these children. EBV causes chronic active hepatitis in HIV-infected children but not usually in adults (Bach et al, 1992). Adenovirus infection may cause fatal hepatic necrosis, and this is more frequently seen in children (Krilov et al, 1990). MAI remains the most common organism identified in liver biopsies of AIDS patients (Cappell, 1991).

Both leiomyomas and leiomyosarcomas of the GI tract and liver occur in children with AIDS and are usually associated with perinatal HIV infection. Virtually all of these tumors have been associated with EBV infection (Clayton & Clayton, 1997; Molle et al, 2000).

Homosexual males with AIDS are at the highest risk of developing AIDS-related lymphoma, a complication rarer in other groups, including children (Cappell, 1991). Burkitt lymphoma is the most common diagnosed malignancy in children with AIDS (Biggar et al, 2000). The liver and GI tract are common sites of involvement by extranodal lymphomas in AIDS patients. These lesions have not been well characterized in children (Cappell, 1991; Poles et al, 1997).

Noninfectious Disorders

Amyloidosis

Amyloidosis in the pediatric population is extremely rare. Most pediatric cases are associated with rheumatoid arthritis, familial Mediterranean fever, and other chronic inflammatory conditions. Patients with GI amyloidosis may present with weight loss, diarrhea, obstipation, and gastrointestinal hemorrhage (Hake et al, 1976). Reactive amyloidosis or secondary amyloidosis has been rarely reported in children with idiopathic inflammatory bowel disease (Kahn et al, 1989). Amyloid has been reported in the lower intestinal tract in association with agammaglobulinemia and a plasma cell dyscrasia in a child (Pick et al, 1977), and primary systemic amyloidosis with GI involvement also occurs in children (Hake et al, 1976). Intestinal amyloid deposits are patchy and predominantly located in the bowel mucosa, although amyloid deposits in the submucosa and blood vessels of the GI tract may also be seen (Kahn et al, 1989; Pick et al, 1977).

The liver is a major site of amyloid deposition in amyloidosis associated with immunocyte dyscrasias (AL amyloid) and those types secondary to other diseases (AA amyloid). The liver is involved in amyloidosis in $>50\%$ of cases (Hake et al, 1976). Hepatomegaly and elevated serum alkaline phosphatase levels often signal hepatic involvement by amyloid, but clinical symptoms of liver disease are seldom present. Severe intrahepatic cholestasis affects a minority of AL amyloid patients but not those with AA amyloidosis. Amyloid deposition is seen in hepatic sinusoids with associated compression and atrophy of hepatocytes, and deposition in blood vessel walls is also frequently seen. Associated nonspecific findings in AL and AA amyloidosis include portal fibrosis, portal lymphocytic inflammatory infiltrates, cholangiolar proliferation, steatosis, and reactive Kupffer cells (Chopra et al, 1984).

Inherited Metabolic Disorders

Many inherited metabolic disorders affect the hepatic mononuclear phagocyte system. The spectrum of hepatic involvement ranges from inconsequential to severe dysfunction. Gaucher disease is one of the commonest lysosomal storage diseases (Beaudet, 1987; Beutler, 1991). It is an autosomal recessive disorder caused by a deficiency of glucocerebrosidase. Gaucher disease mimics hematopoietic neoplasms because of its clinical presentation of marked hepatosplenomegaly, thrombocytopenia, bone involvement, and neurologic dysfunction.

Gaucher disease is most common in the Ashkenazic Jewish population and is caused by a number of genetic mutations. The absence of the enzyme glucocerebrosidase causes the insoluble glucocerebroside to accumulate in the central nervous system as well as in macrophages within the liver, spleen, marrow, and, rarely, lung. Three clinical subtypes have been defined. Type 1, the adult or nonneuropathic type, constitutes $>99\%$ of cases and does not cause neurologic involvement. These patients generally have few symptoms, and the diagnosis is often made in middle or older age (Beutler, 1991). Type 1 Gaucher disease is the commonest lysosomal storage disease (Beaudet, 1987). Type 2, the acute neuronopathic type, is a fulminant disease characterized by severe central nervous system involvement (including oculomotor apraxia, strabismus, and hypertonicity) and causes death by age 2 years. Type 3, the juvenile or subacute neuronopathic type, is a juvenile form in which there is a later onset of neurologic symptoms and a longer disease course (Beutler, 1991).

Type 1 Gaucher disease is associated with a wide clinicopathologic spectrum of liver involvement. Hepatosplenomegaly is often present, but the clinical stigmata of liver disease are only rarely reported. Increased fibrosis and progression to cirrhosis have been rarely encountered, as have esophageal varices, portal hypertension, and ascites. Transaminase and alkaline phosphatase levels are often normal. Glucocerebroside accumulates in portal macrophages and Kupffer cells, resulting histologically in aggregates of macrophages with small round nuclei and abundant cytoplasm with a striated or "tissue paper" appearance (Fig. 19–14). Their pattern of distribution may be focal, diffuse, or concentrated in central or peripheral zones.

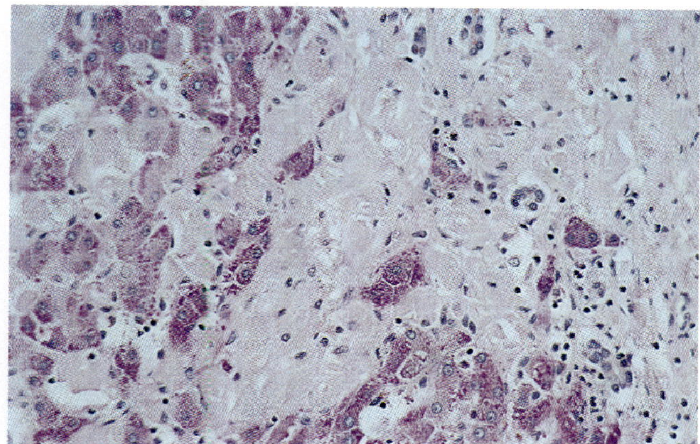

Figure 19–14

Gaucher disease, liver. Aggregates of macrophages contain abundant cytoplasm with the classic "tissue paper" or striated appearance of the Gaucher cell. Periodic acid–Schiff stain.

Gaucher cells are highlighted by periodic acid–Schiff, Masson trichrome, or aldehyde fuschin stains, and acid phosphatase activity may be demonstrated. Numbers of inflammatory cells, predominantly lymphocytes, are slightly increased in association with the Gaucher cells, and pericellular fibrosis is common. Erythrophagocytosis and mild hemosiderosis may also be present. Acidophil bodies, cholestasis, and cholangiolar proliferation are rarely found. In general, the severity of liver disease parallels the severity of extrahepatic disease (Ishak, 1986; James et al, 1981).

NEOPLASTIC DISEASES OF THE LIVER

Lymphoma

Primary Hepatic Lymphoma

B and T cell lymphomas frequently involve the liver, but primary hepatic lymphoma is exceedingly rare in adults and even rarer in children. Pediatric patients with primary hepatic lymphoma present with abdominal pain and hepatomegaly, often including a large liver mass or multiple masses. Enlarged lymph nodes at the porta hepatis are frequently seen as well. Transaminase levels are often normal in children, and may be accompanied by hyperbilirubinemia and jaundice (Collins et al, 1993; Miller et al, 1983; Ramos et al, 1997). In the few cases reported, there is a male predominance, and patients are usually between 7 and 13 years of age. These tumors behave aggressively, disseminate despite treatment, and are often rapidly fatal (Miller et al, 1983; Ramos et al, 1997).

On gross examination, the liver is seen to be enlarged, with either a single mass or multiple firm, white-tan nodules (Aozasa et al, 1993). The vast majority of primary hepatic lymphomas in children are large–B cell lymphomas, although primary hepatic Burkitt lymphoma has been reported (Collins et al, 1993; Huang et al, 1997; Miller et al, 1983). Histologically, the neoplastic lymphocytes expand portal triads and replace the adjacent parenchyma to form nodular masses. Sinusoidal involvement may also occur (Osborne et al, 1985). Plasmacytic differentiation is often noted (Miller et al, 1983; Osborne et al, 1985). Several cytogenetic abnormalities, including t(8;14), occur in pediatric primary hepatic lymphomas (Collins et al, 1993). Chronic hepatitis, including hepatitis B and C, is associated with primary hepatic B cell lymphomas to the extent that a pathogenetic role has been suggested (Aozasa et al, 1993; Huang et al, 1997; Mizorogi et al, 2000; Rubbia-Brandt et al, 1999).

Peripheral T cell lymphomas are very rare in childhood. Most express surface receptors of the α/β type, but very rarely hepatosplenic γ/δ T cell lymphomas occur in childhood (Garcia-Sanchez et al, 1995). Histologically, T cell lymphomas involving the liver usually exhibit marked sinusoidal infiltration (Fig. 19–15) by abnormal lymphocytes that line up in a "beads on a string" pattern or form small aggregates. Associated portal infiltration (see Fig. 19–15), portal fibrosis, hepatocellular atrophy, and hepatocellular necrosis may also be seen (Gaulard et al, 1986). This lymphoma may be difficult to distinguish from an inflammatory process, and multiparameter studies, including gene rearrangement, may be required for diagnosis.

Secondary Involvement by B and T Cell Lymphomas

Secondary lymphomatous involvement of the liver is common and is usually accompanied by splenic involvement. Approximately 50% of patients (mostly adults) had hepatic

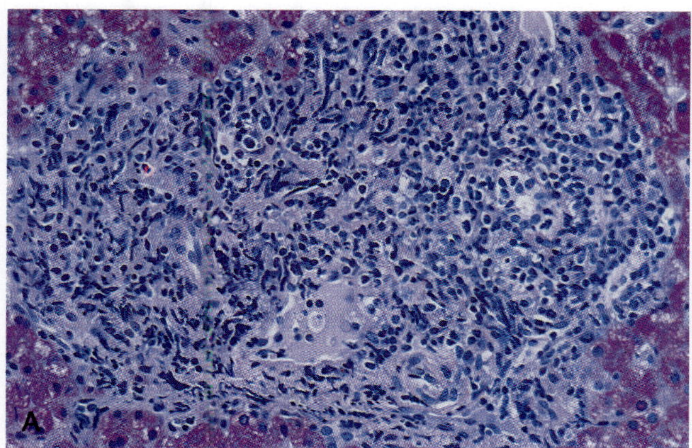

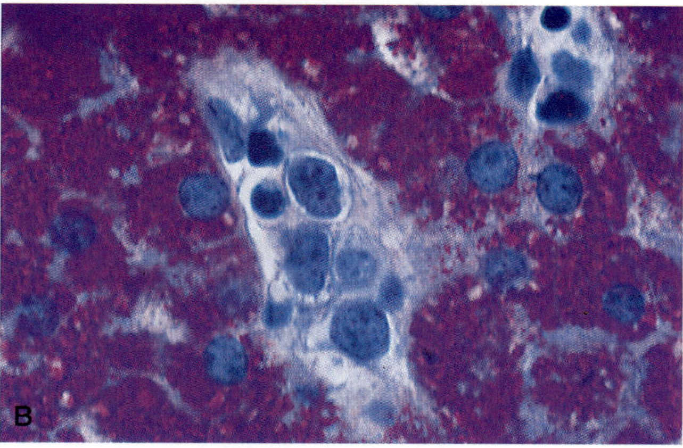

Figure 19–15

Hepatosplenic T cell lymphoma. *A*, Neoplastic lymphocytes expand portal triads. *B*, Hepatic sinusoids are involved. Neoplastic cells expressed $\alpha\beta$ T cell receptors.

involvement in a large autopsy series of disseminated B and T cell lymphoma (Ryan et al, 1988). However, the detection rate of hepatic involvement in vivo by needle biopsy is much lower. Hepatic lymphomatous involvement is usually seen with low-grade processes that do not occur in children. Chronic hepatitis C infection has also been associated with secondary hepatic B and T cell lymphomas (Higuchi et al, 1997; Izumi et al, 1997; Zuckerman et al, 1997), but this association has not been conclusively documented in children. Extranodal non-Hodgkin lymphomas are well described in children with AIDS (see previous section on AIDS).

Secondary Involvement by Hodgkin Disease

Hodgkin disease (HD) is uncommon in young children and even rarer in infants. There is a striking male predominance in children, and Caucasians are affected more often than other races (Lynch, 1975). The liver is often sampled in staging HD, since hepatic involvement indicates stage IV disease. HD was present in the liver in 33% of patients in a large series (Dich et al, 1989). The recognition of HD in the liver is problematic, since "diagnostic" Reed-Sternberg cells are often sparse. Furthermore, the liver often contains inflammatory and granulomatous lesions in the presence or absence of concomitant lymphoma, as discussed later.

HD may produce large masses or multiple small nodules in the liver. In these lesions the infiltrate is characteristically portal, consisting of Reed-Sternberg cells or mononuclear variants in a polymorphous background of eosinophils, lymphocytes, histiocytes, plasma cells, and neutrophils. Mononuclear Reed-Sternberg variants are sufficient for the diagnosis of hepatic HD (Fig. 19–16) (Apt et al, 1974; Dich et al, 1989) when the diagnosis of HD has been previously established in a lymph node.

In HD there are often "nonspecific" portal inflammatory infiltrates that consist predominantly of lymphocytes but may also contain numerous eosinophils and histiocytes. Inflammatory changes of this type should prompt a very careful search for features more diagnostic of HD, especially when the infiltrate is large, contains transformed lymphocytes, or is accompanied by acute cholangitis, portal edema, or marked cholestasis (Dich et al, 1989). Both the diagnostic changes of HD and nonspecific changes in these livers often have a focal distribution. Seventy-five percent of patients with HD in one large study had both positive and negative liver biopsy results over their disease course (Dich et al, 1989). Whether or not the liver is involved by HD, various nonspecific findings may be present, including lobular lymphocytic aggregates, hemosiderosis, steatosis, capsular or subcapsular fibrosis, and granulomas (Apt et al, 1974; Leslie & Colby, 1984).

Noncaseating, epithelioid granulomas are found in portal tracts in approximately 9% of livers in patients with HD (Sacks et al, 1978). By definition, they do not contain dysplastic lymphocytes or Reed-Sternberg cells. These granulomas, in the liver or elsewhere, do not signify involvement by HD. Although the clinical significance of hepatic granulomas is unknown, patients with them have a significantly higher 5-year survival rate, regardless of stage of disease, than do patients without granulomas (Sacks et al, 1978). Epithelioid granulomas have also been reported in the portal tracts of patients with B and T cell lymphomas, often preceding the demonstration of the lymphoma. The histopathologic features of these lesions are similar to those of the granulomas associated with HD (Aderka et al, 1984).

HD has been associated with idiopathic jaundice in adults and, rarely, in adolescents. Jaundice may occur either before or after the detection of HD. Liver function tests show an "obstructive" pattern, but liver biopsy specimens are free of HD, livers appear normal on gross examination at staging laparotomy, and cholangiograms are normal. Some patients may have involvement of the porta hepatis nodes without compression of the biliary tree (Perera et al, 1974). Severe jaundice has also been associated with B and T cell lymphomas without evidence of hepatic involvement. Liver biopsies have demonstrated canalicular cholestasis with varying degrees of inflammation (Perera et al, 1974; Watterson & Priest, 1989).

Hepatic Involvement by Leukemia

The liver is a frequent site of involvement in acute lymphocytic and myelogenous leukemias (Swerdlow et al, 1985). There are rare reports of fulminant hepatic failure in children with acute lymphoblastic leukemia. These patients usually present with jaundice, abdominal pain and distention, hepatomegaly, and a viral-like prodrome. At autopsy, there is massive infiltration of the hepatic sinusoids and portal triads by leukemic cells, with associated subcapsular hemorrhage (Conway et al, 1992). Hepatic involvement by juvenile or

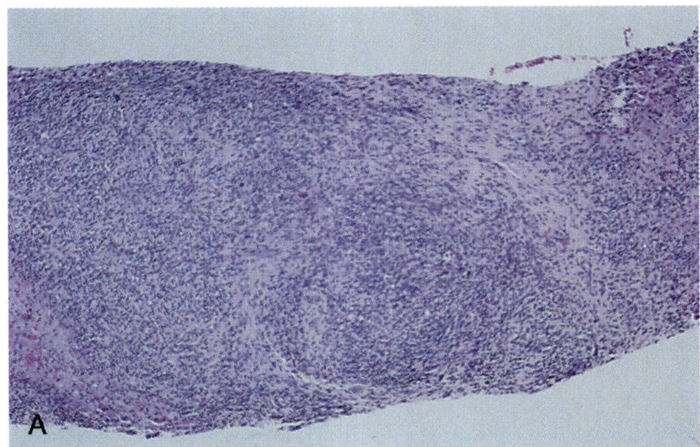

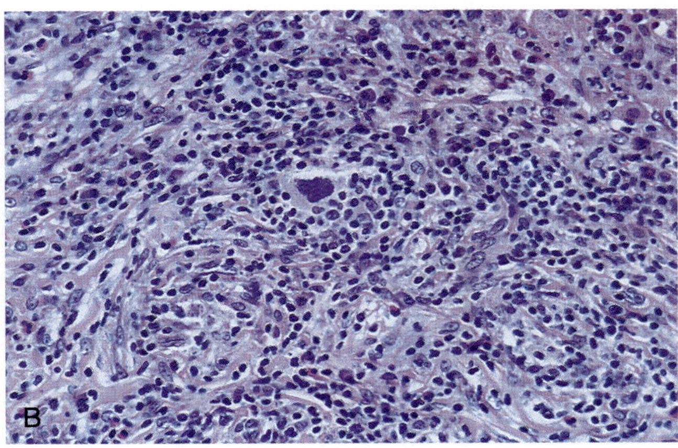

Figure 19–16

Hodgkin disease, liver. *A,* A liver biopsy specimen contains multiple noncaseating granulomas. *B,* At higher magnification a mixed infiltrate and scattered mononuclear Reed-Sternberg cells are seen.

adult-type chronic myelogenous leukemia in children has not been well characterized.

Posttransplant Lymphoproliferative Disorder

The term *posttransplant lymphoproliferative disorder* (PTLD) refers to abnormal proliferations of lymphocytes after solid organ transplants and reflects an imprecise understanding of these often aggressive processes. Some of these proliferations meet the pathologic criteria for lymphoma but regress with diminished immunosuppression. (See the more extensive discussion of PTLD in Chap. 12.) The majority of PTLD cases may be attributed to EBV infection or reactivation (Basgoz & Preiksaitis, 1995), although EBV-negative PTLD cases are well-documented (Basgoz & Preiksaitis, 1995; Nelson et al, 2000). Heart-lung transplant recipients have the highest risk of PTLD, followed by heart, liver, and kidney transplant recipients. The risk of developing PTLD is highest within the first year posttransplant (Basgoz & Preiksaitis, 1995). Primary immunosuppressive therapy with tacrolimus has a higher risk of PTLD in pediatric liver transplant patients than does this therapy with cyclosporine (Younes et al, 2000).

The risk of developing PTLD is significantly higher in children and adults who have primary infection with EBV after transplant than in those who have reactivation of EBV (Ho et al, 1988). The incidence of EBV-associated PTLD in children following solid organ transplant has been reported as 4% compared with 0.8% in adults. Children are at an increased risk of complications of EBV infection posttransplant, since they are more likely to be seronegative pretransplant.

Three major forms of PTLD are recognized. Many patients have a self-limited illness similar to infectious mononucleosis in immunocompetent patients, including pharyngitis, fever, lymphadenopathy, and hepatosplenomegaly. A second group of patients present similarly but within months develop a polymorphous form of PTLD that may involve multiple organ systems and result in death. The third form of PTLD tends to occur later and is associated with development of extranodal large-cell lymphomatous masses. PTLDs involving the GI tract and liver have been reported to be both polymorphous and monomorphous in pediatric series (Basgoz & Preiksaitis, 1995; Ho et al, 1988).

B cell, T cell, mixed B and T cell, and natural killer cell immunophenotypes have been described (Dror et al, 1999; His et al, 1998). Most cases of PTLD involving the GI tract are B-cell processes, and light chain restriction is often present (Guettier et al, 1992). The liver and GI tract are frequent sites of involvement by PTLD. Jaundice, liver failure, diarrhea, GI hemorrhage, hypoalbuminemia, protein-losing enteropathy, and intestinal perforation may be seen in these children (Younes et al, 1999). The GI tract is the commonest site of presentation of PTLD in patients treated with cyclosporin A (Basgoz & Preiksaitis, 1995). PTLD of the intestine is commoner in the small bowel and usually consists of multiple intramural discrete nodules containing a diffuse, deeply infiltrative lymphocytic process with associated ulceration. These tumors may be polymorphous, containing lymphocytes in all stages of transformation with plasma cells and other inflammatory cells, or monomorphous, resembling a large cell or immunoblastic lymphoma (Fig. 19–17). Angiocentrism, a high mitotic rate, and focal lymphoepithelial lesions may be seen. Surrounding lymphocytic hyperplasia is rare.

PTLDs involving the liver may also be polymorphous or monomorphous. Lesions may be solitary or multifocal and may contain extensive necrosis and prominent mitotic activity. Hepatic PTLDs are almost exclusively B cell processes, and light-chain restriction may be present (Purtilo et al, 1992; Raymond et al, 1995).

Malignant Histiocytosis

The term *malignant histiocytosis* (MH) refers to malignancies of the mononuclear phagocyte system. Even this broad term is somewhat controversial in concept and in application to specific diseases, partly because of the rarity of MH (and consequently the inexperience of individual laboratories in recognizing it) and partly because of imprecise criteria for recognition and classification of mononuclear phagocyte system (MPS) subpopulations and the derivative neoplasms. For a general discussion, see Chap. 10. The following discussion is related specifically to GI and liver involvement in these diseases.

In MH there is an infiltration of morphologically atypical cells involving multiple organ systems. Patients may present with persistent fever, hepatosplenomegaly, jaundice, generalized lymphadenopathy, rash, pancytopenia, and hemorrhagic diathesis. Abnormal laboratory findings include hypocholesterolemia, elevated transaminase levels, hyperbilirubinemia, hypoalbuminemia, and elevated lactic dehydrogenase levels (Favara,

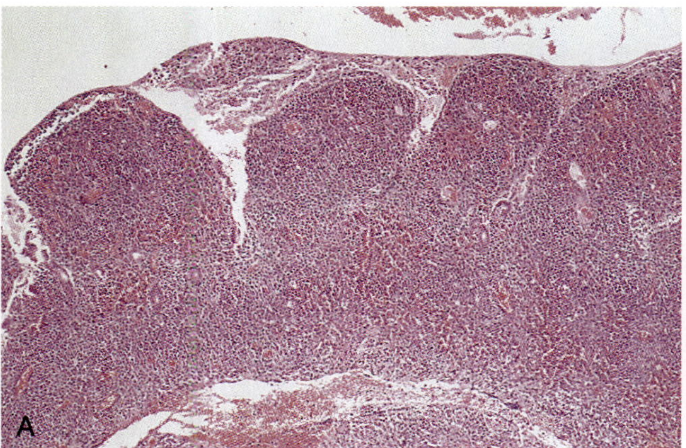

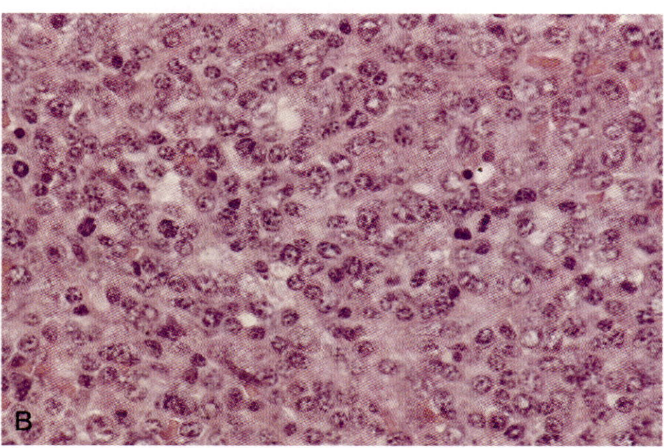

Figure 19–17

Posttransplant lymphoproliferative disorder, small intestine. *A,* This monomorphous infiltrate distends the villi and extends through the bowel wall to the serosal surface (serosa not shown). *B,* The monomorphic B cell process resembles an immunoblastic lymphoma and showed light-chain restriction.

1996; Hibi et al, 1988). These diseases occur in children of any age but are commoner under 2 years of age (Heyn et al, 1990; Hibi et al, 1988). Involvement of the GI tract has been reported in approximately 13–48% of patients (Aosaza et al, 1985; Geissman et al, 1996), and hepatic involvement is present in a majority of cases (Favara, 1996; Hibi et al, 1988).

Although the presence of liver dysfunction at the time of diagnosis is considered a sign of poor prognosis, deaths in MH are rarely attributable to liver disease (Heyn et al, 1990). The most common hepatobiliary complications in pediatric patients with MH include cirrhosis and portal hypertension. Other hepatobiliary complications of MH include a clinical and pathologic picture resembling sclerosing cholangitis, with fibrosis and stenosis of the intra- and extrahepatic biliary tree and associated cholestasis. In addition, the extrahepatic biliary tree may be compressed by enlarged nodes in the porta hepatis. Patients with only triaditis at the time of diagnosis are less likely to have liver dysfunction or progressive hepatic involvement than are patients with fibrohistiocytic or cirrhotic changes. However, there is no correlation between portal changes and the progression of disease in other organ systems (Heyn et al, 1990). Patients with treated histiocytosis may have residual liver dysfunction related to remaining fibrosis even when histiocytes are not demonstrable (Grosfeld et al, 1976).

On gross examination, the liver is often firm and enlarged but without focal lesions (Hibi et al, 1988). Histologically, several patterns of involvement have been described that may coexist. Some cases exhibit an expansion of portal triads by a mixed infiltrate of neutrophils, eosinophils, histiocytes, and mononuclear cells. This triaditis may be the only abnormality seen. The collections of histiocytes and inflammatory cells may progress to form large masses with parenchymal destruction (Kaplan et al, 1999). Cholestasis and cholate stasis are variable along with cholangiolar proliferation. Small bile duct destruction as well as cholangitis-related large duct destruction is well-described (Kaplan et al, 1999). Some degree of periportal or bridging fibrosis is often present and may progress to established "biliary"-type cirrhosis (Kaplan et al, 1999). Occasionally, the histologic features of histiocytosis overlap with infection-associated hemophagocytic syndrome, as discussed earlier. For a description of the infiltrate in Langerhans cell histiocytosis, see the following section.

Digestive tract involvement by MH may be manifested as diarrhea (often bloody), failure to thrive, vomiting, malabsorption, protein-losing enteropathy, or a combination of these symptoms. The spectrum of endoscopic observations in these patients is broad, ranging from normal to findings of enteritis, ulceration, stricture formation, and perforation (Geissman et al, 1996; Mead et al, 1987). Histologically, the histiocytic infiltrate is predominantly in the lamina propria and may be composed of single cells or aggregates of cells, most with abundant cytoplasm. Those cases of MH arising from the Langerhans granule cell typically have grooved nuclei (Fig. 19–18). There is an associated infiltrate of eosinophils, lymphocytes, and macrophages. Histiocytes may focally infiltrate glands, and glandular necrosis may be present. Overall, villous architecture is normal. Enlarged villi containing an inflammatory infiltrate and histiocytes are seen occasionally. Digestive tract involvement may be observed anywhere from stomach to rectum. Gut involvement is strongly associated with skin and mucosal involvement at other sites, and digestive tract involvement may be the first or even the predominant manifestation of extracutaneous involvement. Severe diarrhea and the need for parenteral nutrition are correlated with poor prognosis (Aozasa et

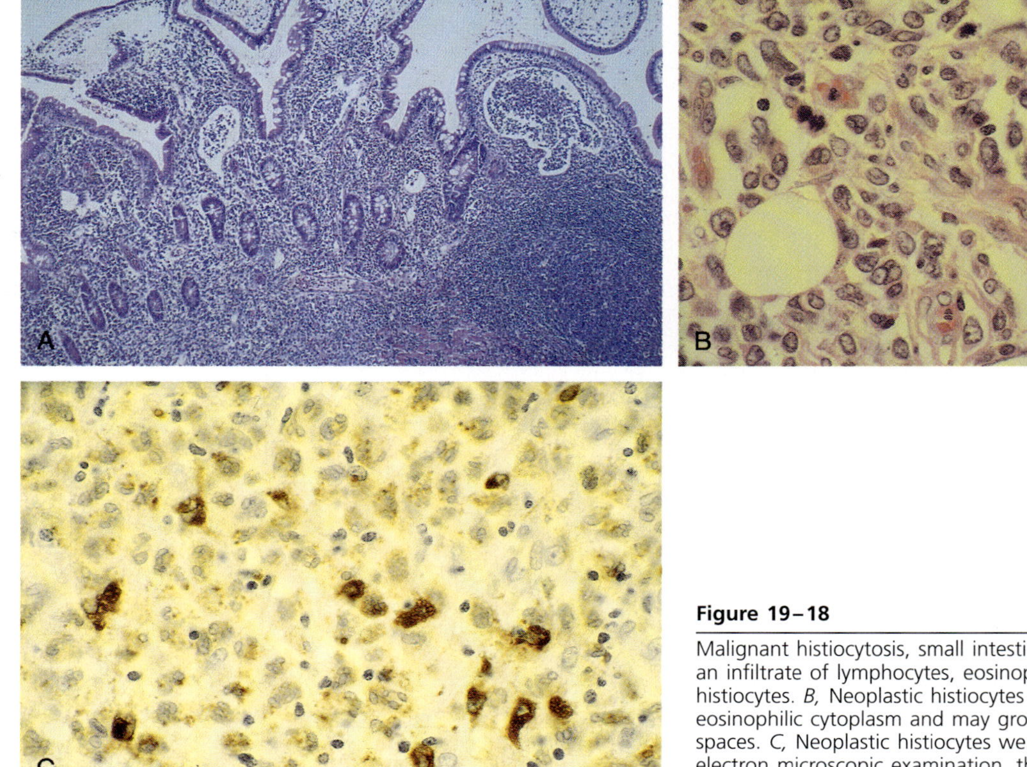

Figure 19–18

Malignant histiocytosis, small intestine. *A,* Distended villi contain an infiltrate of lymphocytes, eosinophils, and neoplastic histiocytes. *B,* Neoplastic histiocytes usually have abundant eosinophilic cytoplasm and may grow in aggreates or lymphatic spaces. *C,* Neoplastic histiocytes were KP-1+ (CD68+). By electron microscopic examination, the cytoplasm was shown to contain haloed granules typical of histiocytes.

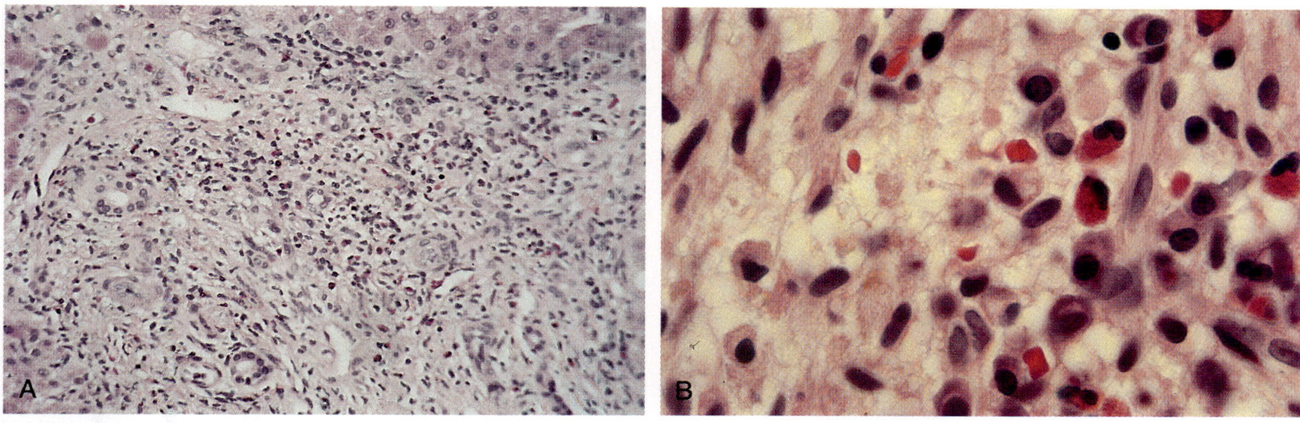

Figure 19–19

Mastocytosis, liver. *A,* A portal triad in mastocytosis often becomes fibrotic, as shown here, and contains a mixed infiltrate. *B,* On high magnification, lymphocytes, eosinophils, and scattered mast cells are present. Mast cells may be plump or spindly and usually have oval or bean-shaped, bland nuclei.

al, 1985; Geissman et al, 1996). Chemotherapy in patients with gastrointestinal MH may result in severe GI bleeding and/or perforation (Mead et al, 1987).

Numerous antibodies are available for the evaluation of histiocytosis in paraffin-embedded, formalin-fixed tissue, and frozen tissue. They include S-100, CD68, CD1a, α_1-antitrypsin, α_1-antichymotrypsin, nonspecific cross-reacting antigen (NCA), concanavalin A receptors (ConAR), HLA-DR antigens, and lysozyme (Favara, 1996; Geissman et al, 1996; Heyn et al, 1990; Hibi et al, 1988). The prevalence of S-100-positive histiocytes in these diseases is apparently higher in children than in adults (Hibi et al, 1988). S-100-positive cases are expected to exhibit Birbeck granules in ultrastructural studies. Most cases of MH involving the liver have few or no Birbeck granules (Heyn et al, 1990).

Mastocytosis

Mastocytosis may involve numerous organ systems, including skin, liver, spleen, lymph nodes, GI tract, marrow, and the skeletal system. In approximately 55% of patients, mastocytosis develops between birth and 2 years of age. An additional 10% are symptomatic before age 15. Pruritus is the commonest presenting symptom, and additional symptoms include flushing, headache, asthma, and GI symptoms (Kettelhut & Metcalfe, 1991). Plasma histamine levels are almost always elevated.

Up to 80% of patients with mastocytosis have GI complaints, including hemorrhage, vomiting, abdominal pain, diarrhea, malabsorption, weight loss, peptic ulcer disease, and, rarely, steatorrhea (Fishman et al, 1979; Kettelhut & Metcalfe, 1991; Lewin et al, 1992). Occasionally, GI symptoms may be present in the absence of skin lesions (Fishman et al, 1979). Rarely, infants may develop a fulminant illness consisting of bullous skin eruptions and GI hemorrhage (Kettelhut & Metcalfe, 1991). Endoscopically, the GI tract may show erosion, ulceration, thickened folds, and nodular lesions or an urticaria-like mucosal lesion (Lewin et al, 1992; Marney, 1992). Histologically, the mast cell infiltrate is found principally in the mucosa and submucosa, with an associated mixed inflammatory infiltrate containing numerous eosinophils. Erosive gastritis, mucosal congestion, and hemorrhage may be secondary to the release of histamine and other vasoactive substances from mast cells (Lewin et al, 1992).

Hepatic involvement occurs in approximately 60% of patients with mastocytosis and is associated with elevated transaminase and serum alkaline phosphatase levels and hepatomegaly. Histologically, liver biopsies may be normal or contain varying numbers of mast cells that predominate in the hepatic sinusoids but may also involve portal areas and aggregate concentrically around vessels. Mast cells have pale cytoplasm and irregular, oval nuclei with small nucleoli. They are usually accompanied by a mixed inflammatory infiltrate in the portal triads, containing numerous eosinophils, lymphocytes, and histiocytes (Fig. 19–19). Steatosis may be seen, and cholestasis is rare (Metcalfe, 1991). Portal fibrosis is present in a majority of cases, and some patients occasionally progress to cirrhosis with ascites and other stigmata of portal hypertension. Mast cells mark well with toluidine blue and other special stains, including chloroacetate esterase (Mican et al, 1995). Immunostaining with antibodies against tryptase, chymase, and the c-kit oncoprotein may also be useful (Horny et al 1997; Maruyama et al, 1998).

Fibrosis of the biliary tree and clinical and cholangiographic changes similar to primary sclerosing cholangitis have been reported in adults with mastocytosis (Baron et al, 1995). Rarely, nodular regenerative hyperplasia and hepatic veno-occlusive disease may be associated with hepatic mastocytosis (Mican et al, 1995).

REFERENCES

Abramowsky CR, Sorensen RU: Regional enteritis-like enteropathy in a patient with agammaglobulinemia: histologic and immunocytologic studies. Hum Pathol 19:483–486, 1988.

Adal KA, Cockerell CJ, Petri WA: Cat-scratch disease, bacillary angiomatosis, and other infections due to *Rochalimaea*. N Engl J Med 330:1509–1515, 1994.

Aderka D, Kraus M, Avidor I, et al: Hodgkin's and non-Hodgkin's lymphomas masquerading as "idiopathic" liver granulomas. Am J Gastroenterol 79:642–644, 1984.

Agha FP, Schnitzer B: Esophageal involvement in lymphoma. Am J Gastroenterol 80:412–416, 1985.

Ament ME, Ochs HD: Gastrointestinal manifestations of chronic granulomatous disease. N Engl J Med 288:382–387, 1973.

Aozasa K, Mishima K, Ohsawa M: Primary malignant lymphoma of the liver. Leuk Lymphoma 10:353–357, 1993.

Aozasa K, Tsujimoto M, Inoue A: Malignant histiocytosis: report of twenty-five cases with pulmonary, renal, and/or gastrointestinal involvement. Histopathology 9:39–49, 1985.

Apt AB, Kirschner RH, Belliveau RE, et al: Hepatic pathology associated with Hodgkin's disease. Cancer 33:1564–1571, 1974.

Autenrieth IB, Firsching R: Penetration of M cells and destruction of Peyer's patches by *Yersinia enterocolitica*: an ultrastructural and histological study. J Med Microbiol 44:285–294, 1996.

Bach N, Theise ND, Schaffner F: Hepatic histopathology in the acquired immunodeficiency syndrome. Semin Liver Dis 12:205–212, 1992.

Barcos M, Lane W, Gomez GA, et al: An autopsy study of 1206 acute and chronic leukemias (1958 to 1982). Cancer 60:827–837, 1987.

Baron TH, Koehler RE, Rodgers WH, et al: Mast cell cholangiopathy: another cause of sclerosing cholangitis. Gastroenterology 109:1677–1681, 1995.

Basgoz N, Preiksaitis JK: Post-transplant lymphoproliferative disorder. Infect Dis Clin North Am 9:901–923, 1995.

Beaudet AL: Gaucher's disease. N Engl J Med 316:619–621, 1987.

Berry CL, Keeling JW: Gastrointestinal lymphoma in childhood. J Clin Pathol 23:459–463, 1970.

Beutler E: Gaucher's disease. N Engl J Med 325:1354–1360, 1991.

Biggar RJ, Frisch M, Goedert JJ. Risk of cancer in children with AIDS. JAMA 284:205–209, 2000.

Boeck A, Buckley RH, Schiff RI: Gastroesophageal reflux and severe combined immunodeficiency. J Allergy Clin Immunol 99:420–424, 1997.

Buckley PJ, O'Laughlin S, Komp DM: Histiocytes in familial and infection-induced/idiopathic hemophagocytic syndromes may exhibit phenotypic differences. Pediatr Pathol 12:51–66, 1992.

Buret A, Curtis GH, Gall DG: Effect of acute *Yersinia enterocolitica* infection on small intestinal ultrastructure. Gastroenterology 98:1401–1407, 1990.

Cappell MS: Hepatobiliary manifestations of the acquired immune deficiency syndrome. Am J Gastroenterol 86:1–11, 1991.

Carstensen H, Widding E, Storm K, et al: Hepatosplenic candidiasis in children with cancer. Pediatr Hematol Oncol 7:3–12, 1990.

Chopra S, Rubinow A, Koff RS, et al: Hepatic amyloidosis. Am J Pathol 115:186–193, 1984.

Clayton F, Clayton CH: Gastrointestinal pathology in HIV-infected patients. Gastroenterol Clin North Am 26:191–240, 1997.

Collins MG, Orazi A, Bauman M, et al: Primary hepatic B-cell lymphoma in a child. Am J Surg Pathol 17:1182–1186, 1993.

Conley ME, Ziegler MM, Borden ST, et al: Multifocal adenocarcinoma of the stomach in a child with common variable immunodeficiency. J Pediatr Gastroenterol Nutr 7:456–460, 1988.

Conway EE, Santorineou M, Mitsudo S: Fulminant hepatic failure in a child with acute lymphoblastic leukemia. J Pediatr Gastroenterol Nutr 15:194–197, 1992.

Craft JC: *Giardia* and giardiasis in childhood [review]. Pediatr Infect Dis 1:196–211, 1982.

Cunningham-Rundles C: Clinical and immunologic analyses of 103 patients with common variable immunodeficiency. J Clin Immunol 9:22–33, 1989.

Cunningham-Rundles C, Lieberman P, Hellman G, et al: Non-Hodgkin lymphoma in common variable immunodeficiency. Am J Hematol 37:69–74, 1991.

Davidson GP, Barnes GL: Structural and functional abnormalities of the small intestine in infants and young children with rotavirus enteritis. Acta Paediatr Scand 68:181–186, 1979.

Deutsch J, Wolf H, Becker H, et al: Demonstration of Epstein-Barr virus DNA in a previously healthy boy with fulminant hepatic failure. Eur J Pediatr 145:94–98, 1986.

Dhesi I, Marsh MN, Kelly C, et al: Morphometric analysis of small intestinal mucosa: 2. Determination of lamina propria volumes: plasma cell and neutrophil populations within control and coeliac disease mucosae. Virchows Arch A Pathol Anat Histopathol 403:173–180, 1984.

Dich NH, Maj MC, Goodman ZD, et al: Hepatic involvement in Hodgkin's disease. Cancer 64:2121–2126, 1989.

Dobbins WO III: Human intestinal intraepithelial lymphocytes. Gut 27:972–985, 1986.

Dror Y, Greenberg M, Taylor G, et al. Lymphoproliferative disorders after organ transplants in children. Transplantation 67:990–998, 1999.

El-Maraghi NR, Mair NS: The histopathology of enteric infection with *Yersinia pseudotuberculosis*. Am J Clin Pathol 71:631–639, 1979.

Eltumi M, Brueton MJ, Francis N: Ulceration of the small intestine in children with coeliac disease. Gut 39:613–614, 1996.

Farthing MJ: Giardiasis [review]. Gastroenterol Clin North Am 25:493–515, 1996.

Faurschou M, Nielsen OJ, Hensen PB, et al. Fatal virus-associated hemophagocytic syndrome associated with coexistent chronic active hepatitis B and acute hepatitis C virus infection. Am J Hematol 61:135–138, 1999.

Favara BE: Histopathology of the liver in histiocytosis syndromes. Pediatr Pathol Lab Med 16:413–433, 1995.

Ferguson A, Kingstone K: Coeliac disease and malignancies. Acta Paediatr Suppl 412:78–81, 1996.

Filipovich AH, Mathur A, Kersey JH, et al: Lymphoproliferative disorders and other tumors complicating immunodeficiencies. Immunodeficiency 5:91–112, 1994.

Fine KD: The prevalence of occult gastrointestinal bleeding in celiac sprue [see comments]. N Engl J Med 334:1163–1167, 1996.

Fishman RS, Fleming CR, Li CY: Systemic mastocytosis with review of gastrointestinal manifestations. Mayo Clin Proc 54:51–54, 1979.

Garcia-Sanchez F, Menarguez J, Cristobal E, et al: Hepatosplenic gamma-delta T-cell malignant lymphoma: report of the first case in childhood, including molecular minimal residual disease follow-up. Br J Haematol 90:943–946, 1995.

Gaulard P, Zafrani ES, Mavier P, et al: Peripheral T-cell lymphoma presenting as predominant liver disease: a report of three cases. Hepatology 6:864–868, 1986.

Geissman F, Thomas C, Emile JF, et al: Digestive tract involvement in Langerhans cell histiocytosis. J Pediatr 129:836–845, 1996.

Gerber MA, Thung SN: Histology of the liver. Am J Surg Pathol 11:709–722, 1987.

Givler RL: Esophageal lesions in leukemia and lymphoma. Am J Dig Dis 15:31–36, 1970.

Gleason TH, Patterson SD: The pathology of *Yersinia enterocolitica* ileocolitis. Am J Surg Pathol 6:347–355, 1982.

Greenstein AJ, Lowenthal D, Hammer GS, et al: Continuing changing patterns of disease in pyogenic liver abscess: a study of 38 patients. Am J Gastroenterol 79:217–226, 1984.

Grosfeld JL, Fitzgerald JF, Wagner VM, et al: Portal hypertension in infants and children with histiocytosis X. Am J Surg 131: 108–113, 1976.

Guettier C, Hamilton-Dutoit S, Guillemain R, et al: Primary gastrointestinal malignant lymphomas associated with Epstein-Barr virus after heart transplantation. Histopathology 20:21–28, 1992.

Hake H, Goll U, Thoenes W: Primary perireticulin amyloidosis in a 14-year-old girl. Eur J Pediatr 124:43–49, 1976.

Hermaszewski RA, Webster AD: Primary hypogammaglobulinaemia: a survey of clinical manifestations and complications [see comments]. Q J Med 86:31–42, 1993.

Heyn RM, Hamoudi A, Newton WA: Pretreatment liver biopsy in 20 children with histiocytosis X: a clinicopathologic correlation. Med Pediatr Oncol 18:110–118, 1990.

Hibi S, Esumi N, Todo S, et al: Malignant histiocytosis in childhood. Hum Pathol 19:713–719, 1988.

Hill SM, Milla PJ, Bottazzo GF, et al: Autoimmune enteropathy and colitis: is there a generalised autoimmune gut disorder? Gut 32:36–42, 1991.

Ho M, Jaffe R, Miller G, et al: The frequency of Epstein-Barr virus infection and associated lymphoproliferative syndrome after transplantation and its manifestations in children. Transplantation 45:719–727, 1988.

Holmes GKT: Non-malignant complications of coeliac disease. Acta Paediatr Suppl 412:68–75, 1996.

Horny HP, Ruck P, Krober S, Kaiserling E. Systemic mast cell disease (mastocytosis). Histol Histopathol 12:1081–1089, 1997.

Hsi ED, Picken MM, Alkan S. Posttransplantation lymphoproliferative disorder of the NK-cell type: a case report and review of the literature. Mod Pathol 11:479–484, 1998.

Huang CB, Eng HL, Chuang JH, et al: Primary Burkitt's lymphoma of the liver: report of a case with long-term survival after surgical resection and combination chemotherapy. J Pediatr Hematol Oncol 19:135–138, 1997.

Ishak KG: Granulomas of the liver. In Ioachim HL (ed): Pathology of Granulomas. Raven Press, New York, pp 307–369, 1983.

Ishak KG: Hepatic morphology in the inherited metabolic diseases. Semin Liver Dis 6:246–258, 1986.

James SP, Stromeyer FW, Chang C, et al: Liver abnormalities in patients with Gaucher's disease. Gastroenterology 80:126–130, 1981.

Johnson TL, Barnett JL, Appelman HD, et al: *Candida* hepatitis. Am J Surg Pathol 12:716–720, 1988.

Kahn E. Gastrointestinal manifestations in pediatric AIDS. Pediatr Pathol Lab Med 17:171–208, 1997.

Kahn E, Markowitz J, Simpser E, et al: Amyloidosis in children with inflammatory bowel disease. J Pediatr Gastroenterol Nutr 8:447–453, 1989.

Kaplan KJ, Goodman ZD, Ishak KG. Liver involvement in Langerhans' cell histocytosis: a study of nine cases. Mod Pathol 12:370–378, 1999.

Katz JA, Wagner ML, Gresik MV, et al: Typhlitis: an 18-year experience and postmortem review. Cancer 65:1041–1047, 1990.

Kemper CA, Lombard CM, Dereskinski SC, et al: Visceral bacillary epitheloid angiomatosis: possible manifestations of disseminated cat-scratch disease in the immunocompromised host. Am J Med 89:216–222, 1990.

Kettelhut BV, Metcalfe DD: Pediatric mastocytosis. J Invest Derm 96:15S–17S, 1991.

Kilpatrick ZM: Structural and functional abnormalities of liver in infectious mononucleosis. Arch Intern Med 117:47–53, 1966.

Kother R, Marsh F Jr, Posner G, et al: Endoscopic leukemic polyposis [review]. Am J Gastroenterol 85:884–886, 1990.

Krilov LR, Rubin LG, Frogel M, et al: Disseminated adenovirus infection with hepatic necrosis in patients with human immunodeficiency virus infection and other immunodeficiency states. Rev Infect Dis 12:303–307, 1990.

Lamps LW, Gray GF, Scott MA: The histologic spectrum of hepatic cat-scratch disease. Am J Surg Pathol 20:1253–1259, 1996.

Laszewski MJ, Kemp JD, Goeken JA, et al: Clonal immunoglobulin gene rearrangement in nodular lymphoid hyperplasia of the gastrointestinal tract associated with common variable immunodeficiency. Am J Clin Pathol 94:338–343, 1990.

Lau YL, Srivastava G, Lee CW, et al: Epstein-Barr virus associated aplastic anemia and hepatitis. J Paediatr Child Health 30:74–76, 1994.

Lavillia P, Gil A, Rodriguez MCG, et al: X-linked agammaglobulinemia and gastric adenocarcinoma. Cancer 72:1528–1531, 1993.

Laxer RM, Roberts EA, Gross KR, et al: Liver disease in neonatal lupus erythematosus. J Pediatr 116:238–242, 1990.

Lederman HM, Winkelstein JA: X-linked agammaglobulinemia: an analysis of 96 patients. Medicine 64:145–156, 1985.

Lee EY, Clouse RE, Aliperti G, et al: Small intestinal lesion resembling graft-vs-host disease: a case report in immunodeficiency and review of the literature. Arch Pathol Lab Med 115:529–532, 1991.

Lemos LB, Baliga M, Benghuzzi HA, et al: Nodular hematopoiesis of the liver diagnosed by fine-needle aspiration cytology. Diagn Cytopathol 16:51–54, 1997.

Leonard N, Feighery CF, Hourihane DOB: Peptic duodenitis: does it exist in the second part of the duodenum? J Clin Pathol 50:54–58, 1997.

Lerner A, Kumar V, Iancu TC: Immunological diagnosis of childhood coeliac disease: comparison between antigliadin, antireticulin and antiendomysial antibodies. Clin Exp Immunol 95:78–82, 1994.

Leslie KO, Colby TV: Hepatic parenchymal lymphoid aggregates in Hodgkin's disease. Hum Pathol 15:808–809, 1984.

Lewin KJ, Riddell RH, Weinstein WM: Gastrointestinal manifestations of extraintestinal disorders and systemic disease. In: Lewin KJ, Riddell RH, Weinstein WM (eds): Gastrointestinal Pathology and Its Clinical Implications. Igaku-Shoin, New York, p366, 1992.

Lloyd-Still JD, Scott JP, Crussi F: The spectrum of Epstein-Barr virus hepatitis in children. Pediatr Pathol 5:337–351, 1986.

Lucas SB: Other viral and infectious diseases and HIV-related liver disease. In MacSween RNM, Anthony PP, Scheuer PJ et al (eds): Pathology of the Liver, 3rd ed. Churchill Livingstone, Hong Kong, pp 269–315, 1994.

Lynch RG: Blood and bone marrow. In Kissane JM (ed): Pathology of Infancy and Childhood, 2nd ed. CV Mosby, St Louis, pp 887–888, 1975.

Machida HM, Catto Smith AG, Gall DG, et al: Allergic colitis in infancy: clinical and pathologic aspects [see comments]. J Pediatr Gastroenterol Nutr 19:22–26, 1994.

MacSween RNM, Scothorne RJ: Developmental anatomy and normal structure. In MacSween RNM, Anthony PP, Scheuer PJ, Burt AD, Portmann BC, (eds): Pathology of the Liver, 3rd ed. Churchill Livingstone, Hong Kong, p 6, 1994.

Maluenda C, Phillips AD, Briddon A, et al: Quantitative analysis of small intestinal mucosa in cow's milk-sensitive enteropathy. J Pediatr Gastroenterol Nutr 3:349–356, 1984.

Mantle M, Atkins E, Kelly J, et al: Effects of *Yersinia enterocolitica* infection on rabbit intestinal and colonic goblet cells and mucin: morphometrics, histochemistry, and biochemistry. Gut 32: 1131–1138, 1991.

Marney SR: Mast cell disease. Allergy Proc 13:303–310, 1992.

Maryuama H, Sugihara S, Ishihara K, et al. Systemic mast cell disease with splenic infarction: a case report. Pathol Int 48:403–411, 1998.

McLoughlin LC, Nord KS, Joshi VV, et al: Severe gastrointestinal involvement in children with the acquired immunodeficiency syndrome. J Pediatr Gastroenterol Nutr 6:517–524, 1987.

Mead GM, Whitehouse JM, Thompson J, et al: Clinical features and management of malignant histiocytosis of the intestine. Cancer 60:2791–2796, 1987.

Metcalfe DD: The liver, spleen, and lymph nodes in mastocytosis. J Invest Dermatol 96:45S–46S, 1991.

Mican JM, Di Bisceglie AM, Fong TL, et al: Hepatic involvement in mastocytosis: clinicopathologic correlations in 41 cases. Hepatology 22:1163–1170, 1995.

Mike N, Hansel TT, Newman J, et al: Granulomatous enteropathy in common variable immunodeficiency: a cause of chronic diarrhoea [see comments]. Postgrad Med J 67:446–449, 1991.

Miller ST, Wollner N, Meyers PA, et al: Primary hepatic or hepatosplenic non-Hodgkin' lymphoma in children. Cancer 52:2285–2288, 1983.

Mirakian R, Richarson A, Milla PJ, et al: Protracted diarrhoea of infancy: evidence in support of an autoimmune variant. BMJ 293:1132–1136, 1986.

Mizorogi F, Hiramoto J, Nozato A, et al. Hepatitis C virus infection in patients with B-cell non-Hodgkin's lymphoma. Intern Med 39:112–117, 2000.

Molle ZL, Moallem H, Desai N, et al. Endoscopic features of smooth muscle tumors in children with AIDS. Gastrointestinal Endosc 52:91–94, 2000.

Nelson BP, Nalesnik MA, Bahler DW, et al. Epstein-Barr virus–negative posttransplant lymphoproliferative disorders: a distinct entity? Am J Surg Pathol 24:375–385, 2000.

Oberhuber G, Kastner N, Stolte M: Giardiasis: a histologic analysis of 567 cases. Scand J Gastroenterol 32:48–51, 1997.

Odze RD, Wershil BK, Leichtner AM: Allergic colitis in infants. J Pediatr 126:163–170, 1995.

Okano M, Gross TG: Epstein-Barr virus–associated hemophagocytic syndrome and fatal infectious mononucleosis. Am J Hem 53:111–115, 1996.

Osborne BM, Butler JJ, Guarda LA: Primary lymphoma of the liver. Cancer 56:2902–2910, 1985.

Perera DR, Greene ML, Fenster LF: Cholestasis associated with extrabiliary Hodgkin's disease. Gastroenterology 67:680–685, 1974.

Pick AI, Versano I, Schreibman S, et al: Agammaglobulinemia, plasma cell dyscrasia, and amyloidosis in a 12-year-old child. Am J Dis Child 131:682–686, 1977.

Poles MA, Lew EA, Dieterich DT: Diagnosis and treatment of hepatic disease in patients with HIV. Gastroenterol Clin North Am 26:291–321, 1997.

Prolla JC, Kirsner JB: The gastrointestinal lesions and complications of the leukemias. Ann Inter Med 61:1084–1103, 1964.

Purtilo DT, DeFlorio D, Hutt LM, et al: Variable phenotypic expression of an X-linked recessive lymphoproliferative syndrome. N Engl J Med 297:1077–1080, 1977.

Purtilo DT, Stroback RS, Okano M, et al: Epstein-Barr virus–associated lymphoproliferative disorders. Lab Invest 67:5–19, 1992.

Ramos G, Murao M, de Oliveira BM, et al. Primary hepatic non-Hodgkin's lymphoma in children: a case report and review of the literature. Med Pediatr Oncol 28:370–372, 1997.

Raymond E, Tricottet V, Samuel D, et al: Epstein-Barr virus–related localized hepatic lymphoproliferative disorders after liver transplantation. Cancer 76:1344–1351, 1995.

Reyes E, Hernandez J, Gonzalez A: Typhoid colitis with massive lower gastrointestinal bleeding: an unexpected behavior of *Salmonella typhi*. Dis Colon Rectum 29:511–514, 1986.

Risdall RJ, McKenna RW, Nesbit ME, et al: Virus-associated hemophagocytic syndrome: a benign histiocytic proliferation distinct from malignant histiocytosis. Cancer 44:993–1002, 1979.

Rowland HAK: Typhoid fever and other *Salmonella* infections. Br J Hosp Med 10:54–62, 1974.

Roy J, Snover D, Weisdorf S, et al: Simultaneous upper and lower endoscopic biopsy in the diagnosis of intestinal graft-versus-host disease. Transplantation 51:642–646, 1991.

Rubbia-Brandt L, Brundler MA, Kerl K, et al. Primary hepatic diffuse lar380ge B-cell lymphoma in a patient with chronic hepatitis C. Am J Surg Pathol 23:1124–1130, 1999.

Ryan J, Straus DJ, Lange C, et al: Primary lymphoma of the liver. Cancer 61:370–375, 1988.

Sacks EL, Donaldson SS, Gordon J, et al: Epithelioid granulomas associated with Hodgkin's disease. Cancer 41:562–567, 1978.

Salazar de Sousa J, da Silva A, Pereira MV, et al: Cow's milk protein–sensitive enteropathy: number and timing of biopsies for diagnosis. J Pediatr Gastroenterol Nutr 5:207–209, 1986.

Sale GE, McDonald GB, Shulman HM, et al: Gastrointestinal graft-versus-host disease in man: a clinicopathologic study of the rectal biopsy. Am J Surg Pathol 3:219–229, 1979.

Salim AF, Phillips AD, Walker-Smith JA, et al: Sequential changes in small intestinal structure and function during rotavirus infection in neonatal rats. Gut 36:231–238, 1995.

Scott H, Nilsen E, Sollid LM, et al: Immunopathology of gluten-sensitive enteropathy. Springer Semin Immunopathol 18:535–553, 1997.

Shanahan F: A gut reaction: lymphoepithelial communication in the intestine. Science 275:1897–1898, 1997.

Shaw NJ, Evans JH: Liver failure and Epstein-Barr virus infection. Arch Dis Child 63:432–433, 1988.

Shulman HM, Sharma P, Amos D, et al: A coded histologic study of hepatic graft-versus-host disease after human bone marrow transplantation. Hepatology 8:463–470, 1988.

Shulman HM, Sullivan KM, Weiden PL, et al: Chronic graft-versus-host syndrome in man: a long-term clinicopathologic study of 20 Seattle patients. Am J Med 69:204–217, 1980.

Sloan JM, Cameron CH, Maxwell RJ, et al: Colitis complicating chronic granulomatous disease: a clinicopathological case report. Gut 38:619–622, 1996.

Snover DC: Mucosal damage simulating acute graft-versus-host reaction in cytomegalovirus colitis. Transplantation 39:669–670, 1985.

Snover DC, Filipovich AH, Ramsay NKC, et al: Graft-versus-host disease–like histopathological findings in pre-bone marrow transplantation biopsies of patients with severe T cell deficiency. Transplantation 39:95–97, 1985.

Snover DC, Weisdorf SA, Ramsay NL, et al: Hepatic graft versus host disease: a study of the predictive value of the liver biopsy in diagnosis. Hepatology 4:123–130, 1984.

Steiner MS, Morton RA: Nutritional and gastrointestinal complications of the use of bowel segments in the lower urinary tract. Urol Clin North Am 18:743–754, 1991.

Stenhammar L, Masreliez V: T-cell–rich B-cell lymphoma in a child with celiac disease. J Pediatr Gastroenterol Nutr 17:337–338, 1993.

Stephan JL, Galambrun C. Reactive hemophagocytic syndrome in children. Arch Pediatr 7:278–286, 2000.

Stern M, Dietrich R, Muller J: Small intestinal mucosa in coeliac disease and cow's milk protein intolerance: morphometric and immunofluorescent studies. Eur J Pediatr 139:101–105, 1982.

Swerdlow SH, Glick AD, Cousar JB, et al: Acute leukemias of childhood: pathologic features. Hematol Oncol 3:99–131, 1985.

Takahashi H, Hansmann ML: Primary gastrointestinal lymphoma in childhood (up to 18 years of age): a morphological, immunohistochemical and clinical study. J Cancer Res Clin Oncol 116: 190–196, 1990.

Teahon K, Webster AD, Price AB, et al: Studies on the enteropathy associated with primary hypogammaglobulinemia. Gut 35:1244–1249, 1994.

Tsui WMS, Wong KF, Tse CCH: Liver changes in reactive hemophagocytic syndrome. Liver 12:363–367, 1992.

van der Meer JW, Weening RS, Schellekens PT, et al: Colorectal cancer in patients with X-linked agammaglobulinaemia. Lancet 341:1439–1440, 1993.

Verdi CJ, Grogan TM, Protell R, et al: Liver biopsy immunotyping to characterize lymphoid malignancies. Hepatology 6:6–13, 1986.

Ward H, Jalan KN, Maitra TK, et al: Small intestinal nodular lymphoid hyperplasia in patients with giardiasis and normal serum immunoglobulins. Gut 24:120–126, 1983.

Washington K, Bentley RC, Green A, et al: Gastric graft-versus-host disease: a blinded histologic study. Am J Surg Pathol 21:1037–1046, 1997.

Washington K, Gossage DL, Gottfried MR: Pathology of the liver in severe combined immunodeficiency and DiGeorge syndrome. Pediatr Pathol 13:485–504, 1993.

Washington K, Stenzel TT, Buckley RH, et al: Gastrointestinal pathology in patients with common variable immunodeficiency and X-linked agammaglobulinemia. Am J Surg Pathol 20:1240–1252, 1996.

Watterson J, Priest JR: Jaundice as a paraneoplastic phenomenon in a T-cell lymphoma. Gastroenterology 97:1319–1322, 1989.

Weisdorf D, Arthur D, Rank J, et al: Gastric recurrence of acute lymphoblastic leukemia mimicking graft-versus-host disease. Br J Haematol 71:559–564, 1989.

Weiss RL, Lazarus KH, Macon WR, et al: Natural killer–like T-cell lymphoma in the small intestine of a child without evidence of enteropathy. Am J Surg Pathol 21:964–969, 1997.

Whang EE, Dunn JC, Joffe H, et al: Enterocyte functional adaptation following intestinal resection. J Surg Res 60:370–374, 1996.

Younes BS, McDiarmid SV, Martin MG, et al. The effect of immunosuppression on posttransplant lymphoproliferative disease in pediatric liver transplant patients. Transplantation 70:94–99, 2000.

Younes BS, Ament ME, McDiarmid SV, et al. The involvement of the gastrointestinal tract in posttransplant lymphoproliferative disease in pediatric liver transplantation. J Pediatr Gastroenterol Nutr 28:380–385, 1999.

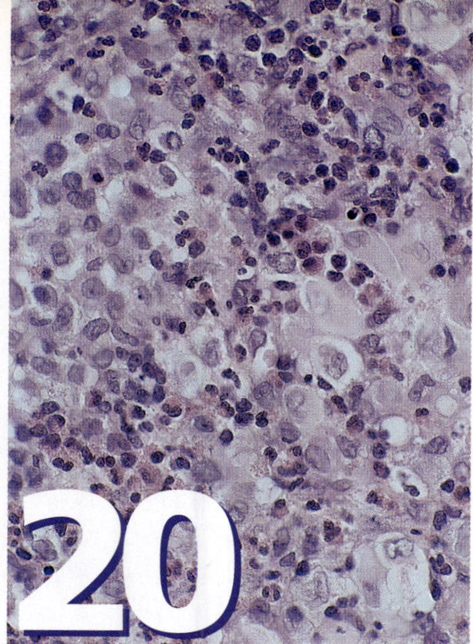

Andras Khoor

LUNG

NORMAL STRUCTURE AND FUNCTION

The respiratory tract contains aggregates of lymphocytes beneath the bronchial mucosa in the visceral pleura and interlobar septa. These aggregates have close structural and functional similarities to other forms of mucosa-associated lymphatic tissue and are usually referred to as bronchus-associated lymphatic tissue (BALT). BALT is not prominent in the normal human lung but often permeates the overlying epithelium. BALT plays an important role in antigen uptake, initiating immune responses and disseminating primed lymphocytes throughout the respiratory tract (Pabst & Gehrke, 1990). Abnormal lymphocytic infiltrates often follow the normal distribution of BALT in the lung.

REACTIVE PROLIFERATIONS OF LYMPHOCYTES

Follicular Bronchitis or Bronchiolitis

Follicular bronchitis or bronchiolitis is defined as hyperplasia of lymphatic tissue within the bronchovascular bundles in patients who do not have underlying bronchiectasis, cystic fibrosis, and common chronic infections (Yousem et al, 1985a). In children, follucular bronchitis or bronchiolitis may be associated with systemic autoimmune diseases, such as juvenile rheumatoid arthritis (Athreya et al, 1980; Franchi et al, 1992; Yousem et al, 1985a), congenital and acquired immunodeficiency states (Yousem et al, 1985a), or previous viral infections (Bramson et al, 1996), or it may be idiopathic (Kinane et al, 1993). Patients with follicular bronchitis or bronchiolitis usually present with cough and tachypnea, and physical examination reveals diffuse fine crackles or coarse rhonchi. Chest radiographs demonstrate bilateral reticular or reticulonodular infiltrates. Response to corticosteroid therapy is minimal. Children with juvenile rheumatoid arthritis have presented between the ages of $3\frac{1}{2}$ and 9 years and have developed either stable or progressive lung disease (Athreya et al, 1980; Yousem et al, 1985a). Patients with immunodeficiency often have recurrent pneumonia and a poor long-term prognosis (Yousem & Colby, 1992; Yousem et al, 1985b). Children with previous viral infections or idiopathic follicular bronchitis or bronchiolitis are often symptomatic by 6 weeks of age (Bramson et al, 1996; Kinane et al, 1993), but at 3 years of age the radiographs begin to return to normal. By 8 years of age clinical symptoms have disappeared, and pulmonary function tests demonstrate only mild residual obstructive lung disease.

Histologically, follicular bronchitis or bronchiolitis is characterized by the presence of abundant germinal centers around bronchi and bronchioles. These follicles, located between bronchioles and juxtaposed pulmonary arteries, often compress bronchiolar lumens. Bronchioles are also surrounded by an infiltrate of lymphocytes and plasma cells, and lymphocytes may be present in the bronchiolar epithelium. Changes less frequently seen include luminal purulent exudates, peribronchial fibrosis, focal bronchiolitis obliterans, and lymphoplasmacytic infiltration of vessel walls.

Since bronchiectasis, cystic fibrosis, and common chronic infections elicit a similar histologic reaction, these conditions should be excluded before a diagnosis of follicular bronchitis or bronchiolitis is made (Yousem et al, 1985a). Lymphocytic hyperplasia commonly extends along the lymphatic routes in follicular bronchitis or bronchiolitis (Yousem et al, 1985a), and its distinction from lymphocytic interstitial pneumonia may become arbitrary. Cases with overlapping features should be classified according to the dominant component (Nicholson et al, 1995).

Lymphocytic Interstitial Pneumonia

Lymphocytic interstitial pneumonia, also known as diffuse lymphoid hyperplasia (Kradin & Mark, 1983), was initially described as a chronic interstitial pneumonia that is rich in lymphocytes and plasma cells (Liebow & Carrington, 1973). By current definition, the lymphocytic infiltrate is histologically polymorphous and is polyclonal (Colby, 1994). In children, lymphocytic interstitial pneumonia is associated with juvenile rheumatoid arthritis (Athreya et al, 1980), but it is most commonly associated with HIV infection. It is one of the most prevalent AIDS-defining conditions (Nielsen et al, 1997).

Clinically, HIV-infected patients present with cough, dyspnea, and hypoxemia (Teirstein & Rosen, 1988) as well as digital clubbing and parotid gland enlargement (Rubinstein et al, 1986). Dysproteinemias (hyper- and hypogammaglobulinemia) are found in $>60\%$ of cases (Fishback & Koss, 1996). CD8+ lymphocytosis may be present in the peripheral blood, bronchoalveolar lavage fluid, lung tissue, and salivary gland tissue. Radiographically, most patients have diffuse reticulonodular infiltrates, and some have patchy areas of consolidation. Computed tomographic scans reveal nodular or "ground-glass" patterns. Reduced lung volumes and diffusing capacities are consistently demonstrated. Lung biopsies are often necessary to establish the diagnosis, since the clinical presentation is also

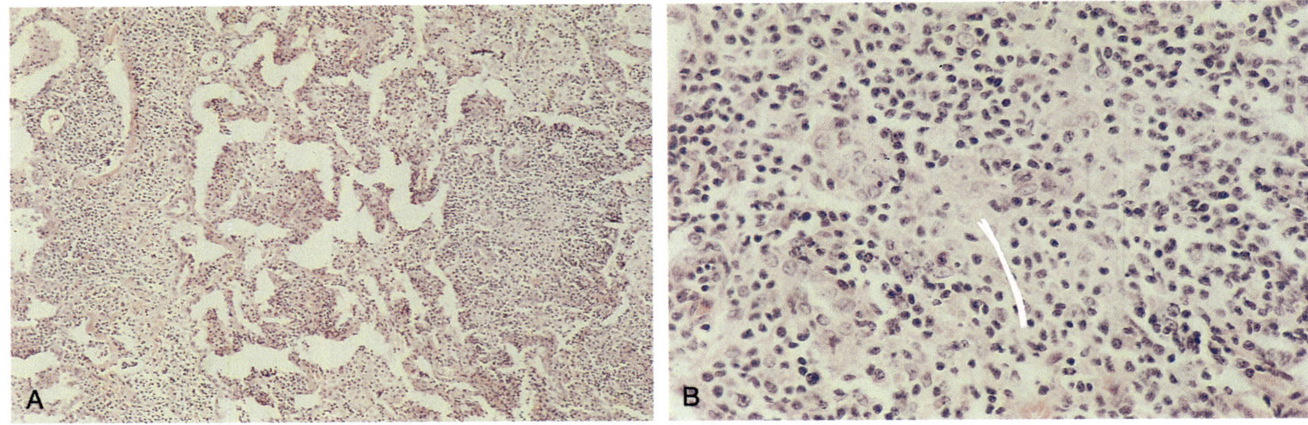

Figure 20–1

Lymphocytic interstitial pneumonia, lung. *A*, A marked interstitial infiltrate of mononuclear cells and numerous germinal centers are apparent. *B*, The infiltrate is polymorphous.

suggestive of *Pneumocystis carinii* pneumonia. Some HIV-infected patients with lymphocytic interstitial pneumonia respond dramatically to corticosteroid therapy, but others improve with no treatment. Most patients eventually succumb to other complications of HIV infection.

Histologic sections in lymphocytic interstitial pneumonitis exhibit a diffuse interstitial infiltrate of small lymphocytes, plasma cells, and histiocytes that widens the alveolar septa and involves bronchovascular bundles, interlobular septa, and pleura (Fig. 20–1) (Nicholson et al, 1995). Variable amounts of fibrosis may accompany the interstitial infiltrate. Secondary follicles, vaguely formed granulomas, and type 2 cell hyperplasia are often seen. Immunohistochemical studies reveal numerous T cells, particularly T helper cells, and a polyclonal population of B cells (Koss et al, 1987).

The patterns of lymphocytic interstitial pneumonitis and follicular bronchitis or bronchiolitis commonly overlap. The diagnosis in these cases is based on the dominant component (Nicholson et al, 1995). The differential diagnosis of lymphocytic interstitial pneumonitis includes low-grade B cell lymphoma, a malignancy vanishingly rare in children, that produces monomorphic large nodules of clonal lymphocytes. The pathogenesis of lymphocytic interstitial pneumonitis is not known, but there is evidence that many cases associated with AIDS are due to HIV and/or Epstein-Barr viruses (EBVs) (Koss, 1995; Rubinstein et al, 1986). Eight of 10 lung biopsy specimens from children have contained EBV DNA (Andiman et al, 1985).

Angiofollicular Hyperplasia (Castleman Disease)

Angiofollicular hyperplasia, rarely seen in children (Salisbury, 1990), classically involves the mediastinum but may also occur in the hilar region of the lung. Angiofollicular hyperplasia produces an asymptomatic mass or constitutional symptoms of fever, weight loss, and anemia. Surgical excision is curative in most pediatric cases (Salisbury, 1990).

The lung is usually involved by the hyalin vascular form, in which there are numerous small follicular centers with prominent central blood vessels that exhibit hyalinized walls and plump endothelial cells. Concentric layers of small lymphocytes and plasma cells surround the follicular centers. The interfollicular areas display vascular proliferation and variable numbers of lymphocytes and plasma cells.

Inflammatory Pseudotumor

Inflammatory pseudotumor, also known as inflammatory myofibroblastic tumor or plasma cell granuloma, is the commonest benign pulmonary mass in children (Hartman & Shochat, 1983). It is discussed here, with reactive lymphocytic proliferations, but it may be a low-grade neoplasm of myofibroblastic cells that has elicited a marked inflammatory reaction (Su et al, 1998). Males and females are equally affected. Most patients are asymptomatic, but some have chest pain and dyspnea. Radiographs reveal solitary masses that may be calcified (Kaufman, 1988). The prognosis is usually excellent after complete surgical excision (Pettinato et al, 1990). Aggressive lesions may involve the mediastinum, recur locally, or metastasize (Biselli et al, 1996; Kim et al, 1992; Maier & Sommers, 1987; Spencer, 1984). Some aggressive "inflammatory pseudotumors" may actually be misdiagnosed inflammatory fibrosarcomas (Meis & Enzinger, 1991).

Inflammatory pseudotumors are usually well-circumscribed, albeit unencapsulated, masses and may measure 1.2–15 cm in greatest dimension (Pettinato et al, 1990). Microscopically, they are fibrosing processes composed of varying numbers of inflammatory cells (mainly lymphocytes and plasma cells) as well as spindled fibroblasts and myofibroblasts commonly arranged in fascicles. The spindle cells have plump or oval nuclei, small nucleoli, and eosinophilic cytoplasm. Lymphocytes or plasma cells are interspersed among the spindle cells and may form clusters or linear arrays. Lymphatic follicles may be found at the periphery of the lesion, and foci of organizing pneumonia may also be seen (Matsubara et al, 1988). In immunohistochemical studies, the spindle cells are reactive focally for vimentin, actin, and desmin (Pettinato et al, 1990) but not for p53 protein (Ledet et al, 1995). The latter finding may help distinguish inflammatory pseudotumors from some sarcomas. Immunoreactivity for epithelial markers may be present if there are entrapped epithelial cells (Colby et al, 1994). The plasma cells are polyclonal. Ultrastructurally, the spindle cells resemble fibroblasts and myofibroblasts (Pettinato et al, 1990). Cytogenetic analysis may demonstrate clonal chromosomal aberrations in the spindle cells (Su et al, 1998).

Inflammatory pseudotumors must be distinguished from inflammatory fibrosarcoma, a neoplasm that also contains proliferating spindle cells and admixed inflammatory cells (Coffin et al, 1998; Meis & Enzinger, 1991; Meis-Kindblom et al, 1998). Inflammatory fibrosarcoma is recognized by its increased cellularity and significant atypia (Colby et al, 1994), features that may be focally distributed and found only by thorough sampling.

LYMPHOMAS

Hodgkin Disease

Hodgkin disease commonly involves the lung by direct extension from the mediastinum, but pulmonary involvement also occurs at dissemination. In 105 patients with Hodgkin disease under 14 years of age, radiographic evidence of lung involvement was present in 14.3% of cases (Kolygin & Vesnin, 1976). The likelihood of pulmonary involvement is correlated with the histologic subtype and is highest in the lymphocyte-depletion category. Primary pulmonary Hodgkin disease is rare in adults (Yousem et al, 1986) and even rarer in children. Only 2 children were included in a series of 61 patients with primary pulmonary Hodgkin disease (Radin, 1990). These 2 children, included in separate reports, were a 12- and a 13-year-old male who presented with cough, chest pain, dyspnea, fatigue and weight loss (Ball et al, 1982; Demos et al, 1982). The chest radiograph of the 12-year-old boy revealed lingular nodules and a left-sided effusion (Demos et al, 1982). The other patient had an unusual pattern of bilateral pulmonary infiltrates (Ball et al, 1982).

The histologic appearance of Hodgkin disease in the lung is similar to that in lymph nodes, with Reed-Sternberg cells in the appropriate cellular milieu required for the diagnosis. Lesions may form large masses or small nodules, the latter with a lymphatic distribution. A diffuse pneumonic pattern has also been described (Ball et al, 1982). Vascular infiltration and necrosis are common, and a granulomatous reaction may also be seen (Colby et al, 1994). Immunoreactivity of the large cells for CD15 and CD30 may help confirm the diagnosis by differentiating Hodgkin disease from infectious or noninfectious granulomas and other lymphomas.

Low-Grade B Cell Lymphoma

Low-grade B cell lymphomas of mucosa-associated lymphatic tissue (MALT) are the most common primary lymphoma of the lung in adults. These tumors are very rare in children and appear to be limited to the HIV-positive population. A pulmonary low-grade B cell lymphoma of MALT in a 7-year-old, HIV-positive girl manifested as a 4-cm left upper lobe mass was resected surgically (Teruya-Feldstein et al, 1995). The cut surface of this lymphoma was pale tan, smooth, and homogeneous.

Histologically, the pulmonary parenchyma contained numerous germinal centers surrounded by a dense infiltrate of irregular small lymphocytes ("centrocyte-like") and plasma cells. Lymphocytes were also present in the respiratory epithelium. The nearby pulmonary parenchyma exhibited lymphocytic interstitial pneumonitis, which may represent a predisposing factor (Teruya-Feldstein et al, 1995).

In adults, immunohistochemical analysis demonstrating monoclonal light-chain expression and coexpression of CD43 (Leu-22) by the tumor cells supports the diagnosis of lymphoma. Monoclonal immunoglobulin heavy- and light-chain gene rearrangements may be shown by Southern blot analysis. Pathologists are cautioned against diagnosing lymphomas in small lesions or needle biopsy specimens of larger processes on the basis of clonality alone. All lymphomas are clonal, but the converse is not true (Collins, 1997). Lymphoepithelial "lesions" have also been touted as evidence of extranodal lymphoma, although lymphocytes normally traverse mucosal linings, as noted earlier.

Lymphomatoid Granulomatosis

Lymphomatoid granulomatosis is an angiocentric lymphoproliferative disorder with prominent pulmonary involvement (Liebow et al, 1972) that usually effects middle-aged adults (Myers et al, 1995). Rare cases have also been described in children (Drut, 1988; Ilowite et al, 1986; Pearson et al, 1983; Shen et al, 1981). Some of these children had underlying malignant neoplasms or severely depressed immune function (Drut, 1988; Ilowite et al, 1986; Shen et al, 1981). Fever, cough, malaise, and weight loss were common at presentation. Virtually all patients demonstrated pulmonary nodules, but the skin and central nervous system may also be involved. Chest radiographs demonstrated bilateral multiple nodules, most of which were in the lower and peripheral lung fields. Optimal therapy is unknown, but chemotherapy is often used. α_{2b}-Interferon may be effective in some cases (Wilson et al, 1996).

Histologically, arteries and veins are infiltrated by variable numbers of large cells as well as small or medium-sized lymphocytes, plasma cells, and histiocytes. The endothelium is characteristically pushed up by dysplastic cells. Large areas of necrosis are often seen. Immunohistochemical studies reveal a background population of T lymphocytes. The scattered large cells are immunoreactive for B cell markers in most cases and exhibit nuclear labeling for EBV RNA by *in situ* hybridization (Guinee et al, 1994; Myers et al, 1995; Wilson et al, 1996). Immunoglobulin light-chain restriction and immunoglobulin gene rearrangement may also be detected. In a few cases, the large cells are reactive for T cell markers and not for EBV RNA (Myers et al, 1995).

The results of the immunohistochemical and *in situ* hybridization studies indicate that some cases of lymphomatoid granulomatosis resemble T cell–rich B cell lymphomas that are associated with EBV infection (Guinee et al, 1994; Myers et al, 1995; Wilson et al, 1996). The association of immune defects and EBV infection is similar to the pathogenesis of posttransplant lymphoproliferative disorders (PTLDs) (Koss, 1995). Rare cases of lymphomatoid granulomatosis appear to be T cell lymphomas unrelated to EBV infection (Myers et al, 1995).

Anaplastic Large-Cell Lymphoma (Ki-1+)

Anaplastic large-cell lymphoma (ALCL) is a rare, distinct type of high-grade lymphoma associated with peripheral lymphadenopathy and frequent extranodal disease in children and young adults. Skin lesions occur in >20% of patients. Other extranodal sites are bone, soft tissue, gastrointestinal tract, lung, and pleura (Kadin, 1994). The radiographic features of ALCL are usually similar to those of lymphomatoid granulomatosis. Patients with ALCL have a good prognosis when treated with multiagent intensive chemotherapy, with 5-year survival and progression-free survival rates as high as 84 and 72%, respectively (Massimino et al, 1995). However, lung involvement is an unfavorable prognostic indicator.

Most cases of ALCL produce mass lesions that may be necrotic or cavitated. The microscopic features of ALCL in the lung parallel those in the lymph nodes (see Chap. 15). Large anaplastic tumor cells with lobulated, convoluted, or wreath like nuclei and relatively pale cytoplasm are present (Close et al, 1993). Other features include high mitotic rate, necrosis, and a reactive cellular infiltrate at the edge of the lesion. Approximately 70% of Ki-1+ ALCL cases are of T cell lineage, 15% are of B cell lineage, and 15% are undefined (Kadin, 1994).

Morphologic variants of ALCL resemble carcinoma, syncytial variant of nodular sclerosing Hodgkin disease, malignant histiocytosis or interdigitating cell sarcoma, and mycosis fungoides (Kadin, 1994). ALCL may be distinguished from these morphologically similar disorders by immunophenotypic features, since ACLCs are typically CD30+, CD45+, CD15−, CD68−, EMA positive, and keratin negative.

Langerhans Cell Histiocytosis

Langerhans cell histiocytosis (LCH), a disease complex previously known as histiocytosis X, is characterized by the proliferation of Langerhans cells in one or more organs and is classified according to the extent of disease (Egeler & D'Angio, 1995). In children, the lung is usually involved as part of acute disseminated LCH (Letterer-Siwe disease) or multifocal LCH (Knutsen & Goodman, 1993; Smets et al, 1997). Isolated lung involvement (pulmonary eosinophilic granuloma) typically occurs in adult smokers but occurs infrequently in children (McDowell et al, 1988; Nondahl et al, 1986; O'Donnell et al, 1987). Tachypnea with rib retraction is often the only clinical evidence of pulmonary involvement, but fever and weight loss may also be prominent (Egeler & D'Angio, 1995). Radiographic findings include reticular or micronodular opacities as well as large nodules or honeycombing.

Histologically, lung lesions in multifocal LCH and isolated pulmonary eosinophilic granuloma are similar (Colby & Lombard, 1983). Early lesions are often centered on bronchioles and appear as interstitial infiltrates of Langerhans cells, a variable number of eosinophils, and other inflammatory cells. Later the cellular infiltrates enlarge, and their center is gradually replaced by fibroblastic proliferation and scarring. Lesions at various stages of development may be observed in biopsy specimens. The most characteristic lesion is a stellate scar with an active, cellular zone at the periphery. In most cases, the lesions "burn out" and appear as scattered, nondescript scars. In progressive disease, parenchyma is progressively involved, and the scars become confluent. The interstitial infiltrates in Letterer-Siwe disease are diffuse, monomorphic, and rarely associated with fibrosis (Fig. 20–2).

Clusters of Langerhans cells in the pulmonary interstitium are pathognomonic of LCH, but it should be emphasized that scattered Langerhans cells may be identified in a wide variety of conditions (Casolaro et al, 1988; Colasante et al, 1993; Hammar et al, 1986; Kawanami et al, 1981; Soler et al, 1989). Langerhans cells are large mononuclear cells with bland-appearing, folded nuclei, often with a central groove. The chromatin is usually finely dispersed, and the nucleus may contain a small nucleolus. Immunohistochemical staining for either CD1a antigen or S-100 protein highlights the presence of Langerhans cells. Immunoreactivity for the CD1a antigen is more specific, since it is absent in other histiocytic disorders (Emile et al, 1995). Ultrastructurally, Langerhans cells contain characteristic racquet-shaped Birbeck granules.

Leukemic Infiltrates

Involvement of the lung by leukemia is usually seen in previously diagnosed patients (Colby, 1994) and is rarely a presenting manifestation of leukemia. At autopsy, pulmonary involvement is frequent, but clinically significant leukemic infiltrates during life are uncommon, since respiratory symptoms in leukemia are most often due to complicating infections. Chest radiographs of patients with leukemic infiltrates reveal a diffuse interstitial pattern (Georgitis et al, 1979) or, rarely, a mixed interstitial and nodular pattern (Corbaton et al, 1984). Radiographic distinction between leukemic infiltration and infection may be difficult, requiring lung biopsy to establish the diagnosis.

Microscopically, leukemic infiltrates are present along the lymphatic routes and in the interstitium (Colby et al, 1994). Infiltration of the alveolar walls is usually inconspicuous in comparison with perivascular and peribronchiolar infiltration. Infection may elicit similar infiltrates in patients with leukemia. Patients with very high peripheral blast counts may develop pulmonary leukostasis. Chemotherapy may produce necrosis of leukemic blasts that become lodged in the pulmonary vasculature and lead to secondary thrombosis, pulmonary edema, and hemorrhage (Myers et al, 1983). Rarely, patients with massive tumor lysis after treatment develop pulmonary vascular obstruction by fragments of leukemic cells and DNA (Swerdlow et al, 1985).

Posttransplant Lymphoproliferative Disorders

Posttransplant lymphoproliferative disorder (PTLD) is a serious EBV-related complication of organ transplantation that is

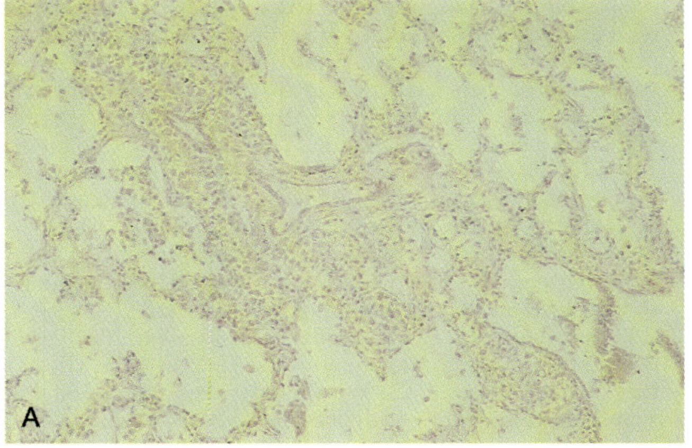

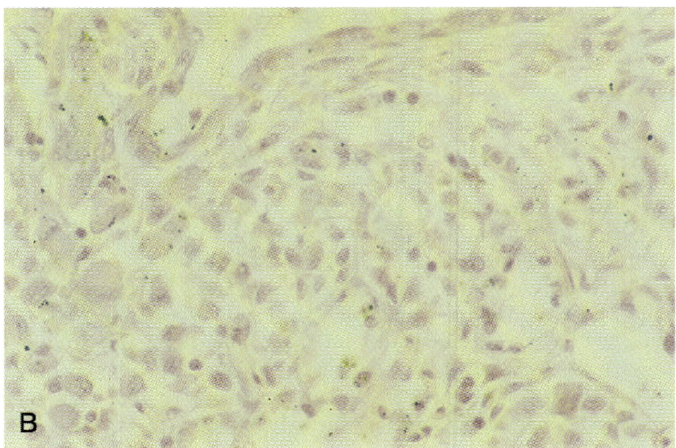

Figure 20–2

Letterer-Siwe disease, lung. *A*, A monomorphous interstitial infiltrate is present. There is no significant fibrosis. *B*, At higher magnification the infiltrate is seen to be composed principally of Langerhans cells, some of which appear multinucleated.

commonest among thoracic organ recipients, who require relatively high levels of immunosuppression (Randhawa et al, 1989). PTLD also occurs with greater frequency in children than in adults, with its incidence among pediatric heart-lung and lung transplant patients as high as 19.5% (Boyle et al, 1997). The lung is one of the extranodal sites most commonly affected by PTLD. Presentation is variable, ranging from asymptomatic nodules on chest radiograph to respiratory failure. Multiple, well-circumscribed pulmonary nodules with or without mediastinal adenopathy are highly suggestive of PTLD (Dodd et al, 1992), but pathologic examination is usually necessary for diagnosis.

PTLDs exhibit a wide spectrum of histologic changes and are classified as polymorphous or monomorphous (Craig et al, 1993). The polymorphous type exhibits a mixture of small lymphocytes, plasma cells, and transformed lymphocytes, whereas the monomorphous type resembles large-cell lymphoma, since it is composed principally of large cells. Vascular invasion and necrosis are often present. With reduced immunosuppression, PTLDs may involute, leaving behind ghost outlines of proliferating cells and a peripheral granulomatous reaction (Yousem & Colby, 1992). Polymorphous PTLD responds more frequently to reduced immunosuppression than does monomorphous PTLD. In immunohistochemical studies, the proliferating cells are usually found to be of B cell lineage. Polymorphous lesions usually display a polyclonal mixture of light chains, whereas monomorphous lesions are usually monoclonal. By molecular techniques, EBV may be demonstrated in most cases.

Pulmonary Complications in Children with Hematologic Malignancies

Children with hematologic malignancies are predisposed to a variety of infections as a consequence of their compromised immune status. Pulmonary pathogens encountered in immunocompromised hosts include gram-positive and gram-negative bacteria, fungi, and viruses (Shorter et al, 1988; Stokes et al, 1989; Winer-Muram et al, 1997). Clinically, infected patients usually present with pulmonary distress. Chest x-rays show diffuse alveolar, interstitial, or localized infiltrates. Histologically, infections are commonly represented by nonspecific reactions that replace the normal inflammatory response (Katzenstein, 1997). Aspergillosis is the most frequently diagnosed fungal infection (Logan et al, 1995). It is often invasive, producing extensive necrosis and hemorrhage in which fungi are difficult to see on routine stains. However, the branching, septate hyphae are readily recognizable with methenamine silver stains. Infection by *Pneumocystis carinii* usually elicits diffuse alveolar damage in children with hematologic malignancies. Typical foamy intraalveolar exudates are rarely seen. The most common viral pathogen is cytomegalovirus, which commonly produces diffuse alveolar damage (Crawford et al, 1989). Characteristic viral inclusions are not always present, and immunohistochemical, in situ hybridization, or polymerase chain reaction studies may be required for diagnosis (Barbera et al, 1996; Burgart et al, 1991).

Diffuse alveolar hemorrhage constitutes a heterogeneous group of disorders with various causes that may develop in children with hematologic malignancies. Especially common after marrow transplantation (Agusti et al, 1995; Winer-Muram et al, 1994), it is often seen in association with pulmonary infection or diffuse alveolar damage (Agusti et al, 1995). Patients usually present with acute respiratory failure, and their mortality rate is high. Chest radiographs show a diffuse alveolar pattern. Histologically, diffuse alveolar hemorrhage is manifested by intraalveolar red blood cells, fibrin, and hemosiderin-laden macrophages. Since extravasation of red blood cells may be secondary to the surgical procedure in a biopsy specimen, diffuse alveolar hemorrhage should not be diagnosed without the presence of hemosiderin-laden macrophages or an appropriate clinical history.

Diffuse alveolar damage is the usual histologic finding in patients with adult respiratory distress syndrome. In children with hematologic malignancies, similar alveolar damage may be associated with pulmonary infection, drug toxicity, shock, sepsis, and leukemic cell lysis (Tryka et al, 1982). The prognosis is generally poor, but surviving patients demonstrate little or no pulmonary function abnormalities. Histologically, the acute phase of diffuse alveolar damage, the first week of injury, is characterized by alveolar and interstitial edema as well as hyaline membranes. Mild interstitial mononuclear cell infiltrate and type 2 cell hyperplasia may also be observed. The organizing phase, after the first week, is distinguished by a fibroblastic proliferation that involves predominantly the alveolar septa. Type 2 cell hyperplasia is still present, but only remnants of hyaline membranes are seen. Tests with special stains should always be performed to exclude underlying infection. The presence of focal necrosis is particularly suggestive of an infectious agent. Abundant neutrophils usually mark bacterial infection or superinfection. Otherwise, there are no specific features to suggest a particular cause, and many cases of diffuse alveolar damage remain unresolved. Although it is difficult to prove, the majority of unresolved cases may represent drug reactions (Logan et al, 1995).

Bronchiolitis obliterans organizing pneumonia is a well-defined clinicopathologic entity that may be idiopathic. When seen in children with hematologic malignancies, it may be related to drug toxicity or unidentified infectious agents (Battistini et al, 1997). Patients usually develop low-grade fever and cough. Imaging studies reveal bilateral patchy opacities (Mathew et al, 1994; Winer-Muram et al, 1997). The treatment of choice is steroids in most cases. The prognosis is generally excellent, but fatalities have been reported (Mathew et al, 1994). The histologic hallmark of bronchiolitis obliterans organizing pneumonia is the presence of pale-staining fibroblastic plugs filling the bronchiolar lumina and extending into the peribronchiolar air spaces (Fig. 20–3). The lesions are patchy and are sharply demarcated from the adjacent pulmonary parenchyma. Sometimes, features of both diffuse alveolar damage and bronchiolitis obliterans organizing pneumonia coexist. Such cases may be diagnosed as acute lung injury pattern (Katzenstein, 1997), but the prognosis is usually determined by the diffuse alveolar damage.

Constrictive bronchiolitis obliterans, or obliterative bronchiolitis, is a common complication of marrow transplantation and is usually associated with chronic graft-versus-host disease (Sargent et al, 1995; Schultz et al, 1994). Patients present with nonproductive cough, wheezing, and dyspnea. Pulmonary function tests demonstrate obstructive lung disease. The clinical course is variable, but the process is often fatal, particularly when the obstruction is severe or rapidly progressive (Crawford & Clark, 1993). Interventions are directed at immuno suppression and at diagnosing and treating secondary infections. Histologically, the bronchiolar lumens are narrowed by concentric mural fibrosis. Intraluminal fibroblastic plugs, characteristic of bronchiolitis obliterans organizing pneumonia, are not seen in constrictive bronchiolitis obliterans.

The lung may also be the site of leukemic relapse, which should be considered among the differential diagnostic possibilities in a child with history of leukemia (Georgitis et al, 1979). Chest radiographs reveal nondescript interstitial or nodular patterns, and a lung biopsy may be necessary for diagnosis (Corbaton et al, 1984).

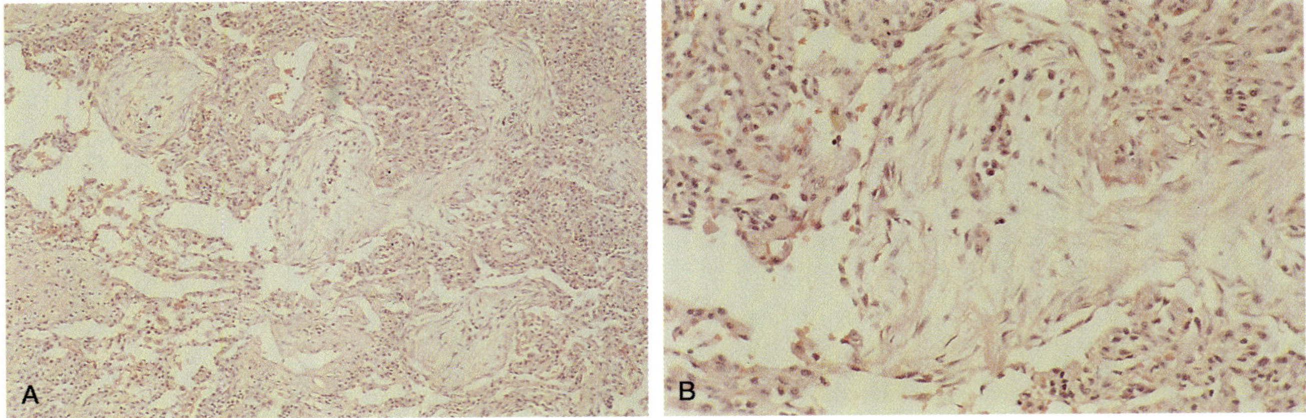

Figure 20–3

Bronchiolitis obliterans organizing pneumonia, lung. *A*, Fibroblastic plugs are prominent even at low magnification. Mild inflammation of alveolar septeum is also present. *B*, Fibroblastic plugs are located within the air spaces and are composed of fibroblasts and pale-staining matrix.

Pulmonary Complications in Children with Immunodeficiencies

Pulmonary complications commonly occur in children with congenital immunodeficiencies as well as those with iatrogenic immunodeficiencies and AIDS (Deerojanawong et al, 1997; Marolda et al, 1991). Infections are the commonest type of pulmonary pathologic condition (Grattan-Smith et al, 1992; Izraeli et al, 1996; Moran et al, 1994). The infectious complications in this group of patients are similar to those in children with hematologic malignancies (discussed earlier), with some differences (Foglia et al, 1989; Joshi et al, 1990; Logan et al, 1995; McSherry, 1996). *Pneumocystis carinii* usually produces diffuse alveolar damage in children with hematologic malignancies but causes the more typical frothy exudates in patients with AIDS. Mycobacterial infections are more common in patients with AIDS than in those with hematologic malignancies (Martinez-Arroyo et al, 1996; Taylor et al, 1995).

The spectrum of pulmonary lymphatic lesions associated with congenital or acquired immunodeficiency states includes follicular bronchitis or bronchiolitis (Yousem et al, 1985a), lymphocytic interstitial pneumonia (Joshi et al, 1997; Nielsen et al, 1997; Scott et al, 1989), and low-grade B cell lymphoma (Teruya-Feldstein et al, 1995). EBV-associated lymphoproliferative disorders also occur and are apparently analogous to PTLDs (Elenitoba-Johnson & Jaffe, 1997; Joshi et al, 1987). Diffuse alveolar damage is a common complication of immunosuppression and may be due to combination of such factors as opportunistic infection and oxygen therapy (Joshi et al, 1985). Desquamative interstitial pneumonia–like reaction, characterized by large intraalveolar collections of mononuclear cells and type 2 cell hyperplasia, has also been described in children with AIDS (Joshi et al, 1985).

REFERENCES

Agusti C, Ramirez J, Picado C, et al: Diffuse alveolar hemorrhage in allogeneic bone marrow transplantation: a postmortem study. Am J Respir Crit Care Med 151:1006–1010, 1995.

Andiman WA, Eastman R, Martin K, et al: Opportunistic lymphoproliferations associated with Epstein-Barr viral DNA in infants and children with AIDS. Lancet 2:1390–1393, 1985.

Athreya BH, Doughty RA, Bookspan M, et al: Pulmonary manifestations of juvenile rheumatoid arthritis: a report of eight cases and review. Clin Chest Med 1:361–374, 1980.

Ball DG, Herman TE, Variakojis D, et al: Primary pulmonary Hodgin's disease: a case report. Arch Intern Med 142:1941–1943, 1982.

Barbera JA, Martin-Campos JM, Ribalta T, et al: Undetected viral infection in diffuse alveolar damage associated with bone marrow transplantation. Eur Respir J 9:1195–200, 1996.

Battistini E, Dini G, Savioli C, et al: Bronchiolitis obliterans organizing pneumonia in three children with acute leukaemias treated with cytosine arabinoside and anthracyclines. Eur Respir J 10: 1187–1190, 1997.

Biselli R, Ferlini C, Fattorossi A, et al: Inflammatory myofibroblastic tumor (inflammatory pseudotumor): DNA flow cytometric analysis of nine pediatric cases. Cancer 77:778–784, 1996.

Boyle GJ, Michaels MG, Webber SA, et al: Posttransplantation lymphoproliferative disorders in pediatric thoracic organ recipients. J Pediatr 131:309–313, 1997.

Bramson RT, Cleveland R, Blickman JG, et al: Radiographic appearance of follicular bronchitis in children. AJR 166:1447–1450, 1996.

Burgart LJ, Heller MJ, Reznicek MJ, et al: Cytomegalovirus detection in bone marrow transplant patients with idiopathic pneumonitis: a clinicopathologic study of the clinical utility of the polymerase chain reaction on open lung biopsy specimen tissue. Am J Clin Pathol 96:572–576, 1991.

Casolaro MA, Bernaudin JF, Saltini C, et al: Accumulation of Langerhans' cells on the epithelial surface of the lower respiratory tract in normal subjects in association with cigarette smoking. Am Rev Respir Dis 137:406–411, 1988.

Close PM, Macrae MB, Hammond JM, et al: Anaplastic large-cell Ki-1 lymphoma: pulmonary presentation mimicking miliary tuberculosis. Am J Clin Pathol 99:631–636, 1993.

Coffin CM, Dehner LP, Meis-Kindblom JM: Inflammatory myofibroblastic tumor, inflammatory fibrosarcoma, and related lesions: an historical review with differential diagnostic considerations. Semin Diagn Pathol 15:102–110, 1998.

Colasante A, Poletti V, Rosini S, et al: Langerhans cells in Langerhans cell histiocytosis and peripheral adenocarcinomas of the lung. Am Rev Respir Dis 148:752–759, 1993.

Colby TV: Lymphoproliferative diseases. In Dail DH, Hammar SP (eds): Pulmonary Pathology. Springer-Verlag, New York, pp 1097–1122, 1994.

Colby TV, Koss MN, Travis WD: Tumors of the lower respiratory tract. In Atlas of Tumor Pathology, 3rd series, fascicle 13. Armed Forces Institute of Pathology, Washington, DC, 1994.

Colby TV, Lombard C: Histiocytosis X in the lung. Hum Pathol 14:847–856, 1983.

Collins RD: Is clonality equivalent to malignancy: specifically, is immunoglobulin gene rearrangement diagnostic of malignant lymphoma? Hum Pathol 28:757–759, 1997.

Corbaton J, Munoz A, Madero L, et al: Pulmonary leukemia in a child presenting with infiltrative and nodular lesions. Pediatr Radiol 14:431-432, 1984.

Craig FE, Gulley ML, Banks PM: Posttransplantation lymphoproliferative disorders. Am J Clin Pathol 99:265–276, 1993.

Crawford SW, Clark JG: Bronchiolitis associated with bone marrow transplantation. Clin Chest Med 14:741–749, 1993.

Crawford SW, Hackman RC, Clark JG: Biopsy diagnosis and clinical outcome of persistent focal pulmonary lesions after marrow transplantation. Transplantation 48:266–271, 1989.

Deerojanawong J, Chang AB, Eng PA, et al: Pulmonary diseases in children with severe combined immune deficiency and DiGeorge syndrome. Pediatr Pulmonol 24:324–330, 1997.

Demos PA, Johnson BL, Putnam WD, et al: Unusual presentation of Hodgkins disease in a twelve-year-old boy with left pleural effusion and weight loss of four months duration. S D J Med, 35:17–22, 1982.

Dodd GDD, Ledesma-Medina J, Baron RL: Posttransplant lymphoproliferative disorder: intrathoracic manifestations. Radiology 184:65–69, 1992.

Drut R: Angiocentric B-cell lymphoma of the lung in an immunocompromised boy. Pediatr Pathol 8:395–400, 1988.

Egeler RM, D'Angio GJ: Langerhans cell histiocytosis. J Pediatr 127:1–11, 1995.

Elenitoba-Johnson KS, Jaffe ES: Lymphoproliferative disorders associated with congenital immunodeficiencies. Semin Diagn Pathol 14:35–47, 1997.

Emile JF, Wechsler J, Brousse N, et al: Langerhans' cell histiocytosis: definitive diagnosis with the use of monoclonal antibody O10 on routinely paraffin-embedded samples. Am J Surg Pathol 19:636–641, 1995.

Fishback N, Koss M: Update on lymphoid interstitial pneumonitis. Curr Opin Pulm Med 2:429–433, 1996.

Foglia RP, Shilyansky J, Fonkalsrud EW: Emergency lung biopsy in immunocompromised pediatric patients. Ann Surg 210:90–92, 1989.

Franchi LM, Chin TW, Nussbaum E, et al: Familial pulmonary nodular lymphoid hyperplasia. J Pediatr 121:89–92, 1992.

Georgitis J, Eigen H, Provisor D, et al: Isolated pulmonary leukemic relapse following successful bone marrow transplant in a child with acute lymphoblastic leukemia. Pediatrics 64:913–917, 1979.

Grattan-Smith D, Harrison LF, Singleton EB: Radiology of AIDS in the pediatric patient. Curr Probl Diagn Radiol 21:79–109, 1992.

Guinee D Jr, Jaffe E, Kingma D, et al: Pulmonary lymphomatoid granulomatosis: evidence for a proliferation of Epstein-Barr virus infected B-lymphocytes with a prominent T-cell component and vasculitis. Am J Surg Pathol 18:753–764, 1994.

Hammar S, Bockus D, Remington F, et al: The widespread distribution of Langerhans cells in pathologic tissues: an ultrastructural and immunohistochemical study. Hum Pathol 17:894–905, 1986.

Hartman GE, Shochat SJ: Primary pulmonary neoplasms of childhood: a review. Ann Thorac Surg 36:108–119, 1983.

Ilowite NT, Fligner CL, Ochs HD, et al: Pulmonary angiitis with atypical lymphoreticular infiltrates in Wiskott-Aldrich syndrome: possible relationship of lymphomatoid granulomatosis and EBV infection. Clin Immunol Immunopathol 41:479–484, 1986.

Izraeli S, Mueller BU, Ling A, et al: Role of tissue diagnosis in pulmonary involvement in pediatric human immunodeficiency virus infection. Pediatr Infect Dis J 15:112–116, 1996.

Joshi VV, Gagnon GA, Chadwick EG, et al: The spectrum of mucosa-associated lymphoid tissue lesions in pediatric patients infected with HIV: a clinicopathologic study of six cases. Am J Clin Pathol 107:592–600, 1997.

Joshi VV, Kauffman S, Oleske JM, et al: Polyclonal polymorphic B-cell lymphoproliferative disorder with prominent pulmonary involvement in children with acquired immune deficiency syndrome. Cancer 59:1455–1462, 1987.

Joshi VV, Oleske JM, Connor EM: Morphologic findings in children with acquired immune deficiency syndrome: pathogenesis and clinical implications. Pediatr Pathol 10:155–165, 1990.

Joshi VV, Oleske JM, Minnefor AB, et al: Pathologic pulmonary findings in children with the acquired immunodeficiency syndrome: a study of ten cases. Hum Pathol 16:241–246, 1985.

Kadin ME: Primary Ki-1-positive anaplastic large-cell lymphoma: a distinct clinicopathologic entity. Ann Oncol 5(suppl 1): 25–30, 1994.

Katzenstein A-LA: Katzenstein and Askin's Surgical Pathology of Non-Neoplastic Lung Disease, vol. 13. Major Problems in Pathology. W.B. Saunders Company, Philadelphia, 1997.

Kaufman RA: Calcified postinflammatory pseudotumor of the lung: CT features. J Comput Assist Tomogr 12:653–665, 1988.

Kawanami O, Basset F, Ferrans VJ, et al: Pulmonary Langerhans' cells in patients with fibrotic lung disorders. Lab Invest 44:227–233, 1981.

Kim I, Kim WS, Yeon KM, et al: Inflammatory pseudotumor of the lung manifesting as a posterior mediastinal mass. Pediatr Radiol 22:467–468, 1992.

Kinane BT, Mansell AL, Zwerdling RG, et al: Follicular bronchitis in the pediatric population. Chest 104:1183–1186, 1993.

Knutsen AP, Goodman GM: A 13-month-old child with chronic diarrhea, weight loss, and tachypnea [clinical conference]. Ann Allergy 71:352–356, 1993.

Kolygin BA, Vesnin AG: Hodgkin's disease in children: clinicoroentgenologic features of the lesion in the chest. Pediatr Radiol 4:144–148, 1976.

Koss MN: Pulmonary lymphoid disorders. Semin Diagn Pathol 12:158–171, 1995.

Koss MN, Hochholzer L, Langloss JM, et al: Lymphoid interstitial pneumonia: clinicopathological and immunopathological findings in 18 cases. Pathology 19:178–185, 1987.

Kradin RL, Mark EJ: Benign lymphoid disorders of the lung, with a theory regarding their development. Hum Pathol 14:857–867, 1983.

Ledet SC, Brown RW, Cagle PT: p53 immunostaining in the differentiation of inflammatory pseudotumor from sarcoma involving the lung. Mod Pathol 8:282–286, 1995.

Liebow AA, Carrington CB: Diffuse pulmonary lymphoreticular infiltrations associated with dysproteinemia. Med Clin North Am 57:809–843, 1973.

Liebow AA, Carrington CR, Friedman PJ: Lymphomatoid granulomatosis. Hum Pathol 3:457–558, 1972.

Logan PM, Primack SL, Staples C, et al: Acute lung disease in the immunocompromised host: diagnostic accuracy of the chest radiograph. Chest 108:1283–1287, 1995.

Maier HC, Sommers SC: Recurrent and metastatic pulmonary fibrous histiocytoma/plasma cell granuloma in a child. Cancer 60: 1073–1076, 1987.

Marolda J, Pace B, Bonforte RJ, et al: Pulmonary manifestations of HIV infection in children. Pediatr Pulmonol 10:231–235, 1991.

Martinez-Arroyo L, Ramos Amadon JT, Cela de Julian E, et al: Fatal Mycobacterium avium complex disease in a patient with acute nonlymphoblastic leukemia. J Pediatr Hematol Oncol 18: 218–222, 1996.

Massimino M, Gasparini M, Giardini R: Ki-1 (CD30) anaplastic large-cell lymphoma in children. Ann Oncol 6:915–920, 1995.

Mathew P, Bozeman P, Krance RA, et al: Bronchiolitis obliterans organizing pneumonia (BOOP) in children after allogeneic bone marrow transplantation. Bone Marrow Transplant 13:221–223, 1994.

Matsubara O, Tan-Liu NS, Kenney RM, et al: Inflammatory pseudotumors of the lung: progression from organizing pneumonia to fibrous histiocytoma or to plasma cell granuloma in 32 cases. Hum Pathol 19:807–814, 1988.

McDowell HP, Macfarlane PI, Martin J: Isolated pulmonary histiocytosis. Arch Dis Child 63:423–426, 1988.

McSherry GD: Human immunodeficiency-virus–related pulmonary infections in children. Semin Respir Infect 11:173–183, 1996.

Meis JM, Enzinger FM: Inflammatory fibrosarcoma of the mesentery and retroperitoneum: a tumor closely simulating inflammatory pseudotumor. Am J Surg Pathol 15:1146–1156, 1991.

Meis-Kindblom JM, Kjellstrom C, Kindblom LG: Inflammatory fibrosarcoma: update, reappraisal, and perspective on its place in the spectrum of inflammatory myofibroblastic tumors. Semin Diagn Pathol 15:133–143, 1998.

Moran CA, Suster S, Pavlova Z, et al: The spectrum of pathological changes in the lung in children with the acquired immunodeficiency syndrome: an autopsy study of 36 cases. Hum Pathol 25:877–882, 1994.

Myers JL, Kurtin PJ, Katzenstein AL, et al: Lymphomatoid granulomatosis: evidence of immunophenotypic diversity and relationship to Epstein-Barr virus infection. Am J Surg Pathol 19:1300–1312, 1995.

Myers TJ, Cole SR, Klatsky AU, et al: Respiratory failure due to pulmonary leukostasis following chemotherapy of acute nonlymphocytic leukemia. Cancer 51:1808–1813, 1983.

Nicholson AG, Wotherspoon AC, Diss TC, et al: Reactive pulmonary lymphoid disorders. Histopathology 26:405–412, 1995.

Nielsen K, McSherry G, Petru A, et al: A descriptive survey of pediatric human immunodeficiency virus-infected long-term survivors. Pediatrics 99:593–594, 1997.

Nondahl SR, Finlay JL, Farrell PM, et al: A case report and literature review of "primary" pulmonary histiocytosis X of childhood. Med Pediatr Oncol 14:57–62, 1986.

O'Donnell AE, Tsou E, Awh C, et al: Endobronchial eosinophilic granuloma: a rare cause of total lung atelectasis. Am Rev Respir Dis 136:1478–1480, 1987.

Pabst R, Gehrke I: Is the bronchus-associated lymphoid tissue (BALT) an integral structure of the lung in normal mammals, including humans? Am J Respir Cell Mol Biol 3:131–135, 1990.

Pearson AD, Kirpalani H, Ashcroft T, et al: Lymphomatoid granulomatosis in a 10 year old boy. Br Med J 286:1313–1314, 1983.

Pettinato G, Manivel JC, De Rosa N, et al: Inflammatory myofibroblastic tumor (plasma cell granuloma): clinicopathologic study of 20 cases with immunohistochemical and ultrastructural observations. Am J Clin Pathol 94:538–546, 1990.

Radin AI: Primary pulmonary Hodgkin's disease. Cancer 65:550–563, 1990.

Randhawa PS, Yousem SA, Paradis IL, et al: The clinical spectrum, pathology, and clonal analysis of Epstein Barr virus–associated lymphoproliferative disorders in heart-lung transplant recipients. Am J Clin Pathol 92:177–185, 1989.

Rubinstein A, Morecki R, Silverman B, et al: Pulmonary disease in children with acquired immune deficiency syndrome and AIDS-related complex. J Pediatr 108:498–503, 1986.

Salisbury JR: Castleman's disease in childhood and adolescence: report of a case and review of literature. Pediatr Pathol 10:609–615, 1990.

Sargent MA, Cairns RA, Murdoch MJ, et al: Obstructive lung disease in children after allogeneic bone marrow transplantation: evaluation with high-resolution CT. AJR 164, 693–696, 1995.

Schultz KR, Green GJ, Wensley D, et al: Obstructive lung disease in children after allogeneic bone marrow transplantation. Blood 84:3212–3220, 1994.

Scott GB, Hutto C, Makuch RW, et al: Survival in children with perinatally acquired human immunodeficiency virus type 1 infection. N Engl J Med 321:1791–1796, 1989.

Shen SC, Heuser ET, Landing BH, et al: Lymphomatoid granulomatosis-like lesions in a child with leukemia in remission. Hum Pathol 12:276–280, 1981.

Shorter NA, Ross AJD, August C, et al: The usefulness of open-lung biopsy in the pediatric bone marrow transplant population. J Pediatr Surg 23:533–537, 1988.

Smets A, Mortel E, Praeter GD, et al: Pulmonary and mediastinal lesions in children with Langerhans cell histiocytosis. Pediatr Radiol 27:873–876, 1997.

Soler P, Moreau A, Basset F, et al: Cigarette smoking–induced changes in the number and differentiated state of pulmonary dendritic cells/Langerhans cells. Am Rev Respir Dis 139:1112–1117, 1989.

Spencer H: The pulmonary plasma cell/histiocytoma complex. Histopathology 8:903–916, 1984.

Stokes DC, Shenep JL, Parham D, et al: Role of flexible bronchoscopy in the diagnosis of pulmonary infiltrates in pediatric patients with cancer. J Pediatr 115:561–567, 1989.

Su LD, Atayde-Perez A, Sheldon S, et al: Inflammatory myofibroblastic tumor: cytogenetic evidence supporting clonal origin. Mod Pathol 11:364–368, 1998.

Swerdlow SH, Glick AD, Cousar JB, et al: Acute leukemias of childhood: pathologic features. Hematol Oncol 3:99–131, 1985.

Taylor IK, Coker RJ, Clarke J, et al: Pulmonary complications of HIV disease: 10 year retrospective evaluation of yields from bronchoalveolar lavage, 1983–93. Thorax 50:1240–1245, 1995.

Teirstein AS, Rosen MJ: Lymphocytic interstitial pneumonia. Clin Chest Med 9:467–471, 1988.

Teruya-Feldstein J, Temeck BK, Sloas MM, et al: Pulmonary malignant lymphoma of mucosa-associated lymphoid tissue (MALT) arising in a pediatric HIV-positive patient. Am J Surg Pathol 19:357–363, 1995.

Tryka AF, Godleski JJ, Fanta CH: Leukemic cell lysis pneumonopathy: a complication of treated myeloblastic leukemia. Cancer 50:2763–70, 1982.

Wilson WH, Kingma DW, Raffeld M, et al: Association of lymphomatoid granulomatosis with Epstein-Barr viral infection of B lymphocytes and response to interferon-alpha 2b. Blood 87:4531–4537, 1996.

Winer-Muram HT, Arheart KL, Jennings SG, et al: Pulmonary complications in children with hematologic malignancies: accuracy of diagnosis with chest radiography and CT. Radiology 204:643–649, 1997.

Winer-Muram HT, Rubin SA, Fletcher BD, et al: Childhood leukemia: diagnostic accuracy of bedside chest radiography for severe pulmonary complications. Radiology 193:127–133, 1994.

Yousem SA, Colby TV: Pulmonary lymphomas and lymphoid hyperplasias. In Knowles DM (ed): Neoplastic Hematopathology. Williams & Wilkins, Baltimore, pp 979–1007, 1992.

Yousem SA, Colby TV, Carrington CB: Follicular bronchitis/bronchiolitis. Hum Pathol 16:700–706, 1985a.

Yousem SA, Colby TV, Carrington CB: Lung biopsy in rheumatoid arthritis. Am Rev Respir Dis 131:770–777, 1985b.

Yousem SA, Weiss LM, Colby TV: Primary pulmonary Hodgkin's disease: a clinicopathologic study of 15 cases. Cancer 57:1217–1224, 1986.

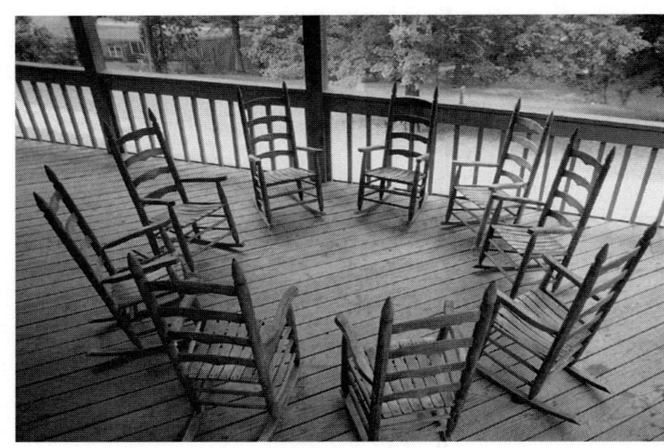

Camp Horizon, near Nashville. Porch scene.

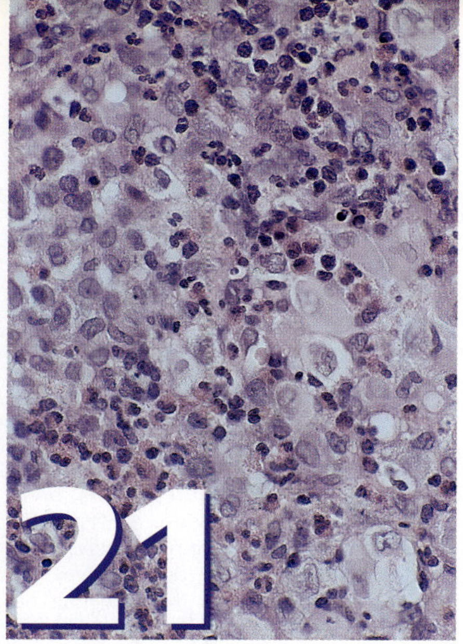

Todd Murry
Kathy Hamilton
Robert D. Collins

Skin and Subcutaneous Tissue

STRUCTURE AND FUNCTION OF SKIN AS AN IMMUNE ORGAN

The principal function of the skin is to provide a barrier between the external and internal environments, a function chiefly accomplished by the formidable mechanical barrier of the stratum corneum. The skin also has well-developed immunologic defenses capable of reacting to and removing foreign antigens that have penetrated this layer. Some of the cells involved in this immunologic shielding have structural and functional features that are unique to the skin. The immunologic responses in the skin follow the same general course as those in other parts of the body. Beginning with antigen presentation, a complex cascade of signals and events follows, resulting, it is hoped, in the removal of the offending agent. The cells involved are briefly described here.

Langerhans Cells

The Langerhans cell, a marrow-derived histiocyte, is the major antigen-presenting cell in the skin (Choi, 1986; Katz et al, 1997). Located in the suprabasal epithelium, Langerhans cells have dendritic processes that extend upward toward the granular layer of the epidermis, forming a net poised to catch antigenic material penetrating the epidermis. After exposure to a soluble antigen or hapten, Langerhans cells migrate to regional lymph nodes and present the foreign material to naive T lymphocytes (Hauser et al, 1991; Katz, 1985).

Lymphocytes

T lymphocytes are the principal immunoreactive cell of the skin (Katz, 1985). Upon antigen presentation by Langerhans cells, naive T cells proliferate clonally, producing memory T cells, which circulate and concentrate at the antigen presentation site in the skin via adhesion molecules expressed on the "activated" vascular endothelium (Santamaria Babi et al, 1995). This process is referred to as sensitization. The vascular activation is mediated, at least in part, by antigen-specific degranulation of mast cells (Klein et al, 1989). On all subsequent challenges (or a persistent challenge with the same antigen), these T cells initiate a complex feedback-controlled elaboration of cytokines, resulting in the recruitment of other immunologic cells (Issekutz et al, 1988). This immune response should result in phagocytosis and removal of the offending agent. Appropriate immune reactions in the skin serve as an important host defense, but inappropriate responses may produce diseases such as eczematous dermatitis.

B lymphocytes as the humoral arm of immune reactions usually proliferate only in regional nodes. However, in certain instances, B cell proliferation may be localized, usually in the deeper dermis, where germinal centers may form (Murphy & Mihm, 1986). Plasma cells are seen in significant numbers in the skin in reaction to some infectious and neoplastic processes. In some cases plasma cells are presumably produced by nearby germinal centers and in others perhaps by differentiation of small lymphocytes.

Mast Cells

Mast cells are marrow derived and are usually present in the skin in small numbers (Kitamura et al, 1977). These cells apparently function by degranulation in response to a range of stimuli, including thermal and mechanical stimuli and IgE surface binding. Their intracytoplasmic granules release a variety of substances with vasoactive (e.g., histamine), immunologic (e.g., tumor necrosis factor), and mitogenic (e.g., β-fibroblast growth factor) properties (Kobayosi & Asboe-Hansen, 1969). These substances apparently mediate portions of several diverse and complex reactions, including leukocyte adhesion and vascular reaction in the T cell immunologic response, edema in urticarial reactions, and epithelial proliferation in response to nevus evolution (Klein et al, 1989; Unvas, 1991).

Other Hematopoetic and Immunologic cells

Neutrophils are found in a number of reactive conditions (e.g., psoriasis), as the predominant cell in certain conditions (e.g., Sweet syndrome), or as a collection of cells in an abscess. Eosinophils are especially frequent in reactive states involving drugs and arthropods and are the predominant reactive cell in certain autoimmune disorders (e.g., pemphigoid) or within spongiotic vesicles (e.g., incontinentia pigmenti). Macrophages are found in varying numbers in virtually all lymphocyte-rich infiltrates as well as in a host of reactive disorders (e.g., Rosai-Dorfman disease).

REACTIVE STATES

This discussion is restricted to those reactive skin diseases that are likely to be seen in children and that are of particular interest to hematopathologists because of clinical confusion with malignant disease and those in which hematopoietic or immune cells have a central role in pathogenesis or diagnosis.

Blueberry Muffin Syndrome

Definition

The term *blueberry muffin* refers to a clinical appearance characterized by multiple violaceous papulonodular lesions seen in various underlying conditions, including metastatic disease (e.g., neuroblastoma) (Hawthrone et al, 1970); leukemic infiltration (Gottesfield et al, 1989); or, most characteristically, extramedullary hematopoiesis in neonates in response to viral infection (Brough et al, 1967), hemolytic disease (Hebert et al, 1985), or twin-twin transfusions (Schwartz et al, 1984). The term *blueberry muffin syndrome* refers to the presence of these lesions when caused by extramedullary hematopoiesis in newborns.

Clinical Features

Blueberry muffin syndrome is characterized by generalized, multiple violaceous papules and nodules, and other clinical features that vary with the underlying disease. The commonest neoplasm associated with this presentation is neuroblastoma, but leukemia (Gottersfeld et al, 1989), alveolar rhabdomyosarcoma (Kitagawa et al, 1989), and Langerhans cell histiocytosis (Enjolras et al, 1992) may also produce similar lesions. Neonatal viral infections causing this syndrome include rubella, coxsackievirus, and cytomegalovirus (Brough et al, 1967). Erythroblastosis fetalis is almost always accompanied by extramedullary hematopoiesis that may be dermal and widespread (Hebert et al, 1985). Donor twins in twin-twin transfusions likewise have a high incidence of dermal hematopoiesis, which may produce this clinical appearance (Schwartz et al, 1984).

Histopathologic Features

The microscopic features depend on the underlying cause, and biopsy specimens of metastatic lesions and leukemic infiltrates resemble the primary tumors. Dermal extramedullary hematopoiesis is characterized by a polymorphous infiltrate that is predominantly perivascular, is present in the superficial and deep dermis, and consists mostly of myelocytic and erythrocytic elements. Numerous megakaryocytes may occasionally be seen.

Pathogenesis

Extramedullary hematopoiesis presumably is caused by profound and widespread stimulation of hematopoietic elements through feedback mechanisms triggered by massive hemolysis, as in hemolytic disease, or severe marrow injury from viral infections.

Arthropod Bite Reaction

Definition

An exaggerated cutaneous reaction may occur to the bite of a parasite, usually an arthropod, although other organisms, such as mites, may generate a similar reaction. The epidermis must be breached and some persistent antigenic material, such as a segment of proboscis in a mosquito bite or fecal material in scabies, deposited in the skin or subcutaneous tissue.

Clinical Features

Arthropod bite reactions may be seen in patients of any age, sex, or race. The species of the offending organism depends on geographic and socioeconomic factors as well as the nature of outdoor and sexual activities. Clinical appearance also varies, but commonly there are multiple erythematous pruritic papules with a punctate hemorrhagic center and with or without secondary changes, such as excoriation and crusting. Lesions usually begin as papules, but may evolve to bullae or foci of epidermal necrosis. Especially exuberant reactions may be clinically difficult to distinguish from lymphoma (Allen, 1948). This type of lesion is more often seen with tick bites and recently treated scabies infestations.

Histopathologic Features

Epidermal changes often seen are a punctum (epidermal break at the site of injury) and surrounding spongiosis. Parts of the offending organism and necrosis are seen more rarely. Early urticarial and neutrophilic infiltration of the dermis gives way to a wedge-shaped, dense lymphohistiocytic infiltrate that begins around vessels and tends to become diffuse (Fig. 21–1). In most cases, the infiltrate is admixed with eosinophils and plasma cells, although this may not be true in cases of first-contact reactions. Certain arthropods, especially fleas and fire ants, may produce neutrophil-rich infiltrates, while others, especially bees, wasps, and certain spiders and ticks, may produce varying degrees of necrosis (Horen, 1972).

Pathogenesis

The characteristic lesion occurs because of the persistence of antigen, followed by recruitment of immune cells with liberation of cytokines that increase the severity of the infiltrate. Further changes may be caused by superinfection, either primary (if the arthropod itself carries bacterial organisms, as in fire ant bites) or secondary, due to the epidermal defect. Necrotic changes may be caused by direct toxic effects of secreted substances, such as venom in bee stings, or by particularly intense inflammation at the site of contact, as with tick bites. Each type of organism may cause a slightly different reaction pattern.

Tick Bites Specific histologic features are associated with tick bites, including the presence of mouth parts, fibrin plugging of capillaries, necrosis of peripunctum epidermis (Fig. 21–2), and granulomatous inflammation and panniculitis (Krinski, 1983). Furthermore, tick bites are associated with a number of systemic reactions related to infectious agents carried by the tick (Marshall, 1967). The two most clinically important are Lyme

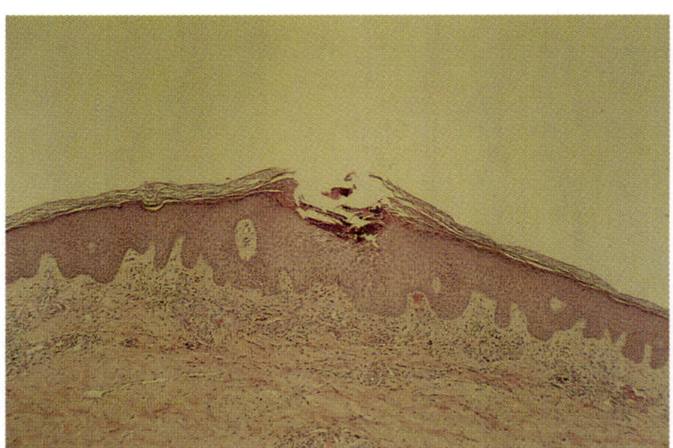

Figure 21–1

Insect bite, skin. At low magnification the punctum and underlying inflammation are visible. The inflammation is wedge shaped, tapering toward the subcutaneous tissue. Plasma cells, lymphocytes, and numerous eosinophils are usually present in insect bites.

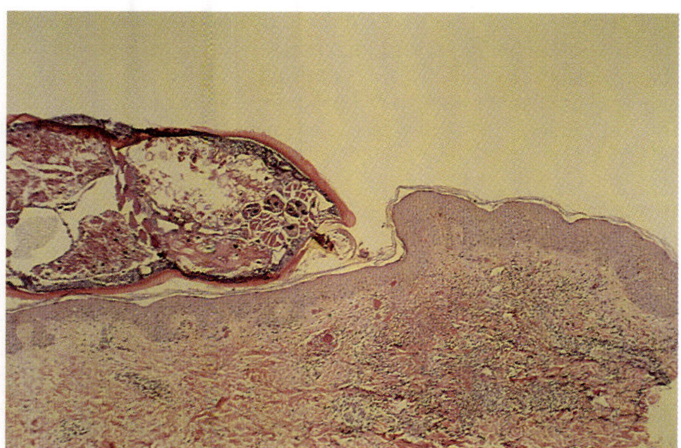

Figure 21–2

Tick bite, skin. The head of the tick is seen, still imbedded within the epidermis. Note the dermal inflammatory reaction.

disease and Rocky Mountain spotted fever. Erythema chronicum migrans is the skin lesion of Lyme disease and is characterized by a dense polymorphous angio-, neuro-, and eccrinotropic infiltrate with spongiotic surface changes. On careful inspection, approximately one or two spirochetal organisms may be seen per section. They are best visualized with Warthin-Starry or Steiner stains. The rash spreads from a central point, in contrast to the persistent nodule produced by a standard arthropod bite. The causative organism is a spirochete *(Borrelia burgdorferi)* that may cause atrophic and sclerotic cutaneous reactions in long-term infections (Berger, 1984). Rocky Mountain spotted fever, caused by *Rickettsia rickettsii*, causes a necrotizing vasculitis that progresses as a disseminated purpuric rash.

Angiolymphoid Hyperplasia with Eosinophilia and Kimura Disease

Definition

Angiolymphoid hyperplasia with eosinophilia, also referred to as epithelioid hemangioma, is characterized by focal proliferation of small to medium-sized arteries lined by epithelioid-appearing endothelial cells (with a "cobblestone" appearance histologically) and a characteristic surrounding inflammatory reaction containing lymphocytes and eosinophils (Wells & Whimster, 1969). Kimura disease is similar to angiolymphoid hyperplasia with eosinophilia except that it occurs in the Far Eastern population as well as having a wider age range, more extensive lesions, and slight histologic differences (Kimura et al, 1948).

Clinical Features

Angiolymphoid hyperplasia with eosinophilia is clinically subdivided into superficial and deep forms. The former affects younger females, producing numerous, unilateral, erythematous pruritic papules that are characteristically periauricular in location (Olsen & Helwig, 1985). Deeper lesions affect slightly older patients of either sex with (usually solitary) firm nodules of the head and neck. Lesions are uncommon on the trunk and almost never found on the extremities. Either of these types of lesion may persist for years and yet rarely progress. Kimura disease predominantly affects Oriental males of a wide age range, with spread beyond the head and neck.

Histopathologic Features

Angiolymphoid hyperplasia with eosinophilia is characterized by a lobular proliferation of small to medium-sized arteries lined by plump endothelial cells, giving the inner surface of the vessels an epithelioid, "cobblestone" appearance. Occlusion of medium-sized vessels by endothelial proliferation is also often seen. Surrounding these vessels is a moderate lymphocytic and eosinophilic infiltrate (5–15% eosinophils) in which germinal centers often form in areas away from the vessels. These changes (Fig. 21–3) are seen in the deep dermis and subcutaneous tissue in the superficial form of the disease, whereas the deep form involves the deeper tissues. Kimura disease has similar histologic features (Fig. 21–4) except that the epithelioid vascular changes are less robust and sometimes absent, vascular occlusive areas are not seen, and dermal fibrosis may be present around the lesion.

Pathogenesis

The lesions may represent a response to traumatic injury in which there is exaggerated vascular proliferation with an additional allergic inflammatory component (Fetsch & Weiss,

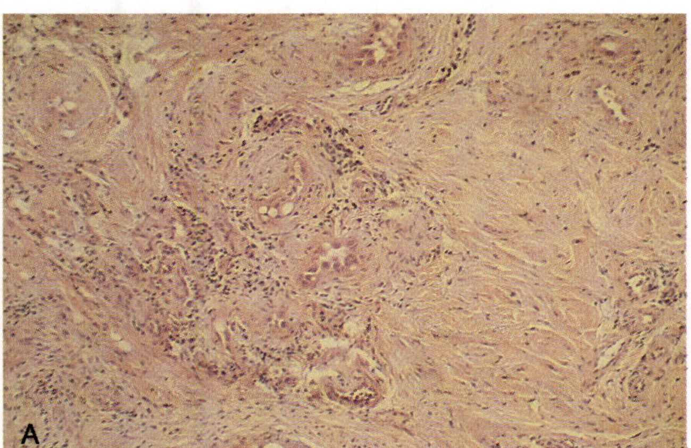

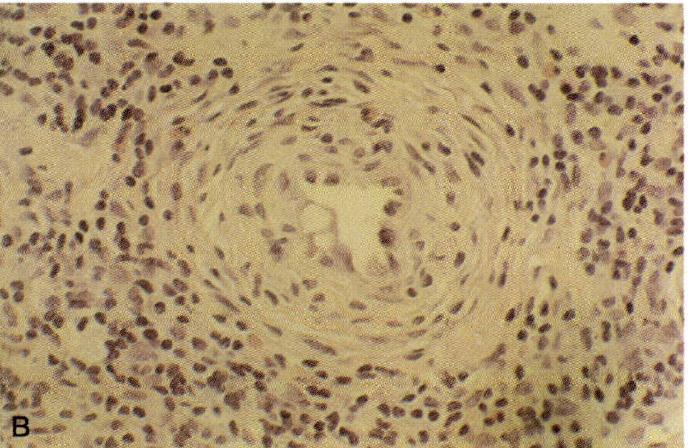

Figure 21–3

Angiolymphoid hyperplasia with eosinophilia, skin. *A*, At intermediate magnification inflammation is centered around a network of proliferating vascular channels in the dermis. *B*, Closer examination reveals that the infiltrate is composed of lymphocytes and numerous eosinophils, with capillary endothelial cells that exhibit a "hobnail" appearance.

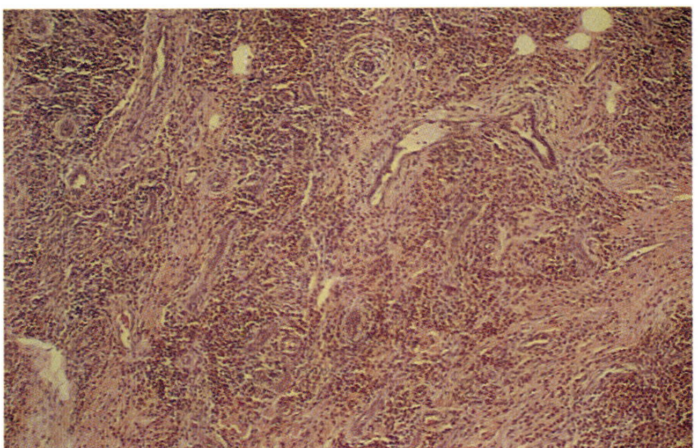

Figure 21–4

Kimura disease, skin. Subtle differences from angiolymphoid hyperplasia with eosinophilia include attenuated vascular changes and increased dermal fibrosis.

1991), but the actual pathobiology is unknown. The inflammatory component is present even when there are minimal vascular changes, suggesting that inflammation is the central event in formation of the lesion.

Sinus Histiocytosis with Massive Lymphadenopathy (Rosai-Dorfman Disease)

Definition

Sinus histiocytosis with massive lymphadenopathy is a rare disease characterized by lymphadenopathy that is usually painless, bilateral, and cervical (Rosai & Dorfman, 1969). It is most often self-limiting but may progress to involve the upper airways or other organs. (For additional details, see Chap. 16.)

Clinical Features

Sinus histiocytosis with massive lymphadenopathy affects males and females equally. Although it may be seen in patients of any age, 80% of cases occur in children and adolescents. Isolated skin involvement is present in about 10% of patients and is characterized by single or multiple brown-red nodules, papules, or plaques that may be larger than 4 cm and usually are located on the malar face and eyelids (Thaweroni et al, 1978).

Histologic Features

Lesions of skin resemble those in lymph nodes and other sites. There is a proliferation of histiocytes containing abundant pink cytoplasm, with an admixture of neutrophils, lymphocytes, and plasma cells (Fig. 21–5). Occasional histiocytes demonstrate emperipolesis. Within the skin, histiocytes form a dense infiltrate that fills the deep reticular dermis, may extend into the subcutaneous fat, and may stretch or rupture the overlying epidermis.

Immunophenotype

Histiocytes express S-100 protein, similarly to Langerhans-type histiocytes, but do not contain Birbeck granules. They express several other macrophage markers, including Mac-387, CD68, and CD14 (Paulli et al, 1992).

Pathogenesis

The cause of sinus histiocytosis with massive lymphadenopathy is unknown, although there is some evidence that it is an aberrant response to chronic infection.

Graft-versus-Host Disease

Definition

Graft-versus-host disease (GVHD) is a systemic disorder caused by circulating immunocompetent T cells that identify host cells as foreign. GVHD most commonly occurs after heterologous marrow transplantation due to the engraftment of donor T cells (Anderson & Weinstein, 1990). However, it may also occur after transfusion of blood that has not been filtered to remove leukocytes. Rarely, maternal lymphocytes cross the placenta and cause GVHD in the neonate (Morhenm & Marbach, 1974). In all cases, host cells, especially those in liver, gastrointestinal tract, and skin, are attacked and killed.

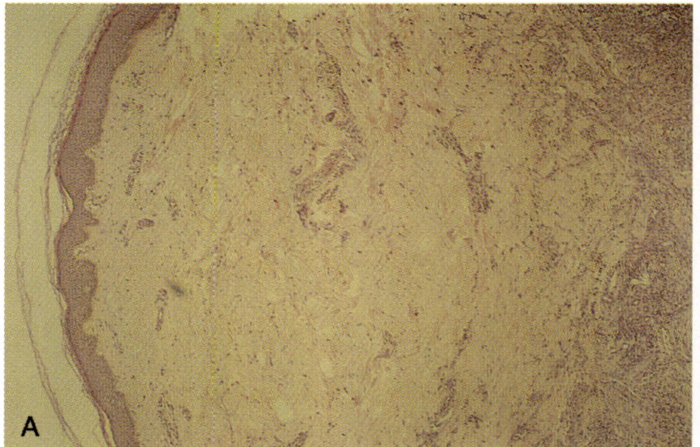

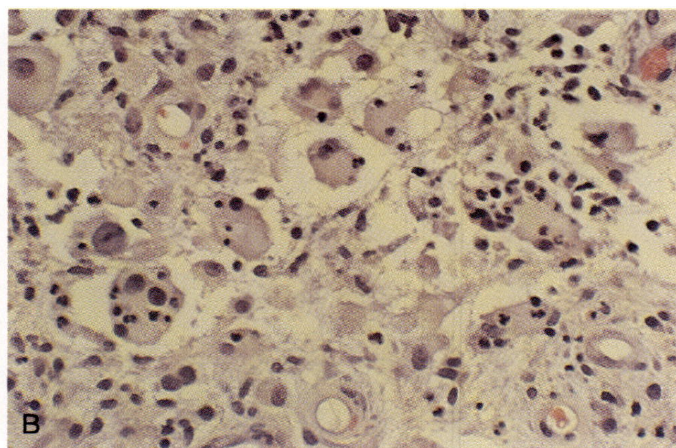

Figure 21–5

Sinus histiocytosis with massive lymphadenopathy, skin. *A*, A dense lymphohistiocytic infiltrate is present in the lower dermis, forming a nodule. *B*, High magnification reveals a dense collection of epitheliod histiocytes that contain well-preserved lymphocytes and other inflammatory cells.

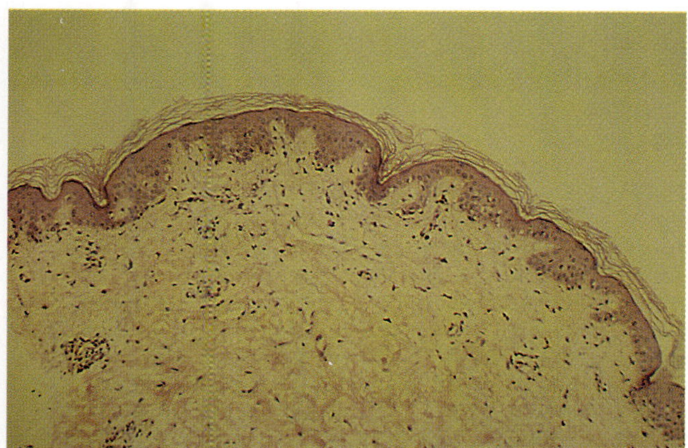

Figure 21–6

Graft-versus-host disease, grade I, skin. In mild acute lesions, the only detectable abnormalities may be a slight lymphocytic infiltrate and basal vacuolar change.

Clinical Features

GVHD has acute and chronic forms. The acute form is usually manifested by a circumscribed erythematous or purpuric rash that may progress to vesiculation and full-thickness necrosis. Severely affected patients develop systemic symptoms, including diarrhea and jaundice. The rash occurs in a mantle distribution (neck, shoulders, and upper chest) as well as on the face and acral regions. GVHD may occur as early as 10–11 days posttransplant. Similar-appearing reactions before this time probably represent the effects of chemotherapy. The disease usually peaks at about 18 days posttransplant. Although the mortality rate is high (up to 30% in some studies), the lesions gradually clear in the survivors (Darmstadt et al, 1992). The chronic form, beginning at any time after 100 days posttransplant, is characterized by erythema and hyperpigmentation that may appear lichenoid and that ultimately progress to sclerosis and epidermal atrophy (Saurat et al, 1975).

Histologic Changes

Acute GVHD is characterized by a sparse perivascular and interface lymphocytic infiltrate and evidence of epidermal damage. The latter should be characterized carefully, since it determines the grade of GVHD and ultimately the prognosis (Deebarats et al, 1994). In all grades there is a perivascular lymphocytic infiltrate, which may be quite mild. In addition, grade I lesions exhibit vacuolar degeneration of the basal layer (Fig. 21–6). Grade II lesions also display dyskeratotic epidermal cells (Fig. 21–7) that are often surrounded by lymphocytes, a process called satellite cell necrosis. Spongiosis is seen as well. In grade III disease, the basal degeneration has evolved into a subepidermal split (Fig. 21–8). Grade IV lesions are characterized by complete epidermal necrosis or loss of the epidermis. Histopathologic changes should be evaluated in the context of time after transplant and treatment, as similar changes may also result from chemotherapy. Because GVHD does not occur unless the marrow has engrafted, success of engraftment should be evaluated by leukocyte counts before analysis of skin biopsy specimens.

The histologic features of chronic GVHD are similar to those of lichen planus. There is a lichenoid inflammatory infiltrate, with pigment dropout, dyskeratotic cells (occasionally with satellite cell necrosis), acanthosis, and hypergranulosis. Ultimately, chronic lesions may progress to resemble scleroderma by developing full-thickness dermal sclerosis with overlying atrophic epithelium and pigment dropout.

NEOPLASMS AND PROLIFERATIONS

Mast Cell Disease

The term *mast cell disease* encompasses several distinct disorders that have as a common feature the proliferation of mast cells, most commonly in the skin. Mast cell diseases include the childhood and adult types of urticaria pigmentosa, systemic mastocytosis, and mast cell leukemia. The adult type of disease is mentioned here only in contrast to the pediatric forms.

Definitions

In urticaria pigmentosa, mast cell proliferation is limited to the skin. Rarely, there is progression to systemic mastocytosis, in which other organs are extensively involved. Mast cell leukemia is an extremely rare condition in which malignant mast cells extensively involve the marrow and peripheral blood (Friedman et al, 1958).

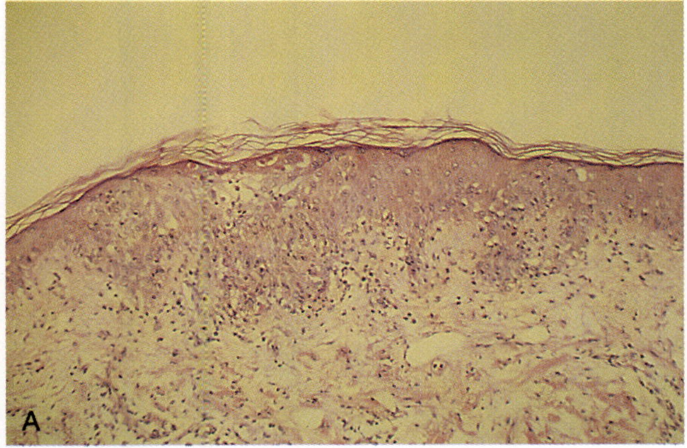

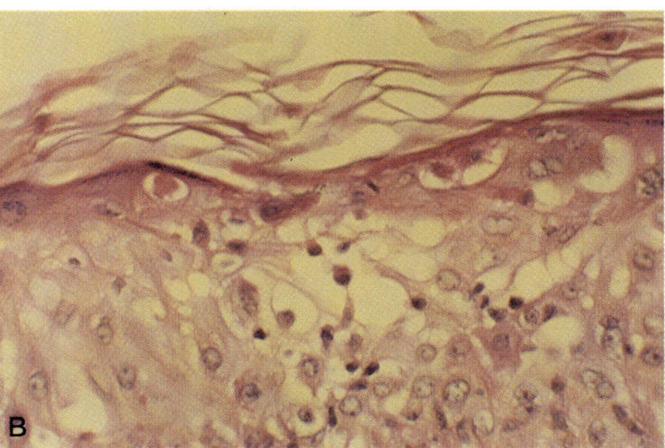

Figure 21–7

Graft-versus-host disease, grade II, skin. *A*, This illustration shows increased interface damage, with vacuolization of the epidermis and lymphocytic infiltrate. *B*, The presence of dyskeratotic cells in addition to the changes seen in *A* are the hallmarks of grade II disease.

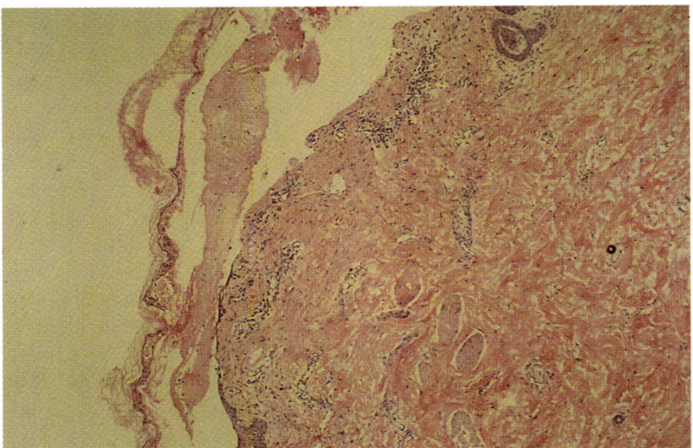

Figure 21–8

Graft-versus-host disease, grade III, skin. Subepidermal splitting characterizes grade III disease. The most severe type (grade IV, not shown) is characterized by full-thickness epidermal necrosis that may result in complete sloughing, leaving only exposed dermis.

Clinical Features

Urticaria pigmentosa is manifested in children with specific skin lesions. If the mast cell infiltration is extensive, there may be systemic symptoms, such as episodic flushing, diarrhea, or transient arrhythmias. The skin lesions include brown maculopapular or nodular lesions, seen also in adults, that demonstrate a wheal and flare reaction when mechanically stimulated (Darier sign); solitary, large cutaneous nodules that form bullae when stroked (mastocytoma, usually seen in infants); and, infrequently, a vesiculating erythroderma (bullous mastocytosis, seen almost exclusively in infants) (Klaus & Wenkeliman, 1962). Infants with the latter presentation may occasionally die suddenly from histaminergic shock owing to massive mast cell degranulation (Allison, 1967). All lesions usually clear by puberty, in contrast to adult-type disease, which is persistent albeit indolent (Kettlehut & Metcalfe, 1994). Systemic mastocytosis produces lesions of other organ systems. Since the total mast cell burden is generally higher than in skin-restricted disease, the incidence of systemic symptoms is much higher.

Histologic Features

All of the mast cell diseases exhibit an increased number of mast cells within the dermis. Mast cells are mononuclear, with a characteristic gray cytoplasm containing granules that are almost invisible on hematoxylin-eosin–stained sections but conspicuously purple on Giemsa or toluidine blue staining (Fig. 21–9*A* & *B*). Mast cells may have degranulated, leading to a falsely negative result on staining, if the biopsy is performed on the same lesion used to test for the Darier sign. In the maculopapular lesions, mast cells are perivascular or dispersed through the interstitum, and thus the use of the above mentioned stains may be necessary to differentiate them from histiocytes. However, in the nodular lesions, a clearly defined dermal mass is produced, a process that is readily recognized without special stains. Changes may occur in the overlying epidermis, including spongiosis and subepidermal bulla formation (e.g., in the bullous mastocytosis–type lesions), and the dermis may exhibit the pigment dropout that gives these lesions both their brown color and the name *pigmentosa*.

T CELL PROLIFERATIONS AND NEOPLASMS INVOLVING THE SKIN AND SUBCUTANEOUS TISSUE

Skin and subcutaneous tissue involvement by T cell lymphoproliferations is exceedingly rare in children. Since general pathologists may have very limited experience with these lesions in children or adults, they are not likely to consider such disorders in the differential diagnoses when examining skin biopsy specimens from a child. The T cell proliferations and neoplasms considered in this section are T cell acute lymphocytic leukemia or lymphoblastic lymphoma, anaplastic large-cell lymphoma and lymphomatoid papulosis, cutaneous T cell lymphoma (mycosis fungoides), and other peripheral T cell lymphomas (subcutaneous panniculitic and natural killer like).

T Cell Acute Lymphocytic Leukemia or Lymphoblastic Lymphoma

Involvement of the skin of children by T cell acute lymphocytic leukemia or lymphoblastic lymphoma is extremely unusual. Most lymphoblastic processes manifested as skin lesions have a B phenotype (see "B Cell Lymphomas," later in this

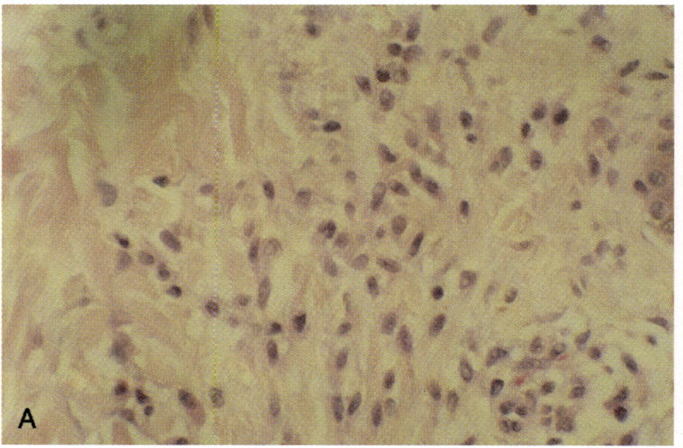

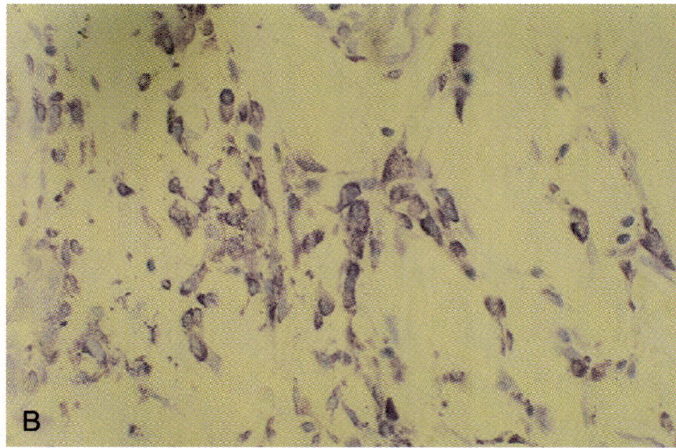

Figure 21–9

Urticaria pigmentosa, maculopapular, skin. *A*, High magnification reveals a mononuclear infiltrate that may be difficult to characterize without special stains. *B*, Staining reveals that the infiltrate is composed of numerous mast cells. Toluidine blue.

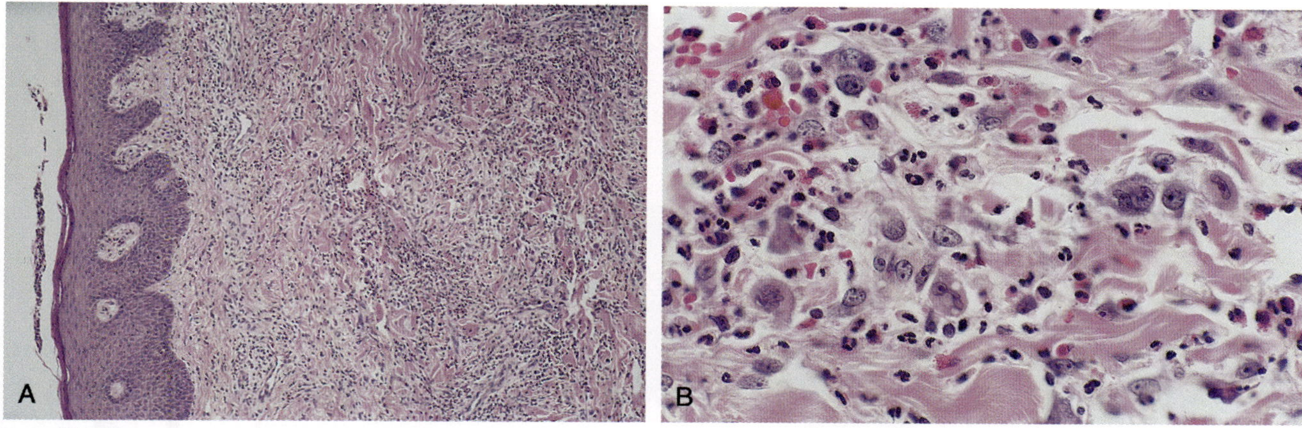

Figure 21–10

Lymphomatoid papulosis, skin. *A*, At low magnification there are a superficial dermal infiltrate, hypervascularity, and hyperkeratosis. *B*, High magnification shows an infiltrate of eosinophils, neutrophils, macrophages, and scattered transformed lymphocytes. A few dysplastic, mutinucleated cells with prominent nucleoli are seen. The low-magnification appearance certainly favors diagnosis of a reactive process, but the dysplastic cells (in some cases present in greater numbers than shown here) explain the choice of the term *lymphomatoid*.

chapter). In a review of lymphoblastic lymphoma occurring in cutaneous sites there were only six cases (Sander et al, 1991). The two children had a pre-B immunophenotype. Only one of these six cases had a clear T phenotype. This patient was a 25-year-old man with multiple scalp nodules, a mediastinal mass, pleural effusion, and no marrow involvement.

Lymphomatoid Papulosis

Clinically and histologically, lymphomatoid papulosis in children is similar to that in adults (Zirbel et al, 1995), with the exception of its rarity in children. Fewer than 50 cases have been described in children in the English-language literature. Twenty-eight of these cases are summarized and an additional 6 presented in the review by Zirbel and associates (1995). The age range was 13 months to 17 years. Children seemed to have three clinical patterns unusual for lymphomatoid papulosis: outbreaks that dwindled in frequency and number of lesions, lesions localized in one area for long periods before generalization, and crops of >100 papules or nodules (2 cases) (Zirbel et al, 1995). The disease remits in most cases under treatment or because of treatment. Two adults have developed lymphomas after having lymphomatoid papulosis as children. Healing lesions may ulcerate, may be covered by eschar, and may scar with hyperpigmentation.

Histopathologic Features

Dense, typically wedge-shaped infiltrates extend from the epidermis into the dermis (Fig. 21–10). Overlying epithelium is often hyperplastic or may be ulcerated. Lymphocytes far outnumber reacting cells, such as neutrophils or eosinophils, and take the form of transformed lymphocytes with prominent nuclei and basophilic cytoplasm (type A) or smaller, hyperchromatic cells with scant cytoplasm (type B). Some cells in type A resemble Reed-Sternberg cells in their nuclear configuration and overall appearance, whereas the lymphocytes in type B may be cerebriform and resemble Sézary cells.

Immunophenotypic Features

The large cells in lymphomatoid papulosis have the immunophenotype of activated T cells, usually of the helper type. Positivity for both CD30 and CD15 is usual. The predominant cells often express CD2 and CD3 while lacking some T cell antigens, such as CD5 and/or CD7. Rare cases have been CD8+ (Hellman et al, 1990). Clonality has been demonstrated in this T cell population. In a remarkable longitudinal study, lymphomatoid papulosis lesions over a 26-year period were shown to be derived from a single T cell clone (Chott et al, 1996). Overall, lesions separate in location and time were clonal in five of six patients studied (Chott et al, 1996).

Anaplastic Large-Cell Ki-1+ Lymphoma

In 1986, Kadin and associates provided the first comprehensive review of the clinicopathologic syndrome of childhood Ki-1+ lymphoma manifested as skin lesions and peripheral lymphadenopathy. Patient populations were multiracial, were of both sexes, and ranged in age from 8 to 19 years. Four of the six patients presented with rapidly growing, painful nodular lesions of the skin, neck, and chest as well as upper or lower extremities. Several patients presented with tender adenopathy, and they noticed cutaneous nodules in the region, often attributed to insect bites or cat scratches. In three cases there was temporary spontaneous regression, further delaying the correct diagnosis. Several lesions had been incorrectly diagnosed as regressing atypical histiocytosis.

Since 1986, it has become apparent that there is a *primary* cutaneous CD30+ anaplastic large-cell lymphoma (Beljaards et al, 1992; Krishnan et al, 1993). The diagnosis is made when patients have cutaneous lymphomas with no extracutaneous disease at presentation, there is no evidence of concurrent lymphomatoid papulosis or mycosis fungoides, and the cutaneous lymphoma contains large cells that are immunoreactive (75–90%) with CD30. Virtually all primary cutaneous CD30+ anaplastic large-cell lymphomas occur in older adults, with one 2-year-old in the series of 47 patients (Beljaards et al, 1992). Skin involvement also occurs concurrently with nodal disease or in patients with bone and/or soft tissue lesions (Kadin et al, 1986; Reiter et al, 1994). Nine of a total of 62 patients with anaplastic large-cell lymphoma had skin involvement (Reiter et al, 1994). Analysis of the response to treatment of those with primary involvement, as opposed to the response

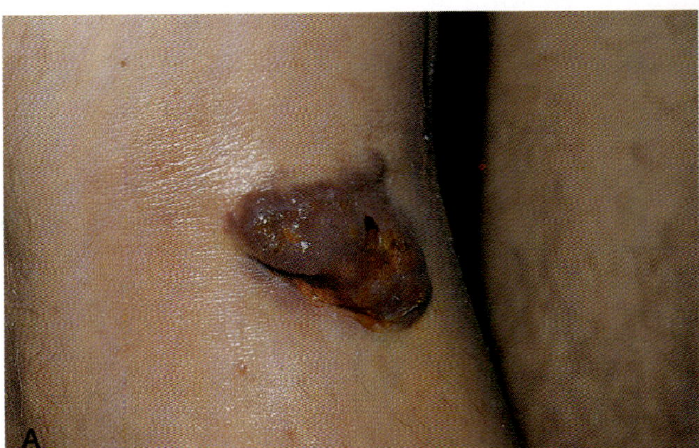

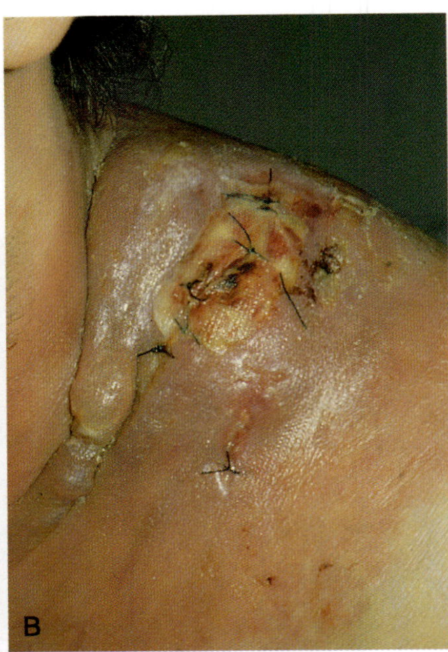

Figure 21–11

Anaplastic large-cell Ki-1+ lymphoma, skin. *A*, Patients with these lymphomas often present with skin ulcers on the upper extremity or shoulder. A typical lesion is shown in this photograph. *B*, Late lesions may become very indurated, as in this case, in which several biopsies were required before the lymphoma was recognized. Superficial biopsies of this lesion revealed dense fibrous tissue with no evident tumor.

of those with secondary or concurrent disease elsewhere, reveals a far more favorable response in the primary group (Beljaards et al, 1992).

In most patients, anaplastic large-cell lymphomas form single red or skin-colored nodules or may produce several nearby nodules on virtually any skin site (Kaudewitz et al, 1994). Lesions develop over several weeks, range in size from 1–10 cm in diameter, may ulcerate (Fig. 21–11*A*), indurate (Fig. 21–11*B*), or "spontaneously regress." The morphologic features of these lesions resemble those in nodes (see Chap. 15). Multinucleated giant tumor cells may be seen. A small-cell variant of anaplastic large-cell lymphoma has proved particularly difficult to recognize in its initial phase (Kinney et al, 1993). Skin lesions may be very subtle with infiltrates of small, irregular lymphocytes in a perivascular and periappendageal distribution extending from the superficial dermis to subcutaneous tissue (Fig. 21–12). Large cells may be rare in such infiltrates. Transformation of this variant to the more typical large-cell form has been described in a five-year-old child (Hodges et al, 1999). This child initially had a skin lesion. After 96 months, transformation was shown in a node biopsy specimen. Although the clinical and morphologic features are often distinctive in anaplastic large-cell lymphoma, the diagnosis should certainly be confirmed by immunohistology. Large tumor cells in paraffin sections typically have distinct membrane and dot Golgi positivity with CD30 (Fig. 21–12*C*). Most are T cell processes of helper subtype. Very few are EMA positive, in contrast to nodal anaplastic large-cell lymphoma.

The differential diagnosis of primary cutaneous anaplastic large-cell lymphoma in children is essentially limited to the exclusion of lymphomatoid papulosis. Features clearly favoring lymphomatoid papulosis include multiple lesions, lesions <1 cm in diameter, lack of extension into subcutaneous tissue, many mixed inflammatory cells, and scattered single or small clusters of CD30+ cells (Kinney & Kadin, 1998).

Mycosis Fungoides

Mycosis fungoides is a rare cutaneous T cell lymphoma in adults, and only a handful of cases have been described in children. Despite the small number of cases, most of the presenting manifestations seen in adults have been described in children (Hickham et al, 1997), including patch, plaque, and tumor stages; alopecia mucinosa; and Sézary syndrome. Hyperpigmented forms have been seen in black patients. Both aggressive and indolent forms of mycosis fungoides apparently occur in children. In a series of five cases occurring in patients under 20 years of age and accumulated over a 20-year period, the duration of skin disease prior to diagnosis ranged from 1.5 to 13 years. Various biopsies during these years revealed nonspecific changes lichenoid changes, and eczematous changes.

Diagnosis in the late stages is not difficult, owing to the presence of dense infiltrates of hyperchromatic cells with cerebriform nuclear outlines. In the earlier stages, B5 fixation enhances cytologic detail and thus facilitates detection of dysplastic cells. Transformation to a large-cell lymphoma, a phenomenon seen in adults in 10–15% of cases, must be very rare in children and would require differentiation from an anaplastic large-cell lymphoma.

Angiocentric Cutaneous T Cell Lymphoma

Assuming that it is not underdiagnosed, angiocentric cutaneous T cell lymphoma is extremely rare. Most patients have been children from Asia or Latin America (Magaña et al, 1998). There seems little question that the lesion is lymphomatous, given its histopathologic features and clinical course, and the neoplastic cells in the few cases studied have had T features. The clinical presentation indicates a cutaneous origin, and its pathogenesis is not known. The natural history is not established, but several patients have had internal dissemination.

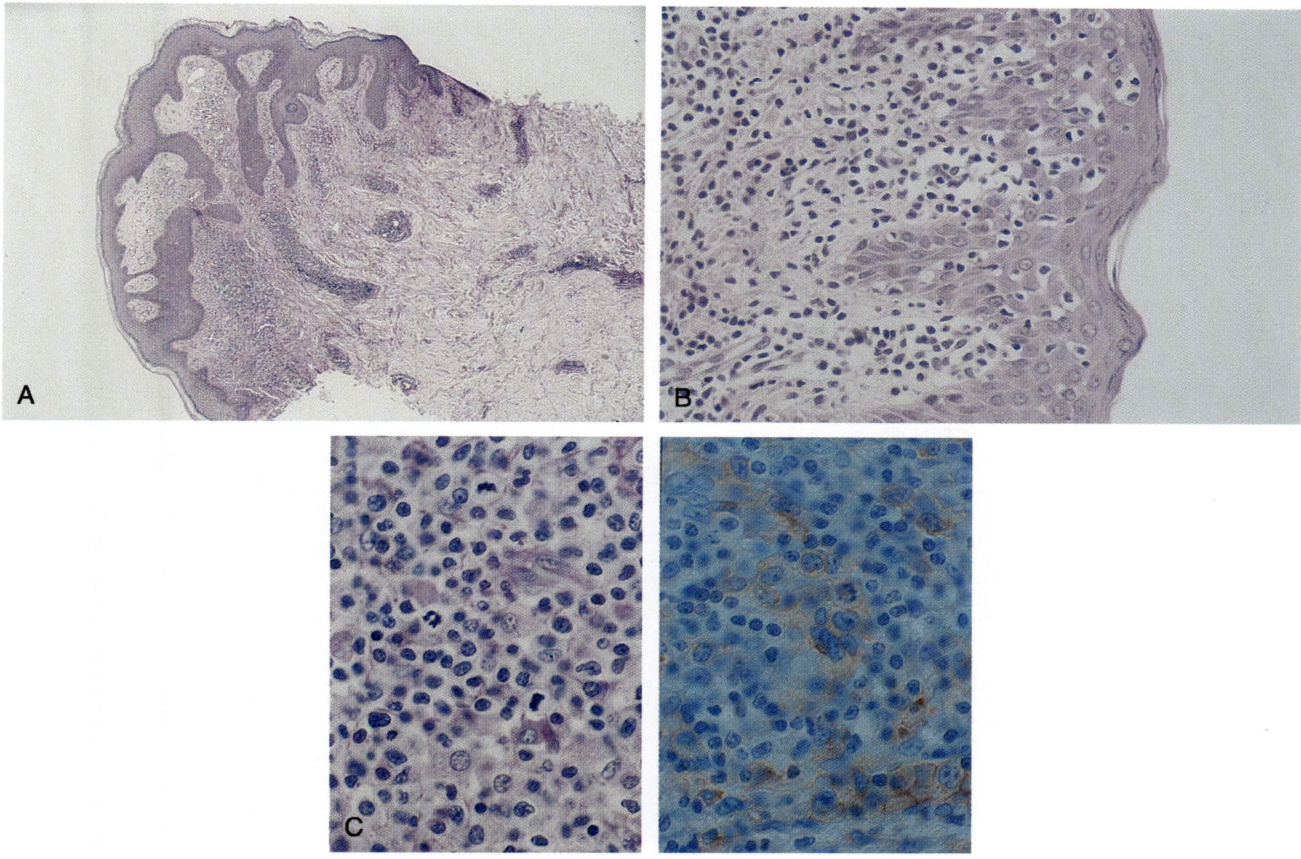

Figure 21–12

Small-cell variant, anaplastic large-cell Ki-1+ lymphoma, skin. *A*, A low-magnification photomicrograph shows a scant lymphocytic infiltrate in the upper and mid-dermis. Infiltrates this subtle may be very difficult to identify as lymphomatous, even after immunoperoxidase studies. Identification of the ALK protein in nuclei of small lymphocytes establishes the diagnosis of the small-cell variant. This possibility should be suspected, particularly if there is lymphadenopathy. *B*, Intermediate magnification reveals a sparse superficial dermal and epidermal infiltrate. Epithelial hyperplasia with and without epidermotropism may be seen in these cases. *C*, This composite shows a monomorphous infiltrate of small lymphocytes at high magnification, but the adjacent immunoperoxidase preparation shows scattered large Ki-1+ cells.

Patients have had vesicles, necrotic areas, scars, and associated edema. Some lesions have been so large and deep that disfigurement resulted (Fig. 21–13*A*). Lesions are seen in sun-exposed and protected areas and are not exacerbated by sun exposure.

Histologically, there are dense lymphocytic infiltrates throughout the dermis, often under ulcers. Angiocentricity is a prominent feature (Fig. 21–13*B* to *D*), and vasculitis or panniculitis has been noted in some cases (Magaña et al, 1998). Neoplastic lymphocytes described as "atypical," with enlarged, pleomorphic nuclei, have been demonstrated within and around blood vessels. A few histiocytes and eosinophils may be present. Immunophenotyping in a few cases (Magaña et al, 1998) has shown reactivity of neoplastic cells with CD3 but not with natural killer cell marker CD56. CD30 positivity has been noted in more than 40% of neoplastic cells.

The differential diagnosis involves other extranodal angiocentric lymphomas. Although there may be some overlap, the angiocentric lymphomas involving the nose usually express CD56 (Chan et al, 1999; Kanavaros et al, 1993). Since panniculitic processes involve the deep dermis, with minimal epithelial extension, epithelial necrosis and vesicles are not found. Cutaneous Ki-1+ lymphomas are also included in the differential diagnosis. Such lymphomas often produce single or closely approximated large lesions in which neoplastic cells with abundant cytoplasm as well as multinucleated forms are prominent. Angiocentric features are not typically seen.

T Cell Lymphoma Involving Subcutaneous Tissue

T cell lymphomas may also arise in and principally affect the subcutaneous tissue. Most cases have been reported in adults, with a mean age of 35 years. The youngest patient in the initial series was 19 (Gonzalez et al, 1991). Both blacks and whites were affected. Patients presented with 1- to 12-cm subcutaneous nodules, often in the extremities. All patients developed some evidence of hemophagocytosis (Gonzalez et al, 1991). Aggressive chemotherapy put three patients into remission, but the remaining five died with lymphoma and hemophagocytic syndrome.

Inflammatory panniculitis was suggested clinically and pathologically, as the neoplastic component often produced an interstitial infiltrate, with aggregates or sheets of lymphocytes seen focally. Panniculitis was further suggested by the presence of fat necrosis or karyorrhexis in all cases, coupled with giant cells and granulomas. The neoplastic infiltrate was concentrated in the subcutaneous adipose tissue, rarely extending up to the papillary dermis. Neoplastic cells were small to large, hyperchromatic lymphocytes with scant cytoplasm and irregu-

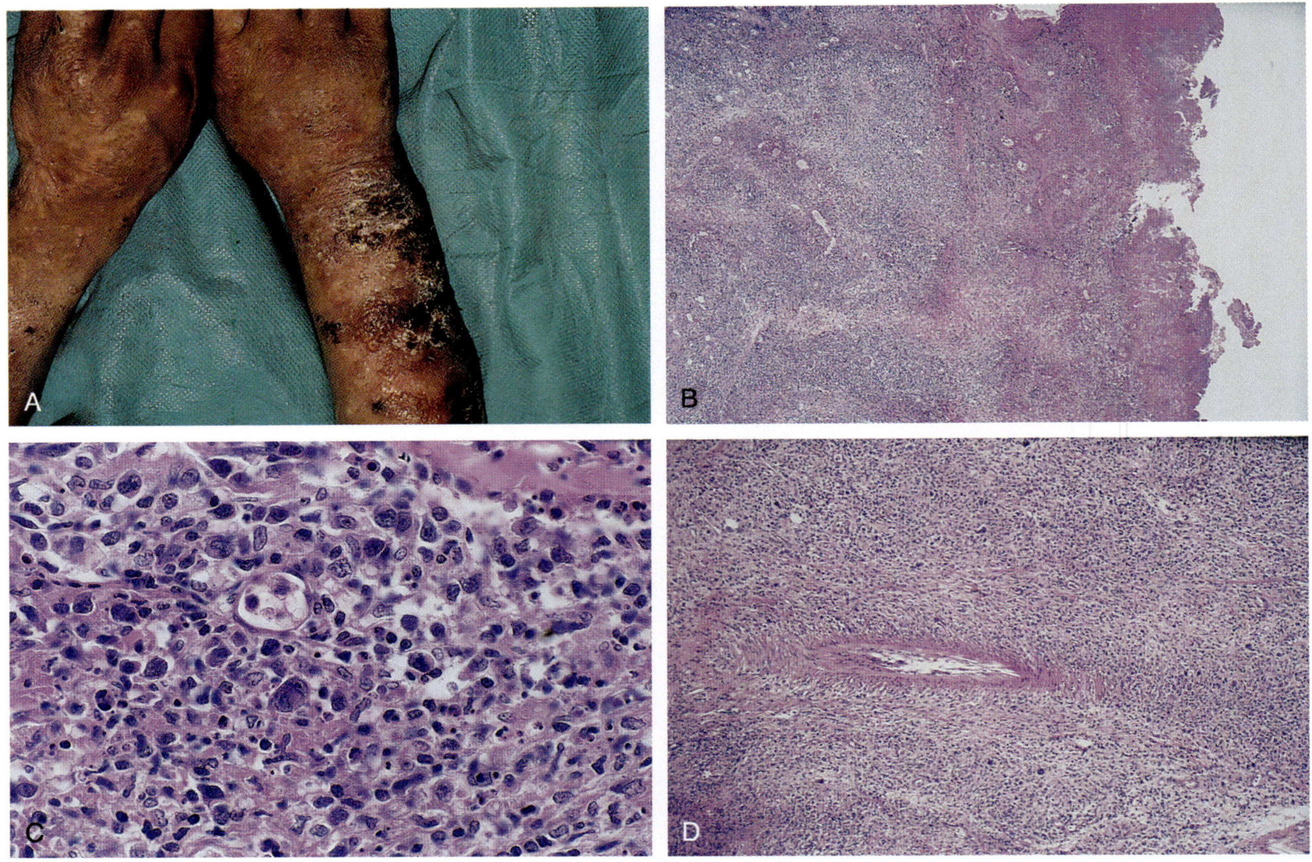

Figure 21–13

Angiocentric cutaneous T cell lymphoma, skin. *A*, Deforming, ulcerative lesions are found in this rare lymphoma. *B*, At low magnification ulceration with extensive necrosis can be seen. There is a dense lymphocytic infiltrate involving arteries and veins. *C*, At high magnification a polymorphous process is evident, with small and transformed lymphocytes predominating. *D*, Vessel walls are infiltrated. Here a small artery is surrounded by tumor. (Courtesy Dr. Omar P. Sangueza, Associate Professor of Pathology and Medicine, Medical College of Georgia.)

lar nuclear outlines. The infiltrate was not angiocentric, although some small veins were infiltrated.

Most cases expressed a mature T cell phenotype that was usually CD4+ (Gonzalez et al, 1991). Two of the cases studied were CD30−. In one case (of three studied) the T cell receptor β chain was clearly rearranged. The biology of the T cell population giving rise to this lymphoma is not known, and its pathogenesis is not understood.

B CELL LYMPHOMAS

B cell neoplasms—including lymphoblastic lymphoma, acute lymphoblastic leukemia, and small transformed (noncleaved) cell lymphoma of the Burkitt and non-Burkitt type—occasionally occur as cutaneous lesions in children. These neoplasms are all high grade and aggressive. Low-grade B cell neoplasms are not seen in pediatric patients, in sharp distinction to the situation in adults.

B Lymphoblastic Lymphoma

B cell lymphoblastic lymphoma (B-LBL) is the most common pediatric B cell neoplasm that involves the skin. B-LBL is most often seen in the first and early second decades, with several neonatal cases reported. Slightly more females than males are affected. Cutaneous lesions may predate evidence of systemic or marrow disease by a few days to many months. Some patients present with simultaneous cutaneous lesions and systemic or marrow involvement, including lymphocytosis and lymphadenopathy. The cutaneous lesions are usually asymptomatic, indurated papules or nodules that are red-brown or purple and without excoriation or ulceration. The size of the lesions ranges from 0.5–6.5 cm. The commonest site of involvement is the head, including the scalp, forehead, and face (Millot, 1997; Sander, 1991). Other reported sites of involvement include the neck, trunk, arms, and legs.

Histologically, the lesions of B-LBL are characterized by a diffuse infiltration of the entire dermis and superficial subcutaneous fat with sheets of mononuclear cells (Fig. 21–14*A*), although the neoplastic cells may infiltrate through the dermis in a single-cell fashion in early lesions and at the edge of older lesions. The epidermis is uninvolved, and there is a small Grenz zone. Deeper, the infiltrate surrounds appendages and vessels. The neoplastic cells are intermediate in size, smaller than most histiocytes and larger than normal small lymphocytes. The nuclei are oval, with finely distributed chromatin and scant cytoplasm. Small, indistinct nucleoli and nuclear convolutions may be present. Scattered mitotic figures are often seen (Fig. 21–14*B*).

Immunophenotypically, the tumor cells usually have features of pre–B cells, expressing surface CD19, CD10, and TdT. They contain cytoplasmic IgM, but no surface immunoglobulin

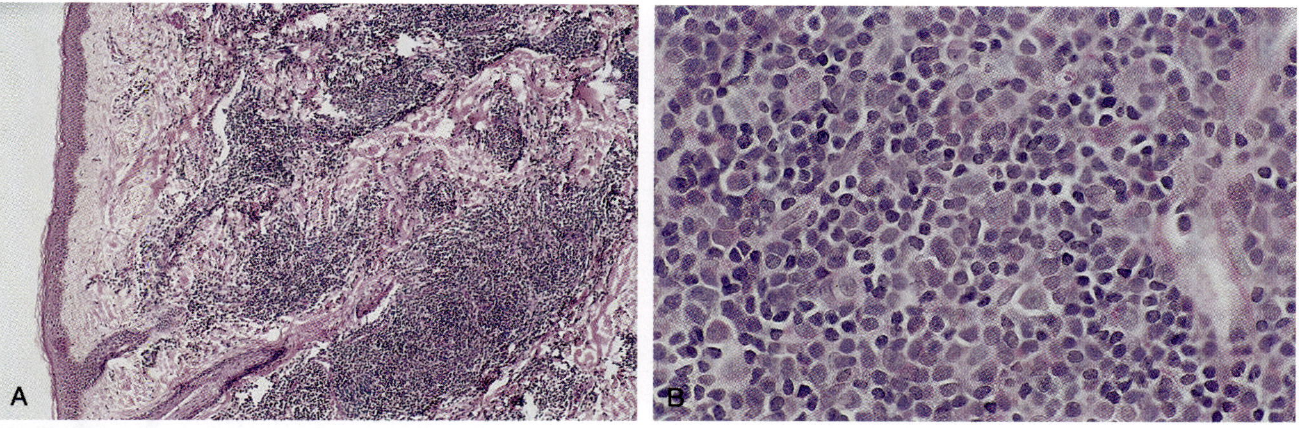

Figure 21–14

B lymphoblastic lymphoma, skin. *A*, Low magnification reveals a monomorphic infiltrate in the dermis and subcutaneous tissues. *B*, At high magnification the infiltrate is seen to be composed of intermediate-sized cells with oval nuclei and a minimal amount of cytoplasm. Mitotic figures are common.

is produced (Grumayer et al, 1988). However, pre–pre-B phenotypes without cytoplasmic or surface immunoglobulin and mature B-cell phenotypes with surface immunoglobulin have also been reported. Cytogenetic abnormalities in the short arm of chromosome 9 have been observed in lymphoblastic lymphomas (Chilcote et al, 1985), but no specific chromosomal abnormality has been linked with cutaneous involvement. Limited studies indicate that the presence of cutaneous involvement at presentation likely does not affect prognosis, and the relapse rate in these patients is similar to that in patients with disease of a similar stage but without cutaneous involvement (Millot et al, 1997). However, the number of cases examined is too few to draw conclusions about the prognostic significance of cutaneous involvement at the time of presentation.

B Cell Acute Lymphoblastic Leukemia

Overall, only 1–2% of pediatric acute lymphoblastic leukemia (ALL) cases involve the skin, most of them of B cell lineage. At presentation, there is usually lymphocytosis and organomegaly, likely reflecting widespread dissemination. In rare cases, a single skin lesion predates by months the diagnosis of marrow involvement (Millot et al, 1997).

Histologically, the cutaneous lesions of B-ALL are very similar to those of lymphoblastic lymphomas, with a dense mononuclear dermal infiltrate extending from the superficial dermis into the deep reticular dermis and often into the subcutis (Fig. 21–15*A*). Epidermotropism is not seen. The infiltrate is monomorphic, composed of intermediate-sized cells with round to oval nuclei, dispersed chromatin, and a minimal amount of cytoplasm. Small, indistinct nucleoli and nuclear convolutions may be present. Mitoses are often numerous (Fig. 21–15*B*).

Immunophenotypic studies of cutaneous ALL cases reveal that the neoplastic cells are most often pre–B cells. They express CD19, CD10, TdT, and cytoplasmic IgM. Specific cytogenetic abnormalities have not been correlated with cutaneous involvement by ALL. Cases of pre–B cell ALL with the t(1;19)(q23;p13.3) translocation occurred in patients with an

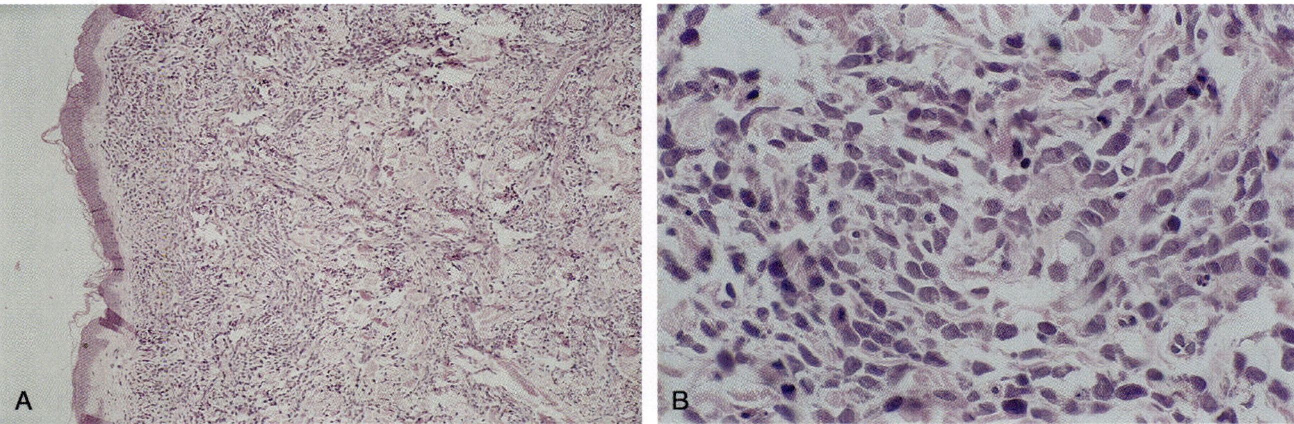

Figure 21–15

Acute lymphoblastic leukemia B, skin. *A*, Low magnification shows a dense mononuclear infiltrate extending from the reticular dermis to the subcutaneous fat. *B*, At high magnification the infiltrate is seen to be composed of large mononuclear cells with scant cytoplasm, some of them infiltrating in a single-file fashion.

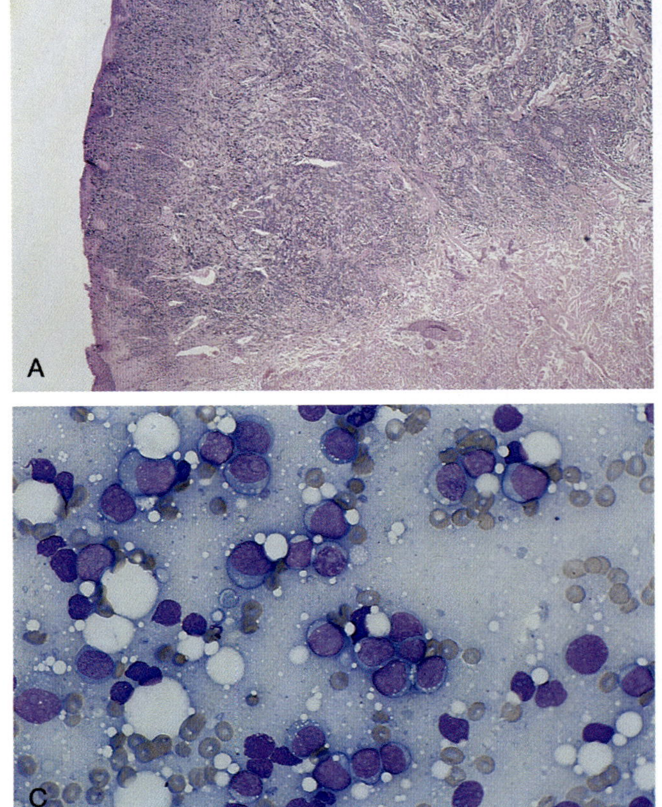

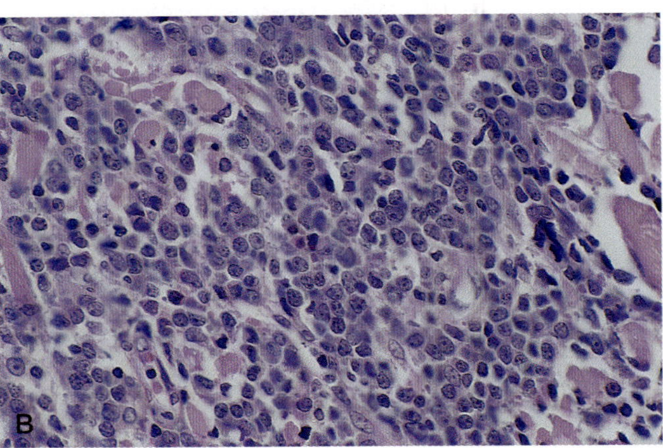

Figure 21–16

Malignant lymphoma, small transformed (noncleaved) cell type, skin. *A*, Low magnification shows a dense lympocytic infiltrate in the dermis and subcutaneous tissue, with adjacent necrosis. *B*, High magnification reveals that the neoplastic cells are small transformed cells with oval nuclei, prominent nucleoli, and a minimal amount of cytoplasm. Scattered mitoses are present. *C*, High magnification of a stained touch preparation shows neoplastic cells with deep-blue cytoplasm and numerous cytoplasmic vaculoes. Wright stain.

increased leukocyte count. These patients often have central nervous system involvement and have a worse prognosis than do patients with pre–B cell ALL without the translocation. Other translocations linked with B cell ALL, such as t(9:22)(q34;q11) and t(8:14)(p13;q11), are not linked with cutaneous involvement (Pui, 1995).

Small Transformed (Noncleaved) Cell Lymphomas of Burkitt and Non-Burkitt Types

Isolated cases of small transformed cell lymphoma with cutaneous involvement have all had extensive systemic involvement by tumor at the time of diagnosis (Banks, 1975; Riyat, 1995). The lesions were described as nodules, but their site was not reported. Following cytotoxic therapy, the nodules resolved. Approximately 10% of the children with Burkitt lymphoma also complained of generalized pruritus at the time of presentation.

Histologically, the nodular lesions consist of a dense monomorphic infiltrate that is predominantly in the dermis, extending from the upper dermis into the subcutaneous fat (Fig. 21–16*A*). A "starry sky" appearance is often seen, with numerous macrophages containing apoptotic debris scattered among the neoplastic cells. Epidermotropism is minimal. The neoplastic cells are small transformed cells, with round to oval nuclei, prominent and often multiple nucleoli, and scant cytoplasm (Fig. 21–16*B*). Numerous mitotic figures are seen. Wright-stained touch or imprint preparations reveal that the tumor cells have deep-blue cytoplasm with multiple clear vacuoles (Fig. 21–16*C*).

Flow cytometric studies demonstrate that the small transformed cells express the pan–B cell antigens CD19, CD20, and CD22 as well as CD10, CD21, and CDw32. In addition, they express monotypic surface immunoglobulin, with IgM and IgD being the commonest heavy chains and either κ or λ light chain (Garcia et al, 1987). The cytogenetic findings in small transformed cell lymphoma have been well described (see Chap. 2 for more details).

Myelomonocytic Leukemias

Leukemias involving newborns or infants are often myelocytic and/or monocytic in differentiation. Thirty to 50% of the former (Resnik & Brod, 1993) and 18% of latter (van Wering & Kamps, 1986) have cutaneous involvement at presentation. The cutaneous lesions are firm red, blue, purple, or brown nodules or plaques. They are often multiple and are generalized in distribution. Oral mucosal involvement at presentation very rarely occurs in newborns and infants, in contrast to the frequency in monocytic leukemias in older children and adults. Systemic disease is usually seen at the time of diagnosis in the form of hepatosplenomegaly and lymphadenopathy, but cutaneous lesions precede other signs of leukemia in 7% of cases (Canioni et al, 1996).

Histologically, these lesions consist of a dense monomorphic dermal infiltrate that extends from the superficial dermis into the subcutaneous fat. The epidermis is uninvolved but thinned, with flattening of the rete ridges (Fig. 21–17*A*). A small zone in the upper dermis (Grenz zone) is spared. The infiltrate is composed of mononuclear cells with large, often

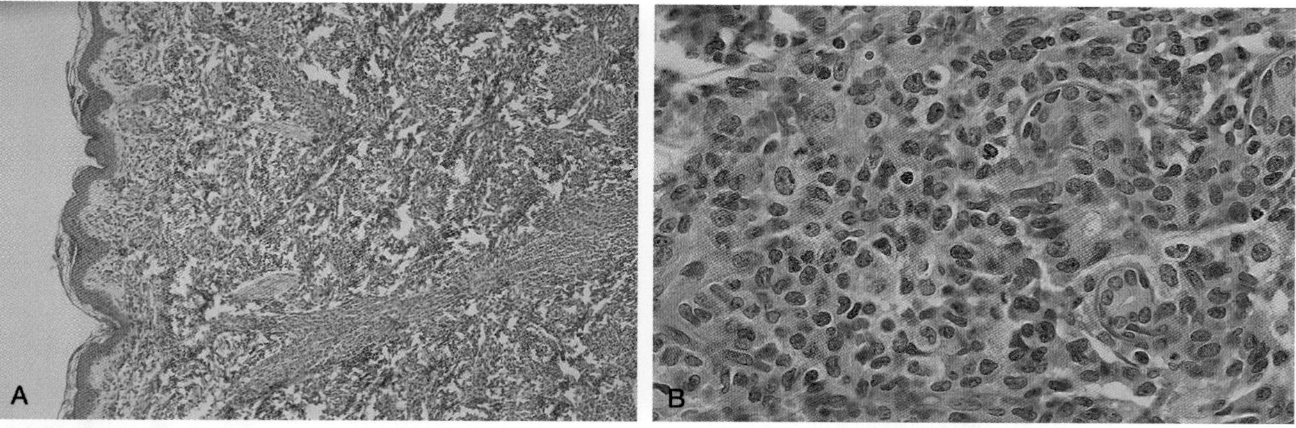

Figure 21–17

Acute myelomonocytic leukemia, skin. *A*, Low magnification shows a monomorphic dermal infiltrate that flattens the rete ridges but spares the epidermis. *B*, High magnification reveals that the infiltrate consists of mononuclear cells with folded nuclei, prominent nucleoli, and abundant cytoplasm. A skin appendage is present on the left side.

folded or vesicular nuclei, prominent nucleoli, and minimal to moderate amounts of pale or granulated cytoplasm. Mitotic figures may be rare or common (Fig. 21–17*B*).

Immunophenotypically, the neoplastic cells usually express the monocytic markers CD68, CD13, and CD14. In addition, the blasts may express CD45 (leukocyte common antigen), CD4, and CD13 (Canioni et al, 1996). Eighty to 90% of these leukemias have associated karyotypic abnormalities. The karyotypic abnormalities seen in these cases are polytypic, but the commonest abnormality, a 11q23 rearrangement, is often seen with central nervous system involvement and coagulation disorders (Pui, 1995).

When they do occur in neonates and infants, myelomonocytic leukemias often involve extramedullary sites, including the skin. Rare cases of spontaneous remission have been described, but all of these patients relapsed within a few months. If untreated, the disease is uniformly fatal, and the patients usually die within 2 months. As in the cases of lymphoblastic lymphoma, cutaneous involvement by myelomonocytic leukemia reflects widespread systemic involvement, and the cutaneous involvement alone does not appear to affect prognosis (Resnik & Brod, 1993).

Histiocytoses

The proliferations and neoplasms of histiocytes involving the skin are described in Chap. 10.

REFERENCES

Allen AC: Persistent "insect bites" (dermal eosinophilic granulomas) simulating lymphoblastomas, histiocytoses, and squamous cell carcinomas. Am J Pathol 24:367, 1948.

Allison J: Skin mastocytosis presenting as neonatal bullous eruption. Aust J Dermatol 9:83, 1967.

Anderson KC, Weinstein HJ: Transfusion associated graft-versus-host disease. N Engl J Med 323:315, 1990.

Banks PM, Arseneau JC, Gralnick HR, et al. American Burkitt's lymphoma: a clinicopathologic study of 30 cases. II. Pathologic correlations. Am J Med 58:322–329, 1975.

Beljaards RC, Kaudewitz P, Berti E, et al: Primary cutaneous CD30-positive large cell lymphoma: definition of a new type of cutaneous lymphoma with a favorable prognosis. Cancer 71:2097, 1993.

Berger BW: Erythema chronicum migrans of Lyme disease. Arch Dermatol 120:1017, 1984.

Brough AJ, Jones D, Page RH, et al: Dermal erythropoesis in neonatal infants: a manifestation of intrauterine viral disease. Pediatrics 40:627, 1967.

Canioni D, Fraitag S, Thomas C, et al: Skin lesions revealing neonatal acute leukemias with monocytic differentiation: a report of 3 cases. J Cutan Pathol 23:254, 1996.

Chan AC, Ho JW, Chiang AK, Srivastava G. Phenotypic and cytotoxic characteristics of peripheral T-cell and NK-cell lymphomas in relation to Epstein-Barr Virus association. Histopathology 34:16–24, 1999.

Chilcote RR, Brown E, Rowley JD: Lymphoblastic leukemia with lymphomatous features associated with abnormalities of the short arm of chromosome 9. N Engl J Med 313:286, 1985.

Choi KL: The role of the Langerhans cell and keratinocyte in epidermal immunity. J Leukocyte Biol 39:343, 1986.

Chott A, Vonderheid EC, Olbricht S, et al: The dominant T cell clone is present in multiple regressing skin lesions and associated T cell lymphomas of patients with lymphomatoid papulosis. J Invest Dermatol 106:696, 1996.

Darmstadt GL, Donnenberg AD, Vogelsang GB, et al: Clinical, laboratory, and histopathologic indicators of progressive graft-versus-host disease. J Invest Dermatol 99:397, 1992.

Desbarats J, Seemayer TA, Lapp WS: Irradiation of the skin and systemic graft-versus-host disease synergise to produce cutaneous lesions. Am J Pathol 144:883, 1994.

Enjolras O, Leibowitch M, Bonacini F, et al: [Congenital cutaneous Langerhans histiocytosis: apropos of 7 cases]. Ann Dermatol Venereol 119:111, 1992.

Fetsch JF, Weiss SW: Observations concerning the pathogenesis of epithelioid hemangioma (angiolymphoid hyperplasia). Mod Pathol 4:449, 1991.

Friedman BL, Will JJ, Friedman DG, et al: Tissue mast cell leukemia. *Blood* 13:70, 1958.

Garcia CF, Weiss LM, Warnke RA: Small noncleaved cell lymphoma: an immunophenotypic study of 18 cases and comparison with large cell lymphoma. Hum Pathol 17:454, 1986.

Gonzales CL, Medeiros LJ, Braziel RM, et al: T-cell lymphoma involving subcutaneous tissue. AM J Surg Pathol 15:17, 1991.

Gottesfeld E, Silverman RA, Coccia PF, et al: Transient blueberry muffin appearance of a newborn with congenital monoblastic leukemia. J Am Acad Dermatol 21:347, 1989.

Grumayer ER, Landenstein RL, Slavc I, et al: B-cell differentiation pattern of cutaneous lymphomas in infancy and childhood. Cancer 61:303, 1988.

Hauser C, Elbe A, Stingl E: The Langerhans cell. In Goldsmith LA (ed): Physiology, Biochemistry, and Molecular Biology of the Skin, 2nd ed. Oxford University Press, New York, pp 1144, 1991.

Hawthorne HC, Nelson JS, Witzleben CL, et al: Blanching subcutaneous nodules in neonatal neuroblastoma. J Pediatr 77:297, 1970.
Hebert AA, Esterly NB, Gardner TH: Dermal erythropoiesis in Rh hemolytic disease of the newborn. J Pediatr 5:799, 1985.
Hellman J, Phelps RG, Baral J, et al: Lymphomatoid papulosis with antigen deletion and clonal rearrangement in a 4-year-old boy. Pediatr Dermatol 7:42, 1990.
Hickham PR, McBurney EI, Fritzgerald RL: CTCL in patients under 20 year of age: a series of five cases. Pediatr Dermatol 14:93, 1997.
Hodges KB, Collins RD, Greer JP, et al. Transformation of the small cell variant Ki-1+ lymphoma to anaplastic large cell lymphoma: pathologic and clinical features. Am J Surg Pathol 23:49–58, 1999.
Horen WP: Insect and scorpion sting. JAMA 221:894, 1972.
Issekutz TB, Stoltz JM, van der Meide P: The recruitment of lymphocytes into the skin by T cell lymphokines: the role of gamma-interferon. Clin Exp Immunol 73:70, 1988.
Kadin ME, Sako D, Berliner N, et al: Childhood Ki-1 lymphoma presenting with skin lesions and peripheral lymphadenopathy. Blood 68:1042, 1986.
Kanavaros P, Lescs M-C, Briere J, et al. Nasal T-cell lymphoma: a clinicopathologic entity associated with peculiar phenotype and with Epstein-Barr virus. Blood 81:2688, 1993.
Katz SI: The skin as an immunologic organ. J Am Acad Dermatol 13:530, 1985.
Katz SI, Tamaki K, Sachs DH: Epidermal Langerhans cells are derived from cells originating in bone marrow. Nature 282:324, 1979.
Kaudewitz P, Kind P, Sander CA: CD30+ anaplastic large cell lymphomas. Semin Dermatol 13:180, 1994.
Kettlehut BV, Metcalfe DD: Pediatric mastocytosis. Ann Allergy 73:197, 1994.
Kimura T, Yoshimura S, Ishikawa E: Unusual granulation combined with hyperplastic change of lymphatic tissue. Trans Soc Pathol Jpn 37:179, 1948.
Kinney MC, Collins RD, Greer JP, et al. A small-cell-predominant variety of primary Ki-1 (CD30)+T-cell lymphoma. Am J Surg Pathol 17:859–868, 1993.
Kinney MC, Kadin ME: The pathologic and clinical spectrum of anaplastic large cell lymphoma and correlation with *ALK* gene dysregulation. Am J Pathol 111(suppl 1):S56, 1999.
Kitagawa N, Arata J, Ohtsuki Y, et al: Congenital alveolar rhabdomyosarcoma presenting as a blueberry muffin baby. J Dermatol 16:409, 1989.
Kitamura Y, Shimada M, Hatanaka K, et al: Development of mast cells from grafted bone marrow cells in irradiated mice. Nature 268:442, 1977.
Klaus SN, Winkelmann RK: Course of urticaria pigmentosa in children. Arch Dermatol 86:68, 1962.
Klein LM, Lavker RM, Matis WL, et al: Degranulation of human mast cells induces an endothelial antigen central to leukocyte adhesion. Proc Natl Acad Sci USA 86:8972, 1989.
Kobayasi T, Asboe-Hansen G: Degranulation and regranulation of human mast cells. Acta Derm Venereol (Stockh) 49:369, 1969.
Krinsky WL: Dermatoses associated with the bites of mites and ticks (Arthropoda: Acari). Int J Dermatol 22:75, 1983.
Krishnan J, Tomaszewski MM, Kao GF: Primary cutaneous CD30-positive anaplastic large cell lymphoma: report of 27 cases. J Cutan Pathol 20:193, 1993.
Langerhans P: Über die Nerven der menschlichen haut. Virchows Arch Pathol Anat 44:325, 1886.
Marshall J: Ticks and the human skin. Dermatologica 135:60-65, 1967.
Metcalfe DD, Horan RF, Austin KF, et al: Chemistry and storage function of mast cell granules. J Invest Dermatol 96:1, 1991.
Millot F, Robert A, Bertrand Y, et al: Cutaneous involvement in children with acute lymphoblastic lymphoma. Pediatrics 100:60, 1997.
Morhenn VB, Maibach HI: Graft vs host reaction in a newborn. Acta Derm Venereol (Stockh) 54:133, 1974.
Murphy GF, Mihm MC: Benign, dysplastic, and malignant lymphoid infiltrates of the skin: an approach based on pattern analysis. In Murphy GF, Mihm MC (eds): Lymphoproliferative Disorders of the Skin. Butterworth, Boston, p 123, 1986.
Olsen TG, Helweg EB: Angiolymphoid hyperplasia with eosinophilia: a clinicopathologic study of 116 patients. J Am Acad Dermatol 12:781, 1985.
Paulli M, Rosso R, Kindl S, et al: Immunophenotypic characterization of the cell infiltration in five cases of sinus histiocytosis with massive lymphadenopathy (Rosai-Dorfman disease). Hum Pathol 23:647, 1992.
Pui CH: Childhood leukemia. N Engl J Med 332:1618, 1995.
Ramón G, Sangüeza OP: Angiocentric cutaneous T-cell lymphoma of childhood (hydroa-like lymphoma): a distinctive type of cutaneous T-cell lymphoma. J Am Acad Dermatol 38:574, 1998.
Reiter A, Schrappe M, Tiemann M, et al: Successful treatment strategy for Ki-1 anaplastic large-cell lymphoma of childhood: a prospective analysis of 62 patients enrolled in three consecutive Berlin-Frankfurt-Munster group studies. J Clin Oncol 12:899, 1994.
Resnik KS, Brod BB: Leukemia cutis in congenital leukemia. Analysis and review of one world literature with report of an additional case. Arch Dermatol 129:1301, 1993.
Riyat MS: Mucocutaneous manifestations of lymphomas and leukemias in black Kenyan children. Int J Dermatol 34:249, 1995.
Rosai J, Dorfman RF: Sinus histiocytosis with massive lymphadenopathy: a newly recognized benign clinicopathologic entity. Arch Pathol 87:63, 1969.
Sander CA, Medeiros LJ, Abruzzo LV, et al: Lymphoblastic lymphoma presenting in cutaneous sites. J Am Acad Dermatol 25:1023, 1991.
Santamaria Babi LF, Moser R, Perez Soler MT, et al: Migration of skin-homing T cells across cytokine-activated human endothelial cell layers involves interaction of the cutaneous lymphocyte–associated antigen (CLA), the very late antigen-4 (VLA-4), and the lymphocyte function–associated antigen-1 (LFA-1). J Immunol 154:1543, 1995.
Santamaria Babi LF, Moser R, Perez Soler MT, et al. Circulating allergen-reactive T cells from patients with atopic dermatitis and allergic contact dermatitis express the skin-selective homing receptor, the cutaneous lymphocyte-associated antigen. J Exp Med 181:1935–1940, 1995.
Saurat JH, Gluckman E, Russel A, et al: The lichen planus–like eruption after bone marrow transplantation. Br J Dermatol 93:675, 1975.
Schwartz JL, Maniscalco WM, Lane AT, et al: Twin transfusion syndrome causing cutaneous erythropoiesis. Pediatrics 14:527, 1984.
Thawerani H, Sanchez RL, Rosai J, et al: The cutaneous manifestations of sinus histiocytosis with massive lymphadenopathy. Arch Dermatol 114:191, 1978.
vanWering ER, Kamps WA: Acute leukemia in infants, a unique pattern of acute nonlymphoblstic leukemia. Am J Pediatr Hematol Oncol 8:220, 1986.
Wells GC, Whimster IW: Subcutaneous angiolymphoid hyperplasia with eosinophilia. Br J Dermatol 81:1, 1969.
Zaatari GS, Chan WC, Kim TH, et al: Malignant lymphoma of the skin in children. Cancer 59:1040, 1987.
Zirbel GM, Gellis SE, Kadin ME, et al: Lymphomatoid papulosis in children. J Am Acad Dermatol 33:741, 1995.

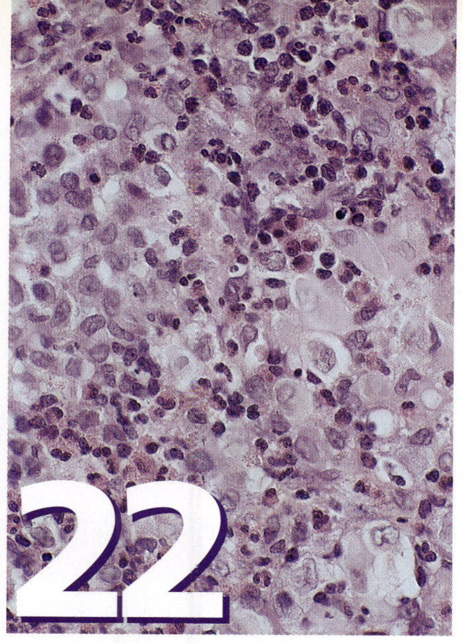

Sanya Sukpanichnant

Other Extranodal Sites

The extranodal sites discussed in this chapter are the heart, testes, ovaries, kidneys, and central nervous system (CNS), including the eyes. All of these extranodal sites are protected from contact with the environment and are therefore mostly devoid of lymphocytic tissue in "physiologic" states. Reactive and neoplastic hematopathologic disorders affecting these extranodal sites are discussed selectively. The reactive disorders include orbital inflammatory pseudotumor, Rosai-Dorfman disease of the ocular adnexa, and Kawasaki disease of the heart. The neoplastic disorders include extranodal lymphoma and leukemic infiltration. Langerhans cell histiocytosis and mastocytosis are discussed in Chaps. 10 and 8, respectively.

ORBITAL INFLAMMATORY PSEUDOTUMOR

Equivalent Terms

Orbital inflammatory pseudotumor is also known as idiopathic inflammatory orbital pseudotumor in childhood.

Definition

Orbital inflammatory pseudotumor is an inflammatory lesion of unknown cause that occurs within the orbit and clinically simulates a neoplasm.

Clinical Features

Lymphocytic proliferation in the ocular adnexa rarely occurs in childhood, but inflammatory pseudotumor occurs in children as well as in adults. There is no sex predilection. Patients typically develop sudden onset of periocular pain, swelling, chemosis, conjunctival injection, proptosis, a palpable mass, and ophthalmoplegia. Visual acuity is only slightly affected initially. Bilateral orbital involvement may occur, as may papilledema and iritis. No orbital bone changes or associated sinus diseases are observed. Simultaneous occurrence of painful ophthalmoplegia and positive antinuclear antibody test results are described in Tolosa-Hunt syndrome. Most cases respond dramatically to high doses of systemic corticosteroids (Mottow & Jakobiec, 1978).

Histopathologic Features

The lesion is typically hypocellular, with prominent fibrosis and edema. Widening of interlobular septa of lacrimal tissue is observed (Fig. 22–1). Only slight lymphocytic infiltration is noted, predominantly around capillaries and postcapillary venules. A few reactive lymphocytic follicles may be seen. No true vasculitis is detected. Tissue eosinophilia is occasionally seen, as is a lipogranulomatous response to damaged fat cells. No atypical cells are noted (Mottow-Lippa et al, 1981).

Differential Diagnosis

The hypocellular and inflammatory appearance of inflammatory pseudotumor distinguish it from ocular adnexal lymphocytic hyperplasia, malignant lymphoma, granulocytic sarcoma, and other tumors (Knowles & Jakobiec, 1992). Rosai-Dorfman disease should be considered if many histiocytes with emperipolesis are present.

ROSAI-DORFMAN DISEASE OF THE OCULAR ADNEXA

Equivalent Terms

Rosai-Dorfman disease is also known as sinus histiocytosis with massive lymphadenopathy (SHML).

Definition

SHML is a benign histiocytic proliferation of unknown cause seen mainly in lymph nodes but sometimes involving extranodal sites.

Clinical Features

SHML of the orbit is rare. Patients may present with isolated ocular involvement or with concurrent nodal and extranodal disease. Pain, proptosis, ptosis, decreased visual acuity, and ophthalmoplegia are observed (Wenig et al, 1993). Constitutional symptoms may be present, but hepatosplenomegaly is uncommon. Spontaneous remission may occur, but

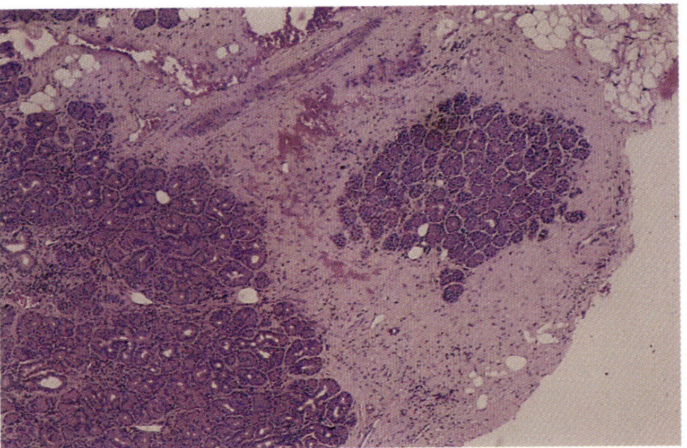

Figure 22–1

Inflammatory pseudotumor, eye. Incisional biopsy of an orbital mass demonstrates prominent fibrosis with widening of interlobular septa of lacrimal tissue. The surrounding adipose tissue is also involved. Mild chronic inflammation is present.

a minority of patients require treatment. The results of various kinds of treatment are controversial. Patients with an aggressive course tend to have involvement of many lymph nodes as well as extranodal sites (Foucar et al, 1990).

Histopathologic Features

The histologic features are similar to those described in lymph nodes, with dilated sinuses containing histiocytes. The characteristic histiocytes showing emperipolesis are usually fewer and less prominent than in the nodal lesion, whereas fibrosis is generally greater. Plasma cells are numerous. Paraffin-section immunoperoxidase studies demonstrate that the characteristic histiocytes express S-100 protein (Fig. 22–2).

Differential Diagnosis

Inflammatory pseudotumor is the most important differential diagnostic consideration.

KAWASAKI DISEASE INVOLVING THE HEART

Equivalent Terms

Kawasaki disease is also known as mucocutaneous lymph node syndrome.

Definition

Kawasaki disease is an acute febrile illness with systemic vasculitis of unknown etiology mainly affecting infants and young children.

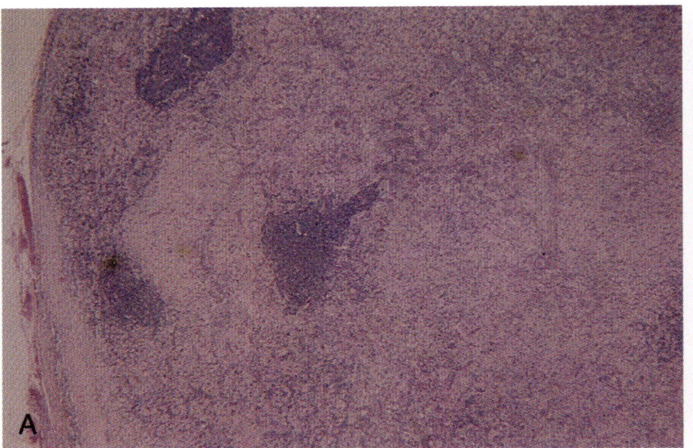

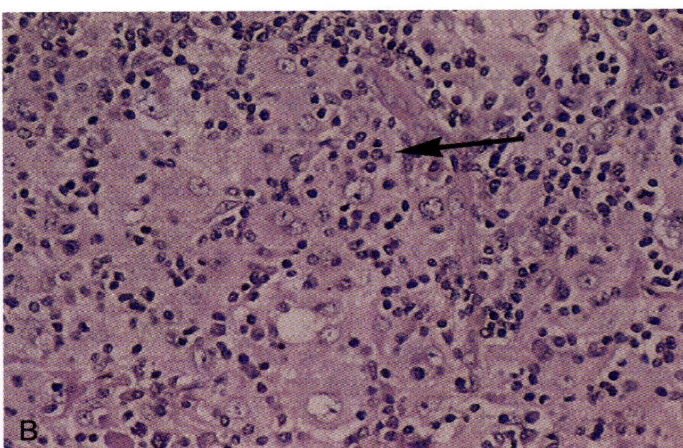

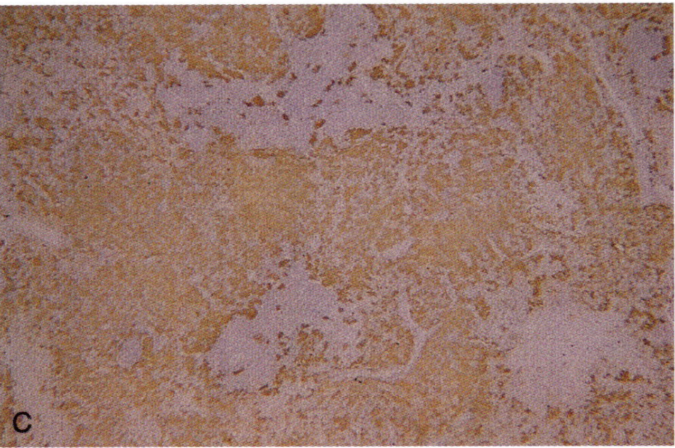

Figure 22–2

Rosai-Dorfman disease, eye, adnexa. *A,* An encapsulated mass is noted, with lymph node sinus–like pale eosinophilic areas separating aggregates of small lymphocytes and plasma cells. *B,* Accumulation of histiocytes. Typical emperipolesis is demonstrated (*arrow*). *C,* Lymph node sinus–like areas due to accumulation of S-100+ histiocytes are demonstrated. S-100 protein by paraffin-section immunoperoxidase.

Clinical Features

The manifestations of Kawasaki disease are fever persisting 5 days or more; erythema of the palms and soles, desquamation of the fingers and toes, and peripheral nonpitting edema; polymorphous exanthema; bilateral conjunctival congestion; lesions of the lips and oral cavity; and acute nonpurulent cervical lymphadenopathy (see Chap. 16). The diagnosis is usually based on the presence of at least five of these clinical criteria or four criteria if coronary artery aneurysms are demonstrable. Involvement of the coronary arteries is found in 20–40% of cases. Coronary thrombosis leading to myocardial infarction and death occurs in a small number of cases (Tizard et al, 1991).

Histopathologic Features

Histopathologic changes in Kawasaki disease include acute perivasculitis and vasculitis of smaller arteries, including major coronary arteries, arterioles, capillaries, and venules, often complicated by aneurysm and thrombosis, especially in epicardial coronary arteries. Pericarditis, myocarditis, endocarditis or valvulitis, and inflammation of the atrioventricular conduction system are also present. These changes usually disappear after 4 weeks. However, scarring, with severe stenosis of coronary arteries, fibrosis of myocardium, and endocardial fibroelastosis, may develop (Fujiwara & Hamashima, 1978). The mononuclear cells in the cardiac lesions are mainly macrophages and activated helper T cells. HLA-DR expression has been demonstrated on these mononuclear cells and endothelium of coronary artery at the infiltration sites (Terai et al, 1990).

LYMPHOMA INVOLVING OTHER EXTRANODAL SITES

Lymphomas in children frequently involve extranodal sites. The three common types of childhood lymphomas have a propensity for specific anatomic sites of involvement. Lymphoblastic lymphoma occurs in the anterior mediastinum in >50% of cases. Small noncleaved cell lymphomas of both Burkitt and non-Burkitt types occur in the abdomen in approximately 50% of cases, with the most common sites of involvement the distal small intestine, ovaries, and other pelvic organs. Large-cell lymphomas involve the central nervous system, bone, soft tissue, gonad, and upper respiratory tract, including the nasopharynx and paranasal sinuses, and are rarely seen in the anterior mediastinum. Childhood lymphomas also exhibit early, wide, noncontiguous dissemination and early marrow involvement. Hodgkin disease rarely involves extranodal sites (Kjeldsberg et al, 1983).

Lymphoma of the Central Nervous System

CNS involvement by lymphoma is common in advanced lymphoma or at relapse, but primary lymphomas of the CNS are rare, accounting for 1–2% of all malignant lymphomas and 0.5–1.5% of all CNS neoplasms. In adults, polymorphous high-grade B cell lymphoma is the predominant type (Schwechheimer et al, 1994). The incidence of primary CNS lymphoma in children is not known. Only 1 of 83 cases of primary CNS lymphoma from the Armed Forces Institute of Pathology series occurred in a child (Henry et al, 1974). Pediatric patients were not included in a large series of 105 cases of CNS involvement in B and T cell lymphomas (only 8 cases were primary CNS lymphoma) (MacKintosh et al, 1982). Five pediatric cases with CNS lymphoma were included in 91 CNS lymphomas with immunophenotypic studies (Murphy et al, 1989; Simon et al, 1987; Smith et al, 1988; Taylor et al, 1978).

Prognosis depends on the specific site of CNS involvement, stage of disease, tumor size, and histologic type. Survival was greatest in patients <30 years of age with primary CNS lymphoma who were treated by whole-brain irradiation and intrathecal chemotherapy (MacKintosh et al, 1982).

Lymphoma of the Eye and Ocular Adnexa

Primary lymphoma very rarely involves the eye or ocular adnexa in childhood. In two large series of 118 cases of malignant lymphoma of the ocular adnexa, the youngest patient was 17 years old, and the peak incidence was in the sixth and seventh decades (Knowles et al, 1990; Medeiros & Harris, 1989). Ocular lymphoma is closely associated with primary CNS lymphoma (Peterson et al, 1993). The orbital "histiocytic lymphomas" in old reports were probably granulocytic sarcomas or embryonal rhabdomyosarcomas (Jakobiec & Font, 1986).

Lymphoma of the Heart

Primary lymphoma of the heart is very rare. From a 20-year experience with 12,485 consecutive autopsies, there were 7 cases of primary and 154 cases of secondary cardiac tumors. No primary lymphoma of the heart was found, but secondary involvement represents the most common malignant tumor involving the heart (Lam et al, 1993). Most lymphomas involve the heart by local extension from the mediastinum or as a late manifestation of advanced lymphoma (Petersen et al, 1976). Among 196 autopsy cases of malignant lymphomas, 48 had cardiac involvement (24%), with an average age of 46 years. Few details have been reported about patient age, but a 7-year-old girl with lymphosarcoma has been described (Roberts et al, 1968). Most cases of childhood lymphoma are high-grade lymphomas of either the lymphoblastic lymphoma (Bagby et al, 1972) or the small noncleaved cell type (Cole et al, 1975). Most patients do not have signs or symptoms directly attributable to cardiac lymphoma, but cardiac tamponade, acute myocardial infarction, or arrhythmias may occur.

Lymphoma of the Gonad

Testicular involvement by lymphoma is rare in children. Nine of 131 cases (6.9%) of advanced childhood lymphoma exhibited testicular involvement (Kellie et al, 1989). Six were small noncleaved cell lymphoma, one lymphoblastic, and the other two unclassifiable. In 195 cases of primary testicular lymphomas (Duncan et al, 1980; Ferry et al, 1994; Martenson et al, 1988; Paladugu et al, 1980; Turner et al, 1981; Wilkins et al, 1989), there was 1 pediatric case (0.5%) of small noncleaved cell lymphoma. An angiocentric T cell lymphoma involving the testis was described in a child with T cell acute lymphoblastic leukemia during remission (Hsueh et al, 1993). Follicular center cell lymphomas are very rare in childhood, with 1 large-cell lymphoma reported. It is of interest that *BCL2* expression or gene rearrangement was not detected (Moertel et al, 1995).

Ovarian involvement by small noncleaved cell lymphoma is expected. In 19 pediatric cases from series of 109 cases of lymphoma involving the ovary, 15 cases were small noncleaved cell, 3 diffuse large cell, and 1 lymphoblastic type (Chorlton et al, 1974; Monterroso et al, 1993; Osborne & Robboy, 1983; Paladugu et al, 1980). Almost all of them were secondary.

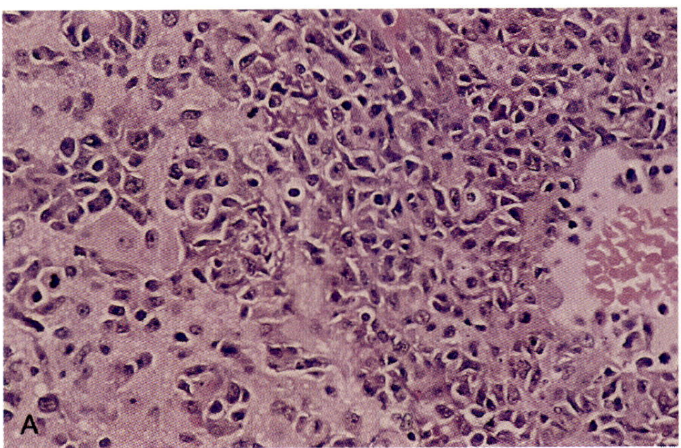

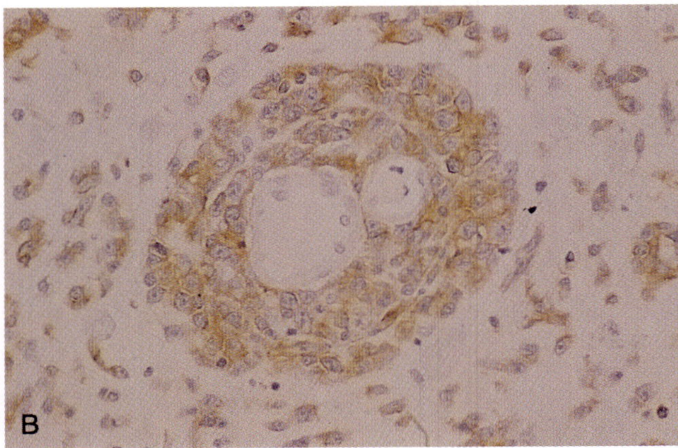

Figure 22–3

Lymphoma, central nervous system. *A,* Perivascular infiltration by lymphoma cells is a distinctive feature. These lymphoma cells are somewhat polymorphous and intermediate to large sized. *B,* CD20 positivity is demonstrated, indicative of B cell lymphoma. CD20 (L-26) by paraffin-section immunoperoxidase.

Lymphoma of the Kidney

Primary lymphoma of the kidney is very rare, with only a few cases involving kidney at presentation (Capps & Das Narla, 1995; Sumboonnanonda et al, 1994; Vujanic et al, 1995). Secondary lymphoma, particularly small noncleaved cell lymphoma, often involves the kidneys and retroperitoneal structures (Kjeldsberg et al, 1983).

Histopathologic Features

The histologic features of various types of lymphomas have been described in the previous chapters, but some extranodal lymphomas have typical growth patterns. Perivascular distribution is striking in both primary and secondary CNS lymphomas (Fig. 22–3) Pericardium and subepicardial fatty tissue as well as myocardium commonly exhibit lymphomatous involvement.

Lymphoma involving the testis demonstrates diffuse infiltration and peritubular invasion. Many atrophic or sclerotic seminiferous tubules are observed, and invasion of the tubules by lymphoma cells may be seen. Lymphoma involving the ovary also exhibits diffuse infiltration, with frequent destruction of ovarian follicles. Lymphoma cells may be arranged in a single-file pattern in the ovarian stroma, especially at the periphery of the ovarian cortex. Lymphoma often spreads along the serosal surface and infiltrates the adjacent structures, including fallopian tubes, uterus, rectum, bowel, and omentum (Fig. 22–4). Lymphoma of the kidney demonstrates an interstitial infiltrating pattern with destruction of the normal structures (Fig. 22–5).

Diagnostic Criteria

Extranodal lymphomas in childhood may be readily diagnosed if there are mass lesions produced by high-grade lymphoma. Polymorphous lesions may occur after transplantation (see Chap. 3) or after viral infection in patients with various immune deficits.

Differential Diagnosis

Leukemic infiltration is the most important differential diagnostic consideration. Clinical correlation, cytologic evaluation of the peripheral blood and marrow aspirate films, and immunophenotyping may be required for distinction. CNS lymphomas may resemble the more common primary CNS tumors, especially medulloblastoma. Seminoma of the testis may resemble large-cell lymphoma, although lymphoma often exhibits interstitial infiltration that is different from the pushing borders seen in most seminomas. Immunohistochemical studies are rarely required to distinguish between these two neoplasms.

Pathogenesis

Two explanations have been proposed for the origin of lymphoma cells in extranodal sites normally devoid of specially localized lymphocytic tissue (e.g., absence of bronchus-associated lymphoid tissue). One is that inflammatory cells may be recruited into an extranodal site by an infection, and then a clone of the inflammatory cells may be locally transformed

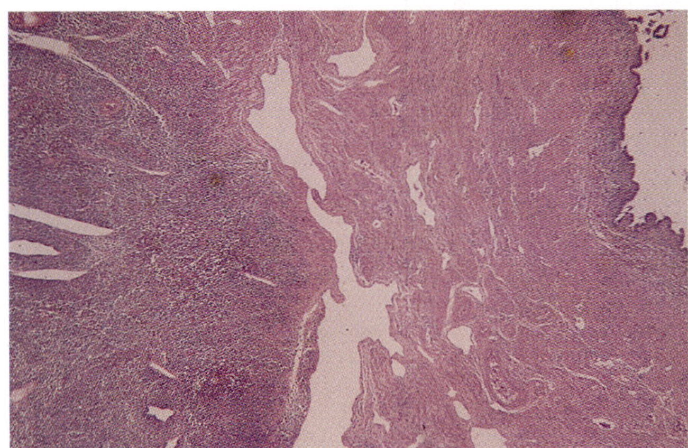

Figure 22–4

Lymphoma, parametrium and uterus. A small noncleaved cell lymphoma of the Burkitt type involved both ovaries and the omentum (not shown) and had spread along the serosal surface to involve the parametrium and the outer part of the uterine wall. Note the normal (inactive) endometrium on the right.

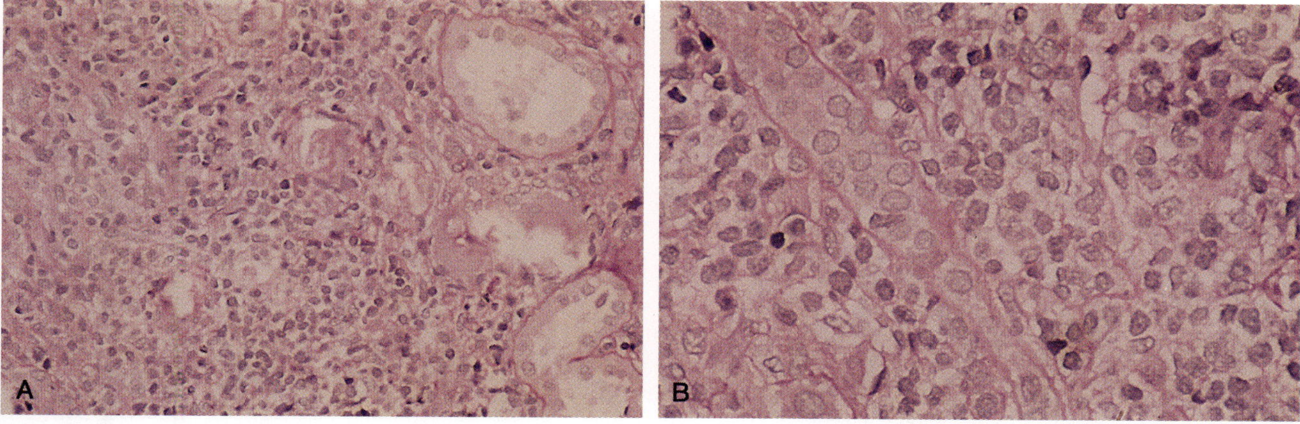

Figure 22–5

Lymphoma, kidney. *A,* Interstitial infiltration by small to intermediate-sized lymphoma cells is noted. *B,* Lymphoblastic appearance of lymphoma cells is demonstrated. A residual renal tubule is also noted. Periodic acid–Schiff stain.

into neoplastic cells (Hochberg & Miller, 1988). For instance, a primary diffuse large–B cell lymphoma of the brain was reported in a 12-year-old boy after a 5-year history of encephalitis. The evidence of Epstein-Barr virus infection demonstrated by polymerase chain reaction techniques and in situ hybridization suggested that Epstein-Barr virus infection occurred before the lymphoma (Aozasa et al, 1993). Lymphoma cells with specific binding sites may also migrate to particular extranodal sites after developing within a lymph node or elsewhere. In this regard, the homing cell adhesion molecule CD44 has been demonstrated in the blood vessels of the CNS parenchyma (Aho et al, 1993). The first speculation is generally assumed to explain most adult extranodal lymphomas and probably applies to children as well. Proving the site of origin of any lymphoma often is difficult, even in autopsy material from untreated patients. The pathogenesis of extranodal lymphomas will probably not be understood until there is a much broader comprehension of lymphocyte trafficking and more specific techniques for measuring lymphocyte adhesion molecules.

LEUKEMIC INFILTRATION

Equivalent Terms

Leukemic infiltration by acute myelogenous leukemia (AML) is also known as granulocytic sarcoma.

Definition

Leukemic infiltration of extramedullary structures may occur without evidence of leukemia in peripheral blood or marrow. Virtually any organ may be involved during advanced stages of leukemia. Organs outside the hematopoietic and lymphocytic system that are commonly involved include the CNS, lungs, kidneys, testes, and gums.

Leukemic infiltration of the CNS is common in acute lymphoblastic leukemia (ALL). More than half of CNS relapses show no evidence of marrow relapse (Swerdlow et al, 1985). Leukostasis is commonly observed in leukemic patients with a high leukocyte count. Although rarely seen, some patients with AML have intravascular leukocyte thrombi and aggregates producing infarction, edema, and hemorrhage (McKee & Collins, 1974).

Leukemic infiltration of the eye and periorbital tissue is uncommon. However, orbital granulocytic sarcoma has been reported from Turkey, Africa, and the Middle and Far East, ranging from 3–46% of patients with AML of all French-American-British classification subtypes. Most cases involve both eyes. Patients may have proptosis, conjunctival hemorrhage, and chemosis. Although most cases occur during the active phase of the disease, a few patients do not develop overt leukemia for months. The tumor mass responds well to chemotherapy, and patients with such presentations do not have a poorer prognosis (Shome et al, 1992).

Leukemic infiltration of the heart has been found in 37% of 420 autopsy cases of acute leukemia in all age groups (Roberts et al, 1968). Forty-four percent of 116 children dying of acute leukemia had at least one focus of cardiac leukemic infiltration. A significantly higher incidence of cardiac infiltration was found in AML than in ALL (66% versus 35%). There is a significant increase in cardiac infiltration in patients with a peripheral leukocyte count of 50,000/mm^3 or more. Cardiac hypertrophy found in acute leukemia may be the result of chronic anemia (Sumners et al, 1969).

Leukemic infiltration of the gonad is quite common. The testis and brain may represent protected sites not fully accessible to chemotherapeutic agents, and testicular relapse is common. A Southwest Oncology Group study reported occult testicular leukemia in 8.5% of 59 cases of ALL patients who were in complete remission (Askin et al, 1981). Approximately half or more of the testicular relapses in ALL occur without evidence of marrow relapse (Swerdlow, 1985). Leukemic infiltrations of the testis and the ovary were observed in 65 and 66%, respectively, of childhood leukemias in one postmortem survey (Reid & Marsden, 1980). Leukemic infiltration of the kidneys is commonly seen in ALL. Presentation with renal involvement may lead to the diagnosis (Bunchman et al, 1992).

Clinical Features

In addition to evidence of a local tumor mass, patients may have signs and symptoms associated with marrow failure, a high leukocyte count, cytopenia, or a previous history of treated leukemia or other neoplasms following systemic chemotherapy or irradiation. It is important to emphasize that leukemic infiltration, particularly granulocytic sarcoma, may occur without marrow evidence of leukemia.

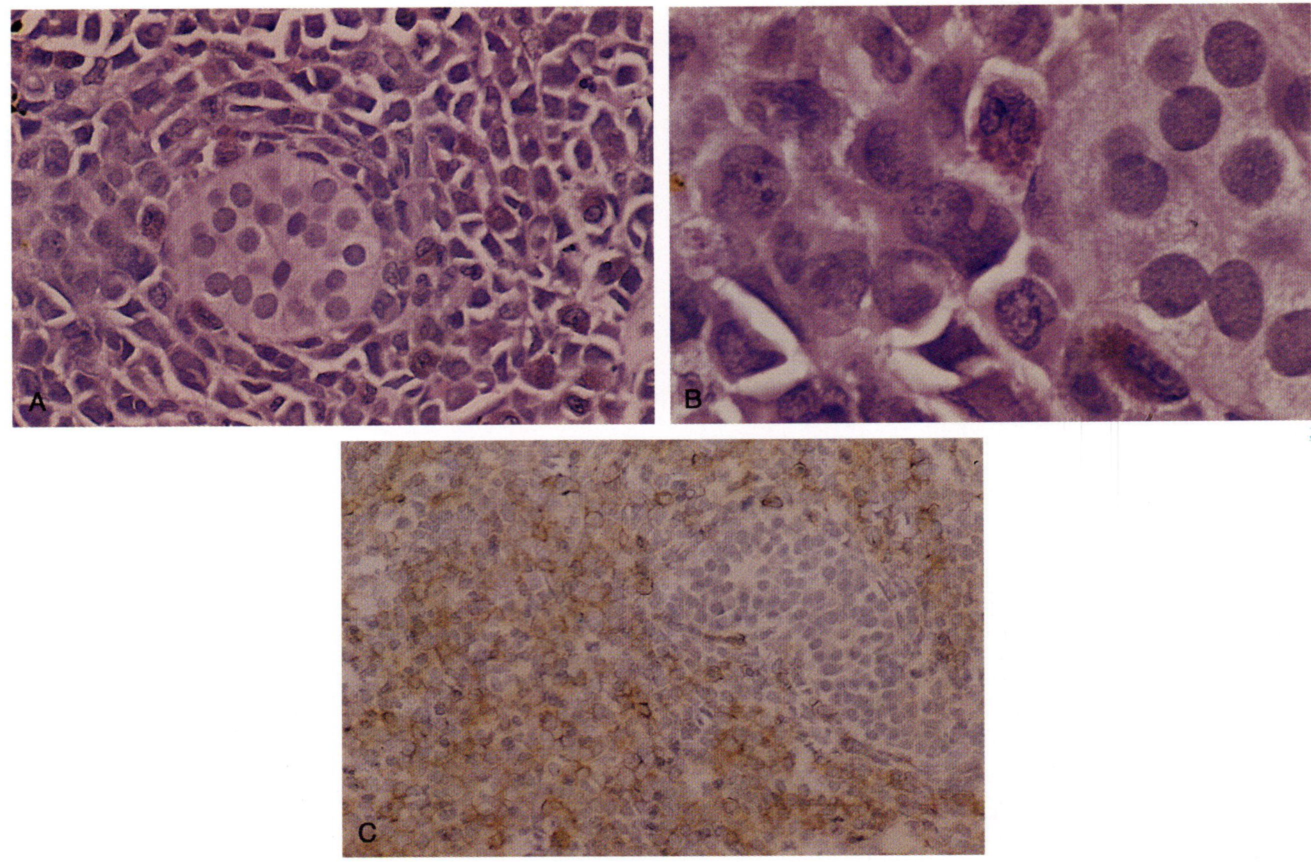

Figure 22–6

Leukemic infiltration, testis. *A,* Extensive interstitial infiltration by leukemic cells is noted, along with the residual seminiferous tubule, in acute myeloblastic leukemia. *B,* Leukemic cells on the left show delicate nuclear chromatin with some nuclear irregularity compared with the benign bland nuclei of the cells in the seminiferous tubule on the right. Eosinophils are also noted. *C,* CD43+ myeloblasts are demonstrated. Note the negative residual seminiferous tubule. CD43 by paraffin-section immunoperoxidase.

Histopathologic Features

Leukemic cells may be found in the blood vessels of affected tissues but are not impressive in most cases. Leukemic infiltrations are generally interstitial and may be focal or diffuse, destroying the normal structures of the affected organ (Fig. 22–6). Leukemic infiltration in the CNS commonly involves the leptomeninges and tends to be perivascular. Rare cases with leukostasis may be associated with hemorrhage, edema, and infarction. Most cases of CNS involvement in leukemia are recognized by cytologic studies of cerebrospinal fluid. Leukemic infiltrates of the heart are focal, are usually few in number, are most frequently located in the pericardium and walls of the left ventricle and right atrium, and occasionally extend through the cardiac wall. Leukemic infiltration of the testis is usually diffusely interstitial. Instances of focal involvement may be difficult to distinguish from crushed hyperchromatic tubular cells (Swerdlow et al, 1985).

Diagnostic Criteria

Interstitial infiltration by mononuclear cells with dispersed nuclear chromatin and occasional nucleoli (a blastic appearance) should raise the possibility of leukemia. Occasionally, the presence of immature eosinophils or megakaryoblasts allows a morphologic diagnosis of granulocytic sarcoma. In most cases, evaluation of peripheral blood and marrow aspirate smears establishes an underlying leukemia. In cases without evidence of leukemia in the marrow or peripheral blood, immunophenotypic or ultrastructural studies of the extranodal lesion are needed to make a diagnosis of leukemia.

REFERENCES

Orbital Inflammatory Pseudotumor

Knowles DM, Jakobiec FA: Malignant lymphomas and lymphoid hyperplasias that occur in the ocular adnexa (orbit, conjunctiva, and eyelids). In Knowles DM (ed): Neoplastic Hematopathology. Williams & Wilkins, Baltimore, pp 1009–1046, 1992.

Mottow LS, Jakobiec FA: Idiopathic inflammatory orbital pseudotumor in childhood. Arch Ophthalmol 96:1410–1417, 1978.

Mottow-Lippa L, Jakobiec FA, Smith M: Idiopathic inflammatory orbital pseudotumor in childhood: II. Results of diagnostic tests and biopsies. Ophthalmology 88:565–574, 1981.

Rosai-Dorfman Disease of the Ocular Adnexa

Foucar E, Rosai J, Dorfman R: Sinus histiocytosis with massive lymphadenopathy (Rosai-Dorfman disease): review of the entity. Semin Diagn Pathol 7:19–73, 1990.

Wenig BM, Abbondanzo SL, Childers EL, et al: Extranodal sinus histiocytosis with massive lymphadenopathy (Rosai-Dorfman disease) of the head and neck. Hum Pathol 24:483–492, 1993.

Kawasaki Disease Involving the Heart

Fujiwara H, Hamashima Y: Pathology of the heart in Kawasaki disease. Pediatrics 61:100–107, 1978.

Terai M, Kohno Y, Namba M, et al: Class II major histocompatibility antigen expression on coronary arterial endothelium in a patient with Kawasaki disease. Hum Pathol 21:231–234, 1990.

Tizard EJ, Suzuki A, Levin M, et al: Clinical aspects of 100 patients with Kawasaki disease. Arch Dis Child 66:185–188, 1991.

Lymphoma Involving Other Extranodal Sites

Kjeldsberg CR, Wilson JF, Berard CW: Non-Hodgkin's lymphoma in children. Hum Pathol 14:612–627, 1983.

Lymphoma of the Central Nervous System

Henry JM, Heffner RR, Dillard SH, et al: Primary malignant lymphomas of the central nervous system. Cancer 34:1293–1302, 1974.

MacKintosh FR, Colby TV, Podolsky WJ, et al: Central nervous system involvement in non-Hodgkin's lymphoma: an analysis of 105 cases. Cancer 49:586–595, 1982.

Murphy JK, O'Brien CJ, Ironside JW: Morphologic and immunophenotypic characterization of primary brain lymphomas using paraffin-embedded tissue. Histopathology 15:449–460, 1989.

Schwechheimer K, Braus DF, Schwarzkopf G, et al: Polymorphous high-grade B cell lymphoma is the predominant type of spontaneous primary cerebral malignant lymphomas. Am J Surg Pathol 18:931–937, 1994.

Simon J, Jones EL, Trumper MM, et al: Malignant lymphomas involving the central nervous system: a morphological and immunohistochemical study of 32 cases. Histopathology 11:335–349, 1987.

Smith WJ, Garson JA, Bourne SP, et al: Immunoglobulin gene rearrangement and antigenic profile confirm B cell origin of primary cerebral lymphoma and indicate a mature phenotype. J Clin Pathol 41:128–132, 1988.

Taylor CR, Russell R, Lukes RJ, et al: An immunohistological study of immunoglobulin content of primary central nervous system lymphomas. Cancer 41:2197–2205, 1978.

Lymphoma of the Eye and Ocular Adnexa

Jakobiec FA, Font RL: Orbit: lymphoid tumors. In Spencer WH, Font RL, Green WR, et al (eds): Ophthalmic Pathology: An Atlas and Textbook, 3rd ed. W.B. Saunders Company, Philadelphia, pp 2663–2737, 1986.

Knowles DM, Jakobiec FA, McNally L, et al: Lymphoid hyperplasia and malignant lymphoma occurring in the ocular adnexa (orbit, conjunctiva, and eyelids): a prospective multiparametric analysis of 108 cases during 1977 to 1987. Hum Pathol 21:959–973, 1990.

Medeiros LJ, Harris NL: Lymphoid infiltrates of the orbit and conjunctiva: a morphologic and immunophenotypic study of 99 cases. Am J Surg Pathol 13:459–471, 1989.

Peterson K, Gordon KB, Heinemann M-H, et al: The clinical spectrum of ocular lymphoma. Cancer 72:843–849, 1993.

Lymphoma of the Heart

Bagby GC, Jr, Goldman RD, Newman HC, et al: Acute myocardial infarction due to childhood lymphoma. N Engl J Med 28:338–340, 1972.

Cole TO, Attah EB, Onyemelukwe GC: Burkitt's lymphoma presenting with heart block. Br Heart J 37:94–97, 1975.

Lam KY, Dickens P, Chan ACL: Tumors of the heart: a 20-year experience with a review of 12,485 consecutive autopsies. Arch Pathol Lab Med 117:1027–1031, 1993.

Petersen CD, Robinson Wa, Kurnick JE: Involvement of the heart and pericardium in the malignant lymphomas. Am J Med Sci 272:161–165, 1976.

Roberts WC, Glancy DL, DeVita VT Jr: Heart in malignant lymphoma (Hodgkin's disease, lymphosarcoma, reticulum cell sarcoma and mycosis fungoides): a study of 196 autopsy cases. Am J Cardiol 22:85–107, 1968.

Lymphoma of the Gonad

Chorlton I, Norris HJ, King FM: Malignant reticuloendothelial disease involving the ovary as a primary manifestation: a series of 19 lymphomas and 1 granulocytic sarcoma. Cancer 34:397–407, 1974.

Duncan PR, Checa F, Gowing NFC, et al: Extranodal non-Hodgkin's lymphoma presenting in the testicle: a clinical and pathologic study of 24 cases. Cancer 45:1578–1584, 1980.

Ferry JA, Harris NL, Young RH, et al: Malignant lymphoma of the testis, epididymis, and spermatic cord. A clinicopathologic study of 69 cases with immunophenotypic analysis. Am J Surg Pathol 18:376–390, 1994.

Hsueh C, Gonzalez-Crussi F, Murphy SB: Testicular angiocentric lymphoma of postthymic T-cell type in a child with T-cell acute lymphoblastic leukemia in remission. Cancer 72:1801–1805, 1993.

Kellie SJ, Pui C-H, Murphy SB: Childhood non-Hodgkin's lymphoma involving the testis: clinical features and treatment outcome. J Clin Oncol 7:1066–1070, 1989.

Martenson JA Jr, Buskirk SJ, Ilstrup DM, et al: Patterns of failure in primary testicular non-Hodgkin's lymphoma. J Clin Oncol 6:297–302, 1988.

Moertel CL, Watterson J, McCormick SR, et al: Follicular large cell lymphoma of the testis in a child. Cancer 75:1182–1186, 1995.

Monterroso V, Jaffe ES, Merino MJ, et al: Malignant lymphomas involving the ovary: a clinicopathologic analysis of 39 cases. Am J Surg Pathol 17:154–170, 1993.

Osborne BM, Robboy SJ: Lymphomas or leukemia presenting as ovarian tumors: an analysis of 42 cases. Cancer 52:1933–1943, 1983.

Paladugu RR, Bearman RM, Rappaport H: Malignant lymphoma with primary manifestation in the gonad. A clinicopathologic study of 38 patients. Cancer 45:561–571, 1980.

Turner RR, Colby TV, MacKintosh FR: Testicular lymphomas: a clinicopathologic study of 35 cases. Cancer 48:2095–2102, 1981.

Wilkins BS, Williamson JMS, O'Brien CJ: Morphological and immunohistological study of testicular lymphomas. Histopathology 15:147–156, 1989.

Lymphoma of the Kidney

Capps GW, Das Narla L: Renal lymphoma mimicking clear cell sarcoma in a pediatric patient. Pediatr Radiol 25(suppl 1):S87–S89, 1995.

Kjeldsberg CR, Wilson JF, Berard CW: Non-Hodgkin's lymphoma in children. Hum Pathol 14:612–627, 1983.

Sumboonnanonda A, Veerakul C, Sukpanichnant S, et al: Clinical quiz (lymphoma involving the kidney with tumor lysis syndrome). Pediatr Nephrol 8:641–643, 1994.

Vujanic GM, Webb D, Kelsey A: B-cell non-Hodgkin's lymphoma presenting as a primary renal tumour in a child. Med Pediatr Oncol 25:423–426, 1995.

Pathogenesis

Aho R, Ekfors T, Haltia M, et al: Pathogenesis of primary central nervous system lymphoma: invasion of malignant lymphoid cells into and within brain parenchyme. Acta Neuropathol (Berl) 86:71–76, 1993.

Aozasa K, Saeki K, Horiuchi K, et al: Primary lymphoma of the brain developing in a boy after a 5-year history of encephalitis: polymerase chain reaction and in situ hybridization analyses for Epstein-Barr virus. Hum Pathol 24:802–805, 1993.

Hochberg FH, Miller DC: Primary central nervous system lymphoma. J Neurosurg 68:835–853, 1988.

Leukemic Infiltration

Askin FB, Land VJ, Sullivan MP, et al: Occult testicular leukemia: testicular biopsy at three years continuous complete remission of childhood leukemia: a Southwest Oncology Group study. Cancer 47:470–475, 1981.

Bunchman TE, Gale GB, O'Connor DM, et al: Renal biopsy diagnosis of acute lymphocytic leukemia. Clin Nephrol 38:142–144, 1992.

McKee LC, Collins Rd: Intravascular leukocyte thrombi and aggregates as a cause of morbidity and mortality in leukemia. Medicine 53:463–478, 1974.

Reid H, Marsden HB: Gonadal infiltration in children with leukemia and lymphoma. J Clin Pathol 33:722–729, 1980.

Roberts WC, Bodey GP, Wertlake PT: The heart in acute leukemia: a study of 420 autopsy cases. AM J Cardiol 21:388–412, 1968.

Shome DK, Gupta NK, Prajapati NC, et al: Orbital granulocytic sarcomas (myeloid sarcomas) in acute nonlymphocytic leukemia. Cancer 70:2298–2301, 1992.

Sumners JE, Johnson WW, Ainger LE: Childhood leukemia heart disease: a study of 116 hearts of children dying of leukemia. Circulation 40:575–581, 1969.

Swerdlow SH, Glick AD, Cousar JB, et al: Acute leukemias of childhood: pathologic features. Hematol Oncol 3:99–131, 1985.

INDEX

Page numbers in *italics* refer to figures. Page numbers followed by t refer to tables.

A

Abdominal lymph node(s), metastatic neuroblastoma in, 318
Abscess(es), hepatic, *371,* 371–372
  in chronic granulomatous disease, 37, *352*
  splenic, 352–353
Acquired immunodeficiency disorder (AIDS). See *Human immunodeficiency virus (HIV) infection.*
Actinomycosis, and lymphadenitis, 293, *293*
Acute lymphocytic leukemia (ALL), classification of, 69–70, 74t–75t
  cytogenetic abnormalities in, 73t
  diagnosis of, cerebrospinal fluid examination in, 6–7, *6–7*
  granular, 81–82, *83*
  hyperdiploid, 63–64, 79, *80*
  L3, with Burkitt lymphoma, 80–81, *81*
    immunophenotypic evaluation in, 66–67, 72t, *72*
      pathology of, marrow biopsy in, *67*
  Philadelphia chromosome–positive, 80
  pre-B, with t(1;19), 80
  T cell, 81
    skin disorders from, 394–395
  vs. Burkitt lymphoma, 238, *238*
  with cryptic t(12;21), 79–80
  with eosinophilia, and t(5;14), 81, *82*
Acute myelogenous leukemia (AML), "biologic" subgroups of, 70, 75t
  classification of, 69–70, 74t–75t
  diagnosis of, flow cytometry in, 62, *63*
  epidemiology of, 61
  extranodal infiltration of, 407–408, *408*
  mediastinal germ cell tumors with, 338, *338*
  multidrug-resistant, 79
  pathology of, blasts in, 63, *65–66*
    cytochemical evaluation in, 65, 68t, *69*
    morphologic features of myeloblasts and, *63*
  promyelocytic, 72–73, 76t, *77*
  therapy-related, 78t, 78–79, *79*
  vs. T lymphoblastic lymphoma/leukemia, 332, *333*
  with inv(16)(p13q22), 74–75, 76t, *78*
  with monosomy 7 syndrome, 76–78
  with myelodysplastic features, 75–77
  with t(8,21), 73–76, *77*
Acute promyelocytic leukemia (APL), 72–73, 76t, *77*
ADA (adenosine deaminase), deficiency of, 31
Adenocarcinoma, in hyper-IgM syndrome, 25t
Adenosine deaminase (ADA), deficiency of, 31
Agammaglobulinemia, and splenic function, 351
  X-linked, 27
    gastrointestinal manifestations of, 363
Age, and incidence of Hodgkin disease, 211
  and weight of thymus, 323, 324t
Agnogenic myeloid metaplasia, 148, *150,* 150t
Agranulocytosis, genetic, infantile, 128
AIDS (acquired immunodeficiency disorder). See *Human immunodeficiency virus (HIV) infection.*
ALCL. See *Anaplastic large-cell lymphoma (ALCL).*
ALK antibody(ies), in anaplastic large-cell lymphoma, 254
Alkylating agent(s), and leukemia, 78t, 78–79
ALL. See *Acute lymphocytic leukemia (ALL).*
Allergic proctocolitis, 364
Allergy(ies), in IgA deficiency, 24
Allograft, rejection of, vs. posttransplant lymphoproliferative disorders, 56
Amastigote(s), in leishmaniasis, 312, *313*
AML. See *Acute myelogenous leukemia (AML).*
Amyloidosis, hepatic manifestations of, 372
Anaplastic large-cell lymphoma (ALCL), 249–254, *251–257,* 258t–259t
  and overlap with Hodgkin disease, 251–252
  clinical features of, 249–250
  diagnostic criteria for, 253, 259t
  differential diagnosis of, 253–254
  epidemiology of, 199–200, 249–250
  fine-needle aspiration biopsy in, *17,* 17–18
  genotypic features of, 202
  histopathologic features of, 250–253, *251–257*
  immunophenotypic features of, 253, 258t
  Ki-1+, 395–396, *396–397*
  monomorphic variant of, 250, *251*
  pathogenesis of, 254
  pleomorphic, *251*
  prognosis in, 250
  pulmonary, 383–384
  sarcomatoid variant of, 251, *255*
  skin lesions in, 252, *256*
  small-cell variant of, 250–251, *252–255, 257*
  treatment of, 250
  vs. Hodgkin disease, 214, 216t
  vs. lymphomatoid papulosis, 252
Anemia, aplastic, 126–127, 126t–127t, *127*
  cardiac disease and, 161
  collagen vascular disease and, 162
  Cooley. See *Thalassemia.*
  Diamond-Blackfan, 125–126, 125t–126t
Anemia *(Continued)*
  differential diagnosis of, 118t
  dyserythropoietic, congenital, 115–116, 116t, *117*
    vs. thalassemia, 144
  erythroblastic. See *Thalassemia.*
  Fanconi, 126
  from reduced red cell production, in neonates, 175, 177t
  from viral infections, 158
  gastrointestinal disorders and, 161
  glucose-6-phosphate dehydrogenase deficiency and, 113–115, 114t–116t, *115*
  hemolytic, 122–124, 123t–124t, *124*
    causes of, 123t
    clinical features of, 122–123
    IgG and, 122
    in neonates, 175, 177t
    laboratory studies in, 123, 123t
    prosthetic heart valves and, 161
    splenectomy for, 344, *347*
  in bacterial infection, 157
  in human immunodeficiency virus infection, 159
  in neonates, 174–175, 177t
    from blood loss, 174, 177t
  inherited, 105–112, *106–112,* 106t–112t
    and elliptocytosis, 111, 112t
    and pyropoikilocytosis, 112, *112*
    and sickle cell disease, 105–106, *106,* 106t. See also *Sickle cell disease.*
    and spherocytosis, 109–112, 110t
    and xerocytosis, 112–113
  lead-associated, 121–122, *122,* 122t
  megaloblastic, 119–121, 120t, *121*
    etiology of, 119–121, 120t
    laboratory studies in, 120t, 121, *121*
  nutritional/toxic, 116–122, *117–122,* 118t–122t
    iron deficiency, laboratory studies in, 117–118, 118t
      vs. anemia of chronic disease, 160, 161t
      vs. thalassemia, 144
    megaloblastic, 119–121, 120t, *121*
    nutritional/toxic, iron deficiency, 116–118, *117,* 118t
    sideroblastic, 118–119, *119,* 119t
      vs. thalassemia, 144
  of chronic disease, 160, 161t
  pyruvate kinase deficiency and, 113, *113,* 114t
  refractory, in myelodysplasia, 150–151
  renal disease and, 161–162

Angiocentric cutaneous T cell lymphoma, 396–397, *398*
Angiocentric natural killer cell lymphoma, 266–267, *267*, 267t
Angiofollicular hyperplasia, 283–287, *284–286*, 286t
  clinical features of, 283–284
  definition of, 283
  diagnostic criteria for, 286
  differential diagnosis of, 286t, 287
  fine-needle aspiration biopsy in, 16
  genotypic studies of, 285–286
  histopathologic features of, 284–285, *284–286*
  hyaline vascular, 283, *284–285*
  in lungs, 382
  in thymus, 329, *329–330*
  markers for, 285
  multifocal, in spleen, 354
  pathogenesis of, 287
  plasma cell, 283–284, *286*
  variants of, 283–284
  vs. interfollicular mixed cellularity Hodgkin disease, 216, *218*
  vs. progressive transformation of germinal centers, 281t
Angioimmunoblastic lymphadenopathy-like T cell lymphoma, 254–257, *258*, 258t
Angiolymphoid hyperplasia, with eosinophilia, *391*, 391–392
Angioma, littoral cell, of spleen, 348
Angiosarcoma, of spleen, 348
Anisocytosis, in thalassemia, *141*
Antibody deficiency(ies), classification of, 23t
Antibody titer(s), in immunodeficiency disorders, 22
Antigen(s), CD. See *CD antigen(s).*
Antigen-presenting cell(s) (APCs), in Hodgkin disease, 220-221
APL (acute promyelocytic leukemia), 72–73, 76t, *77*
Aplastic anemia, 126–127, 126t–127t, *127*
Appendix, *Yersinia* infections of, 366, *366*
Argyrophilic inclusion(s), in red cells, and splenic function, 344, *345*
Arthropod bite(s), skin reactions from, 390–391, *390–391*
Aspergillosis, and lymphadenitis, 301–302, *302*
  pulmonary, 385
Ataxia-telangiectasia, 34–35
Autoimmune disorder(s), and splenic function, 352
  gastrointestinal manifestations of, 364–365, *365*
Autoimmune enteropathy, 365
AZT (zidovudine), hematologic effects of, 159

B

B cell(s), abnormalities of, in combined variable immunodeficiency disorders, 28–29
  deficiency of, and splenic function, 351
    in X-linked agammaglobulinemia, 27
  disorders of, in severe combined immunodeficiency disorder, 29, 30t, 31
  immunophenotypic features of, 70t
B7, expression of, in Reed-Sternberg cells, 203
Babesiosis, vs. malaria, 171–172
Bacterial infection(s), 157–158, 158t, *158–159*
  hepatic, *371*, 371–372
BALT (bronchus-associated lymphatic tissue), 381
Basophil(s), stippling of, in thalassemia, 142, *142*
    lead poisoning and, 122, *122*
Basophilia, 129–130, 130t
Basophilic cytoplasm, in Burkitt lymphoma, 237, *238*
BCL2, and prognosis in acute leukemia, 87
BCL6, in anaplastic large-cell lymphoma, 202
  in Burkitt lymphoma, 201
    mutations in, in posttransplant lymphoproliferative disorders, 54–55
Bernard-Soulier syndrome, 132, *132*
Biopsy, advances in, 2–3
  bone marrow. See *Bone marrow, biopsy of.*
  fine-needle aspiration. See *Fine-needle aspiration (FNA) biopsy.*
Birbeck granule(s), in Langerhans cell histiocytosis, 189
Bite(s), arthropod, skin reactions from, 390–391, *390–391*
Bite cell(s), in glucose-6-phosphate dehydrogenase deficiency, 114, *115*
Blast(s), in acute leukemia, morphologic features of, 63, 64t, *64–66*
    relapse of, 85, *87*
  in cerebrospinal fluid, in acute lymphoblastic leukemia, 6, *6*
  in extramedullary leukemia, 319, *319*
  in lymphoblastic lymphoma, T cell lineage, 247, *248*
"Blast count," low, 85
Blast crisis, in chronic myelogenous leukemia, 96–97, *98–100*, 99t
Blastomyces dermatitidis lymphadenitis, 299–300
Blood loss, anemia from, in neonates, 174, 177t
Blood study(ies). See under specific disorder(s), e.g., *Chronic myelogenous leukemia (CML).*
Blueberry muffin syndrome, 390
Body fluid(s), examination of, 5–11
    cerebrospinal, 5-6
    serous, 6, 8–11, *9–11*
    specimen handling in, 5
  hematologic disorders in, 6–8, *6–8*
Bone, Langerhans cell histiocytosis in, 190
Bone marrow. See *Marrow* entries.
Bordetella pertussis infection, lymphocytosis in, 157, *158*
Bowel. See *Intestine(s).*
Break-bone fever, 169–170
Bronchiolitis, follicular, 381
Bronchiolitis obliterans, 385, *386*
Bronchitis, follicular, 381
Bronchus-associated lymphatic tissue (BALT), 381
Brucella lymphadenitis, *297*, 297–298
BTK gene, defects in, and X-linked agammaglobulinemia, 27
Bubonic plague, and lymphadenitis, 295
Burkholderia pseudomallei melioidosis, 313–314, *314*
Burkitt lymphoma, 235–239, 236t, *236–239*
  classification of, 235
  clinical features of, 235–236, 236t
  cytogenetic features of, 239
  definition of, 235
  differential diagnosis of, 239
  discovery of, 1
  epidemiology of, 199–200, 235–236, 236t
  fine-needle aspiration biopsy in, 17, *17*
  genotypic features of, 200–201
  histopathologic features of, 236–238, *236–238*
  historical perspective on, 235
Burkitt lymphoma *(Continued)*
  immunophenotypic features of, 238–239, *239*
  pathogenesis of, infection in, 204
  peritoneal effusion in, *9*, 9–10
  skin disorders in, 400, *400*
  vs. acute lymphocytic leukemia, 238, *238*
  vs. intestinal T cell lymphoma, 268–269
  vs. T lymphoblastic lymphoma/leukemia, 331, 331t, *332*
  with L3 acute lymphocytic leukemia, 80–81, *81*

C

CAE (chloracetate esterase), naphthol, 68t
Candidal infection(s), in severe combined immunodeficiency disorder, 29
Candidal lymphadenitis, 301
Cardiac. See also *Heart* entries.
Cardiac disease, hematologic effects of, 160–161, *161*
Castleman disease. See *Angiofollicular hyperplasia.*
Cat-scratch disease, 295–296, *296*
  and granulomatous lymphadenitis, 15, *15*
  hepatic, 371, *371*
CD antigen(s), and CD4 lymphopenia, idiopathic, 32
  CD3, in natural killer cell leukemia/lymphoma, 264
    in thymus, *325*
  CD15, in Reed-Sternberg cells, 220, *221*
  CD18, mutations in, in leukocyte adhesion deficiency, 36–37
  CD20, in Burkitt lymphoma, 238, *239*
    in large B cell lymphoma, 333, *334*
    in Reed-Sternberg cells, 221, *222*
  CD22, expression of, in acute leukemia, 66, *67*
  CD30, in anaplastic large-cell lymphoma, 202, *251*, 253, 258t
    in Hodgkin disease, of thymus, 337, *337*
    in Ki-1+ anaplastic large-cell lymphoma, 396
    in Reed-Sternberg cells, 220, *221*
  CD34, expression of, in acute leukemia, 66–67
  CD40L, abnormalities of, in hyper-IgM syndrome, 26–27
  CD43, in Wiskott-Aldrich syndrome, 35
  CD56, in angiocentric lymphoma, 267
    in precursor natural killer cell leukemia/lymphoma, 269
  expression of, in T cell lineage lymphoblastic lymphoma, 247–248, 249t
Celiac disease, 364–365, *365*
  IgA deficiency and, 24, 363
Celiac lymph node(s), Hodgkin disease in, staging of, *228*
Cell-mediated defect(s), congenital, and infectious lymphadenitis, 292
Central nervous system (CNS), lymphoma of, 405
Cerebriform cell(s), in mycosis fungoides, 259–260, *259–260*
Cerebrospinal fluid (CSF), examination of, 5–6
  leukemic cells in, 6–8, *6–8*
  lymphoma in, 8, *8*
  red cell contamination of, 7, *8*
Ceroid storage disease, splenomegaly in, 357
Cervical lymph node(s), lymphoblastic lymphoma in, T cell lineage, *248*
  metastatic nasopharyngeal carcinoma in, *319*
  metastatic rhabdomyosarcoma in, *318*
Chédiak-Higashi syndrome, 38, 128, *129*

Chemotherapy, for posttransplant lymphoproliferative disorders, 51
hematologic effects of, 163–164, *163–164,* 164t
Chloracetate esterase (CAE), naphthol, 68t
Cholesterol ester storage disease, splenomegaly in, 356–357
Chromosomal defect(s), immunodeficiency disorders from, classification of, 23t
Chromosome(s), 22q, microdeletion in, and DiGeorge anomaly, 34
Chronic granulomatous disease, 37–38, 291–292, *292*
and splenic function, 351–352, *352*
gastrointestinal manifestations of, 363–364
Chronic myelogenous leukemia (CML), 95–99, *96–100,* 96t, 99t–100t
blood and marrow findings in, 95, 96t, *97–98*
clinical features of, 95
course of, 96–97, *98–100,* 99t–100t
cytogenetic molecular features of, 95–96, *98*
differential diagnosis of, 97–99, 100t
incidence of, 95
Clear cell lymphoma, 333
Clonality, demonstration of, in diagnosis of lymphoma, 198
CML. See *Chronic myelogenous leukemia (CML).*
CMV (cytomegalovirus) infection, and lymphadenitis, 306, *306*
CNS (central nervous system), lymphoma of, 405
Coagulation disorder(s), cardiac disease and, 161
Cobalamin, deficiency of, and megaloblastic anemia, 119–120, 120t
"Cobblestone" appearance of nodes, in angiolymphoid hyperplasia, with eosinophilia, 391, *391*
Coccidioides immitis lymphadenitis, 300, *300*
Colitis, in common variable immunodeficiency, 362–363
Collagen, sclerosis of, in large B cell lymphoma, 333, *334*
in T lymphoblastic lymphoma/leukemia, *330*
Collagen band(s), in Hodgkin disease, nodular sclerotic, 217, *218–219*
Collagen vascular disease(s), hematologic effects of, 162
Colon, graft-versus-host disease in, *368*
Combined variable immunodeficiency disorder (CVID), *28,* 28–29, 30t, 31
gastrointestinal manifestations of, 362–363, *362–363*
Communication, between pathologists and other physicians, 3
Complement disorder(s), classification of, 23t
Cooley anemia. See *Thalassemia.*
Corynebacterium diphtheriae lymphadenitis, 294
Cow's milk–sensitive enteropathy, 364
Crypt cell(s), in graft-versus-host disease, 367, *368*
Crypt hyperplasia, in celiac disease, 364, *365*
Cryptococcus neoformans lymphadenitis, 300, *301*
CSF. See *Cerebrospinal fluid (CSF).*
Cutaneous T cell lymphoma. See *Mycosis fungoides.*
CVID (combined variable immunodeficiency disorder), *28,* 28–29, 30t, 31
gastrointestinal manifestations of, 362–363, *362–363*
Cyst(s), splenic, 347
thymic, 327–329, *328,* 328t
Cystic fibrosis, hematologic effects of, 162
Cytocentrifugation, for cerebrospinal fluid examination, 6
for serous effusion examination, 6
Cytochemical study(ies), in acute leukemia, 65, 68t, *69*
of cerebrospinal fluid, in diagnosis of leukemia, 7
Cytogenetic abnormality(ies). See specific disease, e.g., *Burkitt lymphoma.*
Cytokine(s), defects of, in severe combined immunodeficiency disorders, 30t, 30–31
hematologic effects of, 165–167, *166,* 166t
in Reed-Sternberg cells, 221–222
Cytomegalovirus (CMV) infection, and lymphadenitis, 306, *306*
Cytoplasm, blebbing of, in neonates with Down syndrome, 179, *181*

D

Dendritic cell(s), biology of, 189–190
Dendrocyte(s), dermal, and xanthogranuloma, 191–192, *193*
benign cutaneous disorders from, *193,* 193–194
Dengue hemorrhagic fever, 169–170
Dermal dendrocyte(s), and xanthogranuloma, 191–192, *193*
benign cutaneous disorders from, *193,* 193–194
Diamond-Blackfan anemia, 125–126, 125t–126t
Diarrhea, from severe combined immunodeficiency disorder, 363
Diff-Quik stain, of lymph node fine-needle biopsy aspirate, 14
Diffuse lymphoid hyperplasia, 381–382, *382*
DiGeorge syndrome, *33,* 33–34, 292
Direct antibody testing, in hemolytic anemia, 123, 123t
Döhle body(ies), cytokine administration and, 165, *166*
in bacterial infections, 157, *158*
Down syndrome, and acute leukemia, 72, *76*
incidence of, 61
in neonates, hematologic diseases with, 178–179, 179t–180t, *180–181*
Drug(s), and hemolytic anemia, 123, 124t
and toxic anemia, 122t
Dyserythropoiesis, in myelodysplasia, 149–150, *152*
Dyserythropoietic congenital anemia, 115–116, 116t, *117*
vs. thalassemia, 144
Dyspoiesis, in chronic myelogenous leukemia, 96, *98*

E

EBV. See *Epstein-Barr virus (EBV).*
Ectopic thymus, *328*
11q23 translocation, and congenital leukemia, 71, *75*
and leukemia, in neonates, 181t, 181–182, *182*
Elliptocytosis, hereditary, 111, 112t
End-stage renal disease (ESRD), erythropoietin for, hematologic effects of, 166–167
Enteric fever, *316,* 316–317
Enterocolitis, neutropenic, 367, *367*
Enteropathy, autoimmune, 365
intestinal T cell lymphoma with, 268–269, *269,* 269t
Enteroviral infection(s), in X-linked agammaglobulinemia, 27
Enzyme deficiency(ies), with immunodeficiency disorders, 31
Eosinophil(s), in skin, 389
Eosinophil peroxidase, deficiency of, 38
Eosinophilia, 129, *129,* 129t
acute lymphocytic leukemia with, and t(5;14), 81, *82*
angiolymphoid hyperplasia with, *391,* 391–392
Eosinophilic cytoplasm, in typhoid fever, *316*
Eosinophilic granuloma, in Langerhans cell histiocytosis, 190, *191*
Epithelial cell(s), in thymus, 323–324, *324*
in large B cell lymphoma, *333*
Epithelioid histiocyte(s), in Hodgkin disease, 215, *216*
in *Toxoplasma gondii* lymphadenitis, 308, *308*
Epstein-Barr virus (EBV), 159
and angiofollicular hyperplasia, 285
and Burkitt lymphoma, 236
and hepatitis, 369–370, *370*
and Hodgkin disease, 211, 222–223, *223*
and lymphadenitis, 304–305, 304t, *305*
and lymphoma, 204–205
anaplastic large-cell, 254
in posttransplant lymphoproliferative disorders, 50, *52,* 57
in X-linked lymphoproliferative disorders, 46–47
serologic testing for, 304t
vs. angioimmunoblastic lymphadenopathy-like T cell lymphoma, 257
vs. juvenile myelomonocytic leukemia, 101–102
Erythroblast(s), in neonates with Down syndrome, 179, *180*
Erythroblastic anemia. See *Thalassemia.*
Erythroblastopenia, transient, vs. Diamond-Blackfan anemia, 126, 126t
Erythrocyte(s). See *Red cell(s).*
in malaria, 171, *171,* 171t
Erythrophagocytosis syndrome, infection-associated, *309,* 309–310
Erythropoietin, for end-stage renal disease, hematologic effects of, 166–167
Esophagus, normal mucosa of, 361
Essential thrombocythemia, 147, *149,* 149t
Ethanolaminosis, splenomegaly in, 356–357
Extramedullary hematopoiesis, 354
in graft-versus-host disease, *369*
in liver, 370
in spleen, 343
Extramedullary leukemia, *319,* 319–320
acute, 82–84, *83–86,* 85t
diagnosis of, 84, 85t, 86
misdiagnosis of, 83, *84,* 85t
Eye(s), leukemic infiltration of, 407
lymphoma of, 405

F

FAB classification. See *French-American-British (FAB) classification.*
Familial hemophagocytic lymphohistiocytosis, 357
Fanconi anemia, 126
FAS mutation(s), and autoimmune lymphoproliferative disorders, 354
Fat overload syndrome, 345

Fatal infectious mononucleosis. See *Lymphoproliferative disorder(s), X-linked.*
Febrile paroxysm(s), in malaria, 170
Fever, dengue hemorrhagic, 169–170
Fibrosarcoma, inflammatory, in lung, 382–383
FICTION (fluorescent immunophenotyping and interphase cytogenetic analysis), in Hodgkin disease, 202
Filter technique(s), for cerebrospinal fluid examination, 6
Fine-needle aspiration (FNA) biopsy. See also specific disorder(s), e.g., *Angiofollicular hyperplasia.*
  of lymph nodes, 12-19
    accuracy of, 13, 13t
    advantages of, 12, 13t
    contraindications to, 12
    disadvantages of, 12-13
    results of, inaccurate, 12–13, 13t
    technique of, 13–14
    vs. surgical biopsy, 12, 12t
  technique of, 19
FISH (fluorescent *in situ* hybridization), in Hodgkin disease, 202
Flow cytometry, in acute leukemia, 66, 70t–71t, *72*
  in acute myelogenous leukemia, 62, *63*
  in lymphoma, 197–198
Fluorescent immunophenotyping and interphase cytogenetic analysis (FICTION), in Hodgkin disease, 202
Fluorescent in situ hybridization (FISH), in Hodgkin disease, 202
FNA biopsy. See *Fine-needle aspiration (FNA) biopsy.*
Folate, deficiency of, and megaloblastic anemia, 119–120, 120t
Follicular bronchitis, 381
Follicular bronchiolitis, 381
Follicular hyperplasia, in Epstein-Barr virus lymphadenitis, 304, *305*
  in human immunodeficiency virus lymphadenitis, 307, *307*
  in hyper-IgM syndrome, 26, *26*
  in IgA deficiency, 24
  in thymus, 326, *326*
  vs. follicular lymphoma, 242
Follicular lymphoma, vs. follicular hyperplasia, 242
  vs. progressive transformation of germinal centers, 281t
Francisella tularensis lymphadenitis, 296–297, *297*
French-American-British (FAB) classification, of acute leukemia, 70, 74t
  of myelodysplasia, 149, 151t
Fungal infection(s), 160
  hepatic, 371–372
Fungal lymphadenitis, 298–301, *299–301*

G

G6PD. See *Glucose-6-phosphate dehydrogenase (G6PD).*
Gastrointestinal tract, anatomy of, 361
  disorders of, autoimmune, 364–365, *365*
    hematologic effects of, 161
    iatrogenic, 367–369, *367–369*, 369t
    IgA deficiency in, 24
    infectious, in leukocyte adhesion deficiency, 36
    neoplastic, 369–370, *370*
  histology of, 361
Gastrointestinal tract *(Continued)*
  immunodeficiency and, 361–364, 362t, *362–363*
  infections of, 365–367, *366–367*
  obstruction of, from chronic granulomatous disease, 363–364
Gaucher disease, hepatic manifestations of, 372–373, *373*
  splenomegaly in, *356,* 356–357
G-CSF. See *Granulocyte colony–stimulating factor (G-CSF).*
Genotypic study(ies), of acute leukemia, 67–69, 70t–73t
  of anaplastic large-cell lymphoma, 202
  of angiofollicular hyperplasia, 285–286
  of Burkitt lymphoma, 200–201
  of Hodgkin disease, 202–204
  of lymphoma, 200–204, 201t
Germ cell tumor(s), mediastinal, with acute myelogenous leukemia, 338, *338*
  vs. Hodgkin disease, in thymus, 337
Germinal center(s), enlargement of, in combined variable immunodeficiency disorders, 28, *28*
  in Hodgkin disease, lymphocyte-predominant, *224,* 225
  in interfollicular mixed cellularity Hodgkin disease, vs. angiofollicular hyperplasia, 216, *218*
  progressive transformation of, 279–280, *280,* 281t
  regressive transformation of, in angiofollicular hyperplasia, 329, *329*
Giardiasis, 365–366, *366*
Glanzmann thrombasthenia, 132
Globin biosynthesis ratio, in thalassemia, 143–144
Globin chain, synthesis of, defective, in thalassemia, 144–145
Glucose-6-phosphate dehydrogenase (G6PD), deficiency of, 38, 113–115, 114t–116t, *115*
    classification of, 115, 115t
    clinical features of, 114, 114t
    laboratory studies in, 114–115, *115,* 115t–116t
Glutathione synthetase, deficiency of, 38
Gluten-sensitive enteropathy, 364–365, *365*
Glycolytic pathway, 113, *113*
GM-CSF (granulocyte-macrophage colony-stimulating factor), hematologic effects of, 165–167, *166,* 166t
Gonad(s), lymphoma of, 405, *406*
Graft-versus-host disease (GVHD), 345
  gastrointestinal manifestations of, 367–368, *368–369,* 369t
  skin disorders from, 392–393, *393–394*
Granular acute lymphocytic leukemia, 81–82, *83*
Granulation, in bacterial infections, 157, *158*
Granulocyte(s), hyperplasia of, in chronic myelogenous leukemia, 95, *97*
Granulocyte colony–stimulating factor (G-CSF), hematologic effects of, 165–167, *166,* 166t
Granulocyte-macrophage colony-stimulating factor (GM-CSF), hematologic effects of, 165–167, *166,* 166t
Granulocytic sarcoma, *319,* 319–320, 407–408, *408*
  vs. Burkitt lymphoma, 239
Granuloma, eosinophilic, in Langerhans cell histiocytosis, 190, *191*
  noncaseating, in Hodgkin disease, 374, *374*
Granuloma *(Continued)*
  of spleen, 353
    in Hodgkin disease, 228, *229*
  plasma cell, 382–383. See also *Lymph node(s), inflammatory pseudotumor of.*
Granulomatosis, lymphomatoid, pulmonary, 383
Granulomatous disease, chronic, 37–38, 291–292, *292*
    and splenic function, 351–352, *352*
    gastrointestinal manifestations of, 363–364
Granulomatous inflammation, in *Mycobacteria* infection, 157–158, *159*
Granulomatous lymphadenitis, cat-scratch disease and, 15, *15*
  fine-needle aspiration biopsy in, 15, *15*
  in melioidosis, 313, *314*
  with stellate microabscesses, 295, *296*
Griscelli syndrome, 32
Growth retardation, immunodeficiency disorders with, classification of, 23t
Gum(s), leukemic infiltration of, 61, *62*
GVHD (graft-versus-host disease), 345
  gastrointestinal manifestations of, 367–368, *368–369,* 369t
  skin disorders from, 392–393, *393–394*

H

Haloed granule(s), in histiocytosis, *188*
Hamartoma, of spleen, 347
Hand-Schüller-Christian disease, 189
Hashimoto-Pritzker disease, 190–191, *192*
Hassall corpuscle(s), 323–324, *324–325*
Heart. See also *Cardiac* entries.
  Kawasaki disease of, 404–405
  leukemic infiltration of, 407
  lymphoma of, 405
  prosthetic valves for, and hemolytic anemia, 161
Heinz body(ies), and unstable hemoglobin, 108, *109*
Hemangioendothelioma, of spleen, 348
Hemangioma, of spleen, 348
Hematogone(s), after myeloablative chemotherapy, 164, *164*
  in neonates, 177–178, *178,* 178t
  vs. acute leukemia, 85–87, *87,* 87t
  vs. lymphoblasts, 164t
Hematologic disease(s), in neonates, See also specific disease(s), 173–183, 176t
    assessment of, 174, 176t
    factors associated with, 176t
    with Down syndrome, 178–179, 179t–180t, *180–181*
  organs affected by, 5
Hematologic malignancy(ies), pulmonary complications of, 385, *386*
Hematologic profile(s), of neonates, 173–174, *174–175*
Hematopathology, principles of, 5
  superspecialization in, 1
Hematopoiesis, disorders of, 105–133. See also *Anemia; Hemoglobinopathy.*
    and aplastic anemia, 126–127, 126t–127t, *127*
    and mastocytosis, *131,* 130–131
    and red cell aplasia, 124–126, *125,* 125t–126t
  extramedullary, 354
    in graft-versus-host disease, 369
    in liver, 370
    in spleen, 343
Hematopoietic cell(s), in skin, 389

Hemoglobin, electrophoresis of, in thalassemia, 143
unstable, 108, *109*
Hemoglobin Bart, hydrops fetalis with, 141, 141t
Hemoglobin C disease, 107, 107t, *107–108*
Hemoglobin E disease, 107–108, 108t, *108–109*
Hemoglobin F, in sickle cell disease, 106
Hemoglobin S, and sickle cell disease, 105, 106t
and thalassemia, *349–350*
Hemoglobinopathy, 105–108, *106–109*, 107t–108t
and sickle cell disease, 105–107, *106*, 106t. See also *Sickle cell disease.*
and splenic function, 349–350, *349–350*
mixed, 107
vs. thalassemia, 144
Hemoglobinuria, diseases associated with, 115t
Hemolysis, drugs causing, 124t
in elliptocytosis, 111
in glucose-6-phosphate dehydrogenase deficiency, 114, 114t
in pyruvate kinase deficiency, 113, 114t
in spherocytosis, 109–110
Hemolytic anemia, 122–124, 123t–124t, *124*. See also *Anemia, hemolytic.*
Hemolytic crisis, in sickle cell disease, 105
Hemolytic disease of newborn, 123
Hemophagocytic lymphohistiocytosis, familial, 357
Hemophagocytic syndrome, 160, *160*
infection-associated, 370–371, *371*
Hemophagocytosis, infection-associated, splenomegaly in, 357
Hemorrhagic fever, dengue, 169–170
Hemosiderosis, with thalassemia, 142, *143*
HEMPAS (hereditary erythroblastic multinuclearity with positive acidified serum test), 116
Hepatic. See also *Liver* entries.
Hepatic lymphoma, primary, 373, *373*
Hepatic necrosis, in X-linked lymphoproliferative disorders, 43–44, *43–44*, 45, *47*
Hepatitis, Epstein-Barr virus and, 369–370, *370*
vs. graft-versus-host disease, 368
Hereditary erythroblastic multinuclearity with positive acidified serum test (HEMPAS), 116
Herpes simplex virus (HSV), and lymphadenitis, *305*, 305–306
Herpesvirus 8, and angiofollicular hyperplasia, 285
Histiocyte(s), epithelioid, in Hodgkin disease, 215, *216*
in *Toxoplasma gondii* lymphadenitis, 308, *308*
proliferation of, in spleen, 353
Histiocytosis, 185–194
classification of, 185, 186t
in bone, 190
indeterminate-cell, 191
Langerhans cell, 187–188, 188t, 320
biology of, 189–190
clinical features of, 188, 190
cytochemical markers of, 189
histopathologic features of, 188–190, *190–191*
in thymus, 337–338, *338*
literature review of, 188t
prognosis in, 189
pulmonary, 384, *384*
vs. sinus histiocytosis, 278t, 279
Histiocytosis *(Continued)*
malignant, diagnosis of, 185–186, *186–189*
hepatic manifestations of, 375–377
macrophage type, 188–189
of childhood, 187
sinus, with massive lymphadenopathy, 277–279, *278*, 278t, 310, *310*
fine-needle aspiration biopsy in, 15, 16
in ocular adnexa, 403–404, *404*
skin disorders from, 392, *392*
splenomegaly in, *357–358*
with mastocytosis, hepatic manifestations of, 377, *377*
Histoplasma capsulatum lymphadenitis, 298–299, *299–300*
Histoplasmosis, vs. penicilliosis, 315–316
HIV infection. See *Human immunodeficiency virus (HIV) infection.*
"Hobnail" appearance, in angiolymphoid hyperplasia, with eosinophilia, 391, *391*
Hodgkin disease, 211–230
and overlap with anaplastic large-cell lymphoma, 251–252
and progressive transformation of germinal centers, 279
and therapy-induced secondary malignancy, 213
classification of, 196–197, 197t, 213–220, *214–220*, 215t–217t
comparison of systems for, 213, *215*
lymphocyte-depletion, 219–220, *220*
lymphocyte-predominant, 223–227, *224–226*
clinical features of, 223
differential diagnosis of, 225
diffuse variant of, 225, *225*
in spleen, 355
nodular variant of, *224*, 224–225
pathologic features of, 224–225, *224–225*
phenotypic studies of, 226, *226*
with large-cell lymphoma, 226–227
mixed cellularity, 214–217, *215–218*, 216t–217t
immunophenotypic studies in, 214–215, 216t–217t
interfollicular, 216–217, *217–218*
lymphocyte-rich, 215, *216*
nodular sclerotic, 217–219, *218–220*
clinical features of, 211–212
diagnostic criteria for, 213
epidemiology of, 199–200, 211
Epstein-Barr virus and, 211, 222–223, *223*
fine-needle aspiration biopsy in, 17–18, *18*
genotypic features of, 202–204
hepatic manifestations of, 374, *374*
in hyper-IgM syndrome, 25t
in marrow, *229*, 229–230
in spleen, 354–355
staging of, 228–229, *228–229*
in thymus, 335–337, *336–337*
clinical features of, 335, *336*
differential diagnosis of, 336–337, *337*
histopathologic features of, 335–336, *336*
karyotypic studies in, 222
lymphoproliferative, vs. progressive transformation of germinal centers, 279, 280t
molecular genetic studies in, 222
pathogenesis of, infection in, 204–205
phenotypic studies in, 220–222, *221–222*, 222t
pleural effusion in, 10, *10*
prognosis in, 212–213
pulmonary, 383
Hodgkin disease *(Continued)*
staging of, 227, 227t
specimens from, evaluation of, 227–230, *228–229*
vs. anaplastic large-cell lymphoma, 214, 216t, 253
vs. angiofollicular hyperplasia, 286t, 287
vs. angioimmunoblastic lymphadenopathy-like T cell lymphoma, 257
vs. B and T cell lymphoma, 222t
vs. mediastinal large B cell lymphoma, 335, *335*
with human immunodeficiency virus infection, 212–213
HSV (herpes simplex virus), and lymphadenitis, *305*, 305–306
HTLV-1, and T cell lymphoma/leukemia, 262–263, *263*
Human immunodeficiency virus (HIV) infection, 159–160
and lymphadenitis, 306–307, *307–308*
infectious, 292
mycobacterial, 303, *304*
and thymic atrophy, 327, *327*, 327t
and thymic cysts, 328, *329*
hepatic manifestations of, 372
Hodgkin disease with, 212–213
pulmonary complications of, 386
Humoral defect(s), congenital, and infectious lymphadenitis, 292
Hyaline vascular angiofollicular hyperplasia, 283, *284–285*
Hydrops fetalis, with hemoglobin Bart, 141, 141t
Hyperdiploid acute lymphocytic leukemia, 68, 73t, 79, *80*
Hypereosinophilia, *129*
Hyper-IgM syndrome, 25t, 25–27, *26*
clinical features of, 25, 25t
definition of, 25
diagnosis of, 26
histopathologic features of, 26, *26*
pathogenesis of, 26–27
Hypersplenism, 344
Hypertransfusion therapy, for thalassemia, 141, *141*
Hypogammaglobulinemia, and splenic function, 351
Hyposplenism, 343–344, *345–346*

I

IgA. See *Immunoglobulin(s) A IgA.*
Immunization, lymphadenitis after, 307–308
Immunoblast(s), atypical, in posttransplant lymphoproliferative disorders, 52, *55*
proliferation of, in spleen, 353
transformation of, in posttransplant lymphoproliferative disorders, 48–49
Immunoblastic large B cell lymphoma, 240, *241*
Immunocompromised patient(s), mycobacterial lymphadenitis in, 303, *303–304*
Immunocytochemical study(ies), of serous effusion, 11
Immunodeficiency disorder(s), 21–38
and splenic function, 350–351
classification of, 21, 22t–23t
combined, 29–32, 30t
classification of, 23t
Griscelli syndrome, 32
idiopathic CD4 lymphopenia, 32
Nezelof syndrome, 32
rare lymphocytic syndrome, 31–32
reticular dysgenesis, 32

Immunodeficiency disorder(s) *(Continued)*
severe. See *Severe combined immunodeficiency disorders (SCIDs).*
with enzyme deficiency, 31
with phenotypic findings, *33,* 33–35
ataxia-telangiectasia, 34–35
classification of, *235*
DiGeorge anomaly, *33,* 33–34
Wiskott-Aldrich syndrome, 35
combined variable, *28,* 28–29
gastrointestinal manifestations of, 362–363, *362–363*
diagnosis of, 22–24
epidemiology of, 21–22, *22*
from chromosomal defects, classification of, 23t
gastrointestinal manifestations of, 361–364, 362t, *362–363*
of phagocytic system, 35–38, *36.* See also *Phagocytic disorder(s).*
predominantly immunoglobulin, 24t, 24–29, *26, 28.* See also *Immunoglobulin(s), disorders of.*
pulmonary complications of, 386
secondary, classification of, 23t
thymus and, 326–327, 327t
with dermatologic defects, classification of, 23t
with growth retardation, classification of, 23t
with hereditary metabolic defects, classification of, 23t
with skeletal abnormalities, classification of, 23t
X-linked agammaglobulinemia, 27
Immunoglobulin(s), disorders of, 24t, 24–29, *26, 28*
hyper-IgM syndrome as, 25t, 25–27, *26*
hypercatabolism of, 23t
IgA, deficiency of, 21–22, 24t, 24–25
gastrointestinal manifestations of, 363
selective, 24t, 24–25
IgG, and hemolytic anemia, 122
deficiency of, in X-linked lymphoproliferative disorders, 46
Immunology, evolution of, available information and, 1, *3*
Immunoperoxidase technique(s), in acute leukemia, 72t
extramedullary, 85t
Immunophenotypic study(ies), of acute leukemia, 66–67, 70t–72t, *71–72*
of anaplastic large-cell lymphoma, 253, 258t
of angioimmunoblastic lymphadenopathy-like T cell lymphoma, 257
of Burkitt lymphoma, 238–239, *239*
of Hodgkin disease, 214–215, 216t–217t
of lymphoblastic lymphoma, T cell lineage, 247–248, 249t
of mycosis fungoides, 261
of natural killer cell leukemia/lymphoma, 264
Immunosuppressive drug(s), dosage of, decrease in, for posttransplant lymphoproliferative disorders, 51
Infantile genetic agranulocytosis, 128
Infection(s), 157–160, 158t, *158–160.* See also specific type, e.g., *Human immunodeficiency virus (HIV) infection.*
and hemophagocytic syndrome, 160, *160*
and Hodgkin disease, 211
and lymphoma, 204–205
bacterial, 157–158, 158t, *158–159*
fungal, 160
parasitic, 160
viral, 158–160, *159*
Infection-associated erythrophagocytosis syndrome, *309,* 309–310
Infectious mononucleosis. See *Mononucleosis.*
Inflammatory cell(s), in Hodgkin disease, 213
Inflammatory fibrosarcoma, in lung, 382–383
Inflammatory pseudotumor(s), of lungs, 382–383
of lymph nodes. See *Lymph node(s), inflammatory pseudotumor of.*
orbital, 403, *404*
Insect bite(s), skin reactions from, 390–391, *390–391*
Interfollicular mixed cellularity Hodgkin disease, 216–217, *217–218*
Interfollicular vascularization, in human immunodeficiency virus lymphadenitis, 307, *307*
Interleukin(s), in Reed-Sternberg cells, 221–222
Interleukin-6 (IL-6), increased synthesis of, in angiofollicular hyperplasia, 287
Interstitial pneumonia, lymphocytic, 381–382, *382*
Intestinal T cell lymphoma, 268–269, *269,* 269t
Intestine(s), malignant histiocytosis of, *186–188*
small, common variable immunodeficiency and, 362–363, *362–363*
malignant histiocytosis of, *186–188,* 376, *376*
normal mucosa of, 361
Iron deficiency anemia, 116–118, *117,* 118t
laboratory studies in, 117–118, 118t
vs. anemia of chronic disease, 160, 161t
vs. thalassemia, 144
Iron study(ies), conditions affecting, 118t

J

Jaundice, in glucose-6-phosphate dehydrogenase deficiency, 114, 114t
Jejunum, T cell lymphoma in, 268, *269*
JMML. See *Juvenile myelomonocytic leukemia (JMML).*
Juvenile myelomonocytic leukemia (JMML), 99–102, 101t, *101–102*
clinical features of, 99–100, *101–102*
cytogenetic features of, 100–101
differential diagnosis of, 101–102
Juvenile xanthogranuloma, splenomegaly in, 358

K

Karyotypic study(ies), in Hodgkin disease, 222
in lymphoma, 198, 200–204, 201t
Kawasaki disease, 309
cardiac, 404–405
Ki-1+ anaplastic large-cell lymphoma, 395–396, *396–397*
Kidney(s), disorders of, hematologic effects of, 162. See also *Renal.*
lymphoma of, 406, *407*
Kikuchi-Fujimoto necrotizing lymphadenitis, 309
Kimura disease, 391–392, *392*
Kostmann syndrome, 128

L

L and H cell(s), in Hodgkin disease, lymphocyte-predominant, *224,* 224–226, *226*
L3 acute lymphocytic leukemia, with Burkitt lymphoma, 80–81, *81*
Lacrimal tissue, interlobular septa of, in orbital inflammatory pseudotumor, 403, *404*
Lacunar cell(s), in Hodgkin disease, nodular sclerotic, 217, *218–219*
Langerhans cell(s), in skin, 389
Langerhans cell histiocytosis. See *Histiocytosis, Langerhans cell.*
Large granular lymphocytic leukemia, natural killer cell type, 264–265, *264–266,* 265t–266t
Large-cell lymphoma, pleural effusion in, 9, *9–10*
with lymphocyte-predominant Hodgkin disease, 226–227
Lead, and anemia, 121–122, *122,* 122t
Left shift, physiologic, in neonates, 173, *174–175*
Leishmaniasis, 312–313, *313*
Letterer-Siwe disease, 189
pulmonary, 384, *384*
Leukemia, acute, 61–88. See also *Acute lymphocytic leukemia (ALL); Acute myelogenous leukemia (AML).*
classification of, 69–70, 74t–75t
clinical features of, 61, *62*
congenital, 71, *75*
definition of, 61
differential diagnosis of, 85–87, *87,* 87t
epidemiology of, 61
extramedullary, 82–84, *83–86,* 85t
diagnosis of, 84, 85t, *86*
histopathologic features of, 319, *319*
misdiagnosis of, 83, *84,* 85t
genotypic features of, 67–69, 70t–73t
histopathologic features of, 62–69, *63–72,* 63t–73t
cytochemical evaluation in, 65, 68t, *69*
establishment of lineage and, 62
establishment of maturation stage and, 62, *63,* 63t
immunoperoxidase techniques in, 72t
immunophenotypic evaluation in, 66–67, 70t–72t, *71–72*
morphologic evaluation in, 63–65, 64t, *64–67*
historical perspective on, 61–62, *62*
in spleen, *355,* 355–356
megakaryoblastic, 72, *76*
"mixed lineage," 82
monocytic, 82, *83*
myelomonocytic, 82, *83*
prognosis in, 87–88, 88t
relapse of, 85, *87*
vs. hematologic effects of cytokine administration, 165–166, 166t
residual, 84–85, 86t
treatment of, myeloablative chemotherapy in, and bone marrow toxicity, 163, *163*
with Down syndrome, 72, *76*
in neonates, 179, 180t
chronic, 95–102
in spleen, 355
myelogenous. See *Chronic myelogenous leukemia (CML).*
congenital, in neonates, 179–182, 181t, *182*
biologic subsets of, 181t, 181–182, *182*
diagnosis of, cerebrospinal fluid examination in, 6–8, *6–8*
change in methods of, 2–3
early, 1–2
extramedullary, *319,* 319–320
extranodal, 407–408, *408*
gastrointestinal manifestations of, 369
hepatic manifestations of, 374–375

Leukemia *(Continued)*
in hyper-IgM syndrome, 25t
lymphoblastic. See also *Lymphoma/leukemia, T lymphoblastic.*
monocytic, vs. malignant histiocytosis, 185–186
myelomonocytic, skin disorders in, 400–401, *401*
pulmonary, 384
T cell, adult, 261–262, *263*
Leukemia/lymphoma. See *Lymphoma/leukemia.*
Leukocyte(s), adhesion deficiency disorders of, *36,* 36–37
Leukocytosis, in chronic myelogenous leukemia, 95, 96t
in neonates with Down syndrome, 179, *180*
Leukoerythroblastic reaction, to marrow metastatic disease, 162
Leukopenia, in acute leukemia, 61, *62*
in viral infections, 158
Listeria monocytogenes lymphadenitis, 294
Littoral cell angioma, of spleen, 348
Liver. See also *Hepatic* entries.
abscesses in, *371,* 371–372
amyloidosis in, 372
anatomy of, 370
extramedullary hematopoiesis in, 370
graft-versus-host disease in, 367, *369*
histiocytosis in, malignant, 375–377
with mast cell disease, 377, *377*
in Gaucher disease, 372–373, *373*
infections of, 370–372, *371*
leukemia in, 374–375
lymphoma in, 373–377, *373–377*
primary, 373, *373*
secondary, in B and T cell lymphoma, 373–374
in Hodgkin disease, 374, *374*
mastocytosis in, 377, *377*
necrosis of, in X-linked lymphoproliferative disorders, 43, *43–44,* 45, *47*
physiology of, 370
Liver disease, and splenomegaly, 348
hematologic effects of, 161
Liver transplantation, lymphoproliferative disorders after, 375, *375*
"Low blast count," 85
Lung(s). See also *Pulmonary* entries; specific disorder(s), e.g., *Pneumonia.*
angiofollicular hyperplasia in, 382
hematologic malignancies and, 385, *386*
immunodeficiency and, 386
Langerhans cell histiocytosis in, 190
Letterer-Siwe disease in, 384, *384*
leukemia in, 384
lymphoma in, 383–386, *384, 386*
normal histology of, 381
posttransplant lymphoproliferative disorders in, 384–385
reactive proliferation of lymphocytes in, 381–383, *382*
Lyme disease, skin reactions in, 390–391, *391*
Lymph node(s), abdominal, metastatic neuroblastoma in, *318*
architecture of, in X-linked lymphoproliferative disorders, 44–46, *44–45, 47*
biopsy of, in infections, 289–290, *290*
blast crisis in, in chronic myelogenous leukemia, *100*
Burkitt lymphoma in, *237*
cervical, lymphoblastic lymphoma in, T cell lineage, *248*
metastatic nasopharyngeal carcinoma in, *319*

Lymph node(s) *(Continued)*
metastatic rhabdomyosarcoma in, *318*
fine-needle aspiration biopsy of, 12–19. See also *Fine-needle aspiration (FNA) biopsy.*
in Hodgkin disease. See *Hodgkin disease.*
inflammatory pseudotumor of, 280–283, *282,* 283t
clinical features of, 280–281
definition of, 280
diagnostic criteria for, 282
differential diagnosis of, 282, 283t
histopathologic features of, 281–282, *282*
pathogenesis of, 282–283
prognosis in, 280–281
large-cell lymphoma in, 240, *240*
melioidosis in, 313–314, *314*
metastatic disease in, fine-needle aspiration biopsy in, 18, *18*
reactive hyperplasia of, fine-needle aspiration biopsy in, *14,* 14–15
Lymphadenitis, fine-needle aspiration biopsy in, 15–16, *15–16*
granulomatous, cat-scratch disease and, 15, *15*
fine-needle aspiration biopsy in, 15, *15*
with stellate microabscesses, 295, *296*
in melioidosis, 313, *314*
infection-associated erythrophagocytosis syndrome and, *309,* 309–310
infectious, 289–310
bacterial, 292–298, *293–298*
gram-negative, 294–295, *295*
gram-positive, 293–294, *293–294*
congenital cell-mediated defects and, 292
congenital humoral defects and, 292
congenital phagocytic defects and, 291–292
diagnosis of, 289–290, *290,* 290t–291t
from opportunistic mycosis, 301–302, *302*
fungal, 298–301, *299–301*
in immunocompetent children, 290
in immunocompromised children, 290–292
mycobacterial, 302–303, *303–304*
viral, 303-308, 304t, *305–308*
necrotizing, Kikuchi-Fujimoto, 309
postimmunization, 307–308
protozoan, *308,* 308–309
toxoplasmic, vs. lymphocyte-predominant Hodgkin disease, 225
Lymphadeno-hepatosplenomegaly syndrome, 354
Lymphadenopathy, benign, fine-needle aspiration biopsy in, 14–16, *14–16*
in Hodgkin disease, 211–212
in Kawasaki disease, 309
in progressive transformation of germinal centers, 279
massive, sinus histiocytosis with, 277–279, *278,* 278t, 310, *310*
in ocular adnexa, 493–404, *404*
skin disorders from, 392, *392*
neoplastic, fine-needle aspiration biopsy in, 16–18, *16–18*
Lymphangioma, of spleen, 347
Lymphatic disease(s), organs affected by, 5
Lymphoblast(s), in acute lymphocytic leukemia, 63–64, *67*
vs. hematogones, 164t
Lymphoblastic lymphoma. See *Lymphoma, lymphoblastic.*

Lymphocyte(s), in hyper-IgM syndrome, 26, *26*
in serous effusion, benign, transformation of, 10–11, *11*
in skin, 389
proliferation of, reactive, in lungs, 381–383, *382*
Lymphocyte-depletion Hodgkin disease, 219–220, *220*
Lymphocyte-predominant Hodgkin disease, 223–227, *224–226*
clinical features of, 223
differential diagnosis of, 225
diffuse variant of, 225, *225*
nodular variant of, *224,* 224–225
pathologic features of, 224–225, *224–225*
phenotypic studies of, 226, *226*
with large-cell lymphoma, 226–227
Lymphocyte-rich multicellularity Hodgkin disease, 216, *217*
Lymphocyte-rich thymoma, vs. T lymphoblastic lymphoma/leukemia, 331, 331t, *332*
Lymphocytic interstitial pneumonia, 381–382, *382*
Lymphocytic syndrome, rare, 31–32
Lymphocytosis, in *Bordetella pertussis* infection, 157, *158*
in neonates, 177–178, 178t, *178–179*
in viral infections, 158
Lymphoepithelioma, metastatic, fine-needle aspiration biopsy in, 18, *18*
Lymphoglandular body(ies), in reactive lymph node hyperplasia, 14, *14*
Lymphohistiocytosis, hemophagocytic, familial, 357
Lymphoid hyperplasia, diffuse, 381–382, *382*
Lymphoid nodule(s), paracortical, in typhoid fever, 316, *316*
Lymphoma, anaplastic large-cell. See *Anaplastic large-cell lymphoma (ALCL).*
B cell, Burkitt. See *Burkitt lymphoma.*
hepatic manifestations of, 373–374
in skin, 398–401, *399–401.* See also *Skin disorder(s) in B cell lymphoma.*
in spleen, 355
inheritance of, 200
large, 239–241, *240–241*
classification of, 239–240
clinical features of, 240
cytogenetic features of, 241
definition of, 239
differential diagnosis of, 241–243
mediastinal, 240–241, *241,* 332–335, *333–334*
pathologic features of, 240–241, *240–241*
low-grade, in lung, 383
lymphoblastic, 242, *242,*
fine-needle aspiration biopsy in, *16,* 16–17
genotypic features of, 201–202
in skin, 398–399, *399*
pleural effusion in, 9, *9*
skin disorders in, 394–395, *399,* 399–400
rare, 242
small transformed cell, 235–239, 236t, *236–239,* 400, *400.* See also *Burkitt lymphoma.*
vs. Hodgkin disease, 222t
lymphocyte-predominant, 225
cardiac, 405
classification of, 196–197, 197t
clonal nature of, 195

Lymphoma *(Continued)*
diagnosis of, clonality demonstration in, 198
common vs. rare forms and, 195, 196t
early, 1–2
flow cytometry in, 197–198
karyotypic studies in, 198, 200–204, 201t
key clinical features in, 195–196
optimal tissue processing in, 195
differential diagnosis of, 198
epidemiology of, 199–200
extranodal. See also specific site(s), e.g., *Heart.*
differential diagnosis of, 406
histopathologic features of, 406, *406–407*
pathogenesis of, 406–407
follicular, vs. follicular hyperplasia, 242
vs. progressive transformation of germinal centers, 281t
genotypic features of, 202–204, 204t
gonadal, 405, *406*
growth patterns of, factors affecting, 197
hepatic. See *Liver, lymphoma in.*
Hodgkin. See *Hodgkin disease.*
in cerebrospinal fluid, 8, *8*
in hyper-IgM syndrome, 25t
in IgA deficiency, 24
in posttransplant lymphoproliferative disorders, 50
in serous effusions, 8–10, *9–10*
in spleen, 355
in subcutaneous tissue, 397–398
in X-linked lymphoproliferative disorders, 43
inheritance in, 200
large-cell, anaplastic, fine-needle aspiration biopsy in, *17,* 17–18
pleural effusion in, 9, *9–10*
with lymphocyte-predominant Hodgkin disease, 226–227
malignant, gastrointestinal manifestations of, 369, *370*
in spleen, 354–355
of central nervous system, 405
of eye, 405
oncogenic genomic changes and, 195
pathogenesis of, infectious agents in, 204–205
primary, serous effusions in, 10, *10*
pulmonary, 383–386, *384, 386*
renal, 406, *407*
small noncleaved cell. See *Burkitt lymphoma.*
T cell, adult, 261–262, *263*
anaplastic large cell. See *Anaplastic large cell lymphoma (ALCL).*
angiocentric cutaneous, 396–397, *398*
angioimmunoblastic lymphadenopathy-like, 254–257, *258,* 258t
classification of, 254–256
clinical features of, 256
diagnostic criteria for, 257, 259t
differential diagnosis of, 257
histopathologic features of, 256, *258*
immunophenotypic features of, 257
pathogenesis of, 257
classification of, 245
clinical features of, 246–247
diagnosis of, 245–246
differential diagnosis of, 249,250t
hepatosplenic $\gamma\Delta$, 267–268, *268,* 268t
histopathologic features of, 247, *248*
Hodgkin disease and, 213
immunophenotypic features of, 247–248, 249t
intestinal, 268–269, *269,* 269t

Lymphoma *(Continued)*
lymphoblastic, 247–249, *248,* 249t–250t. See also *Lymphoma, B cell, lymphoblastic.*
clinical features of, 330
definition of, 329
differential diagnosis of, 331–332, 331t, *332–333*
histopathologic features of, 330, *330–331*
phenotypic features of, 330–331, *331*
mycosis fungoides, 258–261, *259–260,* 260t
clinical features of, 258–259
diagnostic criteria for, 260, 260t
differential diagnosis of, 261
histopathologic features of, 259–260, *259–260*
immunophenotypic features of, 261
pathogenesis of, 261
prognosis in, 258–259
skin disorders in, 396
natural killer cell. See *Natural killer cell lymphoma/leukemia.*
pathogenesis of, 249
pleomorphic, 261
prognosis in, 247
staging of, 246–247
subcutaneous panniculitis-like, 261, *262*
treatment of, 247
vs. Burkitt lymphoma, 239
vs. Hodgkin disease, 222t
Lymphoma/leukemia, natural killer cell. See *Natural killer cell lymphoma/leukemia.*
vs. acute myelogenous leukemia, 332, *333*
Lymphomatoid granulomatosis, pulmonary, 383
Lymphomatoid papulosis, 395, *395*
vs. anaplastic large-cell lymphoma, 252
Lymphopenia, CD4, idiopathic, 32
in immunodeficiency disorders, 22
Lymphophagocytosis, with sinus histiocytosis, *278*
Lymphoproliferative disorder(s), in spleen, 354
posttransplant, 48–57
after liver transplantation, 375, *375*
after marrow transplantation, 49–50
BCL6 mutations in, 54–55
classification of, 48–49, 49t
clinical features of, 49–51
definition of, 48
diagnostic criteria for, 56
differential diagnosis of, 56–57
histopathologic features of, 51–54, *52–56*
in lung, 384–385
incidence of, 49–50
markers for, 54–56
monomorphic, 53, *55*
pathogenesis of, 57
prognosis in, 50–51
T-cell type, 54, *56*
treatment of, 51
Reed-Sternberg cells and, 223
vs. lymphoma, 198
X-linked, 42–48
clinical features of, 42–44, *43–47*
definition of, 42
histopathologic features of, 44–46
laboratory studies in, 46
pathogenesis of, 46–48

M

M cell(s), intestinal, 361
Macrophage(s), starry sky, in Burkitt lymphoma, *236*
Macrophage-type histiocytosis, 188–189
Major histocompatibility complex (MHC), in thymus, 324
Major histocompatibility complex (MHC) antigen, deficiency of, 31–32
Malabsorption, in IgA deficiency, 24
Malaria, 170–172, *170–171,* 171t
clinical features of, 170
definition of, 170
diagnostic criteria for, 171
differential diagnosis of, 171–172
laboratory studies in, 170–171, *170–171,* 171t
pathogenesis of, 172
Marrow, anaplastic large-cell lymphoma in, small-cell variant, 252, *257*
biopsy of, in acute lymphocytic leukemia, 63–64, *67*
in chronic myelogenous leukemia, 95, 96t, *97–98*
in juvenile myelomonocytic leukemia, 100, *102*
in metastatic disease, *162,* 162–163, 163t
depletion of, in X-linked lymphoproliferative disorders, 44, *44,* 45, *46*
fibrosis of, conditions associated with, 150t
Hodgkin disease in, *229,* 229–230
in neonates, 173–174
metastatic tumors in, *162,* 162–163, 163t
necrosis of, in acute lymphocytic leukemia, 64, *67*
neoplasms of, and splenic function, *355,* 355–356
"Marrow exhaustion," in neonates, 175
Marrow toxicity, myeloablative chemotherapy and, *163,* 163–164
radiation therapy and, 164
Marrow transplantation, failure of, 165
for aplastic anemia, 127
for myelodysplasia, 153
hematologic effects of, 164–165
lymphoproliferative disorders after, 49–50
Mast cell(s), in skin, 389
Mast cell disease, 393–394, *394*
Mastocytosis, hepatic manifestations of, 377, *377*
vs. inflammatory pseudotumor of lymph nodes, 282, 283t
MDRI (multidrug-resistant protein I), and leukemia, 79
M/E (myelocyte/erythrocyte) ratio, cytokine administration and, 165
Mediastinum, germ cell tumors in, with acute myelogenous leukemia, 338, *338*
large B cell lymphoma in, 240–241, *241,* 332–335, *333–334*
Megakaryoblast(s), in neonates with Down syndrome, 179, *180*
Megakaryoblastic leukemia, 72, *76*
acute, pathology of, 66–67, 70t–72t, *71–72*
Megakaryocyte(s), disorders of, 131t, 131–133, *132*
in neonates, 178
in chronic myelogenous leukemia, 95, *97*
mononuclear, in myelodysplasia, *152*
Megaloblastic anemia, 119–121, 120t, *121*
etiology of, 119–121, 120t
laboratory studies in, 120t, 121, *121*
Melanoma, *vs.* anaplastic large-cell lymphoma, 253
Melioidosis, 313–314, *314*
Meningitis, viral, vs. lymphoma, in cerebrospinal fluid, 8, *8*
Metabolic disorder(s), inherited, hepatic manifestations of, 372–373, *373*
immunodeficiency disorders with, 23t

Microabscess(es), stellate, with granulomatous lymphadenitis, 295, *296*
"Micro-Heinz bodies," in sickle cell disease, 105
Microscopy, advantages of, 3
Mixed cellularity Hodgkin disease. See *Hodgkin disease, classification of, mixed cellularity.*
"Mixed lineage" acute lymphocytic leukemia, 82
MLL gene, in congenital leukemia, 71
Molecular genetic study(ies), in Hodgkin disease, 222
Monocyte(s), deficiency of, and splenic function, 351–352, *352*
  disorders of, 127–130, 127t–130t, *129*
  in acute leukemia, 63, *64*
  plasmacytoid, in angiofollicular hyperplasia, 284, *285*
Monocytic leukemia, acute, 82, *83*
  vs. malignant histiocytosis, 185–186
Monocytosis, 129–130, 130t
  in bacterial infections, 157
Monomorphic anaplastic large-cell lymphoma, 250, *251*
Monomorphic posttransplant lymphoproliferative disorders, 53, *55*
Mononucleosis, 159, *159*
  and lymphadenitis, 304, *305*
  fatal. See *Lymphoproliferative disorder(s), X-linked.*
  fine-needle aspiration biopsy in, 16, *16*
  in posttransplant lymphoproliferative disorders, 50
Monosomy 7 syndrome, acute myelogenous leukemia with, 76–78
  infantile, 152–153, 153t
  with juvenile myelomonocytic leukemia, 100–101
Mucocutaneous lymph node syndrome, 309
  of heart, 404–405
Multicentric angiofollicular hyperplasia, 284
Multidrug-resistant protein I (MDRI), and leukemia, 79
Multilobated large B cell lymphoma, 240, *241*
Multinuclearity, in congenital dyserythropoietic anemia, 116, *117*
Mummified cell(s), in Hodgkin disease, 213
Mumps, and lymphadenitis, 306
MYC gene translocation, in Burkitt lymphoma, 200–201, 201t, 239
Mycobacteria infection(s), granulomatous inflammation in, 157–158, *159*
Mycobacterial lymphadenitis, 302–303, *303–304*
Mycosis, opportunistic, and lymphadenitis, 301–302, *302*
Mycosis fungoides. See *Lymphoma, T-cell, mycosis fungoides.*
Myeloblast(s), morphologic features of, *63*
Myeloblastic sarcoma, in acute leukemia, 61, *62*
Myelocyte(s), disorders of, 127–130, 127t–130t, *129*
  in chronic myelogenous leukemia, 95, *97*
Myelocyte/erythrocyte (M/E) ratio, cytokine administration and, 165
Myelodysplasia, 148–153, 151t, *152*, 153t
  acute myelogenous leukemia with, 75–77
  bone marrow transplantation for, 153
  classification of, 149, 151t
  genetic factors in, 153
  morphologic features of, 149, 151t
  prognosis in, 153
  secondary, 153
Myeloid metaplasia, agnogenic, 148, *150*, 150t
Myelomonocytic leukemia, acute, 82, *83*
  juvenile, 99–102, 101t, *101–102*. See also *Juvenile myelomonocytic leukemia (JMML).*
  skin disorders in, 400–401, *401*
Myeloperoxidase, deficiency of, 38
  in acute leukemia, 68t
Myelophthisic pattern, in *Mycobacteria* infection, 158, *159*
Myeloproliferative disorder(s), 128–129, 147–148, 148t–150t, *150*
  and agnogenic myeloid metaplasia, 148, *150*, 150t
  and essential thrombocythemia, 147, *149*, 149t
  in spleen, 355
  polycythemia vera and, 147, 148t
  transient, in neonates with Down syndrome, 178–179, 179t–180t, *180–181*
  vs. bacterial infections, 157, 158t
  vs. chronic myelogenous leukemia, 99
Myofibroblastic tumor(s), inflammatory, in lung, 382–383

N

NADPH oxidase system. See *Nicotinamide adenine dinucleotide phosphate (NADPH) oxidase system.*
Naphthol ASD chloracetate esterase (CAE), in acute leukemia, 68t
Nasal angiocentric natural killer cell lymphoma, 266–267, *267*, 267t
Nasopharyngeal carcinoma, 318–319, *319*
  metastatic, to lymph nodes, fine-needle aspiration biopsy in, 18, *18*
Natural killer cell lymphoma/leukemia, 263–269, *264–269*, 264t–268t
  angiocentric, 266–267, *267*, 267t
  biologic characteristics of, 263–264, 264t
  histopathologic features of, 264
  immunophenotypic features of, 264
  in spleen, 355
  pathogenesis of, infection in, 204
  precursor, 269
  with large granular lymphocytic leukemia, 264–266, *264–266*, 265t–266t
NBT testing, in chronic granulomatous disease, 37
Necrotizing lymphadenitis, Kikuchi-Fujimoto, 309
Neonate(s), Down syndrome in, hematologic disease with, 178–179, 179t–180t, *180–181*
  hematologic profile of, 173–174, *174–175*
Neuroblastoma, 317, *318*
  fine-needle aspiration biopsy in, 18
  in neonates, 183, *183*
  metastatic, in marrow, *162*
  pleural effusion in, 9, *9*
Neutropenia, 127t, 127–128
  and enterocolitis, 367, *367*
  in acute leukemia, 61, *62*
  in bacterial infections, 157
  in neonates, 175, 177
Neutrophil(s), absence of, in leukocyte adhesion deficiency, 36, *36*
  deficiency of, and splenic function, 351–352, *352*
  disorders of, 127–129, 127t–128t, *129*
  hypersegmented, in megaloblastic anemia, *121*
  in acute myelogenous leukemia, *65*
  in Chédiak-Higashi syndrome, 128, *129*
Neutrophil(s) *(Continued)*
  in myelodysplasia, *152*
  in skin, 389
Neutrophilia, in neonates, 175, 177
  physiologic, in neonates, 173, *174*
  reactive, vs. chronic myelogenous leukemia, 97, 99, 100t
Nezelof syndrome, 32
Nicotinamide adenine dinucleotide phosphate (NADPH) oxidase system, defects of, in chronic granulomatous disease, 37
Niemann-Pick disease, splenomegaly in, 356–357
Nocardia lymphadenitis, 293
Nodular sclerotic Hodgkin disease, 217–219, *218–220*
  histologic grading of, 218–219
  of spleen, 354–355
  syncytial variant of, 218, *218*, *220*
Noncaseating granuloma, in Hodgkin disease, 374, *374*
Noncleaved cell lymphoma, small. See *Burkitt lymphoma.*
Normoblast(s), intranuclear bridging in, in congenital dyserythropoietic anemia, 115, *117*
NPM, in anaplastic large-cell lymphoma, 202
Nuclear inclusion(s), in cytomegalovirus lymphadenitis, 306, *306*
  in herpes simplex virus lymphadenitis, *305*
Nutritional disorder(s), and anemia, 116–122, *117–122*, 118t–122t. See also *Anemia, nutritional/toxic.*

O

Ocular adnexa, lymphoma of, 405
  Rosai-Dorfman disease of, 403–404, *404*
Omenn syndrome, 351
Opportunistic mycosis, and lymphadenitis, 301–302, *302*
Orbit, inflammatory pseudotumor of, 403, *404*
Osmotic fragility test, for spherocytosis, 110–111, *111*, 111t
Osteopetrosis, in neonates, 182–183
Ovary(ies), lymphoma of, 405
"Owl's eye" nuclear inclusion(s), in cytomegalovirus lymphadenitis, 306, *306*

P

p53, in Hodgkin disease, 203
p80, in anaplastic large-cell lymphoma, 254
Pagetoid reticulosis, 259, *260*
Pancytopenia, after marrow transplantation, 165
  in acute leukemia, 61, *62*
  in aplastic anemia, 127, *127*
Panniculitis-like T cell lymphoma, subcutaneous, 261, *262*
Papanicolaou stain, for body fluid examination, 6
Papulosis, lymphomatoid, 395, *395*
  vs. anaplastic large-cell lymphoma, 252
Paracortex, lymphoid nodules in, in typhoid fever, 316, *316*
Parasitic infection(s), 160
Paroxysmal nocturnal hemoglobinuria (PNH), 123–124, 124t
Parvovirus infection, and anemia, 122
  and red cell aplasia, 125, *125*
PAS stain (periodic acid–Schiff stain), in acute lymphocytic leukemia, 65, 68t, *69*
Pathologist(s), communication with other physicians, 3

Pathology, future of, 4
Peliosis, 348
Penicilliosis, 314–316, *315*
biologic characteristics of, 316
clinical features of, 314–315
definition of, 314
diagnostic criteria for, 315
differential diagnosis of, 315–316
laboratory studies in, 315, *315*
Pericardial effusion, examination of, 6
Periodic acid–Schiff (PAS) stain, in acute lymphocytic leukemia, 65, 68t, *69*
Peritoneal effusion, in Burkitt lymphoma, 9, 9–10
Petriellidium lymphadenitis, 302
Phagocytic disorder(s), 35–38, *36*
Chédiak-Higashi syndrome as, 38
chronic granulomatous disease as, 37–38
classification of, 23t
congenital, and infectious lymphadenitis, 291–292
eosinophil peroxidase deficiency as, 38
glucose-6-phosphate dehydrogenase deficiency as, 38
glutathione synthetase deficiency as, 38
leukocyte adhesion deficiency as, *36,* 36–37
myeloperoxidase deficiency as, 38
specific granule deficiency as, 38
Phenotypic immunodeficiency disorder(s), 21, 22t
classification of, 23t
Phenotypic study(ies). See under specific disorder(s), e.g., *Hodgkin disease.*
Philadelphia chromosome, in acute lymphocytic leukemia, 80
in chronic myelogenous leukemia, 95–96, *98*
Plasma cell angiofollicular hyperplasia, 283–284, *286*
Plasma cell granuloma, 382–383. See also *Lymph node(s), inflammatory pseudotumor of.*
Plasmacytic hyperplasia, in posttransplant lymphoproliferative disorders, 51, *52–53*
Plasmacytoid monocyte(s), in angiofollicular hyperplasia, 284, *285*
Plasmodium falciparum infection, 170–171, *170–171,* 171t
Platelet(s), disorders of, 131t, 131–133, *132*
in neonates, 178
Platelet count, after marrow transplantation, 165
Platelet peroxidase, in acute leukemia, 68t
Pleocytosis, nonspecific, in cerebrospinal fluid, in leukemia, 7–8, *8*
Pleomorphic lymphoma, 261
anaplastic large-cell, *251*
Pleural effusion, examination of, 6
in Hodgkin disease, 10, *10*
in large-cell lymphoma, 9, *9–10*
in lymphoblastic lymphoma, 9, *9*
in neuroblastoma, 9, *9*
Pneumocystis carinii lymphadenitis, 308
Pneumonia, interstitial, lymphocytic, 381–382, *382*
with bronchiolitis obliterans, 385, *386*
PNH (paroxysmal nocturnal hemoglobinuria), 123–124, 124t
PNP (purine nucleoside phosphorylase), deficiency of, 31
POEMS syndrome, 284
Poikilocytosis, in thalassemia, *141*
Polycythemia, in neonates, 175
Polycythemia vera, 147, 148t
Polymerase chain reaction (PCR), in infectious lymphadenitis, 291t
in leukemia, acute, residual, 84–85, 86t
Polymorphic proliferation(s), in posttransplant lymphoproliferative disorders, 48–49, 49t, 52, *54*
Postimmunization lymphadenitis, 307–308
Posttransplant lymphoproliferative disorder(s). See *Lymphoproliferative disorder(s), posttransplant.*
Pre-B acute lymphocytic leukemia, with t(1;19), 80
Preleukemia. See *Myelodysplasia.*
Proctocolitis, allergic, 364
Promyelocyte(s), cytokine administration and, 165
Promyelocytic leukemia, acute, 72–73, 76t, *77*
Pronormoblast(s), in red cell aplasia, 125, *125*
Prosthetic heart valve(s), and hemolytic anemia, 161
Protozoan lymphadenitis, *308,* 308–309
Pruritus, in Hodgkin disease, 212
Pseudallescheria lymphadenitis, 302
Pseudomonas lymphadenitis, 294–295, *295*
Pseudotumor(s), inflammatory, of lung, 382–383
of lymph nodes. See *Lymph node(s), inflammatory pseudotumor of.*
orbital, 403, *404*
Pulmonary disease, hematologic effects of, 162
Purine nucleoside phosphorylase (PNP), deficiency of, 31
Pyronophilia, in Burkitt lymphoma, 237, *238*
Pyropoikilocytosis, hereditary, 112, *112*
Pyruvate kinase, deficiency of, and anemia, 113, *113,* 114t

R

Radiation therapy, and marrow toxicity, 164
for lymphoblastic lymphoma, T cell lineage, 247
Rare lymphocytic syndrome, 31–32
Rash, in graft-versus-host disease, 393
Reactive hyperplasia, of lymph nodes, fine-needle aspiration biopsy in, *14,* 14–15
Red cell(s), aplasia of, 124–126, *125,* 125t–126t
etiology of, 125, 125t
laboratory studies in, 125
argyrophilic inclusions in, and splenic function, 344, *345*
contamination of cerebrospinal fluid by, 7, *8*
deformability of, 109
hyperplasia of, in thalassemia, 142, *142*
osmotic fragility of, in spherocytosis, 110–111, *111,* 111t
precursors of, dysplasia of, in myelodysplasia, *152*
production of, reduced, in neonates, 175, 177t
Red cell count, after marrow transplantation, 165
Red cell inclusion(s), in thalassemia, 143, *143*
Reed-Sternberg cell(s), and lymphoproliferative disorders, 223
B7 expression in, 203
cytokines in, 221–222
histopathologic features of, 213, *214*
immunophenotypic features of, 214–215, 216t
Reed-Sternberg cell(s) *(Continued)*
in Hodgkin disease, 202–203
fine-needle aspiration of, 18, *18*
lymphocyte-depletion, 220, *220*
in marrow, *229,* 229–230
in thymus, 336, *336*
phenotypic studies of, 220–222, *221–222,* 222t
Rejection, of allograft, vs. posttransplant lymphoproliferative disorders, 56
Renal. See *Kidney(s).*
Reticular dysgenesis, 32
Reticular fibrosis, in acute lymphocytic leukemia, 64
Reticulohistiocytosis, congenital self-healing, 190–191, *192*
Reticulosis, pagetoid, 259, *260*
Retroviral agent(s), for human immunodeficiency virus infection, 307
Rhabdomyosarcoma, 317–318, *318*
Rhodococcus equi lymphadenitis, 293–294, *294*
Rosai-Dorfman disease, 277–279, *278,* 278t, 310, *310*
fine-needle aspiration biopsy in, 15, *16*
of ocular adnexa, 403–404, *404*
skin disorders in, 392, *392*

S

Salmonella lymphadenitis, 295
Sarcomatoid anaplastic large-cell lymphoma, 251, *255*
SCIDs. See *Severe combined immunodeficiency disorders (SCIDs).*
Sea-blue histiocytosis, splenomegaly in, 357
Seminoma, vs. mediastinal large B cell lymphoma, 335, *335*
Serous effusion(s), benign lymphocytes in, transformation of, 10–11, *11*
examination of, 6, 8–11, *9–11*
immunocytochemical studies of, 11
in primary lymphoma, 10, *10*
malignant, 8–10, *9–10*
Severe combined immunodeficiency disorders (SCIDs), 29–31, 30t
clinical features of, 29, 30t
definition of, 29
gastrointestinal manifestations of, 363
pathogenesis of, 30–31
X-linked, 30t, 31
Sézary syndrome, 259
SHML (sinus histiocytosis with massive lymphadenopathy), 277–279, *278,* 278t, 310, *310*
fine-needle aspiration biopsy in, 15, *16*
in ocular adnexa, 403–404, *404*
skin disorders from, 392, *392*
Shock syndrome, dengue, 169–170
Short bowel syndrome, 369
Sickle cell disease, 105–107, *106,* 106t
clinical features of, 105
laboratory studies in, 106–107, *106,* 106t
pathogenesis of, 105
splenic pathology in, 348–350, *349–350*
Sickle trait, 107
Sideroblastic anemia, 118–119, *119,* 119t
vs. thalassemia, 144
Sideroblastosis, in hemoglobin S thalasssemia, *349*
Sieve apparatus, in spleen, 343, *344*
Sinus histiocytosis with massive lymphadenopathy (SHML), 277–279, *278,* 278t, 310, *310*
fine-needle aspiration biopsy in, 15, *16*

Sinus histiocytosis with massive lymphadenopathy (SHML) *(Continued)*
in ocular adnexa, 403–404, *404*
skin disorders from, 392, *392*
Skeletal abnormality(ies), immunodeficiency disorders with, classification of, 23t
Skin, physiology of, 389
Skin disorder(s). See also specific disorder(s), e.g., *Mast cell disease.*
benign, from dermal dendrocytes, *193,* 193–194
immunodeficiency disorders with, classification of, 23t
in acute lymphocytic leukemia, T cell, 394–395
in anaplastic large-cell lymphoma, 252, *256*
in angiocentric cutaneous T cell lymphoma, 396–397, *398*
in B cell lymphoma, 398–401, *399–401*
lymphoblastic, 398–399, *399*
in Burkitt lymphoma, 400, *400*
in histiocytosis, *193,* 193–194
Langerhans cell, 190, *190*
in mastocytosis, 130, *131*
in mycosis fungoides, 258–260, *259–260*
in severe combined immunodeficiency disorder, 29
neoplastic, 393–398, *394–398*
reactive, 389–393, *390–394*
Slide preparation, for fine-needle aspiration biopsy, 19
Small intestine. See *Intestine(s), small.*
Small noncleaved cell lymphoma. See *Burkitt lymphoma.*
Socioeconomic status, and incidence of Hodgkin disease, 211
Specific granule deficiency, 38
Spectrin, defects of, in spherocytosis, 109
Spherocytosis, 109–112, 110t
clinical features of, 109–110
hereditary, 109, 110t
laboratory studies in, 110–111, *110–111,* 110t–111t
Spindle cell(s), in inflammatory pseudotumor of lymph nodes, 281–282, 283t
proliferation of, in spleen, 353
Spirillum minus lymphadenitis, 298
Spirochete lymphadenitis, 298, *298*
Spleen, abscesses of, 352-353
anatomy of, 343, *344*
angiofollicular hyperplasia in, multifocal, 354
angioma of, littoral cell, 348
angiosarcoma of, 348
blast crisis in, in chronic myelogenous leukemia, *99*
calcification of, 353–354
congenital abnormalities of, 345–347, 347t
cysts of, 347
function of, autoimmune diseases and, 352
B cell deficiency and, 351
bone marrow neoplasms and, *355,* 355–356
hemoglobinopathy and, 349–350, *349–350*
immunodeficiency and, 350–351
monocyte deficiencies and, 351–352, *352*
neutrophil deficiencies and, 351–352, *352*
T cell deficiency and, 351
hamartoma of, 347
Hodgkin disease of, 354–355
staging of, 228–229, *228–229*
Spleen *(Continued)*
immunoblast proliferation in, 353
infarction of, 353
in sickle cell disease, 105
infections of, 352–354, 353t
lymphangioma of, 347
lymphoproliferative disorders in, 354
malignant lymphoma in, 354–355
myeloproliferative disorders in, 355
necrosis of, 353
in X-linked lymphoproliferative disorders, 44, *43, 45, 47*
physiology of, 343, *344*
rupture of, 354
sequestration of, in sickle cell disease, 349–350, *350*
trauma to, 348
vascular tumors of, 347–348
Splenectomy, indications for, 344, *347*
Splenomegaly, in chronic myelogenous leukemia, *95, 96*
in combined variable immunodeficiency disorders, 28, *28*
in Gaucher disease, *356,* 356–357
in histiocytosis, 357–358
in hyper-IgM syndrome, 26, *26*
in Waterhouse-Friderichsen syndrome, *346*
liver disease and, 348
Sporotrichum lymphadenitis, 302
Sprue, nontropical, 364–365, *365*
Staphylococcal lymphadenitis, 293
Starry sky macrophage(s), in Burkitt lymphoma, *236*
Stellate microabscess(es), with granulomatous lymphadenitis, 295, *296*
Stenotrophomonas maltophilia lymphadenitis, 297
Stomatocytosis, 112
Storage disease(s), splenomegaly in, *356, 356–357*
Subcutaneous panniculitis-like T cell lymphoma, 261, *262*
Subcutaneous tissue, B cell lymphoma in, 398–399, *399*
T cell lymphoma in, 397–398
Sudan black B, in acute myelogenous leukemia, 65, 68t, *69*
Superspecialization, in hematopathology, 1
Syndecan-1, in Hodgkin disease, 203
Syphylitic lymphadenitis, 298, *298*
Systemic disease(s), hematologic manifestations of, 160–162, *161,* 161t

T

T cell(s), abnormalities of, in combined variable immunodeficiency disorders, 29
biology of, 245, 246t
deficiency of, and splenic function, 351
disorders of, in IgA deficiency, 25
in severe combined immunodeficiency disorder, 29, 30t, 31
in Wiskott-Aldrich syndrome, 35
in X-linked lymphoproliferative disorders, 47–48
immunophenotypic features of, 70t
in posttransplant lymphoproliferative disorders, 55
in thymus, 323–326, *324–325*
T cell antigen receptor(s), in lymphoblastic lymphoma, 201
T cell leukemia, acute lymphocytic, 81
adult, 261–262, *263*
T cell lymphoma. See *Lymphoma, T cell.*
T cell lymphotrophic virus, and adult T cell leukemia/lymphoma, 205
T cell receptor (TCR), expression of, in severe combined immunodeficiency disorders, 30
gene rearrangements of, in acute lymphocytic leukemia, 69, 73t
TAL1, in lymphoblastic lymphoma, 201
TdT. See *Terminal deoxynucleotidyl transferase (TdT).*
Terminal deoxynucleotidyl transferase (TdT), in cerebrospinal fluid, in leukemia, 7
Testes, leukemic infiltration of, 407, *408*
lymphoma of, 405
Th1 response, in X-linked lymphoproliferative disorders, 47–48
Th2 response, in X-linked lymphoproliferative disorders, 47–48
Thalassemia, 140–145
classification of, 140–141, 141t
clinical features of, 140–141, 141t
definition of, 140
diagnostic criteria for, 144
differential diagnosis of, 144
globin biosynthesis ratio in, 143–144
hemoglobin electrophoresis in, 143
hemoglobin S, *349–350*
hypertransfusion therapy for, 141, *141*
laboratory studies in, 141–144, *141–143*
molecular pathology of, 144, 144t
pathogenesis of, 144–145
red cell inclusions in, 143, *143*
Thrombasthenia, Glanzmann, 132
Thrombocythemia, essential, 147, *149,* 149t
Thrombocytopenia, 131t, 131–133, *132*
in neonates, 178
Thrombocytosis, in bacterial infections, 157
in thrombocythemia, 147, *149,* 149t
Thrombopoietin, hematologic effects of, 167
Thymoma, lymphocyte-rich, *vs.* T lymphoblastic lymphoma/leukemia, 331, 331t, *332*
vs. angiofollicular hyperplasia, 286t, 287
vs. Hodgkin disease, in thymus, 337
Thymus, anatomy of, 323–326, 324t, *324–325*
and immunodeficiency, 326–327, 327t
angiofollicular hyperplasia in, 329, *329–330*
atrophy of, 327, *327,* 327t
in X-linked lymphoproliferative disorders, 44, *46*
cysts of, 327–329, *328,* 328t
dysplasia of, 327, 327t
ectopic, *328*
embryology of, 323
histology of, 323, *324–325*
Hodgkin disease in, 335–337, *336–337*
clinical features of, 335, *336*
differential diagnosis of, 336–337, *337*
histopathologic features of, 335–336, *336*
hyperplasia of, 326, *326,* 326t
Langerhans cell histiocytosis in, 337–338, *338*
mediastinal large B cell lymphoma in, 332–335, *333–334*
T lymphoblastic lymphoma/leukemia in, 329–332. See also *Lymphoma/leukemia, T lymphoblastic.*
undescended, in DiGeorge anomaly, 33, *33*
weight of, age and, 323, 324t
Tick bite(s), skin reactions from, 390–391, *391*
T/NK-cell lymphoma, 266–267

Topoisomerase II inhibitor(s), and leukemia, 78t, 78–79, *79*
Torulopsis glabrata lymphadenitis, 301
Touton giant cell(s), and xanthogranuloma, 192, *193*
Toxin(s), and anemia, 119, 122, 122t
Toxoplasmic lymphadenitis, *308*, 308–309
  vs. lymphocyte-predominant Hodgkin disease, 225
Transferrin, and iron absorption, 116
Transferrin saturation, in iron deficiency anemia, 118
Transfusion(s), malaria from, 172
Transient myeloproliferative disorder, in neonates with Down syndrome, 178–179, 179t–180t, *180–181*
Transplantation, lymphoproliferative disorders after, 48–57. See also *Lymphoproliferative disorder(s), posttransplant.*
  marrow. See *Marrow transplantation.*
Trauma, to spleen, 348
Treponema pallidum lymphadenitis, 298, *298*
t(1;19) translocation, in acute lymphocytic leukemia, pre-B, 80
t(1;22) translocation, and leukemia, in neonates, 181t, 182
t(2,5) translocation, in anaplastic large-cell lymphoma, 202
t(2;5) translocation, in anaplastic large-cell lymphoma, 254
t(5;14) translocation, in acute lymphocytic leukemia, with eosinophilia, 81, *82*
t(8;14) translocation, in Burkitt lymphoma, 239
t(8;21) translocation, in acute myelogenous leukemia, 73–76, *77*
t(12;21) translocation, cryptic, in acute lymphocytic leukemia, 79–80
Tuberculosis, and lymphadenitis, 302, *303*
  fine-needle aspiration biopsy in, *15*
Tuberous sclerosis, splenomegaly in, 357
Tuftsin, production of, 343
Typhlitis, 367, *367*
Typhoid fever, *316*, 316–317
  gastrointestinal manifestations of, 366

U

Ulcer(s), in angiocentric cutaneous T cell lymphoma, 397, *398*
Urticaria pigmentosa, 393–394, *394*
  in mast cell disease, 130, *131*
Uterus, lymphoma of, *406*

V

Vascular tumor(s), of spleen, 347–348
Vasculitis, in inflammatory pseudotumor of lymph nodes, 281, *282*
Viral infection(s), 158–160, *159*
Viral lymphadenitis, 303–308, 304t, *305–308*
Viral meningitis, vs. lymphoma, in cerebrospinal fluid, 8, *8*
Vitamin B_{12}, deficiency of, and megaloblastic anemia, 119–121, 120t
  hematologic effects of, 161

W

Waterhouse-Friderichsen syndrome, splenomegaly in, *346*
White blood cell (WBC) count, in acute leukemia, 61
  in immunodeficiency disorders, 22
Whitmore disease, 313–314, *314*
WHO (World Health Organization), classification of immunodeficiency disorders, 21, 23t
  classification of lymphproliferative disorders, 48–49
Wiskott-Aldrich syndrome, 35, 132–133, 351
Wolfram syndrome, 118–119
Wolman disease, splenomegaly in, 356–357
Woringer-Kolopp disease, 259, *260*
World Health Organization (WHO), classification of immunodeficiency disorders, 21, 23t
  classification of lymphoproliferative disorders, 48–49
Wright-Giemsa stain, for body fluid examination, 6

X

Xanthogranuloma, 191–192, *193*
  juvenile, splenomegaly in, 358
Xerocytosis, hereditary, 112–113
X-linked agammaglobulinemia (XLA), 27
  gastrointestinal manifestations of, 363
X-linked lymphoproliferative disorder(s). See *Lymphoproliferative disorder(s), X-linked.*

Y

Yersinia infection(s), and lymphadenitis, 297, *297*
  gastrointestinal manifestations of, 366–367, *366–367*
Yersinia pestis lymphadenitis, 295

Z

Zidovudine (AZT), hematologic effects of, 159